Multiple Organ Failure

Springer-Science+Business Media, LLC

Arthur E. Baue, MD
Professor Emeritus, Department of Surgery,
St. Louis University Hospital, St. Louis, Missouri, USA

Eugen Faist, MD
Professor, Department of Surgery, Klinikum Grosshadern,
University of Munich, Munich, Germany

Donald E. Fry, MD
Professor and Chairman, Department of Surgery, School of Medicine,
University of New Mexico, Albuquerque, New Mexico, USA

Editors

Multiple Organ Failure

Pathophysiology, Prevention, and Therapy

With 188 Figures

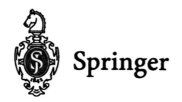

Arthur E. Baue, MD
Department of Surgery
St. Louis University Hospital
St. Louis, MO 63110
USA

Eugen Faist, MD
Department of Surgery
Klinikum Grosshadern
University of Munich
D-81377 Munich
Germany

Donald E. Fry, MD
Department of Surgery
School of Medicine
University of New Mexico
Albuquerque, NM 87131
USA

Library of Congress Cataloging-in-Publication Data
Multiple organ failure : pathophysiology, prevention, and therapy /
  edited by Arthur E. Baue, Eugen Faist, Donald E. Fry.
    p. cm.
  Includes bibliographical references and index.
  ISBN 978-1-4612-7049-2   ISBN 978-1-4612-1222-5 (eBook)
  DOI 10.1007/978-1-4612-1222-5
  1. Mutiple organ failure. I. Baue, Arthur. II. Faist, E.
(Eugen) III. Fry, Donald E.
  [DNLM: 1. Multiple Organ Failure—physiopathology. 2. Multiple
Organ Failure—therapy. 3. Sepsis Syndrome—physiopathology.
4. Sepsis Syndrome—therapy.   QZ 140 M9612 2000]
RB150.M84M89 2000
616.07—dc21
DNLM/DLC
for Library of Congress   99-39600

Printed on acid-free paper.

© 2000 Springer Science+Business Media New York
Originally published by Springer-Verlag New York in 2000
All rights reserved. This work may not be translated or copied in whole or in part without the written permission of the publisher (Springer-Science+Business Media, LLC), except for brief excerpts in electronic adaptation, computer connection with reviews or scholarly analysis. Use in connection with any form of information storage and retrieval, software, or by similar or dissimilar methodology now known or hereafter developed is forbidden.

The use of general descriptive names, trade names, trademarks, etc., in this publication, even if the former are not especially identified, is not to be taken as a sign that such names, as understood by the Trade Marks and Merchandise Marks Act, may accordingly be used freely by anyone.
While the advice and information in this book are believed to be true and accurate at the date of going to press, neither the authors nor the editors nor the publisher can accept any legal responsibility for any errors or omissions that may be made. The publisher makes no warranty, express or implied, with respect to the material contained herein.

Production coordinated by Chernow Editorial Services, Inc., and managed by Terry Kornak; manufacturing supervised by Jerome Basma.
Typeset by Scientific Publishing Services (P) Ltd., Madras, India.

9 8 7 6 5 4 3 2 1

ISBN 978-1-4612-7049-2

Preface

> Inflammation in itself is not to be considered as a disease . . . and in disease, where it can alter the diseased mode of action, it likewise leads to a cure; but where it cannot accomplish that solitary purpose . . . it does mischief.
> — John Hunter, *A Treatise on the Blood, Inflammation, and Gunshot Wounds* (London, 1794)[1]

As we reached the millennium, we recognized the gap between our scientific knowledge of biologic processes and our more limited clinical capabilities in the care of patients. Our science is strong. Molecular biology is powerful, but our therapy to help patients is weaker and more limited. For this reason, this book focuses on the problems of multiple organ failure (MOF), multiple organ dysfunction syndrome (MODS), and systemic inflammatory response syndrome (SIRS) in high-risk patients, that is, patients who have severe injuries; require major, overwhelming operations; or have serious illnesses requiring intensive care; patients who have diseases elsewhere, in other organs or systems, that limit their capabilities to survive a new insult; and patients who are elderly or at high risk for sepsis or other complications. These are the patients who need our help. They need the advances in science, in molecular biology, immunology, pathophysiology, biochemistry, genetics, high technology, and other areas of maximum support at the bedside. These advances could potentially have the greatest impact on improving patient care.

We hope that this book will provide information for clinicians to provide up-to-date care of their patients with everything that is known in science that has been tested and is valid for the care of patients. Although the basic sciences are important in understanding biology and medicine, this is not a basic science book. It is a book for clinicians written by experts in the field who have assessed what we presently know and presently can do. The basic science background needed to understand the processes leading to organ failure is presented. These pages contain no predictions of care by therapy and methods that have not been evaluated clinically. In that sense, we separate the wheat from the chaff, or vice versa.

The mortality rates associated with MODS and MOF remain high no matter what the cause of the problem. Many scientific reports in the literature have begun with an introductory statement such as, "MOF is the leading cause of death in the intensive care unit."[2] Another introductory statement is, "The systemic inflammatory response syndromes (SIRS) is a leading cause of morbidity and mortality during critical illness or following severe injury."[3] A third such statement is, "MODS remains a leading cause of death in the intensive care unit."[4] The incidence of MODS and MOF varies with the severity of the illness or the insult. There have been many classifications, or scores, for MOF, and these are reviewed.

Three books have already been published on the general subject of multiple organ failure. In the first, *Multiple Organ Failure: Patient Care and Prevention* (1990), all but one chapter was written by Arthur E. Baue; the exception was the chapter on "Ethics of the Intensive Care Unit" written by

Preface

Rosemary Baue. Later in 1990, Edwin Deitch edited a 17-chapter textbook, *Multiple Organ Failure: Pathophysiology and Basic Concepts of Therapy*. The third, *Multiple Organ Failure* (1991), was edited by Donald E. Fry. The present book is an amalgamation of those three books in which the information about what is known and what can be done has been brought up to date. We have been fortunate in gathering an outstanding international group of authors, including scientists, clinicians, intensivists, and surgeons from around the world, all of whom have written extensively about the areas they cover in this book.[5-7]

This book will lead into this year's Fifth World Congress in Munich, which was developed by Professor Eugen Faist. This book, and the meeting in Munich, will set the stage for what can be accomplished in the new millennium. Where will we go? What can we do? How will our powerful science help us to better care for our patients? Are we winning the battle against SIRS, MODS, and MOF? Perhaps we are, but it is going very slowly. We hope that this book will appeal to general, trauma, vascular, plastic, and cardiothoracic surgeons; intensivists, orthopedists, urologists, gynecologists, pulmonologists, cardiologists, internists, and all those who care for sick patients and who do research related to human biology. We also hope that residents, medical students, and nurses will be interested in many of the topics covered in this book.

The key features of the book include comprehensive coverage of MOF, authoritative authorship, presentation of practical guidelines that are supported by scientific data, discussion of the importance of prompt and appropriate treatment for the prevention of MOF, the basic understanding of the processes presented in the sections on mechanisms of MOF and the mediators and effectors, the organization of supportive care for easy understanding and retrieval of information, presentation of and rationale behind accepted treatment strategies, discussion of ethical issues that are so prevalent in the intensive care unit, review of the pros and cons of emerging and controversial therapies, and supplemental illustrations, tables, charts, and algorithms.

Multiple Organ Failure will be a thorough, but practical, reference for those who manage the care of critically ill patients in the intensive care setting. It will provide (1) the basic science background necessary to understand the processes of organ failure and (2) practical guidance on how to manage patients to prevent organ failure and implement strategies to improve the outcome of patients with organ failure.

It is important to remember that SIRS, MODS, and MOF are concepts, or constructs, not diseases. They are not even true syndromes, because a syndrome is defined as "a number of symptoms occurring together and characterizing a specific *disease*." The disorders causing MODS and MOF are infection, inflammation, injury, ischemia, reperfusion, immune reaction, iatrogenic factors, intoxication, or poisoning and idiopathic causes. Each of these diseases, illnesses, or injuries requires specific therapy to cure the patient. Early effective treatment of an inflammatory problem, such as pancreatitis, will decrease the possibility of MODS and MOF occurring and will decrease mortality. Thus, prevention is the key. Once MODS and MOF develop, all we can do is support organ functions and hope that they improve while still trying to treat the underlying cause.

Exciting studies on inflammation and mediators can help us to better understand, treat, or prevent such developments. The search for a magic bullet for treating inflammation and sepsis has so far been unsuccessful. It is impossible to predict where the next breakthrough will occur in the attempt to control an overwhelming inflammatory response and altered host immune responses. Much has been learned about the prevention of MOF, MODS, and SIRS. Excellent resuscitative care of the injured patient, or appropriate and timely operative intervention, careful zero-defect operations, and vigorous organ support intraoperatively and in the intensive care unit decrease the likelihood of organ failures. Important steps in support of organs before they fail are described herein and represent advances in the care of our patients. Thus, the frequency of MODS, MOF, and SIRS seems to be decreasing, even though mortality remains high once multiple organs fail.

We thank our colleagues for their contributions to this book. Preparing chapters for books are labors of love devoted to better care of our patients. We hope that more frequent prevention of MOF, MODS, and SIRS will result.

St. Louis, MO	*Arthur E. Baue, MD*
Munich, Germany	*Eugen Faist, MD*
Albuquerque, NM	*Donald E. Fry, MD*

References

1. Hunter J. Treatise on the Blood, Inflammation, and Gunshot Wounds, 2nd ed. Philadelphia, James Webster, 1823;205.
2. Tamura DY, Moore EE, Patrick DA, Johnson JL, Offner PJ, Sillman CC. Acute hypoxemia in humans enhances the neutrophil inflammatory response. Surg Forum 1998:107–109.
3. Ali MR Jr, Hills JS, Ogawa M, Hebra A. Interleukin-11 upregulates cytokine expression. Surg Form 1998:97–99.
4. Fanning NF, Kell MR, Kirwan WO, Cotter TG, Redmond HP. Plasma from patients with systemic inflammatory response syndrome inhibits neutrophil apoptosis. Surg Forum 1998:19–22.
5. Baue AE. Multiple Organ Failure: Patient Care and Prevention. St. Louis, Mosby, 1990.
6. Deitch EA. Multiple Organ Failure: Pathophysiology and Basic Concepts of Therapy. New York, Thieme, 1990.
7. Fry DE. Multiple System Organ Failure. St. Louis, Mosby, 1991.

Contents

Preface	v
Contributors	xv

Part I Development of SIRS, MODS, and MOF

1.	History of MOF and Definitions of Organ Failure *Arthur E. Baue*	3
2.	SIRS, MODS, and the Brave New World of ICU Acronyms Have They Helped Us? *John C. Marshall*	14
3.	Systemic Inflammatory Response and Multiple Organ Dysfunction Syndrome: Biologic Domino Effect *Donald E. Fry*	23
4.	Risk Factors for MOF and Pattern of Organ Failure Following Severe Trauma *Patrick J. Offner and Ernest E. Moore*	30
5.	Risk and Setting for Multiple Organ Failure in Medical Patients *Kang Lee and Derek C. Angus*	44
6.	Epidemiology, Risk Factors, and Outcome of Multiple Organ Dysfunction Syndrome in Surgical Patients *Philip S. Barie and Lynn J. Hydo*	52

Part II Mechanisms of SIRS and Organ Failure

7.	Systemic Inflammation After Trauma, Infection, and Cardiopulmonary Bypass: Is Autodestruction a Necessary Evil? *E.E. de Bel and R.J.A. Goris*	71
8.	Cardiopulmonary Bypass for Cardiac Surgery: An Inflammatory Event: Can It Be Modulated? *Arthur E. Baue*	82
9.	Gut: Clinical Importance of Bacterial Translocation, Permeability, and Other Factors *Andrew M. Munster*	86
10.	Microcirculatory Arrest Theory of SIRS and MODS *Donald E. Fry*	92

11. Infection, Bacteremia, Sepsis, and the Sepsis Syndrome: Metabolic Alterations, Hypermetabolism, and Cellular Alterations.. 101
    Matthias Majetschak and Christian Waydhas

12. Ischemia and Reperfusion as a Cause of Multiple Organ Failure 108
    H. Gill Cryer

13. Endotoxin in Human Disease and Its Endogenous Control 114
    Alexander Shnyra, Michael Lucchi, Jiangjun Gao, Christopher J. Papasian, David L. Horn, Richard Silverstein, and David C. Morrison

14. Untimely Apoptosis in Human SIRS, Sepsis, and MODS 131
    Timothy G. Buchman

15. Immunosuppression with Injury and Operation and Increased Susceptibility to Infection 134
    Eugen Faist and Martin K. Angele

Part III Mediators and Effectors

16. Emerging Evidence of a More Complex Role for Proinflammatory and Antiinflammatory Cytokines in the Sepsis Response 145
    Lyle L. Moldawer, Rebecca M. Minter, and John E. Rectenwald III

17. Counterregulation of Severe Inflammation: When More Is Too Much and Less Is Inadequate 155
    Vishnu Rumalla and Stephen F. Lowry

18. Reactive Oxygen Species in Clinical Practice.. 167
    Aruna Nathan and Mervyn Singer

19. Nitric Oxide as a Modulator of Sepsis: Therapeutic Possibilities 176
    A. Neil Salyapongse and Timothy R. Billiar

20. Mast Cells 188
    Donald E. Fry

21. Eicosanoids 196
    Geoffrey T. Manley, Mary J. Vassar, and James W. Holcroft

22. Platelet-Activating Factor 204
    M. Poeze, W.A. Buurman, G. Ramsay, and J.W.M. Greve

23. Therapeutic Complement Inhibition 214
    Katrin Jurianz and Michael Kirschfink

24. Leukocyte–Endothelial Cell Interactions: Review of Adhesion Molecules and Their Role in Organ Injury 224
    Milind S. Shrotri, James C. Peyton, and William G. Cheadle

Part IV Prevention and General Therapy

25. Care of Injured Patients in the Field, During Transport, and in the Emergency Department 243
    Steffen Ruchholtz, Christian Waydhas, and Dieter Nast-Kolb

26. Intensive Care Monitoring 254
    Orlando C. Kirton and Joseph M. Civetta

27. Peritonitis: Management of the Patient with SIRS and MODS 264
    Donald E. Fry

28. Hypothermia–Coagulopathy–Acidosis Syndrome: When to Operate/When to Stop Operating 273
    Asher Hirshberg and Kenneth L. Mattox

29. Early Definitive Fracture Fixation with Polytrauma: Advantages Versus Systemic/Pulmonary Consequences 279
    Hans-Christoph Pape and Harald Tscherne

30. Abdominal Compartment Syndrome 291
    Eduardo Bumaschny and Alejandro Rodríguez

31. SIRS and MODS: Indications for Surgical Intervention? 303
    Donald E. Fry

32. Nosocomial Infections in the ICU 309
    Gina Quaid and Joseph S. Solomkin

33. Modulation of the Hypermetabolic Response After Trauma and Burns 322
    Art Sanford and David N. Herndon

Part V Specific Remote Organ Failures

34. Circulation 333
    Jean-Louis Vincent

35. Effect of Inflammatory Conditions on the Heart 340
    A.B.J. Groeneveld and L.G. Thijs

36. Lung 353
    R. Phillip Dellinger

37. Renal Function and Dysfunction in Multiple Organ Failure 365
    Richard J. Mullins

38. Metabolic Depletion and Failure: Muscle Cachexia During Injury and Sepsis 378
    Timothy A. Pritts, David R. Fischer, and Per-Olof Hasselgren

39. Immunomodulation of Cell-Mediated Responses: Is It Feasible? 389
    Eugen Faist and M.W. Wichmann

40. Central Nervous System Failure: Neurotrauma Trials 398
    Jamie S. Ullman and Anthony H. Sin

41. Stress Gastritis: Is It a Disappearing Disease? 411
    Rodney M. Durham and Kelly Dreste

42. Gut and the Immune System: Enteral Nutrition and Immunonutrients 420
    Stig Bengmark

43. Disseminated Intravascular Coagulation 438
    J. Heinrich Joist

44. Refunctionalization of the Gut 447
    Stig Bengmark

45. Liver: Multiple Organ Dysfunction and Failure 459
    Arthur E. Baue

46. Liver: Hepatic Support and the Bioartificial Liver 462
    Walid S. Arnaout and Achilles A. Demetriou

Part VI Therapeutic Horizons

47. Laboratory Markers to Support Early Diagnosis of Infection and Inflammation 477
    Franz J. Wiedermann, Wolfgang Schobersberger, Bernhard Widner, Dietmar Fries, Barbara Wirleitner, Georg Hoffmann, and Dietmar Fuchs

48. Endotoxin Antagonists 492
    David L. Dunn

49. Blood Purification Therapy to Prevent or Treat MOF 501
    Hiroyuki Hirasawa and Arthur E. Baue

50. Antithrombin III and Tissue Factor Pathway Inhibitor: Two Physiologic Protease Inhibitors of the Coagulation System 505
    Gerhard Dickneite and Axel Mescheder

51. Rationale for Glucocorticoid Treatment in Septic Shock and Unresolving ARDS 514
    G. Umberto Meduri

52. Pathophysiologic and Clinical Importance of Stress-Induced Th1/Th2 T Cell Shifts 524
    Siegfried Zedler and Eugen Faist

53. Pathophysiologic and Clinical Role of Interferon-γ and Its Release Triggering Cytokines IL-12 and IL-18 531
    Eugen Faist, C. Schinkel, and C. Kim

54. Interleukin-11: Potential Therapeutic Activity in Systemic Inflammatory States 539
    Steven M. Opal and James C. Keith, Jr.

55. Minimal Surgical Procedures to Decrease the Stress Response and New Potential Therapeutic Agents 545
    Arthur E. Baue

56. Wound Healing: Physiology, Clinical Progress, Growth Factors, and the Secret of the Fetus 553
    David T. Efron, Maria B. Witte, and Adrian Barbul

57. Problems with Magic Bullets: Future Trials and Multiagent Therapy 562
    Arthur E. Baue

Contents

58. Maximizing Oxygen Delivery and Consumption: In Whom and for Whom? 571
    Robert F. Wilson and James G. Tyburski

59. Gut Decontamination: Prevention of Infection and Translocation 580
    M. Poeze, J.W.M. Greve, and G. Ramsay

60. Myocardial Depression: Is It Clinically Relevant? 591
    Fred Bongard

61. Infection: Cause or Result of Organ Failure? 598
    Donald E. Fry

62. Hypertonic Solutions 605
    Mauricio Rocha e Silva and Luiz F. Poli de Figueiredo

63. Blood Substitutes 613
    A. Gerson Greenburg and Hae Won Kim

64. Growth Factors G-CSF and GM-CSF: Clinical Options 621
    Thomas Hartung, Sonja von Aulock, and Albrecht Wendel

65. Anabolic Effects of Growth Hormone in Critically Ill Patients 630
    Douglas W. Wilmore

66. Immunoglobulin Therapy: Where Does It Stand Clinically? 638
    Günter Pilz

67. Horizons in the Anesthetic Care of Injured, Operated, and Stressed Patients 641
    Antonino Gullo, Giorgio Berlot, and Giovanni Galimberti

68. Integrative Biology and Genetic Variability: MODS' Next Frontiers 651
    Timothy G. Buchman

69. Are We Making Progress in Preventing and Treating MOF? 656
    Arthur E. Baue

70. Ethical Considerations of MODS, SIRS, and MOF 663
    Rosemary Dysart Baue

71. Socioeconomic Impact of Multiple Organ Failure 672
    Carol R. Schermer and Donald E. Fry

72. Future Directions in the Treatment of SIRS and MODS 678
    Donald E. Fry

73. Summary and Overview: What Does the Future Hold? 689
    Arthur E. Baue, Donald E. Fry, and Eugen Faist

Index 693

Contributors

Martin K. Angele, MD
Department of Surgery, Klinikum Grosshadern, University of Munich, D-81377 Munich, Germany

Derek C. Angus, MD
Critical Care Medicine, University of Pittsburgh, Pittsburgh, PA 15213, USA

Walid S. Arnaout, MD
Department of Surgery, Cedars-Sinai Medical Center, Los Angeles, CA 90048, USA

Adrian Barbul, MD
Department of Surgery, Sinai Hospital of Baltimore, Baltimore, MD 21215, USA

Philip S. Barie, MD
SICU, Department of Surgery, New York Hospital-Cornell Medical Center, New York, NY 10021-4873, USA

Arthur E. Baue, MD
Department of Surgery, St. Louis University Hospital, St. Louis, MO 63110, USA

Rosemary Dysart Baue, MM, M.Div
Fishers Island, New York, NY 06390, USA

E.E. de Bel, MD
Department of Intensive Care, University Hospital Nijmegen, 6500 HB Nijmegen, The Netherlands

Stig Bengmark, MD, PhD
Department of Surgery, University of Lund, Beta House IDEON Research Center, S-22370 Lund, Sweden

Giorgio Berlot, MD
Department of Anaesthesia and Intensive Care, Trieste University School of Medicine, Alpha Studio, 1-34125 Trieste, Italy

Timothy R. Billiar, MD
Department of Surgery, University of Pittsburgh, Pittsburgh, PA 15261, USA

Fred S. Bongard, MD
Division of Trauma and Critical Care, Professor of Surgery, Harbor-UCLA Medical Center, Torrance, CA 90502, USA

Timothy G. Buchman, MD, PhD
Burn, Trauma, Critical Care Section, Department of Surgery, Washington University School of Medicine, St. Louis, MO 63110-1093, USA

Eduardo Bumaschny, MD, PhD
Department of Surgery, University of Buenos Aires, Hospital Israelita "Ezrah," Buenos Aires 1416, Argentina

W.A. Buurman, PhD
Department of Surgery, University Hospital Maastricht, 6202 Maastricht, The Netherlands

William G. Cheadle, MD
Department of Surgery, University of Louisville School of Medicine, Louisville, KY 40292, USA

Joseph M. Civetta, MD
Department of Surgery, University of Connecticut, Farmington, CT 06030-3955, USA

H. Gill Cryer, MD
Department of Surgery, UCLA Medical Center, Los Angeles, CA 90024, USA

R. Phillip Dellinger, MD
Section of Critical Care Medicine, Rush-Presbyterian-St. Luke's Medical Center, Chicago, IL 60612-3833, USA

Achilles A. Demetriou, MD
Cedars-Sinai Medical Center, Los Angeles, CA 90048, USA

Gerhard Dickneite, MD
Department of Preclinical Pharmacology and Toxicology, Centeon Pharma BmbH, D-35041 Marburg, Germany

Kelly Dreste, PharmD
St. Louis University Health Sciences Center, St. Louis, MO 63110, USA

David L. Dunn, MD
Department of Surgery, University of Minnesota, Minneapolis, Minnesota 55455, USA

Rodney M. Durham, MD
Department of Surgery, St. Louis University School of Medicine, St. Louis, MO 63110, USA

David T. Efron, MD
Department of Surgery, Sinai Hospital of Baltimore and the Johns Hopkins Medical Institutions, Baltimore, MD 21215, USA

Eugen Faist, MD
Department of Surgery, Klinikum Grosshadern, University of Munich, D-81377 Munich, Germany

David R. Fischer, MD
Department of Surgery, College of Medicine, University of Cincinnati, Cincinnati, OH 45267, USA

Dietmar Fries, MD
Division for General and Surgical Intensive Care Medicine, Department of Anesthesiology and Intensive Care Medicine, University of Innsbruck, A-6020 Innsbruck, Austria

Donald E. Fry, MD
Department of Surgery, School of Medicine, University of New Mexico, Albuquerque, NM 87131, USA

Dietmar Fuchs, MD
University of Innsbruck, Institute of Medical Chemistry and Biochemistry, and Ludwig Boltzmann Institute for AIDS Research, A-6020 Innsbruck, Austria

Giovanni Galimberti, MD
Department of Anesthesia and Intensive Care, Trieste University School of Medicine, President Club, APICE, Alpha Studio, 1-34125 Trieste, Italy

Jiangjun Gao, PhD
Department of Pathology, University of Kansas Medical Center, Kansas City, KS 66160, USA

R.J.A. Goris, MD
Algemeine Chirurgie, Academisch Ziekenhuis Nijmegen, 6500 HB Nijmegen, The Netherlands

A. Gerson Greenburg, MD
Department of Surgery, Miriam Hospital, Providence, RI 02906, USA

J.W.M. Greve, MD, PhD
Department of Surgery, University Hospital of Maastricht, 6202 Maastricht, The Netherlands

A.B.J. Groeneveld, MD, PhD
Medical Intensive Care Unit, Free University Hospital, 1081 Amsterdam, The Netherlands

Antonino Gullo, MD
Department of Anaesthesia and Intensive Care, Trieste University School of Medicine, President Club APICE, Alpha Studio, I-34125 Trieste, Italy

Thomas Hartung, MD, PhD
Biochemical Pharmacology, University of Konstanz, D-78457 Konstanz, Germany

Per-Olof Hasselgren, MD, PhD
Department of Surgery, College of Medicine, University of Cincinnati, Cincinnati, OH 45267-0558, USA

David N. Herndon, MD
Shriners Burn Institute, Galveston, TX 77550-2725, USA

Hiroyuki Hirasawa, MD, PhD
Department of Emergency and Critical Care Medicine, Chiba University School of Medicine, 1-8-1 Inohana, Chuo, Chiba 260, Japan

Asher Hirshberg, MD
Department of Surgery, Baylor College of Medicine, Houston, TX 77030, USA

Kang Lee Hoe, MD
Department of Medicine, National University Hospital, Singapore 0511, Republic of Singapore

Georg Hoffmann, PhD
Department of Physiology I, University of Bonn, D-53115 Bonn, Germany

James W. Holcroft, MD
Department of Surgery, University of California at Davis Medical Center, Sacramento, CA 95817, USA

David L. Horn, MD
U.S. Human Health, Merck and Co., Inc., West Point, PA 19486, USA

Lynn J. Hydo, BS, RN, CCRN
Anne and Max A. Cohen Surgical Intensive Care Unit, New York Presbyterian Hospital, New York, NY 10021, USA

J. Heinrich Joist, MD
Pathology and Medicine, St. Louis University Hospital, St. Louis, MO 63110, USA

Katrin Jurianz, MD
Institute of Immunology, University of Heidelberg, D-69120 Heidelberg, Germany

James C. Keith, Jr., DVM, PhD
Department of Preclinical Research and Development, Genetics Institute of Wyeth-Ayerst Research, Andover, MA 01810, USA

C. Kim, MD
Klinikum Grosshadern, University of Munich, D-81377 Munich, Germany

Hae Won Kim, MD
Department of Surgery, Brown University School of Medicine, The Miriam Hospital, Providence, RI 02906, USA

Michael Kirschfink, DVM, PhD
Institute of Immunology, University of Heidelberg, D-69120 Heidelberg, Germany

Orlando C. Kirton, MD
Department of Surgery, Department of Surgery, University of Connecticut, Farmington, CT 06030-3955, USA

Kang Lee, MA
National University Hospital, Kent Ridge Road, Singapore 119074, Republic of Singapore

Stephen F. Lowry, MD
Department of Surgery, University of Medicine and Dentistry of New Jersey, Robert Wood Johnson Medical School, New Brunswick, NJ 08903, USA

Michael Luchi, MD
Department of Medicine, Division of Infectious Diseases, University of Kansas Medical Center, Kansas City, KS 66160, USA

Matthias Majetschak, MD
Department of Trauma Surgery, University of Essen, D-45147 Essen, Germany

Geoffrey T. Manley, MD, PhD
Department of Neurosurgery, San Francisco University School of Medicine, San Francisco General Hospital, San Francisco, CA 94143-0807, USA

John C. Marshall, MD
Department of Surgery, General Division, The Toronto Hospital, Toronto, Ontario M5G 1X5, Canada

Kenneth L. Mattox, MD
Baylor College of Medicine, Houston TX 77030, USA

G. Umberto Meduri, MD, FCCP
Department of Medicine, Director of the Memphis Lung Research Program, University of Tennessee at Memphis, Memphis, TN 38163, USA

Axel Mescheder, MD
Department of Preclinical Pharmacology and Toxicology, Centeon Pharma BmbH, D-35041 Marburg, Germany

Rebecca M. Minter, MD
Department of Surgery, University of Florida College of Medicine, Gainesville, FL 32610, USA

Lyle L. Moldawer, PhD
Department of Surgery, University of Florida College of Medicine, Gainesville FL 32610, USA

Ernest E. Moore, MD
Department of Surgery, Denver Medical Center, Denver CO 80204-4507, USA

David C. Morrison, MD
Cancer Center, University of Kansas Medical Center, Kansas City, KS 66160-7385, USA

Richard J. Mullins, MD
Department of Surgery, Oregon Health Sciences University, Portland, OR 97201, USA

Andrew M. Munster, MD
Francis Scott Key Medical Center, Baltimore, MD 21224, USA

Dieter Nast-Kolb, MD
Department of Trauma Surgery, University of Essen, D-45147 Essen, Germany

Aruna Nathan, MB, BS, FRCA
Bloomsbury Institute of Intensive Care Medicine, University College, London Medical School, London WC1 E65J, United Kingdom

Patrick J. Offner, MD
Department of Surgery, University of Colorado Health Sciences Center, Chief, Surgical Critical Care, Denver Health Medical Center, Denver, CO 80204, USA

Steven M. Opal, MD
Infectious Disease Division, Memorial Hospital of Rhode Island, Pawtucket, RI 02860, USA

Christopher J. Papasian, PhD
Department of Basic Medical Science, University of Missouri-Kansas City School of Medicine, Kansas City, MO 64108, USA

Hans-Christoph Pape, PhD
Unfallchirurgusche Klinik, Medizinische Hochschule Hannover, D-30625 Hannover, Germany

James C. Peyton, MD
Department of Surgery, University of Louisville School of Medicine, Louisville, KY 40292, USA

Günter Pilz, MD
Oberarzt-Leiter des Herzkatheterlabors, Krankenhaus Agatharred, Hausham, Germany

M. Poeze, MD
Department of Surgery, University Hospital Maastricht, 6202 Maastricht, The Netherlands

Luiz F. Poli de Figueiredo, MD
Department of Cardiopneumology, Heart Institute, University of São Paulo, 05403-00, São Paulo, Brazil

Timothy A. Pritts, MD
Department of Surgery, University of Cincinnati, Cincinnati, OH 45267, USA

Gina Quaid, MD
Department of Surgery, University of Cincinnati, Cincinnati, OH 45267, USA

G. Ramsay, MD, PhD
Department of Surgery, University Hospital Maastricht, 6202 Maastricht, The Netherlands

John E. Rectenwald III, MD
Department of Surgery, University of Florida, College of Medicine, Gainesville, FL 32610, USA

Mauricio Rocha e Silva, MD, PhD
Department of Physiology, Director, Research Division, Instituto do Coracao, Faculdade de Medicina, Universidade de São Paulo, 05403-00 São Paulo, Brazil

Alejandro Rodríguez, MD
Intensive Care Unit, Universidad Hebrea Argentine Bar Ilan, Buenos Aires 1416, Argentina

Steffen Ruchholtz, MD
Department of Trauma Surgery, University of Essen, D-45147 Essen, Germany

Vishnu Rumalla, MD
Department of Surgery, University of Medicine and Dentistry of New Jersey, Robert Wood Johnson Medical School, New Brunswick, NJ 08901, USA

A. Neil Salyapongse, MD
Department of Surgery, University of Pittsburgh Medical Center, Pittsburgh, PA 15261, USA

Art Sanford
Shriners Burn Institute, Galveston, TX 77550-2725, USA

Carol R. Schermer, MD
Department of Surgery, University of New Mexico School of Medicine, Albuquerque, New Mexico 87131, USA

C. Schinkel, MD
Department of Surgery, Klinikum Grosshadern, University of Munich, D-81377 Munich, Germany

Wolfgang Schobersberger, MD
Division for General and Surgical Intensive Care Medicine, Department of Anesthesiology and Intensive Care Medicine, University of Innsbruck, A-6020 Innsbruck, Austria

Alexander Shnyra, MD, PhD
Department of Microbiology, Molecular Genetics and Immunology, University of Kansas Medical Center, Kansas City, KS 66160, USA

Milind S. Shrotri, FRCS
Department of Surgery, University of Louisville School of Medicine, Louisville, KY 40292, USA

Richard Silverstein, PhD
Department of Biochemistry, University of Kansas Medical Center, Kansas City, KS 66160, USA

Anthony H. Sin, MD
Department of Neurosurgery, Mount Sinai School of Medicine–Elmhurst Hospital Center, Elmhurst, NY 11373, USA

Mervyn Singer, MD
Bloomsbury Institute of Intensive Care Medicine, University College of London Medical School, London WC1 E6, United Kingdom

Joseph S. Solomkin, MD
Department of Surgery, University of Cincinnati College of Medicine, Cincinnati OH 45267, USA

L.G. Thijs, MD
Medical Intensive Care Unit, Free University Hospital, 1081 Amsterdam, The Netherlands

Harald Tscherne, MD
Unfallchirurgusche Klinik, Medizinische Hochschule Hannover, D-30625 Hannover, Germany

James G. Tyburski, MD
Wayne State University, Detroit Receiving Hospital, Detroit, MI 48201, USA

Jamie S. Ullman, MD
Department of Neurosurgery, Mount Sinai School of Medicine, New York, NY 10029, USA

Mary J. Vassar, MS
Department of Surgery, San Francisco University School of Medicine, San Francisco General Hospital, San Francisco, CA 94143-0807, USA

Jean-Louis Vincent, MD
Department of Intensive Care, Erasme Hospital, Free University of Brussels, B-1070 Brussels, Belgium

Sonja von Aulock, MD
Biochemical Pharmacology, University of Konstanz, D-78457 Konstanz, Germany

Christian Waydhas, MD
Klinik und Poliklinik für Unfallchirurgie, Universitätsklinikum Essen, D-45147 Essen, Germany

Albrecht Wendel, PhD
Biochemical Pharmacology, University of Konstanz, D-78457 Konstanz, Germany

M.W. Wichmann, MD
Department of Surgery, Kinikum Grosshadern, University of Munich, D-81377 Munich, Germany

Bernhard Widner, DSc
University of Innsbruck, Institute of Medical Chemistry and Biochemistry, and Ludwig Boltzmann Institute for AIDS Research, A-6020 Innsbruck, Austria

Franz J. Wiedermann, MD
Division for General and Surgical Intensive Care Medicine, Department of Anesthesiology and Intensive Care Medicine, University of Innsbruck, A-6020 Innsbruck, Austria

Douglas W. Wilmore, MD
Department of Surgery, Brigham and Women's Hospital, Boston, MA 02115, USA

Robert F. Wilson, MD
Wayne State University, Detroit Receiving Hospital, Detroit MI 48201, USA

Barbara Wirleitner, MSc
University of Innsbruck, Institute of Medical Chemistry and Biochemistry, and Ludwig Boltzmann Institute for AIDS Research, A-6020 Innsbruck, Austria

Maria B. Witte, MD
Department of Surgery, Sinai Hospital of Baltimore, Baltimore, MD 21215, USA

Siegfried Zedler, MD
Department of Surgery, Klinikum Grosshadern, University of Munich, D-81377 Munich, Germany

Part I
Development of SIRS, MODS, and MOF

1
History of MOF and Definitions of Organ Failure

Arthur E. Baue

History of Multiple Organ Failure and the Importance of Prevention

A chain is only as strong as its weakest links. When links are strengthened where the chain has broken previously, new weak spots appear simply because the chain holds to test them. The obvious weak link in the severely wounded in this war [World War II] was the kidney—
                                Edward D. Churchill, M.D.[1]

Throughout the short history of modern medicine, whether one begins with Ambrose Paré, John H. Hunter, or Theodor Billroth, there have been limits to surgical capability. Whether imposed by pain (calling for the development of anesthesia), by hemorrhage and fluid loss (calling for hemostasis and intravenous fluids), or by infection (calling for antisepsis and then asepsis), these limits have challenged physicians to develop the technical resources and biologic understanding to go beyond their existing capability. This striving by the practitioner, the academician, and the investigator to extend the limits of our capability is part not only of our heritage but of our responsibility to our patients and our profession.

Certainly, limits in treating various types of disease exist, with extirpation of cancer and bypass grafting of artherosclerotic occlusions serving as prime examples. We are also limited in our overall ability to care for patients after severe injury, major life-threatening operations, and catastrophic illnesses requiring operations for treatment and prolonged intensive care, or those with significant chronic illnesses who face any of these problems. Reviewing recent progress on an organ or organ system basis can best elucidate our present limitations.

Organizing clinical thinking and patient care on the same basis is helpful. Just as the systems review in the patient's history helps to ensure complete evaluation, so can such methods assist in overall patient care. Weed[2] proposed using problem orientation for medical records, particularly when, as with most patients, multiple problems exist. Even better for surgical patients is a system- or organ-structured method of record-keeping and management. As the problem of patients after injury and operation become increasingly complex and affect a number of body systems, we must develop methods of recording information about the patient's course in the hospital record. Katz and Ottinger[3] developed an approach that requires writing follow-up notes and orders to consider each system and document the patient's course. The physician analyzes the function of each system and defines a plan for each. Data are displayed by systems rather than by problems and are thus compatible with computer analysis. This approach also provides a constant frame of reference applicable to all acutely ill patients.

Development of the MOF Concept

In recent surgical history, one or another single, limiting organ system has stood out as the primary factor in morbidity and mortality after injury. I use the generic meaning of "injury," which includes both trauma (accidental trauma) and an operation (planned trauma in the operating room). At the beginning of World War II the cardiovascular system and shock comprised the major problems. Patients who died after injury or operation frequently died of circulatory failure or inadequacy or of shock. Our understanding of hypovolemic shock and volume replacement was incomplete. As our knowledge of these concepts and problems developed, the treatment of shock greatly improved. Hemodynamic studies eliminated the mystique of wound shock. Fluid resuscitation and volume replacement eliminated shock as the single most important limiting factor or system contributing to morbidity and mortality after injury. The use of whole blood transfusions during World War II was a major contribution of E.D. Churchill.[1]

By the end of World War II and through the Korean conflict, the kidneys became the limiting organ system.[1] The US Army Surgical Research Unit in Korea used the term "posttraumatic renal insufficiency" to describe a condition that occurred 20–30 times more commonly in Korea than it did later in the Vietnam conflict.[4] Their studies demonstrated that the most common cause of delayed death in patients who had been successfully resuscitated from severe injury was acute renal failure. At that time acute renal failure developed in 1 in 200 seriously injured soldiers, with a mortality rate close to 90%. B. Rush (personal communication, 1960), who was part of the research team in Korea, indicated that this was the time when we were recognizing sodium retention as part of the biologic response to injury. Surgeons hesitated to give sodium solutions in any great quantity to injured and postoperative patients because these fluids would be retained. Thus injured and operated patients were given blood and plasma, but they were not given sufficient fluid and electrolyte solutions, particularly sodium ions. They were kept dry. Recognizing the problem of posttraumatic renal insufficiency and the need for larger volumes of intravenous water and sodium for injured patients led to better support of this organ system. As our understanding of the factors producing renal insufficiency developed, we often prevented this problem by rapid fluid resuscitation, supporting the kidneys by improving renal blood flow and promoting adequate urine output. We could also treat renal failure, when it did occur, more satisfactorily.

As the circulation and renal function received better support after injury, a new problem came into focus: pulmonary failure. During the Vietnam War it was called "posttraumatic pulmonary insufficiency."[5] Soon the lungs became the limiting organ system after injury, in both civilian and military practice. None of the four volumes of reports by the US Army Surgical Research Team in Korea mentioned the lungs;[4,6] they were not a problem at that time. Did pulmonary failure develop because of better resuscitation and support of the cardiovascular and renal systems or because aggressive and perhaps, on occasion, excessive fluid resuscitation jeopardized the lungs? Probably both these problems occurred. Adequate (not excessive) fluid resuscitation after injury and recognition of the lung as a limiting organ system after injury contributed to more frequent prevention of respiratory failure. Even when we cannot prevent respiratory failure, often we can treat it much more satisfactorily. Today mortality caused solely by ventilatory failure should be fairly low. Thus posttraumatic pulmonary insufficiency is no longer the single most important limiting organ system after injury.

The next limiting organ system that appeared was not a single organ but the complex or syndrome of multiple organ failure. When I read Professor Churchill's book in 1972, the concept of "weak links in the chain" fascinated me. At that time we were developing a cardiac surgical program in St. Louis at the Jewish Hospital of St. Louis and the Washington University School of Medicine. The support of failed organs had come into being with peritoneal dialysis and renal dialysis. There were early ventilators for support of the lungs and drugs for support of the cardiovascular system, but the concept of remote organ failure had not yet developed fully. Low cardiac output was a frequent postoperative problem. This was prior to the development of the intraaortic balloon pump for patients during and after cardiac surgery.

The concept of "weak links in the chain" led me to question what our weak links were in our intensive care units (ICUs) following operations in 1972. I reviewed the autopsy reports on all patients who died after prolonged period of resuscitation and support in our ICU. The problems detailed by these reports suggested a pattern of damage in organs remote from the primary site of injury or pathologic condition. One example was a patient who, following a colon resection, had a breakdown of the anastomosis with peritonitis. The anastomosis was exteriorized, but the patient died after 6 weeks of progressive difficulty. At autopsy we found pulmonary congestion and edema, focal organizing pneumonia, thrombi in the renal glomerular capillaries with acute tubular necrosis at a stage of early healing, icterus with massive acute centrilobular hepatic necrosis, multiple infarcts of the spleen, and autolysis of the adrenal glands. This patient, although dying essentially of peritonitis, thus had the findings of multiple organ failure, with evidence of failure of the lungs, liver, kidneys, and adrenal glands.

In another patient who died after a prolonged period of care for hemorrhagic pancreatitis, the findings at autopsy indicated generalized jaundice, pleural fluid, aspiration pneumonia, tubular necrosis, extensive necrosis of the liver, and ulcerations of the gut. This patient also died of multiple remote organ problems. A third patient, at autopsy, had necrotizing bacterial arteritis, interstitial pulmonary edema with hilar membranes, acute renal failure at a stage of healing, massive acute centrilobular necrosis of the liver, and passive congestive of the spleen. This patient died about 6 weeks after aortic and mitral valve replacements with continuous low cardiac output after operation. Again, in this patient the primary problem was an inadequate circulation, but the patient died of multiple organ problems. These patients had different initial diseases, but the final problem that led to their deaths was similar.

These findings led me to describe this problem in an editorial in the *Archives of Surgery* in July 1975 entitled, "Multiple progressive, or sequential systems failure: a syndrome of the 1970s."[7] As I searched for an appropriate name for this entity, I came across a 1973 article by Tilney et al. with the title "Sequential system failure after rupture of abdominal aortic aneurysms: an unsolved problem in postoperative care."[8] The term "sequential system failure" was unique. I wished that I had thought of it first, and I cited their observation about patients with abdominal aortic aneurysms in my 1975 editorial.

Tilney et al. described patients who required hemodialysis after surgical treatment of ruptured abdominal aortic aneurysms. They found a similar progression of organ system failure that began with pancreatic or pulmonary disease and progressed to upper gastrointestinal bleeding. They explained the lethality of renal failure after a ruptured aneurysm as a superimposition of preexisting, chronic cardiovascular disease on the mechanical and metabolic consequences of the operation. The mortality in their patients was more than 90%.[8]

Many other physicians have contributed to the development of these concepts and to our knowledge of remote organ failure. It is often as difficult to determine the exact origin of ideas and concepts as it is to recognize all of those who have contributed. Claude Welch, one of the senior attending surgeons at the Massachusetts General Hospital when I was a resident, taught us the concept of refunctionalization of the gastrointestinal tract.[9] Welch noted that if bowel function allowing oral intake did not return in approximately 2 weeks in an otherwise normal patient with peritonitis immediate operation could help the gut function and could decrease mortality. If there was delay, by 3 weeks the patient would deteriorate and eventually die. This was before the era of total parenteral nutrition to prevent or delay metabolic failure.

Burke et al. then described high output respiratory failure in patients with peritonitis.[10] Most of these patients eventually died of renal failure, but in the process they exhibited overbreathing (hypoxic hyperventilation) and respiratory failure. Skillman et al. found a high mortality rate in patients with peritonitis who developed respiratory failure,[11] as did Clowes and his group[12] and Border et al.[13] Siegel et al. described myocardial failure with sepsis.[14] Skillman et al. found that respiratory failure, hypotension, sepsis, and jaundice led to lethal hemorrhage due to acute gastric stress ulcers.[15] Thus the beginning of concepts of remote organ problems, particularly with sepsis, were coming into focus.

After my report in 1975, Eiseman et al. described patients with organ failure, emphasizing hepatic failure. They coined the expression "multiple organ failure" (MOF), which has continued to be popular today.[16] Polk and Shields found remote organ failure to be a sign of occult intraabdominal infection.[17] They pointed out that if a patient developed remote organ failure the chances were at least 50% that the cause of the problem would be in the peritoneal cavity and would require surgical therapy. They recommended that a patient with remote organ failure should undergo exploratory laparotomy to find the problem and correct it. The concept of a blind laparotomy for sepsis and remote organ failure developed. Patients without abdominal infection or a necrotic organ such as acalculous cholecystitis (a frequent finding) would likely die anyway, so the blind laparotomy seemed justified. Now this blind approach is no longer necessary because of better means of detecting intraabdominal problems by ultrasonography and computed tomographic (CT) scanning. Inflammation, or a nonbacteremic septic state defined by Meakins and Marshall,[18] is the cause about half the time, and laparotomy is not helpful. The emphasis on the role of uncontrolled infection in organ failure came from Fry et al.[19] along with Polk and Shields.[17] Border et al.[20] provided extensive observations and measurements of metabolic alterations in patients with multiple systems organ failure, as they now called it.

Many have contributed to our knowledge of MOF, including Trunkey and Miller,[21] Marshall and Dimick,[22] Cassone,[23] Border et al.,[24] Cerra et al.,[25] Carrico,[26] the late George Clowes et al.,[12] and Deitch et al.[27] Faist et al. described early and late MOF after trauma and referred to it as an early hit/late hit, or two-hit, phenomenon.[28] Clear definitions of organ failure and the factors contributing to it emerged.[29,30]

Soon it became apparent to Goris et al.[31] that severe inflammation itself, associated with tissue necrosis or other problems without infection, could produce or activate mediators that depressed the circulation and altered organ function. Patients with limited function of one or more organ systems, such as vascular occlusive disease, chronic obstructive lung disease, hepatic damage, immunosuppression due to various disease processes or organ transplantation, and cardiac disease before operation or injury, were more susceptible to MOF than were otherwise normal persons.

Morbidity and death after an operation, injury, or illness still occur owing to various complications such as thromboembolism, acute vascular occlusions or infarction, shock, posttraumatic renal failure, posttraumatic pulmonary failure, sepsis, peritonitis, and others. We can often treat each of these problems successfully when it occurs by itself. Renal failure associated with sepsis and respiratory or hepatic failure still has a grave prognosis, but renal failure alone is no longer a critical event. The incidence of renal failure in the injured in Vietnam was only 0.1–0.2%, but the mortality of those whose kidneys failed was high (63–77%) because of associated injuries and sepsis rather than renal failure per se.[32] We are now recognizing liver problems (hepatomegaly and jaundice) with trauma or sepsis more frequently (posttraumatic hepatic insufficiency). Likewise, the gastrointestinal tract, which seemed to wait quietly during starvation and sepsis, is now recognized as causing problems due to bleeding or perforation, translocation of organisms, or altered immune function. The occurrence of these problems of organ failure in combination or in sequence may exceed the limits of our present capabilities for supporting and providing survival of such patients.

The central nervous system (CNS) remains a major limitation after accidental injury. Baker et al.[33] at the San Francisco General Hospital, Faist et al.,[28] at the University of Munich, and Baker and our group[34] at Yale documented that primary CNS problems are the cause of death in 50% of patients dying after accidental injury. The CNS presents a major challenge to preventing injury and caring for the injured. Patients with primary CNS injury may die of the CNS injury itself or of multiple organ problems. Nonetheless, the CNS remains the major single limiting organ system after injury. The recognition of multiple or sequential systems or organ failure as a current problem is prompting study of how some of these sequences or simultaneous events occur and how they might be prevented.

Defining Multiple Organ Failure

When more than one system or organ cannot support its activities spontaneously, MOF is present. Detailed definitions of organ failure may be found in the second part of this chapter. Failure of the *ventilatory system* is defined as the requirement for assisted ventilation to maintain adequate gas exchange, including oxygenation and eliminating carbon dioxide. *Cardiovascular system* failure is reflected in hypotension, low or marginal cardiac output, or in general terms inadequate circulation that requires pharmacologic or mechanical circulatory assistance (or both). *Renal failure* is the inability of the kidneys to regulate volume, maintain electrolyte concentrations, and remove waste products. The definition of *hepatic failure* is inexact but is reflected in an elevated bilirubin level, elevated hepatic enzyme levels, and end-stage hepatic coma.

Coagulation system failure includes diffuse intravascular coagulation on one hand and primary bleeding problems on the other. *Gastrointestinal failure* is the inability of the gut to function and maintain nutrition by oral intake; it may be reflected in gastrointestinal bleeding that becomes life-threatening, perforation due to acute or stress ulceration, translocation of bacteria, or altered immune function. Failure of the *metabolic and musculoskeletal systems* is a twofold problem: (1) failure to provide for protein synthesis and prevent the central metabolic alterations of catabolism; and (2) catabolism of skeletal muscle, with loss of strength-producing problems with ventilation, ambulation, decubitus ulcers, and others. Failure of the *immune system* is exemplified by the development of sepsis that is unexpected or difficult to control or that cannot be eliminated. Failure of the *central nervous system* is defined as decreased or depressed sensorium or coma. Injury to the CNS, however, frequently becomes the limiting factor that prevents survival. Whether several organs fail progressively, sequentially, or all at once depends on the severity of the insult and the individual's preinjury or preoperative state.

Several organs failing together may cause death because of certain specific relations. Simultaneous renal and ventilatory failure is potentially lethal because as renal failure occurs or is diagnosed large fluid loads may be administered, overloading the lungs. Only peritoneal dialysis or hemodialysis can get rid of this fluid quickly. Another difficult combination is ventilatory and metabolic failure. Weaning a patient who is catabolic with decreased muscular strength from a ventilator may be difficult or impossible because he or she cannot breathe spontaneously. An example is the patient with end-stage valvular heart disease and cardiac cachexia. We can replace cardiac valves and provide good cardiovascular function, but the muscle mass loss is so great that spontaneous ventilation is impossible and complications occur. Renal failure in a patient with a ruptured aneurysm is particularly lethal because of shock, problems with cross-clamping the aorta, arteriosclerotic embolization, and vascular disease of the kidneys. Some patients with this problem now survive, particularly if we can prevent all complications (especially sepsis) while they undergo a prolonged period of anuria or oliguria and dialysis. Cardiac failure and ventilatory failure occurring together present a difficult problem because the treatment of ventilatory failure (including high levels of positive end-expiratory pressure) may adversely influence cardiac function. Finally, the combination of peritonitis with organ failure—whether ventilatory failure, cardiovascular instability, hepatic problems, or renal failure—is common and often lethal unless the primary problem of peritonitis can be controlled.

Five clinical characteristics may produce this sequence of events ending in MOF: (1) a severe metabolic insult, injury, operation, or both; a major operation or multiple systems injury in a normal individual can set the stage for MOF; (2) clinical or technical errors that escape recognition initially, such as continued bleeding, inadequate wound closure, a difficult anastomosis that leaks, a collection in the chest or the peritoneal cavity, or massive bacterial contamination; (3) infection, especially peritonitis or pneumonia, is often the underlying problem, initiating organ failure or developing as one or more organs fail; (4) severe inflammation, particularly when associated with tissue necrosis, may produce or activate mediators that depress the circulation and alter organ function; and (5) an individual with functional limitations in one or more organs before operation or injury is more susceptible to MOF. Patients with vascular occlusive disease, chronic obstructive lung disease, hepatic damage, immunosuppression from various diseases or organ transplantation, or cardiac disease are especially susceptible. A common thread in all these problems is altered circulation, reduced blood flow, inadequate tissue perfusion, and ischemia or reperfusion injury (or both). Each of these diseases, illnesses, or injuries requires specific therapy to cure the patient. Early and effective treatment of an inflammatory problem, such as pancreatitis, decreases the possibility of MOF and so decreases mortality. Once multiple organ dysfunction syndrome (MODS) and MOF develop, all we can do is support organ functions and hope that they improve while still trying to do something specific about the underlying cause.[35-39]

Concept of Limits and the Importance of Prevention

Multiple organ failure is not a disease but a concept in the care and study of injured patients. It is not even a true syndrome, as a syndrome is defined as "a number of symptoms occurring together and characterizing a specific *disease*." At any point in time, limits in our capability to care adequately for injured operated or sick patients can be defined. Defining our limitations helps us to overcome them and often prevent MOF; and it provides a framework for clinical problem solving that should be an important activity for all physicians whether working individually or collectively. Observations of one's own limitations or limitations within a hospital and the limits set by the patient's problems challenge everyone to do better the next time.

Although we strive to support the organs that have failed—especially with long-term support of failed kidneys, lungs, and the circulation—the primary approach I emphasize is preventing MOF during the initial phase of treatment, operation, or injury. Such prevention requires increased understanding in four areas: (1) defining and recognizing the problem; (2) identifying the setting in which these problems occur and the disease processes, abnormalities, and sequences that produce it; (3) determining the relations among the various systems that can lead to a domino effect of one system triggering problems in another; and (4) ensuring that currently available methods to support organs and systems do not fail individually or trigger problems and failure in other systems. The concept of limits includes defining our present biologic, scientific, technical, and personal limits and trying to exceed them. I hope readers can expand their personal limits by developing and contributing to the biologic and scientific arena within which we work. To achieve this one must have a clear understanding of all that is involved in the care of surgical patients, and it is to this end that we have dedicated this book.

The mortality associated with MOF is high no matter what the cause of the problem. Many reports begin with an introduction such as "MOF is the leading cause of death in the ICU." As documented by Zimmerman et al.[40] MOF remains the major contributor to death for patients in ICUs with no change in incidence or outcome over the past 8 years. This confirms my contention that the secret to MOF is prevention.[41]

Each organ or system must be supported. MOF often begins with a single organ failure and progresses as a domino effect with deleterious relations among the various organs and systems. These interrelations are still not completely understood. Gradually, however, I believe we are preventing MOF more frequently. Throughout this book is information for the clinician about support of organ function and the prevention of MOF.

What Is Organ Failure?

Definitions and Classifications

At what point is an abnormality in organ function considered organ failure? For both conceptual and quantifying purposes, we need some general agreement. Such a consensus would also help us develop preventive methods. Any classification is of necessity arbitrary. One might render a simplistic definition—organ failure occurs when the organ must be supported artificially—but such a definition is overly strict if cardiac failure by definition would require a ventricular assist device. Alternatively, one might define organ failure as failure to support life; but again this definition is too rigid for the liver in a patient with hepatic coma. I recommend the following classifications.[28,42]

Pulmonary failure: the need for ventilatory assistance for at least 72 hours and the need for fraction of inspired oxygen (FiO_2) of 0.40 or more and positive end-expiratory pressure (PEEP) of 5–10 cm H_2O or more. Using this definition we identified three grades of posttraumatic pulmonary insufficiency (Table 1.1).

Cardiac failure: high filling pressures with inadequate circulation and arrhythmias, with the need for drugs to support the circulation (autopsy findings of cardiac damage)

Shock: systolic blood pressure less than 80 mmHg

Kidney failure: serum creatinine levels ≥2 mg/dl regardless of polyuria or oliguria (dialysis required for late failure)

Liver failure: serum bilirubin level >2 mg/dl for 48 hours, with elevation of glutamate dehydrogenase level to >10 mU/ml (twice normal)

TABLE 1.1. Posttraumatic Pulmonary Insufficiency.

Grade I	FiO_2	PEEP (cm H_2O)
I	>0.4	5
II	≥0.4	5–10
III	>0.5	>10

Ventilatory support is required for all grades. Grades II and III signify ventilatory failure.

Coagulation failure: thrombocytopenia with <60,000 platelets/mm^3, declining prothrombin index, and need for administration of clotting factors because of abnormal bleeding.

Immune system: usually not evaluated but characteristics could include (1) anergy or (2) infection in a previously normal person with *Staphylococcus epidermidis*, *candida*, or *Pseudomonas*

Gastrointestinal failure: endoscopically confirmed bleeding from the gastrointestinal tract, requiring replacement of 2 units of blood or more, due to (1) perforation or (2) inability to take enteral nutrition within 5–7 days after injury or operation.

Metabolic failure: no clinically measurable criteria other than weight loss, cachexia, and inanition

Neuroendocrine failure: need for hormonal support; presence of adrenal failure

Central nervous system: Glasgow Coma Scale (see Chapter 7) of 6 or less

Pancreas: shock, pulmonary failure, and gastrointestinal failure

Wound failure: poor healing and little granulation tissue, which usually indicate metabolic failure

Many complex physiologic and biochemical measurements would better define failure of various processes and systems. Other definitions we have used include the following.

Massive blood transfusions: 8–10 or more units of blood during the first 6 hours of injury or after operation

Sepsis: (three to five of these criteria are required)
  Temperature >39°C for several days
  Leukocytosis >10,000 cells/ml
  Positive blood culture
  Circulatory instability requiring dopamine, 10 mg/h
  Focus of infection

Knaus et al.[43] provided other definitions of organ failure (Table 1.2); and Goris et al.[44] provided a third list (Table 1.3). However we define failure, we must keep in mind that any organ or system can fail and frequently does (Table 1.4). Other chapters address why organs fail and how to remedy the problems.

Classification of MOF

Is the incidence of MOF or MODS changing? Is the mortality of MOF decreasing? Are we making a difference? The answers to these questions are imponderable. There are no exact answers. If more and more sick, septic, injured, or operated patients survive the initial insult, the incidence of MOF may increase or stay the same. This is true even if MOF is prevented more frequently. The incidence of MOF depends on how it is defined, what classification is used, what criteria are used, how many organs are involved, and how much better early patient care has become (better triage, emergency care, diagnostic capabilities, and operations). There are a number of MOF and MODS classifications (Table 1.5). The most commonly used MOF score today is that of Knaus et al., who studied the

TABLE 1.2. Definitions of Organ System Failure.

If the patient had one more of the following during a 24-hour period (regardless of other values), organ system failure existed on that day.

1. *Cardiovascular failure* (presence of *one or more* of the following)
   a. Heart rate $\leq$ 54 beats/min
   b. Mean arterial blood pressure $\leq$ 49 mmHg
   c. Ventricular tachycardia, ventricular fibrillation, or both
   d. Serum pH $\leq$ 7.24 with $PaCO_2$ of $\leq$ 49 mmHg
2. *Respiratory failure* (presence of *one or more* of the following)
   a. Respiratory rate $\leq$ 5 or $\geq$ 49 breaths/min
   b. $PaCO_2 \geq$ 50 mmHg
   c. $AaDO_2 \geq$ 350 mmHg ($AaDO_2 = 713\ FiO_2 - PaCO_2 - PaO_2$)
   d. Dependent on ventilator on the fourth day of organ system failure (e.g., *not* applicable for the initial 72 hours of organ system failure)
3. *Renal failure* (presence of *one or more* of the following)[a]
   a. Urine output $\leq$ 479 ml/24 hr or $\leq$ 159 ml/8 hr
   b. Serum blood urea nitrogen $\geq$ 100 mg/dl
   c. Serum creatinine $\geq$ 3.5 mg/dl
4. *Hematologic failure* (presence of *one or more* of the following)
   a. White blood cell count $\leq 1000/mm^3$
   b. Platelets $\leq 20,000/mm^3$
   c. Hematocrit $\leq$ 20%
5. *Neurologic failure*
   a. Glasgow Coma Score $\leq$ 6 (in absence of sedation at any one point in day)
   b. Glasgow Coma Score: sum of best eye-opening, best verbal, and best motor responses; scoring of responses as follows (points)
      (i) Eye: opens spontaneously (4), to verbal command (3), to pain (2), no response (1)
      (ii) Motor: obeys verbal command (6); response to painful stimuli, localizes pain (5); flexion-withdrawal (4); decorticate rigidity (3); decerebrate rigidity no response (1); movement without any control (4)
      (iii) Verbal: oriented and converses (5); disoriented and converses (4); inappropriate words (3); incomprehensible sound (2); no response (1). If intubated, use clinical judgement for verbal responses as follows: patient generally unresponsive (1); patient's ability to converse in question (3); patient appears able to converse (5)

Modified from Knaus et al.,[43] with permission.
[a] Excluding patients undergoing chronic dialysis before hospital admission.

TABLE 1.3. Definitions of Organ Failure.

Several classification systems of organ failure have been described. Based on these systems, a scoring method was developed for each organ failure with a severity grading of 0 not present, 1 moderate, and 2 severe. The following criteria were also established for specific organ failures.

1. *Pulmonary failure*: 0, no mechanical ventilation; 1, mechanical ventilation with a positive end-expiratory pressure (PEEP) of 10 cm H_2O or less and a fraction of inspired oxygen (FiO_2) of 0.4 or less; 2, mechanical ventilation with a PEEP >10 cm H_2O and/or FiO_2 > 0.4.
2. *Cardiac failure*: 0, normal blood pressure with no vasoactive substances necessary; 1, periods with hypotension necessitating manipulations, such as volume loading, to keep blood pressure >100 mmHg, dopamine hydrochloride infusion of $\leq$ 10 μg/kg/min or nitroglycerin of 20 μg/min; and 2, periods with hypotension <100 mmHg, and/or dopamine hydrochloride >10 μg/kg/min, and/or nitroglycerin >20 μg/min.
3. *Renal failure*: 0, serum creatinine <20 mg/dl; 1, serum creatinine $\geq$ 2 mg/dl; 2, hemodialysis or peritoneal dialysis necessary.
4. *Hepatic failure*: 0, serum glutamic-oxaloacetic transaminase (SGOT) <25 units/L and total bilirubin <2 mg/dl; 1, bilirubin $\geq$ 2 mg/dl <6 mg/dl or SGOT $\geq$ 25 units/L and <50 units/L; 2, bilirubin $\geq$ 6 mg/dl or SGOT $\geq$ 50 units/L.
5. *Hematologic failure*: 0, normal counts of thrombocytes and leukocytes; 1, thrombocyte count < 50×10^9/L and/or leukocyte count $\geq 30 \times 10^6$/L and < 60×10^6/L; 2, hemorrhagic diathesis or a leukocyte count < 2.5×10^6/L or 60×10^6/L.
6. *Gastrointestinal tract failure*: 0, normal functioning; 1, acalculous cholecystitis or stress ulcer; 2, bleeding from stress ulcer necessitating transfusion of > 2 units of blood per 24 hours, necrotizing enterocolitis, and/or pancreatitis, and/or spontaneous perforation of the gallbladder.
7. *Central nervous system failure*: 0, normal functioning; 1, clearly diminished responsiveness; 2, severely disturbed responsiveness and/or diffuse neuropathy.

Modified from Goris et al.,[44] with permission.

prognosis of acute organ system failure and developed a scoring system for organ failure.[43] They developed objective definitions for five organ system failures and found in 1985 that single-organ system failure was associated with 40% mortality, two-organ system failures 60% mortality, and three or more organ system failures lasting for more than 3 days 98% mortality. Advanced age increased the possibility of organ system failure and resulting death. The Goris classification has been used by some. Moore et al. continue to use their classification for trauma patients.[58] The Goris, Knaus, and Moore classifications are similar. The reason so many classifications were developed was to describe the differing populations studied by each author(s). They are now of historic interest only. Ralph Waldo Emerson put it well when he wrote, "Though old the thought and oft expressed, tis his at last who says it best." Multiple organ dysfunction scores with a number of approaches have now been developed. The first, by Marshal, has been used by many.[63] Who knows where this will end: Everyone seems to develop his or her favorite approach. It reminds us of attempts years ago to develop a uniform shock model to be used by all, which of course never happened.

One potential use for these severity of illness scores is to evaluate therapy. Thus if a certain agent in a randomized trial decreased the severity of illness score, it might be interpreted as a positive result. Knaus has urged the use of his scoring system to determine entry criteria for clinical trials, which could ensure that only very sick patients would be enrolled. Whether this would be useful remains to be determined.

Three approaches can be used to try to answer the original question: Are we winning the battle? (1) Reviews of injury and severity of illness scoring may allow comparison of results over the

TABLE 1.4. Organs and Systems That Can Fail After Trauma.

Circulatory failure → shock
Low cardiac output
Renal failure
Pulmonary insufficiency
Hepatic failure
Coagulation problems
Immunosuppression → immune failure
Gastrointestinal failure
Metabolic failure
Neuroendocrine failure
Musculoskeletal failure
Central nervous system failure

1. History of MOF and Definitions of Organ Failure

TABLE 1.5. Sources for Definitions and Scoring Systems of Multiple Organ Failure and Multiple Organ Dysfunction Syndrome.

Author	Year
Knaus et al.[43]	1985
Goris et al.[44]	1985
Faist et al.[28]	1993
Norton et al.[45]	1985
Pine et al.[46]	1983
Carrico et al.[47]	1986
Marshall et al.[48]	1988
Bihari et al.[49]	1987
Bell et al.[50]	1983
Darling et al.[51]	1988
Rubin et al.[52]	1990
Saffle et al.[53]	1993
Kollef et al.[54]	1994
Hebert et al.[55]	1993
Ruokenen et al.[56]	1991
Manship et al.[57]	1984
Moore et al.[58]	1991
Fry et al.[59]	1980
Dorinsky & Gadek[60]	1990
Dobb[61] (Royal Perth Hospital Criteria)	1991
Eiseman et al.[62]	1977

years. (2) If care improves, certain clinical problems should decrease in frequency—is it happening? (3) Reviews of clinical advances that seem to make sense or have had a positive impact on the care of certain patients may contribute, and there may be extensive experimental animal background or clinical research.[64]

Today there are a number of organ dysfunction scores. They are reviewed by Marshall in Chapter 2.[63,65–67]

Severity of Illness or Injury: Stratification and Outcome Prediction

> Predictions are tricky particularly about the future.—Sam Goldwyn, Hollywood, California

Wright et al., considering the measurements in surgical clinical research, described the issues involved in measurement and the development of an index.[68] First is the definition of the purpose of the index. Feinstein classified four objectives or purposes:[69] (1) evaluation of patients at a single point in time (status index); (2) measurement of clinical change (change index); (3) prediction of an outcome (prognostic index); and (4) description of clinical change (clinical guidelines). Second is the focus or areas of interest of the index. The focus can be objective outcomes, subjective evaluations, or generic health status measurements. Third is the type of measurement, or multiitem indexes. This is followed by scale development for item generation and item reduction. After the instrument has been developed, it must be evaluated. Wright et al. described the evaluation criteria as sensibility, reliability, validity, and responsiveness.[68] Feinstein defined sensibility as "a mixture of ordinary common sense plus a reasonable knowledge of pathophysiology and clinical reality."[69] Reliability means that the same result is obtained when the same phenomenon is measured repeatedly by the same or different physicians. Validity means that the measure represents what is being sought, which can be criterion or construct validity. Finally responsiveness is the ability to measure clinical change. It has also been called sensitivity.

It is helpful to review first where we have been. The history of scoring begins with attempts to quantitate our activities (Table 1.6). Indices or scores have been developed to determine the status of a situation at a point in time; and there are indices of change, prognostic indices, and indices used as clinical guidelines. Scoring systems have been developed for a number of health-related matters (Table 1.6).

A number of excellent classifications were developed after my initial description of MOF.[7] It was soon recognized by Knaus and his group that there is a wide distribution of severity of illness in patients with similar organ failure classifications.[43] Thus MOF scales were imprecise. There could be a little or a lot of organ failure. Certain combinations of organ failures are more lethal than others.[42] This led to the development of the Acute Physiology and Chronic Health Evaluation (APACHE) concept on one hand[70] and the systemic inflammatory response syndrome (SIRS)/MODS approach on the other.[71]

What is the purpose of a score? Why score? What are the issues: to predict outcome (measure prognosis), describe or classify the severity of illness; set criteria for clinical trials of new therapies; assist, guide or stop therapy? Can these measures improve care? Are the various programs interactive for therapy? Can a worsening score allow one to stop therapy or organ support, or can an improved score indicate survival? We can describe metabolic and cardioventilatory characteristics consistent with illness or survival, but can they contribute to clinical research and other trials? As we compare survival or death and continuity of care, probability may not be a certainty. Finally, should we strive for consensus and a single universal scoring system? Can we ever all speak the same language?

TABLE 1.6. History of Scoring.

Game Scores
Romantic conquest by women and men
Wellness scores
Neonatal score: APGAR
Sepsis scores
SIRS and MODS scores
TISS-76 (Therapeutic Intervention Scoring System)
Health Status Evaluation
Severity of Illness
Sepsis
MOF scores
Disease scores
Injury scores
TISS-28
TRISS (Trauma and Injury Severity Score)
PISS (Predicted Injury Severity Score)
Injury severity
Futility
Injured extremity

TABLE 1.7. Sepsis Scoring.

Sepsis score—sepsis severity score (Elebute-Stoner)
Complete septic shock score
Simplified septic shock score
Risk of operative site infection formula
Surgical stratification system for intraabdominal infections
Delayed-type hypersensitivity (DTH) skin test score
Lipopolysaccharide (LPS) cytokine score:LPS, tumor necrosis factor-α (TNFα), interleukins (IL-1β, IL-6)

Many scores have been developed for each area of medical activity. Thus for sepsis there are numerous scoring systems (Table 1.7); for severity of illness scoring there are a multitude of systems (Table 1.8); and at least 19 methodologies have been proposed to document the severity of injury and compare trauma results (Table 1.9).

I have not attempted to provide references for each of these efforts. The major programs are cited and include APACHE II and III.[40,72] Simplified Acute Physiology Score (SAPS II),[73] Mortality Probability Models (MPM II),[74–76] the Therapeutic Intervention Scoring System (TISS),[77] the Multiple Organ Dysfunction Score (MODS)[63] developed by Marshall et al., and the Sepsis-related Organ Failure Assessment Score (SOFA) developed by Vincent.[66] The emphasis of these methods is on ideal variables that are (1) objective, simple, easily available, and reliable; (2) obtained routinely and regularly in every institution; (3) specific for the function of the organ considered; and (4) a continuous variable independent of the type of patient and the therapeutic interventions.

LeGall and his group developed two instruments for probability determination. The first approach is to customize existing models such as SAPS II or MPM II for subgroups of patients such as those with early severe sepsis.[75,78] They proposed this technique as an adjunct for clinical trials of new therapeutic agents. More recently LeGall et al. developed a way to assess organ dysfunction in the ICU. They call it the Logistic Organ Dysfunction System (LODS).[67] On the patient's first day in the ICU LeGall et al. identify one to three levels of organ dysfunction for six organ systems and the relative severity among organ systems.

There have been a number of studies and publications comparing many of these scoring systems, including a guide to

TABLE 1.8. Severity of Illness Scoring (Predictors of Mortality).

Acute Physiology and Chronic Health Evaluation (APACHE I, II, III)
Simplified Acute Physiology Score (SAPS I and II)
Mortality Probability Mode (MPM 11, 0, 24)
Clinical Assessment, Research scoring system (CARE)
Probability of death score (PODS)
MOF score
Multiple Systems Organ Failure (MSOF) score
MODS score
Hospital prognostic index
Therapeutic Intervention Scoring System (TISS)
Prognostic nutritional index
Pediatric Risk of Mortality (PRISM)

TABLE 1.9. Injury Severity Scoring.

ISS—Injury Severity Score
AI—Anatomic Index, HICDA-8 code
PEBL—Penetrating and Blunt Injury Code
ASCOT
OIS—Organ Injury Scales
AIS—Abbreviated Injury Score
GCS—Glasgow Coma Scale
TS—Trauma Score
TI—Trauma Index
MTOS—Major Trauma Outcome Study
HTI—Hospital Trauma Index
CRAMS—Circulation, Respiration, Abdomen, Motor, Speech
MESS—Managed Extremity Severity Score

prognostic scoring systems by Seneff and Knaus.[79] Castella et al. led a multicenter, multinational study and concluded that APACHE III, SAPS II, and MPM II perform better than their predecessors; and all three showed good discrimination and calibration.[80] Roumen et al. compared seven scoring systems, including APACHE II and the Injury Severity Score (ISS), in severely traumatized patients.[81] They concluded that the ISS, for example, predicted complications such as adult respiratory distress syndrome (ARDS) and MOF, whereas APACHE predicted mortality. Barie et al. found that the combined use of APACHE III and the MODS score predicted a prolonged stay in the ICU but could not predict outcome adequately in individual patients.[82] Rutledge raised the question as to whether the ISS can differentiate between severe injury and poor care.[83] Lewis pointed out that the timing of the measurement makes a difference.[84] Comparison of APACHE II and TRISS in trauma patients indicated that both accurately predicted group mortality in ICU trauma patients, but neither was accurate enough for prediction of outcome in individual patients.[85]

Can we develop a scoring system accurate enough for individual patients to predict mortality with complete certainty. I doubt it, and it is dangerous to make absolute predictions. The vagaries and complexities of human disease are a source of continuous wonderment. All we can do is keep trying.[86]

Risk Factors

Sauaia et al. found the early predictors of postinjury MOF to be age >55 years, ISS ≥ 25, and transfusion of ≥ 6 units of red blood cells during the first 12 hours. A base deficit >8 mEq/L and lactate >2.5 mmol/L added to the predicted value.[87] This emphasized the importance of the initial insult as a major risk factor. Tran et al. found the risk factors for MOF and death to be advancing age, prior chronic disease, malnutrition, ISS, coma on admission, the number of blood transfusions, and the use of H_2-receptor antagonist or antacids.[88] Early enteral feeding and gastric mucosal protection without altering the gastric pH (sucralfate) may eliminate this risk factor.[89] In those patients little could be done to prevent MOF other than to prevent the injury. Baker et al. found that the age of the patient,

ISS, and the length and depth of shock were the major risk factors predicting eventual mortality.[34] Because shock and transfusion requirements were important, the initial period of ischemia/reperfusion injury seemed deleterious. More recently Sauaia et al. developed a method to predict the development of MOF within the first 12 hours of admission into the hospital, operating room, or ICU.[90] The most important factor here is for the care givers to determine what they can do to alter this state and improve outcome despite prediction of MOF and its associated high mortality.

Henao et al. found that independent risk factors for MOF were hypovolemic shock, sepsis, and the time from injury to arrival at a trauma center.[91] Hammermeister et al. found that the risk factors for cardiac surgical patients to develop postoperative complications were previous cardiac surgical operations, cardiac status, older age, peripheral vascular disease, and high serum creatine levels.[92]

References

1. Churchill ED: Surgeons to Soldiers. Lippincott, Philadelphia, 1972.
2. Weed LL: Medical records that guide and teach. N Engl J Med 1968;278:593–600, 652–657.
3. Katz NM, Ottinger LW: System-structured management of acutely ill surgical patients. Arch Surg 1976;111:239–242.
4. US Army: Battle Casualties in Korea—Studies of the Surgical Research Team, vol IV. Washington, DC, Army Medical Service Graduate School, Walter Reed Army Medical Center, 1956.
5. Moore FD, Tilney NL, Morgan AP: Post-traumatic respiratory insufficiency. Philadelphia, Saunders, 1969.
6. US Army: Battle Casualties in Korea—Studies of Our Limitations So We Can Overcome Them, the Surgical Research Team, vols I–IV. Washington, DC, Brooke Army Medical Center and Army Medical Service Graduate School, Walter Reed Army Medical Center, 1956.
7. Baue AE: Multiple, progressive, or sequential systems failure: a syndrome of the 1970s. Arch Surg 1975;110:779–781.
8. Tilney NL, Bailev GL, Morgan AP: Sequential system failure after rupture of abdominal aortic aneurysms: an unsolved problem in postoperative care. Ann Surg 1973;178:117–122.
9. Welch CE: Treatment of combined intestinal obstruction and peritonitis by refunctionalization of the intestine. Ann Surg 1955;142:739.
10. Burke JF, Pontoppidan H, Welch CE: High output respiratory failure: an important cause of death ascribed to peritonitis or ileus. Ann Surg 1963;158:581–595.
11. Skillman JJ, Bushnell LS, Hedley-Whyte J: Peritonitis and respiratory failure after abdominal operations. Ann Surg 1969;170: 122–127.
12. Clowes GHA Jr, Zuschneid W, Turner M, et al: Observations on the pathogenesis of the pneumonitis associated with severe infections in other parts of the body. Ann Surg 1968;167:630.
13. Border JR, Tibbets JC, Schenk WG: Hypoxic hyperventilation and acute respiratory failure in the severely stressed patient: massive pulmonary arteriovenous shunts? Surgery 148;64:710.
14. Siegel JH, Greenspan M, DelGuercio LRM: Abnormal vascular tone, defective oxygen transport and myocardial failure in human septic shock. Ann Surg 1967;165:504.
15. Skillman JJ, Bushnell LS, Goldman H, Silen W: Respiratory failure, hypotension, sepsis and jaundice. Am J Surg 1969;117:523–530.
16. Eiseman B, Beart R, Norton L: Multiple organ failure. Surg Gynecol Obstet 1977;144:323–326.
17. Polk HC Jr, Shields CL: Remote organ failure: a valid sign of occult intra-abdominal infection. Surgery 1977;81:310–313.
18. Meakins JL, Marshall JC: The gastrointestinal tract: the 'motor' of MOF (part of SIS panel discussion). Arch Surg 1986;121: 197–201.
19. Fry DE, Pearlstein L, Fulton RL, Polk HC Jr: Multiple system organ failure. Arch Surg 1980;115:136–140.
20. Border JR, Chenier R, McMenamv RH, et al: Multiple systems organ failure: muscle fuel deficit with visceral protein malnutrition. Surg Clin North Am 1976;56:1147–1167.
21. Trunkey DD, Miller CL: Multiple organ failure and sepsis. In: Najarian JS, Delaney JP (eds) Emergency Surgery. Chicago, Year Book, 1982;273–285.
22. Marshall WG Jr, Dimick AR: The natural history of major burns with multiple subsystem failure. J Trauma 1983;23:102–105.
23. Cassone E: Clinical and laboratory signs of multiple organ failure. Infect Surg 1983;2:857–862.
24. Border JR, Hassett J, LaDuca J, et al: The gut origin septic states in blunt multiple trauma (ISS = 40) in the ICU. Ann Surg 1987;206:41–59.
25. Cerra FB, Siegel JH, Colman B, Border J, McMenamy RH: Autocannibalism, a failure of exogenous nutritional support. Ann Surg 1980;192:570.
26. Carrico CJ: Multiple organ failure syndrome [SIS panel discussion]. Arch Surg 1986;121:196–197.
27. Deitch EA, Winterton J, Berg R: Effect of starvation, malnutrition, and trauma on the gastrointestinal tract flora and bacterial translocation. Arch Surg 1987;122:1019–1024.
28. Faist E, Baue AE, Dittmer H, Heberer G: Multiple organ failure in polytrauma patients. J Trauma 1993;23:775–787.
29. Bumaschny E, Doglio G, Pusajo J, et al: Postoperative acute gastrointestinal tract hemorrhage and multiple-organ failure. Arch Surg 1988;123:722–726.
30. Shen P-F, Zhang S-C: Acute renal failure and multiple-organ-system failure. Arch Surg 1987;122:1131–1133.
31. Goris RJA, te Boekhorst TPA, Nuytinck JKS: Multiple organ failure: generalized autodestructive inflammation? Arch Surg 1985;120:1109–1115.
32. Fischer RP: High mortality of post-traumatic renal insufficiency in Vietnam: a review of 96 cases. Am Surg 1974;40:172–177.
33. Baker CC, Trunkey D, Miller C: Epidemiology of trauma deaths. Am J Surg 1980;140:144–150.
34. Baker CC, Trunkey D, Miller C: Impact of a trauma service on trauma care in a university hospital. Am J Surg 1985;149:453–458.
35. Baue AE: Sequential or multiple systems failure. In: Najarian J, Delaney J (eds) Critical Surgical Care. Miami, Symposia Specialists, 1977;293–300.
36. Baue AE, Chaudry IH: Prevention of multiple systems failure. Surg Clin North Am 1980;60:1167–1178.
37. Baue AE: Multiple organ or systems failure. In: Haimovici H (ed) Vascular Emergencies Norwalk, CT, Appleton-Century-Crofts, 1981.
38. Faist E, Heberer G, Baue AE: Das mehrorgan versagen beim polytraumatisierten patienten. Krankenhausarzt 1983;56: 1–14.

39. Baue AE: Multiple organ or systems failure. In: Delaney JP, Najarian JS (eds) Trauma and Critical Care Surgery. Chicago, Year Book, 1987;363–367.
40. Zimmerman JE, Knaus WA, Sun X, Wagner DP: Severity stratification and outcome prediction for multisystem organ failure and dysfunction. World J Surg 1996;20:401–405.
41. Baue AE: Multiple organ failure, multiple organ dysfunction syndrome, and the systemic inflammatory response syndrome: where do we stand? Shock 1994;2:395–397.
42. Baue AE: Multiple Organ Failure: Patient Care and Prevention. St. Louis, Mosby-Year Book, 1990.
43. Knaus WA, Draper EA, Wagner DP, et al: Prognosis in acute organ-system failure. Ann Surg 1985;202:685–693.
44. Goris RJA, te Bockhorst TPA, Nuytinck JKS, Gimbrere JSF: Multiple organ failure. Arch Surg 1985;120:1109–1110.
45. Norton LW: Does drainage of intraabdominal pus reverse multiple organ failure? Am J Surg 1985;149:347–350.
46. Pine RW, Wertz MJ, Lennard ES, et al: Determinants of organ malfunction or death in patient with intra-abdominal sepsis. Arch Surg 1983;118:242–249.
47. Carrico CJ, Meakins JL, Marshall JC, Fry D, Maier V: Multiple-organ failure syndrome. Arch Surg 1986;121:196–208.
48. Marshall JC, Christou NV, Horn R, Meakins JL: The microbiology of multiple organ failure. Arch Surg 1988;123:309–315.
49. Bihari D, Sinithies M, Ginison A, Tinker J: The effects of vasodilation with prostacyclin on oxygen delivery and uptake in critically ill patients. N Engl J Med 1987;317:397–403.
50. Bell RC, Coalson JJ, Smith JD, Johanson WG: Multiple organ system failure and infection in adult respiratory distress. Ann Intern Med 1983;99:293–298.
51. Darling GE, Duff JH, Mustard RA, Finley JR: Multiorgan failure in critically ill patients. Can J Surg 1988;31:172–176.
52. Rubin DB, Wiener-Kronish JP, Murray JF, et al: Elevated von Willebrand factor antigen is an early plasma predictor of acute lung injury in nonpulmonary sepsis syndrome. J Clin Invest 1990;86:474–480.
53. Saffle JR, Sullivan JJ, Tuohig GM, Larson CM: Multiple organ failure in patients with thermal injury. Crit Care Med 1993;21:1673–1683.
54. Kollef MH: Ventilator-associated pneumonia. JAMA 1994;270:1964–1970.
55. Hebert PC, Drummond AJ, Singer J, Bernard GR, Russel JA: A simple multiple system organ failure scoring system predicts mortality of patients who have sepsis syndrome. Chest 1993;104:230–235.
56. Ruokenen E, Takala J, Kari A, Alhava E: Septic shock and multiple organ failure. Crit Care Med 1991;10:1146–1151.
57. Manship L, McMillin RD, Brown JJ: the influence of sepsis and multisystem and organ failure on mortality in the surgical intensive care unit. Am Surg 1984;50:94–101.
58. Moore FA, Moore EE, Pogetti R, et al: Gut bacterial translocation via the protal vein: a clinical perspective with major torso trauma. J Trauma 1991;31:629–638.
59. Fry DE, Pearlstein L, Fulton RL, Polk HC: Multiple system organ failure. Arch Surg 1980;115:136–140.
60. Dorinsky PM, Gadek JE: Multiple organ failure. Clin Chest Med 1990;11:581–591.
61. Dobb GJ: Multiple organ failure: "words mean what I say they mean." Intensive Care World 1991;8:157–159.
62. Eiseman B, Beart R, Norton L: Multiple organ failure. Surg Gynecol Obstet 1977;144:323–326.
63. Marshall JC, Cook DA, Sibbald WJ, Roy PD, Christou NV: The multiple organ dysfunction (MOD) score: a reliable descriptor of a complex clinical outcome. Crit Care Med 1992;20:580.
64. Baue AE, Durham R, Faist E: Systemic inflammatory response syndrome (SIRS), multiple organ dysfunction syndrome (MODS), multiple organ failure (MOF): are we winning the battle? Shock 1998;20(2):79–89.
65. Bernard G: The Brussels Score. Sepsis 1997;1:43–44.
66. Vincent JL: Organ dysfunction as an outcome measure: the sofa score. Sepsis 1997;1:53–54.
67. LeGall F, Klar J, Lemeshow S: How to assess organ dysfunction in the intensive care unit? The logistic organ dysfunction (LOD) system. Sepsis 1997;1:45–47.
68. Wright JG, McLeod RS, Lossing A, et al: Measurement in surgical clinical research. Surg 1996;119:241–244.
69. Feinstein AR: Clinimetrics. New Haven, CT, Yale University Press, 1987.
70. Knaus WA, Zimmerman JE, Wagner DP, et al: APACHE: Acute physiology and chronic health evaluation; a physiologically based classification system. Crit Care Med 1981;9:591–597.
71. AACP/SCCM Consensus Conference Committee: Definitions for sepsis and organ failure and guidelines for the use of innovative therapies in sepsis. Chest 1992;101:1644.
72. Knaus WA, Wagner DP, Draper EA, et al: The APACHE III prognostic system: risk prediction of hospital mortality for critically ill hospitalized adults. Chest 1991;100:1619–1636.
73. LeGall J-R, Lemeshow S, Saulnier F: A new Simplified Acute Physiology Score (SAPS II) based on a European/North American multicenter study. JAMA 1993;270:2957–2486.
74. Lemeshow S, Teres D, Klar J, et al: Mortality probability models (MPM II) based on an international cohort of intensive care unit patients. JAMA 1993;270:2478–2486.
75. Zhu B-P, Lemeshow S, Hosmer DW, et al: Factors affecting the performance of the models in the mortality probability model II system and strategies of customization: a simulation study. Crit Care Med 1996;24:57–63.
76. Lemeshow S, Klar J, Teres D, et al: Mortality probability models for patients in the intensive care unit for 48 or 72 hours: a prospective, multicenter study. Crit Care Med 1994;22:1351–1358.
77. Cullen DJ, Civetta JM, Briggs BA, et al: Therapeutic intervention scoring system: a method for quantitative comparison of patient care. Crit Care Med 1974;2:57–60.
78. LeGall JR, Lemeshow S, Leleu G: Customized probability models for early severe sepsis in adult intensive care patients. JAMA 1995;273:644–650.
79. Seneff M, Knaus WA: Predicting patients outcome from intensive care: a guide to APACHE, MPM, SAPS, PRISM, and other prognostic scoring systems. J Intensive Care Med 1997;5:33–52.
80. Castella X, Artigas A, Bion J, et al: A comparison of severity of illness scoring systems for intensive care unit patients: results of a multicenter, multinational study. Crit Care Med 1995;23:1327.
81. Roumen RMH, Redl H, Schlag G, et al: Scoring systems and blood lactate concentrations in relation to the development of adult respiratory distress syndrome and multiple organ failure in severely traumatized patients. J Trauma 1993;35:349–355.
82. Barie PS, Hydo LJ, Fischer E: Utility of illness severity scoring for prediction of prolonged surgical critical care. J Trauma 1996;40:513–518.
83. Rutledge R: The injury severity score is unable to differentiate between poor care and severe injury. J Trauma 1996;40:944–950.
84. Lewis FR: Editorial comment. J Trauma 1996;40:950.

85. Wong DT, Barrow PM, Gomez M, McGuire GP: A comparison of the acute physiology and chronic health evaluation (APACHE) II score and the trauma-injury severity score (TRISS) for outcome assessment in intensive care unit trauma patients. Crit Care Med 1996;24:1642–1648.
86. Baue AE: Who is keeping score? An overview to introduce a consensus conference on outcome prediction. In: Baue AE, Berlot G, Gullo A (eds) Sepsis and Organ Dysfunction. New York; Springer-Verlag, 1998; 35–44.
87. Sauaia A, Moore FA, Moore EE, et al: Early predictors of postinjury multiple organ failure. Arch Surg 1994;129:39–45.
88. Tran DD, Cuesta MA, van Leeuwen PAM, et al: Risk factors for multiple organ failure and death in critically injured patients. Surgery 1993;114:21–30.
89. Tryba M: Sucralfate vs antacids, H2 antagonist for stress ulcer prophlaxis; a method—analysis on efficacy and pneumonia rate. Crit Care Med 1991;19:942–949.
90. Sauaia A, Moore FA, Moore EE, Norris JM, et al: Multiple organ failure can be predicted as early as 12 hours after injury. J Trauma 1998;45:291–303.
91. Henao FJ, Daes JE, Dennis OJ: Risk factors for multiple organ failure; a case-control study. J Trauma 1991;31:74–80.
92. Hammermeister RE, Burchfield S, Johnson R, Grover F: Identification of patients at greater risk for developing major complications at cardiac surgery. Circulation 1990;82:380–389.

2
SIRS, MODS, and the Brave New World of ICU Acronyms: Have They Helped Us?

John C. Marshall

Physicians like acronyms. Whether they denote a biologic entity such as TNF, a physiologic measurement such as CVP, a classification system such as APACHE, a syndrome such as AIDS, a disease such as TB, a therapy such as a CABG or ECMO, or even an investigative undertaking such as GUSTO, there is something both familiar and authoritative about distilling a complex biomedical concept into a short, manageable, and pronounceable group of initials. Acronyms both clarify and obfuscate, and serve to transform an amorphous clinical problem into one or more recognizable conditions for which the possibilities and limitations are recognized. The patient with acute respiratory failure and a diffuse infiltrate on the chest radiograph is an example: Measure the PCWP—if it is elevated it is CHF, otherwise it is ARDS. The clinical shorthand suggests a rapid diagnostic approach and a simple binary approach to management.

Simplification and classification are necessary preconditions for treatment, and the very essence of diagnosis and clinical decision-making Algorithms, whether implicit or explicit, form the foundation of medical practice. However, in the most complex group of patients encountered in contemporary medical practice—the multiply-traumatized or acutely ill patients who are admitted to an intensive care unit (ICU)—the acronyms have proven to be a particularly inadequate embodiment of clinical reality. SIRS (systemic inflammatory response syndrome), MODS (multiple organ dysfunction syndrome), CARS (compensatory antiinflammatory response syndrome), MARS (mixed antagonistic response syndrome), and ARDS, though reflections of evolving concepts of the nature of critical illness, have proven to have limited utility in identifying groups of critically ill patients who might benefit from a particular approach to therapy. Their limitations point to the need for improved understanding of the process of being critically ill.

Concepts, Syndromes, and Diseases of Critical Illness

A *disease* is a discrete alteration in physiologic function that brings harm to the host. It may have one or many causes. Cancer, for example, is the disease that results when the normal mechanisms limiting cell growth are perturbed, with the result that such growth occurs excessively and autonomously. Meningitis is a disease that arises because of microbial invasion into the cerebrospinal fluid, its life-threatening manifestations reflecting both the local proliferation of microorganisms and the response of the host to their presence. Whereas a disease is defined by derangement of normal function, its treatments are directed at distinct components of that process. When a cancer is localized, it can be treated by surgical resection. If not, cytotoxic therapy given to inhibit the process of pathologic cell growth may be appropriate. However, it is empirically evident that not all cytotoxic agents work equally well for all kinds of cancer and that not all patients with cancer benefit from a particular therapy.

Thus the development of effective treatment requires two more refinements. The disease must be further classified on the basis of biologic variables to delineate more homogeneous subgroups of patients who may respond to a particular therapy (patients with squamous cell carcinoma of the lung versus those with small-cell lung cancer, for example), and it must be staged so treatment is given to those who are most likely to benefit (patients with high grade carotid stenosis versus those with low grade lesions, for example). Within any given group of patients with a disease process that is relatively homogeneous from a biologic perspective, some have disease that is sufficiently early or sufficiently mild that survival following therapy is virtually certain, whereas others have a process that is so advanced therapy cannot be expected to produce a meaningful response.

A *syndrome* is a combination of clinical or biochemical abnormalities thought to be the manifestations of a disease, even when the biologic basis for that disease remains unknown. Prior to identification of the human immunodeficiency virus (HIV), a new syndrome was recognized that was characterized by lymphadenopathy, weight loss, opportunistic infection, and Kaposi's sarcoma; it occurred with increased frequency in certain populations (homosexual men, hemophiliacs, and intravenous drug users).[1] Delineation of this distinctive syndrome aided the search for its cause by focusing attention on a specific group of patients.

Designation of a combination of findings as a syndrome is an arbitrary process: No formal guidelines exist for a particular combination of abnormalities to be denoted as a syndrome. Rather, the acceptance of a new syndrome reflects its perceived utility by a population of practitioners who can use the criteria to categorize patients to understand their illness or to guide their management. One could, for example, define a lung cancer syndrome characterized by cough, weight loss, hemoptysis, and chest radiographic abnormalities. This notion is unlikely to be attractive to clinicians for two reasons. First, not all patients with lung cancer manifest the syndrome; and conversely, not all patients with the syndrome have lung cancer (they might have, for example, tuberculosis, congestive heart failure, or Goodpasture syndrome). Second, and even more importantly, readily available diagnostic tests such as bronchoscopy with biopsy, mediastinoscopy, and computed tomographic (CT) scanning permit the diagnosis to be made with greater sensitivity and specificity than are afforded by the relatively nonspecific clinical criteria of the syndrome. Thus the terminology "syndrome" is useful when it identifies specific groups of patients who might benefit from specific investigations or therapy, or for whom more specific diagnoses cannot be made readily.

There are, however, a large number of disorders whose pathophysiology is unknown or, if it is understood, has not given rise to effective therapy, and whose clinical boundaries are ill-defined. Some are benign, self-limited conditions. The diagnosis of gastroenteritis, for example, encompasses a large number of disease processes, from viral infections to food hypersensitivity to stress-related disorders; the impetus to provide a more precise diagnosis is small, as the consequences are minor and the symptoms generally of short duration. For other diagnoses the consequences may be more severe, yet the lack of an objective basis for differentiating discrete diseases renders the process of diagnosis uncertain and even controversial. In the past, the diagnosis of consumption gave way to the more precise disease diagnoses of tuberculosis or carcinoma of the lung; and that of chronic intestinal stasis[2] was dismissed as a nonentity. Which of these two paths lies in the future of such current conundrums as environmental hypersensitivity or fibromyalgia is unknown.

For still other disorders, the lack of precise understanding that might define a disease stands as a significant impediment to progress in defining more effective therapies. It is ironic that in the ICU, where more physiologic information is available than in any other venue in the health care system, such challenges are particularly common. Entities such as sepsis, acute lung injury, multiple organ failure, and persistent failure to wean are common and readily recognized by all practitioners. Yet the criteria used to delineate these processes are variable; and for any given patient there is less than perfect agreement among clinicians on whether the process, so readily conceptualized in the abstract, is actually present.[3] It is hardly surprising, therefore, that specific therapies are not available, and that attempts to develop therapies have proven so frustrating.

The promulgation of concepts such as that of SIRS or MODS[4] has perhaps served to bring into focus some key aspects of the nature of contemporary critical illness. Whether these acronyms benefit either the patient or the physician is controversial.[5] This chapter argues that they represent initial steps along the complicated road from compelling concepts, to diseases that can be treated, to improve clinical outcome.

Sepsis, SIRS, and the Inflammatory Response in Critical Illness

The word *sepsis* was first used by Hippocrates more than two millennia ago to denote a process of tissue breakdown that resulted in disease, a foul smell, and death. Sepsis was the negative counterpart to *pepsis*, a process of tissue breakdown that was life-giving and embodied in the digestion of food or the fermentation of grapes to produce wine.[6] With the identification of microorganisms as the cause of infectious diseases, the word sepsis was seconded as a synonym for severe microbial infection, and septicemia denoted the presence of bacteria in the circulation.

Prior to the development of effective antimicrobial therapy, the equation of bacterial infection with the clinical response it evoked was a logical step. The introduction of effective antimicrobial therapy exposed a weakness in this assumption, however, as antibiotics did not eliminate the problem of sepsis but merely changed its epidemiology. Studies of the bacteriology of infections in hospitalized patients showed that the introduction of antimicrobial agents was associated with a shift from a predominance of infections with exogenous species to one of infection with endogenous species, with no significant alteration in the prevalence of such infections in hospitalized patients.[7] With the widespread introduction of ICUs during the decade of the 1960s, there was a further shift in the microbial spectrum. Whereas infections with gram-negative organisms had previously been uncommon, these infections emerged as the most common and certainly the most serious infections faced by critically ill patients.[8] The ability to support vital organ function during an acute infection that would otherwise be rapidly lethal also brought an awareness that the physiologic consequences of infection—the acute changes in hemodynamic, respiratory, renal, and gastrointestinal function—represented an unsolved challenge when managing the septic patient.[9] This conceptual shift marked the beginning of studies that focused on trying to improve outcome by modulating the host response.[10,11]

Two large multicenter clinical trials conducted during the early 1980s tested the hypothesis that survival of sepsis could be improved by the concomitant administration of supraphysiologic doses of glucocorticoids.[12,13] Neither of these studies showed benefit for the experimental intervention, but they ushered in a new era in sepsis research by articulating a series of criteria that purported to identify the population of patients most likely to benefit from immunomodulatory therapy: patients manifesting a series of physiologic abnormalities denoted as sepsis syndrome. *Sepsis syndrome* was defined as the occurrence of tachycardia, tachypnea, hyper- or hypothermia, and evidence of altered organ perfusion in a patient suspected of harboring an infection.[14] The rationale for proposing such a syndrome was compelling. Preclinical studies suggested that corticosteroids were most effective when given prior to or as soon as possible after the infectious insult. The results of microbiologic cultures are only slowly obtained, and it was therefore desirable to define a set of clinical parameters, present early in the course of the septic process, that would identify patients who were likely to be infected.

The specific features that define sepsis syndrome were established not through an intensive study of the natural history and clinical epidemiology of critically ill patients with life-threatening infection but, rather, through an ad hoc process of consensus, achieved apparently under somewhat testy circumstances in a hotel room in Las Vegas. It is questionable whether the resulting criteria define a syndrome let alone delineate an appropriate population for a clinical trial of high dose glucocorticoids. Tachycardia and tachypnea are highly nonspecific physiologic responses, and temperature changes may or may not be present in patients with infection; establishment of the presence of infection relies on clinical suspicion, a subjective and poorly reproducible variable. Epidemiologic studies of patients meeting these criteria confirm that the patients comprise a highly heterogeneous group with respect to clinical outcome [14] and the presence of the putative mediators of sepsis.[15] Microbiologically proven infection is present in fewer than half of patients with sepsis syndrome. Sepsis syndrome has been used as the entry criterion for most studies of novel approaches to modulate the inflammatory response.[16] The disappointing outcomes of these studies are well known and reflect, in part, the inadequacy of the entry criterion. In fact, recent work suggests that glucocorticoids can have a beneficial effect on outcome when used in a differently defined population: patients with refractory septic shock, defined as prolonged vasopressor dependence.[17]

Dissatisfaction with the terminology used to describe the process of overwhelming inflammation in the critically ill and, in particular, variability in the use of the word sepsis led to a consensus conference jointly sponsored by the American College of Chest Physicians and the Society of Critical Care Medicine (ACCP/SCCM). That conference suggested that the word sepsis be reserved for those circumstances in which clinical inflammation arises from invasive infection. It defined infection as a microbiologic phenomenon characterized by the invasion of normally sterile host tissues by microorganisms or their products; it suggested that new terminology was needed to describe the process of systemic inflammation, independent of its cause. Thus the acronym SIRS was introduced into the medical lexicon (Fig. 2.1). SIRS describes the occurrence of the physiologic manifestations of systemic inflammation independent of the cause; sterile causes of SIRS include ischemia, tissue injury, sterile inflammation, drug reactions, and autoimmune disorders.[4]

It has been documented in a number of cohort studies that the inflammatory response, independent of the infections that commonly trigger it, is an important determinant of outcome,[18-20] and the concept of SIRS reflects this evolving understanding. SIRS is an attractive concept, but is it a

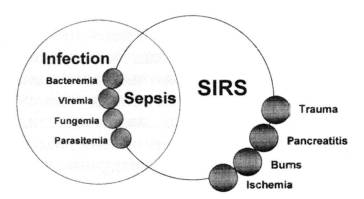

FIGURE 2.1. Interrelation of infection and the host inflammatory response. Infection is a microbial phenomenon characterized by the invasion of normally sterile tissues by microorganisms or their products. Occasionally, those organisms can be isolated from the systemic circulation, giving rise to bacteremia if the organism is a bacterium. The prototypical clinical response that arises in the host in response to serious infection is denoted as the systemic inflammatory response syndrome (SIRS). SIRS is a nonspecific response that is also elicited by trauma, burns, pancreatitis, ischemia/reperfusion injury, drug reactions, and autoimmune disorders. When SIRS arises as a consequence of invasive infection, the process is termed *sepsis*. (Adapted from Bone et al.[4] with permission.)

syndrome? Using the definition proposed above—a combination of clinical or biochemical abnormalities that indicate the presence of disease—it clearly is not: Although SIRS may develop following administration of a bolus of endotoxin to a human volunteer,[21] it may also develop following or during exercise, stress, or lovemaking. The specific criteria used to defined SIRS are similar to those for sepsis syndrome; and like the criteria for sepsis syndrome, they represent an arbitrary constellation of physiologic abnormalities, rather than an empirically derived set of abnormalities that are known to correlate with the pathologic process of interest. Indeed the basis for selecting the four SIRS variables—tachycardia, tachypnea, hyper- or hypothermia, and leukopenia or leukocytosis—is unclear; consideration of specific criteria for SIRS was not part of the ACCP/SCCM consensus conference. The four SIRS criteria are all components of the APACHE II system, suggesting that they are simply generic severity of illness measures, not specific markers of an exaggerated inflammatory response.

The attempt to define a clinical syndrome or a set of diagnostic variables that reflect the systemic activation of a host inflammatory response stems from a well established concept: Infection and other acute insults such as trauma or ischemia produce tissue injury in the host by inducing the release of injurious mediator molecules from host immune cells, and these mediators in turn are responsible for the physiologic and biochemical alterations seen in the clinical setting. However, the definition of a syndrome requires that it first be shown that the elements of the syndrome reliably reflect the presence of the pathologic process underlying it. Because the mediator response is not well defined in biochemical terms, and because the criteria for sepsis syndrome or SIRS lack both sensitivity and specificity for establishing the presence of any discrete component of that response, neither can truly be considered to define a syndrome.

Indeed the concept that the inflammatory response defines a syndrome may be inappropriate. Inflammation is less a pathologic process than an appropriate adaptive response to an acute threat to homeostasis; failure to mount that response can also have adverse consequences for the host.[22] The better conceptual model for systemic inflammation may be that exemplified by either the endocrine or coagulation systems: an adaptive process regulating homeostasis that becomes pathologic when it is deficient or overactive. For both processes, the clinical challenge is to characterize the biochemical abnormality using signs and symptoms to trigger investigations. Easy bruising or inappropriate clotting prompt the physician to define a discrete disorder (e.g., deficiency of factor VIII or protein S). Similarly, tachycardia and heat intolerance, two relatively nonspecific symptoms, prompt the physician to evaluate thyroid hormone levels. In both cases specific therapy is directed toward the abnormality in the level of the factor of interest, and in neither is it a prerequisite that we define either a bleeding syndrome or a syndrome of hyperthyroidism. Yet clinical studies of mediator-targeted therapy have proceeded from precisely the opposite direction: study candidates are selected on the basis of meeting nonspecific criteria for sepsis syndrome or SIRS, and levels of the mediator target of interest are not considered when defining the appropriate population to treat. A retrospective analysis of patients enrolled in a trial of an antiendotoxin therapy[23] showed that evidence of benefit was greatest for those patients in whom levels of endotoxin were highest.

Other systems have been developed to describe or quantify the systemic inflammatory response,[18,24] but none has been shown to correlate with a discrete pathologic process that can be modulated therapeutically. It has also been proposed that the complexities of systemic inflammation can be better described through the adoption of additional acronyms: CARS (compensatory antiinflammatory response syndrome) and MARS (mixed antagonistic response syndrome).[25] Although it is certainly true at a cellular level that the activation of proinflammatory mediator synthesis is accompanied by the synthesis of a number of antiinflammatory and regulatory mediators, there is no evidence at the level of the whole organism that this process occurs separately from activation of a systemic inflammatory response (and therefore merits consideration as an entity distinct from SIRS) or, even if it did, that it can be detected by a panel of parameters, either clinical or biochemical, that would justify its being considered a syndrome.

In summary, then, articulation of the concept of SIRS has served to crystallize an evolving biologic concept: that the morbidity of inflammation arises through the response of the host rather than as a consequence of the particular process that triggered that response. SIRS is a constellation of symptoms, rather than a diagnosis, and should trigger a search for the cause of that symptom complex. The reflex administration of antimicrobial agents to patients with signs and symptoms of inflammation will hopefully become less common as the distinction between infecting and the response to infection becomes appreciated by clinicians. On the other hand, precisely because it is a symptom complex rather than a disease, SIRS does not identify any discrete pathologic process that could reasonably be expected to respond to a given therapy. Until we identify the specific diseases for which SIRS is the clinical manifestation, attempts to modulate the host response will continue to prove frustrating.[26]

Organ Dysfunction, Organ Failure, and the Clinical Sequelae of Inflammation

The evolution of concepts of altered organ function in critical illness mirrors the evolution of ideas regarding sepsis and the inflammatory response. The first ICU was established just over 40 years ago as a locale that could provide specialized, life-sustaining organ system support during a period of otherwise lethal physiologic instability.[27] ICUs became feasible because of the development of techniques of organ system support, including positive-pressure mechanical ventilation, renal dialysis, hemodynamic monitoring with support using fluids and vasoactive agents, and parenteral nutritional support. These advances, all arising within the space of two decades, made possible the prolonged survival of a group of patients who during an earlier era would have died a rapid death. They also established a paradigm for providing such support, by focusing on the particular failing systems whose functions were being supported. Organ system insufficiency requiring support was not only an indication for ICU admission but a complication of the clinical course following that admission.

The first descriptive reports of organ system insufficiency in the ICU focused on isolated organ systems such as the lung[28,29] and viewed the derangements of other systems as a manifestation of failure of a single system, for example, ARDS or disseminated intravascular coagulation (DIC). Skillman et al. were the first to suggest that combinations of failing organ systems might represent a distinct problem in critical care.[30] It remained for Baue in 1975 to articulate the notion that the unsolved problem of critical illness was less the failure of a single organ system than the concomitant failure of multiple organ systems and to emphasize how similar the postmortem findings were in a group of ICU patients dying as a result of highly diverse antecedent conditions.[31] This editorial set the stage for a series of descriptive studies of a phenomenon variously known as multiple organ failure,[32] remote organ failure,[33] and multiple system organ failure,[34] which established three important concepts. First, the syndrome was remarkably similar in its expression, even though its causes were highly diverse. Second, the prognosis for patients manifesting this process was a function of the *number* of failing organ systems. Finally, multiple organ failure commonly arose in the wake of a life-threatening infection and on occasion was the first clinical sign of untreated infection.[33,35]

Subsequent studies showed that the prognosis for patients with organ system failure was a function not only of the number of failing systems but also of the severity of dysfunction within each system.[36,37] Thus the ACCP/SCCM consensus conference proposed that MODS be adopted to describe a process that was not only variable in its severity but potentially reversible following a period of organ system support.[4]

In contrast to SIRS, whose criteria define an appropriate and adaptive physiologic response, the development of organ dysfunction is always detrimental to the host. It is therefore appropriate to consider MODS as a syndrome—not a disease to be treated but an outcome to be prevented. The development of MODS invariably follows an acute threat to life that evokes the physiologic changes of systemic inflammation. MODS can be conceived as the maladaptive outcome of systemic inflammation, the syndrome that reflects the adverse consequences of a potentially life-preserving response. Such a model has important implications for clinical studies of therapies that can modify the expression of inflammation in the critically ill, as the objective of such interventions can be redefined as support of the beneficial aspects of inflammation and minimization of its maladaptive and detrimental consequences. It is of considerable importance therefore that the syndrome be defined optimally.

Approaches to the Description of MODS

If MODS is a syndrome, how should it be characterized? First, although a number of organ systems may show evidence of physiologic dysfunction in the critically ill, there is no convincing evidence to suggest that any particular pattern of organ system involvement characterizes the syndrome. Whereas pulmonary and hematologic dysfunction may arise in one patient, in another the predominant manifestations of organ dysfunction may be cardiovascular, hepatic, and renal dysfunction. It is generally assumed that the specific pattern of organ dysfunction per se has no diagnostic or prognostic significance. Rather, MODS is defined by the concurrence of dysfunction in two or more organ systems; and the severity of the physiologic derangement, rather than its pattern, carries the greatest prognostic importance. Thus descriptive systems for MODS uniformly omit the requirement for involvement of any given organ system but, rather, focus on the multiplicity of systems involved.

The organ systems whose dysfunction is considered to define MODS vary from one report to the next, but a systematic review of all published reports demonstrated that seven organ systems—respiratory, renal, hepatic, gastrointestinal, hematologic, cardiovascular, and neurologic—were included in at least half of all published studies.[38] On the other hand, systems such as the endocrine system[39,40] and the immune system,[41] whose functions can readily be shown to be deranged in critically ill patients, have rarely been included in descriptive reports of MODS. Their omission likely reflects the relative inaccessibility of measures of their dysfunction rather than a belief that this dysfunction portends a fundamentally different clinical process.

As important as the definition of the systems whose dysfunction defines MODS is identification of criteria that characterize dysfunction within a given organ system. In general terms, dysfunction can be defined by one of three approaches.

TABLE 2.1. Differences Between Organ Dysfunction Scales.

Variable	Approaches
Selection of variables	Physiologic variables only
	Combined physiologic and therapeutic variables
Variable describing cardiovascular dysfunction	Pressure-adjusted rate (Heart rate × CVP/MAP)
	Inotrope dose
	Blood pressure (elevation)
	Blood pressure, pH, fluid requirements)
Weighting of variables	Equal weighting based on independent contribution to ICU mortality
	Differential weighting based on aggregate contribution to mortality in logistic model
Value recorded	Worst values
	Representative value

CVP, central venous pressure; MAP, mean arterial pressure.

1. As a single variable that reflects a *physiologic derangement* (e.g., PO_2/FiO_2 ratio)
2. As a single variable that reflects a *therapeutic intervention* in response to a physiologic derangement (e.g., the need for mechanical ventilation)
3. As a combination of variables that in their own right define a *syndrome* (e.g., PO_2/FiO_2 ratio < 200, diffuse fluffy infiltrates on the chest radiograph, and a pulmonary capillary wedge pressure < 18, defining ARDS)

A series of properties of the optimal descriptor of organ dysfunction has been articulated[38] and forms the basis for one system that quantifies the severity of MODS as a score that measures the physiologic derangements of the syndrome.[42] A number of similar systems that measure organ dysfunction as an aggregate score have been proposed.[42–45] They differ in subtle but potentially important ways (Table 2.1), and further refinement of the descriptive process of MODS must focus on resolving or reconciling these differences.

Using Organ Dysfunction Scales to Describe the Course of Critical Illness

Organ dysfunction scores have been developed with the objective of describing the course of a critical illness, rather than predicting its outcome. Their use has been relatively limited to date, but the availability of validated and acceptable measures of organ dysfunction provides a tool that can serve a number of descriptive ends.[46]

Organ Dysfunction as a Risk Factor

The most powerful predictive tools are scoring systems such as APACHE[47] or the Simplified Acute Physiology Score (SAPS),[48] which have been developed to maximize their prognostic

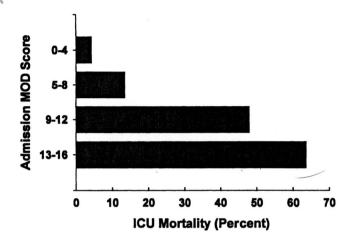

FIGURE 2.2. Severity of organ dysfunction on the day of ICU admission, as reflected in the multiple organ dysfunction (MOD) score, is strongly associated with the probability of ultimate ICU survival. Scores are the aggregate of representative values for dysfunction in each of six organ systems.[42] Data are from a study of 851 patients admitted to a surgical ICU.[49]

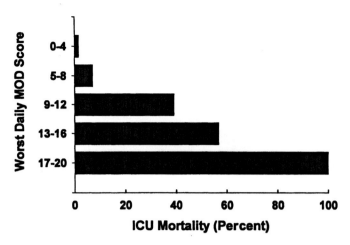

FIGURE 2.3. Severity of organ dysfunction occurring on a given ICU day correlates with the ultimate risk of ICU mortality. Such a point measure of illness severity can be followed to track the response to therapy, or it can be used as a surrogate for the intensity of resource utilization. (From Marshall et al.,[49] with permission.)

capabilities. Nonetheless, an organ dysfunction score that reflects increasing degrees of physiologic derangement early during the patient's clinical course score, by definition, can predict subsequent mortality.

Calculation of an organ dysfunction score on the day of ICU admission provides a measure of the severity of organ dysfunction at the onset of therapy. Such a measure can serve several purposes. As a baseline snapshot of illness severity, it provides the clinician with an indication of the extent of the patient's need for ICU support, which may aid in making decisions regarding staffing or resources and give an indication of the probability that such support will be successful (Fig. 2.2).[49] It cannot predict whether a given patient will live or die; but by providing an objective measure of the challenges faced and the expected outcome, it permits realistic discussions of the need for and limitations of therapy. Calculation of baseline organ dysfunction scores is of benefit for clinicians undertaking ICU research by defining an appropriate population for study (eliminating, for example, those who are either too well or too ill to benefit from therapy). Comparison of baseline scores provides a description of two or more study groups and permits comparison of their similarities and differences at baseline.

Organ Dysfunction as a Point Measure of Illness Severity

Calculating a score on any given day of ICU care provides a point measure of morbidity or illness severity. Such a measure can be followed serially to determine the clinical trajectory of an individual patient or a group of patients, or it can be calculated at a single point in time in a group of patients (e.g., 3 or 14 days after institution of therapy) to determine whether an intervention has altered outcome (Fig. 2.3). The worst single day's score can also be used as an outcome measure for a clinical trial.

Although not explicitly evaluated as such, daily organ dysfunction scores may provide a point estimate of the intensity of resource utilization, analogous to the Therapeutic Intervention Scoring System (TISS).[50]

Organ Dysfunction as a Measure of Aggregate ICU Morbidity

An understanding of the clinical course of an ICU patient cannot adequately be derived from an evaluation of the status of that patient at a single point in time, even if that evaluation is done on the day the patient was most severely ill. By calculating an aggregate organ dysfunction score as the sum of the worst day's values for each isolated organ system, without reference to the day on which that value was obtained, the clinician can obtain a measure of the severity of illness over the entire ICU stay, a measure of global morbidity that occurs during an ICU admission. Such an approach has been taken by organ failure systems that quantify organ dysfunction as the number of failing systems.[34,51,52] A similar approach is readily used with an organ dysfunction score (Fig. 2.4). Aggregate scores may be calculated over any time period (e.g., the ICU stay, the duration of the administration of a novel therapeutic agent, or the same interval for which survival is being evaluated in a clinical trial.

Organ Dysfunction as an Aggregate Measure of Morbidity and Mortality

Organ dysfunction scores minimize the importance of death as an ICU outcome. Although the risk of death increases as the organ dysfunction score increases, it is possible for a given patient to die with a low score or a high score; and regardless of that value, the significance for the patient is the same. If, for example, a new therapy under investigation reduced the severity of organ dysfunction but resulted in an increased risk of fatal

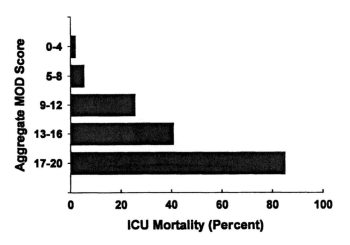

FIGURE 2.4. Aggregate scores are created by summing the worst daily value for each system, irrespective of whether those abnormalities occurred concomitantly or consecutively. They provide an aggregate measure of morbidity over time. The delta score, the difference between aggregate and admission scores, is a measure of morbidity specifically attributable to events occurring within the ICU. (From Marshall et al.,[49] with permission.)

cardiac dysrhythmias or myocardial infarction (complications for which scores would predictably be low), an organ dysfunction score might suggest benefit despite an increased mortality rate. The aggregate score described above can be adjusted to incorporate death as an outcome by assigning a maximal number of points to any patient who dies during the period of ascertainment. Such a mortality-adjusted score is a composite measure of both morbidity and mortality and has been used, for example, to demonstrate the detrimental consequences of transfusion above a trigger of 7 g/dl in critically ill patients.[53]

Measuring Change Over Time

These four basic models for the quantification of organ dysfunction permit the clinician to measure clinical change over time in a variety of ways. The difference between the aggregate score (with or without mortality adjustment) and the admission score (also known as the delta score) is a measure of organ dysfunction that arises after ICU admission and therefore is attributable to events occurring within the ICU and potentially modifiable through the institution of prophylactic or therapeutic measures. The delta score reflects that component of illness that is potentially modifiable and is therefore of particular interest to the physician. It can be calculated, for example, as an outcome measure in a clinical trial. Similarly, because it reflects new morbidity arising after the institution of ICU care, it can serve as a tool to identify cases for closer review for quality assurance processes. Regardless of the baseline severity of organ dysfunction, the risk of mortality in the ICU increases as the delta score increases, suggesting it is a sensitive surrogate outcome measure.

Delta scores can be calculated in other ways. A study of an intervention that may hasten the resolution of organ dysfunction could calculate the difference between baseline scores and the score at a predetermined interval following the resolution of therapy, or it could plot daily scores for two groups in a manner analogous to that used for plotting survival curves.

Conclusions

The ICU is unique in that it provides care for a group of patients who, if endogenous homeostatic processes had taken their normal course, would otherwise be dead. For illness of lesser gravity, survival in the absence of physiologic support is possible, and physiologic mechanisms have therefore evolved to maximize this probability. Evolutionary pressures have never had to contend with the array of interventions we routinely use to support the critically ill patient, and so it is hardly surprising that processes such as inflammation that are life-saving in their milder forms become part of a new problem to be solved in the highly artificial context of the ICU. Moreover, the boundaries of disease are blurred in a cohort of critically ill patients, and the very interventions used to support life become an intrinsic element of the pathologic processes that result in morbidity and death.[54]

The proliferation of acronyms to describe the course of critical illness reflects the efforts of intensivists to understand the complex interaction of disease, illness severity, and therapy that results in morbidity and mortality for the multiply-traumatized or critically ill patient. However, their articulation is a double-edged sword. By describing a process and defining boundaries for that process, the articulation of a new syndrome provides a basis by which workers can focus their investigations on subsets of patients or on a particular aspect of a series of complex physiologic interactions. The downside of such a process is the implicit assumption that by naming a process we have enhanced our understanding of it.

Certain critical care acronyms (e.g., CARS and MARS) describe concepts that have no defined correlate in clinical practice. Although they embody the biologic notion that activation of an inflammatory response is complex and includes intrinsic regulatory processes, they do not delineate a homogeneous group of patients in whom a consistent, unique biologic abnormality can be defined, or who can be shown to benefit from a particular therapeutic intervention. SIRS also defines a concept more than a syndrome, and it is only too well recognized that the criteria proposed for the syndrome lack the specificity necessary to differentiate patients with a disease from those with an appropriate, even pleasurable, physiologic response. The acronyms ARDS and MODS move closer to defining syndromes, as they are specific to processes in the critically ill, and their presence is always detrimental to the host. Their defining criteria remain frustratingly imprecise, however, and fail to discriminate homogeneous subpopulations of patients who might more appropriately be entered into trials of particular prophylactic or therapeutic strategies. The challenge facing critical care research is to move beyond concepts and syndromes to define discrete diseases of critical illness that reflect the derangement of a single, unique biologic process. Only then will we be able to move from nonspecific physiologic support to biology-based therapy.

References

1. Gottlieb MS, Schroff R, Schanker HM, et al: Pneumocystis carinii pneumonia and mucosal candidiasis in previously healthy homosexual men: evidence of a new acquired cellular immunodeficiency. N Engl J Med 1981;305:1425–1431.
2. Lane WA: Chronic intestinal stasis. BMJ 1912;1:989–993.
3. Nathens AB, Marshall JC: Sepsis, SIRS, and MODS. What's in a name? World J Surg 1996;20:386–391.
4. Bone RC, Balk RA, Cerra FB, et al: ACCP/SCCM consensus conference: definitions for sepsis and organ failure and guidelines for the use of innovative therapies in sepsis. Chest 1992;101:1644–1655.
5. Vincent JL: Dear SIRS, I'm sorry to say that I don't like you. Crit Care Med 1997;25:372–374.
6. Majno G: The ancient riddle of (sepsis). J Infect Dis 1991;163:937–945.
7. Rogers DE: The changing pattern of life-threatening microbial disease. N Engl J Med 1959;261:677–683.
8. McCabe WR, Jackson GG: Gram negative bacteremia: clinical, laboratory and therapeutic observations. Arch Intern Med 1962;110:92–100.
9. Maclean LD, Mulligan WG, Mclean APH, Duff JH: Patterns of septic shock in man: a detailed study of 56 patients. Ann Surg 1967;166:543–562.
10. Hinshaw LB, Archer LT, Beller-Todd BK, et al: Survival of primates in LD_{100} septic shock following steroid/antibiotic therapy. J Surg Res 1980;28:151–170.
11. Meakins JL, Christou NV, Shizgal HM, Maclean LD: Therapeutic approaches to anergy in surgical patients: surgery and levamisole. Ann Surg 1979;190:286–296.
12. The veterans administration systemic sepsis cooperative study group: effect of high dose glucocorticoid therapy on mortality in patients with clinical signs of systemic sepsis. N Engl J Med 1987;317:659–665.
13. Bone RC, Fisher CJ, Clemmer TP, Slotman GJ, Metz CA, Balk RA: A controlled clinical trial of high dose methylprednisolone in the treatment of severe sepsis and septic shock. N Engl J Med 1987;317:654–658.
14. Bone RC, Fisher CJ, Clemmer TP, Slotman GJ, Metz CA, Balk RA: The methylprednisolone severe sepsis study group: sepsis syndrome: a valid clinical entity. Crit Care Med 1989;17:389–393.
15. Casey LC, Balk RA, Bone RC: Plasma cytokines and endotoxin levels correlate with survival in patients with the sepsis syndrome. Ann Intern Med 1993;119:771–778.
16. Meade MO, Creery D, Marshall JC: Systematic review of outcome measures in randomized trials of mediator-directed therapies in sepsis. Sepsis 1997;1:27–33.
17. Bollaert PE, Charpentier C, Levy B, Debouvarie M, Audibert G, Larcan A: Reversal of late septic shock with supraphysiologic doses of hydrocortisone. Crit Care Med 1998;26:627–630.
18. Marshall JC, Sweeney D: Microbial infection and the septic response in critical surgical illness: sepsis, not infection, determines outcome. Arch Surg 1990;125:17–23.
19. Rangel-Frausto MS, Pittet D, Costigan M, Hwang T, Davis CS, Wenzel RP: The natural history of the systemic inflammatory response syndrome (SIRS): a prospective study. JAMA 1995;273:117–123.
20. Muckart DJJ, Bhagwanjee S: The ACCP/SCCM consensus conference definitions of the systemic inflammatory response syndrome (SIRS) and allied disorders in relation to critically injured patients. Crit Care Med 1997;25:1789–1795.
21. Suffredini AF: Endotoxin administration to humans: a model of inflammatory responses relevant to sepsis. In: Lamy M, Thijs LG (eds) Mediators of Sepsis. New York, Springer, 1992.
22. Marshall JC: Infection and the host septic response contribute independently to adverse outcome in critical illness: implications for clinical trials of mediator antagonism. In: Vincent J-L (ed) Yearbook of Intensive Care and Emergency Medicine. Berlin, Springer, 1994.
23. Wortel CH, von der Mohlen MA, van Deventer SJ, et al: Effectiveness of a human monoclonal anti-endotoxin antibody (HA-1A) in gram-negative sepsis: relationship to endotoxin and cytokine levels. J Infect Dis 1992;168:1367–1374.
24. Elebute EA, Stoner HB: The grading of sepsis. Br J Surg 1983;70:29–31.
25. Bone RC: Sir Isaac Newton, sepsis, SIRS, and CARS. Crit Care Med 1996;24:1125–1128.
26. Abraham E, Marshall JC: Sepsis and mediator-directed therapy: rethinking the target populations. Mol Med Today 1999;5:56–58.
27. Safar P, De Kornfeld T, Pearson J, et al: Intensive care unit. Anesthesia 1961;16:275.
28. Burke JF, Pontoppidan H, Welch CE: High output respiratory failure: an important cause of death ascribed to peritonitis or ileus. Ann Surg 1963;158:581–595.
29. Ashbaugh DG, Bigelow DB, Petty TL, Levine BE: Acute respiratory distress in adults. Lancet 1967;2:319–323.
30. Skillman JJ, Bushnell LS, Goldman H, Silen W: Respiratory failure, hypotension, sepsis, and jaundice: a clinical syndrome associated with lethal hemorrhage and acute stress ulceration in the stomach. Am J Surg 1969;117:523–530.
31. Baue AE: Multiple, progressive, or sequential systems failure: a syndrome of the 1970s. Arch Surg 1975;110:779–781.
32. Eiseman B, Beart R, Norton L: Multiple organ failure. Surg Gynecol Obstet 1977;144:323–326.
33. Polk HC, Shields CL: Remote organ failure: a valid sign of occult intraabdominal infection. Surgery 1977;81:310–313.
34. Fry DE, Pearlstein L, Fulton RL, Polk HC: Multiple system organ failure: the role of uncontrolled infection. Arch Surg 1980;115:136–140.
35. Meakins JL, Wicklund B, Forse RA, Mclean APH: The surgical intensive care unit: current concepts in infection. Surg Clin North Am 1980;60:117–132.
36. Goris RJA, te Boekhorst TPA, Nuytinck JKS, Gimbrere JSF: Multiple organ failure: generalized autodestructive inflammation? Arch Surg 1985;120:1109–1115.
37. Marshall JC, Christou NV, Horn R, Meakins JL: The microbiology of multiple organ failure: the proximal GI tract as an occult reservoir of pathogens. Arch Surg 1988;123:309–315.
38. Marshall JC: Multiple organ dysfunction syndrome (MODS). In: Sibbald WJ, Vincent J-L (eds) Clinical Trials for the Treatment of Sepsis. Berlin, Springer, 1995;122–138.
39. Rothwell PM, Udwadia ZF, Lawler PG: Thyrotropin concentration predicts outcome in critical illness. Anaesthesia 1993;48:373–376.
40. Baldwin WA, Allo M: Occult hypoadrenalism in critically ill patients. Arch Surg 1993;128:673–676.
41. Christou NV, Meakins JL, Gordon J, et al: The delayed hypersensitivity response and host resistance in surgical patients: 20 years later. Ann Surg 1995;222:534–548.

42. Marshall JC, Cook DJ, Christou NV, Bernard GR, Sprung CL, Sibbald WJ: Multiple organ dysfunction score: a reliable descriptor of a complex clinical outcome. Crit Care Med 1995;23:1638-1652.
43. Vincent JL, Moreno R, Takala J, et al: The sepsis-related organ failure assessment (SOFA) score to describe organ dysfunction/failure. Intensive Care Med 1996;22:707-710.
44. Bernard G, Doig G, Hudson G, et al: Quantification of organ dysfunction for clinical trials in sepsis. Am J Respir Crit Care Med 1995;151:A323.
45. Le Gall JR, Klar J, Lemeshow S, et al: The logistic organ dysfunction system: a new way to assess organ dysfunction in the intensive care unit. JAMA 1996;276:802-810.
46. Marshall JC: Charting the course of critical illness: prognostication and outcome measurement in the ICU. Crit Care Med 1999;27:676-678.
47. Knaus WA, Draper EA, Wagner DP, Zimmerman JE: APACHE II: a severity of disease classification system. Crit Care Med 1985;13:818-829.
48. Le Gall J-R, Lemeshow S, Saulnier F: A new simplified acute physiology score (SAP 11) based on a European/North American multicenter study. JAMA 1993;270:2957-2963.
49. Marshall J, Foster D, McKenna C, et al: Toronto Hospital ICU Research Group: Quantification of the multiple organ dysfunction syndrome (MODS) as a risk, factor, outcome descriptor, and surrogate measure of morbidity in the ICU. Crit Care Med 1996;24:A53.
50. Keene AR, Cullen DJ: Therapeutic intervention scoring system: update 1983. Crit Care Med 1983;11:1-3.
51. Tran DD, Groeneveld ABJ, van der Meulen J, Nauta JJP, Strack van Schijndel RJM, Thijs LG: Age, chronic disease, sepsis, organ system failure, and mortality in a medical intensive care unit. Crit Care Med 1990;18:474-479.
52. Hebert PC, Drummond AJ, Singer J, Bernard GR, Russell JA: A simple multiple system organ failure scoring system predicts mortality of patients who have sepsis syndrome. Chest 1993;104:230-235.
53. Hebert PC, Wells G, Blajchman MA, et al: Transfusion requirements in critical care investigators for the Canadian critical care trials group: a multicentre randomized controlled clinical trial of transfusion requirements in critical care. N Engl J Med 1999;340:409-417.
54. Slutsky AS, Tremblay LN: Multiple system organ failure: is mechanical ventilation a contributing factor? Am J Respir Crit Care Med 1998;157:1721-1725.

3
Systemic Inflammatory Response and Multiple Organ Dysfunction Syndrome: Biologic Domino Effect

Donald E. Fry

Considerable confusion has surrounded the physiologic states of the severely ill surgical patient. Patients who demonstrate tachypnea, tachycardia, fever, diaphoresis, and leukocytosis have a pattern of disease that is commonly associated with severe local clinical infection, bacteremia, or dissemination of microbial cell products (e.g., endotoxin) (or a combination of these entities). Such patients are commonly referred to us with a diagnosis of "sepsis" or "septicemia." The implication of these terms has traditionally been that these clinical manifestations are reflective of uncontrolled invasive infection that have resulted in systemic manifestations of the disease. Implied is that the infectious process itself has passed from a local event to one that is systemic in nature. Precision in the definition of this transition, from a local event to one that is systemic in scope, has been attempted by many authors, but none has been generally accepted. Furthermore, considerable evidence has evolved demonstrating that the systemic "septic" response is not a series of events that arise specifically or uniquely from microbes but is a nonspecific response of a host. Bacterial, fungal, and even viral infections elicit the same systemic response in the host.[1]

Inflammation appears to be the foundation event. Because inflammation is a nonspecific response to any of a series of physiologic perturbations, it is reasonable to assume that any event that activates inflammation locally (e.g., blunt injury, burns), if sufficiently severe or global in scope, could activate the systemic response, producing a clinical syndrome of "sepsis" but lacking microbial pathogens as the instigating event. It has become evident that "sepsis" due to true microbial infection and aseptic "sepsis" due to other stimuli are clinically similar in their clinical presentation, which creates the conundrum of an appropriate description of this systemic response that is independent of the inciting stimulus.

From a consensus conference,[2] the term systemic inflammatory response syndrome (SIRS) has evolved as the descriptive term for this physiologic response of the host to the systemic activation of human inflammation (Table 3.1). The criteria for SIRS have been generally categorized as being too liberal. A temperature over 38°C with a heart rate of more than 90 beats/min meets SIRS criteria but also describes virtually every child with otitis media or any patient with an infection of minimal consequence. Although the criteria are indeed "soft," the concept of inflammation as a beneficial local soft tissue event that becomes activated as a deleterious systemic event is the critical point of emphasis. The occurrence of this transition from a local event to a systemic event is usually evident to the experienced clinician, but precise definition of the transition point with objective clinical measurements has been elusive. Sepsis is thus defined in the contemporary clinical scene as the activation of SIRS by a clinical infectious event. Although this refined definition seems to have provided some order to this complex situation, many patients with severe SIRS have inconclusive evidence that clinical infection is the activating event or that infection becomes a secondary event following the initiation of systemic inflammation by other events such as hemorrhage or severe soft tissue injury (see Chapter 61).

A more detailed discussion of the biology of human inflammation is presented in Chapter 9. The important, beneficial effects that result from local activation of inflammation include (1) local vasodilation of the microcirculation, which increases bulk flow but reduces flow velocity; (2) increased vascular permeability, which facilitates suffusion of the injured or infected tissue with important serum proteins (e.g., opsonins, complement, prekallikrein); and (3) generation of an abundance of chemoattractant signals, which serve as chemical "beacons" to draw neutrophils and monocytes into the midst of the inflammatory milieu. Thus if systemic activation of inflammation becomes the pivotal hallmark of SIRS as a physiologic event, it is reasonable to assume that systemic vasodilatation, systemic increased blood flow, and systemic edema should be objective measures by which to identify when the transition from a local event to SIRS has occurred.

Stages of SIRS

In an important study of a large number of critically ill surgical patients with a septic response (i.e., SIRS), Siegel et al.[3] identified four categories of pathophysiologic hemodynamic and metabolic changes. Although the original report by these authors addressed the response of the host as being the

TABLE 3.1. Current Definition of the Systemic Inflammatory Response Syndrome and Related Terminology.

Systemic inflammatory response syndrome: Systemic inflammatory response to a variety of severe clinical insults. The response is manifested by two or more of the following clinical conditions.

1. Core body temperature >38°C or <36°C
2. Heart rate > 90 beats/min
3. Respiratory rate > 20 breaths/min or $PaCO_2$ < 32 mmHg
4. White blood cell count > 12,000 cells/mm^3 or < 4000 cells/mm^3 or >10% immature (band) forms

Sepsis: Systemic inflammatory response syndrome secondary to infection.

Severe sepsis: Sepsis associated with organ dysfunction, hypoperfusion, or hypotension. Hypoperfusion and perfusion abnormalities may include but are not limited to lactic acidosis, oliguria, and an acute alteration in mental status.

Septic shock: Sepsis with hypotension, despite adequate fluid resuscitation, along with the presence of perfusion abnormalities that may include but are not limited to lactic acidosis, oliguria, and an acute alteration in mental status. Patients who are taking inotropic or vasopressor agents may not be hypotensive when perfusion abnormalities are documented.

Hypotension: Systolic blood pressure of <90 mmHg or a reduction of >40 mmHg from baseline in the absence of other causes of hypotension.

Multiple organ dysfunction syndrome: Presence of altered organ function in an acutely ill patient such that homeostasis cannot be maintained without intervention.

These definitions are frequently used for the critically ill patient but have not achieved standardized and accepted definitions.[2]

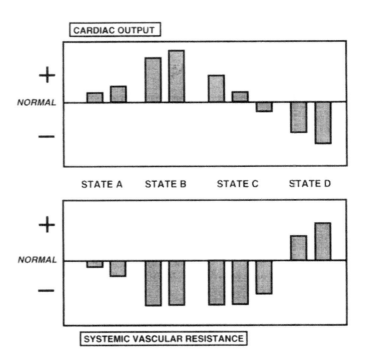

FIGURE 3.1. Relation between cardiac output and systemic vascular resistance during the four states of the systemic inflammatory response syndrome.

consequence of "sepsis," it is equally appropriate to interpret these data as being a prototype of SIRS. In this setting it was concluded that SIRS was the result of infection. Interpretation of the data clearly identifies SIRS as being a continuum of events depending on the response of the host to the inciting event and the physiologic reserve of the patient to respond to these global physiologic changes.

State A, which represents the normal stress response to major operations, injuries, or illness, is characterized by a modest reduction of systemic vascular resistance and a commensurate increase in cardiac output (Fig. 3.1). Such patients might have a calculated systemic vascular resistance of 900–1000 dyne/s/cm^{-5} and a cardiac index of 3.5–4.0 L/m.^{2} The arteriovenous oxygen differences are consistent with the normal physiological condition and, by virtue of the increased cardiac index, reflect an increase in total oxygen consumption in the patient. The increased oxygen consumption represents the hypermetabolic response of the human stress response, but lactate concentrations are normal. This is the normal response seen in every patient after major injury or major surgical procedures. Assuming no intercurrent complications, this transient SIRS response, reflecting the systemic effects of activated human inflammation, resolves as the patient convalesces to the normal physiologic state.

State B represents an exaggerated stress response. The loss of systemic vascular resistance becomes extreme (<800 dyne/s/cm^{-5}), and severe cases may have systemic vascular resistance to levels <400 dyne/s/cm^{-5}. Given appropriate preload support by expansion of the intravascular volume and given excellent left ventricular physiologic reserve, cardiac output increases in a dramatic fashion to meet the demands created by the extreme afterload reduction due to systemic vasodilatation. The combination of vasodilation of the capacitance vessels and extensive expansion of the extracellular space due to systemic edema results in large additional preload volume requirements for state B patients. Failure to achieve appropriate preload (preferentially with crystalloid solutions) may result in hypotension even though the patient has hemodynamic parameters consistent with state B.

In state B a significant transition occurs whereby the arteriovenous oxygen content difference begins to narrow. Does this situation reflect inadequate utilization of oxygen in the periphery, or does it represent oxygen delivery in excess of demand in the peripheral tissues? The evolution of increased lactate concentration suggests that the peripheral utilization of oxygen and substrate is compromised, and that the narrowed arteriovenous oxygen content differences reflect a significant issue in regard to oxygen/substrate delivery or abnormal or defective utilization of oxygen by tissues due to cellular abnormalities of intermediary metabolism (see Chapter 9).

It is in state B that one begins to identify the evolution of multiple organ dysfunction syndrome (MODS). As excess lactate species are seen in the peripheral blood, arterial desaturation is observed. The serum bilirubin level begins to rise above normal. During the years before use of preventive methods to avoid stress ulceration of the gastric mucosa became common practice, the nasogastric tube aspirate showed coffeeground material or frank blood. The serum creatinine level began to rise above 1.0 mg/dl. MODS represents the first evidence of organ dysfunction before the institution of extreme organ support measures, such as pressure-controlled ventilation or positive end-expiratory pressure ventilation, are necessary to avoid pulmonary failure. If the inciting stimulus to state B SIRS is not controlled, a protracted state B leads to the full-blown multiple organ failure (MOF) syndrome and the high probability of death. It is important to emphasize that these end-organ events of MODS and MOF occur during state B while systemic arterial blood pressure appears to be adequately maintained. As is discussed subsequently, MODS and MOF are part of the same continuum of disease and should simply be referred to as MODS collectively to avoid confusion.

State C of SIRS represents decompensation of the exaggerated stress response. The loss of systemic vascular resistance is profound, and the physiologic reserve of the left ventricle is no longer capable of maintaining arterial pressure with this extreme degree of afterload reduction. Cardiac output is normal or even slightly elevated for the patient if one were to assume normal physiologic conditions; but in the face of extreme afterload reduction, arterial pressure cannot be maintained. Hypotension exists even though preload is appropriate. This hypotensive state has traditionally been referred to as septic shock, or the shock state that evolves via the natural history of "sepsis." Clinically, these patients are commonly a paradox, as they are hypotensive but remain warm to the touch.

The summation of bacterial infection and other potential activators of human inflammation may play a synergistic role in the evolution of "septic" shock. Every clinician has seen the bacteremic patient with seemingly normal hemodynamics, whereas other patients with signs of clinical infection but with no bacteria in the blood may have profound shock. The shock state of state C is the summed effects of all potential activators of human inflammation and is likely contributed to by factors other than the bacterial cell. In state C it should come as no surprise that the combined effects of the defective peripheral oxygen utilization of SIRS and the compounding effect of reduced arterial pressure lead to severe lactic acidosis. Patients with true septic shock (i.e., not underresuscitated state B SIRS) exhibiting state C hemodynamics require aggressive, prompt management if survival is to be achieved (Tables 3.2, 3.3).

State D represents the hemodynamic profile of the preterminal patient with SIRS. A hypodynamic circulation is observed with low cardiac output, which seemingly elicits an autonomic vasoconstrictive response as the host attempts to maintain arterial blood pressure. Systemic vascular resistance rises in a dramatic fashion above levels normally observed. State D appears to be superimposition of cardiac failure on the fundamental systemic inflammatory response. Systemic oxygen consumption is now profoundly depressed as the patient experiences the defective peripheral utilization of oxygen identified in SIRS, inadequate cardiac output, and extreme peripheral vasoconstriction. Lactate concentrations are significantly high. Death is imminent for most patients at this point.

Multiple Organ Dysfunction Syndrome/ Multiple Organ Failure

With the development of improved resuscitation measures, more effective anesthetic agents and techniques, and the evolution of intensive care units (ICUs), critically ill and

TABLE 3.2. Management of Patients with Severe SIRS and Septic Shock.

Elements of management	Comments
Source control	Includes resection, plication, exteriorization, or oversewing of intestinal/intraabdominal perforations (e.g., necrotic pancreas) driving the septic process. It may include drainage and debridement of abdominal abscess or chest empyema. Source control can be extended to aggressive pulmonary toilet of severe pneumonias, drainage of the obstructed urinary tract, and removal of infected intravascular devices. In the septic shock patient, source control may need to be timed to follow stabilization of vital signs, but all supportive care is destined to failure without mechanical control of the driving stimulus.
Supportive care	
Respiration	Requires the use of positive, pressure-controlled ventilation, positive end-expiratory pressure, intermittent mandatory ventilation, and other ventilator methods to maintain oxygenation but minimization of the risk of pressure-associated lung injury.
Volume	It requires administration of sufficient volume and red blood cell mass to maintain an adequate preload to optimize cardiac output. The pulmonary capillary wedge pressure may be pushed to levels of 15–18 mmHg. Crystalloid solutions are preferred for volume expansion.
Hemodynamics	Septic shock patient in state C requires elevation of the cardiac output to meet the demands created by the loss of peripheral vascular resistance. In state D, cardiac output similarly needs to be elevated but may require use of a vasodilator to reduce the markedly increased afterload secondary to increased peripheral vascular resistance. Choices of inotropic agents are detailed in Table 3.3.
Renal	It requires the use of any of a number hemofiltration techniques or may require hemodialysis for severe cases.
Stress bleeding	It requires the use of either systemic H_2-antihistamine blockers or the use of sucralfate. Use of antacids via nasogastric tube is discouraged.
Antibiotics	It should be against the documented or likely pathogens to cause infection at the primary site. Intraabdominal infection requires antibiotics against enteric gram-negative rods (e.g., *Escherichia coli*) and obligate anaerobes (e.g., *Bacteroides fragilis*). Pulmonary infection in the ICU requires antibiotics against the resistant gram-negative organisms of that environment (e.g., *Pseudomonas aeruginosa*). Intravascular device bacteremia most commonly is due to a staphylococcal organism.

TABLE 3.3. Potential Inotropic Agents to be Used in Patients with Septic Shock.

Pharmacologic agent	Dosage	Comments
Dobutamine	5–20 μg/kg/min	Principally a β-adrenergic agent that elevates cardiac output and has some vasodilatory effects. It has chronotropic and vasoconstrictive effects only at high doses. It is a good choice for elevating cardiac output without vasoconstriction in the septic shock patient.
Dopamine	2–4 μg/kg/min	This dose has little effect on cardiac output or systemic vascular resistance. It is a dopaminergic dose that presumably increases renal blood flow and is often used in septic, but not shock, patients as a strategy to avoid the development of renal failure.
	4–12 μg/kg/min	This dosage is for β-adrenergic effect. It does not have dopaminergic effects. The β-adrenergic effects are lost at higher doses, which limits the value of dopamine for elevating of cardiac output in the septic shock patient.
	>12 μg/kg/min	At this dose the drug is an α-adrenergic agent. Elevations of arterial blood pressure in the septic shock patient are due to vasoconstriction. Although successful in elevating the blood pressure at high doses (>20 μg/kg/min), vasoconstriction is an undesirable goal in the septic shock patient.
Epinephrine	1–4 μg/min	This is the β-adrenergic dose of this drug and raises cardiac output. At higher doses it has a progressively greater vasoconstrictive effect. It is employed as the agent of last resort because of the undesirable vasoconstrictive effects of the high-dosage regimen.
Norepinephrine	2–8 μg/min	Primarily a vasoconstrictor with β-adrenergic effects at high doses. The marked vasoconstrictive effects make this agent generally undesirable for the septic shock patient.
Isoproterenol	1–4 μg/min	This choice has excellent β-adrenergic effects in raising cardiac output but has a marked chronotropic effect, a vasodilatory effect, and certainly arrhythmia potential.
Phenylephrine	40–100 μg/min	This agent is a pure vasoconstrictor and may reduce cardiac output with vasoconstriction. It has little or no use in the patient with septic shock.

critically injured patients have initially survived cataclysmic events that in prior years resulted in death within a few hours of clinical presentation. The survival of these patients into the postoperative period gave rise to an apparent new pattern of death. Multiple trauma, ruptured aneurysms, and massive gastrointestinal bleeding were not the direct and immediate cause of deaths but, rather, the progressive and relentless loss of homeostatic functions of critical organ systems. Shock lung, shock liver, stress mucosal gastritis, and acute renal failure became expressions of this loss of hemeostatic organ function.

Although apparent failure of organ function was initially identified and reported as individual events, it became apparent that associations existed in the patterns of failure for each of the solitary organ failure events. Skillman et al.[4] noted an association among respiratory failure, jaundice, and acute stress ulceration of the stomach in critically ill surgical patients. They believed these events were sequelae of hypotension and sepsis. Tilney et al.[5] identified "sequential system failure" among a group of patients who survived the acute hemorrhagic event (a ruptured abdominal aneurysm). Many of these patients, who were successfully managed by acute control of the hemorrhagic event and repair of the ruptured aneurysm, proceeded to die from organ failure events that seemed to occur in a "domino" fashion during the postoperative period.

The debate over the various organ failure complexes was intensified by the landmark editorial by Baue,[6] in which the terms "multiple," "progressive," and "sequential" systems failure were used to describe this newly recognized syndrome. Baue summarized the perspectives at that time by identifying numerous clinical conditions, events, or even treatments that were associated with organ failure syndromes. Eiseman et al.[7] used the straightforward term "multiple organ failure" and associated this syndrome with clinical infection. Our group used the phrase "multiple system organ failure" to identify this cascading series of failed functions among critically ill patients.[8–11] As was seen by others,[12–16] organ failure syndromes appeared to occur in a sequential fashion, with the lung being the earliest organ to fail and the kidney being the last in the sequence. More than any other organ system, failure of the kidney appeared to predict a fatal outcome for the patients.

The consequence of the sequential failure of the organ systems to the patient was the increased probability of a fatal outcome. Mortality rates for pulmonary failure and for each of the other organ systems on simple inspection all appear to be more than 50%. However, when the number of organ systems involved is examined, it becomes apparent that it is the additive or synergistic effects of the multiple organ failure syndrome that has the greatest significance. Mortality rates are 30% when a single system is involved; failure of two systems is associated with a 60–70% mortality rate; and in our experience failure of four systems was a uniformly fatal event. Kidney failure usually occurred last and was the greatest predictor of death.

The organ systems most commonly studied in these early reports usually included the lung, heart, liver, gastrointestinal tract (stress mucosal ulceration and bleeding), and kidneys. Other organ systems, such as coagulation (i.e., disseminated intravascular coagulation), metabolism (e.g., hypermetabolism), pancreas (e.g., hyperamylasemia), and the central nervous system (e.g., encephalopathy, coma) were alluded to as potential targets of this syndrome. Similar yet differing definitions were used to characterize the organ failure syndrome. Early studies chose to define patients as having either failure or not having failure (Table 3.4) Subsequent observations have developed graduated organ failure indices of severity for each targeted system and clearly demonstrated gradations of severity of failure when correlated with patient outcome.[13,17–19] (see Chapter 2).

TABLE 3.4. Criteria Used to Define Organ Failure in Early Studies.[8–11]

Pulmonary failure: five or more consecutive days of ventilator support at inspired oxygen content of $FiO_2 \geq 0.4$.

Hepatic failure: presence of both a blood bilirubin concentration higher than 2.0 mg/dl and an increase in serum glutamicoxaloacetic transaminase (SGOT or AST) or lactic dehydrogenase (LDH) to more than twice normal values.

Gastrointestinal failure: upper gastrointestinal hemorrhage due to documented or presumed stress-associated acute gastric ulceration. Presumed bleeding required 2 units of blood transfusion. Documented bleeding was due to endoscopically confirmed bleeding from stress ulcerations of the stomach.

Renal failure: elevation of the serum creatinine higher than 2.0 mg/dl. Urine output was not used as an indicator of renal failure.

Graded severity led to adoption of the term multiple organ dysfunction syndrome (MODS) at a consensus conference, even though individual authors continue to use terms to which they are accustomed. Most consider MODS and multiple organ failure syndrome (MOFS) to be synonyms, but others consider MOFS to be an extremely severe case of MODS.

A clinical event in postinjury, postresuscitation patients, MODS appears to follow two distinctly different pathways. Primary MODS occurs as the direct consequence of the anatomic/physiologic event. Primary MODS occurs early and reflects the direct consequence of hemorrhage, hypoxemia, transfusion, or soft tissue injury. Primary MODS is thought to occur via cellular or microcirculatory events that yield severe loss of critical organ function. Presumably, failure of the delivery of oxygen and substrate and of the circulation to remove the end-products of metabolism result in irreversible injury to the oxidative machinery and other membrane functions of the host's cells. Posttraumatic pulmonary failure, acute tubular necrosis, and early ischemic liver injury due to profound shock are examples.

Secondary MODS is an event that occurs later in the patient's course, often weeks after the acute insult. In the early literature, secondary MODS was most commonly associated with uncontrolled infection, or "sepsis." In our early clinical studies, severe infection was defined as (1) fever and leukocytosis present for a period of 5 days; (2) deep-seated suppurative infection (e.g., abscess or empyema); (3) positive blood cultures; (4) positive cultures from a severe clinical site of infection (e.g., lung cultures); or (5) shock secondary to infection. Although these criteria were thought to be markers for severe infection, in reality they are surrogate markers for SIRS and are not specific for infection.

As contemporary critical care medicine has evolved, clinical manifestations of SIRS appear to occur at earlier times in the patient's management. It is now unclear whether any distinction truly exists between primary MODS being the consequence of the primary event and secondary MODS being secondary to SIRS. Inflammation is a nonspecific response of the host to any of a number of physiologic perturbations. Shock, hemorrhage, ischemia/reperfusion injury, acute global hypoxemia, and massive soft tissue injury all serve as potential stimuli for activating SIRS. With early and aggressive resuscitation, the multiple-trauma patient destined to develop primary MODS demonstrates loss of systemic vascular resistance, increased cardiac output, and increased capillary permeability in much the same fashion as the secondary MODS patient with severe clinical infection. It remains feasible to accept the direct consequences of cellular injury from soft tissue injury, hemorrhagic shock, or profound hypoxemia due to trauma as the principal event for some primary MODS patients, but increasing evidence suggests that SIRS may play a role even in these early postinjury organ failure patients.

SIRS-to-MODS Transition

An element of SIRS can be defined in every patient following a major operation, a significant injury, or even a fairly modest infection. There is clearly a threshold at which the severity of the SIRS response is sufficient to affect end-organ function adversely. Insight into when the transition occurs can be gleaned by a comparison of state A and state B of the SIRS staging system. In state A, increased cardiac output is associated with a normal arteriovenous oxygen content, with increased oxygen consumption the result. In state B the dramatically increased cardiac output is accompanied by narrowing of the arterial venous oxygen content. Oxygen consumption in state B is less than would predicted based on cardiac indices and may be less than that seen in state A. As the arteriovenous oxygen content difference narrows, lactate species accumulate in the patient's blood. This lactic acidemia precedes lactic acidosis, as systemic compensatory mechanisms maintain relatively normal pH values until late in the process. Elevated blood lactate is a consistent predictor of outcome in the septic patient and presumably the patient with SIRS. When lactate species accumulate, organ dysfunction complexes are identified in the patient. Abnormalities in the delivery/utilization of oxygen herald the onset of MODS.

The lactic acidemia of state B SIRS has a unique feature compared to lactic acidosis seen in other clinical settings. With hemorrhagic shock or systemic hypoxemia, lactate increases are dramatic but pyruvate concentrations remain largely unchanged. The regeneration of oxidized nicotinamide adenine dinucleotide (NAD^+) is necessary to maintain energy generation via anaerobic glycolysis, and it results in rapid transition of excess pyruvate to lactate in the absence of oxygen as the electron acceptor for oxidative phosphorylation. The equimolar increase in the concentrations of lactate and pyruvate has led to speculation that pyruvic dehydrogenase activity within the cell is defective and prevents oxidative metabolism in the presence of ample oxygen within the cell's cytoplasm.[3,20–22] An alternative explanation suggests that microcirculatory injury may render some populations of cells ischemic, while other microcirculatory units are unaffected and have normal oxygen delivery and utilization.[23–25] In this circumstance, cell populations with an unaffected microcirculation might serve as a "sink" for the oxidation of excess lactate. Skeletal muscle oxidation of lactate production of visceral lactate has been demonstrated in hemor-

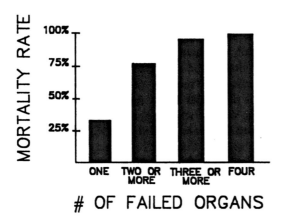

FIGURE 3.2. Temporal relation of failure identified in our early studies[8] of patients with multiple organ failure. It should be noted that clinical "sepsis" was noted to start with the onset of pulmonary failure as the first indicator that multiple organ failure was beginning.

rhagic shock.[26] The lactate-pyruvate balance equilibrates when excess lactate is present and would be the basis for lactic acidosis being accompanied by an equimolar increase in pyruvate. The microcirculatory theory of organ failure is discussed in detail later (see Chapter 9). Whether because of direct cellular dysregulation or microcirculatory arrest, defective oxygen utilization by cells appears to be a seminal event in the transition of SIRS to MODS.

In our studies, MODS appears to be a sequential event with the organ failure complexes occurring in a "domino" fashion[8-11] (Fig. 3.2). Pulmonary failure occurs early in the patient with severe SIRS, hepatic failure follows, and renal failure is the last of the systems to fail. Diffuse cellular or microcirculatory injury would seemingly affect all organ systems uniformly. The sequencing of organ failure may reflect the enhanced vulnerability of one organ system over another with respect to the effects of SIRS. Clinical sensitivity to physiologic changes within the microcirculation of the lung is rapidly translated into clinically relevant arterial desaturation. However, the loss of 30–40% of hepatocyte function might not achieve clinical relevance because of the physiologic reserve of the liver. The recognition of pulmonary failure occurring at an earlier point may simply reflect the greater sensitivity of our clinical indicators to lung changes. In reality, the changes within cells or within the microcirculation of failing organ systems may be similar. Finally, particularly in older patients, variations in the physiologic reserve of each organ system may have relevance to the organ failure sequence. Patients with preexisting liver disease may demonstrate hepatic dysfunction early, whereas others in whom the creatinine clearance is low normally would be far more vulnerable to SIRS-associated renal failure. Many patients defy explanation with organ dysfunction sequences that remain undefined.

The mortality rate due to advanced MODS remains higher than 50%. Many patients with advanced disease are thought not to be salvageable. Whether cellular injury, microcirculatory injury, or a combination of the two, there is a point where clinical recovery is remote. Recovery is unlikely even when the primary event (e.g., hemorrhage) or the sustained event (e.g., invasive infection) has been controlled. The increased mortality rates associated with advanced MODS have been used for the rationale that favors preventive strategies rather than treatment following activation of the process.

Conclusions

Systemic inflammatory response syndrome is the clinical consequence of systemic activation of the human inflammatory cascade. SIRS is most commonly associated with invasive infection but can result from shock, multisystem injury, aseptic inflammation (e.g., acute pancreatitis), and extensive burn injury. Although the source of continued speculation, the phenomenon of microbial translocation from the gut continues to be studied as yet another trigger of SIRS. When the severity of SIRS exceeds a critical threshold, defective oxygen utilization occurs. Failure of the host to utilize available oxygen becomes the defining event in the transition from SIRS to MODS. Failure to control the sustaining activation of SIRS and failure by the host to activate counterinflammatory measures leads to the progressive loss of organ function and death of the patient.

References

1. Deutschman CS, Konstantinides FN, Tsai M, et al: Physiology and metabolism in isolated viral septicemia: further evidence of an organism-independent, host-dependent response. Arch Surg 1987;122:21.
2. American College of Chest Physicians/Society of Critical Care Medicine Consensus Conference: Definition for sepsis and organ failure and guidelines for the use of innovative therapies in sepsis. Crit Care Med 1992;20:864.
3. Siegel JH, Cerra FB, Coleman B, et al: Physiologic and metabolic correlations in human sepsis. Surgery 1979;86:163–193.
4. Skillman JJ, Bushnell LS, Goldman H, Silen W: Respiratory failure, hypotension, sepsis, and jaundice. Am J Surg 1969;117:523–530.
5. Tilney NL, Bailey GL, Morgan AP: Sequential system failure after rupture of abdominal aortic aneurysms: an unsolved problem in postoperative care. Ann Surg 1973;178:117–122.
6. Baue AE: Multiple, progressive, or sequential systems failure. Arch Surg 1975;110:79–81.
7. Eiseman B, Beart R, Norton L: Multiple organ failure. Surg Gynecol Obstet 1977;144:323–326.
8. Fry DE, Pearlstein L, Fulton RL, Polk HC Jr: Multiple system organ failure: the role of uncontrolled infection. Arch Surg 1980;115:136–140.
9. Fry DE, Garrison RN, Heitch RC, et al: Determinants of death in patients with intraabdominal abscess. Surgery 1980;88:517–523.
10. Fry DE, Garrison RN, Polk HC Jr: Clinical implications in bacteroides bacteremia. Surg Gynecol Obstet 1979;149:189–192.
11. Fry DE, Garrison RN, Williams HC: Patterns of morbidity and mortality in splenectomy for trauma. Am Surg 1980;46:28–32.
12. Faist E, Baue AE, Dittmer H, Heberer G: Multiple organ failure in polytrauma patients. J Trauma 1983;23:775–787.

13. Knaus WA, Draper EA, Wagner DP, Zimmerman JE: Prognosis in acute organ-system failure. Ann Surg 1985;202:685–693.
14. Manship L, McMillian RD, Brown JJ: The influence of sepsis and multisystem organ failure on mortality in the surgical intensive care unit. Am Surg 1984;50:94–101.
15. Crump JM, Duncan DA, Wears R: Analysis of multiple organ failure in trauma and non-trauma patients. Am Surg 1988;54:702–708.
16. DeCamp MM, Demling RH: Posttraumatic multisystem organ failure. JAMA 1988;260:530–535.
17. Marshall JC, Cook DJ, Christou NV, et al: The multiple organ dysfunction score: a reliable descriptor of a complex clinical outcome. Crit Care Med 1995;23:1638.
18. Goris RJA, te Boekhurts TPA, Nuytinck JKS, Gimbrere JSF: Multiple-organ failure: generalized autodestructive inflammation? Arch Surg 1985;120:1109.
19. Moore FA, Moore EE, Poggetti R, et al: Gut bacterial translocation via the portal vein: a clinical perspective with major torso trauma. J Trauma 1991;31:629.
20. Cerra FB, Siegel JH, Coleman B, et al: Septic antocannibalism: a failure of exogenous nutritional support. Ann Surg 1980;192:570–574.
21. Vary TC, Drnevich D, Jurasinski C, Brennan WA Jr: Mechanisms regulating skeletal muscle glucose metabolism in sepsis. Shock 1995;3:403–410.
22. Vary TC: Sepsis-induced alterations in pyruvate dehydrogenase complex activity in rat skeletal muscle: effect on plasma lactate. Shock 1996;6:89–94.
23. Fry DE, Silver BB, Rink RD, et al: Hepatic cellular hypoxia in murine peritonitis. Surgery 1979;85:652–661.
24. Townsend MC, Hampton WW, Haybron DM, et al: Effective organ blood flow and bioenergy status in murine peritonitis. Surgery 1986;100:205–213.
25. Schirmer WJ, Townsend MC, Schirmer JM, et al: Galactose elimination kinetics in sepsis: correlation of liver blood flow with function. Arch Surg 1987;122:349–354.
26. Pearce FJ, Connett RJ, Drucker WR: Phase-related changes in tissue energy reserves during hemorrhagic shock. J Surg Res 1985;39:390–398.

4
Risk Factors for MOF and Pattern of Organ Failure Following Severe Trauma

Patrick J. Offner and Ernest E. Moore

Critical care has advanced considerably over the past three decades, allowing patients to survive what previously was uniformly fatal illness or injury. Within this context, multiple organ failure (MOF) emerged as a distinct clinical entity, accounting for most deaths in critically ill patients.[1-3] Early clinical investigation of overwhelming sepsis suggested that death resulted from organ dysfunction unresponsive to treatment.[4,5] Subsequently, Tilney et al. reported sequential organ failure complicating abdominal aortic aneurysm repair following rupture and massive hemorrhage.[6] In this initial description, the authors not only described the pattern of organ failure but also observed that organ failure occurred in initially uninvolved organs. Moreover, organ failure frequently was delayed for days after the original insult. In 1975 Baue proposed that this observation of "multiple, progressive, or sequential systems failure" was a distinct clinical entity.[7] Shortly thereafter, Eiseman et al. introduced the term "multiple organ failure" to describe this syndrome.[8]

A number of issues have hampered the clinical investigation of MOF. The first is the lack of a consistent definition. The criteria used to define individual organ dysfunction or failure and which organ systems are included in the clinical syndrome referred to as MOF vary significantly in the literature.[1,7,9-11] This lack of a consistent definition of MOF has led to confusion with usage of this term to describe a measure of illness severity, a measure of critical illness outcome, or a clinical syndrome.[12] Moreover, an accurate epidemiologic description of MOF, including incidence, risk factors, clinical course, and outcome, remains problematic. Without accurate epidemiologic characterization of MOF, the design and implementation of therapeutic clinical trials is difficult. This problem is further compounded by the inclusion of heterogeneous patient populations in varying descriptive reports of MOF. Emergency surgery and trauma patients may differ significantly from medical intensive care unit (ICU) patients in a number of ways. Furthermore, postinjury MOF may have risk factors, clinical course, and outcome distinct from its medical counterpart. Another factor contributing to the disappointing results of clinical trials to date is the complex pathophysiology of MOF. Despite intense investigation over the past two decades, the mechanisms leading to MOF remain incompletely understood.

Definitions

Recognizing the need for consistent definitions, a consensus conference was sponsored by The Society of Critical Care Medicine (SCCM) and The American College of Chest Physicians (ACCP) in 1991.[13] The primary goal was to define sepsis, particularly with reference to clinical trials. The conference also attempted to define MOF because of its frequent association with sepsis.

Systemic Inflammatory Response Syndrome

Recognizing that a variety of noninfectious and infectious insults can provoke a similar (if not identical) physiologic response, the participants proposed the term systemic inflammatory response syndrome (SIRS) (Fig. 4.1). Diagnostic criteria for SIRS include two or more of the following clinical findings: (1) body temperature >38°C or <36°C; (2) tachycardia, with heart rate >90 beats/min; (3) tachypnea, manifested by a respiratory rate >20 breaths/min or $PaCO_2$ <32 mmHg; and (4) leukocytosis, or white blood cell count (WBC) > 12,000 cells/mm^3, leukopenia (WBC 4000 cells/mm^3), or significant "bandemia" (>10% immature neutrophils). Furthermore, it was recommended that the term sepsis be used only when SIRS is the result of a confirmed infectious process. Although, this terminology was useful in that it emphasizes the common "septic" response to both infectious and noninfectious insults, it has become increasingly evident that the criteria are too sensitive to be clinically helpful.[14-19]

Multiple Organ Failure

The ACCP/SCCM conference further recommended that the term multiple organ dysfunction syndrome (MODS) be adopted and that other terminology, such as multiple organ failure and multiple system organ failure, be abandoned. The participants

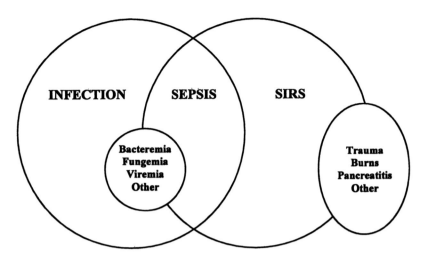

FIGURE 4.1. Inflammatory processes can result in SIRS without evidence of infection. (Adapted from Bone et al.[13])

thought that this term emphasized the continuum of physiologic derangements, rather than an "all or more" phenomenon. This change in terminology has not been universally accepted. We still use the term MOF but recognize that it is both a syndrome and a dynamic process that evolves over time. Moreover, it was implied that MODS would reflect a patient's progress over time. A subsequent prospective study, however, found no difference in mortality prediction comparing a system that defined MODS to one that measured graded organ dysfunction.[20]

MOF Scoring

Our interest in postinjury MOF has been sustained since Eiseman et al. first described the clinical syndrome more than two decades ago.[8] We recognized not only that MOF was an important endpoint but that its clinical investigation suffered because of the lack of unified definitions. Therefore the Denver MOF score was developed based on eight organ systems: pulmonary, renal, cardiac, hepatic, gastrointestinal, hematologic, central nervous (CNS), and metabolic.[21] Organ dysfunction was graded on a scale from zero to three (0 = normal function, 1 = mild dysfunction; 2 = moderate dysfunction; 3 = severe dysfunction) to reflect a continuum of physiologic derangement similar to that later outlined by the ACCP/SCCM consensus conference.[13] The MOF score was the sum of the worst individual organ scores after 48 hours. Organ dysfunction scores obtained during the first 48 hours after injury were not used to define MOF because they might reflect reversible derangements related to the initial injury or to incomplete resuscitation. We began to determine and serially follow MOF scores, allowing us to investigate temporal patterns of MOF occurrence (i.e., early or late) and to quantitate the severity and duration of organ dysfunction.[3]

This original Denver MOF score was later revised and simplified when difficulties were encountered applying the score during a multicenter trial (Table 4.1). Gastrointestinal, hematologic, neurologic, and metabolic failure were excluded because their definitions were subjective; more importantly, they did not

TABLE 4.1. Denver MOF Score.

Dysfunction	Grade 0	Grade 1	Grade 2	Grade 3
Pulmonary (ARDS score)[a]	Normal	>5	>9	>13
Renal (creatinine level, mg/dl)	Normal	>1.8	>2.5	>5.0
Hepatic (bilirubin level, mg/dl)[b]	Normal	1.0	>4.0	>8.0
Cardiac (inotrope level)[c]	Normal	Minimal	Moderate	High

ARDS; adult respiratory distress syndrome.

[a]ARDS score: A + B + C + D + E:
  A. Pulmonary findings by plain chest radiography: 0 = normal; 1 = diffuse, mild interstitial markings/opacities; 2 = diffuse, marked interstitial/mild air-space
  opacities; 3 = diffuse, moderate air-space consolidation; 4 = diffuse, severe air-space consolidation.
  B. Hypoxemia (PaO_2/FiO_2): 0 = >250; 1 = 175–250; 2 = 125–174; 3 = 80–124; 4 = <80
  C. Minute ventilation (l/min): 0 = <11; 1 = 11–13; 2 = 14–16; 3 = 17–20; 4 = >20
  D. Positive end expiratory pressure (cm H_2O): 0 = <6; 1 = 6–9; 2 = 10–13; 3 = 14–17; 4 = >17
  E. Static compliance (ml/cm H_2O): 0 = >50; 1 = 40–50; 2 = 30–39; 3 = 20–29; 4 = <20

[b]Biliary obstruction and resolving hematoma excluded as an etiology.

[c]Cardiac index < 3.0 L/min/m² requiring inotropic support; minimal dose = dopamine or dobutamine < 5 μg/kg/min; moderate dose = dopamine or dobutamine 5–15 μg/kg/min; high dose = more than moderate doses of above agents.

appear to be predictive of MOF. We also revised the definitions of pulmonary, renal, hepatic, and cardiac failure to facilitate objective determination of organ dysfunction at multiple institutions.[22] Individual organ failure is defined as a dysfunction grade ≥ 2, and MOF is defined as the sum of simultaneously obtained organ dysfunction grades ≥ 4 (only scores obtained after 48 hours are used to determine MOF). Patient care protocols determine what and when laboratory data are collected. If laboratory data required for daily organ dysfunction scoring are missing, the most recent prior value is used. If no previous value is available, organ dysfunction is graded zero. MOF is considered early if it is present on hospital day 3 and late if it occurs after day 3.

Alternative MOF scores exist; but, there is still no consensus on which organ systems comprise the syndrome of MOF and how to describe the dysfunction of a given organ system.[1,9,11,23] The recent appearance of several similar MOF scores, suggests the beginning of a consensus on descriptive criteria.[24-26] We recently compared the Denver, Knaus, and Goris MOF scores in 411 consecutive trauma patients with an Injury Severity Score (ISS) >15 who survived longer than 48 hours (Table 4.2). There was no significant difference in the MOF classification between the Denver and Knaus score ($p = 0.66$, McNemar's test). Using the Goris score with (4 $\geq$ indicating MOF), there was a significant difference from the results using the Denver score ($p = 0.0001$, McNemar's test). The Goris score was more sensitive with an MOF rate of 39%, which is higher than that reported in the literature. Moreover, the case-fatality rate was only 20%. Defining MOF with a more restrictive cutoff (Goris score ≥ 6) brought the MOF rate closer to reported levels and lessened the disagreement with the Denver MOF score ($p = 0.71$, McNemar's test). Nonetheless, the absence of a gold standard precludes vigorous validation of any MOF score. Thus lack of a unified definition seriously limits the interpretation of MOF literature.

A second limitation of several MOF scores, including the Denver score, is the treatment of MOF as a categorical variable. It would be ideal to analyze the MOF score as a continuous variable, emphasizing the spectrum of organ dysfunction seen in MOF. The MOF scores, however, are ordinal in nature. The numbers reflect increasingly severe dysfunction, but the intervals are unequal. In other words, the increase in organ dysfunction between a score of 1 and 2 is not the same as that between 2 and 3. Similarly, the same interval change in organ dysfunction score may reflect varying degrees of dysfunction in different organ

systems. Another difficult question is which MOF score to use when measured serially during the ICU stay? Tran et al. proposed using the worst MOF score during the hospital course.[27] Although this approach seems reasonable at first glance, it is problematic because the process of dying leads to progressive organ failure. Therefore the worst MOF score (or MOF scores obtained immediately preceding death) may only represent a description of evolving death.

Models of Postinjury MOF

Although pathophysiology of MOF is beginning to be unraveled, it remains complex and incompletely understood. Although a detailed description is beyond the scope of this chapter, a brief discussion of MOF paradigms serves as a useful construct for identifying potential risk factors.

Initial clinical descriptions of MOF viewed organ failure as the cardinal manifestation of uncontrolled infection.[9,10,28] Subsequent studies, however, observed MOF in the absence of infection.[1,23,29] The term "sepsis syndrome" was introduced to describe a state of systemic inflammation that may exist without overt infection.[30] In the absence of invasive bacterial infection, gut bacterial translocation was proposed as the driving mechanism of MOF.[31,32] Experimental models have failed, however, mechanistically to link bacterial translocation to remote organ injury. We placed portal vein catheters in severely injured patients requiring laparotomy and obtained more than 200 samples of portal venous blood.[21] Cultures were almost uniformly sterile. We subsequently confirmed the infrequent occurrence of bacterial translocation in trauma patients and observed that enteric bacteremia occurred only premortem.[33] Recent clinical observations have failed to identify endotoxin or tumor necrosis factor-α (TNFα) in the serum of patients following severe trauma.[34] Furthermore, selective gut decontamination has failed to reduce either mortality from or occurrence of MOF in the ICU.[35,36] Consequently, alternative hypotheses have proposed that MOF is the end manifestation of uncontrolled systemic inflammation (Fig. 4.2).[23,37,33]

Following major tissue injury, hemorrhagic shock, and resuscitation, patients develop early systemic hyperinflammation, representing what is currently termed SIRS. In most cases SIRS appears to be a beneficial compensatory response leading to patient recovery with supportive care. Two patterns of MOF, however, can emerge (Fig. 4.3). Clearly, a massive traumatic insult can lead to severe SIRS and early MOF (one-hit model). This pattern is what the ACCP/SCCM consensus conference referred to as primary MODS.[13] It seems to occur in patients who cannot be resuscitated into an early hyperdynamic state. Alternatively, MOF may follow multiple sequential insults (two-hit model). Under this paradigm, less severe insults result in a moderate state of SIRS (which may be associated with clinically inapparent organ dysfunction). Certain patients in this state are vulnerable to a second inflammatory stimulus, which results in massive, uncontrolled systemic inflammation and MOF. This has also been termed secondary MODS.[13]

TABLE 4.2. Comparison of the Denver MOF Score with Goris and Knaus MOF Scores.

Denver MOF score	Goris Cutoff ≥ 4		Goris Cutoff ≥ 6		Knaus	
	MOF	No MOF	MOF	No MOF	MOF	No MoF
MOF	78	0	65	13	56	22
No MOF	84	249	15	318	25	308

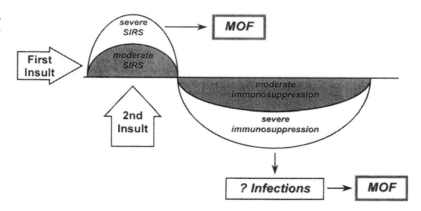

FIGURE 4.2. Inflammatory model of MOF suggests that a variety of initial insults result in dysfunctional hyperinflammation leading to MOF.

Our Trauma Research Center has investigated the priming and activation of polymorphonuclear neutrophils (PMNs) as a laboratory marker for this process.[39] PMN priming is defined as enhancement or amplification of the PMN response to a given stimulus following prior exposure to a different stimulus. Neither stimulus alone elicits a functional PMN response; however, when the activating agent is applied to the primed PMN, a marked response occurs. The response may include superoxide or cytokine production, protease release, and upregulation of PMN adhesion molecule expression. We believe that clinically this priming and activation sequence plays a pivotal role in producing a dysregulated inflammatory response. Specifically, the initial traumatic insult primes the inflammatory response such that a subsequent, otherwise innocuous, inflammatory insult triggers an exaggerated response (severe SIRS), which can evolve into MOF. We and others believe that the two-hit model with multiple sequential insults is the more common clinical scenario leading to MOF.[37,40,41] In fact, it may be difficult to distinguish individual insults, such that what appears to be a single hit may actually be a series of insults (e.g., tissue injury, reperfusion, blood transfusion, general anesthesia, operative trauma).

A variety of clinical conditions may prime the inflammatory response and represent the first hit. In general, the predominant priming events include inadequate tissue perfusion (in particular, splanchnic hypoperfusion), extensive tissue injury, and infection. Implicit in the two-hit model of MOF is the occurrence of a second insult during the vulnerable period (activation). The second insult is presumed to be any untoward event or added stress that overwhelms the host's capacity to generate an appropriate response. Delayed episodes of shock due to any etiology, further tissue injury (e.g., primary or secondary operative procedures such as fracture fixation), pulmonary aspiration, and infection have been implicated.[1,42] Importantly, priming events can also serve as activating insults, which underscores the clinical importance of eradicating infection, vigorously correcting perfusion deficits, and adequately debriding devitalized tissue in surgical patients. As is discussed in more detail later, we have recently identified transfusion of stored blood products as a potential second insult.[43]

Paradoxically, an overzealous inflammatory response to the first insult may result in delayed immunosuppression. The magnitude of the early systemic inflammatory response is related to the severity of the initial insult. Compensatory negative feedback mechanisms downregulate this response in an attempt to limit potentially autodestructive inflammation. These inhibitory cascades may lead to delayed immunosuppression, which is associated with major infectious complications and late MOF. Thus both an early inflammatory insult and a late infectious insult may lead to the same outcome—MOF.

Current Epidemiology of Postinjury MOF

Denver MOF Database

Recognizing the limitations of existing epidemiologic descriptions of postinjury MOF, we established a prospective postinjury MOF database. We identified pertinent data to be collected and established standardized definitions based on an extensive literature review and expert consensus. Inclusion criteria included an ISS >15, age >15 years, and survival >48 hours. Patients were excluded if they were transferred from another institution more than 24 hours after injury. We thought that the trauma population was ideal because it is relatively homogeneous, consisting of mostly young individuals free of significant co-morbidity. Moreover, standardized resuscitation protocols

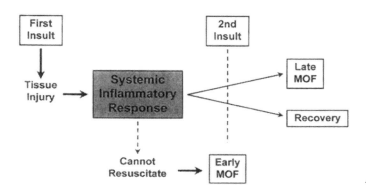

FIGURE 4.3. In the two-hit model of MOF, a second, otherwise innocuous insult can lead to MOF.

TABLE 4.3. Demographic and Outcome Data of Patients with and Without MOF.

Parameter	Total (n = 561)	No MOF (n = 474)	MOF (n = 87)	p
Age (years)	36.3	35.6	39.9	0
Gender (%)				
Male	75.2	75.3	74.7	
Female	24.8	24.7	25.3	0.893
Injury mechanism (%)				
Blunt	78.1			
Penetrating	21.9			
Injury Severity Score	27.0	26.0	32.5	0
Co-morbidity (%)	25	23.2	19.5	0.28
Major Infections (%)	39.8	30.6	89.7	0
Minor Infections (%)	19.3	14.6	44.8	0
Noninfectious complications (%)	24.2	15.6	71.3	0
MOF (%)	15.5			
Mortality (%)	9.1	4.4	34.5	0
ICU length of stay (days)	14.3	11.5	29.5	0
Mechanical ventilation (days)	7.9	5.3	22.4	

have been used at our level I trauma center since the establishment of the MOF database. Therefore treatment variability and patient heterogeneity are kept to a minimum in a patient population at high risk for developing MOF.

The MOF database contains information collected from 1993. Currently, the database contains 561 patients. Table 4.3. depicts demographic data for the population with and without stratification by MOF status. The mean age and gender distribution are typical for an urban level I trauma center (36.0 ± 0.7 years and 75% male). The injury mechanism was predominantly blunt (78%), most commonly the result of a motor vehicle accident. The mean and median ISSs were 27 and 25, respectively, with an overall mortality rate of 9.1%.

Multiple organ failure developed in 87 patients (16%). MOF patients were older; but the frequency of co-morbidity was low and unrelated to the development of MOF. Injury mechanism and gender distributions were not different in MOF and non-MOF patients. In addition to being older, patients developing MOF were more severely injured, with a higher median ISS (29 vs. 25, $p < 0.001$). Not surprisingly, MOF patients experienced significantly more major infections (90% vs. 31%), minor infections (45% vs. 15%), and noninfectious complications (71% vs. 16%). Moreover, MOF patients required longer ventilatory support (22.4 ± 1.8 vs. 5.3 ± 0.4 days), spent more days in the ICU (29.5 ± 2.3 vs. 11.5 ± 1.6 days), and had a higher mortality rate (34.5% vs. 4.4%). Similar to previous reports, mortality increased with an increase in the number of organs that failed: single organ, 11%; two organs 24%; three organs 60%; and four organs 62%.

Between 1991 and 1995 the incidence and mortality due to MOF remained relatively constant (Table 4.4). It appeared that patients were similarly injured during this period. We are currently examining similar data from 1992 through 1998 to confirm these observations. In addition, we are characterizing the patient population in each year group to be sure no major differences in MOF risk factors exist. As it stands, the persistent mortality rates for postinjury MOF underscore the need for continued investigation of MOF and its treatment.

Risk Factors for Postinjury MOF

Developing and testing effective therapeutic interventions for MOF requires identification of patients at risk for developing MOF. We therefore sought to identify early risk factors for the development of postinjury MOF within the paradigm of MOF as a result of systemic hyperinflammation. Risk factors can be categorized based on the two-hit model of MOF, recognizing that some overlap is possible. Early risk factors (e.g., first hit) can be broadly categorized into several categories: (1) severity of tissue injury; (2) severity of shock or ischemia/reperfusion; and (3) severity of the systemic inflammatory response. In the context of postinjury MOF, risk factors associated with the second hit include operative trauma (e.g., orthopedic fixation), transfusion of stored blood products, and infection (in particular, nosocomial pneumonia). In addition, specific host factors such as age, co-morbidity, and host physiology can modify the response to both the first and second insults. Each of these factors is considered in turn.

Risk Factors Associated with the First Insult

Severity of Tissue Injury

A variety of individual injuries have classically been associated with adult respiratory distress syndrome (ARDS) and MOF, including pulmonary contusion, pelvic fractures, and multiple long bone fractures.[9,44,45] Individual injuries, however, fail to account for the potential synergistic effect of multiple trauma.

The ISS is a quantitative measure of anatomic (tissue) injury severity developed by Baker et al. in 1974.[46] The ISS is based on the abbreviated injury scale (AIS), which scores individual injuries on a scale of 1 to 6 (where 1 is a minor injury and 6 is a usually fatal injury). The ISS is calculated as the sum of squares of the highest AIS scores in the three most severely injured body regions. Since its introduction, the ISS has been noted to have several limitations, including failure to account for multiple injuries to the same body region and equal weighting of injuries to disparate body regions. For example, a significant head injury is considered equivalent to a femur fracture, although the outcome from each injury may be vastly different.[47-49]

TABLE 4.4. Temporal Trends in MOF Occurrence and Outcome.

Parameter	1991 (n = 23)	1992 (n = 13)	1993 (n = 18)	1994 (n = 16)	1995 (n = 15)
Age, mean (Years)	41	44	41	37	37
ISS, mean	27	38	30	30	29
Tansfusion > 6 U pRBCs (%)	43	77	67	63	47
Base deficit > 8 (%)	80	73	94	94	71
MOF (%)	15	17	20	12	25
Mortality (%)	43	38	33	31	33

TABLE 4.5. Median NISS and ISS Scores in Patients with and Without MOF.

Test	MOF	No MOF
NISS	42	29
ISS	29	25

In an attempt to address these problems, the anatomic profile (AP) was developed.[49] The AP takes into account multiple injuries to the same body region and more appropriately weights injuries to different body regions. Subsequent comparisons of mortality prediction based on the ISS and AP demonstrated a moderate improvement using the AP.[47,50] Regardless, the ISS remains the most commonly used index of injury severity because of its familiarity and the complexity of the AP.

Despite its limitations, the ISS has been noted to be a consistent risk factor for MOF.[22,27,51] Using our MOF database, we noted that an ISS > 24 was an independent risk factor for MOF (odds ratio 4.0, after controlling for age and shock).[22] Subsequently, we compared the ISS and AP as predictors of MOF and found no significant advantage to the AP.[51] Recently, the "new ISS" (NISS) has been proposed as a more "user-friendly" alternative to the ISS.[52,53] The NISS is calculated based on the sum of squares of the three worst AIS scores regardless of body region. Therefore it accounts (at least in part) for multiple injuries to the same body region. Osler et al.[52] demonstrated that the NISS, as a predictor of survival, was superior to the ISS in two large independent databases. These authors concluded that the NISS should replace the ISS as the standard measure of injury severity following trauma. Subsequently, Brenneman and colleagues confirmed these findings in more than 2000 patients suffering blunt trauma.[53]

We investigated whether the NISS is a better predictor of MOF than the ISS. The NISS was retrospectively calculated in 558 patients at risk for developing postinjury MOF. In fact, the NISS distinguished patients who developed MOF from those who did not better than the ISS (Table 4.5). In 52.8% of the patients the NISS was higher than the ISS (including both blunt and penetrating injuries). This subset of patients had a higher mortality rate and MOF rate than the group in which NISS = ISS (12.8% vs. 4.9% and 27% vs. 8%, respectively). Surprisingly, the median ISS was identical (25) in the two groups. Multiple logistic regression showed improved goodness of fit when the NISS was substituted for the ISS in a predictive model for MOF.

Shock and Ischemia/Reperfusion

In addition to tissue injury, epidemiologic studies have identified overt shock as a predominant risk factor for postinjury MOF.[1,22,27,51] Over the past decade, it has also become apparent that subclinical shock (i.e., tissue oxygen debt) is a major determinant of organ failure.[54-56] We prospectively showed that patients unable to augment oxygen utilization in response to increasing oxygen delivery were at high risk for developing MOF.[56] When oxygen consumption was less than 150 ml/min/m^2 at 12 hours, MOF developed in 12 (80%) of 15 patients. Although this impaired oxygen consumption may be related to persistent flow dependence, we subsequently used near-infrared spectroscopy to demonstrate mitochondrial oxidative dysfunction in severely injured patients who developed MOF.[57]

In our epidemiologic studies of MOF, shock was measured using both clinical and laboratory indicators. Clinical indicators included blood pressure, heart rate, temperature, hourly urine output, volume requirements (including blood products), and vasopressor requirements. Laboratory indicators included hemoglobin, base deficit, and lactate levels. Multivariate analysis identified red blood cell transfusion, lactate level, and moderate inotropic support requirements as independent risk factors for MOF.[51]

The gut is particularly vulnerable to hypoperfusion because splanchnic vasoconstriction is a prominent component of the compensatory response to shock. Moreover, the splanchnic circulation is the last to be restored following resuscitation, which has both pathophysiologic and therapeutic implications. A central theme of our trauma research center has been that the postischemic gut serves as a priming bed for the systemic inflammatory response.[58] As such, splanchnic ischemia/reperfusion may represent the common pathway by which shock serves as an initial insult leading to MOF.

Gut ischemia/reperfusion has the potential to prime the inflammatory response via a variety of mechanisms, including neutrophil priming for augmented cytotoxicity and endothelial cell activation with increased adhesion molecule (ICAM-1) expression. We have found evidence that these effects are both cytokine- and lipid-mediated. We observed platelet-activating factor (PAF) production in the distal small bowel after splanchnic ischemia/reperfusion and noted that neutrophil priming in this setting was inhibited by a PAF receptor antagonist.[59] Clinically, we confirmed that early postinjury neutrophil priming for superoxide production is via a PAF mechanism.[60] More recently we found a correlation between reduced levels of circulating PAF acetylhydrolase (the enzyme responsible for degrading and inactivating PAF) and the development of MOF in severely injured patients.[61]

Interleukin (IL)-6 is considered an integral mediator of the acute-phase response to injury.[62] There is an increasing body of evidence suggesting that IL-6 plays a pivotal role in the systemic hyperinflammation of SIRS.[63,64] An intestinal source for IL-6 following surgery and trauma has been suggested in clinical studies[60,65] and confirmed in animal models.[66,67] The gut may also generate other cytokines, including IL-1 and tumor necrosis factor (TNF);[68,69] although clinical studies have not yet demonstrated their direct involvement following injury. We have serially measured serum IL-6, IL-8, and TNF concentrations in severely injured patients.[21,61] IL-6 and IL-8 levels increase immediately after injury, but TNF levels were no different from those in controls. Similar findings have been reported by several investigators.[34,70]

Bacterial translocation is an alternative mechanism by which splanchnic hypoperfusion can lead to MOF. This concept was first proposed 30 years ago by Fine et al.[71] The theory regained popularity during the 1980s to explain MOF occurring in the absence of invasive infection. Extensive investigation in a variety of animal models documented gut translocation of bacteria or endotoxin following hemorrhagic shock.[72–75] Clinical investigation, however, failed to establish a clear mechanistic role for gut bacterial translocation in the pathogenesis of early-onset MOF. We prospectively placed portal vein catheters in 20 high risk trauma patients who required emergency laparotomy in an attempt to document bacterial translocation; 30% of these patients developed MOF.[21] We did not detect pathogenic bacteria in either the portal or the systemic circulation during the first 5 days after injury. Peitzman et al. reported similar inability to document microbial translocation in severely injured patients.[76]

The focus has shifted from the portal vein to the mesenteric lymph as the preferred route for microbial translocation. Johnston et al.[77] observed that portal blood flow diversion failed to abrogate lung injury after mesenteric ischemia/reperfusion. Sanchez-Garcia and colleagues sampled thoracic duct lymph in patients with MOF and found increased IL-1 and activated T cells.[78] The authors suggested a mechanistic link between MOF and mesenteric lymph. Magnotti et al. demonstrated that mesenteric lymph generated after hemorrhagic shock caused acute lung injury.[79] Moreover, mesenteric lymph diversion ameliorated this lung injury. This same group also demonstrated that after hemorrhagic shock mesenteric lymph is cytotoxic to endothelial cells and enhances neutrophil superoxide generation.[80] We subsequently observed that mesenteric lymph collected after hemorrhagic shock primes neutrophils for superoxide production and CD11b expression.[81] Moreover, we confirmed that lymph diversion attenuated, lung injury following hemorrhagic shock. Identification of the responsible mediators in mesenteric lymph remains an area of active investigation; our preliminary work invokes the lipid component.

Severity of the Systemic Inflammatory Response

Although SIRS is generally accepted as a key component in the pathogenesis of MOF, its measurement and quantification have remained elusive. The concept and definition of SIRS as put forth by the ACCP/SCCM consensus conference may be a step forward in the sense that it emphasizes the generic nature of the inflammatory response and the continuum from SIRS to MOF. Significant limitations exist, however, in the application of these definitions clinical practice. In a prospective survey of mixed ward and ICU admissions to a tertiary care facility, Rangel-Frausto et al.[14] noted that 68% met SIRS criteria. The Italian Sepsis Study observed that more than one-half of patients admitted to 99 ICUs over a 1-year period met SIRS criteria.[82] Moreover, mortality rates were similar in patients with and without SIRS (26.5% vs. 24.0%). Pittet et al.[16] found that SIRS was present in more than 90% of surgical ICU patients and was not useful for predicting severe sepsis and septic shock. Relevant to trauma patients, Smail et al.[15] noted SIRS in 95 of 163 traumatized patients (58%). Although SIRS occurred more frequently in patients who developed MOF, more than 50% of patients without MOF met SIRS criteria. A prospective study of trauma patients in South Africa observed that 87% of patients admitted to the hospital had SIRS.[18] Gando et al. studied 40 trauma patients and noted that the duration of SIRS was associated with MOF.[83] Patients who met SIRS criteria for more than 3 days developed MOF compared to 20% of those with SIRS criteria for less than 2 days. We believe that SIRS, as currently defined, is too sensitive to discriminate patients who develop MOF from those who do not. Moreover, the division of SIRS into "severe" categories based on organ dysfunction or continued hyperinflammation is problematic. These definitions overlap with current definitions of MOF, invalidating their use as risk factors for development of MOF.

A variety of predictive models have been proposed to quantitate SIRS. The Acute Physiology and Chronic Health Evaluation (APACHE) system has been most commonly used.[84] The APACHE score is a composite derived from several components. The first component is the Acute Physiology Score (APS), which is based on the worst values of several physiologic variables. Host factors (e.g., age, gender, co-morbidity) and factors related to the principal diagnosis are also taken into account. The system has undergone revision and currently exists as APACHE III.[85] We chose to use the APS component of APACHE III (APS-APACHE III) as a summary measure of SIRS in our investigation of postinjury MOF. APS-APACHE III was obtained in several time windows, including on admission, between emergency department (ED) discharge and 12 hours, between 13 and 24 hours, and from 25 to 47 hours. Within each of these time windows, the APS-APACHE III was significantly higher in patients who developed MOF (Table 4.6). In subsequent multivariate analysis, however, the APS-APACHE III was not a significant risk factor for MOF until after 24 hours. This unexpected finding has several potential explanations. The APS-APACHE III may not adequately characterize postinjury SIRS; alternatively, SIRS is not an important risk factor for postinjury MOF. Given the clinical and laboratory evidence supporting the inflammatory model of MOF, we favor the former explanation. A third possibility is that tissue injury and shock dominate the clinical picture during the first 24 hours. It is not until resuscitation is complete and injuries are treated that APS-APACHE III becomes a major risk factor.

As the pathophysiology of SIRS is better understood, better ways to identify and quantify systemic inflammation will be developed, such as measurement of neutrophil priming or circulating levels of inflammatory mediators. We have documented early neutrophil priming in severely injured patients.[86] Moreover, we observed that plasma from these injured patients

TABLE 4.6. Mean APS-APACHE III Scores Obtained at Various Time in Patients with and Without MOF.

Time window	MOF	No MOF	p
Admission	47.4 ± 3.2	38.3 ± 1.5	0.01
Post-ED to 12 hours	68.7 ± 3.2	47.5 ± 1.5	0.00001
13–24 hours	49.4 ± 2.5	30.2 ± 1.1	0.00001
25–48 hours	50.8 ± 2.4	31.6 ± 1.1	0.00001

ED, emergency department.

could prime neutrophils from healthy volunteers;[60] and in an animal model this effect was inhibited by pretreatment with WEB 2170 (a PAF antagonist).[58] In a subsequent study, we noted that reduced PAF-acetylhydrolase (PAF-AH) was associated with postinjury MOF.[61]

Cytokines are the physiologic messengers of the inflammatory response, particularly TNF, IL-1, IL-6, and IL-8.[87,88] We investigated serial IL-6 and IL-8 levels in 27 trauma patients at high risk for MOF (ISS >15 and >6 units of blood transfused in 6 hours).[89] MOF developed in one-third of these patients. IL-6 and IL-8 levels were significantly higher in MOF patients within 12 hours of injury and remained elevated for more than 3 days. Predicting outcome in patients on the basis of circulating cytokine levels is potentially problematic for a number of reasons.[90] The physiologic effects of cytokines are most likely related to tissue levels, which may not be accurately reflected in serum or plasma measurements. Moreover, the compensatory elaboration of natural antagonists makes interpretation of serum levels even more difficult. Investigators have documented that other indicators of inflammation (e.g., complement and arachidonic acid metabolites) are early predictors of organ failure in selected patients.[91,92] Continued investigation in large groups of patients is necessary to develop a better measure of SIRS and improve the ability to predict development of postinjury MOF.

Risk Factors Associated with the Second Insult

Infection

Early reports of MOF clearly identified an association between sepsis and MOF.[7,9,10] Though sepsis seems to be found less commonly today, it remains an important factor in the development of MOF. As discussed earlier, postinjury hyperinflammation may result in delayed immunosuppression, which places the patient at risk for subsequent nosocomial infection. This delayed immunosuppression has been postulated to result from the compensatory antiinflammatory response syndrome (CARS), which attempts to control SIRS.[93]

Nosocomial pneumonia is the most common cause of infection in the critically ill[94] and is the principal infection associated with MOF.[95] Recent clinical trials, however, have shown that selective gut decontamination consistently reduced the occurrence of infection (particularly pneumonia) in the ICU but did not decrease MOF or mortality.[35,36] This prompted the hypothesis that infections are frequently symptoms of MOF rather than triggers for MOF. To investigate this point, we evaluated the temporal association between pneumonia and MOF in 123 consecutively injured patients who required mechanical ventilation for more than 24 hours.[96] The diagnosis of pneumonia was temporally related to serial MOF scoring. In particular, the MOF scores obtained on the day of pneumonia diagnosis and 42–72 hours later were compared. Pneumonia was thought to represent a potential trigger if the MOF score was less than 4 and increased by 3 or more following diagnosis. Pneumonia was associated with worsening MOF if the MOF score was >4 on the day of diagnosis and subsequently rose by 3 or more. Pneumonia developed in 43% of patients and was significantly associated with MOF. Moreover, pneumonia was a trigger in patients with late, rather than early, MOF. These findings are similar to those of Waydhas et al.[91] and Faist et al.,[1] and they strengthen the argument that infection is an important second insult leading to postinjury MOF.

Transfusion

We and others have consistently identified blood transfusion as an independent risk factor for postinjury MOF.[22,27,44,51] The basis for this has been twofold. First, transfusion requirement represents an index of blood loss and hemorrhagic shock. It has been difficult, however, to separate transfusion from other measures of shock. Second, transfusions have long been recognized as immunosuppressive and may be responsible for major septic morbidity, which is strongly associated with MOF. The transplant literature clearly demonstrates that kidney transplant rejection is reduced by preoperative blood transfusion.[97] In addition, perioperative blood transfusion has been consistently associated with tumor recurrence following resection of several malignancies.[98,99] After serious injury, blood transfusion has been associated with major infections.[100] In the latter situations, it has been difficult to determine whether the outcome was related to the transfusion or to the underlying reason for which the transfusion was required (i.e., advanced malignancy requiring extensive resection or hemorrhagic shock).

It has been recognized that stored blood components contain proinflammatory mediators (IL-6, IL-8, lipid mediators) that may serve as a second inflammatory stimulus and precipitate MOF.[101–103] We systematically analyzed the MOF database to study in depth the relation between blood transfusion and MOF.[43] We noted a dose-response relation between the number of units of packed red blood cells (pRBCs) transfused during the first 12 hours and subsequent MOF (Fig. 4.4). A series of multiple regression analyses were performed in different time windows; and other shock variables, including base deficit and lactate levels, were progressively added to the analysis in each time window. The procedure was repeated with early and late MOF as the outcome variable. Blood transfusion consistently emerged as an independent risk factor for MOF despite inclusion of other shock indicators. Moreover, the odds ratios of developing MOF following transfusion were consistently high, especially for early MOF (odds ratio = 7.4–13.2). In addition, the correlation between transfusion requirement and other indicators of shock was small, suggesting that blood transfusion is more than just a reflection of shock.

Causation is difficult to prove, although certain factors support a causal relation between blood transfusion and MOF.[104] First, there is both theoretic and biologic plausibility that such a relation exists. There is a clear temporal relation between early blood transfusion and later development of MOF. Second, blood transfusion has consistently emerged as an independent risk factor in multiple studies and multiple subgroup analyses, despite inclusion of other shock indicators. Moreover, the strength of the association, as reflected by the large odds ratios, is high. Finally,

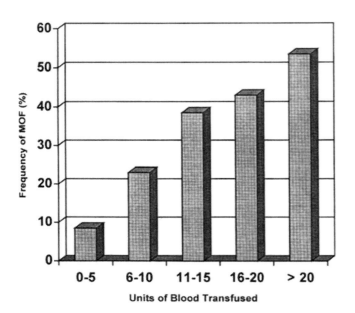

FIGURE 4.4. Units of blood transfused during the first 6 hours after injury and the occurrence of MOF exhibit a dose-response relation.

the dose-response relation between transfusion and MOF strengthens the case for an independent, causal relation.

Our interest in transfusion as a possible second insult originated with the observation that plasma from stored pRBCs primes neutrophils for enhanced superoxide release.[102] This effect seems to be mediated by lipids, particularly lysophosphatidylcholines, generated during storage. Moreover, this priming effect is not seen before 2 weeks of storage, suggesting that the age of transfused blood might be an important risk factor for MOF. Using our MOF database, we identified 26 patients who received 6–20 units of pRBCs during the first 12 hours after injury and who developed MOF; 42 patients with similar ISS and transfusion requirement who did not develop MOF served as a control group.[105] Using blood bank records, the age of each unit of pRBCs transfused during the first 12 hours was determined. The mean age of transfused blood was greater in patients who developed MOF (31 vs. 24 days, $p < 0.05$). The percentage of units transfused that were more than 21 days old was also greater in patients with MOF (98% vs. 80%, $p < 0.05$). Multivariate analysis confirmed that the age of blood transfused during the first 12 hours following injury was an independent risk factor for MOF after controlling for patient age, total transfusion requirement, and base deficit and lactate levels.

We have had the unique opportunity to study a human hemoglobin-based polymerized pyridoxilated stroma-free hemoglobin-solution (Poly-SFH.) In vitro we found that this lipid- and cytokine-free blood substitute is devoid of neutrophil priming effects.[106] Clinically, we noted that substituting Poly-SFH for allogenic blood products avoids transfusion-induced neutrophil priming and upregulation of the CD11b/CD18 receptor complex on the neutrophil.[107] Prospective, randomized clinical trials of Poly-SFH not only will define the role of blood

substitutes in trauma resuscitation but will allow further insights into transfusion as a risk factor for MOF.

Secondary Operative Procedures

Operative procedures represent a form of surgical trauma with consequences similar to those seen with unintentional injury. Specifically, elevations in neutrophil elastase levels, C-reactive protein, IL-6, and other cytokines have been observed to occur in a graded fashion following operative procedures.[108–110] Therefore, secondary operative procedures may represent second insults leading to MOF in "primed" trauma patients.

This issue is perhaps most relevant to timing of skeletal stabilization in multiply-injured patients with major fractures. Studies during the 1980s concluded that operative fracture fixation is superior to nonoperative stabilization with respect to septic and pulmonary complications.[31,111] The timing of fracture fixation, however, is controversial. Early fixation has been suggested to decrease pulmonary complications,[112–114] but others found no benefit to early operative stabilization.[115,116] It has been suggested that early fracture fixation may be detrimental, particularly in patients with blunt chest injury and serious head injury.[117–119] The mechanisms responsible for these adverse effects are not clear. Perioperative hypoxia and hypotension clearly can worsen outcome in head-injured patients.[120–122] Another potential mechanism is exacerbation of neutrophil-mediated systemic hyperinflammation (e.g., a second hit). We have demonstrated that circulating neutrophils are primed for cytotoxicity (superoxide and protease release) 3–24 hours following severe injury.[86] Thus a vulnerable window exists during which secondary operative procedures should be avoided if clinically feasible. Waydhas et al.[123] studied the relation between secondary operations and late MOF in 106 severely injured patients (mean ISS=40.6). The authors measured several indicators of inflammation, including elastase and C-reactive protein prior to operation in each patient; 40 patients (38%) developed organ failure or a worsened existing organ within 2 days of the operation. Preoperative elastase levels and C-reactive protein were significantly higher and the platelet count lower in patients who developed MOF. The authors noted that the combination of neutrophil elastase > 85 ng/ml, C-reactive protein >11 mg/dl, and platelet count <180,000/ml predicted postoperative organ failure with a high degree of accuracy (accuracy 79%, sensitivity 75%, specificity 83%). They concluded that secondary operations might act as a second insult and lead to late MOF in patients with increasing inflammation. Clearly, prospective randomized clinical trials are needed to answer this question definitively.

Host Factors

Age

Patient age is a consistent risk factor for ICU- and trauma-related mortality.[85,124–127] Similarly, age has been recognized as an important risk factor for ARDS and MOF.[22,27,44,45,51] We found that patients older than 45 years of age consistently had a two to three times greater likelihood of developing MOF than their younger counterparts.[51] Morris et al.[128] attributed the worse outcome in elderly patients to the presence of co-morbidity, specifically cirrhosis, ischemic heart disease, obstructive lung disease, and diabetes. The aging process affects all organ systems to a varying degree. The ultimate result is decreased functional reserve that impairs the elderly patient's response to stress.

Preexisting Diseases

Evidence indicates that co-morbidity is an independent risk factor for trauma mortality but is minor compared to age and injury severity.[128,129] In our experience with trauma patients, we did not find co-morbid disease to be independently associated with MOF after controlling for the effect of age.[130] The prevalence of preexisting diseases, however, was only 7% in our predominantly young trauma population. Moss et al.[131] noted that chronic alcohol abuse was a significant risk factor for ARDS in the presence of an identified at-risk diagnosis. Moreover, ARDS mortality was substantially higher in patients with a history of chronic alcohol abuse (60% vs. 36%). We have not yet confirmed a similar relation between chronic alcohol abuse and postinjury MOF. Given the high rate of alcohol abuse in many trauma patient populations, this area deserves further study.

Patterns of Multiple Organ Failure

Tilney et al. first described "sequential organ failure" as a complication of the postoperative course of patients following repair of leaking abdominal aortic aneurysms.[6] The authors reported the sequence of organ failure as pancreas, lungs, liver, central nervous system, gastrointestinal, and finally cardiac failure. Attempts to generalize the specific patterns of MOF development are difficult because there has been no consensus on definitions for individual organ failure. Moreover, considerable individual variation exists in the physiologic reserve of involved organs, both intrinsic and secondary to preexisting disease. Despite these problems, certain common themes emerge from the literature. The sequence of organ failure is similar in numerous reports (Table 4.7).

TABLE 4.7. Sequence of Organ Failure in MOF Based on Literature Review.

	Sequence of organ failure		
	First	Second	Third
Baue[7]	Lung	Kidney	Liver
Border et al.[132]	Lung	Cardiac	Liver
Cerra et al.[133]	Lung	Liver	Kidney
Deitch[134]	Lung	Liver	GI tract
Fry et al.[9]	Lung	Liver	GI tract
Goris et al.[23]	Lung	Liver	GI tract
McMenamy et al.[135]	Lung	Liver	Cardiac
Moore et al.[95]	Lung	Liver	Cardiac
Regel et al.[136]	Lung	Liver	Cardiac

The respiratory system is the main organ system affected in MOF.[1,95,136] Faist and colleagues observed that the respiratory system was the initial and the most frequent organ to decompensate.[1] These authors suggested that MOF without a respiratory component does not occur. Several factors may account for this observed pulmonary predominance in postinjury MOF. Direct lung injury is a frequent cause of early respiratory insufficiency following trauma and is a well recognized risk factor for ARDS.[45] In addition, the pulmonary capillary bed may act as a filter that is exposed to toxins, activated neutrophils, and cytokines. The result is increased vascular permeability and interstitial edema; and the lung is sensitive to these changes. More importantly, clinicians have the means to measure pulmonary dysfunction easily. The liver is generally the second most frequent organ to fail.

Two characteristic patterns of MOF onset have been described: early and late.[1,91,95] More than two decades ago Walker and Eiseman noted that postinjury ARDS presented with early and late forms.[137] Nine of thirteen patients developed classic early-onset ARDS (within 12 hours), and all survived. The remaining patients developed late ARDS (after 5 days) with 100% mortality. In each case ARDS was associated with sepsis. The markedly disparate presentation and outcome led the authors to conclude that the disease processes were distinct. In 1983 Faist et al. similarly noted early and late patterns of MOF following trauma.[1] Early MOF occurred within 12–36 hours in 15 of 34 patients and appeared to be related to severe multisystem trauma and shock. In the remaining 19 patients the onset of MOF was late (average 7.2 days) and was uniformly associated with sepsis. Waydhas et al. noted similar findings in a prospective study of 100 severely injured patients.[91]

We prospectively studied 457 severely injured patients and confirmed a bimodal distribution of MOF.[95] Seventy of these patients developed MOF. In 27 (39%) the occurrence was early (<72 hours), and in 43 (69%) it was delayed (>72 hours). The sequence of organ failure differed with the pattern of onset. On the day of MOF diagnosis early and late MOF had a similar high incidence of pulmonary failure, whereas early MOF had a higher rate of cardiac failure and late MOF was associated with more hepatic failure. Risk factors for early and late MOF differed as well. Indices of shock (e.g., base deficit, lactate levels, transfusion requirements) were more critical risk factors for early MOF, and advanced age was more important for late MOF. Early and late MOF had similar high incidences of major infection, but they appeared to be more important as precipitating factors of late MOF. In aggregate, these studies indicate that postinjury MOF has distinct early and late forms. Further investigation to characterize these forms better is ongoing and may have important epidemiologic and therapeutic implications.

Conclusions

Epidemiologic characterization of postinjury MOF has suffered from the lack of consistent, unified criteria for grading individual organ dysfunction and defining MOF. It is currently accepted

TABLE 4.8. Risk Factors for Postinjury Multiple Organ Failure.

Associated with the first insult
  Severity of tissue injury
  Shock-ischemia/reperfusion
  Severity of the systemic inflammatory response

Associated with the second insult
  Infection
  Transfusion
  Secondary operative procedures

Host factors
  Age
  Preexisting conditions

---

that MOF is the result of dysregulated systemic inflammation following trauma and resuscitation. We have prospectively studied postinjury MOF using consistent criteria for defining organ dysfunction and MOF. Based on the inflammatory paradigm and the two-hit model of MOF, we identified risk factors and categorized them as being associated with the initial insult, the second insult, and host factors (Table 4.8). Refinement of these risk factors will allow early identification of patients prone to develop MOF for inclusion in clinical interventional trials and, hopefully, lend further insight into the complex pathophysiology of postinjury MOF.

References

1. Faist E, Baue AE, Dittmer H, Heberer G: Multiple organ failure in polytrauma patients. J Trauma 1983;23:775–787.
2. Manship L, McMillin RD, Brown JJ: The influence of sepsis and multisystem and organ failure on mortality in the surgical intensive care unit. Am Surg 1984;50:94–101.
3. Sauaia A, Moore FA, Moore EE, et al: Epidemiology of trauma deaths: a reassessment. J Trauma 1995;38:185–193.
4. MacLean LD, Mulligan WG, McLean AP, Duff JH: Patterns of septic shock in man—a detailed study of 56 patients. Ann Surg 1967;166:543–562.
5. Skillman JJ, Bushnell LS, Goldman H, Silen W: Respiratory failure, hypotension, sepsis, and jaundice: a clinical syndrome associated with lethal hemorrhage from acute stress ulceration of the stomach. Am J Surg 1969;117:523–530.
6. Tilney NL, Bailey GL, Morgan AP: Sequential system failure after rupture of abdominal aortic aneurysms: an unsolved problem in postoperative care. Ann Surg 1973;178:117–122.
7. Baue AE: Multiple, progressive, or sequential systems failure. A syndrome of the 1970s. Arch Surg 1975;110:779–781.
8. Eiseman B, Beart R, Norton L: Multiple organ failure. Surg Gynecol Obstet 1977;144:323–326.
9. Fry DE, Pearlstein L, Fulton RL, Polk HC Jr: Multiple system organ failure: the role of uncontrolled infection. Arch Surg 1980;115:136–140.
10. Bell RC, Coalson JJ, Smith JD, Johanson WG Jr: Multiple organ system failure and infection in adult respiratory distress syndrome. Ann Intern Med 1983;99:293–298.
11. Knaus WA, Draper EA, Wagner DP, Zimmerman JE: Prognosis in acute organ-system failure. Ann Surg 1985;202:685–693.
12. Marshall JC: Criteria for the description of organ dysfunction in sepsis and SIRS. In: Fein A, Abraham E, Balk R, et al (eds) Sepsis and Multiorgan Failure. Baltimore: Williams & Wilkins, 1997;286–296.
13. Bone RC, Balk RA, Cerra FB, et al: Definitions for sepsis and organ failure and guidelines for the use of innovative therapies in sepsis; the ACCP/SCCM Consensus Conference Committee, American College of Chest Physicians/Society of Critical Care Medicine. Chest 1992;101:1644–1655.
14. Rangel-Frausto MS, Pittet D, Costigan M, Hwang T, Davis CS, Wenzel RP: The natural history of the systemic inflammatory response syndrome (SIRS): a prospective study. JAMA 1995;273:117–123.
15. Smail N, Messiah A, Edouard A, et al: Role of systemic inflammatory response syndrome and infection in the occurrence of early multiple organ dysfunction syndrome following severe trauma. Intensive Care Med 1995;21:813–816.
16. Pittet D, Rangel-Frausto S, Li N, et al: Systemic inflammatory response syndrome, sepsis, severe sepsis and septic shock: incidence, morbidities and outcomes in surgical ICU patients. Intensive Care Med 1995;21:302–309.
17. Opal SM: The uncertain value of the definition for SIRS: systemic inflammatory response syndrome. Chest 1998;113:1442–1443.
18. Muckart DJ, Bhagwanjee S: American College of Chest Physicians/Society of Critical Care Medicine Consensus Conference definitions of the systemic inflammatory response syndrome and allied disorders in relation to critically injured patients. Crit Care Med 1997;25:1789–1795.
19. Bossink AW, Groeneveld J, Hack CE, Thijs LG: Prediction of mortality in febrile medical patients: how useful are systemic inflammatory response syndrome and sepsis criteria? Chest 1998;113:1533–1541.
20. Barie PS, Hydo LJ, Fischer E: A prospective comparison of two multiple organ dysfunction/failure scoring systems for prediction of mortality in critical surgical illness. J Trauma 1994;37:660–666.
21. Moore FA, Moore EE, Poggetti R, et al: Gut bacterial translocation via the portal vein: a clinical perspective with major torso trauma. J Trauma 1991;31:629–636; discussion 636–638.
22. Sauaia A, Moore FA, Moore EE, Haenel JB, Read RA, Lezotte DC: Early predictors of postinjury multiple organ failure. Arch Surg 1994;129:39–45.
23. Goris RJ, te Boekhorst TP, Nuytinck JK, Gimbrere JS: Multiple-organ failure: generalized autodestructive inflammation? Arch Surg 1985;120:1109–1115.
24. Vincent JL, Moreno R, Takala J, et al: The SOFA (Sepsis-related Organ Failure Assessment) score to describe organ dysfunction/failure: on behalf of the Working Group on Sepsis-Related Problems of the European Society of Intensive Care Medicine. Intensive Care Med 1996;22:707–710.
25. Marshall JC, Cook DJ, Christou NV, Bernard GR, Sprung CL, Sibbald WJ: Multiple organ dysfunction score: a reliable descriptor of a complex clinical outcome. Crit Care Med 1995;23:1638–1652.
26. Bernard GR: Quantification of organ dysfunction: seeking standardization. Crit Care Med 1998;26:1767–1768.
27. Tran DD, Cuesta MA, van Leeuwen PA, Nauta JJ, Wesdorp RI: Risk factors for multiple organ system failure and death in critically injured patients. Surgery 1993;114:21–30.

28. Polk HC Jr, Shields CL: Remote organ failure: a valid sign of occult intra-abdominal infection. Surgery 1977;81:310–313.
29. Marshall WG Jr, Dimick AR: The natural history of major burns with multiple subsystem failure. J Trauma 1983;23:102–105.
30. Balk RA, Bone RC: The septic syndrome: definition and clinical implications. Crit Care Clin 1989;5:1–8.
31. Border JR, Hassett J, LaDuca J, et al: The gut origin septic states in blunt multiple trauma (ISS = 40) in the ICU. Ann Surg 1987;206:427–448.
32. Wilmore DW, Smith RJ, O'Dwyer ST, Jacobs DO, Ziegler TR, Wang XD: The gut: a central organ after surgical stress. Surgery 1988;104:917–923.
33. Moore FA, Moore EE, Poggetti RS, Read RA: Postinjury shock and early bacteremia: a lethal combination. Arch Surg 1992;127:893–897; discussion 897–898.
34. Hoch RC, Rodriguez R, Manning T, et al: Effects of accidental trauma on cytokine and endotoxin production. Crit Care Med 1993;21:839–845.
35. Cerra FB, Maddaus MA, Dunn DL, et al: Selective gut decontamination reduces nosocomial infections and length of stay but not mortality or organ failure in surgical intensive care unit patients. Arch Surg 1992;127:163–167; discussion 167–169.
36. Reidy JJ, Ramsay G: Clinical trials of selective decontamination of the digestive tract: review. Crit Care Med 1990;18:1449–1456.
37. Moore FA, Moore EE: Evolving concepts in the pathogenesis of postinjury multiple organ failure. Surg Clin North Am 1995;75:257–277.
38. Nuytinck HK, Offermans XJ, Kubat K, Goris JA: Whole-body inflammation in trauma patients: an autopsy study. Arch Surg 1988;123:1519–1524.
39. Partrick DA, Moore FA, Moore EE, Barnett CC Jr, Silliman CC: Neutrophil priming and activation in the pathogenesis of postinjury multiple organ failure. New Horiz 1996;4:194–210.
40. Livingston DH, Mosenthal AC, Deitch EA: Sepsis and multiple organ dysfunction syndrome: a clinical-mechanistic overview. New Horiz 1995;3:257–266.
41. Deitch EA: Multiple organ failure: pathophysiology and potential future therapy [see comments]. Ann Surg 1992;216:117–134.
42. Garrison RN, Spain DA, Wilson MA, Keelen PA, Harris PD: Microvascular changes explain the "two-hit" theory of multiple organ failure. Ann Surg 1998;227:851–860.
43. Moore FA, Moore EE, Sauaia A: Blood transfusion: an independent risk factor for postinjury multiple organ failure. Arch Surg 1997;132:620–624; discussion 624–625.
44. Henao FJ, Daes JE, Dennis RJ: Risk factors for multiorgan failure: a case-control study. J Trauma 1991;31:74–80.
45. Hudson LD, Milberg JA, Anardi D, Maunder RJ: Clinical risks for development of the acute respiratory distress syndrome. Am J Respir Crit Care Med 1995;151:293–301.
46. Baker SP, O'Neill B, Haddon W Jr, Long WB: The injury severity score: a method for describing patients with multiple injuries and evaluating emergency care. J Trauma 1974;14:187–196.
47. Champion HR, Copes WS, Sacco WJ, et al: A new characterization of injury severity. J Trauma 1990;30:539–545; discussion 545–546.
48. Copes WS, Champion HR, Sacco WJ, Lawnick MM, Keast SL, Bain LW: The Injury Severity Score revisited. J Trauma 1988;28:69–77.
49. Copes WS, Champion HR, Sacco WJ, et al: Progress in characterizing anatomic injury. J Trauma 1990;30:1200–1207.
50. Markle J, Cayten CG, Byrne DW, Moy F, Murphy JG: Comparison between TRISS and ASCOT methods in controlling for injury severity. J Trauma 1992;33:326–332.
51. Sauaia A, Moore FA, Moore EE, Norris JM, Lezotte DC, Hamman RF: Multiple organ failure can be predicted as early as 12 hours after injury. J Trauma 1998;45:291–301; discussion 301–303.
52. Osler T, Baker SP, Long W: A modification of the injury severity score that both improves accuracy and simplifies scoring. J Trauma 1997;43:922–925; discussion 925–926.
53. Brenneman FD, Boulanger BR, McLellan BA, Redelmeier DA: Measuring injury severity: time for a change? J Trauma 1998;44:580–582.
54. Shoemaker WC, Appel PL, Kram HB: Role of oxygen debt in the development of organ failure sepsis, and death in high-risk surgical patients. Chest 1992;102:208–215.
55. Shoemaker WC, Appel PL, Kram HB: Tissue oxygen debt as a determinant of lethal and nonlethal postoperative organ failure. Crit Care Med 1988;16:1117–1120.
56. Moore FA, Haenel JB, Moore EE, Whitehill TA: Incommensurate oxygen consumption in response to maximal oxygen availability predicts postinjury multiple organ failure. J Trauma 1992;33:58–65; discussion 65–67.
57. Cairns CB, Moore FA, Haenel JB, et al: Evidence for early supply independent mitochondrial dysfunction in patients developing multiple organ failure after trauma. J Trauma 1997;42:532–536.
58. Moore EE, Moore FA, Françoise RJ, Kim FJ, Biffl WL, Banerjee A: The postischemic gut serves as a priming bed for circulating neutrophils that provoke multiple organ failure. J Trauma 1994;37:881–887.
59. Kim FJ, Moore EE, Moore FA, Biffl WL, Fontes B, Banerjee A: Reperfused gut elaborates PAF that chemoattracts and primes neutrophils. J Surg Res 1995;58:636–640.
60. Botha AJ, Moore FA, Moore EE, Peterson VM, Silliman CC, Goode AW: Sequential systemic platelet-activating factor and interleukin 8 primes neutrophils in patients with trauma at risk of multiple organ failure. Br J Surg 1996;83:1407–1412.
61. Partrick DA, Moore EE, Moore FA, Biffl WL, Barnett CC: Reduced PAF-acetylhydrolase activity is associated with postinjury multiple organ failure. Shock 1997;7:170–174.
62. Castell JV, Gómez-Lechón MJ, David M, et al: Interleukin-6 is the major regulator of acute phase protein synthesis in adult human hepatocytes. FEBS Lett 1989;242:237–239.
63. Gennari R, Alexander JW, Pyles T, Hartmann S, Ogle CK: Effects of antimurine interleukin-6 on bacterial translocation during gut-derived sepsis. Arch Surg 1994;129:1191–1197.
64. Simms HH, D'Amico R: Polymorphonuclear leukocyte dysregulation during the systemic inflammatory response syndrome. Blood 1994;83:1398–1407.
65. Wortel CH, van Deventer SJ, Aarden LA, et al: Interleukin-6 mediates host defense responses induced by abdominal surgery. Surgery 1993;114:564–570.
66. Deitch EA, Xu D, Franko L, Ayala A, Chaudry IH: Evidence favoring the role of the gut as a cytokine-generating organ in rats subjected to hemorrhagic shock. Shock 1994;1:141–145.
67. Meyer TA, Wang J, Tiao GM, Ogle CK, Fischer JE, Hasselgren PO: Sepsis and endotoxemia stimulate intestinal interleukin-6 production. Surgery 1995;118:336–342.
68. Altavilla D, Squadrito F, Canale P, et al: Tumor necrosis factor induces E-selectin production in splanchnic artery occlusion shock. Am J Physiol 1995;268:H1412–1417.

69. Welborn MB, III, Douglas WG, Abouhamze Z, et al: Visceral ischemia-reperfusion injury promotes tumor necrosis factor (TNF) and interleukin-1 (IL-1) dependent organ injury in the mouse. Shock 1996;6:171–176.
70. Meade P, Shoemaker WC, Donnelly TJ, et al: Temporal patterns of hemodynamics, oxygen transport, cytokine activity, and complement activity in the development of adult respiratory distress syndrome after severe injury. J Trauma 1994;36:651–657.
71. Fine J, Frank E, Rutenberg S, et al: The bacterial factor in traumatic shock. N Engl J Med 1959;260:217–220.
72. Baker JW, Deitch EA, Li M, Berg RD, Specian RD: Hemorrhagic shock induces bacterial translocation from the gut. J Trauma 1988;28:896–906.
73. Deitch EA, Bridges RM: Effect of stress and trauma on bacterial translocation from the gut. J Surg Res 1987;42:536–542.
74. Koziol JM, Rush BF Jr, Smith SM, Machiedo GW: Occurrence of bacteremia during and after hemorrhagic shock. J Trauma 1988;28:10–16.
75. Sori AJ, Rush BF Jr, Lysz TW, Smith S, Machiedo GW: The gut as source of sepsis after hemorrhagic shock. Am J Surg 1988;155:187–192.
76. Peitzman AB, Udekwu AO, Ochoa J, Smith S: Bacterial translocation in trauma patients. J Trauma 1991;31:1083–1086; discussion 1086–1087.
77. Johnston TD, Fischer R, Chen Y, Reed RL: Lung injury from gut ischemia: insensitivity to portal blood flow diversion. J Trauma 1993;35:508–511.
78. Sanchez-Garcia M, Prieto A, Tejedor A, et al: Characteristics of thoracic duct lymph in multiple organ dysfunction syndrome. Arch Surg 1997;132:13–18.
79. Magnotti LJ, Upperman JS, Xu DZ, Lu Q, Deitch EA: Gut-derived mesenteric lymph but not portal blood increases endothelial cell permeability and promotes lung injury after hemorrhagic shock. Ann Surg 1998;228:518–527.
80. Upperman JS, Deitch EA, Guo W, Lu Q, Xu D: Post-hemorrhagic shock mesenteric lymph is cytotoxic to endothelial cells and activates neutrophils. Shock 1998;10:407–414.
81. Zallen G, Moore E, Johnson J, Biffl W: Post-hemorrhagic shock mesenteric lymph primes circulating neutrophils and provokes lung injury. J Surg Res (in press).
82. Salvo I, de Cian W, Musicco M, et al: The Italian SEPSIS study: preliminary results on the incidence and evolution of SIRS, sepsis, severe sepsis and septic shock. Intensive Care Med 1995;21 (suppl 2):S244–249.
83. Gando S, Kameue T, Nanzaki S, Hayakawa T, Nakanishi Y: Participation of tissue factor and thrombin in posttraumatic systemic inflammatory syndrome. Crit Care Med 1997;25:1820–1826.
84. Knaus WA, Zimmerman JE, Wagner DP, Draper EA, Lawrence DE: APACHE—acute physiology and chronic health evaluation: a physiologically based classification system. Crit Care Med 1981;9:591–597.
85. Knaus WA, Wagner DP, Draper EA, et al: The APACHE III prognostic system: risk prediction of hospital mortality for critically ill hospitalized adults. Chest 1991;100:1619–1636.
86. Botha AJ, Moore FA, Moore EE, Kim FJ, Banerjee A, Peterson VM: Postinjury neutrophil priming and activation: an early vulnerable window. Surgery 1995;118:358–364; discussion 364–365.
87. Davies MG, Hagen PO: Systemic inflammatory response syndrome. Br J Surg 1997;84:920–935.
88. Yao YM, Redl H, Bahrami S, Schlag G: The inflammatory basis of trauma/shock-associated multiple organ failure. Inflamm Res 1998;47:201–210.
89. Partrick DA, Moore FA, Moore EE, Biffl WL, Sauaia A, Barnett CC Jr: The inflammatory profile of interleukin-6, interleukin-8, and soluble intercellular adhesion molecule-1 in postinjury multiple organ failure. Am J Surg 1996;172:425–429; discussed 429–431.
90. Baue AE: Predicting outcome in injured patients and its relationship to circulating cytokines. Shock 1995;4:39–40.
91. Waydhas C, Nast-Kolb D, Jochum M, et al: Inflammatory mediators, infection, sepsis, and multiple organ failure after severe trauma. Arch Surg 1992;127:460–467.
92. Roumen RM, Redl H, Schlag G, et al: Inflammatory mediators in relation to the development of multiple organ failure in patients after severe blunt trauma. Crit Care Med 1995;23:474–480.
93. Bone RC: Immunologic dissonance: a continuing evolution in our understanding of the systemic inflammatory response syndrome (SIRS) and the multiple organ dysfunction syndrome (MODS) [see comments]. Ann Intern Med 1996;125:680–687.
94. Vincent JL, Bihari DJ, Suter PM, et al: The prevalence of nosocomial infection in intensive care units in Europe: results of the European Prevalence of Infection in Intensive Care (EPIC) Study; EPIC International Advisory Committee. JAMA 1995;274:639–644.
95. Moore FA, Sauaia A, Moore EE, Haenel JB, Burch JM, Lezotte DC: Postinjury multiple organ failure: a bimodal phenomenon. J Trauma 1996;40:501–510; discussion 510–512.
96. Sauaia A, Moore FA, Moore EE, Haenel JB, Read RA: Pneumonia: cause or symptom of postinjury multiple organ failure? Am J Surg 1993;166:606–610; discussion 610–611.
97. Opelz G, Terasaki PI: Improvement of kidney-graft survival with increased numbers of blood transfusions. N Engl J Med 1978;299:799–803.
98. Tartter PI: The association of perioperative blood transfusion with colorectal cancer recurrence. Ann Surg 1992;216:633–638.
99. Mickler TA, Longnecker DE: The immunosuppressive aspects of blood transfusion. J Intensive Care Med 1992;7:176–188.
100. Edna TH, Bjerkeset T: Association between blood transfusion and infection in injured patients. J Trauma 1992;33:659–661.
101. Heddle NM, Klama L, Singer J, et al: The role of the plasma from platelet concentrates in transfusion reactions. N Engl J Med 1994;331:625–628.
102. Silliman CC, Thurman GW, Ambruso DR: Stored blood components contain agents that prime the neutrophil NADPH oxidase through the platelet-activating-factor receptor. Vox Sang 1992;63:133–136.
103. Stack G, Snyder EL: Cytokine generation in stored platelet concentrates. Transfusion 1994;34:20–25.
104. Hill AB: The environment and disease: association or causation? Proc R Soc Med 1965;58:295–300.
105. Zallen G, Offner P, Moore E, Silliman C: Age of transfused blood is an independent risk factor for postinjury multiple organ failure. Am J Surg (in press).
106. Partrick D, Moore E, Barnett C, Silliman C: Human polymerized hemoglobin as a blood substitute avoids transfusion-induced neutrophil priming and superoxide and elastase release. Shock (in press)
107. Johnson J, Moore E, Offner P, Silliman C: Resuscitation with a blood substitute attenuates postinjury upregulation of neutrophil CD11b/CD18. Shock 1998;9:S13.

108. Roumen RM, Hendriks T, van der Ven-Jongekrijg J, et al: Cytokine patterns in patients after major vascular surgery, hemorrhagic shock, and severe blunt trauma: relation with subsequent adult respiratory distress syndrome and multiple organ failure. Ann Surg 1993;218: 769–776.
109. Baigrie RJ, Lamont PM, Dallman M, Morris PJ: The release of interleukin-1 beta (IL-1) precedes that of interleukin 6 (IL-6) in patients undergoing major surgery. Lymphokine Cytokine Res 1991;10:253–256.
110. Cruickshank AM, Fraser WD, Burns HJ, Van Damme J, Shenkin A: Response of serum interleukin-6 in patients undergoing elective surgery of varying severity. Clin Sci (Colch) 1990;79:161–165.
111. Lozman J, Deno DC, Feustel PJ, et al: Pulmonary and cardiovascular consequences of immediate fixation or conservative management of long-bone fractures. Arch Surg 1986;121:992–999.
112. Behrman SW, Fabian TC, Kudsk KA, Taylor JC: Improved outcome with femur fractures: early vs. delayed fixation. J Trauma 1990;30:792–797; discussion 797–798.
113. Charash WE, Fabian TC, Croce MA: Delayed surgical fixation of femur fractures is a risk factor for pulmonary failure independent of thoracic trauma. J Trauma 1994;37:667–672.
114. Johnson KD, Cadambi A, Seibert GB: Incidence of adult respiratory distress syndrome in patients with multiple musculoskeletal injuries: effect of early operative stabilization of fractures. J Trauma 1985;25:375–384.
115. Pelias ME, Townsend MC, Flancbaum L: Long bone fractures predispose to pulmonary dysfunction in blunt chest trauma despite early operative fixation. Surgery 1992;111:576–579.
116. Reynolds MA, Richardson JD, Spain DA, Seligson D, Wilson MA, Miller FB: Is the timing of fracture fixation important for the patient with multiple trauma? Ann Surg 1995;222:470–478; discussion 478–481.
117. Jaicks RR, Cohn SM, Moller BA: Early fracture fixation may be deleterious after head injury. J Trauma 1997;42:1–5; discussion 5–6.
118. Pape HC, Auf'm'Kolk M, Paffrath T, Regel G, Sturm JA, Tscherne H: Primary intramedullary femur fixation in multiple trauma patients with associated lung contusion: a cause of post-traumatic ARDS? J Trauma 1993;34:540–547; discussion 547–548.
119. Townsend RN, Lheureau T, Protech J, Riemer B, Simon D: Timing fracture repair in patients with severe brain injury (Glasgow Coma Scale score < 9). J Trauma 1998;44:977–982; discussion 982–983.
120. Pigula FA, Wald SL, Shackford SR, Vane DW: The effect of hypotension and hypoxia on children with severe head injuries. J Pediatr Surg 1993;28:310–314; discussion 315–316.
121. Wald SL, Shackford SR, Fenwick J: The effect of secondary insults on mortality and long-term disability after severe head injury in a rural region without a trauma system. J Trauma 1993;34:377–381; discussion 381–382.
122. Pietropaoli JA, Rogers FB, Shackford SR, Wald SL, Schmoker JD, Zhuang J: The deleterious effects of intraoperative hypotension on outcome in patients with severe head injuries. J Trauma 1992;33:403–407.
123. Waydhas C, Nast-Kolb D, Trupka A, et al: Post-traumatic inflammatory response, secondary operations, and late multiple organ failure. J Trauma 1996;40:624–630; discussion 630–631.
124. Champion HR, Copes WS, Buyer D, Flanagan ME, Bain L, Sacco WJ: Major trauma in geriatric patients. Am J Public Health 1989;79:1278–1282.
125. Evans L: Risk of fatality from physical trauma versus sex and age. J Trauma 1988;28:368–378.
126. Le Gall JR, Lemeshow S, Saulnier F: A new Simplified Acute Physiology Score (SAPS II) based on a European/North American multicenter study. JAMA 1993;270:2957–2963.
127. Lemeshow S, Teres D, Avrunin JS, Gage RW: Refining intensive care unit outcome prediction by using changing probabilities of mortality. Crit Care Med 1988;16:470–477.
128. Morris JA Jr, MacKenzie EJ, Edelstein SL: The effect of pre-existing conditions on mortality in trauma patients. JAMA 1990;263:1942–1946.
129. Milzman DP, Boulanger BR, Rodriguez A, Soderstrom CA, Mitchell KA, Magnant CM: Pre-existing disease in trauma patients: a predictor of fate independent of age and injury severity score. J Trauma 1992;32:236–43; discussion 243–244.
130. Sauaia A, Moore FA, Moore EE, Lezotte DC: Early risk factors for postinjury multiple organ failure. World J Surg 1996;20: 392–400.
131. Moss M, Bucher B, Moore FA, Moore EE, Parsons PE: The role of chronic alcohol abuse in the development of acute respiratory distress syndrome in adults. JAMA 1996;275:50–54.
132. Border JR, Chenier R, McManamy RH, et al: Multiple systems organ failure: muscle fuel deficit with visceral protein malnutrition. Surg Clin North Am 1976;56:1147–1167.
133. Cerra FB, Siegel JH, Coleman B, Border JR, McMenamy RR: Septic autocannibalism: a failure of exogenous nutritional support. Ann Surg 1980;192:570–580.
134. Deitch EA: Multiple organ failure. Adv Surg 1993;26:333–356.
135. McMenamy RH, Birkhahn R, Oswald G, et al: Multiple systems organ failure. I. The basal state. J Trauma 1981;21: 99–114.
136. Regel G, Grotz M, Weltner T, Sturm JA, Tscherne H: Pattern of organ failure following severe trauma. World J Surg 1996;20: 422–429.
137. Walker L, Eiseman B: The changing pattern of post-traumatic respiratory distress syndrome. Ann Surg 1975;181:693–697.

5
Risk and Setting for Multiple Organ Failure in Medical Patients

Kang Lee and Derek C. Angus

In this chapter we approach the assessment of risk factors and the setting for multiple organ failure (MOF) first by considering the overall concepts of primary injury, the host response to injury, complications leading to increased risk, and the ability to modulate the subsequent chain of events. We then examine specific organ systems and settings for MOF in *medical* patients. We use infection with subsequent sepsis as our main illustrative example of primary injury resulting in secondary organ failure, although septic-like states can exist in the absence of a demonstrable infection. Furthermore, although hypotensive states due to major hemorrhage can develop in medical patients (e.g., major gastrointestinal bleeding) and lead to organ failure, we leave the detailed discussion of this topic to the chapter on surgical patients. Although our focus is on medical patients, when appropriate we mention surgical issues in medical patients and medical issues in surgical patients.

Basic Conceptual Model for the Development of Organ Failure

Organ failure develops as a result of severe primary insult or as an event secondary to a systemic process. Examples of severe primary insults are severe pneumonia causing acute respiratory distress syndrome (ARDS), severe rhabdomyolysis causing acute renal failure, and extensive acute myocardial infarction with cardiogenic shock. Organ failure as a secondary event largely results from the biologic response of the host to an initial insult and is a mark of dysregulation of the inflammatory system.[1] An alternative to the term "dysregulation" is "maladaptation": Instead of a beneficial effect of a systemic inflammatory process to clear infection (adaptive response), the persistence, or overexpression, of the host response (characterized both by pro-and antiinflammatory components) leads to further damage (maladaptive).[2] Organ failure in this situation is a reflection of the host response, which may be genetically determined[3] or the result of the patient's prior medical condition (age, previous illness, immunosuppressed condition, drugs). These host factors interact with the initial severity and site of injury along with adequacy of treatment and subsequent complications to cause the development of MOF several days afterward. Persistent perfusion deficits, nosocomial infection, and remaining necrotic tissue during the ensuing days subsequent to the primary injury may tip the patient into MOF.

Genetic Factors

Primary genetic influences on the host response to infection and subsequent fatality are not well appreciated. Interestingly, as far back as 1988, Sorensen et al. had reported that there was a strong genetic component to fatal infections.[4] Enrollees in their study had a fivefold increased risk of fatal infectious disease if a biologic parent had died from infection. Westendorp et al. subsequently examined the capacity to produce tumor necrosis factor-α (TNFα) and interleukin-10 (IL-10) in the relatives of patients with meningococcal disease.[3] The results indicated that families with low TNFα production had a 10-fold increase in risk of fatal outcome from meningococcal disease, whereas high IL-10 production increased the risk 20-fold. Families with both characteristics were at highest risk. Other familial conditions predispose the patients to infections as well (e.g., immunoglobulin deficiencies and severe combined immunodeficiency).

Host Response

One of the most common insults to medical patients that results in organ failure is infection. As proposed at an American College of Chest Physicians and Society of Critical Care Medicine (ACCP/SCCM) consensus conference, the host response has been divided into several categories, depending on the severity of response (Table 5.1).[5] These categories represent a continuum of increasing severity that reflects the vigor of the host response. Although controversy has been raised over the fact that the mildest state, the systemic inflammatory response syndrome (SIRS), may be both too sensitive (capturing many patients who demonstrate only normal physiologic or mild pathologic states with little chance of subsequent organ dysfunction)[6] and too nonspecific (failing to capture patients whose inflammatory dysregulation presents predominantly as an

TABLE 5.1. Definitions of Sepsis, SIRS, Severe Sepsis, Septic Shock.

Systemic inflammatory response syndrome (SIRS): Clinically recognized by the presence of two or more of the following:
Temperature > 38° or < 36°C
Heart rate > 90 beats/min
Respiratory rate > 20 breaths/min or $PaCO_2$ < 32 mmHg
WBC > 12,000 cells/mm^3, < 4000 cells/mm^3, or > 10% immature (band) forms

Sepsis: Systemic response to infection. Thus the clinical signs describing SIRS are present, together with definitive evidence of infection.

Severe sepsis: Severe when it is associated with organ dysfunction, hypoperfusion, or hypotension. The manifestations of hypoperfusion may include, but are not limited to, lactic acidosis, oliguria, or acute alteration in mental status.

Septic shock: Sepsis with hypotension despite adequate fluid resuscitation combined with perfusion abnormalities that may include, but are not limited to, lactic acidosis, oliguria, or acute alteration in mental status. Patients who are on inotropic or vasopressor agents may not be hypotensive at the time perfusion abnormalities are measured.

Hypotension: Systolic blood pressure of >90 mmHg or a reduction of ≥40 mmHg from baseline in the absence of other causes for the fall in blood pressure.

Modified from ACCP/SCCM Consensus Conference Committee,[5] with permission.

TABLE 5.3. Effect of Culture Positivity on the Development of Organ Failure.

Culture result	ARDS (%)	DIC (%)	ARF (%)	Shock (%)
Sepsis				
Culture-positive	6	16*	19*	20*
Culture-negative	3	20	5	27
Severe sepsis				
Culture-positive	8	18	23*	28*
Culture-negative	4	17	16	22

ARDS, acute respiratory distress syndrome; DIC, disseminated intravascular coagulation; ARF, acute renal failure.
*$p < 0.05$.

antiinflammatory clinical picture)[7] it has been tested in a large cohort of patients with informative results.

The University of Iowa conducted a study of both intensive care unit (ICU) and general ward patients,[8] surveying a total of 3708 patients, 68% of whom met the criteria for SIRS. These investigators demonstrated an increasing mortality with the proposed increased severity (Table 5.2), and the risk of developing subsequent organ failure. For example, the risk of developing ARDS was 18% for those with septic shock but only 2% for those with two criteria for SIRS. The presence of bacteremia increased the risk of ARDS from 3% to 6% for those with sepsis. Similarly, the risk of disseminated intravascular coagulation, acute renal failure, and shock were also higher in the bacteremic patients with sepsis (Table 5.3).

Similarly, a Brussels study[9] demonstrated that patients with shock and suspected sepsis have a higher mortality rate and an increased chance of developing MOF if, upon retrospective review, a source of infection is noted. Furthermore, this study showed that cirrhotic patients had increased risk of MOF (67% vs. 30%). In those who subsequently developed MOF or death, the presence of significant persistent elevated serum levels of TNF and IL-6 were also noted. Further evidence that increasing systemic inflammation is correlated with increasing numbers of organ failures was provided by a study in liver cirrhotic patients.[10] Rosenbloom et al. demonstrated that increasing levels of IL-6 and markers of leukocyte activation (CD11b and CD35) are significantly correlated with organ failure.[10] Furthermore, peripheral neutrophils appear to be apoptotic-resistant when they are activated in patients with SIRS.[11] This may lead to persistent inflammation and the development of organ dysfunction.

In addition to cytokine levels as markers of the inflammatory state, endothelium-derived factors have also been studied in the development of MOF. The endothelium is considered "activated" in SIRS. A study of patients with severe infection demonstrated that levels of serum E-selectin, serum intercellular adhesion molecule (sICAM-1), and von Willebrand factor antigen (vWf:Ag) were higher for nonsurvivors and for patients with septic shock or bacteremia, and they correlated with the Simplified Acute Physiology Score (SAPS) and MOF.[12] Survival outcome was predicted with high sensitivity and specificity by initial plasma levels of sICAM-1 and vWf:Ag. In nonsurvivors, sICAM-1 remained at high levels indefinitely. In another study, E-selectin levels were shown to be associated with hemodynamic compromise and were prognostic for survival and organ failure in septic critically ill patients.[13] This area of research was extended to the administration of monoclonal antibodies to E-selectin, which showed impressive results in an initial Brussels study.[14] Shock and organ failure resolved in most patients.

Another measure of host response is the physiologic derangement at admission to the ICU. Such derangement is commonly measured by a variety of severity illness indices. For instance, high Acute Physiology and Chronic Health Evaluation (APACHE II) scores at ICU admission are associated with a high risk of subsequent organ failure.[15] Utilizing severity scoring indices such as APACHE III may allow better prognostication of hospital outcome than definitions of sepsis alone. Knaus et al. demonstrated that in their database of 17,440 ICU admissions 519 patients had clinical sepsis as the primary clinical diagnosis.[16] When they examined the APACHE III scores, it was found that they varied markedly and were associated with widely varying hospital mortality rates (from 40% to 64%). They concluded that utilization of the APACHE III score, the etiology

TABLE 5.2. Mortality Increases with Progression of Host Response.

Host response	Mortality (%)
No SIRS	3
SIRS with two criteria fulfilled	7
SIRS with three criteria fulfilled	10
SIRS with four criteria fulfilled	17
Sepsis	16
Severe sepsis	20
Septic shock	46

of the sepsis, and the treatment location prior to ICU admission provided the greatest degree of discrimination for determining the risk of hospital death.

The evidence therefore supports the model that, with increasing severity of the persistent host response, measured clinically (e.g., SIRS, septic shock, severe sepsis, severity illness indices) or biologically, there is an increased risk of the development of organ failure and death. As the number of organ failures increases, there is correspondingly higher mortality.[17] The persistence of a dysregulatory inflammatory state is related to secondary events, which adds to the risk for organ failure, with infection remaining the most significant factor for organ dysfunction or failure. Whether any specific interventions can modulate the natural process once it is in progress remains a question deserving further exploration.

Secondary Events

Failure to correct secondary defects (oxygenation debt) and the development of various complications (e.g., nosocomial sepsis, stress ulceration, encephalopathy, renal failure) can lead to MOF. The concept of a pathologic supply-dependence of oxygen transport was championed by Shoemaker et al., who initially demonstrated that nonsurviving shock patients had decreased oxygen transport and consumption.[18] One could argue that with persistent oxygen deficits organ dysfunction would develop followed by organ failure, resulting ultimately in the patient's demise. As such, many studies were conducted to correct these oxygen deficits in order to decrease patient mortality by increasing oxygen transport above 600 ml/min/m^2, and oxygen consumption above 170 ml/min/m^2. Shoemaker et al. initially claimed marked improvement in a trial reported in 1988,[19] but subsequent trials in other centers failed to validate this hypothesis[20,21] and even suggested increased mortality associated with such active interventions to increase oxygen transport (in-hospital mortality: control group 34%, treatment group 54%; $p = 0.04$). Organ dysfunction was also not significantly altered in the treatment group with higher oxygen delivery.[22]

As an adjunct for detecting oxygen deficit, gastric tonometry was developed to measure splanchnic ischemia. Although a low gastric pHi (pH intramucosal) may predict MOF in trauma patients,[23] a study in septic children failed to demonstrate any additional benefit of gastric tonometry for predicting mortality or MOF.[24] Part of the basis for gastric tonometry reflects the concern that the "gut is the motor of multiorgan failure."[25] This is related to the phenomenon of bacterial translocation and increased intestinal permeability in patients with SIRS.[26] To address this concern, the concept of selective bowel decontamination has been studied in many trials.[27] Most regimens include oral nonabsorbed agents that selectively remove aerobic gram-negative bacilli from the oropharynx and gastrointestinal tract and a systemic agent to prevent infection while the oral regimen takes effect. A meta-analysis of 11 trials involving 1489 patients showed no difference in mortality, although nosocomial respiratory infections were reduced by an odds ratio of 0.12 (95% confidence intervals of 0.08–0.19).[28] Development of subsequent organ dysfunction and nosocomial infections is also related to the presence of stomach and small bowel colonization with *Candida, Pseudomonas,* or *Staphylococcus epidermidis* in critically ill patients in the ICU.[29]

Nosocomial sepsis is common in critically ill patients, and the risk is increased with the use of invasive catheters. Hence nosocomial pneumonias derived from intubation, linesepsis from central lines, urosepsis from urinary catheterization, and sinusitis from nasogastric tubes are frequent occurrences in ICU patients. Nosocomial pneumonias have an associated crude mortality rate of 30%.[30] Efforts to reduce the incidence of ventilator-associated pneumonia should therefore minimize the risk of further deterioration toward MOF. For instance, patients with ARDS mainly perish because they develop sepsis and MOF, not because of primary respiratory failure. A 1999 review documented several strategies to address this problem, ranging from simple nonpharmacologic interventions (hand washing, protective gowns and gloves, semirecumbent position, avoidance of large gastric volumes, oral intubation rather than nasal intubation, continuous subglottic suctioning, humidification with heat and moisture exchangers, less frequent changes of ventilator circuits, and postural changes) to pharmacologic interventions (stress-ulcer prophylaxis and antibiotics).[31]

Adult respiratory distress syndrome represents the extreme spectrum of acute lung injury and failure. Its associated mortality is high and despite many therapeutic approaches, few have been demonstrated to be effective. Seventy-five percent of patients who develop ARDS have aspiration of gastric contents, trauma, or sepsis.[32] Risk factors are additive. Sepsis syndrome alone is associated with a risk of 38% for ARDS, exhibiting a higher mortality than other causes of ARDS (79% vs. 33%). The most common site of infection is the pulmonary system (62%). Mortality in ARDS is commonly secondary to MOF,[33] which is supported by observations that nonpulmonary organ dysfunction is more severe and rapid in nonsurvivors of ARDS than in survivors.[34]

Ventilation with high pressures and high volumes leads to lung injury,[35] which in turn leads to increased cytokine production in the lungs[36] and release into the bloodstream.[37] It is proposed that bacteria present in the lungs may translocate into the bloodstream when high transpulmonary pressures are present.[38] Whether these mechanisms and consequences lead to further multiple-organ dysfunction is unclear.[39] At present there is no support for this concept in clinical studies of ventilatory strategies for ARDS patients.

Modulation of Events

The search for ways to modulate the development of organ failure and ultimately death has been strewn with multiple costly failures. The basic requirements for prompt, adequate resuscitation to prevent the secondary damage that develops over subsequent days remains undervalued and poorly applied. For instance, a survey from southern England demonstrated that poor pre-ICU care led to a poorer outcome.[40] Another study from the University of Iowa demonstrated a poorer outcome when septic shock occurred in the general ward, rather than the ICU, in part associated with slower intervention (fluid boluses and initiation of inotropic support).[41] Moreover, having appropriately trained intensivists appears to improve septic outcome once the patient is admitted to the ICU.[42]

In cases of infection, along with the requirement for appropriate antibiotics, appropriate drainage or débridement is required to minimize continued systemic inflammation. A prospective study with 2124 bacteremic patients demonstrated that for those who received inappropriate empiric antibiotics the mortality was significantly elevated (34% vs. 18%, $p < 0.05$).[43]

Other, more costly interventions have been targeted at the immune response to infection. Early studies utilized steroids in septic and septic shock patients. A meta-analysis of these trials demonstrated no overall beneficial effects, nor were there increased adverse side effects.[44] Another study, however, has demonstrated the benefit of hydrocortisone (100 mg IV three times daily for 5 days) in reversal of shock and 28-day mortality in patients with no adrenocortical insufficiency.[45] The benefit appeared to be derived from a decreased progression to organ failure in the hydrocortisone group, although the basic mechanism of benefit remains to be elucidated. Subsequent antiendotoxin and anticytokine therapies have demonstrated no benefit; and for some interventions the outcome was poorer. HA-1A, a monoclonal antibody to endotoxin or placebo was given to 621 patients with shock and suspected gram-negative bacteremia.[46] There was no difference in 14-day mortality (placebo 32%, HA-1A 33%). An editorial has summarized most of the recent anticytokine trials and has attempted to examine the reason for their negative impact.[47] Interestingly, antithrombin III supplementation has also been used in an attempt to attenuate the inflammatory response and to modulate cell adhesion.[48]

Immunomodulation with enteral nutrition has been attempted utilizing arginine, purine nucleotides, and ω-3 polyunsaturated fatty acids as immunonutrients (Impact, Novartis Nutrition) for ICU patients.[49,50] These nutrients affect the function of T cells and macrophages, dampening their inflammatory contributions; they are thus postulated to dampen the systemic inflammatory response and ultimately improve patients' organ function and outcome. However, in two studies (one from Britain[50] and one from the United States[49]) there was no difference in hospital outcome, although there was a significant reduction in hospital length of stay. In the British study, those who received early nutritional support (>2.5 liters within 72 hours of ICU admission) had significantly fewer days of SIRS when given Impact.[50] For the subgroup with sepsis in the US study, in addition to the reduction in hospital length of stay there was a reduction in acquired infections for those given Impact.[49]

Another approach to modulate the inflammatory cascade has been application of hemofiltration and plasmapheresis.[51] This "blood purification" approach removes various cytokines[52] that are dependent on the effect of convection and not diffusion.[53] Hemodynamics are generally improved,[54] but prospective studies to demonstrate survival benefit are still lacking.[55]

Specific Organ Dysfunction and Settings for MOF in Medical Patients

The definition of the "medical" patient is somewhat arbitrary. Indeed, the classic picture of an elderly patient with multiple preexisting conditions is increasingly the description of many ICU patients, including those undergoing extensive surgical procedures. Nevertheless, the major concern for the development of MOF in nonsurgical ICU patients is that preexisting illness is often present, frequently in more than one organ system. For example, elderly patients often have preexisting ischemic heart disease, hypertension, diabetes mellitus, cerebrovascular disease, and chronic obstructive pulmonary disease (COPD). These diseases increase the likelihood that a patient may require ICU care, increase the likelihood of the development of single-organ dysfunction, and through decreased organ function reserve compound the chances of developing MOF. Unfortunately, most acute supportive therapies for organ dysfunction are less effective when there is preexisting organ damage and are more likely to worsen function in other organ systems already weakened by prior disease. Thus clinicians must be alert to the possibility of preexisting illness and judicious in the use of aggressive therapies. Coupled with this, a keen sense of when aggressive care is futile is essential, as appropriate withdrawal of support and palliation is often a necessary and vital component of good care.

The multiplicity of organ involvement usually interacts to compound the overall condition as a domino effect or a concurrent effect, and the true impact of specific diseases and organ systems on subsequent mortality is difficult to measure and poorly studied to date. Indeed, there are no comprehensive studies of nonsurgical ICU patients that characterize the distribution of both preexisting illnesses and new organ failure, with determination of the relative contribution of each to subsequent mortality. Despite the multiple interactions between diseases and organ systems, for the convenience of discussion we address each organ system and setting separately.

Cardiac Failure

Heart failure, which is commonly the result of ischemic heart disease, leads to decreased perfusion of other organs. The decreased perfusion results in inadequate oxygenation and consequently cellular energy failure with organ dysfunction, resulting in the common manifestations of hypoxemia, oliguric renal failure, mental obtundation, ischemic hepatitis and colitis, and metabolic acidosis in patients with severe heart failure. Concurrently, widespread atherosclerosis may also compound the perfusion to other organs.

Noncardiac causes of mortality for elderly patients with congestive cardiac failure may be as high as 28%, as reported in a Canadian study involving 2216 patients.[56] Five percent of these patients died from multiple system failure. Improving cardiac output with insertion of a left ventricular assist device, as one would expect, improved noncardiac organ function in patients awaiting cardiac transplantation.[57] Although there are nonischemic causes of heart failure (e.g., viral, parasitic, and idiopathic cardiomyopathies), they are rare in the United States and do not contribute significantly to the overall incidence of organ failure.

The major medical diseases that increase the likelihood of ischemic heart disease are hypertension and diabetes mellitus. Both these conditions are associated with widespread atherosclerosis and renal impairment. Smoking and obesity, major risk factors for ischemic heart disease, are also associated with increased risk for pulmonary disease.

Renal Failure

Chronic renal failure patients with renal replacement therapy usually have other, concomitant medical conditions that increase morbidity (e.g., diabetes mellitus, hypertension, hyperlipidemia). As such, the risk of hospital mortality is increased for such patients compared to those without chronic renal failure. Acute renal failure developing in patients with SIRS is fairly common and delays the resolution of SIRS.[58] Mortality among such patients in the ICU rises with increasing numbers of failing organs and advancing age, reflecting an overall mortality of 58%; but whether renal failure is an independent risk factor for mortality remains controversial.[59]

Liver Failure

Acute liver failure (fulminant or acute decompensation) is commonly associated with dysfunction in other organs. Especially among those with fulminant liver failure, mortality is high once the patient develops MOF; here even liver transplantation does not always succeed. Patients may perish owing to cerebral edema or overwhelming nosocomial infections. Variceal bleeding may be difficult to control and is frequently associated with aspiration pneumonia.

Cirrhosis itself is an independent risk factor for MOF when sepsis is present. It is attributable to decreased function of the Kupffer cells to clear organisms arising from the gastrointestinal tract and hence an increased propensity to develop bacteremia and bacterial peritonitis.[60] Fulminant liver failure is due to a wide variety of diseases, but analgesic abuse is one of the commonest causes. It is also associated with acute dysfunction in other organs due to direct injury from other ingested toxins. For example, patients may have ingested sedative agents, compromising neurologic function, or may have ingested salicylates, inducing renal dysfunction and metabolic consequences. These additional factors could be falsely attributed to the liver failure directly, with delayed diagnosis and inadequate treatment.

Pulmonary Failure

Adult respiratory distress syndrome commonly results in MOF, which is the most common mode of death in these patients, rather than respiratory failure alone. Hypoxemia obviously leads to organ dysfunction, and hypercapnia may reduce splanchnic flow and consequently increased bacterial translocation. Ventilatory strategies that require high positive end-expiratory pressure (PEEP) may reduce cardiac output and increase pulmonary vascular resistance. Furthermore, ARDS patients are especially prone to develop nosocomial pneumonia because of their prolonged ventilatory requirements, leading to the complications of further organ failure, as discussed previously. The most common direct, nonsurgical cause of ARDS is pneumonia.

Patients with pneumonia frequently develop respiratory failure and sepsis syndrome; if they do, the mortality risk becomes much higher. Risk factors for increased mortality include the microbiologic etiology, male gender, hypotension, hypothermia, diabetes mellitus, and bacteremia.[61]

Patients with COPD have a poor prognosis when admitted to the ICU, with a 1-year mortality of 59%.[62] Complications usually relate to the prolonged ventilatory course and the presence of cor pulmonale, with the development of nonpulmonary organ system dysfunction as the major predictor of hospital mortality. Again, the extent to which mortality is directly related to the COPD is unclear, as such patients often have coexisting diseases, especially ischemic heart disease.

Neurologic Failure

Patients with decreased conscious levels owing to various central nervous system (CNS) disorders commonly require ventilatory support for airway protection and hypoventilation. Such support frequently leads to nosocomial infections, which in these frequently elderly patients may spiral to further organ involvement (e.g., renal failure, shock, jaundice, stress ulceration). Aspiration pneumonia is also a frequent complication and may lead to severe MOF with ARDS. In a New Orleans study of acute stroke patients, 38% experienced aspiration within 5 days of the stroke, and most of these events could be detected only by video-fluoroscopy.[63] In a multicenter trial for subarachnoid hemorrhage patients, the data from the placebo arm demonstrated that medical causes of mortality were as high as 23%, with 40% having a life-threatening medical complication.[64] Pulmonary complications were the most frequent and occurred usually 3–7 days after the event. Although cerebrovascular disease is probably the most common neurologic setting for subsequent organ dysfunction, other nonsurgical causes include seizures (especially poorly controlled status epilepticus) and drug overdoses.

Hematology, Cancer, and Immunosuppression

Although rare, patients with hematologic conditions, such as lymphoma, leukemia, and platelet abnormalities (e.g., idiopathic thrombocytopenic purpura) require ICU care and develop MOF. In general, MOF is due to secondary infection, bleeding, and thrombosis; although primary disruption of organ dysfunction can occur with the chronic lymphomas and leukemias.

Many patients with cancer undergo chemotherapy, with resultant neutropenia. It frequently translates into bacteremic episodes; should the neutropenia be prolonged, other organ dysfunction occurs with continued sepsis, and organ failure eventually develops. Furthermore, these patients frequently have invasive catheters in place and have a high propensity for colonization with resistant organisms from their frequent hospital visits and hospitalizations. Chemotherapeutic agents may also have severe deleterious effects on other organ systems (cardiac, pulmonary, liver, renal), which leads to more rapid organ failure.

Patients with human immunodeficiency virus (HIV) frequently develop opportunistic infections, especially with low CD-4 counts. Hospital admissions are infrequent, but for those who develop severe *Pneumocytis carinii* pneumonia and require mechanical ventilation, the outlook is poor.[65]

Conclusions

Development of organ failure results from the initial injury if it is sufficiently severe or from the host's response to the injury, graded according to the initial insult, followed by subsequent care. The host response varies depending on age, premorbid condition, medications, and genetic makeup. The more severe the response (measurable by physiologic derangements or immunologic changes and continuance of the response), the more likely is organ failure to develop, resulting in a correspondingly higher risk of mortality. The ability to alter the risk of subsequent organ failure is currently limited to "good and prompt" clinical care, as the newer, more expensive, more glamorous therapeutic interventions have fallen short.

There are a wide variety of nonsurgical settings in which MOF can develop, and the presence of multiple preexisting conditions may increase the likelihood of the development of organ failure and worsen chances for subsequent survival. Interventions to support one organ may be detrimental to other organs, and improvement in one organ system may lead to the improvement of other organ systems. Much of the current intensive care treatment is limited to organ support. As such, no matter what the initial insult, the host response is common in its manifestation. The only issues are the grade of severity and whether recovery and healing can occur. The main thrust of management is thus focused on prompt treatment of the initiating event while supporting other organ dysfunction to allow sufficient time for repair and recovery to occur. If this is not possible, organ failure develops with ensuing death.

Finally, there is much that remains unanswered about acute organ failure. Even beyond the need to better understand the pathophysiologic processes that both initiate and promulgate organ dysfunction, we must better characterize the relative contribution of the various risk factors to subsequent outcome. As new therapies are targeted at reversing organ dysfunction and not simply providing supportive care, the need to delineate the relative contributions of acute deterioration and preexisting damage to both the course of MOF and subsequent outcome are essential.

References

1. Bone RC: Immunologic dissonance: a continuing evolution in our understanding of the systemic inflammatory response syndrome (SIRS) and the multiple organ dysfunction syndrome (MODS). Ann Intern Med 1996;125:680–687.
2. Nathens AB, Marshall JC: Sepsis, SIRS, and MODS: what's in a name? World J Surg 1996;20:386–391.
3. Westendorp RG, Langermans JA, Huizinga TW, et al: Genetic influence on cytokine production in meningococcal disease. Lancet 1997;349:1912–1913.
4. Sorensen TI, Nielsen GG, Andersen PK, et al: Genetic and environmental influences on premature death in adult adoptees. N Engl J Med 1988;318:727–732.
5. ACCP/SCCM Consensus Conference Committee: American College of Chest Physicians/Society of Critical Care Medicine Consensus Conference: definitions for sepsis and organ failure and guidelines for the use of innovative therapies in sepsis. Crit Care Med 1992;20:864–874.
6. Vincent JL: Dear SIRS, I'm sorry to say that I don't like you. Crit Care Med 1997;25:372–374.
7. Bone RC, Grodzin CJ, Balk RA: Sepsis: a new hypothesis for pathogenesis of the disease process. Chest 1997;112:235–243.
8. Rangel-Frausto MS, Pittet D, Costigan M, et al: The natural history of the systemic inflammatory response syndrome (SIRS): a prospective study. JAMA 1995;273:117–123.
9. Pinsky MR, Vincent JL, Deviere J, et al: Serum cytokine levels in human septic shock: relation to multiple-system organ failure and mortality. Chest 1993;103:565–575.
10. Rosenbloom AJ, Pinsky MR, Bryant JL, et al: Leukocyte activation in the peripheral blood of patients with cirrhosis of the liver and SIRS: correlation with serum interleukin-6 levels and organ dysfunction. JAMA 1995;274:58–65.
11. Jimenez MF, Watson RW, Parodo J, et al: Dysregulated expression of neutrophil apoptosis in the systemic inflammatory response syndrome. Arch Surg 1997;132:1263–1269.
12. Kayal S, Jais JP, Aguini N, et al: Elevated circulating E-selectin, intercellular adhesion molecule 1, and von Willebrand factor in patients with severe infection. Am J Respir Crit Care Med 1998;157:T-84.
13. Cummings CJ, Sessler CN, Beall LD, et al: Soluble E-selectin levels in sepsis and critical illness: correlation with infection and hemodynamic dysfunction. Am J Respir Crit Care Med 1997;156:T-7.
14. Friedman G, Jankowski S, Shahla M, et al: Administration of an antibody to E-selectin in patients with septic shock. Crit Care Med 1996;24:229–233.
15. Knaus WA, Wagner DP: Multiple systems organ failure: epidemiology and prognosis. Crit Care Clin 1989;5:221–232.
16. Knaus WA, Sun X, Nystrom O, et al: Evaluation of definitions for sepsis. Chest 1992;101:1656–1662.
17. Vincent JL, De Mendonca A, Cantraine F, et al: Use of the SOFA score to assess the incidence of organ dysfunction/failure in

intensive care units: results of a multicenter, prospective study. Crit Care Med 1998;26:1793–1800.
18. Shoemaker WC, Montgomery ES, Kaplan E, et al: Physiologic patterns in surviving and nonsurviving shock patients: use of sequential cardiorespiratory variables in defining criteria for therapeutic goals and early warning of death. Arch Surg 1973;106:630–636.
19. Shoemaker WC, Appel PL, Kram HB, et al: Prospective trial of supranormal values of survivors as therapeutic goals in high-risk surgical patients. Chest 1988;94:1176–1186.
20. Hayes MA, Timmins AC, Yau EHS, et al: Elevation of systemic oxygen delivery in the treatment of critically ill patients. N Engl J Med 1994;330:1717–1722.
21. Gattinoni L, Brazzi L, Pelosi P, et al: A trial of goal-oriented hemodynamic therapy in critically ill patients. N Engl J Med 1995;333:1025–1032.
22. Yu M, Levy MM, Smith P, et al: Effect of maximizing oxygen delivery on morbidity and mortality rates in critically ill patients: a prospective, randomized, controlled study. Crit Care Med 1993;21:830–838.
23. Kirton OC, Windsor J, Wedderburn R, et al: Failure of splanchnic resuscitation in the acutely injured trauma patient correlates with multiple organ system failure and length of stay in the ICU. Chest 1998;113:1064–1069.
24. Duke TD, Butt W, South M: Predictors of mortality and multiple organ failure in children with sepsis. Intensive Care Med 1997;23:684–692.
25. Swank GM, Deitch EA: Role of the gut in multiple organ failure: bacterial translocation and permeability changes. World J Surg 1996;20:411–417.
26. Rombeau JL, Takala J: Summary of round table conference: gut dysfunction in critical illness. Intensive Care Med 1997;23:476–479.
27. Van Saene HK, Nunn AJ, Stoutenbeek CP: Selective decontamination of the digestive tract in intensive care patients. Br J Hosp Med 1995;54:558–561.
28. Vandenbroucke-Grauls CM, Vandenbroucke JP: Effect of selective decontamination of the digestive tract on respiratory tract infections and mortality in the intensive care unit. Lancet 1991;338:859–862.
29. Marshall JC, Christou NV, Meakins JL: The gastrointestinal tract: the "undrained abscess" of multiple organ failure. Ann Surg 1993;218:111–119.
30. Leu HS, Kaiser DL, Mori M, et al: Hospital-acquired pneumonia: attributable mortality and morbidity. Am J Epidemiol 1989;129:1258–1267.
31. Kollef MH: The prevention of ventilator-associated pneumonia. N Engl J Med 1999;340:627–634.
32. Pepe PE, Potkin RT, Reus DH, et al: Clinical predictors of the adult respiratory distress syndrome. Am J Surg 1982;144:124–130.
33. Montgomery AB, Stager MA, Carrico CJ, et al: Causes of mortality in patients with the adult respiratory distress syndrome. Am Rev Respir Dis 1985;132:485–489.
34. Bone RC, Balk R, Slotman G, et al: Adult respiratory distress syndrome: sequence and importance of development of multiple organ failure. Chest 1992;101:320–326.
35. Kolobow T, Moretti MP, Fumagalli R, et al: Severe impairment in lung function induced by high peak airway pressure during mechanical ventilation. Am Rev Respir Dis 1987;135:312–315.
36. Tremblay L, Valenza F, Ribeiro SP, et al: Injurious ventilatory strategies increase cytokines and c-fos m-RNA expression in an isolated rat lung model. J Clin Invest 1997;99:944–952.
37. Von Bethmann AN, Brasch F, Nusing R, et al: Hyperventilation induces release of cytokines from perfused mouse lung. Am J Respir Crit Care Med 1998;157:263–272.
38. Verbrugge SJ, Sorm V, van't Veen A, et al: Lung overinflation without positive end-expiratory pressure promotes bacteremia after experimental *Klebsiella pneumoniae* inoculation. Intensive Care Med 1998;24:172–177.
39. Dreyfuss D, Saumon G: From ventilator-induced lung injury to multiple organ dysfunction? Intensive Care Med 1998;24:102–104.
40. McQuillan P, Pilkington S, Allan A, et al: Confidential inquiry into quality of care before admission to intensive care. BMJ 1998;316:1853–1858.
41. Lundberg JS, Perl TM, Wiblin T, et al: Septic shock: an analysis of outcomes for patients with onset on hospital wards versus intensive care units. Crit Care Med 1998;26:1020–1024.
42. Reynolds HN, Haupt MT, Thill-Baharozian MC, et al: Impact of critical care physician staffing on patients with septic shock in a university hospital medical intensive care unit. JAMA 1988;260:3446–3450.
43. Leibovici L, Paul M, Poznanski O, et al: Monotherapy versus beta-lactam-aminoglycoside combination treatment for gram-negative bacteremia: a prospective, observational study. Antimicrob Agents Chemother 1997;41:1127–1133.
44. Lefering R, Neugebauer EA: Steroid controversy in sepsis and septic shock: a meta-analysis. Crit Care Med 1995;23:1294–1303.
45. Bollaert PE, Charpentier C, Levy B, et al: Reversal of late septic shock with supraphysiologic doses of hydrocortisone. Crit Care Med 1998;26:645–650.
46. McCloskey RV, Straube RC, Sanders C, et al: Treatment of septic shock with human monoclonal antibody HA-1A: a randomized, double-blind, placebo-controlled trial. Ann Intern Med 1994;121:1–5.
47. Natanson C, Esposito CJ, Banks SM: The sirens' songs of confirmatory sepsis trials: selection bias and sampling error. Crit Care Med 1998;26:1927–1931.
48. Inthorn D, Hoffmann JN, Hartl WH, et al: Effect of antithrombin III supplementation on inflammatory response in patients with severe sepsis. Shock 1998;10:90–96.
49. Bower RH, Cerra FB, Bershadsky B, et al: Early enteral administration of a formula (Impact) supplemented with arginine, nucleotides, and fish oil in intensive care unit patients: results of a multicenter, prospective, randomized, clinical trial. Crit Care Med 1995;23:436–449.
50. Atkinson S, Sieffert E, Bihari D: A prospective, randomized, double-blind, controlled clinical trial of enteral immunonutrition in the critically ill. Crit Care Med 1998;26:1164–1172.
51. Rodby RA: Hemofiltration for SIRS: bloodletting, twentieth century style? Crit Care Med 1998;26:1940–1942.
52. Bellomo R, Tipping P, Boyce N: Continuous veno-venous hemofiltration with dialysis removes cytokines from the circulation of septic patients. Crit Care Med 1993;21:522–526.
53. Kellum JA, Johnson JP, Kramer D, et al: Diffusive vs. convective therapy: effects on mediators of inflammation in patient with severe systemic inflammatory response syndrome. Crit Care Med 1998;26:1995–2000.
54. Heering P, Morgera S, Schmitz FJ, et al: Cytokine removal and cardiovascular hemodynamics in septic patients with continuous venovenous hemofiltration. Intensive Care Med 1997;23:288–296.

55. Schetz M, Ferdinande P, Van den Berghe G, et al: Removal of pro-inflammatory cytokines with renal replacement therapy: sense or nonsense? Intensive Care Med 1995;21:169–176.
56. Ackman ML, Harjee KS, Mansell G, et al: Cause-specific noncardiac mortality in patients with congestive heart failure—a contemporary Canadian audit. Can J Cardiol 1996;12:809–813.
57. Burnett CM, Duncan JM, Frazier OH, et al: Improved multiorgan function after prolonged univentricular support. Ann Thorac Surg 1993;55:65–71.
58. Karnik AM, Bashir R, Khan FA, et al: Renal involvement in the systemic inflammatory reaction syndrome. Ren Fail 1998;20:103–116.
59. Schwilk B, Wiedeck H, Stein B, et al: Epidemiology of acute renal failure and outcome of haemodiafiltration in intensive care. Intensive Care Med 1997;23:1204–1211.
60. Campillo B, Dupeyron C, Richardet JP, et al: Epidemiology of severe hospital-acquired infections in patients with liver cirrhosis: effect of long-term administration of norfloxacin. Clin Infect Dis 1998;26:1066–1070.
61. Fine MJ, Smith MA, Carson CA, et al: Prognosis and outcomes of patients with community-acquired pneumonia: a meta-analysis. JAMA 1996;275:134–141.
62. Seneff MG, Wagner DP, Wagner RP, et al: Hospital and 1-year survival of patients admitted to intensive care units with acute exacerbation of chronic obstructive pulmonary disease. JAMA 1995;274:1852–1857.
63. Daniels SK, Brailey K, Priestly DH, et al: Aspiration in patients with acute stroke. Arch Phys Med Rehabil 1998;79:14–19.
64. Solenski NJ, Haley ECJ, Kassell NF, et al: Medical complications of aneurysmal subarachnoid hemorrhage: a report of the multicenter, cooperative aneurysm study; participants of the Multicenter Cooperative Aneurysm Study. Crit Care Med 1995;23:1007–1017.
65. Rosen MJ, Clayton K, Schneider RF, et al: Intensive care of patients with HIV infection: utilization, critical illnesses, and outcomes; Pulmonary Complications of HIV Infection Study Group. Am J Respir Crit Care Med 1997;155:67–71.

6
Epidemiology, Risk Factors, and Outcome of Multiple Organ Dysfunction Syndrome in Surgical Patients

Philip S. Barie and Lynn J. Hydo

It has been recognized for several years that organ failure is the leading cause of death in surgical patients.[1] It is believed that most cases of multiple organ dysfunction syndrome (MODS) are precipitated by infection, but it is also recognized that the outcome of organ dysfunction does not correlate well with the microbiology of MODS.[2] The isolated organisms are often avirulent bacterial opportunists, colonizing and sometimes invading hosts who are susceptible owing to debility. Moreover, patients who die with MODS often have no demonstrable active infection on postmortem examination.[3] Indeed, some cases of organ dysfunction have been associated with histologic evidence of multiorgan inflammation in the absence of infection.[4] Therefore it is possible that MODS is precipitated by an insult that causes a massive inflammatory response (systemic inflammatory response syndrome, or SIRS) or a dysregulated balance of proinflammatory and compensatory antiinflammatory responses (CARS).[5]

Examples of initially sterile insults that can activate a systemic response include skeletal/soft tissue injury, ischemia/reperfusion injury, burns, pancreatitis, and gastric aspiration. Other cases are clearly precipitated by infection,[6,7] which in turn results in pro- and antiinflammatory responses. It has been argued that MODS deaths occur in a bimodal distribution in trauma patients,[8] with early deaths being less likely to be precipitated by infection or an endogenous source, such as bacterial translocation.[9] Whether trauma patients and other surgery patients develop MODS by a different mechanism or simply have a different precipitant is a matter of speculation, as is whether the distinction makes a difference in outcome.

The timing and magnitude of the insults may influence the expression of MODS. Some initial insults are so massive that MODS is precipitated as a direct result of the insult ("one-hit" model).[10] Examples of this type of injury include (1) multiple trauma with tissue injury and hemorrhagic shock and (2) embolic occlusion of the superficial femoral artery in a patient with paroxysmal atrial fibrillation, especially if resuscitation or surgical stabilization is delayed in either case for any reason. In contrast, the "two-hit" model involves sequential insults, with an initial "priming" insult followed by a second "activating" event, which may generate an accentuated response as a result.[10] It is believed that the "priming" response is related to activation of circulating and fixed-tissue mononuclear and polymorphonuclear phagocytes, which then respond secondarily in a temporally or magnitude-accentuated manner. This situation is difficult to describe clinically because of the heterogeneity of the response. Moreover, a major phenomenon of the "two-hit" model is purported to be activation of immune responses that have no macroscopic manifestations at the bedside. Furthermore, the sequential insults need not be similar, or they may even be both infectious and noninfectious, making the clinical scenarios almost limitless and the causality difficult to ascribe to any combination of insults. A femoral fracture in an elderly patient could be complicated by pneumonia. Initial nonoperative management of a grade III splenic laceration could be complicated by hypoxemia from a pulmonary contusion, or the strategy could fail, requiring an emergency splenectomy when hypotension develops. Even staged reconstructive procedures may provide the "second hit" stimulus.[11]

Most difficult to describe in clinical terms is a phenomenon that has been called the "sustained-hit" model of organ dysfunction.[12] Here, neither an initial insult of a magnitude sufficient to cause organ dysfunction nor a discrete secondary insult is identifiable. Rather, a process such as persistent gut ischemia might expose the liver to a constant barrage of gut-derived bacteria or mediators, leading to hepatic and then pulmonary dysfunction. Alternatively, a persistent focus of necrotic tissue in a case of necrotizing pancreatitis or microcirculatory disruption[13] in a case of lower extremity ischemia/reperfusion injury is a potential explanation.

Clinical Descriptors of Organ Dysfunction

There are several ways to describe organ dysfunction or failure clinically. The literature is replete with individual reports of the catastrophic failure of organs in patients who succumbed; but for the most part, those reports disappeared when blood banking and improved triage and transportation decreased the likelihood, in both military and civilian injured populations, of early death from unresuscitated shock.

During the Korean War acute renal failure became a major issue. Renal replacement therapy was rudimentary, as were techniques for arterial reconstruction. Fifteen years later the problems were acute respiratory distress syndrome (ARDS) and massive upper gastrointestinal (GI) bleeding.[14,15] During the 1970s several observers—Tilney et al.,[16] Baue,[17] Fry et al.,[18] and others—began to observe that many of these individual episodes of organ failure occurred, in individual patients and often appeared sequentially. Typically, pulmonary failure occurred earliest, most often followed by hepatic and renal failure, and if it occurred, upper GI hemorrhage. By the early 1980s improved nutritional support and prophylaxis with antacids and subsequently cimetidine or ranitidine had essentially eliminated stress-related gastric mucosal hemorrhage, but at the possible cost of an increased incidence of nosocomial pneumonia. Mortality was similar (or perhaps increased),[19] but the precipitant was different.

As the observations became more refined, it became apparent that none of the three features of the classic paradigm were necessarily true: That organ failure was an all-or-nothing phenomenon; that it is of late onset, and that it has a stereotypical, predictable sequence. Several descriptors of organ failure as an all-or-nothing phenomenon had been created,[18,20] but the paradigm was changing and the classic description became obsolescent. It is now recognized that not every organ fails in an affected patient, nor does the function of affected organs become equally deranged.[21] Dysfunction of an individual organ may be modest or may not occur at all.[22] Organ dysfunction may manifest much earlier during the hospital stay and may cause major morbidity in patients who are destined to survive.[22-26] Also, certain combinations of organ involvement may be especially deleterious, such as combined hepatic and pulmonary dysfunction.[27] These observations were followed by the development of several new descriptors of organ dysfunction[23,24,28,29] that recognize the new paradigm and changed the emphasis on various "organs" during the development of the syndrome. Diminished in emphasis was stress-related gastritis and increased were cardiovascular and neurologic failure, components that had been recognized for some time but had not previously been considered a part of MODS.

With the improved understanding of cell and molecular biology that led to the description of proinflammatory cytokines and their relation to derangements of the host response during the late 1980s and early 1990s, many attempts were made to relate biology to these clinical descriptors.[30-32] For example, an elevated interleukin-6 (IL-6) concentration has been associated with mortality in the presence of sepsis,[33] and tumor necrosis factor-α (TNFα) has been associated with outcome in septic burn patients.[34] The concentration of circulating (shed) TNF cell-surface receptors has been associated specifically with organ dysfunction.[35] However, the efforts in this area overall have been disappointing for several reasons. Many cytokines are difficult to measure in clinical specimens or may be present in tissue but evanescent in the circulation. Complex interactions among multiple pathways (kinins, complement, coagulation, eicosanoids) make the actions of individual mediators difficult to sort out, and sample sizes are often too small in published reports to overcome the recognized heterogeneity of individual patients for a specific response. Possibly the "correct" mediator has not yet been sought in the appropriate patient population or may not even have been described to date. It is also possible, given the increasing evidence that the development of MODS is an early phenomenon in critical illness, that the cytokine responses should be considered an outcome of the process, rather than an initiator.[24]

Moreover, the balance between pro- and antiinflammatory regulatory responses is only beginning to be described. The proinflammatory response has a clinical correlate [fever, tachycardia, tachypnea, leukocytosis or leukopenia) in SIRS. The antiinflammatory response is not easy to characterize clinically and is not well described in biologic terms. Certain cytokines (IL-4, IL-10, transforming growth factor-β, granulocyte colony-stimulating factor)[36,37] and some biologic responses (apoptosis, or programmed cell death)[38,39] have been associated with regulation of organ dysfunction. It is debated whether the balance of pro- and antiinflammatory responses is important in the pathogenesis of MODS.[5] It is possible that an ill-timed or inadequate antiinflammatory response activates or potentiates MODS by allowing an unopposed proinflammatory response, that an over-exuberant antiinflammatory response opposes the necessary proinflammatory attributes such as normal wound healing, or that the patient is predisposed to nosocomial infection. In such a scenario, oscillation between pro- and antiinflammatory predominance could be analogous to the "sustained hit" theory, but these mechanisms are speculative and impossible to describe clinically at the bedside with current technology.

What can be described clinically are the manifestations of SIRS and MODS, the latter by several descriptors. These various clinical descriptors have seldom been compared,[40,41] so it is not possible at the present time to say that one is "better" for predicting a defined outcome (classically, mortality). In terms of the description of mortality, the use of a graded quantitative system appears to be similar to that of an all-or-nothing system. However, patients who die with moderate degrees of organ dysfunction tend to have high grade dysfunction of a few organs rather than low grade dysfunction of many organs.[40]

Studies of MODS in a Tertiary Care Surgical Intensive Care Unit

A multiyear observation of the epidemiology of MODS has been undertaken in the surgical intensive care unit (ICU) of New York—Presbyterian Hospital–Cornell Medical Center using the scoring system of Marshall et al.[23] The system was originally developed in surgical patients after a logistic regression model was developed from likely important descriptors derived from a literature review. A randomized split-halves validation was performed on the data set, which was collected during 1988–1990 from 693 critically ill patients. Six "organs" [cardiovascular, central nervous system (CNS), coagulation, hepatic,

TABLE 6.1. Demographics of 938 Consecutive Surgical ICU Patients With Multiple Organ Dysfunction Syndrome.

Parameter	All patients	Survivors	Non survivors
Age (years)	66 ± 1	66 ± 1	70 ± 1*
APACHE III score	60 ± 1	52 ± 1	94 ± 1*
ICU stay (days)	10 ± 1	8 ± 1	17 ± 1*
Cumulative MOD Score	7 ± 1	5 ± 1	13 ± 1*
No. of Affected organs	3 ± 1	3 ± 1	5 ± 1*

APACHE, Acute Physiology and Chronic Health Evaluation.
*$p < 0.05$.

pulmonary, renal] have been evaluated in a quantitative or semiquantitative (CNS) manner, and each "organ" was awarded 0–4 points, for a total of 24 points. Use of a 24-point scoring system means that even an increase in serum creatinine to 1.8 mg/dL for a single day registers, making the system sensitive for use in elective surgical patient populations and for surrogate endpoints, such as length of stay.[25,26] Points can be awarded on a cumulative basis (e.g., a patient develops severe acute lung injury and is awarded 4 points but recovers; the pulmonary score would remain at 4 points for the duration of the hospitalization). The score can also be calculated on a daily basis (the score would decrease as the patient recovers) or on the basis of the change during the ICU stay, so-called Δ MODS.[23] Appreciable mortality can be observed when the cumulative score is >4 points. Higher scores correlate with mortality and prolonged length of stay in the ICU for patients who survive.[26] A larger Δ MODS also correlates with increased mortality in some studies.[23]

The demographics of the Cornell patient cohort are shown in Table 6.1. Approximately 54% of the patients developed some degree of MODS during their ICU stay. Among the patients who developed MODS, the mean age was 66 years, and the mean Acute Physiology and Chronic Health Evaluation (APACHE III) score was 60 points. Two-thirds of the patients who developed MODS has been admitted to the ICU emergently. Ten percent of the patients had sustained multiple injuries. The risk factors for the development of MODS are shown in Fig. 6.1. Hypoperfusion/ischemia without shock was most common, although sepsis without shock and shock regardless of etiology were well represented. Most patients who developed any degree of MODS did so to a modest degree (Fig. 6.2); 45% of affected patients scored only 1–4 points and had approximately 2% mortality (Fig. 6.3). The patients who were affected modestly were largely those with hypoperfusion without shock and those with miscellaneous causes (Fig. 6.1). Only 28% of affected patients (15% of the overall ICU patient population) developed major organ dysfunction (>8 points, where mortality is 30% or more). These patients tended to have shock, although severe MODS was as likely as mild manifestations in trauma patients or those with pancreatitis (Fig. 6.1). Only about 13% of patients with MODS (7% of the patients as a whole) developed it to such a degree (>12 points) that mortality was 70% or more but these patients accounted for most of the mortality (8% overall for the hospitalization) in the group. Compared with patients who did not develop any degree of organ dysfunction, those with MODS had a 20-fold increased risk of mortality (20% vs. 1%) and more than double the length of the ICU stay (Table 6.1).

The development of MODS correlates closely with the severity of illness on admission by both APACHE II and APACHE III, although the correlation is stronger with the latter (Fig. 6.3, Table 6.1). Although the MOD score and APACHE

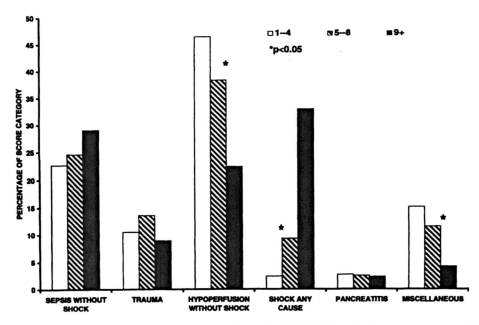

FIGURE 6.1. Risk factors and severity of organ dysfunction in 938 patients with MODS. A predominant cause was ascribed even in cases where multiple risk factors were present, so there is no duplication of cases. Shock was defined as cases in which vasopressor therapy was used.

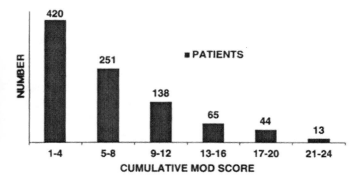

FIGURE 6.2. Distribution of cumulative organ dysfunction scores in the 938 patients with MODS. About 45% of the patients developed only minimal dysfunction.

III are not completely independent variables (some of the same data are used to calculate both scores), a close correlation might not be expected if the classic late-onset paradigm were to hold. It might be expected that the severity of illness on admission would have progressively less relevance to later events as the ICU stay lengthens. However, given that there appears to be relevance, one can postulate that the development of MODS may be regulated by events that occur within the first several hours of the illness (e.g., adequacy of initial resuscitation; see below).

The frequency of organ involvement and the magnitude of organ dysfunction are shown in Fig. 6.4. The incidence of each score is depicted for each of the six systems. Thus hepatic dysfunction was least likely to develop (nearly 60% of patients with MODS had no meaningful increase in serum bilirubin concentration), whereas cardiovascular and pulmonary dysfunction were equally likely to develop (only 38% of patients avoided either). Severe dysfunction (3 or 4 points) was more likely with cardiovascular, CNS, and pulmonary dysfunction. The overall incidence of any degree of dysfunction is shown in Fig. 6.5, where it can be seen that along with cardiovascular and pulmonary dysfunction renal dysfunction is relatively common. Despite this finding, the mortality rates for affected organs are

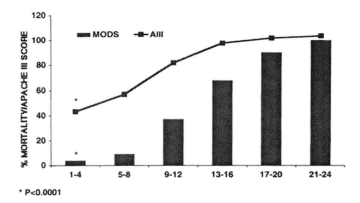

* $P<0.0001$

FIGURE 6.3. Relation between severity of illness on admission (APACHE III) and the subsequent development of organ dysfunction. The statistical analysis is significant across all ranges of MOD scores.

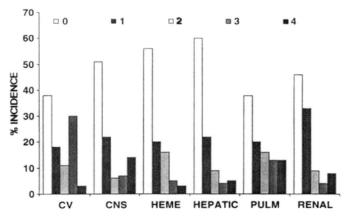

FIGURE 6.4. Distribution of scores (0–4) is depicted for each organ. The incidence of hepatic dysfunction is lowest because the incidence of "0 points" is highest. Conversely, pulmonary and cardiovascular (CV) dysfunction were equally common.

similar. Each of the six organ systems has an independent effect on mortality by multivariate analysis, even when bivariate correlations (e.g., hepatic and coagulation dysfunction) are included in the model because of their inherent relatedness. In fact, CNS dysfunction (encephalopathy leading to stupor or coma) is the most powerful independent predictor of mortality in these patients. The reason for the importance of neurologic dysfunction, as related to outcome, is shown in Fig. 6.6. The difference in MOD scores between survivors and non-survivors was greatest for those with neurologic dysfunction (0.7 ± 0.1 vs. 3.0 ± 1.1 points), which is also reflected in the observation that the difference in mortality rates for patients who score 3 versus 4 points is also highest for neurologic failure. The differences in organ-specific scores between survivors and nonsurvivors were identical for pulmonary and cardiovascular dysfunction (1.1 ± 0.1 vs. 2.6 ± 0.1 points).

Although each of the components of the MOD score has an independent predictive effect on mortality, the effect in aggregate is even more powerful. The receiver operator characteristic (ROC) curve, and example of which is shown in Fig. 6.7,[42] is a method used to assess the sensitivity and specificity of a

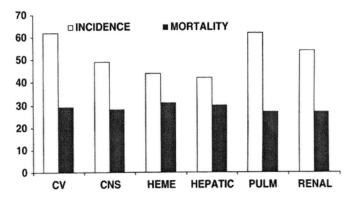

FIGURE 6.5. Although the incidence of organ dysfunction varied, mortality rates for affected patients were similar.

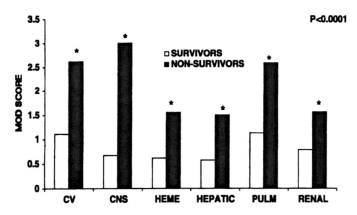

FIGURE 6.6. Difference in scores between survivors and nonsurvivors was greatest for patients with central nervous system (CNS) dysfunction, which is the most powerful independent predictor of mortality by multivariate analysis.

continuous variable for predicting a dichotomous outcome (e.g., mortality). The area under the ROC curve is a measure of system discrimination. An area under the ROC curve of 0.50 represents a chance event, whereas a value of 1.00 indicates perfect calibration. In the Cornell database, the area under the ROC curve is 0.89 for APACHE III versus mortality, indicating that only approximately 10% of the variance in mortality is unexplained by the severity of illness on admission. In contrast, the area under the ROC curve for the MOD score versus mortality in our data set is 0.95, reflecting nearly perfect discrimination. The area under the ROC curve reported by Marshall et al. was 0.93.[23]

The MODS also correlates with ICU length of stay and thus has an important relation to resource utilization.[26,43] The use of surrogate endpoints, such as length of stay or the duration of mechanical ventilation, is problematic because it can be influenced by practitioner preference. More to the point is that critically ill or injured patients sometimes die shortly after admission to an ICU despite maximal support. In such patients the correlation between length of stay and objective measures of severity could be inverse. Therefore the relations between organ dysfunction and ICU length of stay were investigated in survivors,[26] and were found to be highly significant. In the analysis, MODS was the predominant predictor of increased length of stay in the ICU. Because fewer than 5% of patients admitted to surgical ICUs have a truly prolonged stay (>21 days),[43,44] we determined whether significant relations exist between the development of MODS and ICU length of stay even in good-risk patients destined for short stays for postoperative monitoring. This relation exists for both the incidence of MODS (Fig. 6.8) and the magnitude of its expression (Fig. 6.9). Given that short ICU stays are determined by MODS even in good-risk patients, it was hypothesized that events early in the ICU stay were defining the likelihood of developing MODS. To test this hypothesis we examined the relation between SIRS and MODS.[25]

Systemic Inflammatory Response Syndrome

The systemic inflammatory response syndrome (SIRS) has come to represent the clinical manifestations of the proinflammatory host response. As such, it can be stimulated by noninfectious causes or by infection. In the absence of another cause (e.g., recent chemotherapy), SIRS is defined as the presence of at least two of four variables: temperature above or below the range of 36–38°C; white blood cell count above or below the range of 4×10^9 to 12×10^9/L; heart rate > 90 beats/min; respiratory rate > 20 breaths/min (spontaneously) or $PaCO_2$ < 32 mmHg (ventilated). The definition is arbitrary and was reached by consensus without a process of validation.[45] Conceptually, it has been derided as being too sensitive and insufficiently

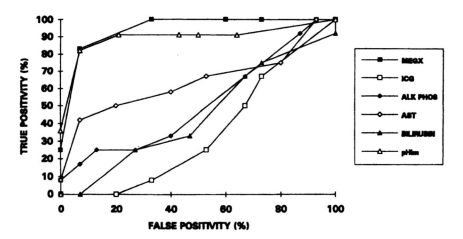

FIGURE 6.7. Receiver-operator characteristic curve of several parameters for the prediction of mortality in 27 critically ill patients with splanchnic ischemia and hepatic dysfunction. Metabolism of lidocaine given as a metabolic indicator (MEGX) and gastric intramucosal pH (pHim) were comparable and effective discriminators of mortality. Indocyanine green clearance (ICG), bilirubin, and hepatic enzymes did not discriminate survivors from nonsurvivors. (From Maynard et al.,[42] with permission.)

6. Epidemiology, Risk Factors, and Outcome of Multiple Organ Dysfunction Syndrome in Surgical Patients

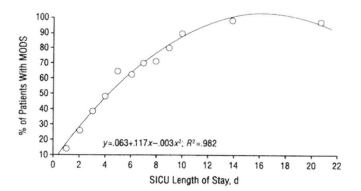

FIGURE 6.8. As the length of stay in the surgical ICU (SICU) increases, so does the incidence of MODS, even for good-risk patients who stay in the ICU for a brief time. (From Talmor et al.,[25] with permission.)

specific.[46,47] For example, many patients with uncomplicated appendicitis present with SIRS. Biologic correlates of quantitated SIRS (i.e., a score of 2–4 points, with 1 point for the presence of each variable) are few.[39,45,48] Opinion is divided as to the usefulness of quantification of SIRS in surgical patients.[23,45,47,49] Of particular concern, other than excessive sensitivity, is that SIRS may be mimicked by certain events that are commonplace during the immediate postoperative period. Aside from activation of proinflammatory cascades, patients may be, for example, tachycardic due to hypovolemia or pain, or they may be tachypneic or hypocarbic due to inappropriate ventilator settings. Waiting for this "pseudo-SIRS" to subside may take several hours after admission to the ICU; by the next day it should have subsided if it is not caused by an underlying physiologic derangement.

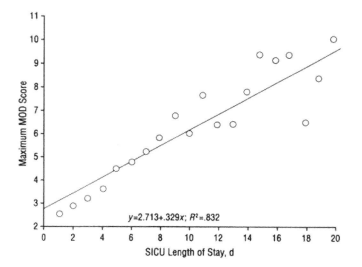

FIGURE 6.9. Mean cumulative MOD scores are depicted as a function of length of stay in the surgical ICU. The relation is especially close for stays in the ICU of 10 days or less. (From Talmor et al.,[25] with permission.)

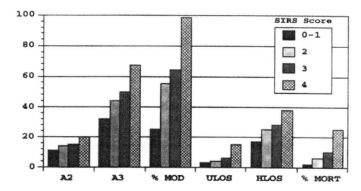

FIGURE 6.10. Increased admission severity of illness (A2, APACHE II; A3, APACHE III) correlated with a higher SIRS score, which in turn was associated with a longer length of stay in the ICU (ULOS) and hospital (HLOS). Mortality was increased in patients with a higher number of SIRS components as well. Each relation is statistically significant at each point ($p < 0.05$).

In our patient population of 2300 subjects, SIRS occurred at some point in 57% of patients,[25] but the distribution of point values among patients with SIRS was identical (18–20% incidence for each group with 2, 3, or 4 points scored). The magnitude of SIRS, without regard to its timing, was related to severity of illness at admission (Fig. 6.10), the incidence of MODS, and its magnitude (Fig. 6.11). Moreover, the magnitude of SIRS was associated with the length of stay in the ICU and the duration of hospitalization, as well as with mortality over an approximate 20-fold range. It was surprising that there was a difference in the magnitude of MODS among patients who did not have SIRS (i.e., no component versus a single positive component). This difference was detectable in terms of admission APACHE scores, length of stay, the incidence of organ dysfunction, and mortality (Table 6.2). The impact of even a single SIRS component being positive is reminiscent of studies that demonstrate how deleterious even brief periods of

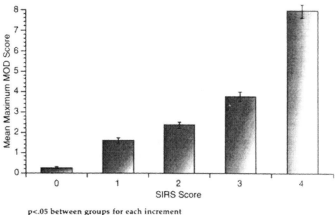

FIGURE 6.11. There is a highly significant ($p < 0.0001$) relation between an increasing SIRS score and the subsequent magnitude of MODS. The patient population is the same as depicted in Fig. 6.10.

TABLE 6.2. Demographics and Outcomes in 958 Patients Without SIRS.

Parameter	SIRS score = 0 (n = 604)	SIRS score = 1 (n = 354)
APACHE III score	24 ± 1	37 ± 1*
ICU length of stay (days)	1.7 ± 0.2	2.8 ± 0.1*
Incidence of MOD (%)	17	40*
Cumulative MOD score	0.2 ± 0.1	1.5 ± 0.2*
Mortality (%)	1.1	2.8*

*$p < 0.05$.

tachycardia can be,[50] although no single component had an independent effect on any outcome.

To evaluate the response of SIRS to being in the ICU under care for the first 24 hours, a study was conducted to focus on the absolute magnitude of the SIRS response on day 2 of the ICU stay compared to that on day 1.[25] Eliminating from consideration those patients who had only an overnight stay before being transferred out of the unit the next morning and who were not evaluated as a consequence, the mean SIRS score decreased 0.8 points regardless of the type of admission (Fig. 6.12). Among those patients who responded to ICU care with a decreased SIRS score on day 2, the hospital mortality rate was only 6% (Fig. 6.13). If there was no change in the SIRS score from day 1 to day 2, the mortality rate increased to 15%. However, if the patient deteriorated by the second day, the mortality rate increased to approximately 20%. Examination of the characteristics of the magnitude of the SIRS score on day 2 is even more revealing (Table 6.3). As the SIRS score increased, so did the APACHE II score from the previous day, the magnitude of MODS, and the mortality rate. Notable is the fact that such an arbitrary and simple score can describe a 10-fold difference in mortality (3.8% vs. 40.0%) as early as the second day in the surgical ICU. Thus although quantitation of SIRS is inappropriate for prognostication in individual patients or small groups,

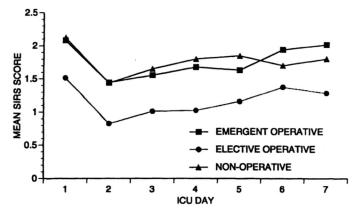

FIGURE 6.12. Regardless of the type of admission, the response of the SIRS score to therapy in the ICU was identical. The mean SIRS score decreased 0.8 points, suggesting that resolution of the proinflammatory response is quantifiable following resuscitation. (From Talmor et al.,[25] with permission.)

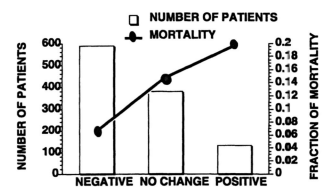

FIGURE 6.13. If the SIRS score declined from the first to the second day, the mortality rate was significantly lower ($p < 0.05$) than if there was no improvement. If the SIRS score increased from day 1 to day 2, mortality was higher still ($p < 0.05$). This analysis excludes patients who were discharged on the morning of the second day.

TABLE 6.3. Characteristics Associated with Day 2 SIRS Scores.

SIRS score	APACHE III score*	ICU length of stay*	MOD score*	%Mortality*
0	48 ± 2	4 ± 1	3.6 ± 0.2	3.8
1	52 ± 2	7 ± 1	4.5 ± 1.2	8.2
2	60 ± 2	11 ± 1	7.0 ± 0.3	18.4
3	58 ± 2	13 ± 1	7.5 ± 0.5	31.2
4	79 ± 5	10 ± 1	8.5 ± 0.6	40.0

*$p < 0.05$.

studies with adequate statistical power indicate clearly that SIRS is a conceptually valid and appropriate way in which to consider the pathogenesis of MODS. Just as some have described organ "dysfunction" as a continuum of severity that culminates as organ "failure" (an arbitrary distinction, to be sure), so too may SIRS lead to MODS. However, the magnitude of organ dysfunction was higher in non-survivors beginning on day 1 and continuing throughout the ICU stay (Fig. 6.14). The data suggest either that the timeline of the SIRS–MODS continuum

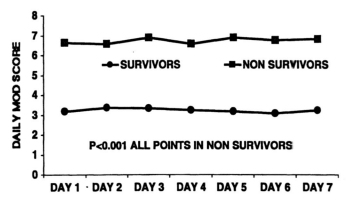

FIGURE 6.14. Magnitude of MODS is higher in nonsurvivors from the first day in the ICU, which belies the notion that MODS is a late-onset phenomenon.

is short, or that the window for successful intervention and resuscitation to prevent or reverse incipient organ dysfunction is narrow and occurs early during critical illness.

Problems and Prospects for MODS Definitions and Risk Factors

Current quantitative concepts of MODS lend themselves well to the description of mortality. One would be hard-pressed to improve on a ROC curve area of 0.95 for predicting mortality by MODS quantitation. Nonetheless, before prognostication by any system can be accepted unquestioningly, some potential users might demand infallibility. An infallible system may be an impossible goal, but it cannot be said that opportunities for improvement should therefore not be sought. The accurate description of MODS depends on the quality of the definitions of its components. Definitions of organ dysfunction are changing constantly, and some concepts (e.g., GI failure) may become unfashionable. Other definitions may be inadequate (e.g., failure of the CNS). Examination of some of the issues related to dysfunction of individual organs and individual risk factors may be enlightening.

Cardiovascular Failure

Cardiovascular failure, defined by Marshall et al.[23] as a product of heart rate and the difference between central venous pressure and arterial blood pressure, is central to the pathogenesis of dysfunction of other individual organs and to the syndrome as a whole. This definition was created to negate the effects of age- or medication-related changes in heart rate and the effects of inotrope or vasopressor therapy when calculating the score. Unrelated to "heart failure" in the classic sense of fluid overload due to congestive heart failure, it is myocardial dysfunction and hypoperfusion that are central to the pathogenesis of MODS.[51] Ischemia with or without reperfusion injury—especially with neutrophil–endothelial cell interactions, endothelial dysfunction, intravascular coagulation, and microvascular flow disruption characteristic of reperfusion injury—are postulated to lead to dysfunction of virtually every organ, including the brain, lungs, stomach, intestine, kidneys, liver, and the heart itself. The injury may be directly to the organ or a response to an anatomically remote insult.

The heart is affected by many toxins, including lipopolysaccharides, TNFα, and reactive oxygen and nitrogen species. Ventricular dilatation occurs as myocardial contractility is impaired[52] even in the absence of irreversible myocyte injury. Given the pathogenesis, some measure of myocardial contractility may be a better indicator of cardiac dysfunction. It is unclear how best to monitor myocardial performance or whether the adequacy of resuscitation or regional indicators of perfusion such as gastric mucosal tonometry are acceptable surrogates. Options for assessing myocardial performance include conventional pulmonary artery catheters, volumetric right heart catheters that assess right ventricular end-diastolic volume, and echocardiography.[53] There is controversy about the many indicators of the adequacy of resuscitation and no certain best option. There is no indicator of cellular oxygenation that can be relied on clinically. An estimator of splanchnic perfusion (gastric mucosal tonometry), despite showing promise in some studies,[54,55] has not been embraced widely because it is cumbersome and subject to error; and confirmatory large-scale multicenter trials have yet to be reported despite the availability of the technology for more than a decade. New techniques using air (gas tonometry) rather than saline to capture CO_2 rather than diffusing H^+ ions may hold promise for increasing the accuracy and ease of use, but the data are scant.

Some investigators, notably Shoemaker's group,[56] championed the concept of a tissue oxygen debt accumulating during hypoperfusion and suggested that prompt "repayment" (during resuscitation) to arbitrary supranormal levels of oxygen delivery with supplemental oxygen and inotrope therapy could ameliorate organ dysfunction and improve survival. This suggestion appeared despite a countervailing belief that excess oxygen introduced to a hypoperfused vascular bed might worsen reperfusion injury by increasing the substrate available for the generation of reactive oxygen species. However, the clinical studies that purported to show a benefit from the strategy generally used as an endpoint oxygen consumption values that were calculated, rather than measured by indirect calorimetry or another method.[57–59] This introduced a bias due to shared measurement error because the two variables—oxygen delivery and consumption—are not independent.[60] Studies in which oxygen consumption was measured failed to show benefit, and the failure of two multicenter trials[61,62] should commit this notion to its final resting place.

Inotrope therapy may not be inherently harmful for the patient when it is used carefully and not at the expense of adequate resuscitation, but a major trial of dobutamine therapy guided by gastric mucosal tonometry showed benefit only in patients who did not have mucosal acidosis,[54] which is counter to expectations. Norepinephrine, perceived to be a more potent vasoconstrictor than dopamine, had been avoided for many years except as "last-ditch" therapy in moribund patients because the vasoconstrictor effect of norepinephrine was postulated to increase the risk of organ failure in general and renal failure in particular. However, data now indicate that mortality may be decreased in patients with septic shock when norepinephrine is used, rather than dopamine.[63] Our evaluation of the use of norepinephrine as the vasopressor of first choice in shock states indicated that mortality was not excessive compared to predicted mortality, and that in patients who succumbed with organ dysfunction the dysfunction was present when vasopressor therapy was started.[64] Moreover, there was no evidence that norepinephrine worsened organ dysfunction once therapy began (Fig. 6.15). Mortality was concentrated in the group of patients with refractory shock who required vasopressor therapy for a week or more.[64]

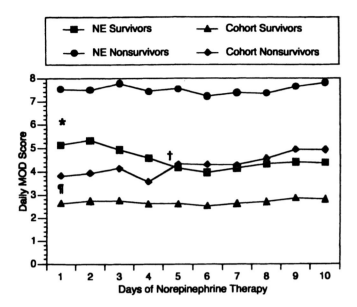

FIGURE 6.15. Norepinephrine (NE) nonsurvivors were admitted to the ICU with more baseline organ dysfunction than NE survivors ($p < 0.0001$). The survivors had an improvement in their organ dysfunction by day 5 ($p < 0.05$). The cohort consisted of comparably severely ill patients who did not have shock and did not require NE therapy. (From Goncalves et al.,[64] with permission.)

Central Nervous System Dysfunction

Neurologic dysfunction poses several major issues and may be better terminology than "CNS dysfunction." It is critical to resolve these issues because neurologic dysfunction is the most powerful predictor of mortality in surgical patients when it is described using the Glasgow Coma Scale (GCS).[65] This predictive power persists even when the possible effects of coexistent renal or hepatic dysfunction are taken into consideration. That neurologic dysfunction is such a powerful predictor of mortality is telling and suggests that evaluation of the neurologic status should have increased importance in the care of critically ill surgical patients. The potential causes of encephalopathy in critically ill surgical patients are many, including disease- and therapy-related causes. Disease-related causes include sepsis (most commonly), subarachnoid hemorrhage or stroke, traumatic brain injury, postoperative edema in neurosurgical patients, liver disease, kidney disease, and ketoacidosis. Therapy-related causes relate largely to pharmacotherapy effects (prolonged emergence from anesthesia, therapeutic sedation) on specific factors, such as air microembolization during cardiopulmonary bypass. Various factors may interact in individual patients (e.g., diabetic ketoacidosis induced by infection, benzodiazepine sedation in a patient with liver disease or traumatic brain injury), which makes it difficult to quantify risk. Moreover, there is disagreement as to the pathogenesis of encephalopathy during sepsis[66] (e.g., hypoperfusion versus microembolization versus cerebral edema caused by a local astroglial cytokine response).[67]

Neurologic dysfunction is usually quantitated using the GCS, which awards points based on the pupillary examination and verbal and motor responses to interrogation (a GCS of 15 represents an intact examination; 3 is the lowest score possible). This definition, although arbitrary, is widely accepted, so it is essentially unknown whether a better system exists or could be developed. Several other coexisting factors can confound calculation of the GCS, including ethanol ingestion (common in the trauma patient), endotracheal intubation (making the verbal responses impossible to quantify), and the issue of emergence from general anesthesia. Quantitation of dysfunction of all other organ systems is based on the worst degree of dysfunction manifested by the patient, and the diagnostic criteria are more objective. Notwithstanding the variation inherent in test methodology, there is usually little disagreement, for example, as to a patient's platelet count on a given day. If neurologic dysfunction were to be quantitated similarly (i.e., using the worst examination of the day in an intubated, sedated patient or one who was emerging from anesthesia or an alcoholic stupor), the degree of dysfunction would likely be overestimated. To eliminate that potential bias we have given patients the "benefit of the doubt" and scored their neurologic dysfunction based on their best neurologic function of the day, rather than their worst. Marshall concurs with this approach (J.C. Marshall, personal communication, 1997). It is a possible that a different bias (i.e., an underestimate) is introduced as a result, but it is certain that neurologic dysfunction remains the most powerful predictor of mortality in surgical patients despite the deliberate minimization of the scores in our patients.

Despite the strong association between encephalopathy and mortality, it is likely that there are other neurologic manifestations of MODS; moreover, it is possible that if they were sought out and quantitated, neurologic dysfunction would be even better described. Candidate neurologic manifestations of MODS include "critical illness polyneuropathy"[66] and changes in autonomic tone manifested by loss of normal sinus heart rate variability.[68–70] These manifestations may be similar in that both involve disruption of neuromuscular signaling and may be analogous to the disrupted cell signaling and intercellular communication that has been described for hepatocytes and Kupffer cells in the pathogenesis of hepatic dysfunction due to sepsis.[71]

Critical illness polyneuropathy has attracted attention for only a few years, although its manifestations have been ever present. Debility, muscle weakness, and atrophy are commonplace but seldom quantitated; they have been variously ascribed to aminoglycoside therapy, prolonged bed rest, electrolyte abnormalities, malnutrition, muscle deconditioning from disuse/lack of exercise, and prolonged neuromuscular blockade. Critical illness polyneuropathy is recognized as a probable peripheral lesion with axonal degeneration that can be diagnosed with nerve conduction studies or electromyography. It is possible that axonal degeneration results from a lack of efferent impulses occasioned by failure of cell–cell interactions during interneuronal or neuromuscular signaling. Although it has been associated prospectively with the development of multiple organ failure,[72] it has yet to be accounted for in quantitative descriptions of the syndrome.

Equally relevant to the possibility of deranged cell–cell signaling and perhaps more important as a potential prognostic tool is the observation that critically ill patients lose their normal sinus heart rate variability. The sinus rate becomes more regular because of cholinergic predominance and relative loss of sympathetic tone. Studies in head-injured patients[68] and general surgical ICU patient populations[69] have shown that decreased heart rate variability and cholinergic predominance are associated with increased mortality. Moreover, the same phenomenon has been documented in normal volunteers who were given a standardized dose of lipopolysaccharide,[70] suggesting an applicability to many clinically relevant manifestations of critical surgical illness. It is unlikely that β-adrenergic blockade can be invoked as an explanation of the increased mortality, given that perioperative β-blockade reduces mortality in surgical patients.[73] It is speculative as to whether this will prove to be a critical manifestation of neurologic dysfunction or if this type of monitoring will be employed widely.

Coagulation System Dysfunction

Failure of the coagulation system is quantitated by the use of the platelet count in the scheme of Marshall et al.[23] This approach has several limitations. Thrombocytopenia is often related to transient bone marrow depression in sepsis but may also be an adverse drug reaction to any of several pharmaceutical agents in active use in critical care units, including H_2-receptor antagonists and β-lactam antibiotics. Platelet function may be abnormal in several circumstances, including therapy with nonselective cyclooxygenase inhibitors or in patients with renal failure, such that the platelet count becomes irrelevant. Use of the platelet count also fails to consider the major role hepatic dysfunction or vitamin K deficiency can play in the coagulation system. Nonetheless, the strong associations between sepsis and organ dysfunction and between sepsis and thrombocytopenia make the platelet count a reasonable estimate of coagulation function, and its use will likely persist unless an equally simple alternative can be identified.

One such possible alternative is the whole-blood D-dimer assay,[74] which is not to be confused with the D-dimer assay performed on serum as part of an evaluation for disseminated intravascular coagulation. The whole-blood assay is qualitative (positive/negative), so if a quantitative result is reported the "wrong" D-dimer assay has been performed. The test is useful in that it has high specificity; if it is negative, the suspicion of venous thromboembolism is diminished.[74] The test may be too sensitive in surgical patients, as it appears possible that surgical bleeding and hemostasis may be sufficient to make the test falsely positive. Nonetheless, use of the whole-blood assay as a screening test upon ICU admission did define a group of patients with increased mortality when the test was positive.[75]

Gastrointestinal Dysfunction

Omitted from consideration in the quantitation system of Marshall et al., GI tract failure was defined historically as an upper GI hemorrhage that required transfusion of ≥ units of blood.[18] GI tract failure manifested during the 1960s and 1970s as a result of incremental improvements in resuscitation from shock. Battlefield casualties no longer succumbed immediately from shock but, rather, survived to sustain complications such as stress-related gastric mucosal injury, or "stress gastritis," which is known to be a manifestation of splanchnic ischemia/reperfusion injury.[76] Vietnam-era military surgical reports are replete with descriptions of massive GI hemorrhage that required subtotal or total gastrectomy for control or resulted in death. Reports in the civilian literature from trauma and neurosurgical units (Cushing's ulcer) and burn units (Curling's ulcer) paralleled the military experience, but few if any data exist from that era that would be helpful for quantifying risk.

A decreased incidence of GI dysfunction in burn patients was associated with aggressive nutritional support during the mid-1970s. Landmark studies around that time demonstrated that antacid prophylaxis could decrease the incidence of bleeding.[77] The introduction shortly thereafter of parenteral H_2-antagonist therapy decreased the incidence further to such a degree that stress gastritis was considered eradicated by some authors.[78] The problem is compounded by endoscopic studies demonstrating that severe gastritis occurs in patients who do not bleed from it,[77] making it difficult to quantify even if the extreme step of performing esophagastroduodenoscopy in all patients at risk is undertaken. Is it correct to exclude gastritis from MODS quantitation schemes because it is unusual and difficult to describe?

Gastritis has not been eradicated in high risk patients, but who should receive prophylaxis and how? A multicenter prospective study of high risk patients demonstrates that patients with coagulopathy or those who are on mechanical ventilation for 48 hours or more are at sufficiently high risk to justify prophylaxis against gastritis.[79] Without either characteristic present, the risk of bleeding was only 0.2%, whereas it was 3.7% if either was present. Prophylaxis reduced the risk of bleeding in high risk patients by 50%.

The choice of drug for prophylaxis has been controversial. Acid-reduction strategies (antacids, H_2-antagonists) are effective; but so is sucralfate, which has a minimal effect on gastric pH and requires the presence of acid to polymerize and form a protective barrier. A study reported in 1987 purported to show an increased incidence of nosocomial pneumonia and increased mortality among patients who were treated prophylactically with an acid-reduction strategy.[80] It was hypothesized that overgrowth of gram-negative bacterial pathogens could occur in the low-acid environment, ready to gain access to the lower respiratory tract should aspiration occur. Numerous follow-up studies were conducted, and discordant meta-analyses were reported. The discrepancy has now been resolved,[81] hopefully in a definitive manner. There is no difference in the incidence of overt bleeding comparing antacids, H_2-antagonists, and sucralfate; nor is there any difference in the incidence of pneumonia. Mortality is lower in patients treated with sucralfate than in those treated with antacids but not when compared to patients given H_2-antagonists.

Other GI manifestations may merit consideration as part of MODS, including small intestinal or colonic ileus, intolerance to enteral feedings (e.g., lack of absorption, diarrhea), or acute acalculous cholecystitis (AAC), which may be increasing in incidence. The pathogenesis of AAC is a paradigm of complexity.[82] Bile stasis, opioid therapy, positive-pressure ventilation, and total parenteral nutrition have been implicated; but ischemia/reperfusion injury and the effects of eicosanoid proinflammatory mediators appears to be the central mechanisms. Ultrasonography of the gallbladder is the most accurate diagnostic modality in the critically ill patient; a gallbladder wall thickness of 3.5 mm or more and pericholecystic fluid are the two most reliable criteria. The mainstay of therapy for AAC has been cholecystectomy, but percutaneous cholecystostomy is gaining acceptance as an alternative to open procedures. The technique controls AAC in about 85% of patients. Rapid improvement should be expected when the procedure is performed properly. The mortality rates associated with percutaneous and open cholecystostomy appear to be similar (both about 30%), reflective of the critically ill population afflicted by AAC.

Hepatic Dysfunction

Hepatic dysfunction is defined by Marshall et al. according to the serum bilirubin concentration,[23] even though a large redundant capacity for bilirubin metabolism means that substantial hepatic injury can occur before the patient becomes icteric. Bilirubin is a waste product of heme metabolism. The substrate for up to 80% of total bilirubin production is hemoglobin of senescent red blood cells. Daily bilirubin production averages 4 mg/kg/day. Transport of bilirubin conjugates from the hepatocyte to the canaliculus for excretion involves an active, saturable, carrier-mediated process that is susceptible to age, hypoxemia, infection, and medications. Total serum bilirubin is less than 1 mg/dL in 95% of adults. Jaundice becomes visible when the serum bilirubin concentration approaches 3 mg/dL. Only conjugated bilirubins are excreted by the kidney (and cleared by hemodialysis). Bilirubinuria is common when the plasma level of esterified ("direct") bilirubin exceeds 2–4 mg/dL. Renal elimination is the predominant route of excretion and largely determines the plasma concentration of bilirubin in patients with severe cholestasis. Hemodialysis can lower the plasma bilirubin level substantially even with severe jaundice.

With the exception of active liver transplant units that manage fulminant hepatic failure (most commonly due to viral hepatitis or drug toxicity) in patients on the transplant list, most jaundice in critically ill surgical patients is reflective of cholestasis. Most clinical cases in the ICU are caused by hepatocyte dysfunction rather than extrahepatic biliary obstruction. Bile flow is an osmotically driven process initiated in large part by active secretion of solutes (primarily bile acids) into the canaliculus. Obstruction to flow can occur at presinusoidal or sinusoidal levels, intracellular sites, the canaliculus, or at the level of the large ducts. Hemodynamic changes can induce cholestasis but not within physiologic limits. The leading causes of hepatocyte dysfunction in the surgical ICU are sepsis, ischemia/reperfusion injury, an overwhelming presentation of heme substrate (e.g., massive transfusion, resorption of a large hematoma), and total parenteral nutrition. Several drugs can cause cholestasis on an ischemic basis, including antiarrhythmic drugs, chlorpromazine, and adrenergic agents.

In experimental animals, portal venous blood flow is increased at an early stage (within 2 hours) in the presence of hyperdynamic sepsis.[83] Hepatocyte dysfunction develops as early as 1.5 hours after the onset of sepsis and persists into the hypodynamic phase; adequate resuscitation does not correct the abnormality. The dysfunction appears to be mediated by the proinflammatory cytokine response (especially TNFα and IL-1). Hepatic oxygen uptake is deranged with sepsis, but the derangements occur after the onset of hepatocellular dysfunction. Hepatic ATP is preserved for up to 10 hours after cecal ligation and puncture (CLP), declining only during the hypodynamic phase. Hypertransaminemia is detectable 10–20 hours after CLP, with the hypodynamic circulation characteristic of late sepsis appearing consistently 20 hours after CLP. Hepatic mitochondrial function is preserved for as long as 18 hours.

In contrast to acute viral hepatitis, where the degree of hyperbilirubinemia does not correlate with outcome, mortality is related to the degree of cholestasis in critical surgical illness. Use of the serum bilirubin concentration to quantitate MODS may therefore be reasonable, but it is certainly insensitive, and there may be more accurate indicators. One such circulating indicator may prove to be Gc-globulin, a vitamin D-binding protein that also is an actin scavenger.[84] Actin is involved in the regulation of hepatic perfusion via the contractile Ito cells that regulate sinusoidal blood flow. Decreased concentrations of Gc-globulin have been correlated with multiple organ failure in humans.[85]

A better approach might be to perform a simple functional test at the bedside. Monoethylglycinexylidide (MEGX) is a easily measured lidocaine metabolite that has been used as an indicator of hepatic metabolism in a prospective study of 27 critically ill patients.[43] There were no differences in bilirubin, aspartate aminotransferase, alkaline phosphatase, or prothrombin concentrations between survivors and nonsurvivors, or in the indocyanine green clearance. On day 3 the median MEGX level was higher in survivors than in nonsurvivors (16 vs. 2.4 ng/mL; $p < 0.001$), and the median MEGX level in nonsurvivors decreased over the 3 days (from 20.6 to 2.4 ng/mL, $p < 0.002$). The MEGX concentration correlated well with gastric intramucosal pH and had comparable discrimination with regard to mortality based on ROC curve analysis (Fig. 6.7). Serum bilirubin predicted outcome no better than chance, but only 63% of those studied were surgical patients.

Pulmonary Dysfunction

The incidence of ARDS varies depending on the risk factors involved but ranges from 1.5 to 5.3 cases/100,000 population per year.[85] Many conditions have been associated with ARDS in surgical patients, some of which are direct insults to the pulmonary parenchyma; others include the pulmonary response to a systemic insult. The risk of developing ARDS from a discrete insult is difficult to define.

Garber et al.[85] undertook a systematic literature overview to evaluate the risk factors associated with ARDS. In the articles they reviewed a definition of ARDS was given in only 49%, and a definition of the potential risk factor was provided in only 64% of reports. Twenty-three percent of published papers provided a definition of neither ARDS nor risk factors. It is difficult to draw inferences from such pervasively poor descriptions of large clinical series. Despite this point, the strongest evidence supporting a cause-effect relation between ARDS and individual risk factors was identified for sepsis, major trauma, multiple transfusions, aspiration of gastric contents, pulmonary contusion, pneumonia, and smoke inhalation. Substantially weaker evidence exists for an association between ARDS and disseminated intravascular coagulation, fat embolism, and cardiopulmonary bypass. Virtually all of the analyzed studies failed to report a relative risk (odds ratio) and, further, failed to control for confounding variables. In a recent review[86] the high risk criteria noted above accounted for almost 80% of ARDS cases. Sepsis appears to be the most prevalent risk factor, accounting for 30-40% of all ARDS cases.[87-89] Conversely, the risk of patients with sepsis developing ARDS has been variably reported between 10% and 25%.[90-92]

Use of the PaO_2/FiO_2 (P/F) ratio to quantify organ dysfunction, according to Marshall et al.,[23] is easy and reasonable, given that the ratio is stable across a wide range of FiO_2 and is not affected by the degree of ventilation/perfusion mismatching. The P/F ratio has been correlated with mortality in prior studies. The problem here, aside from the generally poor quality of the reports, is that improvements in resuscitation and ventilator management may finally be yielding a decrease in mortality due to ARDS.[89] If that is the case historic comparisons may no longer be of value, and the best way to quantitate acute lung injury may need redefinition. Several specific lung injury/ARDS scores exist,[93] but they have not increased diagnostic precision or improved prognostication.

Renal Dysfunction

Acute renal failure is quantitated by the serum creatinine concentration,[23] even though serum creatinine correlates poorly with symptoms of uremia. Creatinine clearance is influenced by many factors, including body mass and the availability of creatine substrate. For example, frail elderly patients, especially women, may have a laboratory picture compatible with prerenal azotemia (high blood urea nitrogen, disproportionately low creatinine) when in fact they are in renal failure and simply do not have the muscle mass to generate creatine. Nonetheless, the serum creatinine assay is objective and does represent a functional assessment, so the criticism is a minor one.

Acute renal failure in surgical patients is usually multifactorial and can be of many etiologies; most of the lesions are either toxic or ischemic to renal tubular cells. Sepsis causes an injury that is both ischemic and toxic, with the ischemia being mediated by TNFα-induced activation of the renin-angiotensin-aldosterone axis and disruption of resting vasomotor tone mediated by eicosanoids. Aminoglycoside injury is primarily due to direct toxicity, but it also has an ischemic component. Pigment-induced injury (myoglobin) can be seen with ischemia/reperfusion injury or crush injury; the toxicity is mediated by ferrihemate production, which also generates reactive oxygen species. Radiocontrast-induced injury remains fairly common; despite the availability of nonionic contrast media, the injury is not prevented by their use. With all potential insults, the likelihood of renal failure is increased when it is superimposed on an already abnormal kidney, although this is best quantitated in patients with diabetic nephropathy.

Regardless of the serum creatinine level, mortality appears to be lower when renal failure is nonoliguric (urine output >400 mL/day in an average-size adult). Electrolyte management may be easier, and there is more flexibility with respect to nutritional support; but both of these putative advantages become moot once renal replacement therapy is undertaken. Moreover, the major causes of death in patients with acute renal failure are no longer fluid overload or critical acid-base or electrolyte abnormalities but, rather, the underlying problem (e.g., sepsis, shock) that caused renal dysfunction. Thus the reports that renal replacement therapy may reduce the mortality of acute renal failure are curious and difficult to interpret.[94,95] Perhaps the improved technology is reducing the frequency of episodes of hemodialysis-associated hemodynamic instability; or some toxin is removed from the circulation by more efficient, more biocompatible membranes.[96,97]

Our data showed that the mortality rate was higher (Fig. 6.6) for patients with a three-point renal score than for those with maximal dysfunction. Despite the inherent objectivity of the use of the serum creatinine concentration, the observation is unique among the assessed organs for two reasons. First, effective renal replacement therapy is available. Second, the data reflect a population of patients with end-stage renal disease. Patients on maintenance hemodialysis have high renal scores even if their admission to the ICU is elective (e.g., monitoring after a peripheral vascular reconstruction). Organ dysfunction scoring systems not distinguish between acute and chronic derangements; perhaps methodology should be developed to address this issue.

Is the Mortality of MODS Decreasing?

Considering that reports indicate that the mortality of ARDS[89] and acute renal failure[94,95] may be decreasing, it is plausible that the mortality associated with MODS is decreasing as well, as these organ failures seldom occur in isolation.[98] Some reports

TABLE 6.4. Comparison of ICU Outcomes for Patients with MODS.

Parameter	Cornell data set	Marshall et al.[23]	p
Subjects (no.)	938	693	
Years of data collection	1992–1995	1988–1990	
Mean APACHE II score	17.9	13.4	
ICU Mortality (%)	12.5	9.4	
Patients with >10 MODS points (%)	19	13	
Hospital mortality (%)			
1–4 Points	3	7	<0.01
5–8 Points	8	16	<0.05
9–12 Points	36	51	<0.05
13–16 Points	67	68	NS
17–20 Points	91	82	NS
21–24 Points	100	100	NS

suggest that the mortality rate associated with ARDS[98] and nosocomial pneumonia[99] is lower in trauma/surgical patients than in medical patients. The incidence of renal failure and ARDS is believed by some to be decreasing as well.[100] It remains difficult to compare heterogeneous populations, and a decrease in mortality may be difficult to discern without correcting for severity of illness, considering that ICU patients are increasingly older and sicker. When comparing the Cornell data set with that of Marshall et al.[23] (Table 6.4), it can be seen that the mortality rate was lower in the Marshall series, but that the Cornell patients were more severely ill and had a higher likelihood of developing severe MODS. Outcomes were significantly better for mild-to-moderately afflicted patients in the Cornell experience, but outcomes were comparable for the severely affected patients. Not only may case mix and severity of illness affect outcomes, but outcomes may be affected by policies for resource utilization, advance directives, and other factors. Large-scale longitudinal studies of outcome may prove that the mortality associated with MODS is decreasing, but few such studies have been reported.[101]

References

1. Carrico CJ, Meakins JL, Marshall JC, et al: Multiple-organ-failure syndrome. Arch Surg 1986;121:196–208.
2. Marshall JC, Christou NV, Horn R, Meakins JL: The microbiology of multiple organ failure: the proximal gastrointestinal tract as an occult reservoir of pathogens. Arch Surg 1988;123:309–315.
3. Sinanan M, Maier RV, Carrico CJ: Laparotomy for intra-abdominal sepsis in patients in an intensive care unit. Arch Surg 1984;119:652–658.
4. Goris RJ, te Boekhorst TP, Nuytinck JK, Gimbrere JS: Multiple-organ failure: generalized autodestructive inflammation? Arch Surg 1985;120:1109–1115.
5. Bone RC: Immunologic dissonance: a continuing evolution in our understanding of the systemic inflammatory response syndrome (SIRS) and the multiple organ dysfunction syndrome (MODS). Ann Intern Med 1996;125:680–687.
6. Kollef MH, Sharpless L, Vlasnik J, et al: The impact of nosocomial infections on patient outcomes following cardiac surgery. Chest 1997;112:666–675.
7. Barie PS, Hydo LJ, Fischer E: Development of multiple organ dysfunction syndrome in critically ill patients with perforated viscus: predictive value of APACHE severity scoring. Arch Surg 1996;131:37–43.
8. Moore FA, Sauaia A, Moore EE, et al: Postinjury multiple organ failure: a bimodal phenomenon. J Trauma 1996;40:501–510.
9. Lemaire LC, van Lanschot JJ, Stoutenbeek CP, et al: Bacterial translocation in multiple organ failure: cause of epiphenomenon still unproven? Br J Surg 1997;84:1340–1350.
10. Moore FA, Moore EE: Evolving concepts in the pathogenesis of postinjury multiple organ failure. Surg Clin North Am 1995;75:257–277.
11. Waydhas C, Nast-Kolb D, Trupka A, et al: Posttraumatic inflammatory response, secondary operations, and late multiple organ failure. J Trauma 1996;40:624–630.
12. Yao YM, Redl H, Bahrami S, Schlag G: The inflammatory basis of trauma/shock-associated multiple organ failure. Inflamm Res 1998;47:201–210.
13. Kirkpatrick CJ, Bittinger F, Klein CL, et al: The role of the microcirculation in multiple organ dysfunction syndrome (MODS); a review and perspective. Virchows Arch 1996;427:461–476.
14. Petty TL: Acute respiratory distress syndrome (ARDS). Dis Mon 1990;36:1–58.
15. Hinchey EJ, Hreno A, Benoit PR, et al: The stress ulcer syndrome. Adv Surg 1970;4:325–392.
16. Tilney NL, Bailey GL, Morgan AP: Sequential system failure after rupture of abdominal aortic aneurysms: an unsolved problem in postoperative care. Ann Surg 1973;78:117–122.
17. Baue AE: Multiple, progressive, or sequential systems failure: a syndrome of the 1970s. Arch Surg 1975;110:779–781.
18. Fry DE, Pearlstein L, Fulton RL, Polk HC Jr: Multiple system organ failure: the role of uncontrolled infection. Arch Surg 1980;115:136–140.
19. Craven DE, Daschner FD: Nosocomial pneumonia in the intubated patient: role of gastric colonization. Eur J Clin Microbiol Infect Dis 1989;8:40–50.
20. Knaus WA, Draper EA, Wagner DP, Zimmerman JE: Prognosis in acute organ-system failure. Ann Surg 1985;202:685–693.
21. Bone RC, Balk RA, Cerra FB, et al: Definitions for sepsis and organ failure and guidelines for the use of innovative therapies in sepsis: the ACCP/SCCM consensus conference committee: American College of Chest Physicians/Society of Critical Care Medicine. Chest 1992;101:1644–1655.
22. Bone RC, Balk R, Slotman G, et al: Adult respiratory distress syndrome: sequence and importance of development of multiple organ failure; the Prostaglandin E_1 Study Group. Chest 1992;101:320–326.
23. Marshall JC, Cook DJ, Christou NV, et al: Multiple organ dysfunction score: a reliable descriptor of a complex clinical outcome. Crit Care Med 1995;23:1638–1652.
24. Cryer HG, Leong K, McArthur DL, et al: Multiple organ failure: by the time you predict it, it's already there. J Trauma 1999;46:597–604.
25. Talmor M, Hydo L, Barie PS: Relationship of systemic inflammatory response syndrome (SIRS) to organ dysfunction, length of stay, and mortality in critical surgical illness: effect of intensive care unit resuscitation. Arch Surg 1999;134:81–87.
26. Barie PS, Hydo LJ: Influence of multiple organ dysfunction syndrome on duration of critical illness and hospitalization. Arch Surg 1996;131:1318–1325.

27. Schwartz DB, Bone RC, Balk RA, Szidon JP: Hepatic dysfunction in the adult respiratory distress syndrome. Chest 1989;95: 871–875.
28. Vincent JL, de Mendonca A, Cantraine F, et al: Use of the SOFA score to assess the incidence of organ dysfunction/failure in intensive care units: results of a multicenter, prospective study; working group on "sepsis-related problems" of the European Society of Intensive Care Medicine. Crit Care Med 1998;26: 1793–1800.
29. Le Gall JR, Klar J, Lemeshow S, et al: The logistic organ dysfunction system: a new way to assess organ dysfunction in the intensive care unit; ICU Scoring Group. JAMA 1996;276: 802–810.
30. Rogy MA, Oldenburg HS, Coyle S, et al: Correlation between Acute Physiology and Chronic Health Evaluation (APACHE) III score and immunological parameters in critically ill patients with sepsis. Br J Surg 1996;83:396–400.
31. Law MM, Cryer HG, Abraham E: Elevated levels of ICAM-1 correlate with the development of multiple organ failure in trauma patients. J Trauma 1994;37:100–110.
32. Roumen RM, Redl H, Schlag G, et al: Inflammatory mediators in relation to the development of multiple organ failure in patients after severe blunt trauma. Crit Care Med 1995;23: 474–480.
33. Patel RT, Deen KI, Youngs D, et al: Interleukin 6 is a prognostic indicator of outcome in severe intra-abdominal sepsis. Br J Surg 1994;81:1306–1308.
34. Marano M, Fong Y, Moldawer L, et al: Serum cachectin/TNF in cricitally ill burn patients correlates with infection and mortality. Surg Gynecol Obstet 1990;170:32–38.
35. Calvano SE, Coyle SM, Barbosa KS, et al: Multivariate analysis of nine disease-associated variables for outcome prediction in patients with sepsis. Arch Surg 1998;133:1347–1350.
36. Neidhardt R, Keel M, Steckholzer U, et al: Relationship of interleukin-10 plasma levels to severity of injury and clinical outcome in injured patients. J Trauma 1997;42:863–870.
37. Simms HH, D'Amico R: Granulocyte colony-stimulating factor reverses septic shock-induced polymorphonuclear leukocyte dysfunction. Surgery 1994;115:85–93.
38. Cobb JP, Hotchkiss RS, Karl IE, Buchman TG: Mechanisms of cell injury and death. Br J Anaesth 1996;77:3–10.
39. Fanning NF, Kell MR, Shorten GD, et al: Circulating granulocyte macrophage colony stimulating factor in plasma of patients with the systemic inflammatory response syndrome delays neutrophil apoptosis through inhibition of spontaneous reactive species generation. Shock 1999;11:167–174.
40. Barie PS, Hydo L, Fischer E: A prospective comparison of two different multiple organ failure/dysfunction scoring systems for prediction of mortality in critical surgical illness. J Trauma 1994;37:660–666.
41. Bertleff MJ, Bruining HA: How should multiple organ dysfunction syndrome be assessed? A review of the variations in current scoring systems. Eur J Surg 1997;163:405–409.
42. Maynard ND, Bihari DJ, Dalton RN, et al: Liver function and splanchnic ischemia in critically ill patients. Chest 1997;111:180–187.
43. Barie PS, Hydo LJ, Fischer E: Utility of illness severity scoring for prediction of prolonged surgical critical care. J Trauma 1996;40:513–519.
44. Buchman TG, Kubos KL, Seidler AJ, Siegforth MJ: A comparison of statistical and connectionist models for the prediction of chronicity in a surgical intensive care unit. Crit Care Med 1994;22:750–762.
45. Muckart DJ, Bhagwanjee S: American College of Chest Physicians/Society of Critical Care Medicine consensus conference definitions of the systemic inflammatory response syndrome and allied disorders in relation to critically injured patients. Crit Care Med 1997;25:1789–1795.
46. Vincent JL: Dear SIRS, I'm sorry to say that I don't like you.... Crit Care Med 1997;25:372–374.
47. Pittet D, Rangel-Frausto S, Li N, et al: Systemic inflammatory response syndrome, sepsis, severe sepsis and septic shock: incidence, morbidities and outcomes in surgical ICU patients. Intensive Care Med 1995;21:302–309.
48. Jimenez MF, Watson RW, Parodo J, et al: Dysregulated expression of neutrophil apoptosis in the systemic inflammatory response syndrome. Arch Surg 1997;132:1263–1269.
49. Haga Y, Beppu T, Doi K, et al: Systemic inflammatory response syndrome and organ dysfunction following gastrointestinal surgery. Crit Care Med 1997;25:1994–2000.
50. Mangano DT, Hollenberg M, Fegert G, et al: Perioperative myocardial ischemia in patients undergoing noncardiac surgery. I. Incidence and severity during the 4 day perioperative period: the Study of Perioperative Ischemia (SPI) research group. J Am Coll Cardiol 1991;17:843–850.
51. Bush HL, Hydo LJ, Fischer E, et al: Hypothermia during elective abdominal aortic aneurysm repair: the high price of avoidable morbidity. J Vasc Surg 1995;21:392–402.
52. Ungureanu-Longrois D, Balligand JL, Kelly RA, Smith TW: Myocardial contractile dysfunction in the systemic inflammatory response syndrome: role of a cytokine-inducible nitric oxide synthase in cardiac myocytes. J Mol Cell Cardiol 1995;27:155–167.
53. Barie PS: Advances in critical care monitoring. Arch Surg 1997;132:734–739.
54. Gutierrez G, Palizas F, Doglio G, et al: Gastric intramucosal pH as a therapeutic index of tissue oxygenation in critically ill patients. Lancet 1992;339:195–199.
55. Ivatury RR, Simon RJ, Havriliak D, et al: Gastric mucosal pH and oxygen delivery and oxygen consumption indices in the assessment of adequacy of resuscitation after trauma: a prospective, randomized study. J Trauma 1995;39:128–134.
56. Bishop MH, Shoemaker WC, Appel PL, et al: Prospective, randomized trial of survivor values of cardiac index, oxygen delivery, and oxygen consumption as resuscitation endpoints in severe trauma. J Trauma 1995;38:780–787.
57. Cryer HG, Richardson JD, Longmire-Cook S, et al: Oxygen delivery in patients with ARDS who undergo surgery: correlation with multiple-system organ failure. Arch Surg 1989;124: 1378–1385.
58. Moore FA, Haenel JB, Moore EE, et al: Incommensurate oxygen consumption in response to maximal oxygen availability predicts postinjury multiple organ failure. J Trauma 1992;33:1–9.
59. Dantzker DR, Foresman B, Gutierrez G: Oxygen supply and utilization relationships: a reevaluation. Am Rev Respir Dis 1991;143:675–679.
60. Stratton HH, Feustel PJ, Newell JC: Regression of calculated variables in the presence of shared measurement error. J Appl Physiol 1987;62:2083–2093.
61. Gattinoni L, Brazzi L, Pelosi P, et al: A trial of goal-oriented hemodynamic therapy in critically ill patients: SvO_2 Collaborative Group. N Engl J Med 1995;333:1025–1032.

62. Alia I, Esteban A, Gordo F, et al: A randomized and controlled trial of the effect of treatment aimed at maximizing oxygen delivery in patients with severe sepsis or septic shock. Chest 1999;115:453–461.
63. Martin C, Papazian L, Perrin G, et al: Norepinephrine or dopamine for the treatment of hyperdynamic septic shock? Chest 1993;103:1826–1831.
64. Goncalves JG Jr, Hydo LJ, Barie PS: Factors influencing outcome of prolonged norepinephrine therapy for shock in critical surgical illness. Shock 1998;10:231–236.
65. Barie PS, Hydo LJ, Fischer E: Development of multiple organ dysfunction syndrome in critically ill patients with perforated viscus: predictive value of APACHE severity scoring. Arch Surg 1996;131:37–43.
66. Nauwynck M, Huyghens L: Neurological complications in critically ill patients; septic encephalopathy, critical illness polyneuropathy. Acta Clin Belg 1998;53:92–97.
67. Sharif SF, Hariri RJ, Chang VA, et al: Human astrocyte production of tumour necrosis factor-α, interleukin-1β and interleukin-6 following exposure to lipopolysaccharide endotoxin. Neurol Res 1993;15:109–112.
68. Winchell RJ, Hoyt DB: Analysis of heart-rate variability: a noninvasive predictor of death and poor outcome in patients with severe head injury. J Trauma 1997;43:927–933.
69. Winchell RJ, Hoyt DB: Spectral analysis of heart rate variability in the ICU: a measure of autonomic function. J Surg Res 1996;63:11–16.
70. Godin PJ, Fleisher LA, Eidsath A, et al: Experimental human endotoxemia increases cardiac regularity: results from a prospective, randomized, crossover trial. Crit Care Med 1996;24:1117–1124.
71. Godin PJ, Buchman TG: Uncoupling of biological oscillators: a complementary hypothesis concerning the pathogenesis of multiple organ dysfunction syndrome. Crit Care Med 1996;24:1107–1116.
72. Leijten FS, Harinck-de Weerd JE, Poortvliet DC, de Weerd AW: The role of polyneuropathy in motor convalescence after prolonged mechanical ventilation. JAMA 1995;274:1221–1225.
73. Mangano DT, Layug EL, Wallace A, Tateo I: Effect of atenolol on mortality and cariovascular morbidity after noncardiac surgery: multicenter study of Perioperative Ischemia Research Group. N Engl J Med 1996;335:1713–1720.
74. Ginsberg JS, Wells PS, Kearon C, et al: Sensitivity and specificity of a rapid whole-blood assay for D-dimer in the diagnosis of pulmonary embolism. Ann Intern Med 1998;129:1006–1011.
75. Kollef MH, Eisenberg PR, Shannon W: A rapid assay for the detection of circulating D-dimer is associated with clinical outcomes among critically ill patients. Crit Care Med 1998;26:1054–1060.
76. Wallace JL: Lipid mediators of inflammation in gastric ulcer. Am J Physiol 1990;258:G1–G11.
77. Marrone GC, Silen W: Pathogenesis, diagnosis and treatment of acute gastric mucosal lesions. Clin Gastroenterol 1984;13:635–650.
78. Reines HD: Do we need stress ulcer prophylaxis? Crit Care Med 1990;18:344.
79. Cook DJ, Fuller HD, Guyatt GH, et al: Risk factors for gastrointestinal bleeding in critically ill patients: Canadian Critical Care Trials Group. N Engl J Med 1994;330:377–381.
80. Driks MR, Craven DE, Celli BR, et al: Nosocomial pneumonia in intubated patients given sucralfate as compared with antacids or histamine type 2 blockers: the role of gastric colonization. N Engl J Med 1987;317:1376–1382.
81. Cook DJ, Reeve BK, Guyatt GH, et al: Stress ulcer prophylaxis in critically ill patients: resolving discordant meta-analyses. JAMA 1996;275:308–314.
82. Barie PS, Fischer E, Eachempati SR: Acute acalculous cholecystitis. Curr Opin Crit Care 1999;5:144–150.
83. Wang P, Chaudry IH: Mechanism of hepatocellular dysfunction during hyperdynamic sepsis. Am J Physiol 1996;270:R927–R938.
84. Schiodt FV, Ott P, Bondesen S, et al: Reduced serum Gc-globulin concentrations in patients with fulminant hepatic failure: association with multiple organ failure. Crit Care Med 1997;25:1366–1370.
85. Garber BG, Hebert PC, Yelle JD, et al: Adult respiratory distress syndrome: a systematic overview of incidence and risk factors. Crit Care Med 1996;24:687–695.
86. Sessler CN, Bloomfield GL, Fowler AA: Current concepts of sepsis and acute lung injury. Clin Chest Med 1996;17:213–235.
87. Moss M, Goodman PL, Heining M, et al: Establishing the relative accuracy of three new definitions of the adult respiratory distress syndrome. Crit Care Med 1995;23:1629–1637.
88. Hudson LD, Milberg JA, Anardi D, et al: Clinical risks for development of the acute respiratory distress syndrome. Am J Respir Crit Care Med 1995;151:293–302.
89. Milberg JA, Davis DR, Steinberg KP, et al: Improved survival of patients with acute respiratory distress syndrome (ARDS): 1983–1993. JAMA 1995;273:306–309.
90. Rangel-Frausto M, Pittet D, Costigan M, et al: The natural history of the systemic inflammatory response syndrome (SIRS): a prospective study. JAMA 1995;273:117–123.
91. Perl TM, Dvorak L, Hwang T, et al: Long-term survival and function after suspected gram-negative sepsis. JAMA 1995;274:338–345.
92. Fisher CJ, Dhainaut JA, Opal SM, et al: Recombinant human interleukin-1 receptor antagonist in the treatment of patients with sepsis syndrome: results from a randomized, double-blind, placebo-controlled trial. JAMA 1994;271:1836–1843.
93. Moss M, Goodman PL, Heinig M, et al: Establishing the relative accuracy of three new definitions of the adult respiratory distress syndrome. Crit Care Med 1995;23:1629–1637.
94. Hakim RM, Wingard RL, Parker RA: Effect of the dialysis membrane in the treatment of patients with acute renal failure. N Engl J Med 1994;331:1338–1342.
95. Schiffl H, Lang SM, Konig A, et al: Biocompatible membranes in acute renal failure: prospective case-controlled study. Lancet 1994;344:570–572.
96. Tani T, Hanasawa K, Endo Y, et al: Therapeutic apheresis for septic patients with organ dysfunction: hemoperfusion using a polymyxin B immobilized column. Artif Organs 1998;22:1038–1044.
97. Koperna T, Vogl SE, Poschl GP, et al: Cytokine patterns in patients who undergo hemofiltration for treatment of multiple organ failure. World J Surg 1998;22:443–447.
98. Ferring M, Vincent JL: Is outcome from ARDS related to the severity of respiratory failure? Eur Respir J 1997;10:1297–1300.
99. Heyland DK, Cook DJ, Griffith L, et al: The attributable morbidity and mortality of ventilator-associated pneumonia in the critically ill patient. Am J Respir Crit Care Med 1999;159:1249–1256.

100. Baue AE, Durham R, Faist E: Systemic inflammatory response syndrome (SIRS), multiple organ dysfunction syndrome (MODS), multiple organ failure (MOF): are we winning the battle? Shock 1998;10:79–89.

101. Zimmerman JE, Knaus WA, Wagner DP, et al: A comparison of risks and outcomes for patients with organ system failure: 1982–1990. Crit Care Med 1996;24:1633–1641.

Part II
Mechanisms of SIRS and Organ Failure

7
Systemic Inflammation After Trauma, Infection, and Cardiopulmonary Bypass: Is Autodestruction a Necessary Evil?

E.E. de Bel and R.J.A. Goris

To survive in nature all animals, including humans, need an efficient defense system to overcome minor trauma and common infections. It had been observed as early as ancient times that limited damage to some part of the body can lead to the collapse of vital organ systems, remote from the original site of impact. Fever and prostration were thought to be caused by "toxins" developing within the wounds. Since the discovery of their pathogenic potential, bacteria seemed to be always present in these cases, suggesting that infection is the decisive factor prohibiting recovery. When effective antimicrobial agents became available, it was originally expected that "killing the bugs" would put an end to disease in serious infections. It was soon experienced, however, that the initial physiologic derangement caused by trauma or infection may progress and kill the host, even when at autopsy no remaining infectious focus can be demonstrated.[1]

During World War II resuscitation of the wounded by transfusing blood and plasma to normalize systolic blood pressure resulted in improved survival. However, the result all to often was renal insufficiency ("shock kidney"). More aggressive fluid resuscitation during the Vietnam war resulted in the prevention of renal failure, but now patients surviving the acute shock phase developed pulmonary edema ("Danang lung"). At first this new problem was attributed to a too generous fluid resuscitation regimen; later this acute respiratory distress syndrome (ARDS) was found to be a consequence of an untoward pulmonary response to shock and nonpulmonary injuries.[2]

Improvements in the initial resuscitation and subsequent management of critically ill patients during the 1970s decreased the incidence of early death from cardiovascular or respiratory failure in patients suffering from trauma, hemorrhage, pancreatitis, or severe infection. Expanding technologic possibilities (e.g., prolonged mechanical ventilation) provided the necessary conditions for the development of new modes of treatment, such as aortocoronary grafting, using the cardiopulmonary bypass technique.

Still, many patients with trauma or sepsis were found to develop progressive neurologic, pulmonary, renal, hepatic, and gastrointestinal dysfunction, even when all infective foci appeared to be eliminated and a normal or even supranormal delivery of oxygen to the tissues had been achieved. The absence of differences in the pattern of organ failure between patients with trauma and abdominal infection led to the hypothesis that the essential cause of multiple organ failure (MOF) might not be infection. Instead, an alternative hypothesis was presented involving massive activation of inflammatory cells, producing mediators resulting in damage to vascular endothelia, permeability edema, and impaired oxygen utilization.[3]

During the 1990s it has become accepted that MOF is the result of a systemic, excessive, self-destructive response to a variety of severe insults, including severe infections, trauma, and pancreatitis. The clinical signs of incipient whole-body inflammation were given the name systemic inflammatory response syndrome (SIRS).[4] In patients with severe trauma (without infection) or peritonitis, systemic levels of various mediators, including the immunomodulatory messenger proteins called cytokines, were found to be predictive of ARDS and MOF.[5] Based on this observation the hypothesis emerged that organ damage in the presence of systemic inflammation is caused by spillover of inflammatory mediators from the focus of injury or infection. The progression from infection to MOF was now presented as a unidirectional cascade of events, starting from the reaction of the host to injury and ending with MOF. This idea inspired the quest for a single medical intervention (a "magic bullet") to interrupt the chain of reactions. Since 1990, many agents that were expected to interfere with unwanted actions of some mediator were investigated in expensive multicenter trials. None was effective in reducing mortality or even morbidity in critically ill patients.[6]

Indeed, it has become apparent that the concept of unopposed autodestruction is an oversimplification, as the persistent presence of high levels of both pro- and antiinflammatory mediators are characteristic for nonsurvivors of MOF.[7] This cacophony of contradictory stimuli may result in dysfunction of immune cells. Immunologic "anergy" is often found in critically ill patients, predisposing to infectious complications.[8] It may be beneficial, therefore, to enhance proinflammatory mechanisms in some patients, whereas antiinflammatory strategies are mandatory in others.[9]

Host Response to Injury

During trauma tissues may be injured (1) directly by mechanical forces; (2) indirectly by disturbances of blood supply causing ischemia followed by necrosis or formation of oxygen radicals after reperfusion; and (3) by physical factors such as heat, cold, and radiation. Infection is the common denominator for damage to the tissues caused by invading microorganisms or their products. Other toxic products that may destroy cells can be exogenous (chemotherapy or environmental intoxication) or endogenous (pancreatic proteases or the by-products of inflammation itself). Contact of blood components with artificial membranes during cardiopulmonary bypass or dialysis may directly activate autotoxic substances.[10] (Table 7.1).

Inflammation is defined as a localized protective response elicited by injury or destruction of tissues that serves to destroy, dilute, or wall off (sequester) both the injurious agent and the injured tissues. Briefly, this response is characterized by the activation of cascade systems (i.e., complement, coagulation, kinins, fibrinolysis), cells (i.e., endothelial cells, leukocytes, monocytes, macrophages, mast cells), and the release of mediators (i.e., oxygen radicals, histamine, eicosanoids, coagulation factors, cytokines). All these processes are interrelated and interconnected by upregulatory and downregulatory mechanisms.

The initial step in any inflammatory reaction to injury involves the intracellular activation of genes expressing cytokines and mediator-producing enzymes in immune effector cells. Studies have shown that some oxidative stress by reactive oxygen species (ROS) on the mitochondria is a necessary condition for this activation.[11,12] The cell type first activated depends on the type of injury (mechanical damage with bleeding, ischemia, presence of bacteria). Irrespective of the cause, however, there is always concomitant activation of the endothelium, polymorphonuclear leukocytes (PMNs), and monocyte/macrophages.

Regulatory Functions of Endothelium During Inflammation

The endothelium (700 m^2 and 1.5 kg/70 kg body weight) is not a passive lining of the vascular lumen. It is constantly processing signals to regulate the flow of substances and cells between the blood and surrounding tissues. It has four key functions that are altered by tissue injury and hemorrhage: (1) regulation of vascular tone; (2) control of hemostasis; (3) control of vascular permeability; and (4) regulation of leukocyte adhesion and trafficking. The highly reactive radical molecule nitric oxide (NO) is constantly synthesized in small amounts from L-arginine by the constitutive form of NO synthase (NOS) in endothelium. It relaxes vascular smooth muscle cells and the endothelium itself by cyclic guanosine monophosphate (cGMP)-mediated removal of intracellular calcium ions. At the luminal side of the endothelium it inhibits adhesion of platelets and leukocytes. NO thus helps keep the healthy vessel open. Because of its short half-life, NO is active only in an autocrine fashion (affecting the producing cell) and paracrine fashion (affecting neighboring cells). NO activity is increased by shear stress to regulate oxygen delivery on the microcirculatory level. Its function is supplemented by the prostaglandins, which act at a greater distance.[13]

Disruption of the endothelial tissue barrier exposes various interstitial molecules to the platelets, thereby initiating their aggregation. Local release of tissue factor further activates the plasma coagulation system via the extrinsic factor VIIa-dependent pathway.[14] At the same time plasminogen activator inhibitor-I and antiplasmin are increased, reducing the propensity of clot lysis.[15]

Activated endothelium, monocytes, and vascular smooth muscle cells express iNOS, the inducible form of the NOS enzyme, which generates massive amounts of NO, limited only by the availability of L-arginine and oxygen. Maximal dilatation of the intact vessels in the inflamed tissues is accomplished in this way, accommodating the passage of sticky leukocytes and platelets.[13] NO production by PMNs and macrophages assist in the killing of microorganisms.

The third reaction of endothelium in inflammation is often described as capillary or microcirculatory leakage. Histamine, a product of interstitial mast cells, and bradykinin, a product of the kallikrein-kinin system, act directly on the postcapillary venular endothelium to open up the tight junctions. Exposure of various foreign surfaces leads to activation of the alternative

TABLE 7.1. Host Response to Injury.

Inflammation
 Complement activation
 Endothelial activation and injury
 Vasodilation
 Microcirculatory leakage, forming protein-rich edema
 Expression of adhesion molecules, cytokines, growth factors
 Extravasation of polymorphonuclear cells and monocytes
 Respiratory burst and phagocytosis
 Removal of debris

Coagulation
 Activation of coagulation
 Inhibition of fibrinolysis
 Systemic enhancement of fibrinolysis

Systemic inflammatory response
 Fever
 Induction of acute-phase proteins, including heat shock proteins
 Stimulation leukocyte proliferation in bone marrow
 Activation and/or proliferation of B and T lymphocytes, depending on stimuli

Metabolic response
 Increased cortisol production
 Activation of the sympathetic nervous system
 Reduction of active thyroid hormones

Repair
 Apoptosis of inflammatory cells
 Regeneration of parenchymal cell (when possible)
 Angiogenesis
 Proliferation of epithelia, fibroblasts

pathway of the complement cascade with formation of anaphylatoxins C3a and C5a,[16] both strong inducers of tissue edema.

Endothelial activation progressing to damage may be the result of a limited number of mechanisms. Endotoxin [lipopolysaccharide (LPS)], cytokines [tumor necrosis factor-α (TNFα), interleukin-1 (IL-1)], and reactive oxygen species, including NO from adherent leukocytes, may act in concert to induce increased cell permeability, detachment, and finally lysis of endothelial cells.[17] Endothelial P-selectin interacts with leukocyte L-selectin and induces rolling of leukocytes, the first stage of leukocyte arrest.[18]

Leukocytes: Main Effector Cells in Acute Inflammation

The complement anaphylatoxins C3a and C5a are strong attractants and stimulants for PMNs. Other activators include TNFα, IL-1, IL-8, leukotrienes, and platelet-activating factor (PAF). Progressive PMN activation is characterized by loss of L-selectin and expression of β_2-integrin (CD11b/CD18).[19] Interaction with adhesion molecules on activated endothelium causes strong adhesion, margination, and sometimes temporary obstruction of the capillary. Various cytotoxic contents from the granula, such as myeloperoxidase and elastase, and reactive oxygen species, particularly hydrogen peroxide, are released into the small crevice between PMNs and endothelium[20] (Fig. 7.1).

Ongoing stimulation induces PMN diapedesis. The respiratory burst in tissue further develops with formation of more oxygen radicals, proteolytic enzymes (e.g., elastase), and a whole array of proinflammatory mediators (most importantly cytokines) and growth factors. Release of granulocyte/macrophage colony-stimulating factor (GM-CSF) and macrophage colony-stimulating factor (M-CSF) as endocrine hormones enhances myelopoiesis and activates circulating leukocytes. Circulating PMNs may then injure otherwise healthy tissues.[21,22]

During a slower response, which may take several days to develop,[23] monocytes are attracted to the site of injury or infection, where they differentiate to macrophages capable of killing bacteria and disposing of necrotic tissue by phagocytosis. Tissue macrophages process antigens and present them to T and B cells, which assist in the eradication of microorganisms. Endotoxin from gram-negative bacteria (lipopolysaccharide, or LPS), especially after combination with LPS-binding protein (LBP) from the plasma is a specifically strong activator of monocytes through binding to monocyte membrane-bound CD14. Macrophages are further elicited/activated by hypoxia and various activating substances, including C5a and IL-1.[24] At the site of injury PMNs and macrophages continue to release proteolytic enzymes, such as elastase and toxic oxygen radicals, which kill native cells and microorganisms alike, resulting in the formation of pus. Other substances, such as PAF, leukotrienes, and cytokines (TNFα, IL-1, IL-6) act in a paracrine way to

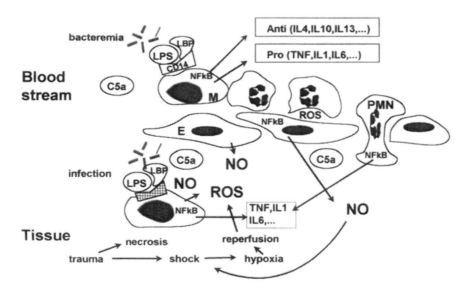

FIGURE 7.1. Trauma and infection activate inflammatory pathways by different routes, but the intracellular mechanisms are rather uniform. Tissue infection and bacteremia induce monocytes/macrophages (M) to produce proinflammatory and antiinflammatory cytokines after complement activation (C5a) or binding the complex of endotoxin (lipopolysaccharide, or LPS) with LPS-binding protein (LBP) to the CD14 molecule. The proinflammatory mediators activate polymorphonuclear leukocytes (PMNs), which begin the synthesis of reactive oxygen species (ROS). Trauma may lead to tissue necrosis, hypoxia, and reperfusion damage, in turn leading to formation of ROS. Rolling, margination, and finally diapedesis through the endothelium (E) of PMNs may take place at the site of injury as well as in remote organs. Endothelium is activated by cytokines and the formation of ROS in the crevice between PMNs and endothelial cells. Nitric oxide (NO) is probably produced by all involved cell types to assist bacterial killing but also inducing vasoplegia, which may lead to shock and further tissue hypoxia. There is a great diversity in mediators, which are involved in communication between different cell types. Intracellular processing of these signals, however, is rather uniform, involving the NFκB pathway.

attract more inflammatory cells to the site. When released into the circulation these factors become endocrine hormones, activating circulating immunocytes.

Systemic Reactions

Systemic release of proinflammatory cytokines induces fever (IL-1) and the production of acute-phase proteins by the liver (IL-6), including C-reactive protein, which may be helpful in injury control. Growth factors (e.g., GM-CSF) stimulate proliferation and early release of leukocytes and platelets. Cytokines also increase the activity of the hypothalamic-adrenal axis with increased synthesis of hydrocortisone, whereas thyroid hormone activity is decreased, leading to the state of "euthyroid sick syndrome."[25] Activation of the sympathetic nervous system serves to meet the increased metabolic demands. These endocrine changes lead to increased hepatic gluconeogenesis, peripheral lipolysis, and protein breakdown, probably to increase the availability of fuel and amino acids to the inflammatory process.

Resolution of Inflammation and Transition to Repair

Antiinflammatory mechanisms and countersignals that dampen the systemic reaction are present from the outset. Direct antiinflammatory cytokines include cytokines IL-4, IL-10, and IL-13. Another antiinflammatory mechanism is the expression of receptor antagonists, such as IL-1 receptor antagonist (IL-1ra). Shedding of soluble receptors for a factor into the circulation [i.e., soluble TNFα receptor (sTNFR)] may decrease the availability of that factor to receptors on target cell membranes.

Neuroendocrine reactions also modulate inflammation. Not only corticosteroids but also catecholamines have a direct antiinflammatory effect. Systemic epinephrine has been shown to inhibit production of TNFα and IL-1, potentiate IL-10 production, and exert antithrombotic effects during human endotoxinemia.[26,27]

The cellular stress response, characterized by transient downregulation of most cellular products and by upregulation of heat-shock proteins (HSPs), is another protective mechanism that may play an important role. HSPs are constitutively present in all cells and can be induced by fever and hypoxia. These proteins play a role in the protection of cell integrity against oxidative stress.[28]

How the inflammation stops at the site of injury is still uncertain. One clue to this question may be that just the disappearance of ongoing stimulation is the main principle of its termination. For example, PMNs have no mechanism by which to retreat from an inflammatory focus; and apoptosis, a controlled program for cell death, is the dominant process leading to the termination of the PMN response.[29]

Tissue repair, characterized by angiogenesis and proliferation of fibroblasts, epithelia, and (when possible) parenchymal cells, is stimulated by growth factors, which form part of the inflammatory repertoire of immune cells. It may be that these reparative processes are initiated as soon as the more "cytotoxic" PMNs and macrophages have stopped to interfere. When low grade proinflammatory forces dominate for a long time over slowly progressing tissue repair, parenchymal regeneration is substituted by excessive filling of the tissue gaps with intercellular matrix, leading to fibrosis.[30]

Pivotal Role of Transcription Factor NFκB in Inflammation

It has become clear that the decisive intracellular step of all inflammatory pathways may reside in activation of a limited set of nuclear factors. Nuclear factor κ-B (NFκB) is a dimer composed of two DNA-binding proteins, mainly P50 (NF-κB1) and P65 (RelA), that is kept dormant by the inhibitory protein IκBA. This complex resides constitutively in the cytoplasm of lymphocytes, granulocytes, monocytes, endothelial cells, and smooth muscle cells.[31] Stimulated cell membrane receptors of a large number of factors, which were long associated with inflammation (Table 7.2), have been found to activate an intracellular tyrosine kinase, which phosphorylates IκBA, the first step leading to its degradation. Some mitochondrial oxidative stress (e.g., the presence of oxygen radicals formed by ischemia/reperfusion) seems to be obligatory for this event. Liberated NFκB then moves into the nucleus, where it promotes the

TABLE 7.2. Factors Activating and Inhibiting NF-κB.

Factors activating NFκB
  Cytokines
    TNFα
    IL-1 and IL-2
    Leukotriene B_4
  Bacterial products
    Endotoxin (LPS)
    Exotoxin B
    Toxic shock syndrome toxin 1
  Viruses
    Many DNA viruses (including HIV-1 and herpes simplex)
    Respiratory viruses
  Oxidants
    Reactive oxygen species
    Hydrogen peroxide (H_2O_2)
  Physical stress
    Radiation

Factors inhibiting NFκB
  Cytokines
    (IL-10)
  Microbiologic
    Endotoxin (LPS)
    Gliotoxin (*Aspergillus*)
  Proteasome inhibitors
    Calpain inhibitor I
    Others
  Antioxidants and radical scavengers
    Superoxide dismutase
    Glutathione
    Acetylcysteine
    Vitamins
  Other
    Glucocorticoids
    Heat shock proteins

transcription of genes encoding for interleukins, interferon, adhesion molecules, acute-phase proteins, growth factors, and iNOS.[12]

Many aspects of inflammation are mirrored in NFκB regulation. For example, bacterial products such as LPS and group B streptococcal cell walls (GBS) both induce NFκB activation and subsequent TNFα production, although interacting with different mediators: LPS activates monocytes after combination with LBP and binding to CD14 on the monocyte cell membrane, whereas GBS acts on NFκB after binding to complement receptors CR3 and CR4.[32]

The end-product of the coagulation cascade, thrombin, has been shown to activate NFκB directly and to potentiate endothelial cell activation by TNFα, providing a molecular explanation for the co-activation of inflammation by coagulation.[15]

Evidence is now accumulating that downregulation of the inflammatory response is closely related to inhibition of NFκB. This inhibition take places in various ways. First, liberated NFκB stimulates the production of its own inhibitor IκBA. Second, regeneration of NFκB after activation by endotoxin is associated with increased synthesis of the P50 monomer, leading to formation of the P50–P50 dimer of NFκB, which is inactive. This process may form the molecular basis of endotoxin tolerance: Exposure of an organism to bacterial endotoxin induces anergy of monocytes to subsequent endotoxin challenge, which may last for days or even weeks.

Heat shock proteins, especially HSP-70, constitute another important counterregulatory mechanism, at least partially acting by inhibiting NFκB.[33] Also, any agent that removes oxygen radicals, such as superoxide dismutase, N-acetylcysteine, glutathione, and vitamins C and E, reduces the rate of NFκB activation.[34,35]

The proteasome is a large cytoplasmatic protein complex involved in protein turnover, including the degradation of IκBA. Calpain I inhibitor and other serine protease inhibitors may be clinically useful in the management of harmful inflammation. Last but not least, all glucocorticoids are potent inhibitors of NFκB activation via both protein–protein interactions and IκBA formation.[36]

Some conclusions about NFκB may be tentatively drawn. First, virulent activation of inflammatory cascades may require a combination of tissue damage or infection and some moment of tissue hypoxia. Second, inflammation has an intrinsic tendency to subside unless the stimulus persists, hypoxia recurs, or both.

MOF: Result of Whole-Body Inflammation

Many of the analogies between local signs of inflammation and the manifestations of progressive MOF are straightforward. In patients with trauma or severe sepsis, there is an early, generalized increase in capillary permeability for water and protein,[3,37] with reduced plasma oncotic pressure, resulting in a positive fluid balance and generalized edema. This clinical capillary leak syndrome is often first observed as pulmonary edema, with the typical radiographic signs of "early" ARDS.

The morphology of the lung during the progression of ARDS has been well characterized, with aggregation and margination of PMNs and subsequent damage to the pulmonary capillary endothelium and the alveolocapillary membrane ('shock lung').[38] Subsequently, an excessive monocyte invasion occurs, extensively so in patients developing MOF.[39] This process can be monitored by repeated bronchoalveolar lavage (BAL).

These alterations, leakage and cellular infiltration, are not confined to the lungs but may also develop in the liver, kidney, heart, spleen, and brain. They may develop after trauma without infection[40] as well as in patients with severe sepsis.[39] Ongoing systemic activation of the coagulation system during endotoxemia and high systemic levels of cytokines (especially IL-1β and IL6) proceeds through the extrinsic tissue factor-mediated pathway. This process, called diffuse intravascular coagulation (DIC), may lead to concurrent thrombosis (gangrene, skin necrosis) and bleeding (petechiae, purpura, spontaneous bleeding) with consumption of both pro- and anticoagulatory factors and platelets. It is more often seen in a mild form with transient thrombocytopenia and abnormal blood coagulation tests without clinical sequelae.[41]

The generalized vasodilation and reduced responsiveness to catecholamines in inflammatory states is closely related to the dramatic, generalized increase in nitric oxide production by iNOS. This vasoplegia leads to a fall in blood pressure, which may or may not be compensated by a sharp rise in cardiac output. The result is hypotension in combination with elevated cardiac output and low peripheral vascular resistance, which sharply differentiates hyperdynamic shock in systemic inflammation from hypovolemic or cardiogenic shock.

Uncompensated vasoplegia results in persistently low perfusion pressure and tissue hypoxemia, especially in the splanchnic organs, which are "sacrificed" by the catecholamine-mediated sympathetic reaction and local release of vasoconstrictors such as endothelin to preserve cardiac and cerebral perfusion. Acute failure of kidney, liver, and gut function is most often seen when vasoplegic shock, capillary leakage, and systemic activation of inflammatory cells are combined. PMN accumulation has indeed been found in the liver, kidneys, spleen, and heart of patients dying after trauma, together with signs of hypoxic cellular necrosis, increasing in severity with the duration of survival after injury.[39]

Leukopenia is an early indicator of PMN sequestration and a prognostic marker for subsequent MOF in trauma and sepsis patients.[42,43] It also holds true in patients undergoing cardiopulmonary bypass in whom PMN counts were elevated in the right atrium but not in the left atrium, whereas significant trapping of PMNs occurred in pulmonary alveolar capillaries.[44] Therefore PMNs in blood samples might represent the immature and senescent populations, not the activated population.[45]

Systemic reaction to injury is associated with the appearance in blood of a vast array of protein and lipid mediators. Elevated plasma levels of the cytolytic terminal complement complex were found in patients with severe blunt trauma,[46] sepsis, or acute limb ischemia, normalizing in some patients but further increasing in patients who developed ARDS.[47] After cardiopulmonary bypass, elevated plasma C3a levels were also predictive of dysfunction of the heart, lungs, kidneys, and clotting system.[48]

Initially, investigators paid most attention to elevations of the proinflammatory mediators, such as TNFα, IL-1, IL-6, and IL-8. However, it has become gradually clear that in patients with unresolving sepsis levels of these proinflammatory and antiinflammatory substances (e.g., IL-1ra, IL-4, IL-10) tumor growth factor-β and soluble receptors to TNFα remain continually high.[7,49]

Of all the cytokines, in many clinical studies TNFα was the first to appear and often the first to disappear from the blood. Sustained high plasma TNFα levels correlated well with severity of illness and mortality, not with positive blood cultures, endotoxin levels, or subsequent septic shock.[50,51] In an experimental model involving induction of sterile peritonitis in rodents by administration of zymosan (the ZIGI model), plasma TNFα levels were elevated on days 1 and 2, were below detection level the following days, and progressively increased from day 8 on. This late peak of plasma TNFα was biologically inactive,[52] but TNFα and IL-6 production by peritoneal macrophages increased steadily throughout the experiment, illustrating a disparity between local and systemic levels of inflammatory mediators.

Administration of IL-1 to rabbits results in hyperdynamic shock with leukopenia and thrombocytopenia.[53] One study reported that persistent elevation of IL-1 concentrations in BAL fluid and plasma appears to be related to outcome in patients developing ARDS,[54] although, others found no consistent correlation between plasma IL-1 levels and the severity of or the mortality associated with ARDS, SIRS, or MOF.[55]

High circulating levels of IL-6 have been found early in patients with sepsis or ARDS. Both the absolute levels and the persistence of elevated levels correlated well with outcome.[56]

Interleukin-10 is a potent inhibitor of monocyte/macrophage proinflammatory cytokine production. In critically ill patients, plasma IL-10 levels were higher in the presence of septic shock.[57] In the lung fluids of patients with ARDS, decreased concentrations of IL-10 and IL-1ra were associated with increased mortality rates.[58]

All these studies of circulating cytokines should be interpreted with caution. Plasma levels of pro- and antiinflammatory substances may not reflect the local situation at all.[52,59] In peritonitis patients the concentrations of TNFα, IL-6, and endotoxin were many times higher in peritoneal fluid than in plasma.[60] In patients with severe brain injury, IL-6 concentrations were 30-fold higher in cerebrospinal fluid (CSF) than in serum, and the high CSF levels correlated with the severity of SIRS.[61] Some cytokines are cell-associated and function by cell contact. For example, high levels of cell-associated IL-1ra and IL-8 could be detected in circulating erythrocytes, mononuclear cells, and PMNs of patients with sepsis but not in their plasma.[62]

Plasma levels of elastase and neopterin, markers for activation of PMNs and macrophages, respectively, have been found to constitute excellent markers of the severity of ARDS, MOF, and sepsis. Persistently elevated neopterin levels accurately predicted nonsurvivors several days before the event.[5,38,63-66]

In conclusion, there is a wide body of clinical and biochemical evidence that shock, sepsis, and organ failure are accompanied by systemic inflammation. Indeed, experimental administration of inflammatory stimuli such as endotoxin, zymosan, or inflammatory mediators may induce SIRS and MOF, in the absence of microorganisms.

Role of Infection

The outcome of many infectious diseases is undeniably related to the invasion of microbial pathogens. The chance of surviving severe systemic infections such as staphylococcal or meningococcal septicemia is dependent on the early administration of effective antimicrobial therapy. Also, abdominal sepsis is associated with high mortality when the primary focus is not eliminated by adequate surgery.

In a classic study comparing the efficacy of antibiotics and cardiovascular support and a combination of these two therapies in dogs with septic shock induced by an intraperitoneal clot containing *Escherichia coli*, survival rates were 0% in the group receiving no therapy (controls), 13% in the group receiving antibiotics alone and the group receiving cardiovascular support alone, but 43% in the group receiving combined therapy.[45] Nosocomial infections, particularly ventilator-associated pneumonia (VAP) are associated with increased morbidity and prolonged stay in the intensive care unit (ICU). Whether this morbidity is a major cause or just a consequence of ongoing MOF has been debated for some time.[67] It is sometimes stated that the critically ill patient dies "with infection, not from infection." Some studies, however, clearly show that inadequate or late antimicrobial coverage of VAP is associated with modest attributable mortality.[68]

The roles of bacteria and endotoxin are less clear in "late" ARDS, sepsis, and MOF.[67] An identical MOF syndrome develops in patients with primarily bacterial (peritonitis) and nonbacterial (pancreatitis, severe trauma) problems; and no clinical, biochemical, or morphologic signs differentiate these patient groups.[66] Moreover, the correlation of sepsis scores to mortality depends on organ failure data, not bacteriologic data.[3] Systemic inflammation as elicited by the extracorporeal circulation during cardiopulmonary bypass is clearly associated with some morbidity, but the outcome is generally excellent. This inflammatory response was previously considered a perfect model of sterile systemic inflammation, mainly caused by complement activation in the extracorporeal circuit.[28] In recent years, however, the severity of postoperative SIRS and the chance of developing MOF were found to be related to the amount of perioperatively circulating endotoxin.[69] In one study, preoperative low levels of immunoglobulin M (IgM) antibodies against endotoxin core antigen were an important independent predictor of an adverse outcome after cardiac surgery, supporting the theory that circulating endotoxin is a cause of postoperative morbidity.[70]

As endotoxemia, but not bacterial infection, could be demonstrated in many patients with ongoing SIRS and shock, the theory was developed that translocation of endotoxin from the gut may contribute to the pathogenesis or perpetuation of the sepsis syndrome.[71] Hypoxic damage to the bowel mucosa from shock and even lower limb ischemia may indeed contribute to increased intestinal permeability followed by endotoxemia and perhaps bacteremia.[40,72] This phenomenon was also demonstrated in patients following cardiac arrest.[73] It is not clear, however, if the finding of increased intestinal permeability is the cause or the effect of ongoing microcirculatory leakage.

Role of Hypoxia

All forms of shock are by definition characterized by insufficient microcirculatory oxygen delivery. As mitochondria are still capable of respiration at a partial oxygen pressure (PO_2) of 1 mmHg, only an insufficient blood flow, not mild hypoxemia by itself, can induce cellular hypoxia.

Prolonged tissue hypoxia leads to depletion of adenosine triphosphate (ATP) and subsequent degradation of adenosine diphosphate (ADP) to adenosine monophosphate (AMP) and finally hypoxanthine. When energy stores fall below a critical level, cells disintegrate after swelling, which is typical for necrosis. Reoxygenation by reperfusion induces the activation of xanthine oxidase, which produces toxic oxygen metabolites such as superoxide, hydrogen peroxide, the highly toxic hydroxyl anion (OH^-), and (in interaction with NO) the highly reactive radical peroxynitrite ($ONOO^-$).[74] Lipid peroxidation and other alterations after oxidative stress induce cell death by a genetically determined scenario characterized by shrinking, a process called apoptosis.[75,76]

Less severe tissue hypoxia is a potent stimulus for activation of immune cells by the NFκB mechanism and subsequent release of proinflammatory mediators. This sequence is well illustrated by an experiment in which infusion of complement-activated plasma into rabbits induces PMN aggregation and sequestration in various organs. These alterations, however, are not severe and are largely reversible. Addition of hypoxia as a second stimulus, however, induces severe morphologic changes, resembling those of early ARDS and MOF in humans.[77]

Another consequence of even mild and transient hypoxia is impaired leukocyte bacterial killing.[78] Activated PMNs must increase their oxygen uptake by a factor of 90 to produce toxic oxygen species for bacterial killing. The risk of wound infection increased exponentially when subcutaneous PO_2 decreased below 90 mmHg.[79]

These sequelae of tissue hypoxia offer a clear explanation for the fact that patients who have been suffering from circulatory shock due to any cause are likely to develop signs of systemic inflammation. After introduction of routine cardiac output measurement during the 1980s it became apparent that a supranormal cardiac output was associated with increased survival of these patients. Maximizing total systemic oxygen delivery (DO_2) to improve oxygen consumption became a therapeutic strategy for treating critically ill patients.[80] The success of this strategy, however, could be proven only in a subgroup of patients admitted with low DO_2 values in whom there was an increase in oxygen consumption during the resuscitation phase. In patients with a high DO_2 at admission to the study, increasing oxygen delivery did not alter oxygen consumption (VO_2) or survival, and oxygen extraction decreased. In a more recent study it was shown that aggressive attempts to increase DO_2 may even lead to increased mortality.[81]

It has been understood that for the entire organism energy metabolism is always completely aerobic. Persistently high levels of blood lactate are associated with a large flux of reducing equivalents from cells in parts of the body where oxygen is available and lactate is used as a main source of energy, thus preserving glucose for nonaerobic ATP regeneration in other cells where the oxygen supply is limited.[82] Indeed, critical global oxygen delivery is probably well below the levels normally achieved during routine resuscitation.[83]

Consequently, persistent lactic acidosis in SIRS leading to MODS implies regional tissue hypoxia despite a supranormal DO_2. For example, after experimental infusion of *Escherichia coli* in dogs, low skeletal muscle PO_2 values were documented in the presence of normal or high DO_2.[84] In this experiment, the only parameter measured correlating with the rapid decrease of tissue PO_2 was a rapid drop in PMN count. From these studies it was concluded that an early microcirculatory injury occurs, during sepsis, that is not dependent on cardiac output. Therefore the focus of studies on tissue-has moved from global oxygen delivery to regulation of the microcirculation.

This regional tissue hypoxia after restoration of global oxygen delivery can be explained by pathologic dilatation of arteriovenous connections (an effect of NO), intermittent microcirculatory interruption of leukocytes and platelet aggregates (caused by cell activation), loss of vasomotion, and disturbed oxygen off-loading due to edema.[85,86] All these mechanisms may account for the variable oxygen concentrations within one and the same organ during septic shock and with the observation that capillary PO_2 can be lower than the PO_2 in veins draining the tissue.[86]

In summary, cellular hypoxia is important in the pathogenesis of MOF. During the early stages hypoxia aggravates the inflammatory insult and may jeopardize leukocyte function. After resuscitation, any drop in oxygen delivery might reinforce NFκB-mediated proinflammatory mechanisms. When microcirculatory disturbances have been established, correction of microcirculatory shunting becomes difficult to achieve.

Systemic Inflammation: Necessary or Autodestructive?

As neutrophil activation seems to be directly responsible for tissue destruction in inflammatory and septic syndromes, it seems logical to investigate the possible beneficial effects of neutrophil inhibition. Inhibition of neutrophil–endothelial interaction by blocking selectin or CD11/CD18 integrin in infectious/inflammatory models has produced conflicting results. It has been beneficial in models using single inflammatory stimuli, such as endotoxin or TNFα, and in ischemia/reperfusion. In models of sepsis, however, the effects of integrin blocking have been beneficial in some experiments but detrimental in others, depending on the species (rats, dogs, rabbits, primates), the site of infection (abdominal sepsis, pneumonia, or bacterial meningitis), the type of infection (*E. coli* vs. meningococci), the stage of disease, and the adequacy of antimicrobial therapy.[9]

The opposite of PMN inhibition—administration of G-CSF to increase the number and activity of PMNs—has also been studied in models of sepsis. This idea is based on the fact that leukopenia due to chemotherapy and functional failure of PMNs as in chronic granulomatous disease are associated with increased mortality due to infection. In studies of murine and rat abdominal sepsis based on cecal ligation and puncture (CLP), early administration of G-CSF improved survival.[87,88] With community-acquired pneumonia, G-CSF administration was associated with significantly faster resolution of infiltrates and fewer complications, but there was no effect on mortality.[89] More clinical data are needed to assess this treatment modality.

Manipulation of macrophages also variably affects outcome. In a study with CLP in mast cell-deficient mice, mortality was 100%, whereas mast cell-reconstituted mice survived the experiment.[90] In the ZIGI model in mice, depletion of peritoneal macrophages by liposome-encapsulated diphosphonates increased early mortality to almost 100%, whereas depletion of liver and splenic macrophages decreased the severity of MOF. Depletion of pulmonary macrophages completely prevented mortality.[91]

An array of clinical studies have assessed the therapeutic value of administering cytokine antagonists such as human anti-TNFα, soluble TNF receptor, IL-1 receptor antagonists, and PAF antagonists. There was no clear benefit to outcome in any of these expensive trials,[92–94] although previously performed studies in homogeneous animal models had predicted a decrease of mortality.

During the 1980s the administration of glucocorticoids was expected to be an easy way to inhibit the detrimental effects of generalized inflammation. Large, randomized trials did not show any decrease in mortality after early, short-course, high-dose intravenous glucocorticoid therapy for sepsis and ARDS.[95,96] Therefore, this therapy was abandoned in clinical practice by many physicians and its use discouraged in textbooks. In 1998 however, two prospective, randomized, double-blind, placebo-controlled trials were reported in which administration of glucocorticoid for late, unresolving sepsis and ARDS resulted in a statistically significant decrease in morbidity and mortality.[97,98] Ongoing studies must be reported, though, before firm conclusions can be drawn about the use of glucocorticoids.

All these experiments confirm the importance of inflammatory cells in preventing or generating mortality in various models. It depends on the type, place, and severity of an injury whether pro- or antiinflammatory treatment strategies are likely to produce beneficial results.

Conclusions

Inflammation and repair are of vital importance for overcoming the minor injuries and infections of normal life. Excessive inflammation may kill some patients after resuscitation. In recent years a large body of knowledge has emerged from clinical and experimental studies on the inter- and intracellular processes regulating the host defense response. These achievements of scientific research have not yet yielded certified new ways of treating the critically ill patient. On the contrary, the importance of focus eradication and avoiding tissue hypoxemia are simply stressed by recent findings.

To develop beneficial therapeutic strategies, we should first extend our knowledge of the regulation of the interlocking, antagonistic or synergistic, complementary, and often apparently redundant mechanisms of the host defense response, which are all active in smaller, not lethal processes, such as a simple bite wound. Second, we need to study the activity of pro- and antiinflammatory mechanisms in our patients at the site of injury and in more remote areas. More knowledge is needed on the intracellular regulating mechanisms responsible for gene transcription and posttranscriptional modulation. Only then may we hope to make any progress in designing immunomodulating treatment strategies that can reduce the autodestructive tendency of the necessary evil called inflammation and improve the prognosis of severe trauma and infection.

References

1. Nuytinck JKS, Offermans XJ, Kubat K, et al: Whole-body inflammation in trauma patients: an autopsy study. Arch Surg 1988;123:1519–1524.
2. Pepe PE, Potkin RT, Reus DH, et al: Clinical predictors of the adult respiratory distress syndrome. Am J Surg 1982;144:124–130.
3. Goris RJ, te Boekhorst TP, Nuytinck JKS, et al: Multiple-organ failure: generalized autodestructive inflammation? Arch Surg 1985;120:1109–1115.
4. Bone RC, Sibbald WJ, Sprung CL: The ACCP-SCCM consensus conference on sepsis and organ failure. Chest 1992;101:1481–1483.
5. Roumen RM, Hendriks T, van der Ven-Jongekrijg J, et al: Cytokine patterns in patients after major vascular surgery, hemorrhagic shock, and severe blunt trauma: relation with subsequent adult respiratory distress syndrome and multiple organ failure. Ann Surg 1993;218:769–776.
6. Foster DM, Doig GS: Clinical trials for the evaluation of sepsis therapies. In: Vincent J-L (ed) Yearbook of Intensive Care and Emergency Medicine 1997. Berlin, Springer, 1997;149–157.
7. Van der Poll T, de Waal Malefyt R, Coyle SM, et al: Antiinflammatory cytokine responses during clinical sepsis and experimental endotoxemia: sequential measurements of plasma soluble interleukin (IL)-1 receptor type II, IL-10, and IL-13. J Infect Dis 1997;175:118–122.
8. Docke WD, Randow F, Syrbe U, et al: Monocyte deactivation in septic patients: restoration by IFN-gamma treatment. Nat Med 1997;3:678–681.

9. Karzai W, Reinhart K: Is it beneficial to augment or to inhibit neutrophil function in severe infections and sepsis? In: Vincent J-L (ed) Yearbook of Intensive Care and Emergency Medicine 1997. Berlin, Springer, 1997;123-132.
10. Gillinov AM, Redmond JM, Winkelstein JA, et al: Complement and neutrophil activation during cardiopulmonary bypass: a study in the complement-deficient dog. Ann Thorac Surg 1994;57:345-352.
11. Sundaresan M, Yu ZX, Ferrans VJ, et al: Requirement for generation of H_2O_2 for platelet-derived growth factor signal transduction. Science 1995;270:296-299.
12. Christman JW, Lancaster LH, Blackwell TS: Nuclear factor kappa B: a pivotal role in the systemic inflammatory response syndrome and new target for therapy. Intensive Care Med 1998;24:1131-1138.
13. Moncada S, Palmer RM, Higgs EA: Nitric oxide: physiology, pathophysiology, and pharmacology. Pharmacol Rev 1991;43:109-142.
14. Biemond BJ, Levi M, Ten Cate H, et al: Complete inhibition of endotoxin-induced coagulation activation in chimpanzees with a monoclonal Fab fragment against factor VII/VIIa. Thromb Haemost 1995;73:223-230.
15. Anrather D, Millan MT, Palmetshofer A, et al: Thrombin activates nuclear factor-kappa B and potentiates endothelial cell activation by TNF. J Immunol 1997;159:5620-5628.
16. Heideman M, Saravis C, Clowes GHA, et al: Effect of non-viable tissue and abscesses on complement depletion and the development of bacteremia. J Trauma 1982;22:527-532.
17. Smedley LA, Tonnessen RA, Sandhaus RA: Neutrophil-mediated injury to endothelial cells. J Clin Invest 1986;77:1233-1243.
18. Dore M, Korthuis RJ, Granger DN, et al: P-selectin mediates spontaneous leukocyte rolling in vivo. Blood 1993;82:1308-1316.
19. Mulligan MS, Varani J, Warren JS, et al: Roles of β_2-integrins of rat neutrophils in complement- and oxygen radical-mediated acute inflammatory injury. J Immunol 1992;148:1847-1857.
20. Gilmont RR, Dardano A, Engle JS, et al: TNF-alpha potentiates oxidant and reperfusion-induced endothelial cell injury. J Surg Res 1996;61:175-182.
21. Wedmore CV, Williams TJ: Control of vascular permeability by polymorphonuclear leukocytes in inflammation. Nature 1981;89:646-650.
22. Anderson BO, Brown JM, Harken AH: Mechanisms of neutrophil-mediated tissue injury. J Surg Res 1991;51:170-179.
23. Nathan C: Secretory products of macrophages. J Clin Invest 1987;79:319-326.
24. Law MM, Cryer HG, Abraham E: Elevated levels of soluble ICAM-1 correlate with the development of multiple organ failure. J Trauma 1994;37:100-110.
25. Baue AE, Gunther B, Hartl W, et al: Altered hormonal activity in severely ill patients after injury or sepsis. Arch Surg 1984;119:1125-1132.
26. Van der Poll T, Lowry SF: Epinephrine inhibits endotoxin-induced IL-1 beta production: roles of tumor necrosis factor-alpha and IL-10. Am J Physiol 1997;273:R1885-90.
27. Van der Poll T, Levi M, Dentener M, et al: Epinephrine exerts anticoagulant effects during human endotoxemia. J Exp Med 1997;185:1143-1148.
28. Kirklin JK, Westaby S, Blackstone EH, et al: Complement and the damaging effects of cardiopulmonary bypass. J Thorac Cardiovasc Surg 1983;86:845-857.
29. Haslett C: Resolution of acute inflammation and the role of apoptosis in the tissue fate of granulocytes. Clin Sci (Colch) 1992;83:639-648.
30. Meduri GU: The role of the host defense response in the progression and outcome of ARDS: pathophysiological correlations and response to glucocorticoid treatment. Eur Respir J 1996;9:2650-2670.
31. Grimm S, Baeuerle PA: The inducible transcription factor NF-kappa B: structure-function relationship of its protein subunits. Biochem J 1993;290:297-308.
32. Medvedev AE, Flo T, Ingalls RR, et al: Involvement of CD14 and complement receptors CR3 and CR4 in nuclear factor-kappa B activation and TNF production induced by lipopolysaccharide and group B streptococcal cell walls. J Immunol 1998;160:4535-4542.
33. De Maio A: The heat-shock response. New Horiz 1995;3:198-207.
34. Chandel NS, Maltepe E, Goldwasser E, et al: Mitochondrial reactive oxygen species trigger hypoxia-induced transcription. Proc Natl Acad Sci USA 1998;95:11715-11720.
35. Wan S, LeClerc JL, Vincent JL: Inflammatory response to cardiopulmonary bypass: mechanisms involved and possible therapeutic strategies. Chest 1997;112:676-692.
36. Blackwell TS, Christman JW: The role of nuclear factor-kappa B in cytokine gene regulation. Am J Respir Cell Mol Biol 1997;17:3-9.
37. Sturm JA, Wisner DH, Oestern HJ, et al: Increased lung capillary permeability after trauma: a prospective clinical trial. J Trauma 1986;26:409-418.
38. Nuytinck JKS, Goris RJ, Redl H, et al: Posttraumatic complications and inflammatory mediators. Arch Surg 1986;121:886-890.
39. Pape HC, Remmers D, Kleemann W, et al: Posttraumatic multiple organ failure: a report on clinical and autopsy findings. Shock 1994;2:228-234.
40. Roumen RM, Hendriks T, Wevers RA, et al: Intestinal permeability after severe trauma and hemorrhagic shock is increased without relation to septic complications. Arch Surg 1993;128:453-457.
41. Van der Poll T, Levi M, van Deventer SJ: Coagulopathy: disseminated intravascular coagulation. In: Fein AM, Abraham EM, Balk RA, et al (eds) Sepsis and Multiorgan Failure. Baltimore, Williams & Wilkins, 1997;255-265.
42. Simms HH, D'Amico R: Increased PMN CD11b/CD18 expression following post-traumatic ARDS. J Surg Res 1991;50:362-367.
43. Botha AJ, Moore FA, Moore EE, et al: Early neutrophil sequestration after injury: a pathogenetic mechanism for multiple organ failure. J Trauma 1995;39:411-417.
44. Howard RJ, Crain C, Franzini DA, et al: Effects of cardiopulmonary bypass on pulmonary leukostasis and complement activation. Arch Surg 1988;123:1496-1501.
45. Natanson C, Danner RL, Reilly JM, et al: Antibiotics versus cardiovascular support in a canine model of human septic shock. Am J Physiol 1990;259:H1440-1447.
46. Roumen RM, Redl H, Schlag G, et al: Inflammatory mediators in relation to the development of multiple organ failure in patients after severe blunt trauma. Crit Care Med 1995;23:474-480.
47. Heideman M, Norder-Hanssen B, Bengtson A, et al: Terminal complement complexes and anaphylatoxins in septic and ischemic patients. Arch Surg 1988;123:188-192.
48. Yodice PC, Astiz ME, Kurian BM, et al: Neutrophil rheologic changes in septic shock. Am J Respir Crit Care Med 1997;155:38-42.

49. Goldie AS, Fearon KC, Ross JA, et al: Natural cytokine antagonists and endogenous anti-cytokine core antibodies in sepsis syndrome. JAMA 1995;274:172–177.
50. Offner F, Phillipe J, Vogelaers D: Serum tumor necrosis factor levels in patients with infectious disease and septic shock. J Lab Clin Med 1990;116:100–105.
51. Meduri GU, Kohler G, Headley S, et al: Inflammatory cytokines in the BAL of patients with ARDS: persistent elevation over time predicts poor outcome. Chest 1995;108:1303–1314.
52. Jansen MJ, Hendriks T, Vogels MT, et al: Inflammatory cytokines in an experimental model for the multiple organ dysfunction syndrome. Crit Care Med 1996;24:1196–1202.
53. Okusawa S, Gelfand JA, Ikejima T, et al: Interleukin 1 induces a shock-like state in rabbits. J Clin Invest 1988;81:1162–1172.
54. Meduri GU, Headley S, Kohler G, et al: Persistent elevation of inflammatory cytokines predicts a poor outcome in ARDS: plasma IL-1-beta and IL-6 levels are consistent and efficient predictors of outcome over time. Chest 1995;107:1062–1073.
55. Blackwell TS, Christman JW: Sepsis and cytokines: current status. Br J Anaesth 1996;77:110–117.
56. Rosenbloom AJ, Pinsky MR, Bryant JL, et al: Leukocyte activation in the peripheral blood of patients with cirrhosis of the liver and SIRS: correlation with serum interleukin-6 levels and organ dysfunction. JAMA 1995;274:58–65.
57. Gomez Jimenez J, Martin MC, Sauri R, et al: Interleukin-10 and the monocyte-macrophage-induced inflammatory response in septic shock. J Infect Dis 1995;171:472–475.
58. Donnelly SC, Strieter RM, Reid PT: The association between mortality rates and decreased concentrations of interleukin-10 and interleukin-1 receptor antagonist in the lung fluids of patients with the adult respiratory distress syndrome. Ann Intern Med 1996;125:191–196.
59. Van Goor H, Borm VJJ, Meer van der J, et al: Coagulation and fibrinolytic responses in human peritoneal fluid and plasma to bacterial peritonitis. Br J Surg 1996;83:113–135.
60. Holzheimer RG, Schein M, Wittman DH: Inflammatory response in peritoneal exudate and plasma of patients undergoing planned relaparotomy for severe secondary peritonitis. Arch Surg 1995;130:1314–1320.
61. Kossmann T, Hans VH, Imhof HG, et al: Intrathecal and serum interleukin-6 and the acute-phase response in patients with severe traumatic brain injuries. Shock 1995;4:311–317.
62. Marie C, Fitting C, Cheval C, et al: Presence of high levels of leukocyte-associated interleukin-8 upon cell activation and in patients with sepsis syndrome. Infect Immun 1997;65:865–871.
63. Duswald KH, Jochum M, Schramm W, et al: Released granulocytic elastase: an indicator of pathobiochemical alterations in septicemia after abdominal surgery. Surgery 1985;98:892–899.
64. Pacher R, Redl H, Frass M, et al: Relationship between neopterin and granulocyte elastase plasma levels and the severity of multiple organ failure. Crit Care Med 1989;17:221–226.
65. Tanaka H, Sugimoto H, Yoshioka T, et al: Role of granulocyte elastase in tissue injury in patients with septic shock complicated by multiple-organ failure. Ann Surg 1991;213:81–85.
66. Waydhas C, Nast-Kolb D, Jochum M, et al: Inflammatory mediators, infection, sepsis, and multiple organ failure after severe trauma, Arch Surg 1992;127:460–467.
67. Headley AS, Tolley E, Meduri GU: Infections and the inflammatory response in acute respiratory distress syndrome. Chest 1997;111:1306–1321.
68. Luna CM, Vujacich P, Niederman MS, et al: Impact of BAL data on the therapy and outcome of ventilator-associated pneumonia. Chest 1997;111:676–685.
69. Oudemans-van Straaten HM, Jansen PG, Hoek FJ, et al: Intestinal permeability, circulating endotoxin, and postoperative systemic responses in cardiac surgery patients. J Cardiothorac Vasc Anesth 1996;10:187–194.
70. Bennett-Guerrero E, Ayuso L, Hamilton-Davies C, et al: Relationship of preoperative antiendotoxin core antibodies and adverse outcomes following cardiac surgery. JAMA 1997;277:646–650.
71. Meakins JL, Marshall JC: The gastrointestinal tract: the "motor" of MOF. Arch Surg 1986;121:197–201.
72. Corson RJ, Paterson IS, O'Dwyer STO, et al: Lower limb ischemia and reperfusion alters gut permeability. Eur J Vasc Surg 1992;6:158–163.
73. Gaussorgues P, Gueugniaud PY, Vedrinne JM, et al: Bacteremia following cardiac arrest and cardiopulmonary resuscitation. Intensive Care Med 1988;14:575–577.
74. Beckman JS, Beckman TW, Chen J, et al: Apparent hydroxyl radical production by peroxynitrite: implications for endothelial injury from nitric oxide and superoxide. Proc Natl Acad Sci USA 1990;87:1620–1624.
75. Van Bebber IPT, Boekholtz WK, Goris RJ, et al: Neutrophil function and lipid peroxidation in a rat model of multiple organ failure. J Surg Res 1989;47:471–475.
76. Wang JH, Redmond HP, Watson RW, Bouchier-Hayes D: Induction of human endothelial cell apoptosis requires both heat shock and oxidative stress responses. Am J Physiol 1997;272:C1543–1551.
77. Nuytinck JKS, Goris RJ, Weerts JG, et al: Generalized microvascular injury by activated complement and hypoxia: the basis of the adult respiratory distress syndrome and multiple organ failure? Br J Exp Pathol 1986;67:537–548.
78. Hopf HW, Hunt TK, West JM, et al: Tissue oxygen tension predicts the risk of wound infection in surgical patients. Arch Surg 1997;132:997–1004.
79. Allen DB, Maguire JJ, Mahdavian M, et al: Hypoxia and acidosis limit neutrophil bacterial killing mechanisms. Arch Surg 1997;132:991–996.
80. Shoemaker WC, Appel PL, Kram HB, et al: Elective trial of supranormal values of survivors as therapeutic goals in high-risk surgical patients. Chest 1988;94:1176–1186.
81. Hayes MA, Timmins AC, Yau EH, et al: Elevation of systemic oxygen delivery in the treatment of critically ill patients. N Engl J Med 1994;330:1717–1722.
82. Leverve XM, Mustafa I, Peronnet F: Pivotal role of lactate in aerobic energy metabolism. In: Vincent J-L (ed) Yearbook of Intensive Care and Emergency Medicine, 1998. Berlin, Springer-Verlag, 1998;588–598.
83. Ronco JJ, Fenwick JC, Tweeddale MG, et al: Identification of the critical oxygen delivery for anaerobic metabolism in critically ill septic and nonseptic humans. JAMA 1993;270:1724–1730.
84. Beerthuizen GIJM, Goris RJ, Beyer HJM, et al: Differences in regional oxygen supply, oxygen consumption and blood flow during the onset of E. coli sepsis. In: Schlag G, Redl H (eds) First Vienna Shock Forum. New York, Liss, 1987;495–502.
85. Lam C, Tyml K, Martin C, et al: Microvascular perfusion is impaired in a rat model of normotensive sepsis. J Clin Invest 1994;94:2077–2083.
86. Ince C, Sinaasappel M: Microcirculatory oxygenation and shunting in sepsis and shock. Crit Care Med 1999 (in press).

87. Lundblad R, Wang MY, Kvalheim G, et al: Granulocyte colony-stimulating factor improves myelopoiesis and host defense in fulminant intra-abdominal sepsis in rats. Shock 1995;4:68–73.
88. Toda H, Murata A, Matsuura N, et al: Therapeutic efficacy of granulocyte colony stimulating factor against rat cecal ligation and puncture model. Stem Cells 1993;11:228–234.
89. Nelson S, Belknap SM, Carlson RW, et al: A randomized controlled trial of filgrastim as an adjunct to antibiotics for treatment of hospitalized patients with community-acquired pneumonia: CAP Study Group. J Infect Dis 1998;178:1075–1080.
90. Echtenacher B, Mannel DN, Hultner L: Critical protective role of mast cells in a model of acute septic peritonitis. Nature 1996;381:75–77.
91. Nieuwenhuijzen GA, Knapen MF, Hendriks T, et al: Elimination of various subpopulations of macrophages and the development of multiple-organ dysfunction syndrome in mice. Arch Surg 1997;132:533–539.
92. Ziegler M, Fisher CJ, Sprung CL: Treatment of gram-negative bacteremia and septic shock with HA-1A human monoclonal antibody against endotoxin. N Engl J Med 1991;324:429–436.
93. Fisher CJ, Agosti JM, Opal SM, et al: Treatment of septic shock with the tumor necrosis factor receptor: Fc fusion protein. N Engl J Med 1996;334:1697–1702.
94. Christman JW, Holden EP, Blackwell TS: Strategies for blocking the systemic effects of cytokines in the sepsis syndrome. Crit Care Med 1995;23:955–963.
95. Bone RC, Fisher CJ Jr, Clemmer TP, et al: A controlled clinical trial of high-dose methylprednisolone in the treatment of severe sepsis and septic shock. N Engl J Med 1987;317:653–658.
96. Bernard GR, Luce JM, Sprung CL, et al: High-dose corticosteroids in patients with the adult respiratory distress syndrome. N Engl J Med 1987;317:1565–1570.
97. Bollaert PE, Charpentier C, Levy B, et al: Reversal of late septic shock with supraphysiologic doses of hydrocortisone. Crit Care Med 1998;26:645–650.
98. Meduri GU, Headley AS, Golden E, et al: Effect of prolonged methylprednisolone therapy in unresolving acute respiratory distress syndrome: a randomized controlled trial. JAMA 1998;280:159–165.

_8_
Cardiopulmonary Bypass for Cardiac Surgery: An Inflammatory Event: Can It Be Modulated?

Arthur E. Baue

The development of cardiopulmonary bypass by Gibbon and its first successful use by him in 1953 was followed by Kirklin popularizing the procedure for cardiac repair in 1955.[1] Following this report came the explosive development of cardiac surgery using cardiopulmonary bypass (CPB). There was also a major development of the technology of CPB, including pumps, oxygenators, filters, heat exchangers, cannulas, suction systems, cell savers, priming solutions, anticoagulation, cardioplegia, and myocardial protective solutions.

During all of these developments there was clinical recognition of remote organ malfunction of the lungs, kidneys, gastrointestinal (GI) tract including the liver, and central nervous system (CNS) with CPB. I remember in the early days the frequent postbypass (postoperative) pulmonary problems that seemed mysterious and were called "pump-lung." Other organ problems were in part related to generalized atherosclerosis in patients who underwent coronary artery bypass grafting (CABG).

Nonpulsatile Perfusion

Part of the problem was considered to be nonpulsatile blood flow with a roller pump. Pulsatile pumping devices were developed but were difficult to use and so were not accepted. We found no difference in brain function or perfusion with pulsatile or nonpulsatile perfusion.[2] There have been many other studies, and Edmunds concluded that there are "no conclusive data indicating nonpulsatile flow is detrimental for short-term perfusions lasting several hours at recommended flow rates."[1,3]

Pulmonary Changes After CPB

Hypoxemia after CPB for aortic valve replacement occurred regularly and was believed due to uneven distribution of ventilation and perfusion.[4] Others found similar changes.[5] McClenahan et al. found anatomic right-to-left shunting along with ventilation perfusion inequality after CPB.[6] Rea et al. measured increased venous admixture and airway and alveolar closure after open cardiac operations.[7] MacNaughton et al. measured deterioration in lung function after CPB, which was characterized by loss of lung volume and CO_2 transfer and an increase in the alveolar–arterial PO_2 gradient.[8] There were many early reports of deleterious effects engendered by CPB that were not seen in patients operated on without CPB.[9]

Inflammation with CPB

One of the earliest observations on abnormalities produced by CPB was the denaturation of plasma proteins, including those of the coagulation system, caused by contact of blood with foreign surfaces and the blood–gas interface.[10,11] These changes were associated with postoperative morbidity. There was also adsorption of plasma proteins onto the surface of the apparatus,[1] and complement levels were found to decrease with CPB, with the complement degradation products C3a and C5a[12,13] produced. These factors cause vasoconstriction and increased capillary permeability,[14] which led Kirklin et al. to propose the hypothesis that "a whole-body inflammatory reaction of variable magnitude develops as a result of CPB and that a transient damaging effect results."[15] They associated the damaging effects of CPB on the heart, lungs, kidneys, and coagulation with changes in the complement system. Pulmonary leukosequestration was a contributor to these effects.[13,15] These changes did not occur during heart or lung operations without CPB. Knowledge of other mediators and further study demonstrated that the inflammatory response to CPB not only activated complement and caused coagulation but activated the fibrinolytic and kallikrein cascades with leukocyte activation and platelet dysfunction.[16] The entire contact system was activated, including factors XII, XI, prekallikrein, and high-molecular-weight kininogen (HK).[1] Both the intrinsic and extrinsic coagulation systems are involved. Elastases are released, and antiproteases increase. Oxygen free radicals contribute to the damage. The cytokines involved include tumor necrosis factor (TNF) and interleukins, (IL-1, IL-6).[16] CPB is associated with high levels of catecholamines, thromboxane, vasopressin, and angiotensin II.[17–20] Endotoxin has also been found to be present

TABLE 8.1. Mediators Activated During CPB.

Catechloamines (epinephrine, norepinephrine)
Vasopressin
Aldosterone
Renin, angiotensin II
Glucagon
Bradykinin
Thyroid, T_4, T_3
Complement
Electrolytes: Ca^{2+}, Mg^{2+}, K^+
Prostaglandins (PGE_2, PGI_2)
Thromboxane H_2
Nitric oxide, endothelin-1
Serotonin
Histamine
Leukotrienes
Proteases
Oxygen radicals
Lysosomal enzymes
Cytokines: interleukins

TABLE 8.2. Control of Inflammatory Complications of CPB.

Surfaces of the tubing and apparatus with heparin binding or coating
Dipyridamole
Prostaglandins
Disintegrins
Aprotinin
Corticosteroids
Neutrophil depletion
Free radical scavengers—Vit C and E
Pentoxifylline
Factors XIIIa: attractive to block
Kallikrein: attractive to block
Factor Xa: attractive to block

during cardiopulmonary bypass.[21] Other mediators may be involved in this inflammatory response as well. (Table 8.1).

Effects of CPB on Organ Function

During bypass there is a reduction in gastric mucosal perfusion, as determined by gastric mucosal tonometry,[22] along with increased gut permeability and gut barrier dysfunction.[23] These changes may contribute to complications with the GI tract, already described.[24] In addition to the lung changes described earlier, there is increased pulmonary vascular permeability.[25] Bleeding may occur related to heparin, platelets, and fibrinolysis. Emboli and thrombi may be produced, and there may be massive fluid retention. Acute renal failure after CPB is most likely the result of preoperative renal limitation and hemodynamic factors, rather than CPB per se.[26] CPB may also alter CNS function, but most problems are due to hypoperfusion, emboli, microemboli, air embolism, and atherosclerotic debris.[1]

The heart may also be affected by CPB, but postoperative myocardial depression is difficult to distinguish from the operative effects on the heart. Cardiac injury may result from anti-heart antibodies, anti-actin antibodies, and anti-myosin antibodies.[27] Both cell-mediated and humoral-mediated immunity are depressed by CPB.[28] Complement activation is part of this process. Increased prostaglandin E_2 (PGE_2) which then decreases IL-2 development, occurs with CPB, as does a shift in T cells from the helper-T1 (Th1) subset to the Th2 subset.[29,30]

Treatment or Prevention of the Inflammatory Complications of CPB

A number of approaches have been evaluated to try to decrease inflammation or the response to it brought about by CPB. Methods evaluated clinically are listed in Table 8.2. A great effort has been devoted to developing a nonthrombogenic surface. Heparin binding or coating to plastics has yielded two commercial products: Duraflo II heparin coating with an ionic bond and Carmeda, a covalently binding coating. These products are useful in certain circumstances and may reduce the heparin dose but do not as yet eliminate anticoagulation.[31,32]

Dipyridamole can weakly inhibit platelet activation and preserve platelet function, but it is long-acting.[33] Prostaglandins and disintegrins are platelet inhibitors but also are powerful vasodilators.[34] They are still being studied.

Aprotinin is a natural serine protease inhibitor that partially inhibits kallikrein activation, complement, and neutrophils. It has reduced bleeding and the need for blood with CPB.[1] Pretreatment with corticosteroids has been reported to decrease lysosomal enzyme release and neutrophil elastase and TNF production. However, steroids do not inhibit complement activation, cellular defense is inhibited, and higher endotoxin levels have been reported.[16]

Neutrophil depletion has been evaluated extensively and protects against lung injury. This combined with platelet depletion also prevents the deterioration of cardiac function after CPB.[35] The need for catecholamines and sodium nitroprusside was also decreased.

Antioxidants such as α-tocopherol (vitamin E) and ascorbic acid (vitamin C) have been given as preoperative supplements to patients before heart operations. They have prevented depletion of the primary lipid-soluble antioxidant in the plasma but did not affect myocardial injury.[36] Superoxide dismutase, catalase, allopurinol, and mannitol may decrease the impact of activated neutrophils.[16]

Pentoxifylline has been effective in many animal studies, but in a clinical study it did not help.[37] IL-8 is known to activate neutrophils, and its level rises up with CPB. However, there was a large decrease in IL-8 binding affinity on neutrophils, suggesting a regulatory mechanism.[38]

Finally, Gott et al. used a multiagent approach to modify the inflammatory response to CPB.[39] Patients in whom heparin-bonded circuits were used had decreased complement activation, and leukocyte filtration reduced postpump leukocytosis. Patients who received aprotinin had less fibrinolysis. A fourth group received methylprenisolone preoperatively. Mortality in all groups was less than half that predicted by risk stratification.

Gott et al. now use leukoreduction for low risk patients, and they use leukocyte filtration for all blood products in all patients. Aprotinin is used for high risk patients and for reoperations. Corticosteroids are given preoperatively to all patients except those with diabetes. Heparin-bonded circuitry is reserved for patients with protamine problems.

Gu et al. studied minimally invasive coronary artery bypass grafting without CPB. They found a reduced inflammatory response, less morbidity, and a shorter hospital stay.[40]

Conclusions

Cardiopulmonary bypass produces a rather severe inflammatory reaction that can be a problem for patients with limited organ function, particularly of the lungs, liver, gut, kidneys, central nervous system, and heart. Many techniques to attenuate this response are now available and can be used. They are described in some detail. They seem to be effective in reducing the morbidity and mortality associated with cardiac operations using CPB.

References

1. Edmunds LH Jr: Cardiopulmonary bypass for open heart surgery. In: Baue AE, Geha AS, Hammond GL, Laks H, Naunheim KS (eds) Glenns Thoracic and Cardiovascular Surgery, 6th ed. Stamford, CT, Appleton & Lamge, 1996;163–165.
2. Geha AS, Salaymeh MT, Abe T, Baue AE: Effect of pulsatile cardiopulmonary bypass on cerebral metabolism. J Surg Res 1972;12:381–387.
3. Edmunds LH Jr: Pulseless cardiopulmonary bypass. J Thorac Cardiovasc Surg 1982;84:800–804.
4. Fordham RMM: Hypoxaemia after aortic valve surgery under cardiopulmonary bypass. Thorax 1965;20:505–509.
5. Hedley-Whyte J, Corning H, Laver MB, et al: Pulmonary ventilation-perfusion relations after heart valve replacement or repair in man. J Clin Invest 1965;44:406.
6. McClenahan JB, Young WE, Sykes MK: Respiratory changes after open-heart surgery. Thorax 1965;20:545.
7. Rea HH, Harris EA, Seelye ER, et al: The effects of cardiopulmonary bypass upon pulmonary gas exchange. J Thorac Cardiovasc Surg 1978;1:104.
8. MacNaughton PD, Braude S, Hunter DN, et al: Changes in lung function and pulmonary capillary permeability after cardiopulmonary bypass. Crit Care Med 1992;20:1289.
9. Anderson NB, Ghia J: Pulmonary function, cardiac status, and postoperative course in relation to cardiopulmonary bypass. J Thor Cardiovasc Surg 1970;59:474.
10. Lee WH Jr, Krumbhaar D, Fonkalsrud EW, et al: Denaturation of plasma proteins as a cause of morbidity and death after intracardiac operations. Surgery 1961;50:29.
11. Kalter RD, Saul CM, Wetstein L, et al: Cardiopulmonary bypass: associated hemostatic abnormalities. J Thorac Cardiovasc Surg 1979;77:427.
12. Parker DJ, Cantrell SW, Karp RB, et al: Changes in serum complement and immunoglobulins following cardiopulmonary bypass. Surgery 1972;71:824.
13. Chenowethy DE, Cooper SW, Hugli TE, et al: Complement activation during cardiopulmonary bypass: evidence for generation of C3a and C5a anaphylatoxins. N Engl J Med 1981;304:497.
14. Dias da Silva V, Eisele JW, Lepow IH: Complement as a mediator of inflammation. III. Purification of the activity with anaphylatoxin properties generated by interaction of the first four components and its identification as a cleavage product of C3. J Exp Med 1967;126:1027.
15. Kirklin JK, Westaby S, Blackstone EH, et al: Complement and the damaging effects of cardiopulmonary bypass. J Thorac Cardiovasc Surg 1983;86:845.
16. Butler J, Rocker GM, Westaby S: Inflammatory response to cardiopulmonary bypass. Ann Thorac Surg 1993;55:552.
17. Reves JG, Karp RB, Buttner EE, et al: Neuronal and adrenomedullary catecholamine release in response to cardiopulmonary bypass in man. Circulation 1982;66:49–55.
18. Davies GC, Sobel M, Salzman EW: Elevated plasma fibrinopeptide A and thromboxane B_2 levels during cardiopulmonary bypass. Circulation 1980;61:808.
19. Faymonville ME, Deby-Dupont G, Larbuisson R, et al: Prostaglandin E_2, prostacyclin, and thromboxane changes during non-pulsatile cardiopulmonary bypass in humans. J Thorac Cardiovasc Surg 1986;91:858.
20. Wu W, Zbuezek VK, Bellevue C: Vasopressin release during cardiac operation. J Thorac Cardiovasc Surg 1980;79:83.
21. Nilsson L, Kulander L, Nystrom SO, Eriksson O: Endotoxin in cardiopulmonary bypass. J Thorac Cardiovasc Surg 1990;100:77.
22. Gaer JA, Shaw AD, Wild R, et al: Effect of cardiopulmonary bypass on gastrointestinal perfusion and function. Ann Thorac Surg 1994;57:371.
23. Jones WG, Barber AE, Fahey TJ, et al: Cardiopulmonary bypass is associated with early gut barrier dysfunction. ACS Surg Forum 1991;42:282–284.
24. Baue AE: The role of the gut in the development of multiple organ dysfunction. Ann Thorac Surg 1993;55:822–828.
25. Messent M, Sinclair DG, Quinlan GJ, et al: Pulmonary vascular permeability after cardiopulmonary bypass and its relationship to oxidative stress. Crit Care Med 1997;25:425.
26. Zanardo G, Michielon P, Paccagnella A, et al: Acute renal failure in the patient undergoing cardiac operation. J Thorac Cardiovasc Surg 1994;107:1489–1495.
27. DeScheerder I, Vandekerckhove J, Robbrecht J, et al: Post-cardiac injury syndrome and an increased humoral immune response against the major contractile proteins (actin and myosin). Am J Cardiol 1985;56:631.
28. Tajima K, Yamamoto F, Kawazoe K, et al: Cardiopulmonary bypass and cellular immunity: changes in lymphocyte subsets and natural killer cell activity. Ann Thorac Surg 1993;55:625.
29. Faist E, Schinkel C, Zimmer S: Inadequate interleukin-2 synthesis and interleukin-2 messenger expression following thermal and mechanical trauma in human is caused by defective transmembrane signaling. J Trauma 1993;6:1–9.
30. Faist E, Schinkel C, Zimmer S: Update on the mechanisms of immune suppression of injury and immune modulation. World J Surg 1996;20:454–459.
31. Videm V, Svennevig JL, Fosse E, et al: Reduced complement activation with heparin-coated oxygenator and tubings in coronary bypass operations. J Thorac Cardiovasc Surg 1992;103:806–813.
32. Borowiec J, Thelin S, Bagge L, et al: Decreased blood loss after cardiopulmonary bypass using heparin-coated circuit and 50%

reduction of heparin dose. Scand J Thorac Cardiovasc Surg 1992;26:177–185.
33. Teoh KH, Chistakis GT, Weisel RD, et al: Dipyridamole preserved platelets and reduced blood loss after cardiopulmonary bypass. J Thorac Cardiovasc Surg 1998;96:332–341.
34. Musial J, Niewiarowski S, Rucinski B, et al: Inhibition of platelet adhesion to surfaces of extracorporeal circuits by disintegrins. Circulation 1990;82:261–273.
35. Chiba Y, Morioka K, Muraoka R, et al: Effects of depletion of leukocytes and platelets on cardiac dysfunction after cardiopulmonary bypass. Ann Thorac Surg 1998;65:107.
36. Westhuyzen J, Cochrane AD, Tesar PJ, et al: Effect of preoperative supplementation with α-tocopherol and ascorbic acid on myocardial injury in patients undergoing cardiac operations. J Thorac Cardiovasc Surg 1997;113:942.
37. Butler J, Baigrie RJ, Parker D, et al: Systemic inflammatory response to cardiopulmonary bypass: a pilot study of the effects of pentoxifylline. Resp Med (in press).
38. Ng T, Gibson F, Nye KE, et al: Desensitization of the inflammatory response in humans: changes in response to cardiopulmonary bypass. Shock 1997;8:159–164.
39. Gott JP, Cooper WA, Schmidt FE Jr, et al: Modifying risk for extracorporeal circulation: trial of four antiinflammatory strategies. Ann Thorac Surg 1998;66:747.
40. Gu YJ, Mariani MA, van Oeveren W, Grandjean JG, Boonstra PW: Reduction of the inflammatory response in patients undergoing minimally invasive coronary artery bypass grafting. Ann Thorac Surg 1998;65:420.

9
Gut: Clinical Importance of Bacterial Translocation, Permeability, and Other Factors

Andrew M. Munster

In 1964 it was observed that small microscopic particles could be absorbed from the intestinal canal into the mesenteric circulation and into the lymphatics of the gastrointestinal tract.[1] This phenomenon was termed "persorption." Shortly after these observations, a technique was developed for the quantitative measurement of endotoxin in human plasma using the lysate technique of the horseshoe crab *Limulus*.[2] It was next demonstrated that tissue homogenates obtained postmortem had measurable levels of endotoxin in 20 of 35 patients, particularly following major trauma, gastrointestinal (GI) bleeding, and liver injury. The findings were explained on the basis of failure of the reticuloendothelial system of the liver to detoxify circulating endotoxin of intestinal origin.

At the same time, in animal experiments involving New Zealand rabbits, it was found that large cutaneous burns caused death due to the absorption of endotoxin from the GI tract, and at death the liver and blood contained endotoxin and gram-negative bacteria. Endotoxemia could be lessened or prevented by resuscitation and by topical treatment of the burned skin with antibiotics. If the GI tract of the rabbit was sterilized, translocational endotoxemia did not occur.[3] It was subsequently shown that resistance to the effects of absorbed endotoxins could be increased by immunization with small doses of endotoxin given prior to the administration of lethal doses.[4]

By the mid-1980s the concept of translocation of gram-negative bacteria and endotoxin from the lumen of the intestine to the mesenteric nodes and then to the portal system and the systemic circulation was well established.[5,6] By the early 1990s it was generally accepted that increases in intestinal permeability allowing translocation of endotoxin and gram-negative bacteria was harmful to the organism and probably played a role in the induction of multisystem failure as a complication of diverse major insults and injuries.[7] There were some negative reports, however; Moore et al. failed to demonstrate the presence of endotoxin or GI bacteria in the portal system of patients who had injuries severe enough to merit surgical exploration.[8]

At the end of the first 20 years of research, the framework encompassing translocation and its consequences was that following conditions of relative intestinal ischemia, whether due to shock induced by hemorrhage, trauma, or major burns or to direct interference with intestinal circulation (e.g., superior mesenteric artery occlusion), intestinal permeability increased; and as part of this pathologic change gram-negative bacterial products normally resident in the intestinal lumen as well as endotoxin would readily translocate submucosally to the mesenteric nodes and from there to the portal circulation, the liver, and the systemic circulation. There was general agreement that this phenomenon of translocation could be at least partially instrumental in the induction of the proinflammatory cytokine cascade with major deleterious effects on the host. Experiments were beginning to show that other variables influenced the occurrence and outcome of translocation as well. There was not, however, clear agreement on whether the phenomenon of translocation was an incidental event or represented a major primary pathogenic event after injury.

Current Status

Increased intestinal permeability following injury, shock, hemorrhage, and burns is now well documented. Ziegler and associates found increased permeability to lactulose in patients with large burns,[9] and this finding was confirmed using an essentially similar technique by Deitch.[10] In most patients with injuries, of course, clinical examination of the intestinal mucosa is not possible; however, when autopsy material was examined in one study, pathologic changes were found in 53% of adults and 61% of children, and it ranged from superficial necrosis to full-thickness mucosal necrosis.[11] Furthermore, this increased permeability seems to have clinical relevance: LeeVoyer et al. studied intestinal permeability in patients with clinical infections and found a significant correlation between the increased rate of infection and increased intestinal permeability, as measured by the lactulose/mannitol ratio.[12] Increased intestinal permeability leads to the translocation of bacteria and bacterial products and the appearance of proinflammatory cytokines in the portal and systemic circulations. Using a rat model of hemorrhagic shock, Jiang and others reported translocation in the small intestinal wall within 30 minutes of resuscitation, a significant increase in lipopolysaccharide (LPS) in the portal vein at 90 minutes, and a simultaneous significant elevation of tumor necrosis factor (TNF) in the portal and systemic circulations.[13] In patients with intestinal ischemia, the clinical course of the disease, as measured by the Acute Physiology and Chronic Health Evaluation (APACHE II) scores and Septic Severity Scores could be correlated with endotoxin concentrations in both peritoneal exudate and plasma.[14]

In addition to passage of bacteria and bacterial products through the mucosa and the intestinal wall itself, absorption into the GI lymphatic circulation appears to be a significant source of systemic endotoxin.[15] That the effect of translocating bacteria and LPS may be dominantly local is supported by the finding that although the thoracic duct of multiple organ failure (MOF) patients did not contain significantly more endotoxin than controls markedly high levels of antiinflammatory cytokines and cytokine antagonists were found in the thoracic duct lymph, suggesting local induction and an attempt at downregulation.[16] In patients with thermal injury, burn size is known to be correlated with the degree of systemic endotoxemia.[17] In addition, endotoxemia has been correlated with the development of MFO.[18] In the absence of other sources of sepsis (e.g., wound, lung), endotoxemia of GI origin, at least in an experimental situation, clears by 96 hours after injury.[19]

Unfortunately, at least from the interventional point of view, it is not clear whether endotoxin or endotoxin-like substances alone, other factors, or both are responsible for the developments and complications seen after portal and systemic endotoxemia have occurred. One of the reasons is that there is a rich mesenteric synthesis of inflammatory cytokines after shock of various types. Tamion et al. investigated the relation between intestinal ischemia/reperfusion and cytokine release in rat models of hemorrhagic and endotoxin shock and found that in hemorrhagic shock proinflammatory cytokines were much increased, but endotoxin was not detectable. Their data suggest that a cytokine-mediated mechanism may be triggered by ischemia/reperfusion injury that is independent of translocation.[20] Similarly, Carsin et al., in a clinical study of patients with large burns, correlated mortality with interleukin-6 (IL-6) and procalcitonin levels but not with endotoxin levels.[21] In a pig model of hemorrhagic and superior mesenteric artery occlusion shock, Schlichting et al. demonstrated mucosal alteration and necrosis, with increased intestinal permeability but no significant elevation in the endotoxin of ascitic fluid,[22] again suggesting that other mechanisms may also be involved. Kelly et al. studied samples of peripheral blood from 10 patients with large burns and 8 trauma patients with an Injury Severity Score (ISS) of 25–57; there was another study using a mouse model with 25% body surface burn injury. There was no increased production of cytokines in either group, nor did measured levels of LPS correlate with complications or mortality in either the human experiments or the animal model.[23] There is some evidence that bacterial translocation in response to LPS challenge may be mediated by inducible nitric oxide synthase.[24]

Finally, the role of the local mucosal T lymphocyte has been investigated, as these cells appear to be responsible for the immunologic protection of the GI mucosa. Mucosal T cells undergo regular apoptosis, and this apoptosis is increased in a septic model. However, increased apoptosis did not occur in Fas ligand-deficient mice, producing some evidence that the mechanism of damage may be mediated through a pathway involving the Fas ligand, rather than a known pathway of binding of endotoxin. The Fas ligand pathway is one of a number of signals leading to the apoptosis of activated T cells; there are many others that remain incompletely studied.[25]

Other factors play a role in bacterial translocation, including some intriguing evidence that genetic influences may be involved. In mice, susceptibility can be correlated not only with the composition of intestinal microflora but their strain.[26] Sepsis of other origin also promotes intestinal translocation,[27] although the mechanism for this effect is not clear. One of the mechanisms may be increased bacterial adherence to the mucosa; protein malnutrition was found to diminish bacterial translocation because of a diminution in mucosa-associated and adherent levels of the bacterial population.[28] In experimental models elevation in gastric pH levels by the administration of H_2-receptor blockers also appears to promote bacterial translocation.[29]

There is evidence that induction of the cytokine cascade following hemorrhage may be independent of translocation endotoxemia. Ayala et al., in a model of hemorrhagic shock in mice, found that markedly elevated TNF levels were not matched by similar elevations in serum endotoxin concentration.[30] More recently, Tamion et al. reported increases in TNF and IL-6 production after hemorrhagic shock and resuscitation; endotoxin remained undetectable.[20] The effects of ischemia/reperfusion injury may therefore act as a second trigger for the induction of cytokines, independent of translocation of bacteria or their products.

Finally, the effect of translocation on prostaglandin metabolism and, conversely, the alterations in prostaglandin synthesis and breakdown following shock, trauma, sepsis, and burns appear to be potentially important. Additionally, there is increasing evidence that not only lymphocyte and macrophage populations of the GI tract but enterocytes in crypts are capable of producing proinflammatory cytokines and prostaglandin E_2 (PGE_2). Culture studies have shown that the most active cells were closer to the crypts away from the tip of the small intestinal villus and produced TNF, IL-1, IL-6, and PGE_2.[31] It has been reported that endotoxin inhibits prostaglandin 15-hydroxydehydrogenase, an enzyme responsible for PGE_2 degradation, leading to sepsis-induced increases in PGE_2 levels, which appear to be deleterious to the host's ability to resist septic complications. Because, in addition to their metabolic effects, the prostaglandins also affect the intestinal microcirculation, these findings may affect interventional approaches.[32] This subject is discussed in the next section.

Potential for Intervention

In view of the nature and effect of bacterial translocation, it is understandable that interventions, particularly in human models, have been remarkably unsuccessful to date in affecting the final clinical manifestation of endotoxemia and cytokinemia, which is multiple organ failure (MOF) and death. The picture is not totally bleak: Several interventional models have been studied, and some appear promising. Recombinant murine granulocyte/macrophage colony-stimulating factor (GM-CSF) improves gut barrier function and enhances killing of translocational organisms, with an improved outcome in a murine cecal ligation and puncture model.[33] Because bactericidal/permeability increasing protein (BT) binds lipopolysaccharide (LPS), attempts have been made to control translocation in a burn model[34] and in a hemorrhage-induced translocation model in rats.[35] In both models, improvements were noted in the incidence of translocation and in organ damage as a result of translocation. In a model of hemorrhage in rats, low-dose polymyxin B, an antibiotic that directly binds LPS, inhibited bacterial translocation and cytokine induction from translocation when used as pretreatment.[36] Depressed Kupffer cell function can be improved and increased inflammatory cytokine release by Kupffer cells significantly downregulated by treating animals subjected to various models of hemorrhage with a number of agents, including chloroquine, ibuprofen, diltiazem, and ATP-$MgCl_2$; whether these effects are due to improved clearance or decreased translocation is not known.[37] In a model of hemorrhagic shock plus LPS administration, monoclonal endotoxin antibody attenuated the mortality and lung injury seen in the controls.[38]

Nitric oxide, as previously mentioned, may also play a role in bacterial translocation. In one report vascular permeability was suppressed for 3 hours after thermal injury to the ear by prophylactic administration of nitric oxide synthase inhibitors.[39] Similarly, inhibition of nitric oxide activity with NG-monomethyl-L-arginine in a rat translocation model prevented endotoxin-induced ileal injury and translocation.[40] From a practical clinical point of view, it would be important to know the effect of vasopressor agents in common clinical usage on bacterial translocation. In a porcine experiment, epinephrine appeared to cause the most reduction in mucosal pH, the most mucosal damage, and the highest level of translocation when compared with norepinephrine and dopexamine.[41] It has been postulated that lactulose, believed to reduce bacterial translocation, could benefit the shock state not only by reducing translocation but also by inhibiting Kupffer cell release of inflammatory mediators.[42] Available data are far more limited for humans. Six burn patients were given the anticholinergic drug anisodamine to reduce splanchnic vasoconstriction due to hypovolemia. Plasma endotoxin and TNF contents were measured at 72 hours and were significantly lower than those of eight burn size-matched controls.[43] Because GI vasoconstriction in the shock state is a recognized cause of increased permeability and translocation, this avenue is certainly an interesting one to pursue.

There has been long-standing interest in the removal of endotoxin from the circulation or its neutralization, the latest strategies for which have focused on extracorporeal absorption. Endotoxin can be removed from the circulation by selective affinity sorbents such as histidine, histamine, or polymyxin B or by nonselective adsorbents such as charcoal.[44] The techniques using such sorbents vary and may include plasmasorption, hemadsorption, or hemoperfusion. Cheadle et al. reported good results with polymyxin B bound to polystyrene fiber, with substantial removal of biologically active endotoxin in a murine model.[45] To reduce toxicity, the continuation of polymyxin B with dextran[46] and with human immunoglobulin G (I_gG)[47] both show sustantial promise. The technique of hemoperfusion using an immobilized polymyxin B-fiber column has gained substantial popularity in Japan.[48]

Direct binding of LPS with anti-LPS antibody has been attempted in 60 patients with large burns. Administration of anti-LPS I_gG resulted in a particularly significant fall in endotoxin levels during the first week and a rise in the anti-endotoxin levels; but it failed to demonstrate a reduction in the mortality rate.[49] At the Baltimore Regional Burn Center, extensive animal and human trials using polymyxin B in small doses have been conducted for a number of years in an attempt to reduce measurable plasma endotoxin levels and subsequent cytokine induction.[50] A clinical sepsis scale was developed; IL-6 levels were measured as the index cytokine; and plasma endotoxin concentrations were assayed. The end result of a series of prospective, randomized trials essentially showed that although systemic endotoxemia was successfully contained by polymyxin B therapy such therapy did not affect the cytokine cascade, the occurrence of clinical septic complications, or the mortality rate. Others have reported a reduction of IL-6 levels with a beneficial effect on postburn catabolism.[51]

More recently, we completed a prospective randomized trial in which all patients with burns of more than 20% of body surface received polymyxin B for 5 days; they were randomized into two prospective groups to receive or not to receive 48 hours of ibuprofen intravenously as well. The results of this trial showed that the administration of ibuprofen significantly reduced IL-6 concentrations and the incidence of septic complications, but translocational endotoxemia, in fact rose by a significant degree. There was again no impact on ultimate outcome in terms of survival or death.[52]

This observation was interestingly confirmed in a different setting. In a group of 50 patients undergoing major abdominal surgery, the effect of mesenteric traction was compared for those who received or did not receive preoperative intravenous ibuprofen; it was found that plasma endotoxin concentrations were significantly higher in the ibuprofen group. This increase appears to be associated with the perioperative release of endogenous prostacyclin and the blockage of this release by the administration of ibuprofen.[53] Here again is evidence of the dissociation between the biologic effects induced by the triggering of the arachidonic acid or cytokine cascades (or both) and the effects induced by bacterial translocation.

Finally, there have been several concerns by investigators and clinicians that the reason reduction of systemic endotoxemia has not successfully controlled the triggering of the inflammatory cascades is that the scenario is played out at the mucosal level, the submucosal level, or perhaps at the level of the lymphatic system of the GI tract. If this is true, one could presume that induction of the cascade in fact takes place at a location where the delivery of antiendotoxin agents in adequate concentrations would be difficult. Following this line of reasoning to a logical conclusion, one is led back inevitably to the concept of intestinal sterilization, an old one, to reduce the load of bacteria that might translocate. Unfortunately, there has never been convincing evidence that reducing the intestinal bacterial load reduces mortality, even though it might reduce translocation.

In a rat model of burn wound sepsis, Jones et al. succeeded in reducing the incidence of bacterial translocation with intestinal decontamination using oral antibiotics but could not affect the 14-day mortality or the incidence of burn wound sepsis.[54] In a more recent study on respirator-dependent patients in a medical-surgical intensive care unit, no substantial benefit could be shown from selective digestive decontamination.[55] Similar findings have been reported by Lingnau et al. for a large group of trauma patients.[56] This approach therefore has not been any more useful to date than systemic control.

Most recently, a new 30-kDa protein has been described, induced in macrophages by TNF and IL-1β and induced to high levels by endotoxin. It may represent a new pathway for triggering or continuing the inflammatory cascade, which may be amenable to intervention.[57] A newly reported class of compounds, the pyridinyl imidazoles, inhibit cytokine biosynthesis. One of these, FR167653, reduces LPS-induced synthesis of PGE_2 by inhibiting cyclooxygenase 2 production as well as IL-1β and TNFα production.[58] These compounds remain to be explored in the clinical arena.

Conclusions

It seems clear, based on work to date, that induction of the potentially lethal proinflammatory cascades following major injury has at least two arms: one related to the wound or the injury itself, and another related to bacterial and endotoxin translocation, at least in part due to the relative vasoconstriction of the intestine that follows major injury. Furthermore, it seems that what is measurable in serum or plasma is only an aftereffect of events occurring at the level of the GI tract and its environs or the wound and its environs. In addition, the long-studied diminution of the ability of the reticuloendothelial system to clear endotoxin and other toxic products, particularly in the liver, probably also plays an important role. For an intervention to be successful, therefore, it follows logically that both systems, or "arms," would have to be manipulated. Although we do not yet fully understand the mechanism by which a wound induces the inflammatory reaction, there is evidence that locally generated neurokinases have a role in macrophage induction, and it is possible that antagonists to this pathway may be found. Alternatively, it may be possible to develop biologic agents with such low toxicity that they can be delivered systemically in high enough concentrations to reach significant concentrations in the mesenteric circulation, or at least in portal venous blood, so endotoxin and other products do not overwhelm the clearing mechanisms of the liver. It may be possible to develop pharmacologic mechanisms for protecting the GI tract against posttraumatic ischemia/reperfusion injury; or at the systemic level, a combination of agents including antiendotoxin and anticytokine agents may be successful in a clinical setting. Intense research in this area must continue, as the price of failure is high.

References

1. Volkheimer G: Der Uebergang kleiner fester theilchen aus dem darmacanal in den milchsaft und das blut. Wien Med Wochenschr 1964;114:915–923.
2. Reinhold RB, Fine J: A technique for quantitative measurement of endotoxin in human plasma. Proc Soc Exp Biol Med 1971;137:334–340.
3. Woodruff PW, O'Carroll DI, Koizumi S, Fine J: Role of the intestinal flora in major trauma. J Infect Dis 1973; 128 (suppl): 290–294.
4. Cuevas P, Fine J, Monaco AP: Successful induction of increased resistance to gram-negative bacteria and to endotoxin in immunosuppressed mice. Am J Surg 1974;127:460–464.
5. Deitch EA, Winterton J, Li M, Berg R: The gut as a portal of entry for bacteremia: role of protein malnutrition. Ann Surg 1985;205:690.
6. Rush BF Jr, Sori AJ, Murphy TF, Smith S, Flanagan JJ Jr, Machiedo GW: Endotoxemia and bacteremia during hemorrhagic shock: the link between trauma and sepsis? Ann Surg 1988;207:549–554.
7. Baue AE: The horror autotoxicus and multiple-organ failure. Arch Surg 1992;127:1451–1462.
8. Moore FA, Moore EE, Puggetti E, et al: Gut bacterial translocation via the portal vein: a clinical perspective with major torso trauma. J Trauma 1991;31:629–638.
9. Ziegler TR, Smith RJ, O'Dwyer ST, Demling RH, Wilmore DW: Increased intestinal permeability associated with infection in burn patients. Arch Surg 1988;123:1313.
10. Deitch EA: Intestinal permeability is increased in burn patients shortly after injury. Surgery 1990;107:411.
11. Desai MH, Herndon DN, Rutan RL, Abston S, Linares HA: Ischemic intestinal complications in patients with burns. Surg Gynecol Obstet 1991;172:257–261.
12. LeeVoyer T, Cioffi WG, Pratt L, et al: Alterations in intestinal permeability after thermal injury. Arch Surg 1992;127:26.
13. Jiang J, Bahrami S, Leichtfried G, Redl H, Ohlinger W, Schlag G: Kinetics of endotoxin and tumor necrosis factor appearance in portal and systemic circulation after hemorrhagic shock in rats. Ann Surg 1995;221:100–106.
14. Schoeffel U, Baumgartner U, Imdahl A, Haering R, von Specht BU, Farthmann EH: The influence of ischemic bowel wall damage on translocation, inflammatory response, and clinical course. Am J Surg 1997;174:39–44.
15. Peng Y, Xiao GX, Ma L: Intestinal lymphatic circulation is one of the important portals for microbial translocation after thermal injury. Chin J Plastic Surg Burns 1996;12(2):83–85.
16. Lemaire LCJM, van Lanschot JB, Stoutenbeek CP, et al: Thoracic duct in patients with multiple organ failure: no major route of bacterial translocation. Ann Surg 1999;229:128–136.
17. Winchurch RA, Thupari JN, Munster AM: Endotoxemia in burn patients: levels of circulating endotoxins are related to burn size. Surgery 1987;102:808.

18. Yao YM, Sheng ZY, Tian HM, et al: The association of circulating endotoxemia with the development of multiple organ failure in burned patients. Burns 1995;21:255–258.
19. Tokyay R, Zeigler ST, Heggers JP, Loick HM, Traber DL, Herndon DN: Effects of anesthesia, surgery, fluid resuscitation and endotoxin administration on postburn bacterial translocation. J Trauma 1991;31:1376.
20. Tamion F, Richard V, Lyoumi S, Daveau M, Bonmarchang G, Leroy J: Gut ischemia and mesenteric synthesis of inflammatory cytokines after hemorrhagic or endotoxic shock. Am J Physiol 1997;273:G314–321.
21. Carsin H, Assicot M, Feger F, et al: Evolution and significance of circulating procalcitonin levels compared with IL-6, TNF alpha and endotoxin levels early after thermal injury. Burns 1997;23:218–224.
22. Schlichting E, Grotmol T, Kahler H, Naess O, Steinbakk M, Lyberg T: Alterations in mucosal morphology and permeability, but no bacterial or endotoxin translocation takes place after intestinal ischemia and early reperfusion in pigs. Shock 1995;3:116–124, .
23. Kelly JL, O'Sullivan C, O'Riordain M, et al: Is circulating endotoxin the trigger for the systemic inflammatory response syndrome seen after injury? Ann Surg 1997;225:530–541.
24. Mishima S, Xu D, Lu Q, Deitch EA: Bacterial translocation is inhibited in inducible nitric oxide synthase knockout mice after endotoxin challenge but not in a model of bacterial overgrowth. Arch Surg 1997;132:1190–1195.
25. Chung C-S, Xu YX, Wang W, Chaudry IH, Ayala A: Is Fas Ligan or endotoxin responsible for mucosal lymphocyte apoptosis in sepsis? Arch Surg 1998;133:1213–1220.
26. Deitch EA, Ma I, Ma J-W, Berg RD: Lethal burn-induced bacterial translocation: role of genetic resistance. J Trauma 1989;29:1480–1487.
27. Jones WG II, Minei JP, Barber AE, et al: Bacterial translocation and intestinal atrophy after thermal injury and burn wound sepsis. Ann Surg 1990;211:399.
28. Katayama M, Xu D, Specian RD, Deitch EA: Role of bacterial adherence and the mucus barrier on bacterial translocation: effects of protein malnutrition and endotoxin in rats. Ann Surg 1997;225:317–326.
29. Avanoglu A, Herek O, Ulman I, et al: Effects of H_2 receptor blocking agents on bacterial translocation in burn injury. Eur J Pediatr Surg 1997;7:278–281.
30. Ayala A, Perrin MM, Meldrum DR, Ertel W, Chaudry IH: Hemorrhage induces an increase in serum TNF which is not associated with elevated levels of endotoxin. Cytokine 1990;2:170–174.
31. Ogle CK, Mao JC, Hasselgren PO, Ogle JD, Alexander JW: Production of cytokines and prostaglandin E_2 by subpopulations of guinea pig enterocytes: effect of endotoxin and thermal injury. J Trauma 1996;41:298–305.
32. Hahn EL, Clancy KD, Tai HH, Ricken JD, He LK, Gamelli RL: Prostaglandin E_2 alterations during sepsis are partially mediated by endotoxin-induced inhibition of prostaglandin 15-hydroxydehydrogenase. J Trauma 1998;44:777–781.
33. Gennari R, Alexander JW, Gianotti L, Eaves-Pyles T, Hartmann S: Granulocyte macrophage colony-stimulating factor improves survival in two models of gut-derived sepsis by improving gut barrier function and modulating bacterial clearance. Ann Surg 1994;220:68–76.
34. Rennekampff OH, Tenenhaus M, Hansbrough J, Kiessig V, Zapata-Sirvent RL: Effects of recombinant bactericidal, permeability-increasing protein on bacterial translocation and pulmonary neutrophil sequestration in burned mice. J Burn Care Rehabil 1997;18:17–21.
35. Yao YM, Bahrami S, Leichtfried G, Redl H, Schlag G: Pathogenesis of hemorrhage-induced bacteria/endotoxin translocation in rats. Effects of recombinant bactericidal/permeability-increasing protein. Ann Surg 1995;221:398–405.
36. Yao YM, Tian HM, Sheng ZY, et al: Inhibitory effects of low-dose polymyxin B on hemorrhage-induced endotoxin/bacterial translocation and cytokine formation in rats. J Trauma 1995;38:924–930.
37. Chaudry IH, Zellweger R, Ayala A: The role of bacterial translocation on Kupffer cell immune function following hemorrhage. Prog Clin Biol Res 1995;392:209–218.
38. Bahrami S, Yao YM, Leichtfried G, Redl H, Schlag G, Di Padova FE: Monoclonal antibody to endotoxin attenuates hemorrhage-induced lung injury and mortality in rats. Crit Care Med 1997;25:1030–1036.
39. Sozumi T: The role of nitric oxide in vascular permeability after a thermal injury. Ann Plast Surg 1997;39:272–277.
40. Mishima S, Xu D, Lu Q, Deitch EA: The relationships among nitric oxide production, bacterial translocation, and intestinal injury after endotoxin challenge in vivo. J Trauma 1998;44:175–182.
41. Sautner T, Wessely C, Riegler M, et al: Early effects of catecholamine therapy on mucosal integrity, intestinal blood flow, and oxygen metabolism in porcine endotoxin shock. Ann Surg 1998;228:239–248.
42. Hartung T, Sauer A, Hermann C, Brockhaus F, Wendel A: Overactivation of the immune system by translocated bacteria and bacterial products. Scand J Gastroenterol Suppl 1997;222:98–99.
43. Sheng CY, Gao WY, Guo ZR, He LX: Anisodamine restores bowel circulation in burn shock. Burns 1997;23:142–146.
44. Anspach FB, Hilbeck O: Removal of endotoxins by affinity sorbents. J Chromatogr A 1995;711:81–92.
45. Cheadle WG, Hanasawa K, Gallinaro RN, Nimmanwudipong T, Kodama M, Polk HC: Endotoxin filtration and immune stimulation improve survival from gram-negative sepsis. Surgery 1991;110:785–792.
46. Doig GS, Martin CM, Sibbald WJ: Polymyxin-dextran antiendotoxin pretreatment in an ovine model of normotensive sepsis. Crit Care Med 1997;25:1956–1961.
47. Drabick JJ, Bhattacharjee AK, Hoover DL, et al: Covalent polymyxin B conjugate with human immunoglobulin G as an antiendotoxin reagent. Antimicrob Agents Chemother 1998;42:583–588.
48. Iwama H, Komatsu T: Effect of an endotoxin-removing column containing immobilized polymyxin B fiber in a patient with septic shock from gram-positive infection. Acta Anaesthesiol Scand 1998;42:590–593.
49. Jones EB: Prophylactic anti-lipopolysaccharide freeze-dried plasma in major burns: a double blind controlled trial. Burns 1995;21:267–272.
50. Munster AM, Smith-Meek M, Dickerson C, Winchurch RA: Translocation: incidental phenomenon or true pathology? Ann Surg 1993;218:321–327.
51. Cone JB, Wallace BH, Lubansky HJ, Caldwell FT: Manipulation of the inflammatory response to burn injury. J Trauma 1997;43:41–45.

52. Smith-Meek M, Munster AM, Dickerson C, Winchurch RA: Ibuprofen increases endotoxemia but downregulates the cytokine cascade in burn patients. Presented at the 31st Annual Meeting of the American Burn Association, Orlando, FL, March 24–27 1999.

53. Brinkmann A, Wolf CF, Berger D, et al: Perioperative endotoxemia and bacterial translocation during major abdominal surgery: evidence for the protective effect of endogenous prostacyclin? Crit Care Med 1996;24:1293–1301.

54. Jones WG II, Barber AE, Minei JP, Fahey TJ, Shires GT III, Shires GT: Antibiotic prophylaxis diminishes bacterial translocation but not mortality in experimental burn wound sepsis. J Trauma 1990;20:737.

55. Wiener J, Itokazu G, Nathan C, Kabins SA, Weinstein RA: A randomized, double-blind, placebo-controlled trial of selective digestive decontamination in a medical-surgical intensive care unit. Clin Infect Dis 1995;20:861–867.

56. Lingnau W, Berger J, Javorsky F, Lejeune P, Mutz N, Benzer H: Selective intestinal decontamination in multiple trauma patients: prospective, controlled trial. J Trauma 1997;42:687–694.

57. Wang H, Bloom O, Zhang M, et al: A 30 kDa protein, p30, is a mediator of lethality during endotoxemia. Presented at the 1999 Annual Meeting of the SUS, February 11–13, New Orleans.

58. Kawano T, Ogushi F, Tani K, et al: Comparison of suppressive effects of a new anti-inflammatory compound, FR167653, on production of PGE_2 and inflammatory cytokines, human monocytes, and alveolar macrophages in response to endotoxin. J Leukoc Biol 1999;65:80–86.

10
Microcirculatory Arrest Theory of SIRS and MODS

Donald E. Fry

Soft tissue injury and soft tissue infection activate the inflammatory response. Indeed, it is the response of the host and not the characteristics of the pathogen in a wound infection that is responsible for the clinical signs of infection in a soft tissue wound.[1] Hyperemia, induration, heat, and pain, the cardinal signs of infection, are representations of elements of inflammation and are not specific to infection. Infection at any anatomic site can be defined as local activation of the human inflammatory response by proliferation of microbial pathogens in soft tissue. Local activation of the human inflammatory response has, as its biologic purpose, the containment and eradication of microbial invaders. Not uncommonly, the pathogenic inoculum may exceed the eradication capacity (i.e., phagocytic capacity) of the response, and abscess is the result. Nevertheless, the foremost response of containment makes abscess of possible and avoids the perilous and commonly fatal systemic access of the pathogens. Whereas local failure phagocytic function is still a resolvable circumstance for the host, in biologic terms systemic access is not, making containment the most critical function of the human inflammatory response.

The systemic inflammatory response syndrome (SIRS) represents the clinical situation where the containment function of inflammation has failed. Such failed containment of a clinical infection may occur when: (1) the microbial pathogen has broken through containment defenses and gained systemic access to the host; (2) pathogenic endotoxins or exotoxins produced by the pathogen have been systemically liberated even though the whole organism per se may be contained at the local site; or (3) the local inflammatory response has successfully contained the microbial cell and cell products, but the intensity of the local response results in the systemic distribution of mediator signals (e.g., chemoattractants, chemokines, or cytokines).

A corollary of the latter mechanism are the proinflammatory events of sufficient intensity that vast quantities of liberated mediator signals could provoke systemic inflammation even without the presence of any microorganisms whatsoever. Examples of the latter scenario include severe multisystem trauma[2], thermal injury[3], and fulminant acute pancreatitis.[4]

Yet another scenario may result in systemic activation of inflammation due to dissemination of microbes or microbial cell products but without clinical infection. Fine et al. proposed the gut as a reservoir for microbial dissemination during shock states.[5,6] The concept has been resurrected, and some experimental and clinical data suggest the existence of microbial translocation as a potential stimulus to SIRS, but as a result of failed containment by the gut barrier rather than by invasive infection.[7-10]

A working definition of SIRS then becomes the systemic activation of the human inflammatory response secondary to the failure of containment of microbes, microbial cell products, or mediator signals from a local inflammatory event. It is the premise of this discussion that all of the salutary benefits of inflammation as a local event become autodestructive when activated systemically,[11] leading to multiple organ dysfunction syndrome (MODS) as the clinical expression of SIRS.[12] All of the biologic mediators activated by the wounding process become the same biologic signals that are crucial to SIRS and ultimately eventuate in MODS.[13] The biology of a wound becomes the paradigm for understanding SIRS and MODS.

Biology of the Wound

Injury of tissue by a clean surgical incision, traumatic injury, or thermal injury serves as a nonspecific stimulus that activates human inflammation. The magnitude and intensity of the inflammatory response is a biologic reflection of the magnitude and intensity of the insult. Thus a clean surgical wound provokes a modest local inflammatory response, whereas more destructive traumatic wounds stimulate a more robust inflammatory response.

Injury of soft tissues activates the five *initiators* of human inflammation. Activation of the five *initiators* provokes the elaboration of secondary mediator or effector signals, which are responsible for the component elements of the human inflammatory response. These five initiators are interactive and redundant in terms of the specific physiologic responses that are generated as the component elements of inflammation.

1. First, activation of *coagulation proteins* becomes a principal, if not the most important, initiator of inflammation.[14,15] Tissue and small vessel injury activates the coagulation cascade to achieve local hemostasis, but the activation of coagulation proteins liberates the cleavage products that initiate inflammation. Activated factor XII (also known as Hageman factor) becomes an important mediator signal that initiates important microcirculatory changes in the wound. Although having a minimal direct effect, activated factor XII assumes major significance in stimulation and amplification of the other initiator events.

2. The second initiator is *activated platelets*.[16,17] Platelets, like the coagulation cascade, are most commonly associated with thrombosis and hemostasis; but activation of platelets results in the release of a host of presynthesized enzyme signals that provoke the inflammatory response. Soluble extracts from lysed platelets are potent activators of inflammation when injected into the soft tissues of experimental animals. The vasoactive role of platelet products are well appreciated, particularly thomboxane A_2 as a potent vasoconstrictor.

3. The third initiator is the *mast cell*.[18,19] Mast cell stimulation by activated factor XII and by platelet products stimulates the release of histamine and other vasoactive signals. Histamine as the prototype signal from mast cells directly relaxes vascular smooth muscle and promotes microcirculatory vasodilation in the tissues about the area of the wound. The vasodilation process results in increased vascular permeability, increased bulk flow, but reduced flow velocity.

4. A fourth initiator is the *contact activating system*.[20,21] (Fig. 10.1) Preformed prekallikrein is a ubiquitous serum protein that awaits activation by an appropriate stimulus. The presence of factor XII results in conversion of prekallikrein to kallikrein, and kallikrein then becomes the catalyst for the synthesis of bradykinin from high-molecular-weight kininogen. Bradykinin is a potent signal that binds to endothelial receptors and induces nitric oxide synthase in the stimulated endothelial cell.[22] This results in the production of the paracrine signal of nitric oxide, which diffuses as a product of the endothelial cell to the adjacent vascular smooth muscle cell and promotes relaxation. The result is similar to that of histamine, with vasodilation and increased microvascular permeability the result, but by a mechanism that is unique and different from the histamine effect.

5. A fifth initiator is the *complement cascade*.[23,24] Activation of complement occurs both through conventional and alternative pathways. Activation of the complement cascade to completion results in a complex protein construct that may lyse offending pathogen cells. More importantly, with inflammation activation of the complement cascade generates a host of cleavage products that have important vasoactive and chemoattractant functions. Of interest, activated complement proteins stimulate activation of coagulation, platelets, mast cells, and indirectly the production of bradykinin.

Thus it appears that activation of any one *initiator* of human inflammation results in the activation of all.[25,26] The summed effect of initiator activation is increased microvascular permeability, increased microcirculatory flow, reduction of microcirculatory flow velocity, and soft tissue edema formation. Importantly, all the cleavage products and enzyme proteins liberated by activation of the initiator events creates a local environment at the site of injury that is rich in chemoattractant signals.[27–30] Table 10.1 identifies the numerous chemoattractants, which are direct or indirect products of the activation of the initiator events. Chemokines (derived from *chemo*attractant cyto*kines*) represents a group of chemically analogous but low

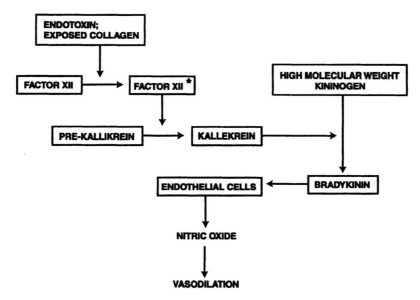

FIGURE 10.1. Pathways for the production of bradykinin. Activation of the coagulation cascade results in the production of activated factor XII, which catalyzes the reaction of prekallikrein that ultimately leads to bradykinin production. Bradykinin becomes the paracrine signal that binds to receptors on the endothelial cell. Nitric oxide production is the result.

TABLE 10.1. Some of the Chemoattractants Presently Known.[a]

Chemoattractant group (abbrevation)	Specific leukocyte group
Complement protein 5 cleavage product (C5a)	Nonspecific
Bacterial formyl peptide (fMLP)	Nonspecific
Platelet activating factor (PAF)	Nonspecific
Leukotriene B$_4$ (LTB$_4$)	Nonspecific
Chemokines; subgroup C-C	Monocytes
Monocyte inflammatory proteins (MIP-1α, MIP-1β)	
Monocyte chemoattractant protein (MCP-1, MCP-2, MCP-3, MCP-4, MCP-5)	
Regulated on activated, normal T expressed and secreted (RANTES)	
I-309	
Eotaxin	
Chemokines, subgroup C-X-C	Neutrophils
Interleukin-8 (IL-8)	
Growth-related oncogene (GRO-α, GRO-β, GRO-γ)	
Granulocyte chemotactic protein-2 (GCP-2)	
Epithelial neutrophil activating protein-78 (ENA-78)	
Platelet basic proteins (PBPs)	
Cleavage products of PBP, including connective tissue activating proteins-III (CTAP-III);	
β-thromboglobulin (β-TG), neutrophil activating protein-2 (NAP-2)	
Platelet factor-4 (PF4)	
Interferon-γ-(IFNγ)-inducible protein (IP-10)	
Monokine induced by IFNγ (MIG)	
Chemokine, subgroup C	
Lymphotactin	??
Chemokine, subgroup C-XXX-C	
Fractalkine	??

[a]The new chemokines are a chemically analogous group of chemoattractant cytokines that have specificity for selected leukocyte groups. The chemokines exceed 40 in number, and the list in the table is not complete.

molecular-weight proteins that appear to have specificity for each leukocyte population. Because chemokines participate in leukocyte rolling, margination, and migration in addition to activation of the luekocyte, specificity of the chemokine for a specific population of luekocyte (e.g., neutrophil, monocyte, eosinophil) may provide an explanation for the predominant leukocyte populations that are seen in various inflammatory conditions.

The biologic objective of the initiators, or phase I of inflammation, is to pave the way for phase II, the phagocytic response. Vasodilation and increased bulk flow increases the rate of delivery of phagocytic cells to the area of injury. Reduced velocity of flow promotes margination of the circulatory phagocytic cell. Increased vascular permeability provides exit routes for marginated phagocytic cells to enter the area of injured soft tissue. Soft tissue edema establishes aqueous conduits through the dense extracellular matrix, allowing phagocytic cell migration directly into the area of injury.

Phase II, the phagocytic phase, of inflammation begins when a criticial threshold of chemoattractant concentration has been eclipsed. Diffusion of the summed chemoattractants from the epicenter of injury allows them initially to bind to specific receptor sites on vascular endothelial cells and activates selection proteins and counterreceptors to match the neutrophil selectins. Neutrophil selectin proteins are constitutively expressed, but transformation of the endothelial counterreceptors initiate the process of neutrophil slowing, or "rolling," on the endothelial cell surface.[31,32] The surface rolling of the neutrophil then permits direct neutrophil effects by the chemoattractant signals to promote completion of the margination process. Chemoattractants result in transformation of the constitutively expressed CD11/18 complex on the surface of the neutrophil that permits adherence to the intercellular adhesion molecule (ICAM) receptor on the endothelial cell surface.[33,34] The result is "docking" of the neutrophil at the surface of the endothelial cell.

The chemoattractant gradient from the epicenter of the injury provides direction for the neutrophil to begin the process of diapedesis. Separation of the junction of endothelial cells from microcirculatory vasodilation exposes receptors that are recognized by the neutrophil, and locomotion through the porous vascular lining into the soft tissue begins. Soft tissue edema not only provides aqueous channels for neutrophil migration; it supplies a rich source of opsonic proteins to facilitate identification of targets for phagocytic activation. An orderly process of phagocytosis is begun with the early arrival of neutrophils into the injury site.

A second critical cell population that participates in phase II of inflammation is the monocyte. Monocytes are "attracted" into the area of injury by mechanisms analogous to those primarily described by the neutrophil. However, the monocyte is a larger cell with a larger cell nucleus. Accordingly, the process of transendothelial migration and diapedesis evolves slower, as the lumbering monocyte requires a longer interval for migration out of the intravascular space and into the area of injury. The intensity of the chemoattractant signal then modulates the monocytic response. Minimal chemoattractant signaling, which may be a quantitative or qualitative effect, may elicit little or no monocyte response. However, chemoattractant effect sufficient to eclipse a critical threshold stimulates a robust proinflammatory cytokine response. The release of the proinflammatory cytokines—tumor necrosis factor (TNF), interleukin-1 (IL-1), interleukin-6 (IL-6), and interleukin-8 (IL-8)— set into motion an array of autocrine, paracrine, and endocrine events that fully activate the phagocytic response.

In efffect, although the monocyte has a critical function in initiating the specific immune response, its most pivotal function in phase II is local orchestration of neutrophil phagocytic function and transformation of the host systemically to a "war time" state. Local effects of TNF on neutrophils is to stimulate aggressive phagocytic activity.[35,36] Such effects promote even extracellular elaboration of reactive oxygen intermediates and acid hydrolases, which among other effects initiate degradation of the tissues about the site of injury and contamination.[37,38] Vigorous phagocytic activity and extracellular liberation of toxic neutrophil products results in liquefaction, necrotic host cells, and dead neutrophils in a protein-rich environment better known as pus.

In a chemoattractant-rich environment that is sufficiently intense to result in local suppuration, the containment function of inflammation extends to the perimeter of the area of injury. Intense chemoattractant signaling may result in full activation of the neutrophils marginated to the vascular endothelium about the site of the injury. Full activation of neutrophils with the release of reactive oxygen intermediates, acid hydrolases, and other lysosomal products results in microcirculatory thrombosis. The microcirculatory thrombosis further facilitates the suppurative process but serves the important role of eliminating portals of egress for bacteria, toxins, and chemoattractants to the systemic circulation.

Oxidative Metabolism and SIRS

The clinical features of SIRS were discussed in Chapter 3. The prototypical SIRS patient has an elevated cardiac output, reduced systemic vascular resistance, and a narrowed arteriovenous oxygen content difference.[39] The blood concentration of lactate, which increases as the prodrome to the emergence of MODS, is a direct reflection of disordered oxygen (or substrate) utilization by the cell. It has been our hypothesis over two decades of investigation that abnormalities of oxygen/substrate delivery or utilization for the production of necessary cellular energy has resulted in SIRS, leading to MODS.[40-43]

Patients with MODS demonstrate interesting histologic findings in the tissues that become dysfunctional, leading to a fatal outcome.[44] Pulmonary tissues in the adult respiratory distress syndrome (ARDS) demonstrate extensive inflammatory exudates within the alveolar spaces and thickened alveolar membranes. Liver histology demonstrates focal areas of cellular necrosis with a "halo" of inflammatory cells about the perimeter of the necrotic epicenter. The gastric mucosa exhibits focal necrosis, and renal tissue demonstrates of acute tubular necrosis. An interesting and consistent observation in the tissues of the MODS patient is that the process is *focal*. It does not have the appearance of diffuse cellular toxicity, as totally normal populations of cells are identified in the lung, liver, and gastric mucosa in immediate proximity to those areas where focal necrotic populations of cells are observed.

Because of speculation that defective oxidative metabolism was fundamental to "sepsis"and organ dysfunction, the mitochondrion and oxidative phosphorylation of organ systems known to fail during the process were studied by experimental methods. Early experimental studies of lethal endotoxemia demonstrated marked uncoupling and inhibition of oxidative phosphorylation in liver mitochondria isolated at several time periods prior to the death of the animal.[45,46] This finding led to speculation that perhaps the endotoxemic process caused the release of cyanide-like or other toxic products that impaired the capacity of the cell to utilize oxygen and substrate. One study even supplied evidence to support the idea that endotoxin might have a direct effect on the mitochondrion.[45] It was interesting that all models employed were severe endotoxemia, that mitochondrial injury effects were similar to those identified during ischemia[47] and hemorrhagic shock,[46] and that experiments with live bacterial infection failed to demonstrate any evidence of mitochondrial injury.[48]

Our studies with severe bacterial peritonitis in the rat failed to identify inhibition or uncoupling of oxidative phosphorylation in isolated hepatic rat mitochondria.[40] In fact, to the contrary, our studies demonstrated increased efficiency of oxidative phosphorylation, which has been reported only in cell populations subject to acute hypoxemia.[49] Because the experimental animals had normal arterial pressures and arterial oxygenation, the issue of microcirculatory abnormalities became the subject of attention. The direct measurement of hepatic tissue PO_2 in peritonitis and gram-negative bacteremia models gave proof of profound tissue hypoxia prior to signs of systemic hypotension or hypoxemia.[40,50] Certainly the idea of a microcirculatory injury or abnormality appeared to be more consistent with the focal necrosis consistently identified in histologic sections of both patients and experimental animals with severe infection or endotoxemia.[44,51]

Further experimental studies provided additional evidence of a microcirculatory injury. Methods to measure cardiac output in the experimental models of peritonitis demonstrated that with appropriate preload the experimental animal had an elevated cardiac output. Measurements of effective hepatic blood flow identified a dissociation of hepatic perfusion from systemic hemodynamics. Measurement of systemic lactate and pyruvate concentrations showed equimolar increases, as had been reported in septic humans, but liver biopsies demonstrated liver lactate to be dramatically elevated with only minimal elevations in pyruvate concentrations. It was concluded that the liver was a major source of lactate production due to the suboptimally perfused tissue, but that systemic lactate/pyruvate ratios were more likely controlled by the adequately perfused and oxygenated skeletal muscle.

Additional studies provided evidence that this microcirculatory arrest was a nonspecific response of the host and was not unique to bacteria or bacterial cell products (e.g., endotoxin). A dilute solution of zymosan was administered systemically to experimental animals,[52] with activation of the complement cascade the result. The rats had a hemodynamic response with complement activation alone that was identical to that seen in experimental animals with peritonitis or endotoxemia. Cardiac output increased, and systemic vascular resistance declined. Effective hepatic blood flow also declined. Septic hemodynamic profiles could be reproduced by activation of one of the *initiators* of inflammation without the presence of bacteria or endotoxin.

Severely injured patients with torso trauma and long bone fractures have comprised a population of patients who especially developed MODS during the postinjury period but also who frequently did not appear to have invasive infection as the triggering event for MODS. With experimental trauma femoral fractures[53] it was demonstrated that traumatic femoral fracture with its attendant soft tissue injury (1) activated the systemic complement cascade, (2) created a hemodynamic profile analogous to that seen in septic rats, and (3) resulted in the decline of effective hepatic blood flow. Based on these studies, our group concluded that any physiologic perturbation that activated the systemic inflammatory response through the *initiator* events would potentially lead to the dissociation of visceral tissue perfusion from systemic hemodynamics and might provide an explanation for the emergence of MODS as a consequence of SIRS.

Microcirculatory Arrest: Consequence of SIRS

It is the hypothesis of the microcirculatory theory of MOF that all of the biologic processes in a simple traumatic wound or seemingly innocent soft tissue infection are the same mediators and effectors responsible for SIRS and its sequelae. The normal and salutary autocrine and paracrine signaling mechanisms of human inflammation become the "horror autotoxicus" when they are endocrine in distribution. Dysregulated, disseminated inflammation is the disease; MODS is the result. Fig. 10.2 shows the 10 component steps of this hypothesis.

Step 1: activators of human inflammation. The same biologic stimuli that can initiate inflammation in a simple wound may provoke systemic activation of inflammation. Severe infection is probably still the most likely candidate to be responsible for the SIRS response. With severe infection the insult is a sustained one, with the active process of microbial proliferation continuing to activate the inflammatory cascade. Unlike a temporally defined traumatic injury, infection is an ongoing process that in all likelihood has a greater prospect for having its summed effects over a period of time reach a critical threshold of severity that is sufficient to activate the systemic response. It is again emphasized that dissemination of the pathogen or its cellular products is not a requirement for activating systemic inflammation.

In recent years considerable interest has focused on the phenomenon of gastrointestinal microbial translocation.[7-10] Can

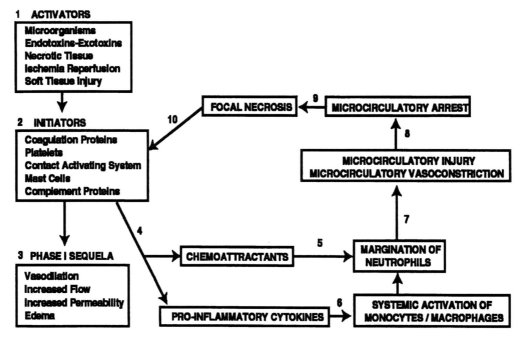

FIGURE 10.2. The 10 steps of the microcirculatory hypothesis of organ failure. Each step is detailed in the text. The important general understanding is that inflammation results in end-organ tissue necrosis, which then becomes the stimulus to reactivate inflammation. Correction of the initiating event may not reverse the inflammatory cycle.

the escape of microbes from the intestinal tract due to failure of the gut barrier elicit a systemic inflammatory response? Although clearly demonstrated as an observed phenomenon in the experimental laboratory, considerably less evidence supports its clinical relevance in critically ill humans. *Candida* spp. have been demonstrated to arise from the gut reservoir and result in candidemia,[54] but bacterial species have been less well documented. All clinicians have had the experience of the critically ill patient with the bacteremia from an unknown site that is temporally associated with the emergence of MODS. Patients with severe catabolic illness and protein-calorie malnutrition may well have a defective gut barrier, and microbes or cell products released from the gut could function as an activator of the inflammatory response. This situation represents microbial dissemination as a function of the failed host rather than an infection in the traditional sense of the term.

Severe but sterile inflammatory foci can be activators of the inflammatory cascade. Most notable in this regard is severe pancreatitis.[4] Pulmonary failure combined with other elements of MODS are frequently seen in the severely ill patient with acute pancreatitis. Organ dysfunction occurs well before there is any evidence of clinical infection in the pancreatic bed. Massive aspiration of acid gastric contents can similarly provide a severe chemical pneumonitis that produces SIRS. Postoperative cardiac bypass patients also demonstrate SIRS and MODS without infection, presumably due to activation of the inflammatory process during use of the membrane oxygenator.[55,56]

Activation of systemic inflammation may require summed insults, commonly referred to as the "two-hit" hypothesis of organ failure.[57,58] This hypothesis would require two sequential activator events before the summed magnitude would be sufficient to provoke systemic inflammation. An initial insult such as a hemorrhagic event, severe injury, or a major operation may prime the inflammatory response so a second activator event (e.g., infection, rebleed, reoperation) within a short interval results in clinical SIRS. The interaction of sequential clinical activators events appears to have real relevance and requires further definition as to mechanism.

Step 2: activation of the initiators. As described in the wound paradigm above, the five major initiator events trigger phase I inflammation at the systemic level. Activation of the coagulation cascade results in disseminated intravascular coagulation with or without clinical bleeding. The patients commonly have prolonged prothrombin times and prolonged activated partial thromboplastin times as a result of consumption of coagulation proteins by the systemic activation. Thrombocytopenia is customary. Systemic activation of complement proteins has been documented. The effects of bradykinin and histamine become fully identified in step 3.

Step 3: systemic consequences of phase I sequelae. The systemic hemodynamic consequences of SIRS are fully explained by the consequences of the initiator events. Vasodilation secondary to systemic effects of bradykinin, histamine, and in all likelihood other mediators results in effects on both the venous and arterial microcirculations. Systemic vascular resistance declines, and vascular capacitance increases. Hypotension may occur early in the process if attention is not given to preload administration because of the relative hypovolemia that is created by capacitance changes. When adequate preload is provided, the cardiac index increases as an function of marked afterload reduction due to vasodilation. Systemic edema especially in the dependent areas of the body are recognized in these patients as evidence of the systemic changes in microcirculatory permeability.

Step 4: systemic distribution of chemoattractants and proinflammatory cytokine signals. Activation of the initiator events at a system level results in a systemic distribution of chemoattractants. Protein cleavage products and cellular enzymes that normally serve as chemoattractants in the soft tissue are now widely disseminated within the extracellular fluid. This generalized distribution results in contact of chemoattractants with all neutrophils that are within the circulation and provides chemoattractant signals for the entire body's population of endothelial cells.

Dissemination of the chemoattractant signals are similarly recognized by the circulating monocytes. In contrast to being drawn to a specific site in injured tissue, the monocyte is bathed in a sea of chemoattractants, which induces production of proinflammatory cytokines directly into the extracellular fluid of the host.

Step 5: generalized margination of neutrophils. The generalized distribution of chemoattractants results in activation of the endothelial cell–neutrophil adhesion process. Unlike the normal response in a wound, the neutrophil does not have a chemoattractant gradient to direct its site of margination for the direction for its subsequent migration. Neutrophil rolling is initiated through the selectin molecule process, and complete margination is achieved via the interaction of CD11/18 complex of the neutrophil and the ICAM on the endothelial cell surface. The process potentially occurs throughout the entire microcirculation but appears to be more prevalent in the visceral circulation than in the somatic circulation. The ultimate organ systems that become the target of MODS (e.g., lung, liver, gut) appear to have the greatest degree of neutrophil margination. An explanation for the preferred tissues for margination can only be speculated, but the preferred site seems to be tissue beds that have fixed macrophage cells. This preference may relate to flow velocity through different tissue beds or to the affinity of receptors from the neutrophil to various endothelial cell populations.

Step 6: full activation of marginated neutrophils of pro-inflammatory cytokines. As was noted in the normal wound above, neutrophils initially have a orderly, controlled pattern of phagocytosis; but stimulation by proinflammatory cytokines such as TNF results in frenzied phagocytic behavior including extracellular release of reactive oxygen intermediates and lysosomal enzymes. This release to toxic substances may occur in areas immediately outside the intravascular compartment, where neutrophils may have migrated, or within the marginated position in the microcirculation. Lipid peroxidation and self-digestion are initiated.

Step 7: microcirculatory injury and microcirculatory vasoconstriction. The release of toxic lysosomal contents by the stimulated neutrophil results in endothelial cell injury and an additional microcirculatory stimulus to activation of the inflammatory cascade. Injury of the endothelial cell results in local loss of regulation of vascular smooth muscle. Coagulation is activated, and platelet aggregation occurs at the sites of chemical injury from the reactive oxygen intermediates and other toxic lysosomal enzymes. Vasoconstriction is the response, perhaps mediated by Thromboxane, A_2.[59,60] Local thrombus is created at the site of endothelial injury within the microcirculation.

Step 8: microcirculatory arrest. The summed effects of microcirculatory vasoconstriction and microcirculatory thrombus formation is dramatic reduction, if not complete cessation, of flow through the microcirculatory unit. Complete thrombosis may occur, but the cell population served by the nutrient vessel so affected experiences a progressive loss of oxygenation and substrate delivery. Although complete thrombosis or microcirculatory vasoconstriction may have been desirable as part of the normal containment strategy of the normal response to wounding and local infection, thrombosis and vasoconstriction can become fundamental to organ dysfunction.

Step 9: focal necrosis. The loss of effective perfusion from vasoconstriction and thrombosis is focal necrosis. The process as described appears to be one that should affect all cell populations and microcirculatory units equally, and it raises the question as to why the process has the appearance of being focal. The answer lies in the fact that the number of endothelial cells is far greater than the number of neutrophils. There would simply not be enough neutrophils to affect all microcirculatory units. However, the response of the host to produce more neutrophils as part of the systemic response to inflammation adds additional neutrophil participants over time and contributes to the progressive and relentless additional loss of functional tissue units as the dysfunction process of MODS continues.

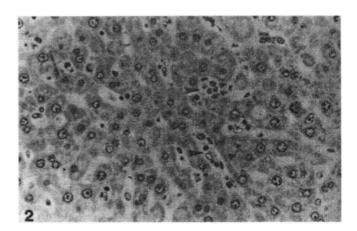

FIGURE 10.4. Rat liver histology 5 hours after administration of intravenous *E. coli*. Note the evidence of neutrophil sequestration within the hepatic sinusoids.

Step 10: self-energizing, self-recycling process. This hypothesis of microcirculatory arrest during organ failure seems relatively simple in that elimination of the stimulus, or activator, should stem the generation of chemoattractants and the whole process should then be downregulated. Unfortunately, systemic inflammation begets tissue injury and necrosis, which begets more systemic inflammation. The outcome of this scenario of metastatic inflammation is that the end-organ lesion becomes itself an activator (Figs. 10.3, 10.4, 10.5). The clinician reaches a point in patient care where even though the instigating activator (e.g., an abdominal abscess) is eradicated and the infectious process totally controlled, a relentless, self-perpetuating process is already beyond what conventional treatment can handle.

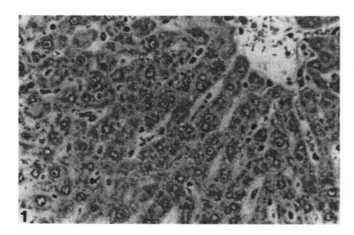

FIGURE 10.3. Normal histology of the rat liver prior to the administration of live intravenous *E. coli*. The sinusoids are clear and without abnormalities.

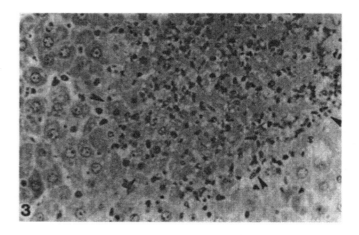

FIGURE 10.5. Rat liver histology 10 hours after administration of intravenous *E. coli*. Focal necrosis with secondary infiltration with additional inflammatory cells can now be seen.

Conclusions

This chapter has explored the hypothesis that SIRS and MODS are the consequences of the normal inflammatory response activated at a systemic, rather than a local, level of organization. Our normal host defense processes that are so beneficial when responding to a soft tissue wound or localized infection become self-destructive when the stimulus results in systemic activation of the process. The true challenge in formulating new treatment strategies for SIRS and MODS is how to modulate the overexuberant response of the systemically activated inflammatory response without at the same time compromising the beneficial effects of local responsiveness of human inflammation.

References

1. Deutschman CS, Konstantinides FN, Tsai M, et al: Physiology and metabolism in isolated viral septicemia: further evidence of an organism-independent, host-dependent response. Arch Surg 1987;122:21–28.
2. Seibel R, LaDuca J, Hassett JM, et al: Blunt multiple trauma (ISS 36), femur traction, and the pulmonary failure-septic state. Ann Surg 1985;202:283–295.
3. Marshall WG, Dimick AR: Natural history of major burns with multiple subsystem failure. J Trauma 1983;23:102–105.
4. Ranson JHC, Rifkind KM, Roses DF, et al: Prognostic signs and the role of operative management in acute pancreatitis. Ann Surg 1974;139:69.
5. Fine J, Frank ED, Ravin HA, et al: The bacterial factor in traumatic shock. N Engl J Med 1959;260:214–220.
6. Ravin HA, Fine J: Biological implications of intestinal endotoxins. Fed Proc 1962;21:65–68.
7. Deitch EA: The role of intestinal barrier failure and bacterial translocation in the development of systemic infection and multiple organ failure. Arch Surg 1990;125:403–404.
8. Wilmore DW, Smith RJ, O'Dwyer ST, et al: The gut: a central organ after surgical stress. Surgery 1988;104:917–924.
9. Deitch EA: Intestinal permeability is increased in burn patients shortly after injury. Surgery 1990;107:411–416.
10. Rush BF, Sori AJ, Murphy TF, et al: Endotoxemia and bacteremia during hemorrhagic shock. Ann Surg 1988;207:549–554.
11. Goris RJ, te Boekhorst TP, Nuytinck JK, Gimbrere JS: Multiple-organ failure: generalized autodestructive inflammation? Arch Surg 1985;120:1109–1115.
12. Baue AE: The horror autotoxicus and multiple organ failure. Arch Surg 1992;127:1451–1462.
13. Border JR: Death from severe trauma: open fractures to multiple organ dysfunction syndrome. J Trauma 1995;39:12–22.
14. Cicala C, Cirino G: Linkage between inflammation and coagulation: an update on the molecular basis of the crosstalk. Life Sci 1998;62:1817–1824.
15. Johnson K, Choi Y, DeGroot E, et al: Potential mechanisms for a proinflammatory vascular cytokine response to coagulation activation. J Immunol 1998;160:5130–5135.
16. Gentry PA: The mammalian blood platelet: its role in haemostasis, inflammation, and tissue repair. J Comp Pathol 1992;107:243–270.
17. Weksler BB: Roles for human platelets in inflammation. Prog Clin Biol Res 1988;283:611–638.
18. Huang C, Sali A, Stevens R: Regulation and function of mast cell proteases in inflammation. J Clin Immunol 1998;18:169–183.
19. Metcalfe DD, Baram D, Mekori YA: Mast cells. Physiol Rev 1997;77:1033–1079.
20. Kaplan AP, Joseph K, Shibayama Y, et al: The intrinsic coagulation/kinin-forming cascade: assembly in plasma and cell surfaces in inflammation. Adv Immunol 1997;66:225–272.
21. Hargreaves KM, Troulles ES, Dionne RA, et al: Bradykinin is increased during acute and chronic inflammation: therapeutic implications. Clin Pharmacol Ther 1998;44:613–621.
22. Ignarro LJ: Biosynthesis and metabolism of endothelium-derived nitric oxide. Annu Rev Pharmacol Toxicol 1990;30:535–560.
23. Mollnes TE, Fosse E: The complement system in trauma-related and ischemic tissue damage: a brief review. Shock 1994;2:301–310.
24. Kaplan AP, Silverberg N: Mediators of inflammation: an overview. Methods Enzymol 1988;163:3–23.
25. Sundsmo JS, Fair DS: Relationships among the complement, kinin, coagulation and fibrinolytic systems in the inflammatory reaction. Clin Physiol Biochem 1983;1:225–284.
26. Kaplan AP, Silverberg M, Dunn JT, Ghebrehiwet B: Interaction of the clotting, kinin-forming, complement, and fibrinolytic pathways in inflammation. Ann NY Acad Sci 1982;389:25.
27. Negus RPM: The chemokines: cytokines that direct leukocyte migration. J R Soc Med 1996;89:312–314.
28. Luster AD: Chemokines—Chemotactic cytokines that mediate inflammation. N Engl J Med 1998;338:436–445.
29. Furie MB, Randolph GJ: Chemokines and tissue injury. Am J Pathol 1995;146:1287–1301.
30. Rollins BJ: Chemokines. Blood 1997;90:909–928.
31. Brown EJ, Lindberg FP: Leukocyte adhesion molecules in host defense against infection. Ann Med 1996;28:210–218.
32. Menger MD, Vollmar B: Adhesion molecules as determinants of disease: from molecular biology to surgical research. Br J Surg 1996;83:588–601.
33. Gahmberg GG: Leukocyte adhesion: CD11/CD18 integrins and intercellular adhesion molecules. Curr Opin Cell Biol 1997;9:643–650.
34. Gahmberg GG, Tolvanen M, Kotovuori P: Leukocyte adhesion—structure and function of human leukocytes beta 2-integrin and their cellular ligands. Eur J Biochem 1997;245:215–232.
35. Klebanoff SJ, Vedes MA, Harlan JM, et al: Stimulation of neutrophils by tumor necrosis factor. J Immunol 1986;136:4220–4225.
36. Larrick JW, Graham D, Toy K, et al: Recombinant tumor necrosis factor causes activation of human granulocytes. Blood 1987;69:640–644.
37. Ferrante A, Nandoskar M, Walz N, et al: Effects of tumor necrosis factor alpha and interleukin 1 alpha and beta on human neutrophil migration, respiratory burst and degranulation. Int Arch Allergy Appl Immunol 1988;86:82–91.
38. Feng L, Xia Y, Garcia GE, et al: Involvement of reaction oxygen intermediates in cyclooxygenase-2 expression induced by interleukin-1, tumor necrosis factor-alpha, and lipopolysaccharide. J Clin Invest 1995;95:1669–1675.
39. Siegel JH, Cerra FB, Coleman B, et al: Physiologic and metabolic correlations in human sepsis. Surgery 1979;86:163–193.
40. Fry DE, Silver BB, Rink RD, et al: Hepatic cellular hypoxia in murine peritonitis. Surgery 1979;85:652–661.

41. Garrison RN, Ratcliffe DJ, Fry DE: Hepatocellular function and nutrient blood flow in experimental peritonitis. Surgery 1982;92:713–719.
42. Townsend MC, Hampton WW, Haybron DM, et al: Effective organ blood flow and bioenergy status in murine peritonitis. Surgery 1986;100:205–213.
43. Schirmer WJ, Townsend MC, Schirmer JM, et al: Galactose elimination kinetics in sepsis: correlation of hepatic blood flow with function. Arch Surg 1987;122:349–354.
44. Fry DE: Multiple system organ failure. In: Fry DE (ed), Multiple System Organ Failure. Chicago, Mosby-Year Book, 1992;14.
45. Schumer W, Das Gupta TK, Moss GS, et al: Effect of endotoxemia on liver cell mitochondria in man. Ann Surg 1970;171:875–879.
46. Mela L, Bacalzo LV, Miller LD: Defective oxidative metabolism of rat liver mitochondria in hemorrhage and endotoxin shock. Am J Physiol 1971;220:571–576.
47. Townsend MC, Yokum MD, Fry DE: Hepatic microsomal adensosine triphosphatase and mitochondrial function: response to cold and warm ischemia. Arch Surg 1987;122:813–816.
48. Decker GA, Danial AM, Blevings D, Maclean LD: Effect of peritonitis on mitochondrial respiration. J Surg Res 1971;11:528–532.
49. Mela L, Olofsson K, Miller LD, et al: Effect of lysosomes and hypoxia on mitochondria in shock. Surg Forum 1971;22:19–21.
50. Fry DE, Kaelin CR, Giammara BL, Rink RD: Alterations of oxygen metabolism in experimental bacteremia. Adv Shock Res 1981;6:45–54.
51. Asher EF, Rowe RL, Garrison RN, Fry DE: Experimental bacteremia and hepatic nutrient blood flow. Circ Shock 1986;20:43–49.
52. Schirmer WJ, Schirmer JM, Naff GB, Fry DE: Systemic complement activation produces hemodynamic changes characteristic of sepsis. Arch Surg 1988;123:316–321.
53. Schirmer WJ, Schirmer JM, Townsend MC, Fry DE: Femur fracture with associated soft tissue injury produces hepatic ischemia. Arch Surg 1988;123:412–415.
54. Stone HH, Kolb LD, Currie CA, et al: Candida sepsis: pathogenesis and principles of treatment. Ann Surg 1974;179:697–711.
55. Nilsson L, Nilsson U, Venge P, et al: Inflammatory system activation during cardiopulmonary bypass as an indicator of biocompatibility: a randomized comparison of bubble and membrane oxygenation. Scand J Thorac Cardiovasc Surg 1990;24:53–58.
56. Wan S, LeClerc JL, Vincnet JL: Inflammatory response to cardiopulmonary bypass: mechanisms involved and possible therapeutic strategies. Chest 1997;112:676–692.
57. Deitch EA: Multiple organ failure: pathophysiology and potential future therapy. Ann Surg 1992;216:117–134.
58. Biffl WL, Moore EE: Splanchnic ischaemia/reperfusion and multiple organ failure. Brit J Anaesth 1996;77:59–70
59. Bernard GR, Reines HD, Halushka PV, et al: Prostacyclin and thomboxane A2 formation is increased in human sepsis syndrome: effects of cyclooxygenase inhibition. Am Rev Respir Dis 1991;144:1095–1101.
60. Schirmer WJ, Schirmer JM, Townsend MC, Fry DE: Imidazole and indomethacin improve hepatic perfusion in sepsis. Circ Shock 1987;21:253–259.

11
Infection, Bacteremia, Sepsis, and the Sepsis Syndrome: Metabolic Alterations, Hypermetabolism, and Cellular Alterations

Matthias Majetschak and Christian Waydhas

The term "sepsis syndrome" describes a systemic inflammatory and hypermetabolic response of the body on the cellular, organ, and organ systems level to a variety of microbial stimuli and to stimuli other than exogenous microbial agents. The latter may include but are not limited to accidental blunt and penetrating injuries, surgical trauma, burns, pancreatitis, inflammatory bowel disease, and others. If bacteria, viruses, or fungi are involved and the sepsis syndrome is caused by these microbes, the term "sepsis" is used. Systemic inflammatory response syndrome (SIRS) is an expression that has been used recently as a common denominator for such inflammatory states independent of their cause. Infection denotes a (locally confined) inflammatory response to the presence of microorganisms or the invasion of normally sterile host tissue by those organisms, and the term "bacteremia" means the presence of bacteria in the bloodstream, indicating an infectious focus with spillover of bacteria into the circulation. Conditions such as viremia and fungemia can be similarly defined.[1,2]

Although the pathophysiologic reaction sequence that eventually results in SIRS may differ depending on the underlying infectious or noninfectious cause, it finally leads to a common pathway characterized clinically by an increased respiratory rate, increased heart rate, and fever. Therefore symptoms and findings of the physical examination and technical and laboratory tests may be similar irrespective of the underlying condition. Potential triggers of SIRS include bacterial toxins (endotoxin, exotoxin), cytokines, arachidonic acid metabolites, humoral cascade systems, and others, discussed in detail elsewhere in this book.

Independent from the underlying disease, the systemic inflammatory response usually leads to a metabolic state characterized by an increase in resting energy consumption, extensive protein and fat catabolism, negative nitrogen balance, hyperglycemia, and increased hepatic glucose production (Fig. 11.1).[3] Hypermetabolism may be defined as a resting energy expenditure of more than 115% of the predicted basal energy expenditure[4] and increased oxygen consumption.

Virtually all cell types are involved in this hypermetabolic response of which immunocompetent, liver, gut, and muscle cells are among the most interesting. The net effect is a progressive loss of body cell mass and finally the development of multiple organ dysfunction or failure.

Metabolism During Inflammation and Sepsis

The resting energy expenditure in critically ill patients is influenced by several endogenous and exogenous factors. Patients' anthropomorphic characteristics, severity of illness, pattern of injury, fever, the type of ventilation and drug treatment, and the type of nutrition, among other factors, have an impact on the resting energy consumption.[4-11] In critically ill patients treated in a modern intensive care unit (ICU), a sustained increase in resting energy expenditure can be found. This increase is associated with a respiratory quotient of 0.8, indicating mixed fuel oxidation.[12-14] Thus compared to starvation, the resting energy expenditure ranges from about 110% of reference values in mechanically ventilated patients after major surgery[15] to about 190% in mechanically ventilated multiply-injured patients suffering from septic complications.[16] In critically ill patients the resting energy expenditure increases within a week after the onset of illness and remains elevated for 3 weeks or more.[17] In trauma patients maximal resting energy expenditure is usually reached within 3–5 days after injury.[5]

In one study the resting energy expenditure was determined in 22 multiply-injured and severely septic patients after the onset of illness.[17] Within the first week the mean resting energy expenditure was 110%. The highest resting energy expenditure was found during the second week after the onset of illness with a mean resting energy expenditure of 160%. The average resting energy expenditure was determined to be 130% over the 3- to 4-week period.

In another study the resting energy expenditure was determined at different stages of infection in medical ICU patients.[18] It was highest in patients with sepsis and those recovering from septic shock with a mean value of about 160%, whereas in patients with sepsis plus organ failure and in those with septic shock it was significantly lower: 124% and 102%, respectively.

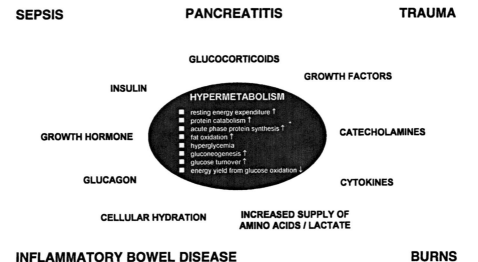

FIGURE 11.1. Scheme of Mediators and metabolic alterations of hypermetabolism.

Because fever is inherent to the definition of SIRS and a close association between fever and hypermetabolism has long been recognized,[19] the two entities appear closely related. This line of reasoning, however, has been questioned by the observation that the increase in resting energy expenditure predominantly correlates with body temperature.[4] In 204 mechanically ventilated critically ill patients the resting energy expenditure was 142% in patients with a body temperature > 38°C versus 124% in afebrile subjects independent of the type or severity of the underlying disease process. Among the 157 individuals with SIRS, 81% presented with fever and 19% had no rise of body temperature with resting energy expenditures of 141% and 123%, respectively. Therefore SIRS without fever may result in a significantly lesser degree of hypermetabolism than SIRS with elevated body temperature.

Calculations of energy requirements showed that about 30 kcal/kg/day are required during the first week and about 50 kcal/kg/day during the second week after the onset of illness to meet energy needs in the critically ill patient.[17] Despite adequate enteral or parenteral feeding, substrate use is significantly impaired in multiple-trauma, burned, or severely septic patients. A state of nutritional resistance with progressive loss of body cell mass develops.

With starvation, fat is the principal energy substrate in both normal and critically ill patients.[20] In healthy subjects in the fed state, insulin secretion, which is stimulated by glucose, inhibits lipolysis and fat oxidation. Although glucose turnover is increased and glucose and insulin levels are often elevated in critically ill patients,[21] fat oxidation is inadequately suppressed. Moreover, the energy yield from glucose oxidation is reduced. In critically ill patients, decreased pyruvate dehydrogenase activity leads to increased conversion of pyruvate to alanine or lactate, with the major proportion originating from skeletal muscle.[22] Therefore even in the absence of hypoxia, blood lactate levels become elevated.[23] Simultaneously, hepatic gluconeogenesis is stimulated by an increased supply of amino acids or lactate. Thus, in contrast to the fasting state in healthy subjects, hepatic glucose production is increased and is less (or not) suppressible by exogenous glucose.[24–27]

In critically ill patients the mixed fuel oxidation persists until progressive organ failure occurs. During these stages the respiratory ratio reaches values of 1.0 and more, indicating lipogenesis, which occurs predominantly in the liver.[12,13]

Although body weight increases during the initial phase in trauma or septic patients, changes in body weight are predominantly caused by accumulation of extracellular body water, which is in the range of 4–14 liters of total body water per patient.[17] It results in a rise of the relative contribution of the extracellular water to the body weight from 36% to 54%.[28] Coincident with the increase in extracellular body water, there is a large loss of total body protein, which can be as high as 1.5 kg, or 20–25% of the total body protein.[17,28–31] Within the first 10 days after onset of trauma or sepsis, most of the protein loss originates from skeletal muscle; at later stages protein is lost predominantly from viscera.[17] The net protein catabolism results from an imbalance of the de novo protein synthesis and breakdown. Although a decrease in protein synthesis and an increase in protein degradation would result in net protein catabolism, there is evidence that in critically ill patients protein catabolism is caused by an increase in protein degradation, especially in skeletal muscle.[32] Protein degradation has been found in several studies to be more than doubled after severe trauma.[33,34] Simultaneously increased protein synthesis has been observed in some studies, increasing the total protein turnover.[33]

Physiologic regulation of selective protein turnover is a highly orchestrated process, with specific protein turnover rates ranging from a few minutes (ornithine decarboxylase) to several days (histones). Up to now, the precise regulation and mechanism of degradation for the mass of intracellular proteins in vertebrate tissues, particularly in inflammatory states, is enigmatic.[35] Nevertheless, inflammatory mediators (e.g., cytokines, glucocorticoids, and growth factors released in inflammatory states) are known inducers of the hepatic acute-phase response, which results in the induction and synthesis of acute-phase proteins. They are thought also to induce protein breakdown simultaneously, (e.g., in skeletal muscle), particularly myofibrillar muscle protein degradation.[36-38]

In addition to the well known lysosomal protein breakdown (cathepsins), other nonlysosomal pathways of protein degradation have been discovered in skeletal muscle, (e.g., Ca^{2+}-dependent proteinases). Protein hydrolysis is usually an exergonic process, and the latter protein degradation systems are energy-independent. Moreover, and somehow contradictory, a nonlysosomal energy (ATP)-dependent proteolytic pathway has been discovered (ubiquitin/proteasome proteolytic pathway), which some investigators regard as the most important pathway of nonlysosomal protein degradation (Fig. 11.2).[35,39-44] Ubiquitin, a highly conserved 8.5-kDa protein, is thought to be covalently linked by an enzyme system (ubiquitin-ligase system; E1, E2, E3) to target proteins (ubiquitylation/formation of ubiquitin-protein conjugate), which then are recognized by the 26S protease (proteasome) for degradation. Finally, after proteolysis of the ubiquitin-protein conjugate, intact ubiquitin is released for reuse in the proteolytic pathway.[35,39,42-44]

Virtually all mammalian tissues studied so far have contained energy-dependent proteolytic activity, which has been identified as being induced by the multicatalytic 26S proteasome. Ubiquitin dependence of the ATP-dependent proteolytic system has not been found in normal mammalian tissues, except in reticulocytes,[45] although some studies have provided evidence of involvement of the ubiquitin-proteasome pathway in muscle protein breakdown in inflammatory situations. In rat soleus muscle, tumor necrosis factor (TNF) has been shown to induce the ubiquitin-proteasome system.[46] Moreover, in experimental animals sepsis has been found to stimulate the nonlysosomal ATP-dependent proteolytic pathway and to increase the ubiquitin mRNA levels in skeletal muscle.[47] Furthermore, a negative nitrogen balance was found to be accompanied by an increase in ubiquitin-proteasome mRNA levels in skeletal muscle from head trauma patients.[48] Based on these data it has been suggested that the increase in energy-dependent muscle proteolysis is, at least in part, responsible for the increase of total energy expenditure in hypermetabolic patients. Nevertheless, several important questions remain unresolved (e.g., the lack of physiologic substrates of the ubiquitin-proteasome pathway in healthy and critically ill subjects). Therefore the relative contribution of the proteolytic pathways in SIRS and sepsis remain to be determined.

Progressive protein catabolism leads to an increase in free amino acids, with flow from the periphery to the liver; and the proportion of energy derived from gluconeogenetic amino acids increases.[49,50] For example, glutamine is used for renal acid excretion, as an energy supply to the gut, and for nucleotide synthesis.[50-53] Although hepatic protein synthesis increases owing to a significant increase in acute-phase protein synthesis, the net proteolytic effect is dominant.

The understanding of factors that determine protein metabolism is further complicated by the type of nutrition given to critically ill patients. The substitution of carbohydrates alone leads to a reduction of the net protein loss compared to that during fasting conditions, which is further attenuated by the additional substitution of amino acids.[54] Administering specific amino acids, such as glutamine, that are not contained in standard nutrition formulas (enteral and parenteral) further reduces the total loss of protein in critically ill patients[55] predominantly by lowering the protein and glutamine flux from skeletal muscle.[56]

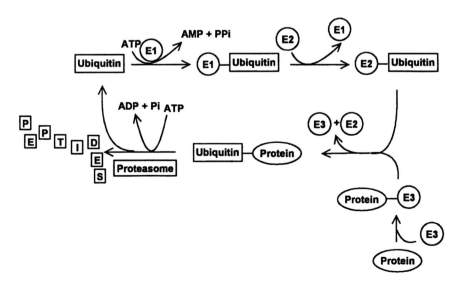

FIGURE 11.2. Ubiquitin-proteasome proteolytic pathway. E1, ubiquitin activating enzyme; E2, ubiquitin carrier or conjugating enzyme; E3, ubiquitin protein ligase.

Mediators During Hypermetabolism

A complex network of primary and secondary mediators involved in inflammation and systemic inflammatory responses have been identified. Among others, some of these mediators have been shown to have an impact on the metabolic alterations described above (Fig. 11.1).

Stress hormones are involved in regulation of the metabolic effects in SIRS and sepsis. Glucocorticoids, catecholamines, and glucagon, whose systemic concentrations are elevated in septic patients, have been shown to act synergistically on metabolic rates when infused in healthy volunteers in a rate sufficient to produce clinically significant concentrations such as those found during moderate infection.[57] In these volunteers, a catabolic effect with increased metabolic rate, increased gluconeogenesis, and nitrogen loss was detectable.

Glucagon has been found to stimulate phenylalanine oxidation in the liver;[58] and the catabolic effect of glucocorticoids on muscle protein metabolism, which can be seen in experimental animals and in human subjects,[59,60] appears to be due to induction of the proteasome system.[61,62] Although catecholamines and insulin are able to increase muscle protein synthesis,[63,64] in critically ill patients, catecholamines seem not to influence protein metabolism because neither propanolol nor metoprolol infusion exerted effects on the net protein turnover, and the anabolic effect of insulin has been found to be impaired.[63,65] More recent work, however, indicates that the endocrine response to trauma, particularly catecholamines, results in a direct interaction with the immune system and immune cells. Although some effects relate to inhibition of immunocompetent cells, stimulation of the activity of lymphocytes and of the antibody and cytokine production by catecholamines has been found,[66–68] indicating hypermetabolic activity on the level of some cell types.

Reduced levels of growth hormone and insulin-like growth factor-1 in critically ill patients may contribute to the catabolic state as well.[29,69–71] However, the role of growth hormone in critically ill patients is not clear, as low levels of somatotropin have been observed during the first week after severe trauma[70] but not in patients with sepsis.[72]

Cytokines are among the pivotal mediators of inflammation, and some were found to exert profound effects on metabolic rates in inflammatory states, particularly in the regulation of hepatic synthesis of acute-phase proteins.

In an oversimplified classification, based on their properties on synthesis of a distinct subset of acute-phase proteins, cytokines can be divided into two groups:[73–78] (1) interleukin-1-type cytokines (e.g., IL-1α, IL-1β), TNFα and TNFβ; and (2) IL-6-type cytokines (e.g., IL-6, IL-11), hepatocyte stimulatory factor (HSF), oncostatin M (OM), and cardiothropin-1 (CT-1). IL-1-type cytokines are inducers of the type 1 acute-phase proteins (e.g., C-reactive protein, complement B, C3, ferritin), whereas IL-6 type cytokines induce synthesis of type 2 acute-phase proteins (e.g., fibrinogen, haptoglobin, α₁-antichymotrypsin). Moreover, IL-6 type cytokines synergize with the IL-1 type cytokines in the induction of type 1 acute-phase proteins, and IL-1 type cytokines have no effect or inhibit type 2 acute-phase protein synthesis.[75,76] Nevertheless, it must be noted that not a single mediator but the individual pattern of mediators released at inflammatory sites is regarded as the main inducer of the hepatic acute-phase response.[77,78] Again, glucocorticoids and growth factors [transforming growth factor β (TGFβ), fibroblast growth factor, hepatocyte growth factor] can modulate hepatic acute-phase protein synthesis and are able to synergize with the action of cytokines.[77] In the context of metabolic changes, in addition to induction of acute-phase protein synthesis, cytokines are involved in the downregulation of synthesis and the decrease in plasma levels of the so-called negative acute-phase proteins. IL-1-type cytokines have been shown to downregulate albumin and transferrin levels.[79] IL-6-type cytokines were found to decrease levels of albumin,[80] and TGFβ reduces albumin and apolipoprotein A-I.[79,81,82]

In addition to induction of the hepatic acute-phase protein synthesis, TNFα appears to have pleiotropic effects on metabolic functions. In experimental animals TNFα has been found to increase triglyceride levels by inhibiting lipoprotein lipase activity and to induce insulin resistance and an increase in glucose blood concentrations.[83] Infused to humans, TNFα is able to evoke the metabolic responses found in sepsis in a dose-dependent manner.[84]

The effect of TNFα on muscle protein breakdown appears to be indirect. With experimental sepsis in animals, anti-TNF antibodies counteracted the sepsis-induced increase in muscle protein catabolism. Treatment with a glucocorticoid receptor antagonist protected the animals from sepsis and from TNF-induced protein breakdown in skeletal muscle. It was concluded that the proteolytic effects of TNFα were secondary and were due to the release of glucocorticoids induced by TNFα.[85,86] Analogous to TNFα, treatment of experimental animals with IL-1 increased muscle protein breakdown; and application of IL-1 receptor antagonist in septic animals reduced protein catabolism.[38,85,87] In contrast to TNFα, the catabolic effect of IL-1 on muscle protein synthesis measured using muscle amino acid uptake is believed to be mediated via a glucocorticoid-independent mechanism because the inhibitory effect on muscle amino acid transport of TNF was blocked by a glucocorticoid receptor antagonist, whereas that of IL-1 remained unaffected.[88,89] A novel, fascinating mechanism of metabolic control is that of cellular hydration.[90] Cellular hydration has been shown to affect both protein synthesis and degradation; cell shrinking is protein catabolic, whereas cell swelling inhibits proteolysis and stimulates synthesis. The cellular hydration is influenced by hormones, ions, and metabolites and can change within minutes.[91–93]

A close relation between total nitrogen balance and cellular hydration has been found in skeletal muscle.[94] In critically ill patients (e.g., with sepsis) muscle glutamine concentrations decrease markedly, and changes in intracellular glutamine concentrations have been found to correlate with protein turnover.[29,95] Moreover, intracellular potassium concentrations are decreased in critically ill patients.[17] It has been shown that amino acid-induced cell swelling occurs in the physiologic concentration range (e.g., for glutamine, half-maximal cell swelling occurs at about 0.7 mM), so the effect of glutamine on protein turnover might be due to changes in cell volume resulting from the extracellular/intracellular glutamine gradient.[91] Moreover, the physiologic actions of insulin and glucagon and the influence of oxidative stress on protein metabolism may, at least in part, be explained by their influence on cellular hydration due to their action on transmembrane ion-transport systems, such as the Na-K-2Cl co-transport and Na^+/K^+-ATPase. Insulin causes cell swelling by an accumulation of Na^+, K^+, and Cl^-, whereas glucagon induces cell shrinking owing to an opening of plasma membrane ion channels. Hydrogen peroxide induces cell shrinking owing to an opening of K^+ channels.[91,92] Although the concept of metabolic control by cellular hydration seems attractive, it implies determination of protein degradation independent from the underlying disease.[91] As the cellular hydration status is certainly multifactorial, the precise role of cell shrinking and swelling in protein metabolism in inflammatory states must be determined.

Conclusions

The clinical consequences of hypermetabolism are as many and varied as are the metabolic responses. In addition to reduced gut function, skeletal and respiratory muscle wasting, impaired wound healing, and other reactions, the host response to infection is impaired and thus promotes the development of hypermetabolism. The extensive loss of total body protein in critically ill patients appears to be of major importance, but we are only at the beginning of understanding the cellular alterations and the inflammation-derived mediator cascades involved.

Current concepts for treating the hypermetabolic patient are predominantly empirical, based on supportive care: aggressive nutritional support,[96–99] oxygen supply, drug treatment (e.g., catecholamines, antibiotics, analgesic-sedatives, muscular relaxants), and fluid therapy. Although supportive care has proved successful,[98] the loss of lean body mass in the critically ill patient is not sufficiently influenced.[29,100] More recent therapeutic approaches (e.g., glutamine administration, growth hormone, or insulin-like growth factor 1 application), pentoxifylline treatment, or application of omega-3-fatty acids, all of which have been shown to exert positive effects on hypermetabolism, must prove their ability to improve clinical outcome in the critically ill patient.[101,102]

Potential new therapeutic approaches to hypermetabolism may develop from the current concepts in protein degradation, in particular by the use of selective proteasome inhibitors [e.g., lactacystin or N-acetyl-leucinyl-leucinyl-norleucinal (LLnL)],[103] although their pharmacologic action in humans is currently unknown. For example, LLnL, an inhibitor of the 20S proteasome, has been shown to protect against the sepsis-induced increase of muscle protein degradation in vitro[104] and to inhibit lipopolysaccharide-induced NF-κB activation, thereby preventing TNFα and IL-6 synthesis in macrophages in co-incubation experiments.[105] The concept of cellular hydration may lead to the discovery of new regulatory mechanisms of metabolic control in inflammatory states, as it has for the cytokine cascades in the development of SIRS in the past.

References

1. American College of Chest Physicians—Society of Critical Care Medicine Consensus Conference: Definitions for sepsis and organ failure and guidelines for the use of innovative therapies in sepsis. Crit Care Med 1992;20:864.
2. Beal AL, Cerra FB: Multiple organ failure syndrome in the 1990s. systemic inflammatory response and organ dysfunction. JAMA 1994;271:222.
3. Nguyen TT, Gilpin DA, Meyer NA, et al: Current treatment of severely burned patients. Ann Surg 1996;223:14.
4. Frankenfield DC, Smith JS, Cooney RN, et al: Relative association of fever and injury with hypermetabolism in critically ill patients. Injury 1997;28:617.
5. Chiolero R, Revelly JP, Tappy L: Energy metabolism in sepsis and injury. Nutrition 1997;13:45S.
6. Jeevanandam M, Young D, Schiller W: Obesity and the metabolic response to severe multiple trauma in man. J Clin Invest 1991;87:262.
7. Wilmore D, Orcutt T, Mason A, et al: Alterations in hypothalamic function following thermal injury. J Trauma 1975;15:697.
8. Viale J, Annat GJ, Bouffard Y, et al: Oxygen cost of breathing in postoperative patients: pressure support ventilation vs. continuous positive airway pressure. Chest 1988;93:506.
9. Boyd O, Grounds M, Bennett D: The dependency of oxygen consumption on oxygen delivery in critically ill postoperative patients is mimicked by variations in sedation. Chest 1992;101:1619.
10. Edwards J, Brown G, Nightingale P: Use of survivors' cardiorespiratory values as therapeutic goals in septic shock. Crit Care Med 1989;17:1098.
11. Allard J, Jeejheebhony K, Whitwell J, et al: Factors influencing energy expenditure in patients with burns. J Trauma 1988;28:199.
12. Giovannini I, Boldrini G, Castagnato M, et al: Respiratory quotient and patterns of substrate utilization in human sepsis and trauma. J Parenter Enteral Nutr 1983;7:226.
13. Elwyn DH, Kinney JM, Juvanandum M: Influence of increasing carbohydrate intake on glucose kinetics in injured patients. Ann Surg 1979;190:117.
14. Carpentier Y, Askanazi J, Elwyn D, et al: The effect of carbohydrate intake on lipolysis rate in depleted patients. Metabolism 1980;29:974.
15. Weissman C, Kemper M: Assessing hypermetabolism and hypometabolism in the postoperative critically ill patient. Chest 1992;102:1566.
16. Frankenfield D, Wiles CB, Bagley S, et al: Relationships between resting and total energy expenditure in injured and septic patients. Crit Care Med 1994;22:1796.
17. Hill GL: Implications of critical illness, injury, and sepsis on lean body mass and nutritional needs. Nutrition 1998;14:557.
18. Kreymann G, Grosser S, Buggisch P, et al: Oxygen consumption and resting metabolic rate in sepsis, sepsis syndrome, and septic shock. Crit Care Med 1993;21:1021.
19. Du Bois EF: The basal metabolism of fever. JAMA 1921;77:352.

20. Klein S, Peters E, Shangraw R: Lipolytic response to metabolic stress in critically ill patients. Crit Care Med 1991;19:776.
21. Elwyn D: Carbohydrate metabolism and requirements for nutritional support. Nutrition 1993;9:50.
22. Cerra FB: Hypermetabolism, organ failure, and metabolic support. Surgery 1987;101:1.
23. Wolfe RR: Substrate kinetics in sepsis. In: Little RA, Frayn KN (eds) The Scientific Basis for the Care of the Critically Ill Patient. Manchester, Manchester University Press, 1986;123.
24. Imamura M, Clowes GH, Blackburn G: Liver metabolism and gluconeogenesis in trauma and sepsis. Surgery 1975;77:868.
25. Rich AJ, Wright PD: Ketosis and nitrogen excretion in undernourished surgical patients. J Parenter Enteral Nutr 1979;3:250.
26. Burke JF, Wolfe R, Mullaney J: Glucose requirements and possible hepatic and respiratory abnormalities following excessive glucose intake. Ann Surg 1979;190:274.
27. Long C, Kinney J, Geiger J: Nonsuppressibility of gluconeogenesis in septic patients. Metabolism 1976;25:193.
28. Shizgal HM: Body composition and nutritional support. Surg Clin North Am 1981;61:729.
29. Wolfe RR, Jahoor F, Hartl WH: Protein and amino acid metabolism after injury. Diabetes Metab Rev 1989;5:149.
30. Streat SJ, Beddoe AH, Hill GL: Aggressive nutritional support does not prevent protein loss despite fat gain in septic intensive care patients. J Trauma 1987;27:262.
31. Cahill GFJ: Starvation in man. N Engl J Med 1970;282:668.
32. Biolo G, Maggi SP, Fleming RYD, et al: Relationship between transmembrane amino acid transport and protein kinetics in muscle tissue of severely burned patients. Clin Nutr 1993;12:4.
33. Birkhahn RH, Long CL, Fitkin D, et al: Effects of major skeletal trauma on whole body protein turnover in man measured by L-[1, ^{14}C]-leucine. Surgery 1980;88:294.
34. Petersen SR, Holaday NJ, Jeevanandam M: Enhancement of protein synthesis efficiency in parenterally fed trauma victims by adjuvant recombinant human growth hormone. J Trauma 1994;36:726.
35. Jennissen HP: Ubiquitin and the enigma of intracellular protein degradation. Eur J Biochem 1995: 231:1.
36. Hasselgren PO, Fischer JE: Sepsis: stimulation of energy-dependent protein breakdown resulting in protein loss in skeletal muscle. World J Surg 1998;22:203.
37. Hasselgren PO, James JH, Benson DW, et al: Total and myofibrillar protein breakdown in different types of rat skeletal muscle: effects of sepsis and regulation by insulin. Metabolism 1989;38:634.
38. Zamir O, Hasselgren PO, von Allmen D, et al: The effect of interleukin-1α and the glucocorticoid receptor blocker RU 38486 on total and myofibrillar protein breakdown in the skeletal muscle. J Surg Res 1991;50:579.
39. Hershko A, Ciechanover A: The ubiquitin system for protein degradation. Annu Rev Biochem 1992;61:761.
40. Michalek MT, Grant EP, Gramm C, et al: A role for the ubiquitin-dependent proteolytic pathway in MHC class I-restricted antigen presentation. Nature 1993;363:552.
41. Chiechanover A, Hod Y, Hershko A: A heat-stable polypeptide component of an ATP-dependent proteolytic system from reticulocytes. Biochem Biophys Res Commun 1978;81:1100.
42. Hershko A, Leshinsky E, Ganoth D, et al: ATP-dependent degradation of ubiquitin-protein conjugates. Proc Natl Acad Sci USA 1984;81:1619.
43. Hough R, Pratt G, Rechsteiner M: Purification of two high-molecular-mass proteases from rabbit reticulocyte lysate. J Biol Chem 1987;262:8303.
44. Hershko A, Chiechaniver A, Heller H, et al: Proposed role of ATP in protein breakdown: conjugation of proteins with multiple chains of the polypeptide of ATP-dependent proteolysis. Proc Natl Acad Sci USA 1980;77:1783.
45. Laub M, Jennissen HP: Synthesis and decay of calmodulin-ubiquitin conjugates in cell-free extracts of various rabbit tissues. Biochim Biophys Acta 1997;1357:173.
46. Tiao G, Fagan JM, Samuels N, et al: Sepsis stimulates non-lysosomal, energy-dependent proteolysis and increases ubiquitin mRNA levels in rat skeletal muscle. J Clin Exp 1994;94:2255.
47. Tiao G, Fagan JM, Samuels N, et al: Sepsis increases proteasome dependent proteolysis and mRNA levels for the proteasome subunit RC2 in skeletal muscle. Surg Forum 1995;46:10.
48. Mansoor O, Beaufrere B, Boirie Y, et al: Increased mRNA levels for components of the lysosomal, Ca^{2+}-activated, and ATP-ubiquitin-dependent proteolytic pathways in skeletal muscle from head trauma patients. Proc Natl Acad Sci USA 1996;93:2714.
49. Cerra FB, Siegel JH, Colman B, Border J, McMenamy RH: Autocannibalism, a failure of exogenous nutritional support. Ann Surg 1980;192:570.
50. Birkhahn R, Long C, Fitkin D, et al: Effects of major skeletal trauma on the whole body protein turnover in man measured by 1, ^{14}C leucine. Surgery 1980;88:294.
51. Garber AJ: Glutamine metabolism in skeletal muscle. In: Mora J, Palacios R (eds) Glutamine: Metabolism, Enzymology and Regulation. San Diego, Academic, 1980;259.
52. Lund P: Metabolism of glutamine, glutamate and aspartate. In: Waterlow JC, Stephen JML (eds) Nitrogen Metabolism in Man. London, Appl. Sci. 1981;155.
53. Meister A: Metabolism of glutamine. Physiol Rev 1955;36:103.
54. Larsson J, Lennmarken C, Martensson J, et al: Nitrogen requirements in severely injured patients. Br J Surg 1990;77:413.
55. Stehle P, Mertes N, Puchstein C, et al: Effect of parenteral glutamine peptide supplements on muscle glutamine loss and nitrogen balance after major surgery. Lancet 1989;1:231-233.
56. Mjaaland M, Unneberg K, Larsson J, et al: Growth hormone after abdominal surgery attenuated forearm glutamine, alanine, 3-methylhistidine, and total amino acid efflux in patients receiving total parenteral nutrition. Ann Surg 1993;217:413.
57. Bessey PQ, Watters JM, Aoki TT, Wilmore DW: Combined hormonal infusion stimulated the metabolic response to injury. Ann Surg 1984;200:264.
58. Tessari P, Inchiostro S, Barazzoni R, et al: Hyperglucagonemia stimulates phenylalanine oxidation in humans. Diabetes 1996;45:463.
59. Kayali AC, Young VR, Goodman MN: Sensitivity of myofibrillar proteins to glucocorticoid-induced muscle proteolysis. Am J Physiol 1987;252:E621.
60. Darmann D, Matthews DE, Bier DM: Physiological hypercortisolemia increases proteolysis, glutamine and alanine production. Am J Physiol 1988;255:E366.
61. Brillon DJ, Zheng B, Campbell RG, et al: Effect of cortisol on energy expenditure and amino acid metabolism in humans. Am J Physiol 1995;268:E501.
62. Price SR, England BK, Baily JL, et al: Acidosis and glucocorticoids concomitantly increase ubiquitin and proteasome subunit mRNAs in rat muscle. Am J Physiol 1994;267:C955.

63. Choo JJ, Horan MA, Little RA, et al: Anabolic effects of clanbuterol on skeletal muscle are mediated by β_2-adrenoreceptor activation. Am J Physiol 1992;92C:135.
64. Biolo G, Flemming RYD, Maggi SP, et al: Effects of hyperinsulinemia on muscle protein kinetics in severely burned patients. Clin Nutr 1994;13:23.
65. Herndon DN, Nguyen TT, Wolfe RR, et al: Lipolysis in burned patients is stimulated by the β_2-receptor for catecholamines. Arch Surg 1994;129:1301.
66. Ader R, Felten DL, Cohen N: Psychoimmunology, 2nd ed. San Diego, Academic, 1991.
67. Reichlin S: Neuroendocrine-immune interactions. N Engl J Med 1993;329:1246.
68. Madden KS, Felten DL: Experimental basis for neural-immune interactions. Physiol Rev 1995;75:77.
69. Jeffries MK, Vance ML: Growth hormone and cortisol secretion in patients with burn injury. J Burn Care Rehabil 1992;13:391.
70. Jeevanandam M, Ramias L, Shamos RF, et al: Decreased growth hormone levels in the catabolic phase of severe injury. Surgery 1992;111:495.
71. Jeevanandam M, Holaday NJ, Peteresen SR: Adjuvant recombinant human growth hormone does not augment endogenous glucose production in total parenteral nutrition-fed multiple trauma patients. Metabolism 1996;45:450.
72. Voerman HJ, Strack van Schijndel RJM, Groeneveld ABJ, et al: Effects of recombinant human growth hormone in patients with severe sepsis. Ann Surg 1992;216:648.
73. Moshage H: Cytokines and the hepatic acute phase response. J Pathol 1997;181:257.
74. Kushner I: The phenomenon of the acute phase response. Ann NY Acad Sci 1982;389:39.
75. Baumann H, Gauldie J: The acute phase response. Immunol Today 1994;15:74.
76. Koj A: Biological functions of acute-phase proteins. In: Gordon AH, Koj A (eds) The Acute Phase Response of Injury and Infection. Amsterdam, Elsevier, 1985;145.
77. Pannen BHJ, Robotham JL: The acute-phase response. New Horiz 1995;3:183.
78. Kushner I: Regulation of the acute phase response by cytokines. Perspect Biol Med 1993;36:611.
79. Perlmutter DH, Dinarello CA, Punsal PI, et al: Cachectin/tumor necrosis factor regulates hepatic acute-phase gene expression. J Clin Invest 1986;78:1349.
80. Koj A, Rokita H, Kordula T, et al: Role of cytokines and growth factors in the induced synthesis of proteinase inhibitors belonging to acute phase proteins. Biomed Biochim Acta 1991;50:421.
81. Andus G, Geiger T, Hirano T, et al: Action of recombinant human interleukin 1β and tumor necrosis factor α on the mRNA induction of acute-phase proteins. Eur J Immunol 1988;18:739.
82. Morrone G, Cortese R, Sorrentino V: Post-transcriptional control of negative acute phase genes by transforming growth factor β. EMBO J 1989;8:3767.
83. Lang CH: Role of cytokines in glucose metabolism. In: Aggarwal BB, Puri RK (eds) Human Cytokines. Their Role in Disease and Therapy. Cambridge, Blackwell, 1995;271.
84. Michie HR, Spriggs DR, Manogue KR, et al: Tumor necrosis factor and endotoxin induce similar metabolic responses in humans. Surgery 1988;104:280.
85. Zamir O, Hasselgren PO, O'Brien W, et al: Muscle protein breakdown during endotoxemia in rats and after treatment with interleukin-1 receptor antagonist (IL-1ra). Ann Surg 1992;216:381.
86. Tiao G, Fagan J, Roegner V, et al: Energy-ubiquitin-dependent muscle proteolysis during sepsis in rats is regulated by glucocorticoids. J Clin Invest 1996;97:339.
87. Zamir O, O'Brien W, Thompson RC, et al: Reduced muscle protein breakdown in septic rats following treatment with interleukin-1 receptor antagonist. Int J Biochem 1994;26:943.
88. Zamir O, Hasselgren PO, James H, et al: Effect of tumor necrosis factor or interleukin-1 on muscle amino acid uptake and the role of glucocorticoids. Surg Gynecol Obstet 1993;177:27.
89. Zamir O, Hasselgren PO, Higashiguchi T, et al: Tumor necrosis factor (TNF) and interleukin-1 (IL-1) induce muscle proteolysis through different mechanisms. Mediat Inflamm 1992;1:247.
90. Häussinger D, Roth E, Lang G, et al: Cellular hydration state: an important determinant of protein catabolism in health and disease. Lancet 1993;341:1330.
91. Häussinger D: Cellular hydratation: an important determinant of protein catabolism. In: Cynober L, Fürst P, Lawin P (eds) Pharmacological Nutrition. Immune Nutrition. Munich: W. Zuckschwerdt Verlag, 1995;50.
92. Häussinger D, Lang F, Häussinger D: Regulation of cell function by the cellular hydration state. Am J Physiol 1994;267:E343.
93. Lang F, Häussinger D: Interaction of Cell Volume and Cell Function. Heidelberg, Springer, 1993.
94. Häussinger D, Roth E, Lang F, et al: Cellular hydration state: an important determinant of protein catabolism in health and disease. Lancet 1993;341:1330.
95. Busch GL, Schreiber R, Dartsch PC, et al: Involvement of microtubules in the link between cell volume and pH of acidic cellular compartments in rat and human hepatocytes. Proc Natl Acad Sci USA 1994;91:9165.
96. Chandra S, Chandra RK: Nutrition and the immune system. Proc Nutr Soc 1993;341:1330.
97. Irving TT: Effects of malnutrition and hyperalimentation on wound healing. Surg Gynecol Obstet 1978;146:33.
98. Streat SJ, Beddoe AH, Hill GL: Aggressive nutritional support does not prevent protein loss, despite fat gain in septic intensive care patients. J Trauma 1987;27:262.
99. Bengmark S, Gianotti L: Nutritional support to prevent and treat multiple organ failure. World J Surg 1996;20:474.
100. Guarnieri G, Toigo G, Situlin R, et al: Muscle-biopsy studies on protein metabolism in traumatized patients. In: Dietze G, Grunert T, Kleinberg A, Wolfram S (eds) Clinical Nutrition and Metabolic Research, Research Proceedings, 7th Congress Espen, Munich, Basel: Karger, 1986;28.
101. Biolo G, Toigo G, Ciocchi B, et al: Metabolic response to injury and sepsis: changes in protein metabolism. Nutrition 1997;13:52S.
102. Michie HR: Metabolism of sepsis and multiple organ failure. World J Surg 1996;20:460.
103. Rock KL, Gramm C, Rothstein L, et al: Inhibitors of the proteasome block the degradation of most cell proteins and the generation of peptides presented on MHC class I molecules. Cell 1994;78:761.
104. Tiao GM, Fagan J, Lieberman M, et al: Sepsis increases proteasome-dependent proteolysis and mRNA levels for the proteasome subunit RC3 in skeletal muscle. Surg Forum 1995;46:10.
105. Schow SR, Joly A: N-Acetyl-leucinyl-leucinyl-norleucinal inhibits lipopolysaccharide-induced NF-kappaB activation and prevents TNF and IL-6 synthesis in vivo. Cell Immunol 1997;175:199.

12
Ischemia and Reperfusion as a Cause of Multiple Organ Failure

H. Gill Cryer

Multiple organ failure continues to be the most common cause of late death after injury. It is also one of the most common causes of mortality in the intensive care unit after major catastrophic medical illnesses and surgical complications. The pathogenesis of the syndrome remains incompletely understood, but it is most likely related to some combination of a dysregulated inflammatory response, maldistribution of microcirculatory blood flow, ischemia-reperfusion injury, and dysregulation of immune function.

Initially the multiple organ system failure syndrome was thought to be the result of sepsis. This idea was based on the observation that the early onset of respiratory failure after some stressful event coincided with a septic response in many patients. The response consisted of fever, leukocytosis, increased cardiac output, and decreased peripheral vascular resistance. Goris and colleagues[1] subsequently demonstrated that up to 50% of all patients developing multiple organ system failure had no evidence of infection. In addition, Nuytinck et al.[2] found that patients with multiple organ system failure who died had evidence of systemic acute and chronic inflammation throughout all of their organs. These findings led to the idea that multiple organ system failure originates with the systemic inflammatory response syndrome (SIRS) and dysregulated systemic hyperinflammatory response rather than sepsis or infection per se. One common inciting event that can lead to this scenario is ischemia/reperfusion injury. The purpose of this review is to explore the idea that ischemia/reperfusion injury is an event that commonly predisposes the clinical syndrome of multiple organ system failure.

Although the term multiple organ failure was first coined during the late 1970s,[3] the clinical syndrome was well described as early as 1960. Haimovici[4] described a 60-year-old man with acute limb ischemia due to a femoral artery embolus. The patient underwent operative removal of the embolus followed by fasciotomies for severe swelling. The procedure was completed 8 hours after the onset of pain. Postoperatively, the patient developed heart failure, renal failure, pulmonary failure, and limb failure; and he ultimately died. Haimovici called this syndrome the myonephropathic-metabolic syndrome, but today we recognize that the local symptoms causing swelling in the extremity were the result of an ischemia/reperfusion injury and the systemic deterioration as SIRS and multiple organ dysfunction or failure. Both the systemic failure and the local failure are now known to be a result of a local and systemic inflammatory response set into motion as a result of the reperfusion of ischemic tissue with oxygenated blood.

The well documented pathophysiology of ischemic injury occurs as a loss of oxygen results in a change from aerobic to anaerobic metabolism at the cellular level. As surgical techniques for restoring flow to such organs improved it became clear that there is a finite period of time that individual organs can tolerate ischemia before irreversible damage occurs. This observation formed the basis for the time-honored surgical therapeutic principle that the outcome of any procedure to restore flow to ischemic tissue is inversely proportional to the time from the onset of ischemia to restoration of flow. However, ischemic cell death alone cannot explain all the features of the disease.

Components of Ischemia/Reperfusion

We now know from basic research studies using models of limb ischemia and reperfusion that two basic problems occur during reperfusion of ischemic skeletal muscle. The first is the no-reflow phenomenon: Upon restoration of flow to the tissue, a certain percentage of capillaries and even small arterial branches remain occluded with thrombus, with obvious persistent ischemic consequences to the cells supplied by those vessels. The second problem is the generalized endothelial cell injury due to reactive oxygen mediators, platelet-activating factor, and polymorphonuclear leukocyte (PMN)-related endothelial cell interactions which leads to edema caused by capillary leak and continued tissue damage from the by-products of PMN activation.

Avoidance of Ischemia/Reperfusion Injury

Quinones-Baldrich and colleagues[5] determined that the fibrinolytic agent urokinase, when administered to an experimental animal at the time of reperfusion, resulted in improved muscle function. The authors combined this technology with the concept of controlled reperfusion in a group of patients undergoing embolectomy for acute vascular occlusion. The authors used isolated limb reperfusion with blood containing 100,000 units of urokinase delivered by an infusion pump at gradually increasing flow rates over 30 minutes. The authors tried this technique in 10 patients who presented with acute severe lower limb ischemia. They were treated with catheter thromboembolectomy followed by isolated limb perfusion using an extracorporeal pump with a heat exchanger and oxygenator to perfuse the isolated extremity at physiologic pressures with autologous blood containing high doses of urokinase. Limb salvage was accomplished in seven of the ten patients. More germane to the current discussion, however, is that none of the patients developed multiple organ system failure or signs of SIRS after reperfusion. Using this technique, the patient's systemic circulation does not see venous drainage from the extremity until the extremity vasculature has been essentially washed out by the extracorporeal pump. Therefore not only does this controlled reperfusion technique alleviate the no-reflow at the local tissue level, it prevents the by-products of the reperfusion injury from washing into the systemic circulation.

Another approach to this clinical problem that may be more effective in preventing the reperfusion injury component was reported by Byersdorf et al.[6] They also used isolated limb reperfusion after thromboembolectomy for ischemic extremities. Their technique differed in that they employed a perfusate solution similar to that used for myocardial preservation during coronary artery bypass instead of the fibrinolytic agents used by Quinones-Baldrich and colleagues. Byersdorf et al. studied 19 patients who had undergone long periods of complete limb ischemia treated by Fogerty catheter clearance of gross thrombus followed by vascular isolation and reperfusion with a reperfusate containing blood/crystalloid, allopurinol, and glutamate aspartate for 30 minutes. It is not clear from the report by Byersdorf et al. if systemic sequelae occurred. The authors stated that there were no systemic complications in the 16 surviving patients, but three patients died, all from cardiogenic shock during the reperfusion procedure. Because the limb was isolated it is doubtful that death was due to sequelae of reperfusion injury, but it cannot be discerned with 100% certainty from their report. Nonetheless, the principles of controlled reperfusion with fibrinolytic agents and pressure-forced flow to prevent the no-reflow phenomenon in concert with reperfusion solutions containing a mix of nutrients, oxygen radical scavengers, and impermeate solutes to prevent reperfusion injury in isolation from the systemic circulation to prevent SIRS represents a major clinical advance.

Similar, more advanced strategies have been employed using controlled reperfusion after ischemia/reperfusion injury incurred during treatment of myocardial infarction and cardiopulmonary bypass for coronary artery bypass grafting or heart transplantation. Reperfusion of ischemic myocardium is associated with a significant risk of multiple organ failure (MOF). Although some of this problem may be secondary to the cardiopulmonary bypass, a significant component is attributable to reperfusion injury.[7] Controlled reperfusion of ischemic myocardium has concentrated on ionic composition, metabolic substrate composition, and the presence of leukocytes and platelets in the reperfusate. Buckberg[7] convincingly demonstrated that improved myocardial functional recovery is achieved in ischemic myocardium when the blood-based reperfusate is hypocalcemic. Byersdorf[8] demonstrated significant improvement in regional myocardial contractility in patients treated with modified reperfusion after emergency coronary artery vascularization for acute coronary occlusion. In this study modified reperfusion consisted of hypocalcemic, glutamate/aspartate-enhanced, hyperosmolor, alkalotic, diltiazem-containing blood cardioplegia delivered at a pressure of 50 mmHg for 20 minutes at the time of reperfusion.

Leukocyte Filtration/Inactivation

More recently measures to filter leukocytes or inhibit their activation have been added to controlled reperfusion techniques and have been quite successful in reducing reperfusion injury. Leukocyte-depleted reperfusion has been shown to reduce infarct size in animal models of regional ischemia and modified reperfusion.[9] Using the combination of leukocyte depletion and aspartate/glutamate enhancement of blood reperfusate, Drinkwater's group[10] initiated a randomized double-blind clinical trial in transplanted human hearts. In their study myocardial biopsy specimens from 16 patients undergoing leukocyte-depleted reperfusion had significantly less ultrastructural injury than 16 patients undergoing whole-blood reperfusion. There were no reported cases of adult respiratory distress syndrome (ARDS) or MOF in this study, but there were two important observations. First, in the control group there was evidence of reperfusion injury 10 minutes after initiation of reperfusion, indicating that this injury begins quickly. Second, leukocyte depletion prevented this early reperfusion injury, suggesting that both the endothelial cell and the leukocyte are somehow primed prior to reperfusion.

Cytokines

Clinical advances in reperfusion of the ischemic limb and myocardium have demonstrated that controlled reperfusion and vascular isolation of the organ to avoid a systemic response can prevent MOF after ischemia and reperfusion. However, it is not always possible to isolate the ischemic organ from the systemic circulation. Under these circumstances cytokines elaborated at reperfusion of the ischemic organ lead to activation of the inflammatory response in distal organs. The classic example is visceral ischemia and reperfusion injury associated with repair of thoracic and abdominal aortic aneurysms. Foulds and associates[11] demonstrated that a rise in intraoperative neutrophil CD11-B expression during supraceliac cross-clamping is a marker for subsequent development of postoperative organ dysfunction. They investigated the relation between visceral ischemia and neutrophil activation, sepsis, and organ dysfunction following visceral reperfusion in 51 patients undergoing supraceliac cross-clamping, 5 with suprarenal clamping, and 8 with infrarenal clamping for repair of aortic aneurysms. There was a significant correlation between visceral clamp time and intraoperative CD11-B expression. Interestingly, there was no difference between bypass- and non-bypass-assisted surgery with regard to neutrophil expression, indicating that differences were due to clamp time alone. More important to the current discussion, there was a significant increase in clamp time and CD11-B expression in patients who developed severe sepsis and postoperative organ dysfunction. These authors also observed that preoperative levels of CD11-B expression were elevated in patients who died intraoperatively and in some patients who went on to develop MOF. Their paper demonstrated that the visceral ischemia/reperfusion injury associated with aneurysm repair leads to upregulation of the adhesion molecule CD11-B on circulating PMNs and is associated with the development of MOF. In addition, the observation that preoperative levels of CD11-B may identify an at-risk subset of patients suggests that under some circumstances PMNs are primed prior to the ischemia/reperfusion episode. The ischemia/reperfusion injury is most severe under these circumstances. These clinical associations suggest that visceral ischemia leads to priming or activation of leukocytes, which cause systemic sequelae in distant organs after reperfusion. This idea has been confirmed in experimental models.

Cell Adhesion Molecules

Endothelial cell adhesion molecules (ECAMS) are thought to play an important role in ischemia/reperfusion injury by causing adhesion of leukocytes to endothelial cells. Intercellular adhesion molecule 1 (ICAM-1) is one of the adhesion molecules that has been shown to be upregulated in response to cytokines. This upregulation leads to leukocyte endothelial cell interaction (adhesion) and to neutrophil infiltration of the affected tissue. Meyer and colleagues[12] measured ICAM-1 expression in the liver and other organs after hepatic ischemia/reperfusion injury in Sprague-Dawley rats using a 45-minute occlusion to the left lateral lobe of the liver followed by 5 hours of reperfusion. After reperfusion, ICAM-1 was upregulated not only in the ischemic lobe of the liver but also in the nonischemic lobe of the liver, the heart, the kidney, the intestine, and the pancreas. Upregulation in the lung was not significant. This study demonstrates that endothelial cells are activated by ICAM-1 upregulation in distant organs after reperfusion of ischemic liver, which may mediate a hyperinflammatory response in these distal organs.

In support of this idea, Sun and associates[13] performed a histologic evaluation of various organs after 8 or 12 hours of ischemia and reperfusion of a single lower extremity in rabbits. Histologic examination showed massive inflammatory destruction of the liver and kidney. The injuries were more obvious in areas with the greatest blood flow during reperfusion. Taken together these papers indicate that ischemia and reperfusion of a single organ causes endothelial activation in remote organs, leading to remote organ inflammatory injury. When possible, strategies to reperfuse ischemic organs in isolation from the systemic circulation should be used. When isolated reperfusion is not possible, strategies to modify the reperfusate to decrease systemic activation of endothelial cells and PMNs must be developed.

One example of such a strategy is demonstrated by Nielsen and colleagues.[14] Using a randomized controlled animal design, the authors hypothesized that multiple organ injury and concentrations of xanthine oxidase would be decreased by the administration of a bolus of colloid solution at reperfusion. Hepatoenteric ischemia was maintained for 40 minutes with a balloon catheter in the thoracic aorta followed by 3 hours of reperfusion. Groups received either a bolus of hetastarch (Hextend), 5% human albumin, or lactated Ringer's solution. Multiple organ injury was assessed by the release of lactate dehydrogenase (LDH) activity into the plasma and by histologic evaluation of gastric and pulmonary injury. Circulating LDH activity was significantly higher in the animals receiving lactated Ringer's solution than in rabbits given either of the colloid solutions. Gastric injury was significantly decreased by administration of both colloid solutions. Lung injury (bronchial alveolar lavage LDH activity) was significantly decreased by hetastarch solution administration. In addition, the hetastarch solution resulted in 50% less xanthine oxidase activity released during reperfusion compared to that seen with albumin or lactated Ringer's solution. Taken together with earlier animal studies[15] that demonstrated decreased PMN adherence to endothelium after ischemia/reperfusion by in vivo videomicroscopy after prophylactic hemodilution with dextran and hetastarch, these data suggest some promise for this strategy.

Systemic Ischemia/Reperfusion Injury

After local isolatable ischemia/reperfusion and nonisolatable local ischemia/reperfusion, systemic ischemia/reperfusion injury such as homorrhagic shock, cardiac arrest, and hypoxia represent the next level of complexity in understanding this complex disease. Hemorrhagic shock is the prototypical systemic ischemia/reperfusion injury. There has been excellent progress in the treatment of hemorrhagic shock over the last 40 years. Major breakthroughs have been made as a result of the experimental finding that, after hemorrhage, restoration of intravascular volume with blood alone does not adequately restore tissue perfusion. This led to adding crystalloid resuscitation to blood transfusion for the treatment of hemorrhagic shock. It markedly improved survival, although, as demonstrated by the following case, certain patients still do poorly.

A 20-year-old man sustained a gunshot wound to the abdomen and arrived in the emergency room with a blood pressure of 80 mmHg. The patient was taken immediately to the operating room where he was found to be bleeding from the splenic hilum and other vessels. The spleen was operatively removed, and several other bleeding vessels were ligated while

10 units of blood were transfused into the patient. The patient's blood pressure was well maintained throughout the procedure. Postoperatively in the recovery room the patient developed severe pulmonary dysfunction due to ARDS and subsequently prolonged MOF requiring 2 months of intensive care unit (ICU) support.

This patient developed multiple organ dysfunction as the result of a reperfusion injury, which initiated SIRS. This case minimizes some but not all of the complicating factors involved with injured patients. Little residual injured tissue remained because the spleen was removed. Therefore the predominant mechanism was prolonged ischemia due to blood loss and reperfusion, and the reperfusion did involve 10 units of banked blood. Blood transfusion after injury is associated with the development of ARDS and MOF.[16,17] It is not known whether this association is due to the transfused blood itself or to the number of blood transfusions, which serves as an indication of the degree of shock suffered by individual patients. However, recent studies in humans and laboratory studies indicate that factors in banked blood, especially blood banked longer than 40 days, may contribute to the development of ARDS and MOF after resuscitation.[18]

As with local limb ischemia/reperfusion injury, much experimental evidence now exists that microvascular blood flow in many organs is not restored to normal after crystalloid resuscitation for hemorrhagic shock, even though total body flow (cardiac output) has returned to normal or above-normal levels.[19,20] These microcirculatory disturbances are undoubtedly related to reperfusion injury and the no-reflow phenomenon. As with visceral reperfusion, isolated controlled reperfusion of the ischemic tissue associated with hemorrhagic shock is not practical. However, the clinical correlate to controlled reperfusion during hemorrhagic shock is seen when oxygen consumption is used as an indication of adequate nutritional blood flow in patients resuscitated from hemorrhagic shock with high levels of oxygen delivery. When patients are monitored carefully and attention is paid to oxygen delivery and oxygen consumption, it has been shown that patients with supernormal levels of oxygen delivery and consumption are more likely to survive and have less organ failure than patients resuscitated to normal oxygen delivery and oxygen consumption levels.[21] Following this observation, the obvious hypothesis was that purposefully pushing cardiac output to supranormal levels would improve survival and decrease organ dysfunction presumably by decreasing the no-reflow phenomenon in various organ systems after resuscitation from hemorrhagic shock. Several prospective randomized studies have been designed to test this hypothesis, with confusing results.[22] Despite problems with the experimental design and the fact that approximately one-third of all patients achieve hyperdynamic supranormal levels of oxygen delivery and consumption on their own with little therapeutic inducement to do so, attempts to achieve supranormal levels of oxygen delivery and consumption have become well accepted endpoints during resuscitation for hemorrhagic shock. On the other hand, although this practice undoubtedly leads to some improvement in morbidity and mortality rates, it is clearly not enough to prevent ARDS and MOF by itself.

Law and colleagues[23] prospectively evaluated 13 severely injured patients in hemorrhagic shock. They were all resuscitated to supranormal values of oxygen delivery and consumption within 24 hours of admission, yet 6 of the 13 patients developed multiple organ dysfunction. In that study we prospectively measured a variety of cytokines in the serum of these patients at various times after admission to the hospital. Of interest, soluble ICAM-1 was significantly elevated by the end of resuscitation in the serum of patients who went on to develop MOF but remained normal in patients who did not. Additionally, when MOF was quantitated with a severity score,[21] there was an excellent correlation between the serum levels of soluble ICAM-1 at the end of resuscitation and the eventual severity of MOF. Serum levels of the proinflammatory cytokines interleukin-6 (IL-6) and IL-8 also increased as the severity of MOF increased over time. These data are consistent with the hypothesis that hyperactivity of the inflammatory response occurs as the result of systemic reperfusion injury leading to MOF in severely injured patients. A more recent study[24] has corroborated these findings.

Seecamp and colleagues[24] measured serum levels of tumor necrosis factor α (TNFα), IL-1, IL-6, the soluble adhesion molecule ICAM-1, E-selectin, IL-1 receptor antagonist (IL-1ra), serum TNF receptor-2 (sTNFr2), and IL-10 in three groups of surgical patients with varying degrees of ischemia/reperfusion. Group 1 included patients undergoing elective limb surgery without a tourniquet. Group 2 included patients subjected to limb surgery with a tourniquet. The third group was composed of accidental trauma patients, who were retrospectively divided into those who subsequently developed multiple organ dysfunction and those who did not. Serial blood samples were obtained for 5 days. There were no elevation in cytokines in group 1. When a tourniquet was applied (mean time 105 minutes) elective limb surgery resulted in significant increases in serum levels of IL-6, IL-1ra, and IL-10 but not TNFr2. On the other hand, tourniquet application did not increase shedding of adhesion molecules. Soluble ICAM-1 and soluble E-selectin remained unchanged throughout the 5-day observation period in groups 1 and 2. All patients with multiple injuries had significant increases of all cytokines early after trauma (up to 10- to 20-fold higher than in elective limb surgery patients). Furthermore, when the accidental trauma patients were divided according to their MOF scores into those who had ($n = 8$) and those who did not have ($n = 22$) multiple organ dysfunction (MOD), a clear difference became evident in the serum IL-6 and IL-1ra levels within the first 4 days and in serum IL-10 levels for the first 2 days after trauma. Serum cytokine levels were significantly higher in the patients developing MOD 3–4 days prior to the onset of the MOD. Unlike the results of our study,[23] although highly elevated, TNFr2 levels did not differentiate between patients developing MOD and those who did not. Similar to the results of our study, the increase in serum cytokine levels was associated with marked expression and shedding of ICAM-1 and E-selectin, with significantly higher levels of serum

ICAM-1 in MOD patients than in non-MOD patients 3–5 days after trauma and increased soluble serum E selectin levels 2–4 days after trauma. These authors confirmed that release of cytokines and soluble adhesion molecules into the circulation correlates well with the degree of trauma and the extent of associated ischemia/reperfusion injury. Furthermore, both groups of mediators are also clearly related to the development of MOD in patients with multiple injuries with generalized ischemia/reperfusion injury caused by hemorrhagic shock. Taken together these studies indicate that the development of MOF after hemorrhagic shock and injury is associated with high levels of circulating proinflammatory cytokines and activation of PMNs early after reperfusion.

As reviewed by Waxman,[20] many strategies to abrogate this systemic reperfusion injury have been tested in experimental models, but few meaningful clinical studies have been reported. In one prospective, randomized trial[25] human recombinant superoxide dismutase (SOD) was given for 5 days after injury to 24 multiply-injured patients. The group receiving antioxidant treatment with SOD had less severe organ failure and shortened stay in the ICU.

Vedder and colleagues[26] prevented PMN activation by the use of monoclonal antibodies to CD11–CD18 and showed a marked decrease in organ injury after hemorrhagic shock and resuscitation in rabbits. Similar findings have been shown in a pig model.[21] A clinical trial in humans using this monoclonal antibody is underway.

With logic similar to what led to using multipronged therapeutic resuscitative fluids to control reperfusion of ischemic limbs and during heart transplantation surgery discussed earlier, Barquist and colleagues[28] attempted resuscitative regimens in seriously injured patients. A treatment algorithm to prevent and ameliorate ischemia/reperfusion injury using antioxidants and splanchnic directed resuscitation was administered to severely injured trauma patients. The xanthine oxidase inhibitor folate and a free radical scavenger mannitol were uniformly administered. Vasoactive agents including isoproterenol, dobutamine, nitroglycerine, nitroprusside, and prostaglandin E were used in sequential order to attempt to correct abnormal gut perfusion as measured by tonometry. Using this treatment regimen the authors found a decrease in the incidence of multiple organ system failure and length of ICU stay compared to that in historical controls. In a later, similar study at the same institution[29] the resuscitative fluid regimen was modified to also include lidocaine, selenium, polymyxin B, and hydrocortisone in addition to glutamine, acetylcysteine, and vitamins A and E. This protocol resulted in normalization of splanchnic blood flow in 90% of patients and a marked reduction in the incidence of multiple organ system failure and ICU length of stay. Although this study is encouraging, it is important to note that the comparison group was historical controls.

An emerging hypothesis is that multiple organ system failure is the result of an exaggerated proinflammatory response coexisting with an exaggerated counterinflammatory response, with the clinical manifestations dependent on the degree of imbalance between the counterregulatory antiinflammatory response and the proinflammatory response. With this hypothesis anticytokines may play an important role in modulating the pathogenesis of ischemia/reperfusion early after reperfusion. If the exaggerated counterinflammatory response persists, a state of immune dysfunction results with an increased susceptibility to infection. Numerous clinical studies support this idea. Law and colleagues[23] demonstrated that early after resuscitation severely injured patients who ultimately develop organ failure have increased levels of soluble ICAM-1, IL-6, and IL-8. The proinflammatory cytokines TNFα and IL-1 could not be found in these patients. However, levels of soluble TNF receptor, thought to be a counterinflammatory cytokine, were elevated in patients developing MOF, and the degree of elevation correlated with the degree of organ failure. Cinat and colleagues[30] showed similar increases in IL-1ra and soluble TNF receptors early after injury. Further complicating this idea, although most reports suggest that sublethal insults are commonly associated with the development of MOF, Miner et al.[31] showed that an initial ischemia/reperfusion episode in the rat small intestine (30 minutes followed by 24 hours of reperfusion) actually protects the intestine from a subsequent ischemia/reperfusion episode. Animals subjected to two insults of ischemia/reperfusion demonstrated significantly less mucosal injury than animals undergoing one episode, despite increased neutrophil infiltration, leukotriene B₄, and activated systemic neutrophils. It appears that the initial episode caused an adaptive response associated with cytoarchitectural preservation following the subsequent insult. Nevertheless, repeated ischemia/reperfusion potentiated the local inflammatory response and the systemic activation of neutrophils. This study supports the idea that episodes of ischemia/reperfusion are associated with an initial hyperinflammatory phase followed by an increase in counterinflammatory cytokines, which blunt the effects of subsequent proinflammatory stimuli. Much work remains to be done to understand and intervene in this delicate balance.

Conclusions

Multiple organ failure after ischemia/reperfusion injury is influenced by a balance of proinflammatory and counterinflammatory cytokines. MOF can occur at either end of the spectrum. If ischemia/reperfusion causes a severe hyperinflammatory response, it can lead directly to MOF. On the other hand, counterinflammatory cytokines result from ischemia/reperfusion as well. Under some circumstances these counterinflammatory cytokines may protect tissue from further episodes of ischemia/reperfusion if the organ recovers from the first episode. On the other hand, in different circumstances these counterinflammatory cytokines may promote MOF. If ischemia/reperfusion occurs in the presence of primed PMNs, the consequences are particularly severe. Similarly, if there are multiple hyperinflammatory stimuli simultaneously, as in the multiply-injured patient with systemic ischemia/reperfusion injury, blood transfusion, and tissue injury, the most severe consequences can occur. Treatment of ischemia/reperfusion injury has relied primarily on controlled reperfusion techniques. They have been well developed for transplantation, vascular, and cardiothoracic surgery and have been initiated in strategies to resuscitate the injured patient. Early response modification of other aspects of shock and injury to modulate the effects of tissue injury and blood transfusion require further research. In addition, an improved understanding of the hypoinflammatory phase is necessary.

References

1. Goris RJA, te Boekhorst TPA, Nuytinck JS, et al: Multiple organ failure: generalized autodestructive inflammation? Arch Surg 1985; 120:1109–1115.
2. Nuytinck HCS, Offermans XJMW, Kubat K, et al: Whole body inflammation in trauma patients: an autopsy study. Arch Surg 1988;123:1519–1524.
3. Eiseman B, Beart R, Norton L: Multiple organ failure. Surg Gynecol Obstet 1977;144:323–326.
4. Haimovici H: Arterial embolism with acute massive ischemic myopathy and myoglobinuria: evaluation of a hither-to unreported syndrome with report of two cases. Surgery 1960;47:739.
5. Quinones-Baldrich WJ, Deaton DH, Ahn SS, Nene S, Cushen C, Moore WS: Isolated fibrinolytic limb perfusion with extra corporal pump in the management of acute limb ischemia. (in press).
6. Beyersdorf F, Mitrev K, Ihken K, et al: Controlled limb reperfusion in patients having cardiac operations. J Thorac Cardiovasc Surg 1996;111:873–881.
7. Buckberg GD: Update on current techniques on myocardial protection. Ann Thorac Surg 1995;60:805–814.
8. Beyersdorf F: Protection of evolving myocardial infarction and failed PTCA. Ann Thorac Surg 1995;60:833–838.
9. Gates RN, Drinkwater DC: Reperfusion injury after heart transplantation. In: Zikria BA (ed) Reperfusion Injuries and Clinical Capillary Leak Syndrome. Armonk, NY, Futura, 1994;259–280.
10. Pearl JM, Laks H, Drinkwater DC, et al: Leukocyte-depleted reperfusion of transplanted human hearts prevents ultrastructural evidence of reperfusion injury. J Surg Res 1992;52:298–308.
11. Foulds S, Mireskandari M, Kalu P, et al: Visceral ischemia and neutrophil activation in sepsis and organ dysfunction. J Surg Res 1998;75:170–176.
12. Meyer K, Brown MF, Zibari G, et al: ICAM 1 up regulation in distant tissues after hepatic ischemia reperfusion: a clue to the mechanism of multiple organ failure. J Pediatr Surg 1998;33:350–353.
13. Sun JS, Tsuang YH, Lou FJ, Lou KS, Hang YS: Biochemical and histopathological changes in the mortality caused by acute ischemic limb injury: a rabbit model. Histol Histopathol 1998;13:47–55.
14. Nielsen VG, Tan S, Bricks AE, Baird MS, Parks DA: Hextend (hetastarch solution) decreases multiple organ injury and xanthine oxidase release after hepatoenteric ischemia reperfusion in rabbits. Crit Care Med 1997;25:1565–1574.
15. Menger MD, et al: Influence of isovolemic hemodilution with dextran and HES on the PMN–endothelium interaction in post ischemic skeletal muscle. Eur Surg Res 1989;21(Suppl 2):74.
16. Sauaia A, Moore FA, Moore EE: Multiple organ failure can be predicted as early as 12 hours after injury. J Trauma 1998;45:291–303.
17. Cryer HG, Leong K, McArthur DL, et al: Multiple organ failure: by the time you predict it, it's already there. J Trauma 1999;46:597–606.
18. Zallen G: Age of transfused blood is an independent risk factor for post injury multiple organ failure. Presented at 21st Annual Resident's Trauma Paper Competition, American College of Surgeons Committee on Trauma, Washington DC, March 18, 1999.
19. Flynn WJ, Cryer HG, Garrison RN: Pentoxifylline but not saralasin restores hepatic blood flow after resuscitation from hemorrhagic shock. J Surg Res 1991;50:616–621.
20. Waxman K: Shock: ischemia, reperfusion, and inflammation. New Horiz 1996;4:153–160.
21. Moore FA, Haemel JB, Moore EE: Incommensurate oxygen consumption in response to maximal oxygen availability predicts post injury multiple organ failure. J Trauma 1992;33:58–63.
22. Yu M, Levy MM, Smith P: Effect of maximizing oxygen delivery on mortality and morbidity rates in critically ill patients: a prospective randomized controlled study. Crit Care Med 1993;21:830–838.
23. Law MM, Cryer HG, Abraham E: Elevated serum levels of I-CAM-1 but not TNF receptor, correlate with the development of multiple organ failure in trauma patients. J Trauma 1994;37:100–110.
24. Seecamp A, Jochum M, Ziegler M, Van Griensbenm, Martin M, Regel G: Cytokines and adhesion molecules in elective and accidental trauma related ischemia reperfusion. J Trauma 1998;44:874–882.
25. Marzi I, Buhren V, Schottler A, et al: Value of superoxide dismutase for prevention of multiple organ failure after multiple trauma. J Trauma 1993;35:110–120.
26. Vedder NB, Winn RK, Rice CL: A monoclonal antibody to the adherence-promoting leukocyte glycoprotein, CD 18, reduced organ injury and improves survival from hemorrhagic shock and resuscitation in rabbits. J Clin Invest 1988;81:939–944.
27. Fabian TC, Croce MA, Stewart RM, et al: Neutrophil CD-18 expression and blockage after traumatic shock and endotoxin challenge. Ann Surg 1994;220:552–563.
28. Barquist E, Kirton O, Windsor J, et al: The impact of antioxidant and splanchnic directed therapy on persistent uncorrected gastric mucosal pH in the critically injured trauma patient. J Trauma 1998;44:355–359.
29. Kirton O, Civetta JM: Ischemia-reperfusion injury in the critically ill: a progenitor of multiple organ failure. New Horiz 1999;7:87–95.
30. Cinat M, Waxman K, Vaziri ND, et al: Soluble cytokine receptors and receptor antagonists are sequentially released following trauma. J Trauma 1995;39:112–120.
31. Miner TJ, Tavaf-Motamen H, Stojadinovic A, Shea-Donohue T: Ischemia reperfusion protects the rat small intestine against subsequent injury. J Surg Res 1999;82:1–10.

# 13
Endotoxin in Human Disease and Its Endogenous Control

Alexander Shnyra, Michael Luchi, Jiangjun Gao, Christopher J. Papasian, David L. Horn, Richard Silverstein, and David C. Morrison

It is impossible to consider the topic of the host systemic inflammatory response and its important role in mediating the pathogenesis of multiple organ failure, a classic outcome of the manifestation of sepsis, without dealing with the potential contribution of endotoxin. From the earliest recognition of the pivotal role of microbes and their products to mortality and morbidity, microbial toxins have served as one of the central foci for both passive and active therapeutic intervention as well as prime candidates for prevention through the development and implementation of immunization programs. Although endotoxin would clearly be included within the collection of microbial toxins capable of causing disease, interest in the pursuit of effective antiendotoxin intervention strategies did not, in the early days, keep pace with the advances made in understanding and treating microbe-based diseases in which exotoxins were positively implicated as causative factors. The reasons for this are complicated but in large part have been attributable to difficulties encountered by investigators in defining the exact chemical structure of this microbial constituent and the remarkable diverse spectrum of biologic activities manifested by endotoxin.

Considerable advances in our understanding of the chemistry and biology of endotoxin have taken place during the last 40–50 years. They include a number of key findings.

1. The toxic portion of the endotoxin being attributable to the relatively highly conserved lipid A domain[1] of the lipopolysaccharide (LPS) constituent of the endotoxin
2. The collective studies of many investigators during the 1960s and 1970s documenting the rather profound and universal capacity of LPS/lipid A to interact with and perturb host inflammatory defense systems[2,3]
3. The discovery and characterization by Sultzer[4] of the inbred endotoxin hyporesponsive C3H/HeJ mouse strain and its value in the elucidation of the pivotal role of systemic inflammation in the in vivo host response to endotoxin as reviewed by Morrison and Ulevitch[5]
4. The pioneering studies of McCabe, Braude, and Ziegler and their colleagues[6] that allowed maturation of the concept that endotoxin was most likely an important factor in gram-negative sepsis
5. The seminal findings of Beutler et al.[7] establishing that antibodies to endotoxin-induced inflammatory cytokines would protect experimental animals against the lethal effects of endotoxin
6. The development by Wolff, Dinarello, and their colleagues of well controlled human volunteer studies that established the fact that purified endotoxin would reproduce in humans many of the clinical and pathophysiologic sequelae seen in patients with the sepsis syndrome[8]
7. The discoveries by Wright and Ulevitch and their colleagues[9] of the important role played by CD14 in LPS-dependent signaling, and the more recent discovery by Yang et al.,[10] Kirschning et al.[11] of the primary role of the Toll-like receptors in LPS-dependent responses

The development of this increased knowledge base regarding structure, function, and potential pathophysiologic manifestations of endotoxin in modulating host immune and inflammatory responses provided basic investigators and clinical researchers with a variety of additional therapeutic strategies by which to intervene in the treatment of gram-negative sepsis. Early on, these approaches were primarily directed at the endotoxin molecule itself through the use of polyclonal and monoclonal antibodies for passive immunotherapy,[12] and a number of clinical trials were designed against the immunologic and immunopharmacologic mediators induced by endotoxin. The failure of virtually all of these approaches to provide substantial levels of protection in the septic patient, despite what was generally viewed as promising (and sometimes even dramatic) protective efficacy in preclinical trials, clearly underscored the complexity of the problems facing the septic patient. These findings clearly indicated the fact that additional studies regarding endotoxin, the control of secretion of inflammatory and antiinflammatory mediators, and a greater appreciation of the conditions that dictate exactly when these factors would be important would be required before truly effective means of dealing with endotoxin could be implemented in the septic patient.

Perhaps one of the more pressing issues that would affect the significance of, and contribution to, the pathogenesis of sepsis of bacterial endotoxin would be the related questions of what endogenous and exogenous factors ultimately dictate the host response to endotoxin. In this respect, it is abundantly clear that if endotoxin is to be considered a relevant target for potential therapeutic intervention and if the consequences of that intervention strategy are to be critically evaluated for efficacy the various conditions under which endotoxin is relevant must be fully understood. This caveat would apply not only to the endotoxin molecule itself but also to the immunologic and immunopharmacologic mediators generated by the host in response to endotoxin. It is the purpose of this chapter to address some of these issues, so their consideration in the design and evaluation of future clinical trials may lead to the most productive and meaningful interpretation of the accumulated data from such studies.

We therefore briefly review five specific, potentially relevant contributing factors that may influence the efficacy of therapies directed against endotoxin and its mediators.

1. Qualitative and quantitative factors important in the release of endotoxin from the gram-negative microbial outer membrane surface (based on the existing experimental evidence that released, or soluble, endotoxin is biologically more active than an equivalent amount of endotoxin associated with the microbe)
2. Potential contribution of other microbial inflammation-inducing factors within the infectious nidus in influencing, via synergistic enhancement or antagonistic suppression, the host response to endotoxin
3. Role of endogenous gut-derived endotoxin controlled by changes in intestinal wall permeability
4. Potential induction of early endotoxin tolerance, hypersensitivity, or both through active "reprogramming" events involving host inflammatory cells
5. Potentially important role of glucocorticoids, endogenous or exogenous, in regulating the host inflammatory response to endotoxin

Although it is likely that each of the above-delineated factors is, under some circumstances, important to a greater or lesser extent depending on specific conditions, the list is certainly not all-inclusive. In this respect, it would be beyond the scope of this chapter to consider other potentially contributing factors, such as genetic differences in host responsiveness to endotoxin, age, and the importance of confounding co-morbidities, the relevance of preclinically used animal models as a means of projecting outcomes in humans, and the criteria of specific outcome assessment requirements on the evaluation of potential therapeutic efficacy of a given treatment intervention. Nevertheless, it is anticipated that these potential factors and those reviewed herein can underscore the real, significant challenges that face the investigator attempting to identify effective therapies to treat the septic patient.

Effects of Antibiotics on Release of Endotoxin from Gram-Negative Bacteria

There is substantial evidence to support the concept that LPS is a potent immunostimulatory molecule and that it can play a key role in the pathogenesis of gram-negative sepsis. However, studies that focus solely on preparations of LPS that have been chemically purified by the hot phenol–water method of Luderitz and Westphal[13,14] do not take into consideration certain differences that might obtain in an infection model. These might include the physical state of the LPS and the presentation of LPS in the context of other bacterial products that are themselves inflammatory and may have additive or synergistic properties with LPS. For example, LPS that is shed from bacteria spontaneously and released through the action of antibody and complement or by antibiotic-mediated killing of gram-negative bacteria, may be present as fragments of the outer membrane when it interacts with host inflammatory cells. Furthermore, unlike chemically purified LPS, endotoxin released from gram-negative bacteria in vivo is likely to act in an environment comprised of other bacterial components that may also induce inflammation, such as DNA, bacterial lipoprotein, lipoteichoic acid, or peptidoglycan.

Studies performed in our laboratory[15] and others[16] indicate that although microbe-associated LPS does have readily measurable biologic activity it is substantially less active than free endotoxin. It is therefore reasonable to focus attention on LPS released from the surface of gram-negative bacteria under conditions of clinical infection. Several mechanisms are responsible for natural "shedding" of LPS from gram-negative bacteria including complement-mediated killing of bacteria,[17–19] ingestion of microbes by host phagocytes and subsequent exocytosis of LPS,[20,21] and LPS release associated with natural bacterial death and bacteriolysis or induced by antibiotic killing of gram-negative bacteria.[22]

These various forms—chemically purified LPS versus LPS released from the bacterial surface as part of a membrane fragment in association with other bacterial products that may be inflammatory—are well served by a useful distinction in terminology. Whereas the term "LPS" should be used to refer to a distinct, relatively homogeneous chemical entity, the term "endotoxin" can more generally be applied to any microbial extract that is enriched in biologic activities characteristic of LPS. Thus the term endotoxin implies an LPS-enriched, though not necessarily chemically purified, product. For this reason "endotoxin" is used here to describe LPS-containing material released from bacterial through the interaction with antibiotics described below.

A great deal of evidence has accumulated that demonstrates the important role antibiotics may have in the release of large quantities of endotoxin from gram-negative bacteria. Several factors might influence the amount of endotoxin released during the interaction of bacteria with antibiotics. Among them are the bacterial strain, the type and concentration of the antibiotic, and the duration of exposure of the bacteria to the antibiotic.[23–26]

The cell wall-active β-lactam antibiotics (in contrast to the aminoglycoside and fluoroquinolone antibiotics, which interrupt protein and DNA synthesis, respectively) are generally considered to be the most potent in releasing bacterial endotoxin. Within this class of antibiotics, however, important associations have been made between the degree to which endotoxin is released and the specific penicillin-binding proteins (PBPs) targeted by the particular antibiotic. PBPs perform an essential role in bacterial cell wall synthesis by catalyzing the crosslinking of the peptidoglycan layers that form the cell wall. Within a given bacterium there may be several forms of PBP. Antibiotic inhibition of various PBPs can have a profound effect on bacterial morphology and endotoxin release. For example, inhibition of PBP-1 is associated with rapid bacteriolysis and the release of relatively small amounts of endotoxin. In contrast, inhibition of PBP-2 causes bacteria to form spheroplasts, and this too is associated with the release of little endotoxin. However, when the function of PBP-3 is selectively inhibited, cell wall synthesis appears to become profoundly disordered. The cell morphology changes from rods to long, filamentous structures, and this change is associated with a marked, quantitative increase in the cell wall biomass and significantly increased endotoxin release.[27]

In vitro studies by Jackson and Kropp[26,27] compared the effects on smooth and rough LPS mutants of *Pseudomonas aeruginosa* of PBP-3-specific ceftazidime (CAZ), a third-generation cephalosporin, and PBP-2-specific imipenem (IMP), a carbapenem antibiotic. Broth cultures were inoculated with 10^5–10^6 CFU of bacteria per milliliter and incubated at 35°C. Antibiotic was added at time 0. After incubation for 4–8 hours, broth was collected and sterile-filtered for determination of free LPS. The minimal inhibitory concentrations (MICs) and bactericidal activity (>99.9% killing) by CAZ and IMP for these strains of *P. aeruginosa* were the same. Importantly, the content of free LPS in the filtered bacterial supernatant, as measured by *Limulus* amebocyte lysate (LAL) assay, was 10- to 40-fold higher in CAZ-treated than IMP-treated cultures. The toxic effects of these filtrates were studied in CD1 mice made hypersensitive to LPS by prior treatment with actinomycin D. IMP-treated culture filtrates were no more lethal than filtrate from cultures that had not been treated with antibiotics. In contrast, CAZ-treated culture-filtrates were about 80-fold more lethal, roughly paralleling the increase in LAL activity detected in vitro.

Dofferhoff et al.[23] generated similar results in their in vitro studies of the effects of several antibiotics on *Escherichia coli*. In this case, even though IMP was associated with more rapid bacterial killing than seen with CAZ, IMP treatment resulted in a 1.8-fold increase in total endotoxin (free plus cell bound) compared to a 5.0-fold increase for CAZ-treated bacteria. Treatment with cefuroxime, a second-generation cephalosporin, or the PBP-3-specific monobactam antibiotic aztreonam, were associated with 22- and 49-fold increases in total endotoxin, respectively, at 4 hours. Increases in free endotoxin were even higher, 118- and 222-fold, respectively. Cefuroxime and aztreonam were associated with the formation of long, filamentous bacteria, readily observed by light microscopy.

The precise composition of antibiotic-released endotoxin remains to be chemically determined, but it is clear that even chemically purified LPS may be contaminated with tightly bound proteins, some of which may themselves have inflammatory properties.[28–31] Other bacterial constituents of the cell wall, such as peptidoglycan, may also have immunostimulatory effects,[32–34] but there is no evidence as yet that they are constituents of antibiotic-released endotoxin.

Nakano and Kirikae have recently characterized endotoxin released from *P. aeruginosa* grown in minimal (M-9) medium at 37°C and treated with CAZ.[35] The authors compared the activity of CAZ-released endotoxin and chemically purified LPS from the same strain of bacteria in the following ways. First, in LAL assays they showed that the two preparations had parallel dose-response curves, suggesting that the endotoxic activity of the two preparations was most likely due to LPS bioactivity. Second, in LPS-normoresponsive C3H/HeN mice sensitized to LPS lethal effects by D(+)-galactosamine, the LD_{50} (dose at which half the mice die) values for CAZ-released endotoxin and chemically purified LPS from *P. aeruginosa* were 10 and 30 ng, respectively, suggesting that CAZ-released endotoxin may be slightly more toxic, although the significance of these differences should not be overstated. In LPS-hyporesponsive C3H/HeJ mice, the LD_{50} values for CAZ-released endotoxin and chemically purified LPS were >1000 and >10,000 ng, respectively. This finding suggests that the toxic effect was mediated by LPS, not by another inflammatory bacterial component.

Finally, peritoneal macrophages derived from these two strains of mice were examined for their ability to trigger the release for inflammatory mediators in vitro in response to purified LPS or CAZ-released LPS. CAZ-released endotoxin and purified LPS induced the production of similar amounts of tumor necrosis factor-α (TNFα) and nitric oxide when incubated with LPS-responsive C3H/HeN macrophages. Significantly higher doses of each preparation were required to elicit the production of TNFα from LPS-hyporesponsive C3H/HeJ macrophages. Interestingly, the addition of polymyxin B, which inhibits LPS-induced responses by binding to the lipid A portion of the molecule,[30] abrogated TNFα production by CAZ-released endotoxin. Together these data strongly suggest that the most important bioactive component of CAZ-released endotoxin in LPS, despite the fact that on a per-weight basis the preparation contains 32 times more protein than LPS.

Thus there are substantial in vitro data to demonstrate that antibiotics specific for PBP-3 induce profound morphologic changes in gram-negative bacteria, and that it is associated with the substantial release of endotoxin. Antibiotic-released endotoxin has activity characteristic of LPS, determined by well defined measures such as LAL activity and toxicity in well characterized ex vivo studies in whole blood to which gram-negative bacteria have been added; and it has been demonstrated to induce the production and release of TNFα and nitricoxide, thought to be key mediators of sepsis, from host macrophages. Norimatsu and Morrison[36] studied the release of endotoxin in whole mouse blood ex vivo that was inoculated with viable *Escherichia coli* and to which either IMP or CAZ had been added. At 4 hours significant increases in number of bacteria were detected in blood not treated with antibiotics, but viable bacteria were undetectable in either the IMP- or CAZ-treated blood. Higher levels of endotoxin, as detected by LAL assay, were identified in CAZ-treated blood samples. Levels of TNFα and interleukin-6 (IL-6) in antibiotic-treated cultures after 8 hours of incubation correlated well with the level of endotoxin detected at 4 hours of incubation.

These data are entirely consistent with the earlier published studies of Arditi et al.,[37] who investigated the production of TNFα from whole human blood ex vivo in response to the release of bacterial products generated by the antibiotic-mediated killing of *Haemophilus influenzae* type B (Hib). In those studies, live Hib (from 10^4–10^7 cfu/ml in log increments) were added to Transwell filter inserts with whole blood and incubated in the presence or absence of ceftriaxone, a third-generation cephalosporin, or IMP. Both antibiotics achieved 98–99% killing, but at each inoculum of Hib ceftriaxone was associated with significantly higher release of TNFα than for IMP (82–187% increase over baseline for ceftriaxone compared to 9–28% for IMP). Polymyxin B inhibited the release of TNFα by 97–99%, indicating that TNFα production was induced by the release of LPS. These data indicate that antibiotics with different binding affinities for PBPs affect free endotoxin release and the generation of proinflammatory cytokines even in whole blood.

Animal models of infection that compare antibiotics with different capacities for endotoxin release also strongly support the concept that there may be a therapeutic advantage in the use of agents associated with the release of relatively less endotoxin. Bucklin and Morrison[38] compared IMP and CAZ in an *E. coli* model of infection of CF-1 mice sensitized to the lethal effects of LPS by administration of D(+)-galactosamine. In control mice treated only with sterile saline, the LD_{50} was determined to be 2×10^4 cfu. The relative efficacy of IMP versus CAZ was studied by simultaneous intraperitoneal injection of bacteria, D(+)-galactosamine, and antibiotic. At a dose of 20 mg/kg for either antibiotic, administration of CAZ resulted in an approximately threefold decrease in the LD_{50}, whereas treatment with IMP resulted in an approximate eightfold decrease. This difference could not be attributed to greater efficacy of the IMP because the MICs for the two antibiotics were identical, and they sterilized blood and peritoneal lavage fluid with virtually the same efficacy. Such differences were heightened when the dose of antibiotic was decreased to 2 mg/kg. Under these conditions, CAZ failed to provide measurable protection, and IMP was almost fully protective. These differences were also found when *P. aeruginosa* was used, but not with *Staphylococcus aureus*. Together these data strongly suggest that the differences in efficacy result from the differential release of endotoxin resulting from treatment with antibiotics that have differing PBP-binding specificities.

To address this question more directly, the authors used C3H/HeJ mice. Although these mice are genetically hyporesponsive to LPS, they remain sensitive to bacterial infection. Consistent with the hypothesis, the authors showed that when treated with antibiotics these LPS-hyporesponsive mice were protected against challenge with significantly higher doses of bacteria than their histocompatible LPS-responsive counterpart, C3Heb/FeJ mice. Finally, the authors demonstrated that a monoclonal antibody directed against the outer core epitope of the LPS from the strain of *E. coli* used in these studies protected CF-1 mice from otherwise lethal challenge with *E. coli*. Thus there is strong evidence to suggest that, with this model of infection, differences in antibiotic efficacy are mediated by the differential release of endotoxin induced by antibiotics that have different PBP-binding characteristics.

In consideration of the important role played by the release of proinflammatory cytokines from LPS-stimulated macrophages in gram-negative sepsis, Jackson and Kropp compared the relative antibiotic efficacy of CAZ and IMP in macrophage-depleted mice.[27] In this model CD-1 mice were treated with a preparation of carrageenam (CGN), an immunosuppressive agent comprised of a heterologous mixture of sulfated polysaccharides isolated from marine algae, which is believed to mediate its effect through its selective cytopathic effects on macrophages.[39] Preliminary studies by the authors indicated that intraperitoneal injection of CGN 1–2 days prior to infection "eliminates a biologically significant number of macrophages without detectable functional effects on a biologically significant number of polymorphonuclear leukocytes" (PMNs).[27] Although endotoxin is generally considered to be one of the most important virulence factors produced by gram-negative bacteria, it is by no means the only one, as demonstrated by the lethality of gram-negative bacteremia in LPS-hyporesponsive C3H/HeJ cells in the saline-treated controls above. The authors first showed that the lethal effects of free endotoxin (filtrates of CAZ-treated *P. aeruginosa* broth cultures) are greatly reduced in CD-1 mice selectively depleted of macrophages by CGN pretreatment, emphasizing the importance of the interaction of endotoxin with macrophages in this mouse model.

The authors then tested the hypothesis that in macrophage-depleted mice the ED_{50} (dose of antibiotic at which 50% of animals survive in a particular model of infection) of antibiotics would depend primarily on their bactericidal activity and be relatively independent of their endotoxin-releasing potential. The ED_{50} of a single dose of antibiotic therapy with either CAZ or IMP were calculated in LPS-normoresponsive CD-1 mice infected intraperitoneally with live *P. aeruginosa*, with or without selective macrophage depletion by CGN pretreatment. In the absence of CGN pretreatment, normal mice required 157- to 227-fold more CAZ than IMP for protection. In contrast, for CGN-treated mice this ratio was decreased to about 8-fold. These data strongly suggest that in macrophage-depleted mice the differential release of free endotoxin is relatively less important than other virulence factors produced by gram-negative bacteria; they emphasize the role played by the interaction of antibiotic-released endotoxin with host macrophages in the toxicity of gram-negative infection.

These more recent studies both support and extend published reports of gram-negative meningitis in animals that address the concept that initiation of therapy with antibiotics that release more endotoxin is associated with worse outcomes. In a rabbit model of *E. coli* meningitis, Tauber et al. earlier demonstrated that treatment with the bactericidal cell wall-active antibiotic cefotaxime was associated with higher endotoxin levels in cerebrospinal fluid (CSF) and more brain edema than treatment with chloramphenicol, a bacteriostatic agent that inhibits protein synthesis.[40] The studies of McCracken and colleagues on *Haemophilus influenzae* meningitis in rabbits and humans are among the most clinically relevant studies examining the role of endotoxin release in the inflammatory response induced by gram-negative infection. Compared to untreated controls, rabbits to whom ceftriaxone had been administered 6 hours after intracisternal injection with *H. influenzae* had a marked increase in CSF levels of free (non-microbe-associated) endotoxin and TNFα. There was also significantly more inflammation as measured by the CSF white blood cell (WBC) count, glucose, protein, and lactate concentrations. Simultaneous administration of dexamethasone with the antibiotic resulted in significantly lower CSF WBC counts and TNFα levels, suggesting that interventions designed to reduce the effect of endotoxin release at the start of antimicrobial therapy may decrease inflammation.[41] These studies formed the basis for a clinical trial in which children with *H. influenzae* meningitis who were given dexamethasone immediately prior to treatment with ceftriaxone had less morbidity than those who did not receive dexamethasone.[42] These data and the observation that serum endotoxin levels drop rapidly after initiation of antimicrobial therapy[43] suggest that interventions designed to reduce the amount of endotoxin release associated with antibiotic treatment must be made early in the course of antimicrobial therapy to have a salutary effect.

One of the first clinical studies to address the issue definitively was reported by Prins et al.[44] in 1995. These investigators compared imipenem with ceftazidime for treatment of patients with urosepsis caused by gram-negative organisms. There were 15 patients in each group. The two antibiotics were equally effective at sterilizing the urine. After 4 hours of treatment, endotoxin levels had declined in all three of the endotoxemic IMP-treated patients but had risen in two of the four endotoxemic CAZ-treated patients. Serum and urine cytokine levels rose 10–40% in the CAZ-treated patients but did not change in the IMP-treated patients. Although there was a trend to slower defervescence in the CAZ-treated patients, a clinically significant advantage for treatment with IMP compared to CAZ was not established. In collaboration with Dr. Steven Opal, we recently concluded a similar trial comparing IMP with CAZ in uroseptic patients. In large part due to extensive patient-to-patient variation, no statistically significant differences in serum or urine cytokine levels or in clinical parameters such as temperature, blood pressure, and heart rate were established (manuscript in preparation). This underscores the profound potential differences that exist in the human population in response to endotoxin that are not yet fully appreciated.

In conclusion, there is ample evidence to suggest that endotoxin released from gram-negative bacterial by a variety of mechanisms may differ from chemically purified LPS in potency. Antibiotic-released endotoxin may be an especially relevant model for studying released endotoxin because of the central role antibiotics play in the treatment of gram-negative infection and because cell wall-active antibiotics with specificity for PBP-3 are associated with the release of relatively large quantities of endotoxin. Antibiotic-released endotoxin is clearly biologically active, as indicated by its ability to induce the production of inflammatory cytokines in whole blood ex vivo. An animal model of infection demonstrates that antibiotics associated with the release of less endotoxin may provide a therapeutic advantage, but this has not yet been demonstrated definitively in human studies of urosepsis. In virtually all studies in which this variable has been tested, it appears that the toxic effects are largely mediated by LPS, as demonstrated by the ability of polymyxin B to inhibit the activity of endotoxin released from gram-negative microbes.

Potential Contribution of Other Microbial Proinflammatory Factors to Host Response to LPS

Despite the fact that LPS is well recognized to play a pivotal role in the pathogenesis of gram-negative bacterial infection-related diseases such as septic shock, the concept that LPS is the sole, primary factor responsible for pathophysiologic manifestation of these diseases in gram-negative infection has not been established unequivocally. Evidence in this regard includes the following: (1) gram-positive bacteria, which generally lack endotoxin, can also cause lethal shock;[45] (2) although LPS does not induce any toxic or lethal effects in LPS-hyporesponsive C3H/HeJ mice, exposure of these mice to live or heat-killed gram-negative bacteria can result in septic shock;[46] and (3) clinical trials employing various anti-LPS therapies have not yet resulted in any significant survival advantage in septic patients.[47] Collectively, these findings strongly support the possibility that gram-negative and gram-positive bacterial components other than LPS may play important roles in septic shock. In fact, a growing body of information has indicated that a number of gram-negative and gram-positive bacterial components are likely to be involved in the pathogenesis of septic shock, including endotoxin-associated proteins (e.g., LAP, EP, EAP),* porins, peptidoglycan, lipoteichoic acid, lipoproteins, and deoxyribonucleic acid (DNA). Because this review focuses on gram-negative bacterial infection-related diseases, the following paragraphs summarize some of the evidence to support a role of components primarily from gram-negative bacteria as potential pathogenic factors.

Protein components that are intimately associated with the lipid A moiety of LPS during mild extraction of endotoxin have been investigated extensively by a number of investigators.[48] Usually these proteins can be removed by more rigorous extraction methods,[49] but this is not always the case, especially

---

*LAP—lipid A associated protein; EP—endotoxin protein; EAP—endotoxin associated protein.

with the so-called rough chemotype LPS (R-LPS). In this respect, although some studies suggested an intrinsic ability of R-LPS to stimulate cells from C3H/HeJ endotoxin-hyporesponsive mice,[50] studies by Manthey and Vogel[51] have shown that such activity can, in fact, be selectively removed if rigorous attention is paid to extraction methodologies. In any event, the biologic activities of proteins associated with LPS have been known for some time to be distinct from those LPS. Furthermore, endotoxin proteins from different gram-negative strains have independently been reported to stimulate lymphocyte proliferation and proinflammatory cytokine production.[18,19,52] Brogden et al.[53] reported that a protein fraction isolated from *Pasteurella haemolytica* induced pulmonary inflammation in vivo in calves and sheep. Earlier studies in our laboratory indicated that immunization of LPS-hyporesponsive C3H/HeJ mice with purified protein–LPS complexes could protect mice against an otherwise lethal dose of *Salmonella typhimurium* infection, suggesting that endotoxin proteins play an important role in protective immunity.[54] The exact mechanism(s) responsible for activities of endotoxin-associated proteins have not been identified, although several in vitro studies indicate that tyrosine phosphorylation is required for macrophage activation in response to endotoxin protein constituents from *S. typhimurium*.[55,56]

In efforts to define more precisely the identification of some of these endotoxin-associated protein constituents, some investigators have evaluated the capacity of purified outer membrane proteins to stimulate the host immune inflammatory response. One such dominant outer membrane protein constituent is the class of porin proteins, exclusively located in the outer membrane of gram-negative bacteria. These proteins are responsible for transport of low-molecular-mass molecules across the permeability barrier of the outer cell membrane. In addition to their transport function, porins from various gram-negative bacteria are also able to stimulate monocytes and lymphocytes to produce proinflammatory and immunomodulatory cytokines such as IL-1, IL-6, TNFα, IL-8, granulocyte/macrophage colony-stimulating factor (GM-CSF), and interferon-γ (IFNγ), which may contribute to their ability to induce infection-related diseases.[57] Porins purified from *S. typhimurium* have been shown to elicit a localized Shwartzman reaction in rabbits and induce lethal shock in D-galactosamine-sensitized LPS-responsive and LPS-hyporesponsive mice. This toxic effect of porins can be completely blocked by preadministration of anti-TNFα serum, indicating that in vivo produced TNFα is a mediator of porin-induced toxic shock.[58] Of particular interest is the fact that a 39-kDa outer membrane protein, OmpA, purified from *Proteus mirabilis*, has been shown to be not only mitogenic for B lymphocytes but also inhibitory of LPS-induced production of IL-1 and oxygen-derived free radicals from murine macrophages.[59,60] Whether porins interact with other bacterial components (e.g., LPS) in an additive or synergistic fashion remains to be investigated. Nevertheless, they are likely to be of considerable potential importance in the overall host response to microbial infection.

Peptidoglycan, present in the cell walls of both gram-negative and gram-positive bacteria, is a dominant constituent of the cell wall, with an important role in maintenance of the structural integrity of the microbe's ultrastructural morphology. Initial studies of the immunoregulatory functions of peptidoglycan were carried out using the synthetic muramyl dipeptide (MDP)-acetyl-muramyl-L-alanyl-D-isoglutamine, the smallest common structural unit of various peptidoglycans. MDP has been shown to induce production of a number of cytokines from a variety of cells and to have both inflammatory and antiinflammatory activities.[61,62] However, because MDP is not a natural degradation product of peptidoglycan, the relation between MDP-bases studies and pathophysiologic effects of peptidoglycan may not always be truly reflective of the biologic activity of the latter.

Peptidoglycan released in vivo is digested by host enzymes to produce breakdown products. One of these naturally occurring breakdown products of peptidoglycan from *E. coli*, G(Anh)MTetra, has been shown to induce synthesis of IL-1β, IL-6, and G-CSF in human monocytes.[32,63] However, whether G(Anh)MTetra plays an important role in infection-related diseases remains to be elucidated.

Although there have been only a few studies regarding peptidoglycan from gram-negative bacteria, peptidoglycan derived from gram-positive bacteria (e.g., *Staphylococcus aureus*) has been shown to have mitogenic effects on B lymphocytes and to be able to stimulate immune cells to produce TNFα, IL-1, and IL-6.[64,65] Furthermore, purified cell wall fragments rich in peptidoglycan have been reported to cause chronic arthritis in experimental models.[66] The molecular mechanism(s) employed by peptidoglycan may involve binding of peptidoglycan to the cell surface receptor CD14, stimulating the mitogen-activated protein (MAP) kinases [e.g., extracellular signal-regulated kinase (ERK) 1, ERK2, p38, and c-Jun NH$_2$-terminal kinase (JNK)] and eventually activating transcription factors such as NF-κB.[34,67]

Furthermore, peptidoglycan has been reported to act, in a synergistic fashion, with another *S. aureus* cell wall component, lipoteichoic acid, to cause multiple organ failure (MOF) and lethal shock in rats. Evidence in support of this concept has derived from the studies of De Kimpe et al.,[68] who reported that in vivo administration of both peptidoglycan and lipoteichoic acid in rats caused systemic release of TNFα and IFNγ, induction of inducible nitric oxide synthase (iNOS), circulatory failure, multiple organ dysfunction syndrome (MODS), and death, despite the fact that neither peptidoglycan nor lipoteichoic acid alone induced these effects. As is elaborated on below, such synergy may well be a common mechanism of inflammatory response induced by microbial constituents.

The evidence to support a potential role of lipoteichoic acid in bacterial infection-related diseases, although it is not a structural component of gram-negative bacteria, is nevertheless of considerable interest from a conceptual perspective. It was first reported by Riesenfeld-Orn et al.[69] that lipoteichoic acid from *Pneumococcus* induced IL-1 but not TNFα from human monocytes. However, both IL-1 and TNFα were reportedly induced in murine mononuclear cells by lipoteichoic acid purified from *Streptococcus faecalis*.[70] Lipoteichoic acids from various strains of gram-positive species may differ in their ability to stimulate cytokine production. It was reported by Bhakdi et al.[71] that lipoteichoic acids purified from a number of enterococcal species were able to stimulate production of IL-1, IL-6, and TNFα in human monocytes, whereas lipoteichoic acids from *S. aureus* and *S. pneumoniae* were not. In addition to the aforementioned cytokines, IL-8,[72] macrophage inflammatory protein-1α,[73] and NO[74] were all reported to be induced by lipoteichoic acid in various cells. Lipoteichoic acid-induced NO has been reported to mediate delayed circulatory failure in rats.[75] Production of NO induced by lipoteichoic acid may involve binding of lipoteichoic acid to cell surface receptor CD14,[76] activation of phosphatidylcholine phospholipase C, tyrosine kinases, and transcription factor NF-κB.[77]

Lipoproteins are abundant bacterial membrane proteins and common constituents of the cell walls of both gram-negative and gram-positive bacteria. In addition to their structural functions and close association with the peptidoglycan in the cell wall/membrane, purified lipoproteins from a number of gram-negative bacteria and their synthetic analogues [e.g., *N*-palmitoyl-*S*-{2,3-bis(palmitoyloxy)-2RS-propyl}-(R)-cysteinyl-alanyl-glycine (Pam3-Cys-Ala-Gly) and CGP 31362] have been reported to have proinflammatory activities that include inducing murine macrophages to release proinflammatory cytokines such as TNFα, IL-1, and IL-6.[78–80] The mechanism(s) responsible for the immunostimulating ability of lipoproteins and their synthetic analogues may involve activation of MAP kinases.[80] Zhang et al.[81] reported that lipoprotein isolated from *E. coli* induced lethal shock in both LPS-responsive and LPS-hyporesponsive mice sensitized with D-galactosamine. In agreement with this result, a mutant *E. coli* strain that lacks lipoprotein was shown to be less effective with respect to their ability to induce lethal shock in C3H/HeJ mice.

Of particular importance is the observation that lipoprotein acted in synergy with LPS in triggering cytokine production and septic shock in mice. In vitro studies indicated that lipoprotein and LPS synergistically induced TNFα and IL-6 production in peritoneal macrophages from both LPS-responsive (C3H/HeOuJ) and LPS-hyporesponsive (C3H/HeJ) mice. Consistent with these in vitro studies, in vivo administration of lipoprotein and LPS caused synergistic induction of TNFα and IL-6 and lethal shock in both LPS-responsive and LPS-hyporesponsive mice.[81]

For decades bacterial DNA has been considered to be immunologically inert except under conditions of autoimmunity, where it stimulates the production of proinflammatory anti-DNA antibody.[82] However, more recent studies indicate that bacterial DNA not only is immunostimulatory but may play an important role in bacterial infection-related diseases. The first strong experimental evidence in support of this hypothesis was the report of Yamamoto et al.[83] in which a DNA fraction from attenuated *Mycobacterium bovis* (BCG) was shown to augment natural killer (NK) cell activity. The molecular properties of bacterial DNA responsible for this activity are thought to be attributable to its content of short sequences with an unmethylated CpG dinucleotide flanked by two 5'-purines and two 3'-pyrimidines.[84] In contrast to the relatively frequent occurrence of such sequences in bacterial DNA, these sequences occur at a much lower frequency in mammalian DNA, and the cytosine present in the CpG dinucleotide is selectively methylated in the latter.[85,86] The immunostimulating ability of bacterial DNA is exemplified by *E. coli* DNA in inducing in vivo synthesis of proinflammatory cytokines and causing inflammation in the lower respiratory tract of mice.[87] Furthermore, DNA from both gram-negative and gram-positive bacteria has been reported to trigger septic shock in D-galactosamine-sensitized mice. This toxic effect of bacterial DNA is due to in vivo induced production of TNFα from macrophages and is mimicked by treatment of mice with synthetic oligonucleotide containing a 5'-Pu-Pu-CpG-Pyr-Pyr-3' sequence.[88] In addition to its potentially detrimental effects, bacterial DNA may also be beneficial to the host in that it activates both innate and acquired immune responses. Bacterial DNA has been reported to induce differentiation of dendritic cells, activation of antigen-presenting cells and NK cells, proliferation of B cells, and maturation of such cells into antibody-producing plasma cells, as well as stimulation of type 1 T-helper (Th1) immune responses.[89,90] Molecular mechanisms of immune activation by bacterial DNA are not yet completely understood, but it is known that activation of stress kinases (e.g., JNK kinase 1, JNK1/2, and p38) and subsequent activation of transcription factor AP-1 is likely to be involved.[91] Bacterial DNA was also able to activate transcription factor NF-κB.[92,93] It has been reported, in this respect, that cellular internalization of bacterial DNA is required for immune stimulation.[84,91,93]

More importantly, bacterial DNA can synergize with LPS in triggering lethal shock by inducing NK cells to produce IFNγ. Cowdery et al.[94] first reported that both *E. coli* DNA and CpG-containing oligonucleotide were able to act in synergy with LPS in the induction of in vivo production of TNFα, IL-6, and IFNγ. Consistent with these results, *E. coli* DNA and LPS were also shown to induce lethality synergistically in normal mice but not in mice that lack the IFNγ gene. Because NK cells were the primary sources of IFNγ,[55] these findings indicate that the synergistic induction of lethal shock by *E. coli* DNA and LPS is mediated, at least in part, by in vivo production of IFNγ from NK cells.

In addition to the constituents mentioned above, other cellular and extracellular components of gram-negative bacteria have been reported to have immunomodulatory activity and to upregulate or even downregulate synthesis of various proinflammatory cytokines. These components include microbial polysaccharides, heat shock proteins, other outer membrane proteins (in addition to porins and LAPs), pili, cell surface-associated proteins, bacterial toxins (e.g., hemolysin from *E. coli*), and proteases. Because the roles of these components in directly addressing the inflammatory response of the host infectious diseases have not been clearly identified, they are beyond the scope of this chapter. For a more comprehensive review about the functions of these components, see Henderson et al.[57]

In summary, a variety of gram-negative bacterial components, in addition to LPS, have been found to possess immunomodulatory ability; and they are likely to be involved in various bacterial infection-related diseases, such as septic shock. The picture of infectious diseases that emerges from this new information, in turn, substantially complicates overall mechanisms of sepsis pathogenesis compared to the one arising from pure LPS-based studies, but they are also more reflective of true bacterial infections. Of particular importance to this emerging concept is the finding of synergistic interactions among various bacterial components. Understanding the interplay of these components and the underlying molecular mechanisms is of key importance in the development of new and effective pharmaceutical agents against bacterial infection-related diseases.

Early Tolerance to Endotoxin

As pointed out earlier in the chapter, a cascade of generalized immunoinflammatory responses in the host characterizes the development of the septic shock syndrome in response to surgical trauma, multiple trauma, thermal injury, hemorrhagic shock, and severe infections; and the persistence of such systemic inflammatory reactions often culminates in the development of MOF.[95] Current concepts of pathogenesis emphasize the pivotal role of macrophage-derived mediators, especially pro- and antiinflammatory cytokines, in the clinical manifestation of different stages of the sepsis.[96] Although cytokines initially serve to limit the magnitude of pathophysiologic impact and ameliorate eradication of microbial pathogen(s) in the infectious nidus, the duration of infection and persisting release of bacterial toxins into the systemic circulation may generalize immunoinflammatory processes in the organism. The excessive systemic cytokine responses can be detrimental and destructive if the immunologic imbalance is not treated appropriately.

Various microbial pathogens and bacterial components are capable of triggering the innate immune responses in the host, among which, as we emphasized in this chapter, endotoxin of gram-negative bacteria is one of the most potent modulators of inflammatory cytokine responses.[97] The potential role of normal microflora and gut-derived endotoxin in perpetuation of the systemic inflammatory responses and development of MOF in noninfective injuries such as burns, hemorrhagic shock, and multiple trauma has yet to be fully defined, as discussed below. Nevertheless, the available experimental evidence supports the concept that the gastrointestinal tract undoubtedly serves as an important immunologic reservoir in the body for exposure to these microbial mediators. In addition, when induced by etiologically different noninfectious insults, changes in the permeability of the gastrointestinal barrier may lead to translocation of bacteria or endotoxin (or both) into the circulation, which would further aggravate the systemic inflammatory responses and promote the development of septic shock and MOF. Because it could have a significant impact on the development of the systemic inflammatory response to endotoxin, the following discussions focus on the cellular and molecular mechanisms involved in endotoxin-dependent activation of the highly orchestrated immunoinflammatory pathways controlling the development of MOF.

It has been estimated that approximately 10^{14} bacterial cells representing 400 bacterial species, many of which are gram-negative, commonly inhabit the normal human gastrointestinal tract.[98] As these bacteria replicate, many release endotoxin-bearing outer membrane fragments that may, under circumstances in which mucosal integrity is somehow compromised, translocate across the intestinal mucosa.[99] This can produce a low-grade endotoxemia within the portal vein that under most conditions is rapidly cleared by the hepatic reticuloendothelial system (RES) without significant detrimental effect. A variety of conditions that alter host defenses can be envisioned, however, that could induce systemic endotoxemia via either enhanced endotoxin translocation or reduced clearance by the hepatic RES. Systemic endotoxemia following endotoxin translocation is distinguished from sepsis following bacterial translocation in that endotoxin translocation does not result in bacteremia or any other readily identifiable bacterial infection.

A physiologically and anatomically intact intestinal mucosa usually provides a highly effective barrier against endotoxin translocation. Clinical conditions that compromise the integrity of the intestinal mucosa have been associated with systemic endotoxemia, presumably owing to increased endotoxin translocation. Endotoxemia without detectable bacteremia is not uncommon in patients with gastrointestinal disorders such as Crohn's disease, acute inflammatory bowel diseases, and necrotizing enterocolitis.[99] Additionally, hypoxemia, ischemia, hyperthermia, and trauma can enhance endotoxin translocation via secondary effects on the intestinal wall. Interestingly, endotoxemia itself has the potential to enhance translocation of endotoxin and viable bacteria (and perhaps other proinflammatory microbial constituents as well) across the gut, perhaps via endotoxin-induced ischemia/reperfusion injury of the intestine.[100] Thus endotoxemia can, at least theoretically, be self-perpetuating by inducing a reciprocal amplification cycle.

Systemic endotoxemia without evidence of gram-negative infection is also common in humans with liver diseases including cirrhosis, fulminant hepatic failure, and obstructive jaundice.[99] Presumably, the reduced capacity of the liver to remove endotoxin from the portal circulation permits passage of this potentially potent microbial mediator into the systemic circulation with an opportunity to induce significant pathologic consequences. Tarao et al. found that 70% of cirrhotic patients had detectable endotoxin in their serum, and that mortality was significantly higher in patients with endotoxemia than in patients without endotoxemia.[101] Bigatello et al. found that 36 of 39 cirrhotic patients had endotoxemia without evidence of sepsis, and that endotoxin concentrations were significantly higher in patients dying with hepatic encephalopathy than in those surviving this condition.[102] Additionally, systemic endotoxemia has often been implicated in the pathogenesis of renal failure and coagulation disorders associated with liver disease.[99] These observations suggest that systemic endotoxemia may exacerbate these conditions, which can also result in increased concentrations of circulating endotoxin.

It is tempting to postulate that in the absence of an identifiable infection systemic endotoxemia resulting from endotoxin translocation contributes to the pathogenesis of the systematic inflammatory response syndrome (SIRS).[103] This contribution could take one of two forms. Systemic endotoxemia might be the "trigger" that initiates SIRS, or SIRS initiated by some other pathogenic mechanism might result in secondary endotoxemia, which could exacerbate SIRS. Conversely, the ability of host inflammatory cells to respond to endotoxin during gram-negative infection might be transiently suppressed by prior exposure to endogenous endotoxin, thereby decreasing the potential contribution of infection-derived endotoxin to the pathogenesis of gram-negative infections. Either or both of these responses would be anticipated to have significant consequences for the host's inflammatory response.

For example, the clinical manifestation and development of endotoxemia and septic syndrome, by endogenous endotoxin or some other mechanism, can be and usually is complicated by the capacity of endotoxin to modulate the transient state of hyporesponsiveness or tolerance to itself. This state can be experimentally induced by a single injection or repeated injections of endotoxin into laboratory animals or healthy volunteers. In pioneer studies carried out in 1938 by Boivin and Mesrobeanu it was demonstrated in experiments using a serum transfer technique that endotoxin or pyrogenic tolerance is, at least in part, mediated by generation of protective antibodies specific to the O-antigen of endotoxin.[104] This concept was further developed in the studies of Beeson[105] and Greisman et al.,[106] who systematically investigated this phenomenon and revealed the existence of two distinct phases of endotoxin tolerance, (i.e., an early cellular refractory phase and a late phase dependent on gradually increasing levels of circulating O-antigen-specific antibodies). The late phase manifests substantial specificity toward the endotoxin serotype used for the primary immunization. The early phase of pyrogenic tolerance appears shortly after endotoxin injection; and before emerging, the detectable levels of serotype-specific antibodies in the serum have the opportunity to develop.

This early refractory phase was shown to manifest the property of cross-tolerance between endotoxins isolated from various gram-negative bacteria and, of importance, could be induced by endotoxins isolated from the O-antigen-deficient mutant bacterial strains. Hence this early state of tolerance "represents an immunologic desensitization to a common toxophore antigen"[106] now recognized as the lipid A-core domain of LPS. The late phase of endotoxin tolerance has potentially beneficial effects in the host, mediated by the capacity of elicited antibodies to neutralize endotoxin and facilitate microbial clearance by phagocytes. Therefore most experimental efforts have focussed on elucidating the regulatory mechanisms and pathways involved in early endotoxin tolerance, characterized as a state of "immunologic paralysis" or endotoxin "hyporesponsiveness."

Significant progress in our understanding of the host cellular and molecular mechanisms underlying both the pathophysiologic responses to endotoxin and early endotoxin tolerance has been achieved. It has been demonstrated, in this respect, that macrophages most likely play a key role in the host responses to endotoxin, as demonstrated by a model of D-galactosamine-induced sensitization to the lethal effects of endotoxin and two histocompatible strains of mice (i.e., endotoxin-sensitive C3H/HeN and endotoxin-hyporesponsive C3H/HeJ).[107] In these seminal studies by Galanos, Freudenberg, and their colleagues, marked susceptibility to endotoxin of otherwise hyporesponsive D-galactosamine-treated C3H/HeJ mice was achieved by adaptive transfer of macrophages isolated from intact C3H/HeN mice. Furthermore, when C3H/HeJ mice that had received via adaptive transfer C3H/HeN macrophages and had been pretreated with nonlethal LPS amounts 1 hour before D-galactosamine injection were challenged with a lethal dose of LPS, the animals developed a state of endotoxin tolerance, as assessed by the lethality assay.[108] Collectively, these studies strongly suggested that macrophages are among the major cellular components of the host RES, mediating both endotoxin lethality and tolerance in experimental animals.

The implication of macrophage-derived cytokines (e.g., TNFα, IL-1, IL-6) as the major mediators initiating and perpetuating the development of pathophysiologic sequelae of sepsis and septic shock had a significant impact on our current understanding of the molecular mechanisms underlying the host inflammatory responses during severe infections.[97] As pointed out earlier in the chapter, administration of recombinant TNFα or IL-1 to experimental animals led to the development of systemic manifestations of disease similar to those seen in septic patients.[109,110] Moreover, in experimental animal models it has been shown that mortality due to septic shock can be reversed by passive immunotherapy with polyclonal or monoclonal antibody against TNFα or IL-1 receptor antagonist (IL-1ra).[7,111,112] Inspired by these early experimental findings, a number of clinical trials were implemented using either anti-TNF-α or anti-IL-1 immunotherapy, which was designed to improve survival of septic patients. However, these therapeutic strategies have failed to demonstrate significant improvement in 28-day survivals in patients with severe sepsis compared to that of control groups.[113–115]

The post hoc evaluation of the results of these clinical trials have identified several potential problems associated with failure of anticytokine immunotherapy in septic patients.[116] Such problems include the important fact that patients enrolled in clinical trials to treat septic shock syndrome can be expected to have a preexisting cytokine-driven immunologic imbalance of inflammatory responses, often associated with endotoxin tolerance mediated by predominant activation of compensatory antiinflammatory responses.[117–119] Depending on the status of the development of the compensatory response, antiinflammatory immunotherapy using TNFα antibodies or IL-1ra may not represent an adequate therapeutic modality for patients with already immunocompromised status due to infections. This notion is supported by many experimental findings that strongly support the hypothesis that moncoytes isolated from septic patients often manifest decreased capacity to produce proinflammatory cytokines such as TNFα, IL-1, and IL-8 upon ex vivo evaluation of LPS-induced cytokine responses.[120–122] Furthermore, it has been demonstrated that monocytes and macrophages isolated from healthy donors and experimental animals can acquire the state of LPS hyporesponsiveness by in vitro pretreatment with low amounts of endotoxin.[123-126]

Although modulation of endotoxin tolerance is currently thought to be mediated by a CD14-dependent mechanism,[127] it appears that the endotoxin refractory state is not controlled by downregulation of CD14 expression on monocytes or macrophages.[127,129] This concept is supported by the findings that expression of CD14 on macrophages isolated from genetically endotoxin-resistant (C3H/HeJ) and endotoxin-sensitive (C3H/HeN) mice are comparable.[9] Further investigation of molecular mechanisms underlying the endotoxin tolerance have demonstrated that downregulation of TNFα production in LPS-hyporesponsive macrophages is, at least in part, mediated by a predominant mobilization of NF-κB transcriptional factor in a p50 homodimer form.[128] These early findings have recently been confirmed in studies using $p50^{-/-}$ knockout mice showing that prolonged LPS treatment of macrophages isolated from these mice failed to modulate endotoxin tolerance as assessed by TNFα production.[130]

Analysis of LPS-induced cytokine responses in the endotoxin-tolerant human promonocytic cell line THP-1 has unveiled downregulation of IL-1β mRNA expression and concomitant overexpression of IκB-α, an inhibitory protein subunit of the NF-κB complex that prevents nuclear translocation of NF-κB transcription factor.[131] Although these data strongly suggest a potential transcriptional pathway(s) in the regulation of TNFα and IL-1β production in LPS-tolerant macrophages, previous studies have also demonstrated that LPS-induced stimulation of macrophages isolated from the congenic LPS-resistant (C3H/HeJ) and LPS-responsive (C3H/HeN) mice exhibits a similar pattern of p50/p65 and p50/c-rel NF-κB heterodimer accumulation in the nuclei.[132] Such discrepancies in the experimental findings characterizing the phenomenon of endotoxin tolerance strongly suggest that regulation of cytokine potential in macrophages and perhaps other cytokine-producing cells represents a complex molecular mechanism(s) controlling cytokine production at both the transcriptional and posttranscriptional level, and that multiple mechanisms may ultimately be found to be involved.

It is becoming increasingly clear, nevertheless, that most if not all immune and inflammatory responses are mediated by the highly coordinated activation of both the proinflammatory and antiinflammatory arms of the cytokine responses. However, with some pathologic conditions, activation of these inflammatory mechanisms may well be reciprocal and mutually exclusive. Conceptually, endotoxin tolerance may represent a compensatory physiologic mechanism(s) that is activated during severe sepsis and other pathophysiologic conditions to limit the extent of uncontrolled (and therefore potentially destructive) proinflammatory immune responses. However, it is becoming evident that acquisition of an endotoxin refractory state is not mediated by complete unresponsiveness of "exhausted" macrophages exposed to continuous LPS stimuli. Rather, considerable experimental evidence indicates that it may reflect a remarkable plasticity of the macrophage inflammatory potential that is controlled by a dynamic balance of proinflammatory and antiinflammatory cytokine responses. Thus it has recently been demonstrated that macrophage-derived antiinflammatory cytokines such as IL-10 and transforming growth factor β (TGFβ) may well modulate endotoxin tolerance in human monocytes.[133] Of importance, the refractory state of LPS responsiveness induced by low LPS doses in isolated human monocytes or experimental animals can be reversed by treatment with recombinant proinflammatory cytokines such as IL-12, IFNγ, and granulocyte/macrophage colony-stimulating factor (GM-CSF).[134,135]

The initial stage of gram-negative infections and the increased permeability of the gastrointestinal barrier owing to noninfectious injuries may well be associated with transient states of low-level endotoxemia, which could be instrumental in modulating the host inflammatory responses via mechanism(s) of differential modulation of cytokine potential in macrophages as effector cells. To support this experimental hypothesis, we have investigated the phenomenon of priming macrophages with low LPS doses and have demonstrated that LPS-dependent desensitization cannot be applied uniformly to all macrophage responses.[136] In vitro priming of naive macrophages with substimulatory LPS doses resulted in biphasic and reciprocal modulation of both TNFα and NO, responses. A significant LPS-dependent modulation of TNFα secretion paralleled the inhibition of NO, whereas in the same macrophages other LPS pretreatment doses resulted in suppression of the TNFα response and enhancement of NO production. To define the mechanism(s) responsible for the observed phenomenon and to underscore its fundamental difference from the endotoxin-refractory state manifested by unresponsiveness of macrophages, we have introduced the term "reprogramming" of macrophage responses. Studies from this laboratory have provided strong experimental support for the concept of multicytokine regulatory mechanism(s) in the modulation of LPS reprogamming effects in macrophages.[137-139]

Specifically, we have shown that LPS reprogramming per se represents polarization of the cellular potential for pro- and antiinflammatory cytokines responses. This polarization is primarily controlled by autocrine/paracrine regulatory pathways of reciprocal induction of IL-12 and IL-10.[139] Using a fibrin-clot model of *E. coli* infection in baboons, we recently confirmed, in collaboration with Fletcher Taylor and his colleagues in Oklahoma City, that a counterbalancing induction of proinflammatory (TNFα, IL-12, IL-18) and antiinflammatory (IL-10) cytokine responses occurs in circulating primate monocytes during the course of a gram-negative infection (unpublished data). Collectively, these data strongly imply that highly orchestrated cytokine regulatory mechanisms control a dynamic balance of proinflammatory and antiinflammatory arms of inflammatory responses in macrophages via autocrine/paracrine regulatory pathways. Exactly how all of this relates to the central hypothesis of this chapter (i.e., that tolerance or reprogramming ultimately dictates the effectiveness of antiendotoxin anticytokine therapies during the treatment of sepsis) remains to be fully investigated.

Role of Glucocorticoid/Hormonal Regulation

Alan Cross, in his keynote address (The Enduring Conundrum) at the Sepsis Symposium of the 1997 ICAAC meetings in Toronto, expressed doubt as to whether progress would be advanced in the treatment of sepsis as much by the introduction of new agents as by a better understanding of the ones already tried.[140] Recent events indicate that this is no less true of glucocorticoids than of other potential therapeutic agents that target endotoxin in particular and bacterial sepsis generally. This would apply to additional consideration of the role of glucocorticoids in the pathogenesis of sepsis and especially the modulation of proinflammatory and inflammatory manifestations.[141] In this regard, it has been reported [142] that a 10 mg/ml dose of staphylococcal toxic shock syndrome toxin 1 (TSST-1) or streptococcal pyrogenic exotoxin A was able to stimulate the release of a glucocorticoid-resistant protein,[143] the macrophage migration inhibitory factor (MIF), from either a murine macrophage-like cell line (RAW cells) or elicited mouse peritoneal macrophages.[142] (Macrophage migration inhibitory factor has been reviewed within the general context of glucocorticoid mechanisms of action.[141] Since that time, a number of developments have emerged, enabling the broader perspective that the present discussion accordingly demands.)

Although the effects of MIF appear at present to be targeted primarily toward the macrophage, MIF has also been shown to be released from T cells in response to proinflammatory agents. First identified in the pituitary, MIF has also been found in the lung, kidney, spleen, adrenal, and skin.[146] Pretreatment of mice with anti-MIF neutralizing antibody was able to protect mice significantly from the lethal effects of these gram-positive bacterial exotoxins in the previously described TNFα-mediated (D-galactosamine) lethality model. Even more recently[144] mice made homozygously deficient in the MIF gene were found to be resistant to the lethal effects of endotoxin (25 mg/kg) in a normal mouse model and to the lethal effects of *Staphylococcus aureus* enterotoxin B in the D-galactosamine lethality model, with correspondingly reduced plasma levels of TNFα. (Noteworthy was the finding that plasma levels of IL-6 and IL-10 appeared to remain normal.) In fact, the relation of glucocorticoid resistance associated with MIF may well extend beyond endotoxin to other bacterial components that are posssibly contained in both gram-positive and gram-negative bacteria. This conclusion receives further support based on an earlier report that exogenously administered glucocorticoid (dexamethasone) attenuates the TNFα response in rats following challenge with lipoteichoic acid plus peptidoglycan.[145]

Studies with MIF have rightfully focused on both broadly based and in-depth attention to glucocorticoid resistance. Such a property, in a somewhat more limited sense, is not new to endotoxin and infectious disease. Long-time students of endotoxin therapy will remember that Berry,[147] more than three decades ago, identified one or more proteins he termed glucocorticoid antagonizing factor(s). He traced the protein(s) to the macrophage, and he and his coworkers demonstrated that the protein(s) had the capacity to antagonize glucocorticoid upregulation of a key gluconeogenic regulatory enzyme (PEPCK) during experimental endotoxemia. More recent studies suggest that this glucocorticoid antagonism may be attributable to one or more cytokines, as previously reviewed.[148]

Glucocorticoid resistance also appears increasingly to be recognized as potentially important to clinical outcome. Notwithstanding the results from several earlier clinical trials that collectively led to the conclusion that glucocorticoids do not provide a meaningful route to effective treatment against sepsis, three trials have provided dramatic encouragement as to the potential efficacy of glucocorticoids in sepsis intervention strategies.[149-151] These developments have been reviewed by Meduri elsewhere in this volume (see Chapter 50). Among the patients who did not survive, there was a marked increase in plasma ACTH and cortisol concentrations, with independent evidence of glucocorticoid resistance.[152] In animal models, it has long been recognized that glucocorticoids given *after* the time of endotoxin challenge lose whatever protective efficacy they might otherwise possess, presumably due at least in part to the development of glucocorticoid resistance. We have observed in published studies, however, that if the dexamethasone dose is raised to 10 mg/kg, it protects normal mice even when given 2 hours after an acute challenge from LPS: 1 of 20 versus 9 of 20 deaths, $p<0.005$ (R. Silverstein et al., unpublished observations).

Thus, it appears that glucocorticoid resistance not only continues to be a subject of important and advancing research in animal sepsis models, but also, based on more recent clinical trials, a continuing problem in septic patients that is in need of resolution. To this end, studies from other laboratories and our own suggest that addressing the problem of glucocorticoid resistance in relation to serious bacterial infection may prove challenging. Our published and unpublished studies suggest that exogenous[153] and endogenous (unpublished data) glucocorticoid may assume a different degree of importance in protecting mice against acute bacterial sepsis, depending directly on whether the challenge is from gram-positive or gram-negative bacterial organisms. For example, when the challenging organism was a gram-negative microbe (e.g., *Escherichia coli*), both exogenous (dexamethasone) and endogenous (with adrenalectomized mice) glucocorticoid appeared to be important in protecting the host, but such was not the case (with endogenous or exogenous glucocorticoid) when the challenge was from a gram-positive microbe (e.g., *Staphylococcus aureus*). Moreover, the sensitivity to exogenous and endogenous glucocorticoid involvement with the *E. coli* challenge was found to parallel that seen with a purified endotoxin challenge. Importantly, these bacterial studies were carried out under comparable conditions, with viable bacterial challenge, and in the absence of any antibiotic treatment.

Experiments demonstrating the lack of endogenous glucocorticoid importance in *S. aureus*-mediated sepsis might at first seem to stand in sharp contrast to the importance of MIF in relation to challenge from gram-positive bacteria. However, the MIF studies were carried out with bacterial components rather than viable organisms. In that regard, unpublished studies from our laboratory have shown that when the viable *S. aureus* is administered along with concomitant and bactericidal-effective imipenem/cilastatin, a carbapenem class antibiotic, dexamethasone protection is in fact potentiated in adrenalectomized or in D-galactosamine-treated mice. This therefore suggests that the capacity of dexamethasone to protect infected mice may be intimately related not only to the classification of the threatening microbe but importantly, also to the consequences of the antibiotic treatment in releasing bacterial components. It is becoming increasingly clear, not only from the above-mentioned studies but from studies of antibiotic-linked differential rates of release of endotoxin and of other proinflammatory mediators,[36,38,154-158] that therapy directed against glucocorticoid resistance may benefit from attention given to corresponding antibiotic therapy and, even so, may prove challenging owing to bacterial identity, choice of antibiotic(s), and the timing and potency of a particular antibiotic regimen.

With increasing evidence that glucocorticoid resistance is not a problem unique to host defense against endotoxin, extending not only to gram-negative but also to gram-positive sepsis, it is essential that horizons regarding the mechanisms via which glucocorticoids and the adrenal and pituitary act against infectious challenge be broadened accordingly. For example, studies with hypophysectomized mice[159] have shown that loss of the pituitary results in increased plasma hemoglobin levels. Hemoglobin had earlier been shown to increase sensitivity to the lethal effects of endotoxin.[160] Endotoxicity has long been associated with abnormalities in metabolism, and one report emphasized a potentially important link to nitrogen metabolism and specifically between endotoxemia, the adrenal, and synthesis of glutamine.[161] There are also reports linking glucocorticoids and endotoxin to such rapidly developing research areas as events associated with leukocyte adhesion[162,163] and the relation of glucocorticoids to the modulation of peroxisome proliferating activated receptors (PPARs).[164,165] The latter reports gain added relevance in light of the finding that another adrenal cortical steriod, dehydroepiandrosterone (DHEA), which has long been seen as a modulator of glucocorticoid action,[166] is a PPARα agonist.[167] PPARs have recently gained attention, not only for their ability to inhibit the action of TNFα but as regulators of macrophage activation.[168]

In conclusion, much has been learned in recent years, and even in recent months, regarding glucocorticoid resistance, particularly with respect to MIF. There has also been a resurgence of clinical interest in glucocorticoids, including that of glucocorticoid resistance based on clinical outcomes. Nevertheless, inherent complexities associated with sepsis, including the choice of the most effective antibiotic treatment, seem to indicate that making maximum use of these new developments remains an awesome but critically important challenge.

Conclusions

The material summarized above has addressed a number of potential contributing factors that influence the role endotoxin plays in the manifestations of the overall host responses during a septic episode. Based on these factors alone, it can be strongly suggested that, although endotoxin is present in all cases of gram-negative sepsis and may well be present in many cases of gram-positive and fungal sepsis (primarily through endogenous sources), its role in the pathophysiology of the overall host inflammatory response, as well as both qualitative and quantitative aspects of exactly what that response is, may not be able to be accurately predicted without a far greater understanding of the specific profile of the septic patient.

As a consequence, if we are to understand the underlying mechanisms operative in the septic patient, increasing emphasis must be placed on a total integrative assessment, not only of the immunologic status of the patient but also of the potential cooperative antagonistic contributions of the various microbial factors that ultimately dictate outcome. In other words, the host response is rarely if ever a well defined singular event that occurs in response to exposure to a specific microbial factor. Rather, it is much more likely, perhaps inevitably, a temporal chain of events that could best be described, at least, as a "two-hit" phenomenon or even a "multi-hit" phenomenon. The potential influence of some of the factors involved in this multi-hit hypothesis have been reviewed herein, but other microbial factors can well be envisioned that are today incompletely understood and may well serve highly influential roles in dictating or orchestrating host responsiveness; these factors have been reviewed in detail by some of the coauthors elsewhere.[169] Until we fully understand the nature of the dominant components responsible, we must conclude that it is unlikely that we can state with any element of certainty why it is that patients die of sepsis.

This conclusion, if in fact justified, would have a significant impact on how to approach the question of assessing new therapeutic intervention strategies in the septic patient. These concerns, in turn, lead to equally important questions as to the current regulations for approval by regulatory agencies of any investigational new drug that targets either endotoxin or the inflammatory mediators generated by the host in response to endotoxin. Nevertheless, it is clear that endotoxin itself usually has the potential to be a contributing factor; therefore, all other things being equal, it might be of value always to assume that endotoxin therapy would be beneficial, provided the economic impact on the patient would not be excessive or prohibitive.

Acknowledgments. The helpful suggestions of Donald C. Johnson, PhD, are acknowledged with gratitude. Support from the National Institutes of Health (AI23447, CA54474, RR11825), Ernest F. Lied Foundation, Kansas University Endowment Association, and Merck & Co. is gratefully acknowledged. The authors also acknowledge the outstanding editorial input of Ms. Kathy Rode.

References

1. Westphal O, Luderitz O: Chemische erforschung von lipopolysacchariden gram-negativer bakterien. Angew Chem 1954;66: 407–417.

2. Morrison DC, Ryan JL: A review: bacterial endotoxins and host immune function. Adv Immunol 1979;28:293–450.
3. Morrison DC, Silverstein R, Luchi M, Shnyra A: Structure/function relationships of bacterial endotoxins and contribution to microbial sepsis. Infect Dis Clin North Am 1999 13:313–340.
4. Morrison DC: The C3H/HeJ mouse strain: its role in the elucidation of host response to bacterial endotoxin. In: Bonventre P (ed) Microbiology. Washington, DC, ASM Publications, 1986;23–28.
5. Morrison DC, Ulevitch RJ: A review: the interaction of bacterial endotoxins with cellular and humoral mediation systems. Am J Pathol 1978;92:527–618.
6. Ziegler EJ: Protective antibody to endotoxin core: the emperor's new clothes? J Infect Dis 1988;158:286–290.
7. Beutler B, Milsark IW, Cerami AC: Passive immunization against cachectin/tumor necrosis factor protects mice from lethal effect of endotoxin. Science 1985;229:869–871.
8. Cannon JG: Endotoxin and cytokine responses in human volunteers. In: Ryan JL, Morrison DC (eds) Bacterial Endotoxic Lipopolysaccharides, vol II: Immunopharmacology and Pathophysiology. Boca Raton, FL, CRC Press, 1992;311–326.
9. Wright SD, Ramos RA, Tobias PS, et al: CD14, a receptor for complexes of lipopolysaccharide (LPS) and LPS binding protein. Science 1990;249:1431–1433.
10. Yang R-B, Wells JD, McCall CA: Interleukin-1 beta expression after inhibition of protein phosphatases in endotoxin-tolerant cells. Clin Diag Lab Immunol 1998;5:281–287.
11. Kirschning CJ, Wesche H, Ayers TM, Rothe M: Human toll-like receptor 2 confers responsiveness to bacterial lipopolysaccharide. J Exp Med 1998;188:2091–2097.
12. Cross AS, Opal S: Therapeutic intervention in sepsis with antibody to endotoxin: is there a future? J Endotoxin Res 1994;57–69.
13. Westphal O, Jann K: Bacterial lipopolysaccharides: extraction with phenol-water and further applications of the procedure. In: Whistler RL (ed) Methods in Carbohydrate Chemistry. Academic Press, 1965;83.
14. Westphal O, Lüderitz: Über die Extraktionen vor Bakterien mit phenol/wasser. Z. Naturforsch, 1952;TeilB7:148–156.
15. Leeson MC, Morrison DC: Induction of proinflammatory responses in human monocytes by particulate and soluble forms of lipopolysaccharide. Shock 1994;2:235.
16. Katz SS, Chen K, Chen S, et al: Potent CD14-mediated signaling of human leukocytes by *Escherichia coli* can be mediated by interaction of whole bacteria and host cells without extensive prior release of endotoxin. Infect Immun 1996;64:3592.
17. Tesh VL, Morrison DC: The interaction of *Escherichia coli* with normal human serum: factors affecting the capacity of serum to mediate lipopolysaccharide release. Microb Pathog 1988;4:175.
18. Tesh VL, Morrison DC: The physical–chemical characterization and biologic activity of serum released lipopolysaccharide. J Immunol 1988;141:3523.
19. Tesh VL, Duncan RL, Morrison DC: The interaction of *Escherichia coli* with normal human serum: the kinetics of serum-mediated lipopolysaccharide release and its dissociation from bacterial killing. J Immunol 1986;137:1329.
20. Duncan RL, Hoffman J, Tesh VL, et al: Immunologic activity of lipopolysaccharide released from macrophages after the uptake of intact *E. coli* in vitro. J Immunol 1986;136:2924.
21. Freudenberg MA, Galanos C: The metabolic fate of endotoxins. Prog Clin Biol Res 1988;272:63.
22. Morrison DC, Bucklin SE, Leeson MC, et al: Contribution of soluble endotoxin released from gram-negative bacteria by antibiotics to the pathogenesis of experimental sepsis in mice. J Endotoxin Res 1996;3:237.
23. Dofferhoff AS, Nijland JH, de Vries Hospers HD, et al: Effects of different types and combinations of antimicrobial agents on endotoxin release from gram-negative bacteria: an in-vitro and in-vivo study. Scand J Infect Dis 1991;23:745.
24. Horii T, Kobayashi M, Sato K, et al: An in vitro study of carbapenem-induced morphological changes and endotoxin release in clinical isolates of gram-negative bacilli. J Antimicrob Chemother 1998;41:435.
25. Jackson JJ, Kropp H, Hurley JC: Influence of antibiotic class and concentration on the percentage of release of lipopolysaccharide from *Escherichia coli*. J Infect Dis 1994;169:471.
26. Jackson JJ, Kropp H: Beta-lactam antibiotic-induced release of free endotoxin: in vitro comparison of penicillin-binding protein (PBP) 2-specific imipenem and PBP 3-specific ceftazidime. J Infect Dis 1992;165:1033.
27. Jackson JJ, Kropp H: Differences in mode of action of beta-lactam antibiotics influence morphology, LPS release and in vivo antibiotic efficacy. J Endotoxin Res 1996;3:201–218.
28. Manthey CL, Vogel SN: Elimination of trace endotoxin protein from rough chemotype LPS. J Endotoxin Res 1994;1:84.
29. Killion JW, Morrison DC: Determinants of immunity to murine salmonellosis: studies involving immunization with lipopolysaccharide-lipid A-associated protein complexes in C3H/HeJ mice. FEMS Microbiol Immunol 1988;1:41.
30. Morrison DC, Betz SJ, Jacobs DM: Isolation of a lipid A bound polypeptide responsible for "LPS-initiated" mitogenesis of C3H/HeJ spleen cells. J Exp Med 1976;144:840–846.
31. Goodman GW, Sultzer BM: Endotoxin protein is a mitogen and polyclonal activator of human B lymphocytes. J Exp Med 1979;149:713–723.
32. Dokter WH, Dijkstra AJ, Koopmans SB, et al: G(Anh)MTetra, a natural bacterial cell wall breakdown product, induces interleukin-1 beta and interleukin-6 expression in human monocytes: a study of the molecular mechanisms involved in inflammatory cytokine expression. J Biol Chem 1994;269:4201. Erratum. J Biol Chem 1994;269:16983.
33. Medvedev AE, Flo T, Ingalls RR, et al: Involvement of CD14 and complement receptors CR3 and CR4 in nuclear factor-kappaB activation and TNF production induced by lipopolysaccharide and group B streptococcal cell walls. J Immunol 1998;160:4535.
34. Dziarski R, Jin YP, Gupta D: Differential activation of extracellular signal-regulated kinase (ERK) 1, ERK2, p38, and c-Jun NH2-terminal kinase mitogen-activated protein kinases by bacterial peptidoglycan. J Infect Dis 1996;174:777–785.
35. Nakano M, Kirikae T: Biological characterization of *Pseudomonas aeruginosa* endotoxin released by antibiotic treatment in vitro. J Endotoxin Res 1996;3:195.
36. Norimatsu M, Morrison DC: Correlation of antibiotic-induced endotoxin release and cytokine production in *Escherichia coli*-inoculated mouse whole blood ex vivo. J Infect Dis 1998;177:1302–1307.
37. Arditi M, Kabat W, Yogev R: Antibiotic-induced bacterial killing stimulates tumor necrosis factor-alpha release in whole blood. J Infect Dis 1993;167:240.
38. Bucklin SE, Morrison DC: Differences in therapeutic efficacy among cell wall-active antibiotics in a mouse model of gram-negative sepsis. J Infect Dis 1995;172:1519–1527.

39. Thomson AW, Fowler EF: Carrageenan: a review of its effects on the immune system. Agents Actions 1981;11:265.
40. Tauber MG, Shibl AM, Hackbarth CJ, et al: Antibiotic therapy, endotoxin concentration in cerebrospinal fluid, and brain edema in experimental *Escherichia coli* meningitis in rabbits. J Infect Dis 1987;156:456.
41. Mustafa MM, Ramilo O, Mertsola J, et al: Modulation of inflammation and cachectin activity in relation to treatment of experimental *Hemophilus influenzae* type b meningitis. J Infect Dis 1989;160:818.
42. Odio CM, Faingezicht I, Paris M, et al: The beneficial effects of early dexamethasone administration in infants and children with bacterial meningitis. N Engl J Med 1991;324:1525.
43. Brandtzaeg P, Kierulf P, Gaustad P, et al: Plasma endotoxin as a predictor of multiple organ failure and death in systemic meningococcal disease. J Infect Dis 1989;159:195.
44. Prins JM, van Agtmael MA, Kuijper EJ, et al: Antibiotic-induced endotoxin release in patients with gram-negative urosepsis: a double-blind study comparing imipenem and ceftazidime. J Infect Dis 1995;172:886.
45. Friedman G, Silva E, Vincent JL: Has the mortality of septic shock changed with time. Crit Care Med 1998;26:2078–2086.
46. Freudenberg MA, Galanos C: Tumor necrosis factor alpha mediates lethal activity of killed gram-negative and gram-positive bacteria in D-galactosamine-treated mice. Infect Immun 1991;59:2110–2115.
47. Barriere SL, Guglielmo BJ: Gram-negative sepsis, the sepsis syndrome, and the role of antiendotoxin monoclonal antibodies. Clin Pharmacol 1992;11:223–235.
48. Hitchcock PJ, Morrison DC: The protein component of bacterial endotoxins. In: Rietschel ET (ed) Handbook of Endotoxin, vol 1: Chemistry of Endotoxin. Amsterdam, Elsevier/North-Holland, 1984;339–374.
49. Skidmore BJ, Morrison DC, Chiller JM, et al: Immunologic properties of bacterial lipopolysaccharide (LPS) II. The unresponsiveness of C3H/HeJ mouse spleen cells to LPS-induced mitogenesis is dependent on the method used to extract LPS. J Exp Med 1975;142:1488–1508.
50. Flebbe L, Vukajlovich SW, Morrison DC: Immunostimulation of C3H/HeJ lymphoid cells by R-chemotype lipopolysaccharide preparations. J Immunol 1989;142:642–652.
51. Manthey CL, Vogel SN: Interactions of lipopolysaccharide with macrophages. Immunol Ser 1994;60:63–81.
52. Reddi K, Poole S, Nair S, et al: Lipid A-associated proteins from periodontopathogenic bacteria induce interleukin-6 production by human gingival fibroblasts and monocytes. FEMS Immunol Med Microbiol 1995;11:137–144.
53. Brogden KA, Ackermann MR, Debey BM: Pasteurella haemolytica lipopolysaccharide-associated protein induces pulmonary inflammation after bronchoscopic deposition in calves and sheep. Infect Immun 1995;63:3595–3599.
54. Killion JW, Morrison DC: Protection of C3H/HeJ mice from lethal *Salmonella typhimurium* LT2 infection by immunization with lipopolysaccharide–lipid A-associated protein complexes. Infect Immun 1986;54:1–8.
55. Abu Lawi KI, Sultzer BM: The tyrosine phosphorylation of a p72syk-like protein in activated murine resident peritoneal macrophages. Cell Mol Biol Res 1995;41:49–58.
56. Abu Lawi KI, Sultzer BM: Induction of serine and threonine protein phosphorylation by endotoxin-associated protein in murine resident peritoneal macrophages. Infect Immun 1995;63:498–502.
57. Henderson B, Poole S, Wilson M: Bacterial modulins: a novel class of virulence factors which cause host tissue pathology by inducing cytokine synthesis. Microbiol Rev 1996;60:316–341.
58. Galdiero F, Sommese L, Scarfogliero P, et al: Biological activities—lethality, Shwartzman reaction and pyrogenicity—of *Salmonella typhimurium* porins. Microb Pathog 1994;16:111–119.
59. Korn A, Kroll HP, Berger HP, et al: The 39-kilodalton outer membrane protein of Proteus mirabilis is an OmpA protein and mitogen for murine B lymphocytes. Infect Immun 1993;61:4915–4918.
60. Weber G, Link F, Ferber E, et al: Differential modulation of the effects of lipopolysaccharide on macrophages by a major outer membrane protein of Proteus mirabilis. J Immunol 1993;151:415–424.
61. O'Reilly T, Zak O: Enhancement of the effectiveness of antimicrobial therapy by muramyl peptide immunomodulators. Clin Infect Dis 1992;14:1100–1109.
62. Zidek Z, Masek K, Sedivy F: Anti-inflammatory effects of muramyl dipeptide in experimental models of acute inflammation. Agents Actions 1984;14:72–75.
63. Dokter WH, Dijkstra AJ, Koopmans SB, et al: G(AnH)MTetra, a naturally occurring 1,6-anhydro muramyl dipeptide, induces granulocyte colony-stimulating factor expression in human monocytes: a molecular analysis. Infect Immun 1994;62:2953–2957.
64. Dziarski R, Dziarski A: Mitogenic activity of staphylococcal peptidoglycan. Infect Immun 1979;23:706–710.
65. Rietschel ET, Schletter J, Weidemann B, et al: Lipopolysaccharide and peptidoglycan: CD14-dependent bacterial inducers of inflammation. Microb Drug Resist 1998;4:37–44.
66. Hazenberg MP, Klasen IS, Kool J, et al: Are intestinal bacteria involved in the etiology of rheumatoid arthritis? Review article. APMIS 1992;100:1–9.
67. Gupta D, Kirkland TN, Viriyakosal S, et al: CD14 is a cell-activating receptor for bacterial peptidoglycan. J Biol Chem 1996;271:23310–23316.
68. De Kimpe SJ, Kengatharan M, Thiemermann C, et al: The cell wall components peptidoglycan and lipoteichoic acid from *Staphylococcus aureus* act in synergy to cause shock and multiple organ failure. Proc Natl Acad Sci USA 1995;92:10359–10363.
69. Riesenfeld-Orn I, Wolpe S, Garcia Bustos JF, et al: Production of interleukin-1 but not tumor necrosis factor by human monocytes stimulated with pneumococcal cell surface components. Infect Immun 1989;57:1890–1893.
70. Tsutsui O, Kokeguchi S, Matsumura T, et al: Relationship of the chemical structure and immunobiological activities of lipoteichoic acid from *Streptococcus faecalis* (*Enterococcus hirae*) ATCC 9790. FEMS Microbiol Immunol 1991;3:211–218.
71. Bhakdi S, Klonisch T, Nuber P, et al: Stimulation of monokine production by lipoteichoic acids. Infect Immun 1991;59:4614–4620.
72. Standiford TJ, Arenberg DA, Danforth JM, et al: Lipoteichoic acid induces secretion of interleukin-8 from human blood monocytes: a cellular and molecular analysis. Infect Immun 1994;62:119–125.
73. Danforth JM, Strieter RM, Kunkel SL, et al: Macrophage inflammatory protein-1 alpha expression in vivo and in vitro: the

73. role of lipoteichoic acid. Clin Immunol Immunopathol 1995; 74:77–83.
74. Keller R, Fischer W, Keist R, et al: Macrophage response to bacteria: induction of marked secretory and cellular activities by lipoteichoic acids. Infect Immun 1992;60:3664–3672.
75. De Kimpe SJ, Hunter ML, Bryant CE, et al: Delayed circulatory failure due to the induction of nitric oxide synthase by lipoteichoic acid from *Staphylococcus aureus* in anaesthetized rats. Br J Pharmacol 1995;114:1317–1323.
76. Hattor Y, Kasai K, Akimoto K, et al: Induction of NO synthesis by lipoteichoic acid from *Staphylococcus aureus* in J774 macrophages: involvement of a CD14-dependent pathway. Biochem Biophys Res Commun 1997;233:375–379.
77. Kengatharan M, De Kimpe SJ, Thiemermann C: Analysis of the signal transduction in the induction of nitric oxide synthase by lipoteichoic acid in macrophages. Br J Pharmacol 1996;117:1163–1170.
78. Radolf JD, Norgard MV, Brandt ME, et al: Lipoproteins of *Borrelia burgdorferi* and *Treponema pallidum* activate cachectin/tumor necrosis factor synthesis: analysis using a CAT reporter construct. J Immunol 1991;147:1968–1974.
79. Hauschildt S, Hoffmann P, Beuscher HU, et al: Activation of bone marrow-derived mouse macrophages by bacterial lipopeptide: cytokine production, phagocytosis and Ia expression. Eur J Immunol 1900;20:63–68.
80. Dong Z, Qi X, Fidler IJ: Tyrosine phosphorylation of mitogen-activated protein kinases is necessary for activation of murine macrophages by natural and synthetic bacterial products. J Exp Med 1993;177:1071–1077.
81. Zhang H, Peterson JW, Niesel DW, et al: Bacterial lipoprotein and lipopolysaccharide act synergistically to induce lethal shock and proinflammatory cytokine production. J Immunol 1997;159:4868–4878.
82. Pisetsky DS: DNA and the immune system [editorial]. Ann Intern Med 1997;126:169–171.
83. Yamamoto S, Kuramoto E, Shimada S, et al: In vitro augmentation of natural killer cell activity and production of interferon-alpha/beta and -gamma with deoxyribonucleic acid fraction from *Mycobacterium bovis* BCG. Jpn J Cancer Res 1988;79:866–873.
84. Krieg AM, Yi AK, Matson S, et al: CpG motifs in bacterial DNA trigger direct B-cell activation. Nature 1995;374:546–549.
85. Bird AP: Functions for DNA methylation in vertebrates. Cold Spring Harbor Symp Quant Biol 1993;58:281–285.
86. Hergersberg M: Biological aspects of cytosine methylation in eukaryotic cells. Experientia 1991;47:1171–1185.
87. Schwartz DA, Quinn TJ, Thorne PS, et al: CpG motifs in bacterial DNA cause inflammation in the lower respiratory tract. J Clin Invest 1997;100:68–73.
88. Sparwasser T, Miethke T, Lipford G, et al: Bacterial DNA causes septic shock. Nature 1997;386:336–337.
89. Heeg K, Sparwasser T, Lipford GB, et al: Bacterial DNA as an evolutionary conserved ligand signaling danger of infection to immune cells. Eur J Clin Microbiol Infect Dis 1998;17:464–469.
90. Pisetsky DS: Immune activation by bacterial DNA: a new genetic code. Immunity 1996;5:303–310.
91. Hacker H, Mischak H, Miethke T, et al: CpG-DNA-specific activation of antigen-presenting cells requires stress kinase activity and is preceded by non-specific endocytosis and endosomal maturation. EMBO J 1998;17:6230–6240.
92. Sparwasser T, Miethke T, Lipford G, et al: Macrophages sense pathogens via DNA motifs: induction of tumor necrosis factor-alpha-mediated shock. Eur J Immunol 1997;27:1671–1679.
93. Stacey KJ, Sweet MJ, Hume DA: Macrophages ingest and are activated by bacterial DNA. J Immunol 1996;157:2116–2122.
94. Cowdery JS, Chace JH, Yi AK, et al: Bacterial DNA induces NK cells to produce IFN-gamma in vivo and increases the toxicity of lipopolysaccharides. J Immunol 1996;156:4570–4575.
95. Tran DD, Groeneveld AB, van der Meulen J, et al: Age, chronic disease, sepsis, organ system failure, and mortality in a medical intensive care unit. Crit Care Med 1990;18:474–479.
96. Bone RC, Gradzin CJ, Balk RA: Sepsis: a new hypothesis for pathogenesis of the disease process. Chest 1997;112:235–243.
97. Dinarello CA: Cytokines as mediators in the pathogenesis of septic shock. Curr Top Microbiol Immunol 1996;216:133–165.
98. Wells CL: Colonization and translocation of intestinal bacterial flora. Trans Proc 1996;2653–2656.
99. Van Leeuwen PAM, Boermeester MA, Houdjik APJ, et al: Clinical significance of translocation. Gut 1994;35(suppl): S23–S34.
100. Xu D, Qi L, Guillory D, et al: Mechanisms of endotoxin induced intestinal injury in a hyperdynamic model of sepsis. J Trauma 1993;34:676–683.
101. Tarao K, So K, Moroi T, et al: Detection of endotoxin in plasma and ascites fluid of patients with cirrhosis: its clinical significance. Gastroenterology 1977;73:539–542.
102. Bigatello LM, Broitman SA, Fattori L, et al: Endotoxemia encephalopathy and mortality in cirrhotic patients. Am J Gastroenterol 1987;82:11–15.
103. Kelly JL, O'Sullivan CO, O'Riordain M, et al: Is circulating endotoxin the trigger for the systemic inflammatory response syndrome seen after injury? Ann Surg 1997;225:530–543.
104. Boivin A, Mesrobeanu L: Recherches sur les Antigenes Somatiques et sur les Endotoxines des Bacteries. Rev Immunol 1938;4:40–52.
105. Beeson PB: Tolerance to bacterial pyrogens. I. Factors influencing its development. J Exp Med 1947;86:29.
106. Greisman SE, Young EJ, Carozza FA: Mechanism of endotoxin tolerance. V. Specificity of the early and late phases of pyrogenic tolerance. J Immunol 1969;103:1223–1236.
107. Freudenberg MA, Keppler D, Galanos C: Requirement for lipopolysaccharide-responsive macrophages in galactosamine-induced sensitization to endotoxin. Infect Immun 1986;51:891–895.
108. Freudenberg MA, Galanos C: Induction of tolerance to lipopolysaccharide (LPS)-D-galactosamine lethality by pretreatment with LPS is mediated by macrophages. Infect Immun 1988;56:1352–1357.
109. Tracey KJ, Lowry SF, Cerami A: Cachectin: a hormone that triggers acute shock and chronic cachexia. J Infect Dis 1988;157:413–420.
110. Okusawa S, Gelfand JA, Ikejima T, et al: Interleukin 1 induces a shock-like state in rabbits: synergism with tumor necrosis factor and the effect of cyclooxygenase inhibition. J Clin Invest 1988;81:1162–1172.
111. Tracey KJ, Fong Y, Hesse DG, et al: Anti-cachectin/TNF monoclonal antibodies prevent septic shock during lethal bacteraemia. Nature 1987;330:662–664.
112. Dinarello CA: Interleukin-1 and interleukin-1 antagonism. Blood 1991;77:1627–1652.

113. Cohen J, Carlet J: INTERSEPT: an international, multicenter, placebo-controlled trial of monoclonal antibody to human tumor necrosis factor-alpha in patients with sepsis; International Sepsis Trial Study Group. Crit Care Med 1996;24:1431–1440.
114. Abraham E, Glauser MP, Butler T, et al: p55 Tumor necrosis factor receptor fusion protein in the treatment of patients with severe sepsis and septic shock: a randomized controlled multicenter trial; Ro 45-2081 Study Group. JAMA 1997;277: 1531–1538.
115. Opal SM, Fisher CJ Jr, Dhainaut JF, et al: Confirmatory interleukin-1 receptor antagonist trial in severe sepsis: a phase III, randomized, double-blind, placebo-controlled, multicenter trial: the Interleukin-1 Receptor Antagonist Sepsis Investigator Group. Crit Care Med 1997;25:1115–1124.
116. Finch RG: Design of clinical trials in sepsis: problems and pitfalls. J Antimicrob Chemother 1998;41(suppl A):95–102.
117. Waage A, Halstensen A, Shalaby R, et al: Local production of tumor necrosis factor alpha, interleukin 1, and interleukin 6 in meningococcal meningitis: relation to the inflammatory response. J Exp Med 1989;170:1859–1867.
118. Van Deuren M, van der Ven Jongekrijg J, Demacker PN, et al: Differential expression of proinflammatory cytokines and their inhibitors during the course of meningococcal infections. J Infect Dis 1994;169:157–161.
119. Keuter M, Dharmana E, Gasem MH, et al: Patterns of proinflammatory cytokines and inhibitors during typhoid fever. J Infect Dis 1994;169:1306–1311.
120. Munoz C, Carlet J, Fitting C, et al: Dysregulation of in vitro cytokine production by monocytes during sepsis. J Clin Invest 1991;88:1747–1754.
121. Van Deuren M, van der Ven Jongekrijg J, Demacker PN, et al: Differential expression of proinflammatory cytokines and their inhibitors during the course of meningococcal infections. J Infect Dis 1994;169:157–161.
122. Schinkel C, Sendtner R, Zimmer S, et al: Functional analysis of monocyte subsets in surgical sepsis. J Trauma 1998;44:743–748; discussion 748–749.
123. Virca GD, Kim SY, Glaser KB, et al: Lipopolysaccharide induces hyporesponsiveness to its own action in RAW 264.7 cells. J Biol Chem 1989;264:21951–21956.
124. Matic M, Simon SR: Tumor necrosis factor release from lipopolysaccharide-stimulated human monocytes: lipopolysaccharide tolerance in vitro. Cytokine 1991;3:576–583.
125. Fahmi H, Chaby R: Selective refractoriness of macrophages to endotoxin-induced production of tumor necrosis factor, elicited by an autocrine mechanism. J Leukoc Biol 1993;53:45–52.
126. Pitton C, Fitting C, van Deuren M, et al: Different regulation of TNF alpha and IL-1ra synthesis in LPS-tolerant human monocytes. Prog Clin Biol Res 1995;392:523–528.
127. Labeta MO, Durieux JJ, Spagnoli G, et al: CD14 and tolerance to lipopolysaccharide: biochemical and functional analysis. Immunology 1993;80:415.
128. Mathison J, Wolfson E, Steinemann S, et al: Lipopolysaccharide (LPS) recognition in macrophages: participation of LPS-binding protein and CD14 in LPS-induced adaptation in rabbit peritoneal exudate macrophages. J Clin Invest 1993;92:2053–2059.
129. Ziegler Heitbrock HW, Wedel A, Schraut W, et al: Tolerance to lipopolysaccharide involves mobilization of nuclear factor kappa B with predominance of p50 homodimers. J Biol Chem 1994;269:17001–17004.
130. Bohuslav J, Kravchenko VV, Parry GC, et al: Regulation of an essential innate immune response by the p50 subunit of NF-kappaB. J Clin Invest 1998;102:1645–1652.
131. LaRue KE, McCall CE: A labile transcriptional repressor modulates endotoxin tolerance. J Exp Med 1994;180: 2269–2275.
132. Ding A, Hwang S, Lander HM, et al: Macrophages derived from C3H/HeJ (Lpsd) mice respond to bacterial lipopolysaccharide by activating NF-kappa B. J Leukoc Biol 1995;57:174–179.
133. Randow F, Syrbe U, Meisel C, et al: Mechanism of endotoxin desensitization: involvement of interleukin 10 and transforming growth factor beta. J Exp Med 1995;181:1887–1892.
134. Randow F, Docke WD, Bundschuh DS, et al: In vitro prevention and reversal of lipopolysaccharide desensitization by IFN-gamma, IL-12, and granulocyte-macrophage colony-stimulating factor. J Immunol 1997;158:2911–2918.
135. Bundschuh DS, Barsig J, Hartung T, et al: Granulocyte-macrophage colony-stimulating factor and IFN-gamma restore the systemic TNF-alpha response to endotoxin in lipopolysaccharide-desensitized mice. J Immunol 1997;158:2862–2871.
136. Zhang X, Morrison DC: Lipopolysaccharide-induced selective priming effects on tumor necrosis factor alpha and nitric oxide production in mouse peritoneal macrophages. J Exp Med 1993;177:511–516.
137. Zhang X, Alley EW, Russell SW, et al: Necessity and sufficiency of beta interferon for nitric oxide production in mouse peritoneal macrophages. Infect Immun 1994;62:33–40.
138. Alipio A, Morrison DC, Shnyra A: Selective immunoregulatory cytokines reproduce low dose LPS reprogramming of mouse macrophages. In: Faist E (ed) Proceedings of the 4th International Congress on the Immune Consequences of Trauma, Shock and Sepsis, 1997;321–326.
139. Shnyra A, Brewington R, Alipio A, et al: Reprogramming of lipopolysaccharide-primed macrophages is controlled by a counterbalanced production of IL-10 and IL-12. J Immunol 1998;160:3729–3736.
140. Cross A: The Enduring Conundrum. Interscience Conference on Antimicrobial Agents and Chemotherapy, Toronto, September 1997.
141. Silverstein R, Johnson DC, Norimatsu M: Glucocorticoid control of endotoxin responses. In: Brade H, Morrison DC, Opal SN, Vogel SN, (eds) Endotoxin in Health and Disease. New York, Marcel Decker, 1999;769–779.
142. Calandra T, Spiegel LA, Metz CN, et al: Macrophage migration inhibitor factor is a critical mediator of the activation of immune cells by exotoxins of gram-positive bacteria. Proc Natl Acad Sci USA 1998;95:11383–11388.
143. Calandra T, Bucala R: Macrophage migration inhibitor factor (MIF): a glucocorticoid counter-regulator within the immune system. Crit Rev Immunol 1997;17:77–88.
144. Bozza M, Satoskar AR, Lin G, et al: Targeted disruption of migration inhibitory factor gene reveals its critical role in sepsis. J Exp Med 1999;189:341–346.
145. Kengatharan KM, Dekimpe SJ, Thiemermann C: Role of nitric oxide in the circulatory failure and organ injury in a rodent model of gram-positive septic shock. Br J Pharmacol 1996;119: 1411–1421.
146. Bacher M, Meinhardt A, Lan HY, et al: Migration inhibitory factor expression in experimentally induced endotoxemia. Am J Pathol 1997;150:235–246.

147. Berry LJ: Glucocorticoid-antagonizing factor. In: Proctor RA (series), Berry LJ (volume) (eds) Cellular Biology of Endotoxin, vol 3. Amsterdam, Elsevier, 1985;123–150.
148. Silverstein R: The endocrine response to endotoxin. In: Ryan JL, Morrison DC (eds) Bacterial Endotoxic Lipopolysaccharides, vol II. Boca Raton, CRC Press, 1992;295–309.
149. Bollaert PE, Charpentier C, Levy B, et al: Reversal of late septic shock with supraphysiologic doses of cortisone. Crit Care Med 1998;26:645–650.
150. Meduri GU, Headley S, Carson SJ, et al: Effect of prolonged methylprednisolone therapy in unresolving acute respiratory distress syndrome. JAMA 1998;159–165.
151. Briegel J, Haller M, Forst H, et al: Effect of hydrocortisone on reversal of hyperdynamic septic shock: a randomized, double-blind, placebo-controlled, single-center study. [abstract 656]. Shock 1997;7:165.
152. Meduri GU, Kanangat S: Glucocorticoid treatment of sepsis and acute respiratory distress syndrome: time for a critical reappraisal. Crit Care Med 1998;26:630–633.
153. Silverstein R, Norimatsu M, Morrison DC: Fundamental differences during gram-positive versus gram-negative sepsis become apparent during bacterial challenge of D-galactosamine-treated mice. J Endotoxin Res 1997;4:173–181.
154. Silverstein R, Wood JG, Johnson DC, et al: Generalized differences in the host inflammatory response to gram-positive and gram-negative sepsis: modulation upon antibiotic treatment in normal, adrenalectomized, and D-galactosamine mouse models. Workshop on Septic Shock Caused by Gram-positive Bacteria, Vibo Valentia, Italy, October 1998.
155. Morrison DC: Endotoxin/antibiotics and gram-negative sepsis. J Endotoxin Res 1996;3:171.
156. Horn DL, Opal SM, Lomastro E: Antibiotics, cytokines, and endotoxin: a complex and evolving relationship in gram-negative sepsis. Scand J Infect Dis Suppl 1996;101:9–13.
157. Schneider CM, Huzly D, Vetter C, et al: Tumor necrosis factor alpha and interleukin 6 release induced by antibiotic killing of *Pseudomonas aeruginosa* and *Staphylococcus aureus*. Eur J Clin Microbiol Infect Dis 1997;16:467–471.
158. Frieling JTM, Mulder JA, Hendriks T, et al: Differential induction of pro- and anti-inflammatory cytokines in whole blood by bacteria: effects of antibiotic treatment. Antimicrob Agents Chemother 1997;41:1439–1443.
159. Bloom O, Wang H, Ivanova S, et al: Hypophysectomy, high tumor necrosis factor levels, and hemoglobinemia in lethal endotoxin shock. Shock 1998;6:395–400.
160. Su D, Roth RI, Yoshida M, et al: Hemoglobin increases mortality from bacterial endotoxin. Infect Immun 1997;65:1258–1266.
161. Lukaszewicz GC, Souba WW, Abcouwer SF: Induction of muscle glutamine synthetase gene expression during endotoxemia is adrenal gland dependent. Shock 1997;7:332–338.
162. Davenpeck KL, Zagorski J, Schleimer RP, et al: Lipopolysaccharide-induced leukocyte rolling and adhesion on the rat mesenteric microcirculation: regulation by glucocorticoids and role of cytokines. J Immunol 1998;161:6861–6870.
163. Panes J, Perry M, Granger DN: Leukocyte endothelial cell adhesion: avenues for therapeutic intervention. Br J Pharmacol 1999;126:537–550.
164. Lemberger T, Staels B, Saladin R, et al: Regulation of the peroxisome proliferator-activated receptor alpha gene by glucocorticoids. J Biol Chem 1994;269:24527–24530.
165. Plant NJ, Horley NJ, Savory RL, et al: The peroxisome proliferators are hepatocyte mitogens in chemically-defined media: glucocorticoid-induced PPARα is linked to peroxisome proliferator mitogeneis. Carcinogenesis 1998;19:925–931.
166. Rook GAW, Hernandez-Pando R, Lightman SL: Hormones, peripherally activated prohormones and regulation of the Th1/Th2 balance. Immunol Today 1994;15:301.
167. Peters JM, Zhou Y-C, Ram PA, et al: Peroxisome proliferator-activated receptor α required for gene induction by dehydroepiandosterone-3-sulfate. Mol Pharmacol 1996;50:67–74.
168. Ricote M, Li AC, Wilson TM, et al: The peroxisome proliferator-activated receptor is a negative regulator of macrophage activation. Nature 1998;391:79–82.
169. Horn DL, Morrison DC, Opal SM, et al: Why do patients with sepsis die? How can we prevent this? Report on a symposium. Clin Infect Dis, 1999 (in press).

14
Untimely Apoptosis in Human SIRS, Sepsis, and MODS

Timothy G. Buchman

Apoptosis refers to a type of cell death characterized by cell shrinkage, cytoconcentration, and DNA fragmentation. Several features distinguish apoptosis from oncosis (death by cell "swelling"), but the two are of special interest to students of MODS.[1] The first feature is that apoptosis does not incite an inflammatory response: The residual components of the newly dead cell are ingested by nearby phagocytic cells without recruiting neutrophils. The second feature is that apoptosis, unlike oncosis, follows explicit biologic signals encoded by every known eukaryotic cell. Apoptosis, often colloquially called "cell suicide," is essential to human gestation and development. For example, without apoptosis humans would have webs instead of separate digits (the interdigital scaffolding would never involute), and we would be hermaphrodites (neither the Müllerian nor the Wolffian apparatus would involute). This apoptosis is also essential to the maintenance of normal physiology; for example, the turnover of gut epithelium and the desquamation of sun-injured skin are but two of many normal apoptotic processes.

The purpose of this brief chapter is to assess how the timing of apoptosis is modified in human systemic inflammatory response syndrome (SIRS), sepsis, and multiple organ dysfunction syndrome (MODS). This review is deliberately restricted to human pathophysiology because the relevance of apoptosis observed in experimental animal models of MODS to apoptosis in human critical illness remains uncertain. This review demonstrates opposing changes in the timing of apoptosis of particular human cells. These changes appear to be characteristic of human inflammation. It is important to emphasize that the biology is purely descriptive; at present, it is uncertain whether these changes in timing of apoptosis cause MODS, are caused by MODS, or merely correlate with MODS.

Neutrophils

Apoptosis is essential to normal neutrophil biology. Given that necrosis triggers an inflammatory response that attracts neutrophils, neutrophil death cannot proceed by typical oncotic pathways. If neutrophils were to die by oncosis, their residua would attract additional neutrophils in a self-sustaining chain reaction. The clinical correlate is that collections of neutrophils, such as those recruited to the site of an abscess, must be rapidly and efficiently lysed if they are not needed to kill an invader, and this lysis must not produce further inflammation. The physiologic correlate is that neutrophils typically survive in the periphery for just a few hours,[2] at which time the genetic code for apoptosis is executed.

Circulating neutrophils are among the easiest cells to obtain from humans: Serial venipuncture is well tolerated, and humans of interest (critically ill humans) often have indwelling vascular cannulas, further simplifying the sampling process. Given the hypothesis that sustained and unbridled inflammation is at least partly responsible for the pathogenesis of MODS, several investigators have recently focused on dysregulation of neutrophil apoptosis as a potential pathogenetic mechanism in MODS.

Interest in apoptosis as a potential mechanism for neutrophil clearance was articulated more than a decade go by Savill and colleagues.[3] By 1992 Haslett recognized apoptosis as an essential mechanism by which neutrophils were cleared after extravasation into tissues.[4] Given the contemporary observation that trauma patients and other critically ill patients died with whole-body inflammation,[5] it was perhaps inevitable that students of critical illness would eventually propose a relation between MODS, sustained inflammation, and neutrophil apoptosis.

Neutrophil apoptosis is modulated by even modest inflammatory responses. Jiminez and her colleagues reported that spontaneous apoptosis was significantly delayed not only in peripheral blood obtained from patients with SIRS (8.6% versus normals of 34.9%) but in patients who had undergone anesthesia and major elective surgery (11.0% in patients immediately following repair of abdominal aortic aneurysms).[6] These authors also used mixing experiments (patient plasma with normal neutrophils) to confirm that plasma-borne factors could contribute to delayed apoptosis.

The list of plasma mediators that have been reported to retard human neutrophil apoptosis is extensive and includes tumor necrosis factor-α,[7] interleukin-1,[8] interleukin-4,[9] interleukin-6,[10] interleukin-8,[11] adenosine,[12] and the "alarmones" diadenosine polyphosphates ApppA and AppppA,[13] granulocyte/macrophage colony-stimulating factor,[14] and glucocorticoids.[15] The effect of Fas ligand–receptor binding is presently unclear.

The list of mediators known to accelerate neutrophil apoptosis is short; among the most interesting observations is that the β_2-integrin CD11b/CD18 is required to accelerate the programmed elimination of their host neutrophils.[16] The collective conclusion is that whereas neutrophils undergo apoptosis by default, upregulation of virtually any member of the network of mediators promoting inflammation retards that process.

Despite rapid progress in unraveling the molecular biology relevant to neutrophil apoptosis, it cannot be determined whether delay in neutrophil apoptosis is a cause, consequence, or epiphenomenon with respect to the evolution of MODS. What is certain, however, is that mild inflammation is sufficient to delay that neutrophil apoptosis.

Other Tissues

For obvious reasons, it is difficult to sample diverse tissues in critically ill patients and, by extension, to assess the importance of apoptosis as a mechanism of cell death in those tissues. Hotchkiss and colleagues completed a comprehensive study of apoptotic cell death in patients with sepsis, shock, and multiple organ dysfunction through analysis of tissues harvested immediately (within minutes to hours) after the death of 20 patients with those diagnoses and comparison with tissues harvested from 19 patients dying of unrelated causes.[17] In the septic patients, apoptosis was detected in diverse organs by three complementary methods, with a marked predominance in lymphocytes and intestinal epithelial cells. Hematoxylin and eosin (HE)-stained specimens from patients dying with sepsis showed at least focal apoptosis in 56% of spleens, 47% of colons, and 28% of ileums. There was also indirect evidence of lymphocyte apoptosis among the septic patients as shown by extensive depletion of lymphocytes in white pulp and a marked peripheral lymphocytopenia in more than three-fourths of the patients. By comparison, HE-stained specimens from nonseptic patients' tissues revealed a low level of apoptosis in a single patient. The TUNEL method, which detects DNA fragmentation, was relatively nonspecific. TUNEL-positive cells increased with delay in tissue fixation, and many TUNEL-positive cells were found in diverse tissues from both septic and nonseptic patients. To identify apoptotic cells more precisely, immunohistochemical staining for the active form of an apoptosis pathway enzyme, caspase-3, showed a marked increase in septic versus nonseptic patients. For example, more than 25–50% of cells stained positive for the activated form of caspase-3 focally in splenic white pulp of several (but not all) septic patients, whereas activated caspase-3 was not similarly detected in patients dying a nonseptic death.

Hotchkiss and coworkers were correct to point out that the apoptotic death of lymphocytes and epithelial cells merely correlates with sepsis and MODS.[17] Although it is attractive to speculate that such lymphocyte depletion is responsible for clinical anergy and predisposes the patient to the overwhelming infections that are typical during the final stages of the disease, those authors clearly articulate the current dilemma. It is increasingly apparent that patients who sustain inflammation, sepsis, and MODS have patterns of cell death that are distinct from those in normal patients and in patients similarly ill but without apparent inflammation. It is decidedly unclear whether interventions aimed at restoring programs of apoptosis to "normal" profiles can have an effect, desirable or adverse.

Conclusions

Despite intense investigation into the molecular mechanisms of apoptosis and the detection and measurement of this process in experimental models of sepsis, little information is presently available concerning altered patterns of apoptosis in human inflammation and consequent organ dysfunction. It appears that even mild inflammation is sufficient to retard neutrophil apoptosis, whereas septic death is associated with accelerated lymphocyte and intestinal epithelial apoptosis. Whether altered patterns of apoptosis are a cause, consequence, or epiphenomenon with respect to human MODS remains unknown. It is likely that human trials of drugs that modulate apoptosis are required to resolve that ambiguity.

References

1. Cobb JP, Hotchkiss RS, Karl IE, Buchman TG: Mechanisms of cell injury and death. Br J Anaesth 1996;77:3–10.
2. Martin TR, Pistorese BP, Hudson LD, Mauder J: The function of lung and blood neutrophils in patients with the adult respiratory distress syndrome: implications for the pathogenesis of lung infection. Am Rev Respir Dis 1991;144:254–262.
3. Savill JS, Wyllie AH, Henson JE, et al: Macrophage phagocytosis of aging neutrophils in inflammation. J Clin Invest 1989;83:865–875.
4. Haslett C: Resolution of acute inflammation and the role of apoptosis in the tissue fate of granulocytes. Clin Sci 1992;83:639–648.
5. Nuytinck HKS, Offerman XJM, Kubat K, Goris JA: Whole-body inflammation in trauma patients: an autopsy study. Arch Surg 1988;123:1519–1524.
6. Jiminez MF, Watson WG, Parodo J, et al: Dysregulated expression of neutrophil apoptosis in the systemic inflammatory response syndrome. Arch Surg 1997;132:1263–1270.
7. Watson RWG, Redmond HP, Wang JH, Bouchier-Hayes DR: Bacterial ingestion, tumor necrosis factor-alpha, and heat induce programmed cell death in activated neutrophils. Shock 1996;5:47–51.
8. Watson RWG, Rotstein OD, Parodo J, Bitar R, Marshall JC: The IL-1 beta converting enzyme (caspase-1) inhibits apoptosis of inflammatory neutrophils through activation of IL-1 beta. J Immunol 1998;161:957–962.
9. Girard D, Paquin R, Beaulieu AD: Responsiveness of human neutrophils to interleukin-4: induction of cytoskeletal rearrangements, de novo protein synthesis and delay of apoptosis. Biochem J 1997;325:147–153.

10. Biffl WL, Moore EE, Moore FA, et al: Interleukin-6 delays neutrophil apoptosis. Arch Surg 1996;131:24–30.
11. Goodman ER, Kleinstein E, Fusco A, et al: Role of interleukin-8 in the genesis of the acute respiratory distress syndrome through an effect on neutrophil apoptosis. Arch Surg 1998;133:1234–1239.
12. Walker BAM, Rocchini C, Boone RH, et al: Adenosine A_{2a} receptor activation delays apoptosis in human neutrophils. J Immunol 1997;158:2926–2931.
13. Gasmi L, McLennan AG, Edwards SW: The diadenosine polyphosphates Ap3A and Ap4A and adenosine triphosphate interact with granulocyte-macrophage colony-stimulating factor to delay neutrophil apoptosis: implications for neutrophil:platelet interactions during inflammation. Blood 1996;87:3442–3449.
14. Brach MA, de Vos S, Gruss HJ, Herrmann F: Prolongation of survival of human polymorphonuclear neutrophils by granulocyte-macrophage colony-stimulating factor is caused by inhibition of programmed cell death. Blood 1992;80:2920–2924.
15. Cox G: Glucocorticoid treatment inhibits apoptosis in human neutrophils: separation of survival and activation outcomes. J Immunol 1995;154:4719–4725.
16. Coxon A, Rieu P, Barkalow FJ, et al: A novel role for the beta 2 integrin CD 11b/CD 18 in neutrophil apoptosis; a homeostatic mechanism in inflammation. Immunity 1996;5:653–666.
17. Hotchkiss RS, Swanson PE, Freeman BD, et al: Apoptotic cell death in patients with sepsis, shock, and multiple organ dysfunction. Crit Care Med 1999;27:1230–1251.

15
Immunosuppression with Injury and Operation and Increased Susceptibility to Infection

Eugen Faist and Martin K. Angele

In the United States, trauma is a leading cause of death during the first three decades of life and ranks as the fourth leading cause of overall mortality, with more than 100,000 deaths each year.[1,2] Much of the mortality observed during the first few hours after trauma is related to irreversible neurologic damage or exsanguination.[3] Assuming the patient survives the initial traumatic insult, he or she is still threatened by subsequent infections (sepsis) and multiple organ failure.[4-7] It has been reported that upward of 50% of trauma patients subsequently die owing to infections and multiple organ failure during the proceeding days to week(s) after trauma.[4-7] In view of this fact, most of the scientific and medical research has been directed toward measuring the progression and interrelations of events that follow trauma and major surgery. These studies indicate that a causal relation exists between the traumatic injury or shock (or both) and the predisposition of these patients to develop septic/infectious complications and multiple organ failure.[8-10] The excessive inflammatory response together with a dramatic paralysis of cell-mediated immunity following trauma or major surgery[8,11] appears to be responsible for the increased susceptibility to subsequent sepsis.

In most clinical studies alterations in immune parameters of patients following trauma or major surgery have been assessed through evaluation of peripheral blood cell function and plasma levels of various mediators. Therefore, it has been advantageous to utilize animal models that simulate the clinical conditions. Such models have allowed us to better define the pathophysiology of the immunoinflammatory response following severe trauma that reduces the trauma victim's capacity to resist subsequent life-threatening infectious complications.

This chapter focuses on the effect of blood loss and injury on cell-mediated immune responses in experimental studies, utilizing models of trauma and hemorrhagic shock that have defined effects on the immunoinflammatory response. Subsequently we discuss how the findings from these experimental studies correlate with data generated from trauma victims and surgical patients. The effect of trauma and major surgeries on the susceptibility to polymicrobial sepsis and infection is then illustrated. Lastly, we point out a few new results demonstrating the effect of gender and sex hormones on cell-mediated immune responses following trauma and major surgery. These studies may generate new approaches to the treatment of immunodepression following trauma and surgery that might be advantageous for decreasing the susceptibility to infection and for increasing the survival rate of the critically ill surgical patient.

Macrophage Function Following Trauma and Hemorrhage

Macrophage Cytokine Release

Several studies have shown markedly depressed cell-mediated immune functions following hemorrhagic shock that were detectable immediately after the hypotensive period.[8,12] Studies have also demonstrated a significantly depressed capacity of splenic, peritoneal, and alveolar macrophages to release interleukins (IL-1, IL-6) and tumor necrosis factor-α (TNFα) following trauma and hemorrhage in vitro.[8,13,14] Studies indicate that the depression of IL-6 release by splenic and peritoneal macrophages persists up to 7 days following trauma and hemorrhage;[15] however, in animals subjected to laparotomy alone (e.g., trauma) or hemorrhage alone, macrophage cytokine production returned to normal by 5 days after the initial insult.[16] These findings suggest additive effects of the traumatic injury and the hemorrhagic shock on the depression of immune responses. Moreover, bone fracture in conjunction with soft tissue trauma and hemorrhagic shock produces more protracted depression of immune function than soft tissue trauma and hemorrhage without bone fracture.[17] Conversely, studies by Nwariaku et al. have shown depressed capacity of alveolar macrophages to release TNFα for up to 5 days following hemorrhage alone in New Zealand White rabbits.[14] The apparent discrepancy between these studies may be due to the anatomic locale of the macrophages studied or the severity of the hemorrhage model utilized.

In contrast to splenic, peritoneal, and alveolar macrophages, Kupffer cells have been shown to have an enhanced capacity to produce pro-inflammatory cytokines (i.e., IL-1, IL-6, TNFα) during the first 24 hours after hemorrhage.[18] Similarly, an increase in cell-associated TNFα has been demonstrated on Kupffer cells but not on splenic macrophages 2 hours after hemorrhagic shock and resuscitation.[19] In this regard, studies by Pellegrini et al.[20] in trauma patients indicated that the ratio of cell-associated TNFα and soluble TNFα receptor levels correlated with the development of multiple organ system failure. Thus the enhanced cell-associated TNFα appears to play an important role in cellular and immunologic alterations following injury.

It should be noted that Kupffer cells and splenic and peritoneal macrophages function in different microenvironments. Thus the data suggest that trauma and hemorrhagic shock might have potentially different effects on different tissue beds. Alternatively, splenic macrophages are in close contact with T cells, and mediators released by these cells following hemorrhage might depress the responsiveness of these macrophages compared to Kupffer cells. Despite the differential cytokine release capacities of macrophages from different microenvironments, a common depression of macrophage ability to present antigen has been demonstrated following severe blood loss.

Macrophage Antigen Presentation Following Trauma and Hemorrhage

Antigen presentation is defined as the process whereby a cell expresses antigen on its surface in a form capable of being recognized by a T cell. The proteinaceous antigen typically undergoes some form of processing in which it is degraded to small peptides, which are capable of associating with major histocompatibility complex (MHC II) for presentation to helper-T (Th) lymphocytes or in association with MHC I to become a target for cytotoxic T lymphocytes.[21] However, for competent antigen presentation to take place, the antigen-presenting macrophage must provide a second costimulatory signal in the form of a membrane or soluble factor (or both).

Several experimental studies have demonstrated marked depression of splenic, peritoneal, and liver macrophage (i.e., Kupffer cells) antigen presentation following severe hypotension of 1 hour.[18,21] This depression occurs as early as 2 hours after hemorrhage and persists up to 5 days.[18,21] Regional hypoxia due to decreased organ blood flow appears to be a trigger for depressing the macrophage antigen-presentation function, as studies indicate that chemically induced hypotension[22] and severe hypoxia (unpublished observation) in the absence of any blood loss also produces depression of macrophage antigen presentation. Studies have shown that depression of the antigen-presentation capacity of macrophages following trauma-hemorrhage was associated with a decrease in MHC II-positive cells and decreased surface density of MHC II antigen on immune cells.[18,21]

Immune deterioration has also been reported in patients after trauma and surgery. In this respect, studies have shown a lack of reactivity of circulating monocytes toward stimulation with bacteria or endotoxin following surgical trauma.[23] This paralysis of monocyte cell function has been reported to persist 3–5 days after trauma[24] and appears to be a potential risk factor for postoperative septic complications.[23] Moreover, MacLean et al.[25] and Christou and Tellado[26] reported that the outcome of trauma patients is worsened when they exhibited a depressed delayed-type hypersensitivity (DTH) reaction. Thus depressed cell-mediated immunity in patients following injury or major surgery associated with increased mortality from subsequent sepsis[27,28] is probably due in part to decreased antigen-presenting capacity by macrophages. Additionally, studies following thermal injury have shown that depressed lymphocyte responsiveness due to depressed MHC II expression was associated with depressed antigen presentation.[29,30]

These findings collectively suggest that the depression of macrophage antigen-presenting capacity following injury or major surgery is an important factor that contributes to the depression of cell-mediated immunity, thereby increasing subsequent susceptibility to infection. Multiple factors including decreased metabolic activity, antiinflammatory cytokines, prostaglandins, and nitric oxide appear to be responsible for the depression of macrophage antigen-presenting capacity.

Lymphocyte Function Following Hemorrhagic Shock, Trauma, and Burns

The central dysregulation of cell-mediated immune responses consists in the dissociation of monocyte (Mϕ)–T cell interactions via overrepresentation of suppressor active Mϕ and underrepresentation of T cell help.[31] A disturbance of lymphocyte systems can be observed following any extensive trauma and presents frequently within an absolute lymphopenia of $CD3^+$ cells and simultaneously with a monocytosis of $CD14^+$ cells.

Successful and protective immune responses are dependent on the activation of adequate T lymphocyte subpopulations that exert characteristic effector functions. Within the T cell subpopulation we observe a shift of the Th $CD4^+$/T-suppressor cytotoxic ($CD8^+$) ratio toward $CD8^+$ cells. It occurs in parallel with a reduction of the proliferative T cell response, reduced IL-2 production, and a disturbance of IL-2 receptor expression.

Both experimental and clinical studies indicate that a wide range of traumatic injuries alter the ability of T lymphocytes to respond to activation by mitogens (i.e., concanavalin A and phytohemagglutinin).[12,32–36] These studies demonstrate decreased mitogenic response of lymphocytes in patients following general surgery, blunt trauma, and thermal injury,[33–36] and the degree of lymphocyte depression correlates with the complexity of the surgery. Similarly, following hemorrhagic shock, decreased splenocyte proliferative capacity in response to the T cell mitogen concanavalin A has been demonstrated extensively in our laboratory.[12,16,32,37] Moreover, the release of Th1 lymphokines [i.e., IL-2, interferon γ (IFNγ)], by splenocytes has been shown to be significantly depressed as early as 2 hours after trauma and hemorrhagic shock,[12,16,32,37] and this depression persists up to 5 days following trauma-hemorrhage.[16] These findings in animal models are supported by several human studies.

Suppressed IL-2 biosynthesis represents the most striking and persistent manifestation of dysregulated cell-mediated immunity. Based on in vitro immunomodulatory experiments, the suppression of IL-2 production is a result of the massive release of immunoreactive prostaglandin E_2 (PGE_2) under stressful conditions.[38-40]

In 1988 Faist et al.[41] and Livingston et al.[42] were the first to detect suppression of IFNγ release from lymphocytes during traumatic stress. During the posttraumatic course the downregulation of IL-2 receptor expression plays a crucial role in the disintegration of adequate Mφ-T cell interactions.[43] The impairment of IL-2 synthesis and gene expression of T lymphocytes following burn trauma let O'Sullivan and coworkers assume a shift within the Th cell population toward the direction of a Th2 phenotype, a phenomenon that could play a central role in the pathogenesis of posttraumatic immunodysfunction.[44] Also the impairment of IFNγ synthesis in human peripheral blood mononuclear cells following major trauma[41] and significantly increased IL-4 production compared to that in healthy controls[44] reconfirm the hypothesis that there must be a dominating Th2 similar cytokine synthesis pattern following major injury. The mechanisms regulating the differentiation of Th cells has not been completely understood until today. For example, it is difficult to decide if an increase of IL-4 or the impairment of IL-12 production is the decisive event responsible for the shift in the Th2 direction following massive trauma, although Hseih et al. in a murine leishmaniasis experiment, found upregulation of IL-4 to be the dominant factor in the process of polarization.[45]

Furthermore, in contrast to Th1 lymphokines, the release of the antiinflammatory Th2 lymphokine IL-10 has been shown to be increased after trauma-hemorrhage. Neutralizing IL-10 by addition of anti-IL-10 monoclonal antibodies to the culture medium restored the depressed splenocyte proliferative capacity in splenocytes harvested from traumatized animals. These findings suggest that increased release of IL-10 following trauma-hemorrhage contributes to the depressed splenocyte Th1 lymphokine release.[12]

In addition to alterations in T lymphocyte function, changes in B cell function have been reported following trauma and shock. The capacity of splenic B cells to produce antibodies is significantly decreased following hemorrhage.[46,47] Moreover, a decrease in overall serum levels of immunoglobulin was seen up to 3 days after hemorrhagic shock.[46,47] It has been suggested that the decreased IL-2 production by T lymphocytes is responsible for the downregulation of antibody production by B cells following severe injury, as T cell lymphokines are a prerequisite for adequate B cell proliferation and immunoglobulin secretion.[8] Whether restoration of T cell function following severe injury and major surgery restores the depressed B cell function remains to be determined.

Circulatory Inflammatory Mediators

The observed immunodeficiency in trauma victims and patients following major surgery has been found to be associated with increased concentrations of inflammatory cytokines, reflecting activated immunocompetent cells in the same patient.[48] Thus it appears that the depressed cell-mediated immune responses in vitro discussed above reflect hyporesponsiveness to a second stimulus following massive activation in vivo.[49]

Elevated plasma levels of TNFα, IL-1, and IL-6 have been well described in animal experiments[8,50,51] and patient studies[10,52-55] following trauma, severe blood loss, and sepsis. The sequence of cytokine release following trauma and hemorrhagic shock includes increased plasma TNFα as early as 30 minutes after the onset of injury, peak TNFα levels by 2 hours after trauma and hemorrhage, and a return toward baseline values at 24 hours[8,50] (Fig. 15.1). In contrast to measurements using a bioassay,[50] elevated plasma TNFα levels were detectable 24 hours after trauma and blood loss by enzyme-linked immunosorbent assay (ELISA).[56] This finding suggests that TNFα detected 24 hours after injury might not be biologically active. Soluble TNFα receptors have been isolated from the plasma that might neutralize the biologic activity of circulating TNFα.[57] Unlike TNFα, plasma IL-6 levels are not significantly elevated until 2 hours after hemorrhage, and levels remain elevated up to 24 hours after the induction of hemorrhage.[58]

Because in vivo administration of IL-1, IL-6, and TNFα[59-62] induces a shock-like syndrome similar to that observed following severe blood loss and sepsis, it has been suggested that these cytokines play a role in initiating the cascade of events that can lead to the development of multiple organ dysfunction following severe hemorrhagic shock.

Furthermore, the increase in the release of proinflammatory cytokines by Kupffer cells following the induction of shock is associated with depressed immune function.[8] This finding suggests that proinflammatory cytokines produced by Kupffer

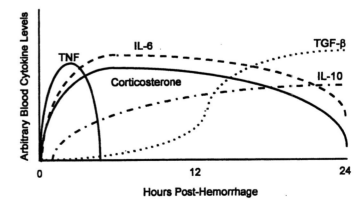

FIGURE 15.1. Arbitrary blood cytokine levels during the first 24 hours following trauma and hemorrhagic shock. Levels of tumor necrosis factor-α (TNF), interleukin-6 (IL-6), and transforming growth factor-β (TGFβ) were determined by specific bioassay. Interleukin-10 (IL-10) was measured by ELISA and corticosterone by radioimmunoassay.

cells following hemorrhage act in both an autocrine and a paracrine fashion to downregulate Kupffer cells and other macrophage populations. Furthermore, Kupffer cells, which represent the largest pool of macrophages in the body, were found to release increased amounts of IL-1, IL-6, and TNFα following shock,[59] and the selective reduction of this macrophage population by injection of gadolinium chloride significantly reduced plasma IL-6 levels following hemorrhage.[63] This leads to the conclusion that Kupffer cells are a significant source of the increased plasma levels of proinflammatory cytokines after trauma and hemorrhage, and these cytokines can depress macrophage function. Whether Kupffer cells are the only contributors to the enhanced proinflammatory plasma levels following severe injury and major surgery remains to be determined.

In contrast to the early increase of proinflammatory cytokines in the plasma following trauma and shock, elevated plasma levels of the antiinflammatory cytokine [i.e., transforming growth factor β (TGFβ)] are not detectable until 24 hours after the insult.[64] Furthermore, this elevation in plasma TGFβ persisted until 72 hours after trauma and hemorrhage.[64] Neutralization of TGFβ using an anti-TGFβ antibody restored depressed antigen presentation to normal levels.[64] These results along with the studies by Miller-Graziano et al.[65] indicate that the enhanced release of TGFβ is an additional factor responsible for the prolonged suppression of macrophage function following hemorrhagic shock.

In addition to pro- and antiinflammatory cytokines, numerous other mediators in the plasma have been reported to contribute to the depression of cell-mediated immune responses following trauma and shock. Eicosanoids have been studied extensively as agents involved in immunologic responses.[66,67] Early after the onset of shock (2 hours) there is increased release of prostaglandins and leukotrienes by macrophages, leading to elevated plasma levels of eicosanoids.[8,68] Moreover, PGE$_2$ has been shown to inhibit cell-mediated immune function.[69,70] Conversely, administration of ibuprofen, an inhibitor of cyclooxygenase, to animals following severe blood loss prevented depression of macrophage function.[71] Ayala and Chaudry[72] demonstrated that rodents prefed a fish oil diet high in omega-3 fatty acids, which are known to inhibit synthesis of PGE$_2$ through inhibition of arachidonic acid metabolism, had normal macrophage functions following hemorrhage.

Increased levels of circulating cytokines have also been reported following a variety of tissue insults in patients, including trauma, sepsis, thermal injury, and surgery.[10,55,73,74] Increased plasma IL-6 levels in patients have been observed during the first week following trauma.[55] Interestingly, levels of proinflammatory cytokines have been shown to be higher in trauma patients with severe blood loss than in patients with trauma alone.[10] Moreover, in septic patients the increase of the proinflammatory cytokines IL-6 and TNFα has been found to be much higher than in trauma victims without septic complications.[55] These findings suggest additive effects of trauma, blood loss, and septic complications on the immunoinflammatory response. Furthermore, proinflammatory cytokine levels and the duration of elevation appear to correlate with the severity of the insult. Elevated cytokine levels have been shown to persist for 5 days after gastrectomy compared to 3 days after mastectomy.[74] Moreover, several clinical studies have shown an association between elevated plasma levels of proinflammatory cytokines and increased infectious complications and higher mortality rates.[10,52,75-79] In this respect, Molloy et al. reported a progressive decline in TNFα levels in survivors of septic shock, whereas TNFα levels remained persistently elevated after the initial diagnosis and attempted treatment in nonsurvivors from septic shock.[80] Furthermore, studies of patients with meningococcal septic shock demonstrated that serum TNFα, IL-1β, and IL-6 levels on admission were a better prognostic parameter for outcome than the leukocyte count, the platelet count, or low blood pressure.[78]

It remains unknown whether increased levels of proinflammatory cytokines correlate with outcome in trauma patients without sepsis. Nonetheless, the above studies suggest the important contribution of proinflammatory cytokines to the pathophysiologic changes seen in trauma victims. Determination of proinflammatory cytokine levels may provide clinicians with an indicator of the intracellular milieu and possibly insight into cellular changes taking place. More refinements toward the rapid and online measurements of cytokines are needed, however, before the full benefits of such information can be effectively translated to better management of trauma patients. Although various cytokine therapies in septic patients so far have not yielded satisfactory results, the lack of beneficial effects might be related to the timing and dose of anticytokine administration. It is our hypothesis that total blockade/neutralization of cytokines is not helpful to the host. Instead, modulation of cytokine production/release by immune cells (i.e., macrophages, T cells) leading to restoration of cellular homeostasis might be a better approach for decreasing the susceptibility of trauma victims and patients following major surgery to subsequent sepsis and infection.

Increased Susceptibility to Infection

Polymicrobial Sepsis

The studies mentioned above indicate depressed immunoresponsiveness after trauma and hemorrhage that persists despite fluid resuscitation. They do not, however, indicate whether these observations translate into an actual reduction in the capacity of these traumatized animals to ward off infection of a clinically relevant nature. To determine this, additional studies were conducted by Stephan et al. in which sepsis was induced 3 days after hemorrhagic shock. The results demonstrated an increased susceptibility of hemorrhaged animals to polymicrobial sepsis as evidenced by an increased mortality rate of these animals following subsequent sepsis (the mortality of hemorrhaged animals following subsequent sepsis was 100% compared to 50% in sham animals subjected to sepsis).[32,81] Similarly, Zapata-Sirvent et al. indicated that the mortality rate in response to a septic challenge was increased in mice.[82] Restoration of the depressed immune responses following trauma and severe blood loss with immunomodulatory agents, specifically flutamide (an androgen receptor blocker) was associated with increased survival rates following subsequent sepsis.[81]

Moreover, an association between the loss of immunocompetence in patients (paralysis of cell-mediated immunity) following traumatic injury and the development of sepsis and late death has been reported[27,28] (Fig. 15.2). Furthermore, alterations in the levels of circulating E-selectin adhesion molecules after trauma and resuscitation have been found to be associated with an increased risk for infectious complications, organ failure, and death.[83] In summary, these studies suggest that the immunodepression following injury and major surgery leads to increased susceptibility to polymicrobial sepsis. Therefore attempts to modulate the depressed immune responses in trauma victims might decrease the development of septic complications and multiple organ failure in those patients.

Wound Infection

In addition to increased susceptibility to polymicrobial sepsis, an increased rate of wound infection has been reported in clinical and experimental studies following severe trauma and blood loss.[84-87] In trauma patients, shock/blood loss and the duration of hypotension have been identified as significant risk factors for the development of wound infection.[88,89] Similarly, significantly more wound complications have been documented following surgery for bleeding peptic ulceration compared to nonbleeding ulceration.[90] Livingston and Malangoni[84] noted increased susceptibility to wound infection following hemorrhagic shock in rats as evidenced by an increased presence of gross purulence at the wound site following *Staphylococcus aureus* injection. Antibiotic prophylaxis failed to reduce the incidence of wound infection.[84] Furthermore, hypovolemic shock or local administration of epinephrine has been shown to increase the virulence of a dermal staphylococcal infection.[85] Studies from our laboratory indicate wound exudate cell hyporesponsiveness to release proinflammatory cytokine (i.e., IL-1β and IL-6) following trauma and hemorrhagic shock for up to 3 days.[91] Furthermore, depressed phagocytic activity of wound exudate cells has been demonstrated under those conditions.[91] The restored wound exudate cell cytokine release on the fifth postoperative day in those studies were associated with an unaltered rate of wound infection in the studies by Livingston and Malagoni.[84] Thus our findings suggest that hyporesponsiveness of wound exudate cells following severe blood loss and trauma contributes to increased susceptibility to wound infection. Therefore attempts to restore immune cell function at the wound site might help decrease the incidence of wound infections in trauma victims and patients following major surgery.

Gender-Specific Immune Responses Following Trauma-Hemorrhage

Despite the fact that gender differences in the susceptibility to and morbidity from sepsis have been observed in several clinical and epidemiologic studies,[4,92-94] little attention has been paid to the influence of gender on immune responses in surgical and trauma patients. Experimental studies investigating alterations in immune functions following trauma have largely used male laboratory animals. Studies initiated by Zellweger et al.[95] however, examined immune functions in female rodents following the induction of sepsis by cecal ligation and puncture (CLP). The results demonstrated maintenance of splenocyte function in females when they were in the proestrous stage of the estrous cycle in contrast to depression of splenocyte function in males following CLP.[95] Furthermore, the preservation of

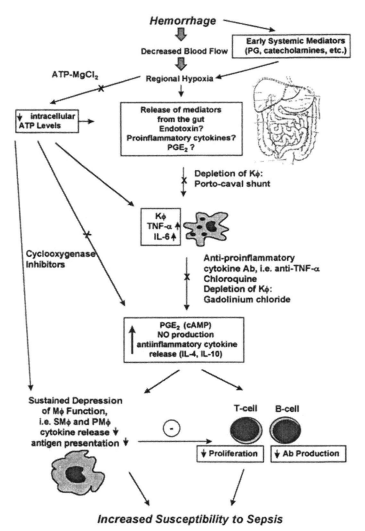

FIGURE 15.2. Hypothesis of the cascade of events following hemorrhagic shock that led to the development of depressed macrophage function (e.g., decreased cytokine release, antigen-presenting capacity), suppression of cell-mediated immunity, and increased susceptibility to sepsis. **X** cascade inhibitors; PG, prostaglandin; Kφ, Kupffer cells; SMφ, splenic macrophages; PMφ, peritoneal macrophages.

immune responses in females was associated with higher survival rates following the induction of sepsis.[95] In light of these findings, further studies were conducted investigating the effect of gender on cell-mediated immunity following trauma and hemorrhage. In particular, females in the proestrous state of the estrous cycle showed enhanced IL-1 and IL-6 release by splenic and peritoneal macrophages and splenocyte IL-2 and IL-3 release, in contrast to depressed macrophage and splenocyte functions in males under such conditions.[96] Higher plasma estradiol, higher plasma prolactin levels, or both in proestrous females might contribute to the enhanced immune responses following hemorrhage in proestrous females.

Administration of estrogen to castrated male mice supplemented with testosterone improved the depressed immune responses in those animals.[97] Similarly, administration of prolactin to male mice following trauma-hemorrhage prevented the depression of immune responses.[98] These findings suggest immunoprotective properties of female sex hormones following trauma-hemorrhage. The lower levels of male sex steroids in female animals compared to those in males might also contribute to the divergent immunoresponsiveness following hemorrhage. Support for the importance of male sex hormones in producing the immune depression in males following hemorrhage comes from studies indicating that castration of male mice 2 weeks prior to hemorrhage prevented the depression of splenic and peritoneal macrophages following the hemorrhagic insult.[13,98] Moreover, depletion of testosterone by castration prior to hemorrhage normalized the IL-6 release by Kupffer cells following hemorrhage.[13,98]

In an attempt to address the issue whether testosterone per se is responsible for the depressed macrophage functions following hemorrhage in males, studies were conducted in which castrated male mice were treated with 5α-dihydrotestosterone prior to trauma-hemorrhage.[97] The results demonstrate that castrated male mice treated with testosterone had elevated plasma testosterone levels (i.e., comparable to that of intact males) and displayed immune responses to hemorrhage similar to those of the normal males (i.e., depression of splenic and peritoneal macrophage function).[97] Similarly, treatment of female mice with 5α-dihydrotestosterone also depressed splenic and peritoneal macrophage function as well as splenocyte responses.[37,99] In addition, gender-specific immune responses have been demonstrated in the thymus, the primary location of T cell lymphopoiesis.[100] The exact mechanism, however, for the immunomodulatory properties of male and female sex steroids following trauma-hemorrhage remains unknown.

Similar observations have been obtained in clinical trials following sepsis. In a retrospective study that incorporated four major sepsis studies, Bone[4] demonstrated a preponderance of morbidity and mortality in males compared to that in females. McGowan et al. also reported a significantly higher incidence of bacteremic infections in males than in females.[93] A prospective study by Schröder et al. confirmed gender differences in human sepsis, with a significantly better prognosis for women.[94] The hospital mortality rate in this study was 70% for male patients and 26% for female patients following the induction of sepsis.[94]

In summary, these studies suggest that gender and the state of the estrous cycle in female subjects should be taken into consideration when designing experimental and clinical studies of the immune response following trauma and shock. Moreover, the results of these studies suggest that administration of sex steroids of treatment with their specific blockers may be a useful approach for modulating the immune responses in those patients.

Conclusions

Studies indicate that injury, trauma, and blood loss produce marked suppression of cell-mediated immunity and increased susceptibility to subsequent sepsis and wound infection. Furthermore, global and differential effects can be observed on macrophages that are dependent on their anatomic location. Nonetheless, the use of a variety of immunomodulatory agents (e.g., dilitiazem, chloroquine, ibuprofen, IFNγ, prolactin, metoclopramide, flutamide) have been shown to help normalize altered immune responses following trauma and hemorrhage.

The use of immunomodulatory agents following hemorrhage in rodent models appears to be promising for the development of new therapeutic concepts for the treatment of immunosuppression and for decreasing the mortality due to subsequent sepsis in humans. However, careful evaluation of both the benefits and potential adverse effects of therapy is needed before widespread clinical use can be envisioned.

The immunoinflammatory response and subsequent sepsis still comprise a major cause of morbidity and mortality following trauma and major surgery. Although significant advances have been made, it is important to define further the pathophysiology and to identify the precise mechanisms responsible for the depression of cell-mediated immunity using experimental animal models. These animal models should take into consideration the various manipulations the patient undergoes as well as such factors as the effect of gender, nutritional status, and preexisting conditions, among others. Only when models of injury begin to consider these factors can effective treatment regimens for patients be developed.

References

1. Shires GT: Principles and management of hemorrhagic shock. In: Shires GT (ed) Principles of Trauma Care 3rd ed. New York, McGraw-Hill, 1985;3–42.
2. Trunkey DD: Trauma. Sci Am 1983;249:28–35.
3. Akiyoshi T, Koba S, Arinaga S, Miyazaki S, Wada T, Tsuji H: Impaired production of interleukin-2 after surgery. Clin Exp Immunol 1985;59:45–49.
4. Bone RC: Toward an epidemiology and natural history of SIRS (systemic inflammatory response syndrome). JAMA 1992;268: 3452–3455.
5. Baue AE: Multiple organ failure. In: Baue AE (ed) Multiple Organ Failure: Patient Care and Prevention. St. Louis, Mosby-Year Book, 1990;421–470.

6. Deitch EA: Multiple Organ Failure: Pathophysiology and Basic Concepts of Therapy. New York, Thieme, 1990;1–299.
7. Goris RJA: Sepsis and multiple organ failure: the result of whole body inflammation. In: Faist E, Meakins J, Schildberg FW (eds) Host Defense Dysfunction in Trauma, Shock and Sepsis. Heidelberg, Springer, 1993;161–170.
8. Chaudry IH, Ayala A: Immunological Aspects of Hemorrhage. Austin, TX: Medical Intelligence Unit, R.G. Landes, 1992;1–132.
9. Stephan RN, Ayala A, Chaudry IH: Monocyte and lymphocyte responses following trauma. In: Schlag G, Redl H (eds) Pathophysiology of Shock, Sepsis and Organ Failure. Berlin: Springer, 1993;131–144.
10. Roumen RM, Hendriks T, van der Ven-Jongekrijg J, et al: Cytokine patterns in patients after major surgery, hemorrhagic shock, and severe blunt trauma. Ann Surg 1993;6:769–776.
11. Faist E, Baue AE, Dittmer H: Multiple organ failure in polytrauma patients. J Trauma 1983;23:775–787.
12. Ayala A, Lehman DL, Herdon CD, Chaudry IH: Mechanism of enhanced susceptibility to sepsis following hemorrhage: interleukin (IL)-10 suppression of T cell response is mediated by eicosanoid induced IL-4 release. Arch Surg 1994;129:1172–1178.
13. Wichmann MW, Ayala A, Chaudry I: Male sex steroids are responsible for depressing macrophage immune function after trauma-hemorrhage. Am J Physiol 1997;273:C1335–C1340.
14. Nwariaku FE, McIntyre KL, Sikes PJ, Mileski WJ: Alterations in alveolar macrophage tumor necrosis factor (TNF) response following trauma-hemorrhagic shock. Shock 1995;4:200–203.
15. Xu YX, Ayala A, Chaudry IH: Prolonged immunodepression following trauma and hemorrhagic shock. J Trauma 1998;44:335–341.
16. Zellweger R, Ayala A, DeMaso CM, Chaudry IH: Trauma-hemorrhage causes prolonged depression in cellular immunity. Shock 1995;4:149–153.
17. Wichmann MW, Zellweger R, Williams C, Ayala A, DeMaso CM, Chaudry IH: Immune function is more compromised following closed bone fracture and hemorrhagic shock than hemorrhage alone. Arch Surg 1996;131:995–1000.
18. Ayala A, Perrin MM, Ertel W, Chaudry IH: Differential effects of hemorrhage on Kupffer cells: decreased antigen presentation despite increased inflammatory cytokine (IL-1, IL-6 and TNF) release. Cytokine 1992;4:66–75.
19. Ayala A, Perrin MM, Wang P, Ertel W, Chaudry IH: Hemorrhage induces enhanced Kupffer cell cytotoxicity while decreasing peritoneal or splenic macrophage capacity: involvement of cell-associated TNF and reactive nitrogen. J Immunol 1991;147:4147–4154.
20. Pellegrini JD, Puyana JC, Lapchak PH, Kodys K, Miller-Graziano CL: A membrane TNF-alpha/TNFR ratio correlates to MODS score and mortality. Shock 1996;6:389–396.
21. Ayala A, Ertel W, Chaudry IH: Trauma-induced suppression of antigen presentation and expression of major histocompatibility class II antigen complex in leukocytes. Shock 1996;5:79–90.
22. Ertel W, Singh G, Morrison MH, Ayala A, Chaudry IH: Chemically induced hypotension increases PGE_2 release and depresses macrophage antigen presentation. Am J Physiol 1993;264:R655–R660.
23. Haupt W, Riese J, Mehler C, Weber K, Zowe M, Hohenberger W: Monocyte function before and after surgical trauma. Dig Surg 1998;15:102–104.
24. Faist E, Storck M, Hultner L, et al: Functional analysis of monocytes activity through synthesis patterns of proinflammatory cytokines and neopterin in patients in surgical intensive care. Surgery 1992;112:562–572.
25. MacLean LD, Meakins JL, Taguchi K, Duignan J, Dhillon KS, Gordon J: Host resistance in sepsis and trauma. Ann Surg 1975;182:207–211.
26. Christou NV, Tellado JM: The impact of preexisting disease conditions for host defense integrity in traumatized and critically ill patients. In: Faist E, Meakins J, Schildberg FW (eds) Host Defense Dysfunction in Trauma, Shock and Sepsis. Heidelberg, Springer 1993;73–82.
27. Levy EM, Alharbi SA, Grindlinger G, Black PH: Changes in mitogen responsiveness lymphocyte subsets after traumatic injury: relation to development of sepsis. Clin Immunol Immunopathol 1984; 32:224–233.
28. Keane RM, Birmingham W, Shatney CM, Winchurch RA, Munster AM: Prediction of sepsis in the multitraumatic patient by assays of lymphocyte responsiveness. Surg Gynecol Obstet 1983;156:163–167.
29. Munster AM: Immunologic response of trauma and burns: an overview. Am J Med 1984;76:142–145.
30. Antonacci AC, Calvano SE, Reaves LE, et al: Autologous and allogenic mixed-lymphocyte responses following thermal injury in man: the immunomodulatory effects of interleukin-1, interleukin-2 and a prostaglandin inhibitor, WY-18251. Clin Immunol Immunopathol 1984;30:304–320.
31. Faist E, Markewitz A, Storkc M, Ertel W, Schildberg FW: Der Einfluss der ausgedehnten operativen Intervention auf die zellvermittelte Immunantwort. Internist 1992;33:370–378.
32. Stephan RN, Kupper TS, Geha AS, Baue AS, Chaudry IH: Hemorrhage without tissue trauma produces immunosuppression and enhances susceptibility to sepsis. Arch Surg 1987;122:62–68.
33. Riddle PR, Berenbaum MC: Postoperative depression of the lymphocyte response to phytohaemagglutinin. Lancet 1967;1:746–748.
34. O'Mahony JB, Palder SB, Wood JJ, et al: Depression of cellular immunity after multiple trauma in the absence of sepsis. J Trauma 1984;24:869–875.
35. Daniels JC, Sakai H, Cobb EK, Lewis SR, Larson DL, Ritzmann SE: Evaluation of lymphocyte reactivity studies in patients with thermal burns. J Trauma 1971;11:595–607.
36. Sakai H, Daniels JC, Lewis SR, Lynch JB, Watson DL, Ritzmann SE: Reversible alterations of nucleic acid synthesis in lymphocytes after thermal burns. J Reticuloendothel Soc 1972;11:19–28.
37. Angele MK, Ayala A, Cioffi WG, Bland KI, Chaudry IH: Testosterone: the culprit for producing splenocyte depression following trauma-hemorrhage. Am J Physiol 1998;274:C1530–C1536.
38. Faist E, Mewes A, Baker CC, et al: Prostaglandin E_2 dependent suppression of interleukin-2 production in patients with major trauma. J Trauma 1987;27:837–848.
39. Wood JJ, Rodrick ML, O'Mahony JB, et al: Inadequate interleukin-2 production: a fundamental immunological deficiency in patients with major burns. Ann Surg 1984;200:311.
40. Abraham E, Chang Y-H: The effects of hemorrhage on mitogen-induced lymphocyte proliferation. Circ Shock 1985;15:141–149.
41. Faist E, Mewes A, et al: Alteration of monocyte function following major injury. Arch Surg 1988;123:287–292.

42. Livingston DH, Appel SH, Wellhausen SR, et al: Depressed interferon gamma production and monocyte HLA-DR expression after severe injury. Arch Surg 1988;123:1309–1312.
43. Ertel W, Faist E, Salmen B, Huber P, Heberer G: Influence of cyclooxygenase inhibition on interleukin-2 receptor (IL-2R) expression after major trauma. Surg Res Commun 1989;5:17–23.
44. O'Sullivan ST, Lederer JA, et al: Major injury leads to predominance of the T helper-2 lymphocyte phenotype and diminished interleukin-12 production associated with decreased resistance to infection. Ann Surg 1995;222:482–490, discussion 490–492.
45. Hseih CS, Macatonia SE, et al: Development of TH1 $CD4^+$ T cells through IL-12 produced by Listeria-induced macrophages. Science 1993;260:547–549.
46. Abraham E, Freitas AA: Hemorrhage in mice induces alterations in immunoglobulin-secreting B-cells. Crit Care Med 1989;17:1015–1019.
47. Abraham E, Freitas AA: Hemorrhage produces abnormalities in lymphocyte function and lymphokine generation. J Immunol 1989;142:899–906.
48. Fuchs D, Gruber A, Wachter H, Faist E: Activated cell-mediated immunity and immunodeficiency in trauma and sepsis. In: Faist E, Baue AE, Schildberg FW (eds) The Immune Consequences of Trauma, Shock and Sepsis: Mechanisms and Therapeutic Approaches. Lengerich, Pabst Science Publishers, 1996;235–239.
49. Fuchs D, Malkovsky M, Reibnegger G, Werner ER, Forni G, Wachter H: Endogenous release of interferon-gamma and diminished response of peripheral blood mononuclear cells to antigenic stimulation. Immunol Lett 1989;23:103–108.
50. Ayala A, Perrin MM, Meldrum DR, Ertel W, Chaudry IH: Hemorrhage induces an increase in serum TNF which is not associated with elevated levels of endotoxin. Cytokine 1990;2:170–174.
51. Ayala A, Wang P, Ba ZF, Perrin MM, Ertel W, Chaudry IH: Differential alterations in plasma IL-6 and TNF levels following trauma and hemorrhage. Am J Physiol 1991;260:R167–R171.
52. Damas P, Reuter A, Gysen P, Demonty J, Lamy M, Franchimont P: Tumor necrosis factor and interleukin-1 serum levels during severe sepsis in humans. Crit Care Med 1989;17:975–978.
53. Damas P, Ledoux D, Nys M, et al: Cytokine serum level during severe sepsis in human IL-6 as a marker of severity. Ann Surg 1992;215:356–362.
54. Romagnani S: Th1 and Th2 in human diseases. Clin Immunol Immunopathol 1996;80:225–235.
55. Martin C, Boisson C, Haccoun M, Thomachot L, Mege JL: Patterns of cytokine evolution (tumor necrosis factor-α and interleukin-6) after septic shock, hemorrhagic shock, and severe trauma. Crit Care Med 1997;25:1813–1819.
56. Ertel W, Morrison MH, Ayala A, Perrin MM, Chaudry IH: Anti-TNF monoclonal antibodies prevent haemorrhage-induced suppression of Kupffer cell antigen presentation and MHC class II antigen expression. Immunology 1991;74:290–297.
57. Porteu F, Nathan C: Shedding of tumor necrosis factor receptors by activated human neutrophils. J Exp Med 1990;172:599–607.
58. Ertel W, Morrison MH, Ayala A, Chaudry IH: Chloroquine attenuates hemorrhagic shock induced suppression of Kupffer cell antigen presentation and MHC class II antigen expression through blockade of tumor necrosis factor and prostaglandin release. Blood 1991;78:1781–1788.
59. Wong GC, Clark SC: Multiple actions of interleukin 6 within a cytokine network. Immunol Today 1988;9:137–139.
60. Okusawa S, Gelfand JA, Ikejima T, Connolly RJ, Dinarello CA: Interleukin-1 induces a shock like state in rabbits: synergism with tumor necrosis factor and the effects of cyclooxygenase inhibition. J Clin Invest 1988;81:1162–1172.
61. Tracey KJ, Lowry SF, Fahey TJI, et al: Cachectin/tumor necrosis factor induces lethal shock and stress hormone responses in the dog. Surg Gynecol Obstet 1987;164:415–422.
62. Lejeune P, Lagadec P, Onier N, Pinnard D, Ohshima Jeannin JF: Nitric oxide involvement in tumor-induced immunosuppression. J Immunol 1994;152:5077–5083.
63. O'Neill PJ, Ayala A, Wang P, et al: Role of Kupffer cells in interleukin-6 release following trauma: hemorrhage and resuscitation. Shock 1994;1:43–47.
64. Ayala A, Meldrum DR, Perrin MM, Chaudry IH: The release of transforming growth factor-β following hemorrhage: its role as a mediator of host immunosuppression [abstract]. FASEB J 1992;6:A1604.
65. Miller-Graziano CL, Szabo G, Griffey K, Metha B, Kodys K, Catalano D: Role of elevated monocyte transforming growth factor beta (TGF-beta) production in posttrauma immunosuppression. J Clin Immunol 1991;11:95–102.
66. Waal Malefyt R, Abrams J, Bennett B, Figdor CG, Vries JE: Interleukin 10 (IL-10) inhibits cytokine synthesis by human monocytes: an autoregulatory role of IL-10 produced by monocytes. J Exp Med 1991;174:1209–1220.
67. Knapp W, Baumgartner G: Monocyte-mediated suppression of human B-lymphocyte differentiation in vitro. J Immunol 1978;121:1177–1183.
68. Johnston PA, Selkurt EE: Effect of hemorrhagic shock on renal release of prostaglandin E. Am J Physiol 1976;230:831–838.
69. Bonta IL, Parnham MJ: Immunomodulatory-antiinflammatory functions of E-type prostaglandins: minireview with emphasis on macrophage mediated effects. Int J Immunopharmacol 1982;4:103–109.
70. Plaut M: The role of cyclic AMP in modulating cytotoxic T lymphocytes. I. In vivo-generated cytotoxic lymphocytes, but not in vitro-generated cytotoxic lymphocytes, are inhibited by cyclic AMP-active agents. J Immunol 1979;123:692–701.
71. Chaudry IH, Ayala A: Immune consequences of hypovolemic shock and resuscitation. Curr Opin Anaesthesiol 1993;6:385–392.
72. Ayala A, Chaudry IH: Dietary n-3 polyunsaturated fatty acid modulation of immune cell function pre- or post-trauma. Nutrition 1995;11:1–11.
73. Beutler B: Tumor necrosis factor and other cytokines in septic syndrome. In: Vincent JL (ed) Sepsis. Berlin, Springer, 1994;107–121.
74. Shirakawa T, Tokunaga A, Onda M: Release of immunosuppressive substances after gastric resection is more prolonged than after mastectomy in humans [in process citation]. Int Surg 1998;83:210–214.
75. Feldbush TL, Hobbs MV, Severson CD, Ballas ZF, Weiler JM: Role of complement in the immune response. Fed Proc 1984;43:2548–2552.
76. Marks JD, Marks CB, Luce JM, et al: Plasma tumor necrosis factor in patients with septic shock. Am Rev Respir Dis 1990;141:94–97.
77. Marano MA, Fong Y, Moldawer LL, et al: Serum cachectin/tumor necrosis factor in critically ill patients with burns correlates with infection and mortality. Surg Gynecol Obstet 1990;170:32–38.

78. Waage A, Halstensen A, Espevik T: Association between tumor necrosis factor in serum and fatal outcome in patients with meningococcal disease. Lancet 1987;1:355–357.
79. Waage A, Brandtzaeg P, Halstensen A, Kierulf P, Espevik T: The complex pattern of cytokines in serum from patients with meningococcal septic shock: association between interleukin 6, interleukin 1, and fatal outcome. J Exp Med 1989;169:333–338.
80. Molloy RG, Mannick JA, Rodrick ML: Cytokines, sepsis and immunomodulation. Br J Surg 1993;80:289–297.
81. Angele MK, Wichmann MW, Ayala A, Cioffi WG, Chaudry IH: Testosterone receptor blockade after hemorrhage in males: restoration of the depressed immune functions and improved survival following subsequent sepsis. Arch Surg 1997;132:1207–1214.
82. Zapata-Sirvent RL, Hansbrough JF, Cox MC, Carter WH: Immunologic alterations in a murine model of hemorrhagic shock. Crit Care Med 1992;20:508–517.
83. Simons RK, Hoyt DB, Winchell RJ, Rose RM, Holbrook T: Elevated selectin levels after severe trauma: a marker for sepsis and organ failure and a potential target for immunomodulatory therapy. J Trauma 1996;41:653–662.
84. Livingston DH, Malangoni MA: An experimental study of susceptibility to infection after hemorrhagic shock. Surg Gynecol Obstet 1989;168:138–142.
85. Miles AA: Nonspecific defense reactions in bacterial infections. Ann NY Acad Sci 1956;66:356–369.
86. O'Keefe GE, Maier RV, Diehr P, Grossman D, Jurkovich GJ, Conrad D: The complications of trauma and their associated costs in a level I trauma center. Arch Surg 1997;132:920–924.
87. Nichols RL: Surgical wound infection. Am J Med 1991;91:54S–64S.
88. Weigelt JA, Haley RW, Seibert B: Factors which influence the risk of wound infection in trauma patients. J Trauma 1987;27:774–781.
89. Polk HC Jr: Factors influencing the risk of infection after trauma. Am J Surg 1993;165:2s–7s.
90. McGinn FP: Effects of hemorrhage upon surgical operations. Br J Surg 1976;63:742–746.
91. Angele MK, Knoferl MW, Schwacha MG, et al: Hemorrhage decreases macrophage inflammatory protein-2 (MIP-2) and IL-6 release: a potential mechanism for increased wound infection. Ann Surg 1999 (in press).
92. Centers for Disease Control: Mortality Patterns — United States, 1989. MMWR1 992;41:121–125.
93. McGowan JE, Barnes MW, Finland N: Bacteremia at Boston City Hospital: occurrence and mortality during 12 selected years (1935–1972) with special reference to hospital-acquired cases. J Infect Dis 1975;132:316–335.
94. Schröder J, Kahlke V, Staubach KH, Zabel P, Stuber F: Gender differences in human sepsis. Arch Surg 1998;133:1200–1205.
95. Zellweger R, Ayala A, Stein S, DeMaso CM, Chaudry IH: Females in proestrous state tolerate sepsis better than males. Crit Care Med 1997;25:106–110.
96. Wichmann MW, Zellweger R, DeMaso CM, Ayala A, Chaudry IH: Enhanced immune responses in females as opposed to decreased responses in males following hemorrhagic shock. Cytokine 1996;8:853–863.
97. Angele MK, Knoferl MW, Ayala A, Cioffi WG, Bland K, Chaudry IH: Male and female sex steroids: do they produce deleterious or beneficial effects on immune responses following trauma-hemorrhage? Surg Forum 1998 (in press).
98. Zellweger R, Zhu X-H, Wichmann MW, Ayala A, DeMaso CM, Chaudry IH: Prolactin administration following hemorrhagic shock improves macrophage cytokine release capacity and decreases mortality from subsequent sepsis. J Immunol 1996;157:5748–5754.
99. Angele MK, Ayala A, Monfils BA, Cioffi WG, Bland KI, Chaudry IH: Testosterone and/or low estradiol: normally required but harmful immunologically for males after trauma-hemorrhage. J Trauma 1998;44:78–85.
100. Angele MK, Xu YX, Ayala A, et al: Gender differences in immune responses: increased thymocyte apoptosis occurs only in males but not in females after trauma-hemorrhage. Surg Forum 1997;48:95–97.

Part III
Mediators and Effectors

16
Emerging Evidence of a More Complex Role for Proinflammatory and Antiinflammatory Cytokines in the Sepsis Response

Lyle L. Moldawer, Rebecca M. Minter, and John E. Rectenwald III

Since the original discovery and cloning of tumor necrosis factor-α (TNFα) and interleukin-1 (IL-1), our understanding of the underlying role that these and other cytokines play in the sepsis response has greatly evolved. The original concept that the sepsis response is a result of a linear cytokine cascade induced by TNFα and IL-1 has given way to the appreciation that sepsis syndromes often result from a more complex interplay between proinflammatory cytokines, antiinflammatory cytokines, and cytokine antagonists. The proinflammatory cytokine-dominated, systemic inflammatory response syndrome is likely an episodic or transient occurrence; and many septic patients present with a compensatory antiinflammatory cytokine response dominated by the release of antiinflammatory cytokines and cytokine antagonists, leading to immune suppression. There is also growing appreciation that other members of the TNFα superfamily, including Fas ligand (FasL) and glucocorticoids, play an increasingly important role in the loss of immune cells during sepsis through apoptotic processes. The cytokine component of the innate immune response to sepsis plays a complex role not only in the inflammatory response syndrome but also in determining the nature and magnitude of the acquired immune response.

Host Cytokine Response to Sepsis

Tumor necrosis factor-α and IL-1 were initially purified and cloned in 1984–1985.[1–5] Within 5 years convincing animal evidence had demonstrated that an exaggerated TNFα and IL-1 response were the prime cause of mortality in bacteremic and endotoxemic shock.[6–8] Since 1993 there have been more than 15 phase II and phase III clinical trials of TNFα and IL-1 inhibitors in patients with sepsis syndromes. The disappointing results of these clinical trials have been the topic of several outstanding reviews[9–12] and are well beyond the scope of this summary.

There is now growing appreciation that the cytokine response to sepsis is not simply a linear cascade initiated by the exaggerated release of proinflammatory cytokines such as TNFα and IL-1. Early studies in primates suggested that in response to gram-negative bacteria or endotoxin there was an immediate systemic TNFα and IL-1 response that initiated the synthesis and release of more distal proinflammatory cytokines, antiinflammatory cytokines, and cytokine inhibitors. Administration of recombinant TNFα to a healthy organism recapitulated the physiologic[13,14] and cytokine responses to endotoxemic or bacteremic shock,[13,15–18] including the release of IL-1, IL-6, IL-8, IL-10, p55, p75, and IL-1 receptor antagonist (IL-1ra). In primate models where gram-negative bacteria or their products were intravenously administered, blocking the endogenous TNFα response suppressed the release of other, more distal proinflammatory cytokines (e.g., IL-1 and IL-8[19,20]), antiinflammatory cytokines (e.g., IL-6 and IL-10), and cytokine antagonists (e.g., IL-1ra and p55).[16,21,22] Although several rodent studies, using cecal ligation and puncture (CLP) to create sepsis, were unable to confirm that blocking TNFα had a positive effect on either outcome or cytokine production,[23–25] clinical trials were initiated in patients with sepsis syndrome.

During the course of those clinical trials, it became evident that a large proportion of critically ill patients with sepsis syndromes do not sustain an exaggerated proinflammatory response but, rather, exhibit what the late Roger Bone called a compensatory antiinflammatory response syndrome and immunosuppression.[26] Plasma cytokine profiles from patients with sepsis or systemic inflammatory response syndromes suggest that fewer than 10% of patients with sepsis syndrome have elevated levels of proinflammatory cytokines (e.g., TNFα, IL-1β, IL-8) at any given time (Table 16.1). As early as 1992 we reported that few patients meeting the clinical criteria of sepsis syndrome had detectable TNFα bioactivity in their serum;[27] rather, most of these patients had net TNF-inhibitory activity in their plasma. In a retrospective analysis of 83 patients from the IL-1ra phase III clinical trial,[28] fewer than 5% of these patients had detectable TNFα or IL-1β in their circulation.[29] Furthermore, blockade of TNFα in patients with sepsis syndrome does not appear to have a significant impact on the concentrations of other proinflammatory or antiinflammatory cytokines,[30] suggesting that in human sepsis TNFα may not be the early, proximal mediator seen in primate models of endotoxin or bacteremic shock.

TABLE 16.1. Plasma Proinflammatory, Antiinflammatory, and Cytokine Antagonists in Patients with Sepsis Syndromes.

Proinflammatory cytokines
  TNFα
  IL-1α, IL-1β
  IL-8
  IL-12 heterodimer
  IL-18
  IFNγ
  IL-6

Antiinflammatory cytokines
  IL-6
  IL-10
  LIF

Cytokine antagonists
  IL-1ra
  p68 (sIL-1RII)
  p55 (sTNFR I)
  p75 (sTNFR II)

TABLE 16.2. Known Antiinflammatory and Immunosuppressive Properties of Interleukin-10.

Antiinflammatory properties
  Suppresses TNFα, IL-1, IL-8, IL-12, GM-CSF, MIP-1, and IFNγ expression
  Increases IL-1ra release, shedding of p55 and p75 receptors
  Inhibits antigen presentation by macrophages and dendritic cells
  Suppresses effector functions of macrophages, T and NK cells
  Blocks phosphorylation of IκB

Immunosuppressive properties
  Suppresses T cell proliferation to mitogen such as concanavalin A
  Suppresses Th1 cell development, reducing cell-mediated immune responses
  Promotes Th2 cell development and antibody formation
  Downregulates IFNγ induced and constitutive expression of MHC class II
  May stimulate lymphocyte apoptosis

In vivo responses
  Exogenous administration prevents endotoxin-induced shock and lethality
  Endogenous production reduces inflammatory response and improves outcome to cecal ligation and puncture and pancreatitis
  Endogenous production after cecal ligation and puncture increases lymphocyte apoptosis and decreases innate immune responses in the lung to Streptococcus and Pseudomonas
  Endogenous production after a burn injury responsible for T cell anergy
  Tolerance to endotoxin is IL-10-dependent

In a large proportion of patients, the clinical manifestations of the sepsis syndrome may not represent a systemic proinflammatory cytokine response but, rather, a refractory antiinflammatory response that leads to anergy and immunosuppression. Indeed, Bone[26,31] argued convincingly that a significant proportion of patients with the sepsis syndrome may be manifesting an unbalanced, compensatory antiinflammatory response that represents the opposite end of the biologic continuum from the proinflammatory response. Indeed, elevated levels of the antiinflammatory cytokine IL-10 have been reported in a large proportion of patients initially with septic shock,[32] and these elevated levels appear to correlate with adverse outcome.[33–35] The apparent immunosuppression seen in some patients with sepsis syndrome has led to the proposition of restoring macrophage deactivation by exogenous administration of interferon-γ (IFNγ).[36,37]

In addition, there is clear evidence that plasma concentrations of cytokine antagonists are elevated in patients with sepsis syndrome; and unlike TNFα and IL-1β, their concentrations remain elevated for sustained periods. In response to an endotoxin or gram-negative bacteremic challenge, TNFα and IL-1β concentrations peak within 1–3 hours and disappear within 4–8 hours,[8,38] whereas IL-1ra, p55, and p75 concentrations remain elevated for up to 24 hours.[39–41]

Interleukin-10

Interleukin-10 has attracted a great deal of attention lately, but its role in the sepsis response remains unclear and complex. Of all the principal antiinflammatory cytokines, IL-10 appears most frequently in the circulation; and modulation of its activity has been shown to have both positive and adverse effects on outcome. IL-10 is produced by macrophages and T cells in response to a variety of stimuli, including endotoxin.[42] The plasma appearance of IL-10 in response to endotoxin stimulation is delayed relative to the proinflammatory cytokines IL-1 and TNFα;[16] IL-10 mRNA transcripts appear 8 hours after endotoxin challenge and peak at 24 hours.[43] In addition, both TNFα[16] and IL-1[44] induce expression of IL-10; and IL-10 has been shown to downregulate its own expression from endotoxin-activated monocytes in an autocrine fashion.[43] IL-10 exhibits direct antiinflammatory and immunosuppressive properties against a variety of cell types including macrophages, endothelial cells, and tissue fibroblasts[42] (Table 16.2). Specifically, IL-10 has been shown to inhibit TNFα, IL-1α, IL-1β, IL-6, IL-8, and macrophage inflammatory protein-1 (MIP-1) expression by endotoxin-stimulated monocytes and neutrophils.[36,37,45,46] In addition, IL-10 promotes shedding of the TNF receptors (p55 and p75) and expression of IL-1ra.[36] In vivo, both Howard et al.[48] and Gerard et al.[49] reported that pretreating mice with IL-10 attenuated the plasma TNFα response and lethality associated with endotoxemic shock. Additionally, intravenously administered IL-10 was shown to block ex vivo endotoxin induction of IL-1 and TNFα in a dose-dependent fashion in normal volunteers, with the effects lasting up to 48 hours.[50,51] These data, in toto, suggest that IL-10 is a natural component of the inflammatory response and serves to shorten its duration and reduce its magnitude. This conclusion is supported by the observation that IL-10 knockout mice and normal mice treated with anti-IL-10 antibodies manifest an exaggerated inflammatory response in response to endotoxin or peritonitis.[52,53]

Experimental studies from our laboratory in the murine visceral ischemia and reperfusion model have examined the potential therapeutic role of IL-10.[54] Pretreatment with human recombinant IL-10 (0.2–20.0 μg) prior to visceral ischemia resulted in a dose-dependent reduction in the resultant lung injury as measured by neutrophil infiltration. Notably, lung injury was reduced with the lower dosages (10–250 μg/kg body weight), but IL-10 was ineffective at the higher dosages

(1–10 mg/kg). Furthermore, no TNFα was detected in the plasma during reperfusion after pretreatment with the lower IL-10 dosages. Similar findings have been reported from our laboratory after pretreatment with IL-10 prior to skeletal muscle ischemia and reperfusion injury in a rat model.[55]

The antiinflammatory properties of IL-10 cannot be distinguished from its immunosuppressive properties, and there is accumulating evidence to suggest that the immune suppression seen after sepsis or thermal injuries is frequently associated with reduced T cell mitogenic responses and increased lymphocyte apoptosis. Kelly et al.[56] demonstrated that systemic release of IL-10 can explain the observed T cell anergy after thermal injury in an experimental model of burn injury. Additionally, Song and colleagues demonstrated that the splenic T cell proliferative responses to concanavalin A were reduced after CLP, due to an endogenous IL-10 response.[57] Similarly, Steinhauser and colleagues demonstrated that after CLP intratracheal instillation of *Pseudomonas* produced an IL-10-dependent increase in mortality.[58] These authors concluded that the septic response substantially impairs the lung's innate immunity to *Pseudomonas*, and this effect is mediated primarily by endogenously produced IL-10. Furthermore, Van der Poll et al.[59] demonstrated that exogenous IL-10 increased the susceptibility to *Streptococcus pneumoniae*-induced acute respiratory distress syndrome (ARDS) in a murine model.

Therapeutic use of IL-10 as an antiinflammatory agent in patients with sepsis and the systemic inflammatory response syndrome (SIRS) remains a highly controversial topic. IL-10 has been or currently is in clinical trials in patients with rheumatoid arthritis, inflammatory bowel disease, human immunodeficiency virus (HIV) infection, hepatitis C infections, and other chronic inflammatory diseases[60,61] (Table 16.3). The safety profile has been good; and despite chronic administration for periods of several months, an increased frequency or severity of infections has not been reported. The primary complications associated with its administration have been minimal and include injection site inflammation, lethargy and headache. There are at present two clinical trials with IL-10 in patients with ARDS and following intestinal ischemia/reperfusion injury after thoracoabdominal aortic injury repair, which will be reported in the near future. The goal of these studies is to determine whether IL-10-mediated suppression of the inflammatory response to ARDS or ischemia/reperfusion injury results in reduced severity and frequency of multisystem organ failure. These studies should go a long way to answering the question of whether the antiinflammatory properties of IL-10 are outweighed by its immunosuppressive properties and if IL-10 has a clinical role as a therapeutic agent in sepsis syndrome.

TNFα and Members of Its Superfamily

TNFα is only one member of an increasingly large superfamily of proteins with structural and functional homology. As shown in Table 16.4, there are multiple members of this family, many of which have functions that are still unknown. Known members of the TNF family [including TNFα, FasL, and apolipoprotein I (Apo I) ligand], and TNF-related apoptosis-inducing ligand (TRAIL, or Apo II ligand) play at least two critical roles in intercellular communication and tissue homeostasis. These proteins signal the presence of inflammation through NFκB-dependent processes and initiate removal of unnecessary or potentially dangerous cells by apoptosis.[62] The proinflammatory properties of TNFα are well known, but it is only during the past few years that the proapoptotic properties of TNFα have been studied, especially in regard to sepsis and SIRS. At present it is unclear why so many distinct members of this cytokine family exist; and the relative contributions played by each in specific inflammatory processes, such as endotoxemic shock and bacterial peritonitis, is uncertain.

The most well known member of the TNF family is TNFα, in part because it is the only member of the TNF family that is readily secreted in a biologically active form. Although 17-kDa TNFα is presumed to play a central role in the vascular changes associated with bacteremic/endotoxemic shock, there is increasing evidence that membrane-associated TNFα also plays a

TABLE 16.3. Diseases for Which IL-10 Therapies Have Been Used and Their Outcome.

Disease	Outcome
Rheumatoid arthritis	Positive results in phase II clinical trials; studies continuing
Inflammatory bowel disease	Positive results in phase II clinical trials; studies continuing
Hepatitis C	Combination therapy with interferon ongoing
ARDS	Results of blinded, randomized phase II trial pending in 1999
Ischemia/reperfusion syndrome	Interim analysis of phase 1A safety trial pending in 1999
OKT3 treatment	Only modest effectiveness
Human volunteers	Antiinflammatory and immunosuppressive properties defined
Psoriasis	Some modest beneficial effects in open label study
Jarisch–Herxheimer reaction	Only modest effectiveness

TABLE 16.4. Known Members of the TNF Superfamily.

Tumor necrosis factor-α (TNFα)
Fas ligand (FasL)
TNF-related apoptosis-inducing ligand (TRAIL)
Lymphotoxin-α, Lymphotoxin-β
Nerve growth factor (NGF)
CD40 ligand, CD27 ligand, CD30 ligand
OX-40 ligand, 4-1BB ligand
Osteoclast differentiation factor (ODF)
TNF-related activation-induced cytokine (TRANCE)
Receptor activator of NFκB ligand (RANKL)
LIGHT
TWEAK
APRIL (a proliferation-inducing ligand)

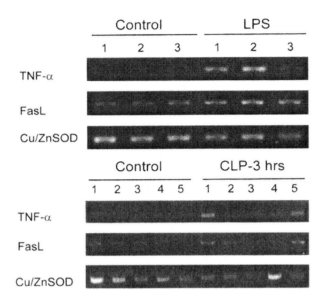

FIGURE 16.1. Reverse transcriptase-polymerase chain reaction (RT-PCR) determination of TNFα and FasL expression in endotoxinemic shock (LPS) and cecal ligation and puncture (CLP). Samples were obtained from mice 2 hours after endotoxemic shock and 3 hours after cecal legation and puncture. (Modified from Tannahill et al.,[69] with permission).

TABLE 16.5. Summary of Cytokine Expression in Various Organs after CLP or Endotoxinemia.

Cytokine	Lung	Liver	Kidney	Spleen
TNFα	++++	++++	+/−	−
FasL	++++	++++	+/−	−
TRAIL	++/−	+/−	+/−	+/−
CD40L	+/−	+/−	+/−	+/−
CD30L	nd	+/−	nd	+/−

CLP, cecal ligation and puncture.
++++, significant increase in expression following CLP and endotoxinemia; −, significant decline in expression after CLP; ++/−, increase in lung expression transiently after endotoxinemia but a progressive decline 24 hour after CLP; +/−, no consistent change in expression; nd, samples were not analyzed.

critical role in inflammation and apoptosis associated with hepatitis and rheumatoid arthritis.[63–65] Other members of the TNF family, including FasL and TRAIL, appear to be almost exclusively membrane-associated, although the adamolysins (which process membrane-associated TNFα) may also process FasL.[66] However, secreted FasL may not be bioactive; rather, it may be an inhibitor of Fas/CD95 signaling.[67]

Members of the TNF family are therefore primarily cell-associated and communicate in a paracrine fashion,[62,68] so it is unlikely that we would detect these proteins in the circulation. Because members of these protein groups often share overlapping biologic activities, the role other members of this family play in the host response to sepsis or SIRS remains unknown. This is particularly the case in rodent CLP models, where the immunologic dissonance and mortality are not dependent on TNFα. In a recently reported study we employed a sensitive, semiquantitative reverse transcriptase-polymerase chain reaction (RT-PCR) technique to quantitate the changes in mRNA levels that occur in response to these inflammatory stimuli[69] (Fig. 16.1). TNFα, FasL, TRAIL, CD30L, and CD40L expression were all evaluated in organs of the reticuloendothelial system in both endotoxemic shock and CLP models.

The results were clear-cut. Of the five members of the TNFα superfamily examined, only expression of TNFα and FasL were increased in both models (Table 16.5). FasL expression was increased in both liver and lung following endotoxinemia and CLP and paralleled the increases in expression of TNFα. Surprisingly, TRAIL expression appeared to be constitutive and was generally unaffected by the presence of inflammation, although expression may have decreased in the lung. CD30L and CD40L expression were highly variable in the organs but did not seem to be affected by either endotoxemia or CLP.

These data suggest that TRAIL, CD30L, and CD40L expression likely do not contribute to organ apoptosis or an inflammatory response after CLP or endotoxinemia. However, TRAIL bioactivity may not be regulated at the level of TRAIL expression but, rather, at the level of receptor signaling. TRAIL can bind to either of two functioning receptors (TRAIL-R1 or TRAIL-R2) or to two decoy receptors (DcR1 and DcR2), which do not transduce a signal.[70] It is the distribution of these receptors that appears to determine the differential responsiveness of normal and malignant cells to TRAIL-mediated apoptosis.

The current findings should help focus research attention on the possible roles played by TNFα and FasL in the host response to acute bacterial infections and endotoxemia. There is growing appreciation that although an exaggerated TNFα response contributes to the organ failure and death associated with bacteremic or endotoxemic shock TNFα does not play a significant contributory role in mortality after CLP. We know, for example, that TNFα through p55 receptor signaling can induce apoptosis in lymphoid, epithelial, and endothelial cells. However, Hiramatsu et al. demonstrated that blocking an endogenous TNFα response had no effect on the increased apoptosis seen in thymus, spleen, lung, and gut.[71] Similarly, Ayala et al. reported increased thymic apoptosis in mice subjected to CLP that was unaffected by TNFα blockade.[72] Although increased TNFα expression appears to be a ubiquitous response to gram-negative bacterial infections and endotoxemia, the findings suggest that other mediators, not TNFα, must contribute to these apoptotic and inflammatory changes.

The current observation that both FasL and TNFα are concordantly increased in liver and lungs from mice following CLP suggests that increased FasL expression may be an additional mediator contributing to the apoptotic processes present in these tissues or organs. We have previously shown that FasL and TNFα expression are concordantly increased in the livers of mice with concanavalin A hepatitis, a T cell-mediated injury, although inhibiting FasL activity with a soluble Fas immunoadhesin had only modest effects.[68]

The role FasL plays in the response to endotoxemia and CLP remains unclear. Nagata's group showed that FasL contributes to the hepatic injury secondary to overexpression of hepatitis B virus (HBV) antigens or endotoxin in a *Corynebacterium parvum*-primed mouse,[73] but that has not been our experience. We demonstrated that FasL played a role in the apoptotic liver injury following administration of concanavalin A only when the processing of FasL was inhibited by a matrix metalloproteinase inhibitor.[68] We could not demonstrate a role for FasL in the apoptotic injury that accompanied concanavalin A administration or after endotoxin-induced shock (unpublished observations).

Role of Cytokines in Organ Apoptosis after Sepsis and Burns

There has been increasing awareness that apoptosis occurs after sepsis and burn injury, but little is known about the organs and cell types affected. We and others have demonstrated that after CLP, endotoxinemia, or a thermal injury increased apoptosis is limited primarily to lymphoid tissues.[71-77] Increased apoptosis is not observed in parenchymal cells of the liver or in epithelial cells of the kidney, although there are modest increases in the lungs. Rather, the increases in organ apoptosis are primarily seen in lymphoid-rich organs (spleen, thymus, small intestine). Hotchkiss et al.[78] also reported increased lymphocyte apoptosis in the lungs of mice after CLP. Such increased apoptosis of lymphoid cell populations, frequently seen following a variety of inflammatory insults, is proposed to contribute to the immune suppression that often results. This increased apoptosis in thymus and spleen is seen in both mature and immature T and B cells; and it appears to be dependent primarily on activation of caspase-3-dependent pathways. We have shown that treatment of mice with a synthetic inhibitor of caspase-3 completely prevented the increased apoptosis seen after a burn injury.[74] Similarly, Hotchkiss et al. reported that mice overexpressing BCL-2 had attenuated apoptosis and increased survival after CLP.[78]

Interestingly, Hotchkiss and colleagues have examined organ apoptosis, caspase-3, and BCL-2 activity in lymphoid organs from patients who had immediately expired from sepsis.[79] Using histologic criteria, these investigators demonstrated that almost 50% of these patients had increased apoptosis and caspase-3 activity in lymphoid cells from spleen and intestine. In contrast, apoptosis was a rare event in patients expiring from nonseptic events. This is the first demonstration of increased apoptosis in lymphoid organs from patients expiring from sepsis and suggests that increased apoptotic loss of immune cells is a real event in human sepsis.

Caspase-3- and BCL-2-dependent apoptosis are hallmarks of TNFα- and FasL-mediated apoptosis, signaling via the p55 and Fas/CD95 receptors, respectively.[62] Activation of the death domains of these two receptors results in concatamerization of death effector molecules, such as TNF-Receptor associated death domain (TRADD) and Fas-associated death domain (FADD), and activation of caspase 8, Mast-associated CED3 Homologue, *MACH* 1, or *FLICE*, FADD-like IL-1-beta converting enzyme. Activation of this early member of the caspase cascade leads to catalysis and autoactivation of caspase-3, a primary effector arm of apoptosis.

Despite convincing evidence that this increased lymphoid apoptosis is caspase-3-dependent, the current evidence to date suggests that neither TNFα nor FasL is responsible for the increased apoptosis in spleen, thymus, and bone marrow. The only exception appears to be in splenic B lymphocytes. Ayala et al. reported that the increased apoptosis of mucosal B lymphocytes seen in mice following bacterial peritonitis was secondary to FasL, as it was markedly reduced in mice expressing defective FasL.[77]

Rather, the data suggest that increased corticosteroid release can explain this increase in apoptosis seen with thermal injuries and CLP, presumably through a caspase-3-dependent process (Table 16.6). There are, in fact, two lines of evidence to suggest a primary role for glucocorticoids in mediating this response. When dexamethasone was administered to healthy mice, similar transient increases in apoptosis were seen in spleen and thymus.[80] Nakamura et al. similarly observed that during glucocorticoid-induced thymocyte death most apoptotic cells aggregated to form clusters being phagocytosed by macrophages.[80] This histologic feature is similar to that observed in thymus and spleen after burn injury. Caspase-3 activity also increases during thymocyte apoptosis induced by dexamethasone; and pretreatment with a caspase-3 inhibitor prevents apoptosis due to corticosteroid administration.[81,82]

Second, blocking endogenous glucocorticoids with mifepristone reduced not only apoptosis in both organs but also caspase-3 activity. We have previously shown that treatment of mice with a caspase-3, but not a caspase-1, inhibitor prevented apoptosis after a burn injury in both spleen and thymus.[74] Treating mice with mifepristone also blocked the increased apoptosis seen in thymus and spleen after a burn injury. These findings are therefore consistent with previous work demonstrating that the increased apoptosis observed in thymus after CLP appeared to be due to glucocorticoids alone.[72] Because suppression of glucocorticoid responses after sepsis is not a viable therapeutic alternative, recent efforts have been directed at blocking organ apoptosis through inhibition of caspase-3 pathways. Synthetic inhibitors of caspase-3 as well as novel pox viral proteins (Crm A and SPI-2) are currently in preclinical testing as a means to reduce the apoptosis of lymphoid organs that accompanies sepsis.

Cell-Associated TNFα Signaling

Although it has been known since the studies of Kriegler et al. that TNFα can exist in both cell-associated and secreted forms, and both forms are bioactive,[83] the role these two species play in organ injury and apoptosis is unclear. We and others have previously shown that it is the secreted 17-kDa TNFα, circulating in a trimeric form, that is primarily responsible for shock and organ injury (for review see Ksontini et al.[62]); but the concept that TNFα signaling of inflammation and apoptosis in vivo

TABLE 16.6. Role of Various Humoral Mediators and Cell Signaling Pathways in Increased Apoptosis after CLP or Thermal Injury.

Mediator/pathway	Role
TNFα	May be associated with hepatocyte apoptosis in models of T cell-mediated liver injury, such as in hepatitis B or C or adenoviral gene therapy, or in macrophage-mediated hepatocyte apoptosis in the presence of transcriptional inhibitors
	Does not appear to play a significant role in lymphoid cell apoptosis in sepsis syndromes or thermal injury
FasL	Does not appear to play a significant role in the mortality due to endotoxoin shock or in liver apoptosis in either macrophage or T cell models of hepatocyte apoptotic injury
	Does not appear to play a significant role in the apoptosis of lymphoid tissues after CLP, with the exception of some gut-associated B cell populations
Granzymes/perforin	Role in mediating apoptosis in sepsis or burn injury unclear
TRAIL	Probably plays little role in organ apoptosis after acute inflammation
Lymphotoxin, CD40L/CD30L, other members of the TNF superfamily	Role in mediating apoptosis in sepsis or burn injury unclear
Glucocorticoids	Major player in the early apoptotic responses by lymphoid tissues to CLP
	Induces apoptosis in several T and B cell classes
	Activates apoptosis through caspase-3-dependent pathways

occurs *solely* through p55 has been challenged by Grell and associates.[84] Grell et al. compellingly demonstrated that the diversity of TNFα actions arises from a differential responsiveness of the two TNFα receptors for the secreted and cell-associated forms of TNFα (Fig. 16.2). We observed that the principal form of TNFα recovered from livers of burned and septic rats was a 26- to 29-kDa protein.[85] TNFα is synthesized as a 26-kDa membrane-associated precursor that is cleaved to the 17-kDa form by TNFα converting enzyme *TACE*, a novel matrix metalloproteinase recently cloned and described.[86] Grell et al. argued that the principal ligand for the p55 receptor is the 17-kDa secreted form of TNFα. The on-off kinetics of the 17-kDa TNFα with p75 receptor are fast. In conditions of low TNFα concentrations, p75 may serve as a ligand passer for the p55 receptor and increase TNFα binding to p55.[87,88] Conversely, close juxtaposition of the 26-kDa cell-associated TNFα to the p75 receptor, as occurs during cell-to-cell contact, allows formation of complexes with increased stability and signaling potential (Fig. 16.2). Grell et al. further proposed that cell-associated TNFα is the prime physiologic activator of the p75 receptor, implying that p75 controls the local TNFα response in tissues.[84]

Data published to date suggest that the 17-kDa secreted TNFα (not the 26-kDa cell-associated form) is primarily responsible for mortality due to endotoxin- or bacteremia-induced shock. Studies conducted in the baboon further suggest that these 17-kDa TNFα actions occur principally through p55 signaling.[13,18] In two recent reports we demonstrated that blocking the secreted form of TNFα with a matrix metalloproteinase inhibitor improves survival after lipopolysaccharide (LPS)/D-galactosamine-induced shock in the mouse but does not protect against the accompanying liver injury.[63,89] In concanavalin A-induced hepatitis, matrix metalloproteinase inhibitors exacerbated hepatocellular necrosis and apoptosis despite more than 90% reduction in plasma TNFα concentrations. Interestingly, treatment with the matrix metalloproteinase inhibitor had minimal effect on the concentration of membrane-associated TNFα in the livers of animals with hepatitis. In contrast, a TNFα-binding protein[90] that neutralized both membrane-associated and soluble TNFα attenuated both LPS/D-galactosamine- and concanavalin A-induced hepatitis in the presence or absence of a matrix metalloproteinase

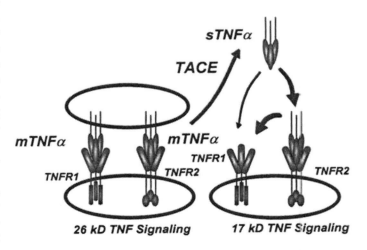

FIGURE 16.2. Proposed TNFα signaling pathways through the p55 and p75 receptor. The primary receptor for the solid 17-kDa TNFα is likely to be p55, whereas low concentrations of TNFα are effectively "passed" from the p75 to the p55 receptor. In contrast, because of steric hindrance, cell-associated 26-kDa TNFα is not easily passed from the p75 receptor to the p55 receptor, and signal transduction through both receptors may occur.

inhibitor. These results suggest that 26-kDa cell-associated TNFα, not the 17-kDa secreted form, plays a critical role in the hepatocellular necrosis and apoptosis that accompany LPS/D-galactosamine- or concanavalin A-induced hepatitis. Therefore the sole blockade of soluble TNFα may be ineffective in preventing this type of injury. Similarly, Georgopolous et al.[91] and Kollias's group[65] demonstrated (using a novel transgenic mouse) that expression of the transmembrane form of TNFα was adequate to produce experimentally induced arthritis.

Although there is now a general consensus that the cell-associated form of TNFα is bioactive and contributes to its juxtacrine effects, confirmation of preferential p75 signaling by cell-associated TNFα remains controversial. Challenging their own hypothesis, Grell and associates demonstrated that endothelial cell apoptosis following irradiation and endotoxemia involved the transmembrane form of TNFα, but that it could be blocked by inhibiting antibodies against the p55, but not the p75, receptor.[92] Similarly, Leist et al. observed that D-galactosamine-sensitized mice expressing a null form of the p55 receptor were resistant to TNFα-induced hepatic injury,[93] suggesting that in experimental hepatitis cell-associated TNFα also signals predominantly through the p55 receptor.

Conclusions

The role of cytokines in the sepsis response has become considerably clearer since the original descriptions of TNFα and IL-1. Although there is agreement that these two cytokines play critical roles in the pathogenesis of sepsis syndrome, interest in them as a therapeutic target in sepsis is waning. A better understanding of the cytokine response to sepsis reveals that several classes of cytokines are induced simultaneously, including proinflammatory and T-helper lymphocyte (Th1)-type cytokines such as TNFα, IL-1, INFγ, and IL-12, as well as antiinflammatory cytokines such as IL-10, and cytokine antagonists such as IL-1ra, p55, p75, and p68. These cytokines not only serve to initiate the innate immune response, but especially IL-10, results in a sustained immunosuppressive response characterized by a Th2-type response and increased lymphoid apoptosis. There is also increasing interest in other members of the TNFα family and the role they play in apoptotic injury. Although FasL expression is increased in animal models of acute inflammation and its expression seems to parallel that of TNFα, its role in the host response to sepsis is unclear. Increased FasL expression does not seem to play a significant role in the mortality or the increased apoptosis in most lymphoid organs. Although progress has been made in understanding the role played by individual cytokines, the lack of a successful therapy for the patient with sepsis suggests that our knowledge of the role cytokines play in the host response to sepsis is still incomplete.

Acknowledgments. Supported in part by grants GM-40586 and HL-59412, awarded by the National Institutes of Health, DHHS. R.M. and J.R. are supported by a research training fellowship (T32 GM-08721), National Institute of General Medical Sciences.

References

1. Pennica D, Nedwin GE, Hayflick JS, et al: Human tumour necrosis factor: precursor structure, expression and homology to lymphotoxin. Nature 1984;312:724–729.
2. Pennica D, Hayflick JS, Bringman TS, Palladino MA, Goeddel DV: Cloning and expression in *Escherichia coli* of the cDNA for murine tumor necrosis factor. Proc Natl Acad Sci USA 1985;82:6060–6064.
3. Lomedico PT, Gubler U, Hellmann CP, et al: Cloning and expression of murine interleukin-1 cDNA in *Escherichia coli*. Nature 1984;312:458–462.
4. Auron PE, Rosenwasser LJ, Matsushima K, et al: Human and murine interleukin 1 possess sequence and structural similarities. J Mol Cell Immunol. 1985;2:169–177.
5. Beutler B, Greenwald D, Hulmes JD, et al: Identity of tumour necrosis factor and the macrophage-secreted factor cachectin. Nature 1985;316:552–554.
6. Tracey KJ, Beutler B, Lowry SF, et al: Shock and tissue injury induced by recombinant human cachectin. Science 1986;234:470–474.
7. Ohlsson K, Bjork P, Bergenfeldt M, Hageman R, Thompson RC: Interleukin-1 receptor antagonist reduces mortality from endotoxin shock. Nature 1990;348:550–552.
8. Fischer E, Marano MA, Van Zee KJ, et al: Interleukin-1 receptor blockade improves survival and hemodynamic performance in *Escherichia coli* septic shock, but fails to alter host responses to sublethal endotoxemia. J Clin Invest 1992;89:1551–1557.
9. Zeni F, Freeman B, Natanson C: Anti-inflammatory therapies to treat sepsis and septic shock: a reassessment [editorial; comment]. Crit Care Med 1997;25:1095–1100.
10. Baue AE: Multiple organ failure, multiple organ dysfunction syndrome, and systemic inflammatory response syndrome: why no magic bullets? Arch Surg 1997;132:703–707.
11. Cain BS, Meldrum DR, Harken AH, McIntyre RC Jr: The physiologic basis for anticytokine clinical trials in the treatment of sepsis. J Am Coll Surg 1998;186:337–350.
12. Vincent JL: Search for effective immunomodulating strategies against sepsis [comment]. Lancet 1998;351:922–923.
13. Welborn MB III, Van Zee K, Edwards PD, et al: A human tumor necrosis factor p75 receptor agonist stimulates in vitro T cell proliferation but does not produce inflammation or shock in the baboon. J Exp Med 1996;184:165–171.
14. Tracey KJ, Lowry SF, Fahey TJ, et al: Cachectin/tumor necrosis factor induces lethal shock and stress hormone responses in the dog. Surg Gynecol Obstet 1987;164:415–422.
15. Van der Poll T, Romijn JA, Endert E, Borm JJ, Buller HR, Sauerwein HP: Tumor necrosis factor mimics the metabolic response to acute infection in healthy humans. Am J Physiol 1991;261:E457–E465.
16. Van der Poll T, Jansen J, Levi M, et al: Regulation of interleukin 10 release by tumor necrosis factor in humans and chimpanzees. J Exp Med 1994;180:1985–1988.
17. Van der Poll T, Jansen PM, Van Zee KJ, et al: Tumor necrosis factor-alpha induces activation of coagulation and fibrinolysis in baboons through an exclusive effect on the p55 receptor. Blood 1996;88:922–927.

18. Van Zee KJ, Stackpole SA, Montegut WJ, et al: A human tumor necrosis factor (TNF) α mutant that binds exclusively to the p55 TNF receptor produces toxicity in the baboon. J Exp Med 1994;179:1185–1191.
19. Fong Y, Tracey KJ, Moldawer LL, et al: Antibodies to cachectin/tumor necrosis factor reduce interleukin 1 beta and interleukin 6 appearance during lethal bacteremia. J Exp Med 1989;170:1627–1633.
20. Van Zee KJ, Moldawer LL, Oldenburg HS, et al: Protection against lethal Escherichia coli bacteremia in baboons (Papio anubis) by pretreatment with a 55-kDa TNF receptor (CD120a)-Ig fusion protein, Ro 45–2081. J Immunol 1996;156: 2221–2230.
21. Jansen J, van der Poll T, Levi M, et al: Inhibition of the release of soluble tumor necrosis factor receptors in experimental endotoxemia by an anti-tumor necrosis factor-α antibody. J Clin Immunol 1995;15:45–50.
22. Van der Poll T, van Deventer SJ, ten Cate H, Levi M, ten Cate JW: Tumor necrosis factor is involved in the appearance of interleukin-1 receptor antagonist in endotoxemia. J Infect Dis 1994;169:665–667.
23. Remick D, Manohar P, Bolgos G, Rodriguez J, Moldawer L, Wollenberg G: Blockade of tumor necrosis factor reduces lipopolysaccharide lethality, but not the lethality of [ceccal ligation and puncture]. Shock 1995;4:89–95.
24. Bagby GJ, Plessala KJ, Wilson LA, Thompson JJ, Nelson S: Divergent efficacy of antibody to tumor necrosis factor-alpha in intravascular and peritonitis models of sepsis. J Infect Dis 1991;163:83–88.
25. Echtenacher B, Falk W, Mannel DN, Krammer PH: Requirement of endogenous tumor necrosis factor/cachectin for recovery from experimental peritonitis. J Immunol 1990;145:3762–3766.
26. Bone RC: Sir Isaac Newton, sepsis, SIRS, and CARS. Crit Care Med 1996;24:1125–1128.
27. Van Zee KJ, Kohno T, Fischer E, Rock CS, Moldawer LL, Lowry SF: Tumor necrosis factor soluble receptors circulate during experimental and clinical inflammation and can protect against excessive tumor necrosis factor alpha in vitro and in vivo. Proc Natl Acad Sci USA 1992;89:4845–4849.
28. Fisher CJ Jr, Dhainaut J-FA, Opal SM, et al: Recombinant human interleukin 1 receptor antagonist in the treatment of patients with sepsis syndrome: results from a randomized, double-blind, placebo-controlled trial. JAMA 1994;271:1836–1843.
29. Pruitt JH, Welborn MB, Edwards PD, et al: Increased soluble interleukin-1 type II receptor concentrations in postoperative patients and in patients with sepsis syndrome. Blood 1996;87:3282–3288.
30. Clark MA, Plank LD, Connolly AB, et al: Effect of a chimeric antibody to tumor necrosis factor-alpha on cytokine and physiologic responses in patients with severe sepsis—a randomized, clinical trial. Crit Care Med 1998;26:1650–1659.
31. Bone RC: Immunologic dissonance: a continuing evolution in our understanding of the systemic inflammatory response syndrome (SIRS) and the multiple organ dysfunction syndrome (MODS). Ann Intern Med 1996;125:680–687.
32. Derkx B, Marchant A, Goldman M, Bijlmer R, van Deventer S: High levels of interleukin-10 during the initial phase of fulminant meningococcal septic shock. J Infect Dis 1995;171:229–232.
33. Marchant A, Deviere J, Byl B, De Groote D, Vincent J-L, Goldman M: Interleukin-10 production during septicaemia. Lancet 1994;343:707–708.
34. Neidhardt R, Keel M, Steckholzer U, et al: Relationship of interleukin-10 plasma levels to severity of injury and clinical outcome in injured patients. J Trauma 1997;42:863–870.
35. Van Dissel JT, Van Sangevelde P, Westendorp RG, et al: Anti-inflammatory cytokine profile and mortality in febrile patients. Lancet 1998;351:950–953.
36. Cassatella MA, Meda L, Bonora S, Ceska M, Constantin G: Interleukin 10 (IL-10) inhibits the release of proinflammatory cytokines from human polymorphonuclear leukocytes: evidence for an autocrine role of tumor necrosis factor and IL-1 beta in mediating the production of IL-8 triggered by lipopolysaccharide. J Exp Med 1993;178:2207–2211.
37. Kasama T, Strieter RM, Lukacs NW, Lincoln PM, Burdick MD, Kunkel SL: Interleukin-10 expression and chemokine regulation during the evolution of murine type II collagen-induced arthritis. J Clin Invest 1995;95:2868–2876.
38. Fong YM, Marano MA, Moldawer LL, et al: The acute splanchnic and peripheral tissue metabolic response to endotoxin in humans. J Clin Invest 1990;85:1896–1904.
39. Fischer E, Van Zee KJ, Marano MA, et al: Interleukin-1 receptor antagonist circulates in experimental inflammation and in human disease. Blood 1992;79:2196–2200.
40. Van Zee KJ, Coyle SM, Calvano SE, et al: Influence of IL-1 receptor blockade on the human response to endotoxemia. J Immunol 1995;154:1499–1507.
41. Calvano SE, Thompson WA, Coyle SN, et al: Changes in monocyte and soluble tumor necrosis factor receptors during endotoxemia or sepsis. Surg Forum 1993;44:114–116.
42. Moore KW, O'Garra A, de Waal Malefyt R, Vieira P, Mosmann TR: Interleukin-10. Annu Rev Immunol 1993;11:165–190.
43. de Waal Malefyt R, Haanen J, Spits H, et al: Interleukin 10 (IL-10) and viral IL-10 strongly reduce antigen-specific human T cell proliferation by diminishing the antigen-presenting capacity of monocytes via downregulation of class II major histocompatibility complex expression. J Exp Med 1991;174:915–924.
44. Wanidworanun C, Strober W: Predominant role of tumor necrosis factor alpha in human monocyte IL-10 synthesis. J Immunol 1996;151:6853–6861.
45. Cassatella MA, Meda L, Gasperini S, Calzetti F, Bonora S: Interleukin 10 (IL-10) upregulates IL-1 receptor antagonist production from lipopolysaccharide-stimulated human polymorphonuclear leukocytes by delaying mRNA degradation. J Exp Med 1994;179:1695–1699.
46. Wang P, Wu P, Anthes JC, Siegel MI, Egan RW, Billah MM: Interleukin-10 inhibits interleukin-8 production in human neutrophils. Blood 1994;83:2678–2683.
47. Van der Poll T, Jansen PM, Montegut WJ, et al: Effects of IL-10 on systemic inflammatory responses during sublethal primate endotoxemia. J Immunol 1997;158:1971–1975.
48. Howard M, Muchamuel T, Andrade S, Menon S: Interleukin 10 protects mice from lethal endotoxemia. J Exp Med 1993;177:1205–1208.
49. Gerard C, Bruyns C, Marchant A, et al: Interleukin 10 reduces the release of tumor necrosis factor and prevents lethality in experimental endotoxemia. J Exp Med 1993;177:547–550.
50. Huhn RD, Radwanski E, O'Connell SM, et al: Pharmacokinetics and immunomodulatory properties of intravenously administered recombinant human interleukin-10 in healthy volunteers. Blood 1996;87:699–705.

51. Chernoff AE, Granowitz EV, Shapiro L, et al: A randomized, controlled trial of IL-10 in humans: inhibition of inflammatory cytokine production and immune responses. J Immunol 1995;154:5492–5499.
52. Standiford TJ, Strieter RM, Lukacs NW, Kunkel SL: Neutralization of IL-10 increases lethality in endotoxemia: cooperative effects of macrophage inflammatory protein-2 and tumor necrosis factor. J Immunol 1995;155:2222–2229.
53. Van der Poll T, Marchant A, Buurman WA, et al: Endogenous IL-10 protects mice from death during septic peritonitis. J Immunol 1995;155:5397–5401.
54. Hess PJ, Seeger JM, Huber TS, et al: Exogenously administered interleukin-10 decreases pulmonary neutrophil infiltration in a tumor necrosis factor dependent model of acute visceral ischemia. J Vasc Surg 1997;26:113–118.
55. Engles RE, Huber TS, Zander DS, et al: Exogenous human recombinant interleukin-10 attenuates hindlimb ischemi-reperfusion injury. J Surg Res 1997;69:425–428.
56. Kelly JL, Lyons A, Soberg CC, Mannick JA, Lederer JA: Antiinterleukin-10 antibody restores burn-induced defects in T-cell function. Surgery 1997;122:146–152.
57. Song GY, Chung CS, Schwacha MG, Jarrar D, Chaudry IH, Ayala A: Splenic immune suppression in sepsis: A role for IL-10-induced changes in P38 MAPK signaling. J Surg Res 1999;83:36–43.
58. Steinhauser ML, Hogaboam CM, Kunkel SL, Lukacs NW, Strieter RM, Standiford TJ: IL-10 is a major mediator of sepsis-induced impairment in lung antibacterial host defense. J Immunol 1999;162:392–399.
59. Van der Poll T, Marchant A, Keogh CV, Goldman M, Lowry SF: Interleukin-10 impairs host defense in murine pneumococcal pneumonia. J Infect Dis 1996;174:994–1000.
60. Keystone E, Wherry J, Grint P: IL-10 as a therapeutic strategy in the treatment of rheumatoid arthritis. Rheum Dis Clin North Am 1998;24:629–639.
61. Van Montfrans C, Camoglio L, van Deventer SJ: Immunotherapy of Crohn's disease. Mediators Inflamm 1998;7:149–152.
62. Ksontini R, MacKay SL, Moldawer LL: Revisiting the role of tumor necrosis factor alpha and the response to surgical injury and inflammation. Arch Surg 1998;133:558–567.
63. Solorzano CC, Ksontini R, Pruitt JH, et al: Involvement of 26-kDa cell-associated TNF-alpha in experimental hepatitis and exacerbation of liver injury with a matrix metalloproteinase inhibitor. J Immunol 1997;158:414–419.
64. Kusters S, Tiegs G, Alexopoulou L, et al: In vivo evidence for a functional role of both tumor necrosis factor (TNF) receptors and transmembrane TNF in experimental hepatitis. Eur J Immunol 1997;27:2870–2875.
65. Alexopoulou L, Pasparakis M, Kollias G: A murine transmembrane tumor necrosis factor (TNF) transgene induces arthritis by cooperative p55/p75 TNF receptor signaling. Eur J Immunol 1997;27:2588–2592.
66. Mariani SM, Matiba B, Baumler C, Krammer PH: Regulation of cell surface APO-1/Fas (CD95) ligand expression by metalloproteases. Eur J Immunol 1995;25:2303–2307.
67. Schneider P, Holler N, Bodmer JL, et al: Conversion of membrane-bound Fas (CD95) ligand to its soluble form is associated with downregulation of its proapoptotic activity and loss of liver toxicity. J Exp Med 1998;187:1205–1213.
68. Ksontini R, Colagiovanni DB, Josephs MD, et al: Disparate roles for TNF-alpha and Fas ligand in concanavalin A-induced hepatitis. J Immunol 1998;160:4082–4089.
69. Tannahill CL, Fukuzuka K, Marum T, et al: Discordant TNF-alpha supefamily expression in bacterial peritonitis and endotoxemic shock. Surgery 1999;126:349–357.
70. Griffith TS, Lynch DH: TRAIL: a molecule with multiple receptors and control mechanisms. Curr Opin Immunol 1998;10:559–563.
71. Hiramatsu M, Hotchkiss RS, Karl IE, Buchman TG: Cecal ligation and puncture (CLP) induces apoptosis in thymus, spleen, lung, and gut by an endotoxin and TNF-independent pathway. Shock 1997;7:247–253.
72. Ayala A, Herdon CD, Lehman DL, Ayala CA, Chaudry IH: Differential induction of apoptosis in lymphoid tissues during sepsis: variation in onset, frequency, and the nature of the mediators. Blood 1996;87:4261–4275.
73. Kondo T, Suda T, Fukuyama H, Adachi M, Nagata S: Essential roles of the Fas ligand in the development of hepatitis. Nat Med 1997;3:409–413.
74. Fukuzuka K, Rosenberg JJ Gaines GC, et al: Caspase-3 dependent organ apoptosis early after burn injury [abstract]. Ann Surg 1999;229:851–858.
75. Hotchkiss RS, Swanson PE, Cobb JP, Jacobson A, Buchman TG, Karl IE: Apoptosis in lymphoid and parenchymal cells during sepsis: a findings in normal and T- and B-cell-deficient mice. Crit Care Med 1997;25:1298–1307.
76. Ayala A, Urbanich MA, Herdon CD, Chaudry IH: Is sepsis-induced apoptosis associated with macrophage dysfunction? J Trauma 1996;40:568–573.
77. Ayala A, Xin XY, Ayala CA, et al: Increased mucosal B-lymphocyte apoptosis during polymicrobial sepsis is a Fas ligand but not an endotoxin-mediated process. Blood 1998;91:1362–1372.
78. Hotchkiss RS, Swanson PE, Knudson CM, et al: Overexpression of Bcl-2 in transgenic mice decreases apoptosis and improves survival in sepsis. J Immunol 1999;162:4148–4156.
79. Hotchkiss RS, Swanson PE, Freeman BD, et al: Apoptotic cell death in patients with sepsis, shock and multiple organ dysfunction [abstract]. Crit Care Med 1999;27:1230–1251.
80. Nakamura M, Yagi H, Ishii T, et al: DNA fragmentation is not the primary event in glucocorticoid-induced thymocyte death in vivo. Eur J Immunol 1997;27:999–1004.
81. Alam A, Braun MY, Hartgers F, et al: Specific activation of the cysteine protease CPP32 during the negative selection of T cells in the thymus. J Exp Med 1997;186:1503–1512.
82. Clayton LK, Ghendler Y, Mizoguchi E, et al: T-cell receptor ligation by peptide/MHC induces activation of a caspase in immature thymocytes: the molecular basis of negative selection. EMBO J 1997;16:2282–2293.
83. Kriegler M, Perez C, DeFay K, Albert I, Lu SD: A novel form of TNF/cachetin is a cell surface cytotoxic transmembrane protein: ramifications for the complex physiology of TNF. Cell 1988;53:45–53.
84. Grell M, Douni E, Wajant H, et al: The transmembrane form of tumor necrosis factor is the prime activating ligand of the 80 kDa tumor necrosis factor receptor. Cell 1995;83:793–802.
85. Keogh C, Fong Y, Marano MA, et al: Identification of a novel tumor necrosis factor alpha/cachectin from the livers of burned and infected rats. Arch Surg 1990;125:79–84.

86. Moss ML, Catherine-Jin SL, Milla ME, et al: Cloning of a disintegrin metalloproteinase that processes precursor tumor-necrosis factor-α Nature 1997;385:733–736.
87. Tartaglia LA, Pennica D, Goeddel DV: Ligand passing: the 75-kDa tumor necrosis factor (TNF) receptor recruits TNF for signaling by the 55-kDa TNF receptor. J Biol Chem 1993;268:18542–18548.
88. Aderka D, Engelmann H, Maor Y, Brakebusch C, Wallach D: Stabilization of the bioactivity of tumor necrosis factor by its soluble receptors. J Exp Med 1992;175:323–329.
89. Solorzano CC, Ksontini R, Pruitt JH, et al: A matrix metalloproteinase inhibitor prevents processing of TNF-alpha and abrogates endotoxin induced lethality. Shock 1997;7:427–431.
90. Solorzano CC, Kaibara A, Hess PJ, et al: Pharmacokinetics, immunogenicity, and efficacy of dimeric TNFR binding proteins in healthy and bacteremic baboon. J Appl Physiol 1998;84:1119–1130.
91. Georgopolous S, Plows D, Kollias G: Transmembrane TNF is sufficient to induce localized tissue toxicity and chronic inflammatory arthritis in transgenic mice. J Inflamm 1996;46:86–97.
92. Eissner G, Kohlhuber F, Grell M, et al: Critical involvement of transmembrane tumor necrosis factor-alpha in endothelial programmed cell death mediated by ionizing radiation and bacterial endotoxin. Blood 1995;86:4184–4193.
93. Leist M, Gantner F, Jilg S, Wendel A: Activation of the 55 kDa TNF receptor is necessary and sufficient for TNF-induced liver failure, hepatocyte apoptosis, and nitrite release. J Immunol 1995;154:1307–1316.

17
Counterregulation of Severe Inflammation: When More Is Too Much and Less Is Inadequate

Vishnu Rumalla and Stephen F. Lowry

The human immune response to infection is orchestrated by complex interactions of soluble mediators and cellular elements. Whereas an attenuated cellular immune defense may lead to poor healing or prolonged infection, a robust response may precipitate shock and multisystem organ failure.[1–3] A proper balance of mediator-driven responses are necessary to regulate both systemic and local immune function properly.

Proinflammatory cytokines have been studied extensively for their potential role in host defense. Many of these mediators have also been implicated as important drivers of the systemic inflammatory response syndrome (SIRS). The diversity of inciting etiologic events that eventuate in SIRS limits the portrayal of a clearly unifying theory of cause and effect in severe SIRS. This potential diversity of mediator activities also challenges effective therapeutic interventions.[4]

The proinflammatory cytokines tumor necrosis factor (TNF) and interleukin-1 (IL-1), among others, are well established as initiators of an inflammatory response. Agents used to blunt and block these cytokines have led to dramatic attenuation of many systemic and organ-specific consequences of an excessive immune response in preclinical trials. Alternatively, studies suggest that the cytokine production response to common antigens may be diminished subsequent to initial injury.[5–7] The variable timing of these disparate responses makes interventions all the more difficult. To elaborate on the above relation, we examine the proinflammatory state and several antiinflammatory and counterregulatory mechanisms that are operative during the initial response to injury.

Proinflammatory Cytokines

Tumor Necrosis Factor

Tumor necrosis factor is released primarily by cells of the macrophage/monocyte lineage in response to soluble antigens or immune complexes. A variety of stimuli including parasites, tumors, and endotoxin stimulate cells to produce TNF.[8–10] TNF is involved in the recruitment and maturation of macrophages and neutrophils,[11] and it is essential for upregulation of cell surface adhesion molecules, which promote the cell-to-endothelium interaction necessary for neutrophil chemotaxis.[12,13] Tissue levels of TNF exert important paracrine effects in initiating proper and expedient healing.[14,15] These effects include hemostasis, increased vascular permeability, increased vascular proliferation, and collagen synthesis.[12] TNF also promotes many cellular metabolic events that contribute to the supply of nutrient substrates and acute-phase protein production.[11]

Excessive production of TNF probably leads to adverse clinical outcomes. Excess circulating TNF has been associated with multisystem organ failure and increased morbidity and mortality in some disease states.[16–20] The consequences of excessive TNF activity may include circulatory collapse and damage to solid organs.[10,21,22] This effect is mechanistically multifactorial. For instance, the procoagulant effect of TNF favors thrombosis of the microcirculation, leading to cellular necrosis and increased vascular permeability. In addition, TNF likely contributes to myocardial depression and the recruitment and activation of macrophages and neutrophils to sites of injury and inflammation.[23,24] Activation of these immune cells may lead to further tissue damage through the production of reactive oxygen and nitrogen metabolites, proteolytic enzymes, and arachidonic acid metabolites.[25,26] The role of TNF in the prolongation of local proinflammatory cell survival is discussed later in the chapter.

Interleukin-1

Interleukin-1 has many of the same physiologic properties as TNF but with less overt capacity to produce shock.[11] This cytokine also activates neutrophils, upregulates adhesion molecules, and promotes chemotaxis.[11] It effects coagulation and tends to favor thrombosis, whereas TNF may promote anticoagulant or fibrinolytic activities.[23,27–29] In addition, IL-1 promotes other cells, such as endothelial cells, to secrete proinflammatory cytokines.[30] In the central nervous system, IL-1 appears to elicit a febrile response and is important in the regulation of the pituitary counterregulatory hormone axis.[31,32] Like TNF, many of the effects of IL-1 are important in wound healing, and an adequate IL-1 response may be essential for longer-term host defense.[2] Although some studies implicate increased IL-1 levels with sepsis, cachexia, and chronic disease, others show that lower levels of circulating IL-1 are associated with greater mortality in some severe injuries (e.g., burns) and may contribute to the immune anergy seen in trauma patients.[33-40]

Interleukin-6

Interleukin-6 promotes stem cell growth, B and T lymphocyte activation, and regulation of the hepatic acute-phase protein response.[41-45] These acute-phase proteins are essential to the host's immune, coagulation, and metabolic response. IL-6 is synthesized by many cells in the body; but like other proinflammatory cytokines, the cells of the macrophage/monocyte line appear to be an important source. IL-6 is released in response to multiple stimuli, with TNF, IL-1, and endotoxin being potent agonists.[46,47]

Circulating levels of IL-6 are increased in vivo during both acute bacteremia and chronic disease states in humans.[48-50] Local tissue levels of IL-6 have been shown to be elevated dramatically at sites of thermal injury.[51] Elevated circulating IL-6 levels are often detected in conditions associated with inflammation, including elective surgery.[2,48-50] Some studies suggest that IL-6 levels correlate with outcome in that higher levels are noted in nonsurvivors than in survivors of burns, pancreatitis, and sepsis.[52] The readily detectable IL-6 concentration in the circulation of patients with severe injury has attracted attention as a surrogate marker for subsequent complications or mortality. At present, this marker lacks sufficient sensitivity and specificity to be of benefit in determining the etiology or outcome of postinjury inflammation.

Interleukin-8

Interleukin-8, along with other members of the chemokine family, is emerging as an important antiinflammatory cytokine in injury. As the most prominent member of the family, IL-8 is secreted primarily by macrophages and has been shown to increase in the circulation soon after IL-6 is detectable.[53] IL-8 has effects that include increased neutrophil and monocyte chemotaxis, increased neutrophil degranulation, and increased expression of endothelial cell adhesion molecules.[54,55] These important influences on leukocyte activities and attraction suggest that cytokines of the IL-8 family may be of importance to the development of multisystem organ failure and especially acute lung injury.[56]

Interferon-γ

Interferon-γ (IFNγ) is a pleotropic cytokine produced primarily by T lymphocytes and macrophages.[56] Its predominant effects include increased macrophage and polymorphonuclear neutrophil (PMN) activation and cytotoxicity. In addition, IFNγ causes lymphocyte proliferation and increases the production of IL-1 and TNF.[56] IFNγ has been found to be essential for survival in some models of bacterial and fungal challenge.[57,53] Similarly, IFNγ administration to septic patients may improve some aspects of immune cell function,[59] although recently terminated phase III trials using IFNγ showed no decrease in the rate of infection or mortality in burn patients.[60,61]

Interleukin-12

Interleukin-12 is a proinflammatory, immunoregulatory cytokine. It is produced primarily by macrophages, and its predominant effects include natural killer (NK) cell and T lymphocyte differentiation.[62,63] Its role in cell-mediated immunity makes it essential in the normal host defense against bacteria and intracellular pathogens. Ertel et al. demonstrated that IFNγ-stimulated IL-12 production is decreased in lipopolysaccharide (LPS)-incubated whole blood of critically ill patients.[64] The authors contended that this inhibition of IL-12 production may in fact make the host more susceptible to infection. Similarly, IL-12 administration restored normal resistance to bacterial challenge after experimental burn injury.[65] Many effects of IL-12 may in fact be related to IL-18 function.[66]

Interleukin-18

Many of the effects of IL-18 are believed to be mediated through the enhancement of IFNγ production.[67,68] IL-18 activates T cells and, in concert with IL-12, promotes T cell differentiation.[66,69] IL-18 administration has been shown to promote clearance of both fungal and bacterial infections in mice. This effect was abrogated through the administration of anti-IL-18 antibodies.[70,71] The role of IL-18 in the response to injury is under study, as is the importance of the IL-18-binding protein as a modifier of IL-18 activity.

Anticytokine Therapy

Given the presumed role that proinflammatory cytokines play in the expression of SIRS and the development of multisystem organ failure, attenuation of an excessive cytokine-driven inflammatory response is an appealing strategy. Both experimental data and theory suggest that effective control of excessive proinflammatory cytokines might benefit patients with severe infection or inflammation. Broad-ranging preclinical and clinical studies have sought to address this concept over the past decade.

Anti-TNF Antibodies

Several experimental studies using specific anti-TNF antibodies during gram-negative sepsis have demonstrated improvement in hemodynamics and survival.[72-75] Decreases in vascular congestion, hemorrhage, leukocyte adhesion, circulatory collapse, and improved left ventricular stroke volume were observed in response to prophylactic therapy with such agents.[74,76] The timing of the administration of this therapy appears crucial. Studies showed that anti-TNF antibody given prior to bacterial or endotoxin challenge was highly effective in preventing circulatory collapse and shock. The benefit of pretreatment seems to be directly related to the kinetics of TNF production: The peak appearance of the bioactive protein occurs within the first 90 minutes of insult, and TNF activity returns to prechallenge levels within 3-4 hours.[9] Thus it appears that any dominant TNF influence occurs early in the inflammatory process. Although some experimental models suggest that a later peak of TNF activity may also contribute to the development of organ injury, this latent effect has proved difficult to confirm directly in clinical studies.[77]

Several experimental studies failed to demonstrate any beneficial effect of anti-TNF therapy, and in some situations it even actually decreased survival. This effect is more readily evident in models of chronic infection/inflammation or with isolated compartmental challenges.[78-80] Similarly, all clinical trials with anti-TNF antibodies in severe SIRS have thus far failed to demonstrate an associated significant decrease in mortality.[81-85]

Soluble TNF Receptors

Soluble TNF receptors (sTNFRs) are derived via cleavage of either of the two cell surface TNF receptors.[84-86] TNFRs have been identified in the blood and urine of acutely septic patients and in chronic disease state.[55,87,88] Following the administration of lipopolysaccharide (LPS), increased levels of sTNFRs are detected in the circulation and persist for several hours beyond the period of TNF ligand detection.[89] We have shown in a primate model that administration of wild-type p55 soluble receptor may have provided some initial improvement in cardiac hemodynamics. This improvement, however, was confined to the period of receptor administration. No overall decrease in mortality was observed once exogenous treatment was terminated.[90]

Recombinant forms of TNFR immunoadhesin-binding proteins have been developed and used in preclinical studies.[91-94] Administration of these proteins has been demonstrated to protect from severe infectious insult. Furthermore, a phase II trial in patients with severe sepsis demonstrated that administration of a p55 TNFR fusion protein, compared to placebo, was associated with a 36% decrease in overall mortality.[94] Unfortunately, more extensive experience with this agent did not demonstrate a significant effect on 28-day mortality. Similarly, clinical studies in humans by Fisher et al. showed that administration of the p75 TNFR fusion protein did not reduce overall mortality, and at higher doses it was associated with increased mortality.[95]

IL-1 Receptor Antagonist

Interleukin-1 binding activity to either IL-1 cell receptor type is effectively prevented by a naturally occurring soluble IL-1 receptor antagonist (IL-1ra).[96,97] IL-1ra is synthesized by many cell lines and binds with high affinity to either of the IL-1 receptors without known agonist activity.[96-99] IL-1ra is released in response to a variety of stimuli including TNF, IL-1β, IL-6, and endotoxin administration in both primate and human models.[100-102] Clinical studies have documented elevated levels of circulating IL-1ra in conditions of trauma, infection, chronic disease, and septic shock.[103,104]

The endogenous production of IL-1ra is insufficient to attenuate the effects of IL-1 fully during severe inflammatory states.[105,106] However, this clinical correlation may not always hold true. For example, in the presence of neonatal sepsis decreased IL-1ra production did not correlate with increased mortality; in fact, higher levels of IL-1ra were detected in adult nonsurvivors than in adult survivors of burn-related sepsis.[107,108]

A recombinant form of the protein has been used extensively in experimental models of infection and other clinically relevant insults. Examples of beneficial effects were the demonstration that IL-1ra administration improved 5-day survival in a murine hemorrhagic shock model and that pretreatment with IL-1ra reduced histologic damage to liver parenchyma in a murine hepatic ischemia/reperfusion model.[109,110]

By contrast, studies in a murine abscess model showed no clinical improvement with IL-1ra administration, and high doses were associated with increased morbidity and mortality.[111] It is now well known that clinical trials of IL-1ra administration in patients with sepsis failed to demonstrate any significant decrease in all-cause mortality compared to controls.[112,113] New isoforms of the receptor antagonist have been cloned and await widespread evaluation.[114]

Antiinflammatory Cytokines

Interleukin-4

Interleukin-4 is produced primarily by T cells, mast cells, and basophils.[115,116] The most prominent effects of IL-4 include B lymphocyte proliferation and immunoglobulin E (IgE) antibody-mediated immunity. IL-4 has been demonstrated to inhibit macrophage production of proinflammatory cytokines, including IL-1, TNF, and IL-6, while promoting IL-1ra production.[117,118] Indeed the production of IL-4 by a subset of CD4$^+$ T cells is believed to define partially an experimental and perhaps clinically significant immune phenotype that may be of consequence in those with severe injury and sepsis. Experimentally, IL-4-deficient mice had increased susceptibility to *Candida* and *Trypanosoma* infections.[60,61] Similarly, exogenous IL-4 administration improved survival of mice infected with gastrointestinal nematodes and pulmonary *Pseudomonas aeruginosa*.[119,120] In contrast, IL-4-deficient mice had improved outcomes compared to those of wild type controls during bacterial septic arthritis and systemic *Salmonella* infection.[57,121] This effect was due in part to an IL-4-mediated decrease in macrophage cytotoxicity. In addition, IL-4 production increased susceptibility of mice to

Leishmania major, and its in vitro administration suppressed neutrophil effector function during systemic fungal infection in both human immunodeficiency virus (HIV)-infected and non-HIV-infected controls.[122,123]

Interleukin-10

Interleukin-10 was isolated from and defined through the study of T-helper (Th2) lymphocytes.[124] IL-10, in part, mediates the inhibition of gene expression and synthesis of several major proinflammatory cytokines, including TNF, IL-1, and IL-6.[106,125] In addition, IL-10 has been shown to enhance IL-1ra synthesis.[118] In vitro studies have shown that IL-10 administration suppresses endotoxin-induced TNF synthesis in monocytes, and IL-10 neutralization led to increased TNF production.[126] More importantly, several studies show that exogenously administered IL-10 or gene transfer in LPS-challenged mice decreases mortality.[127,128] In contrast, in vitro IL-10 administration impaired neutrophil function to fungal challenge in both normal and HIV-infected patients.[124] Plasma levels of IL-10 are often detected in the circulation of patients with sepsis and during experimental and clinical endotoxemia.[104,129–133] The significance of this apparent production and activity to the function of immune effector cells following injury remains under debate.

Macroendocrine Counterregulation

Although more widely studied for its influence on energy regulation and metabolism during severe injury or sepsis, the endocrine system also modulates the postinjury inflammatory environment in important ways. To this end, glucocorticoids and catecholamines have been studied for their role in regulating the pro- and antiinflammatory cytokine response. Glucocorticoids influence the production and modulation of proinflammatory cytokines at multiple levels and blunt the production of IL-1, TNF, and IL-6 at the transcriptional or translational level (or both).[134–138]

Alternatively, proinflammatory cytokines, including TNF and IL-1, also influence the initial (and perhaps subsequent) macroendocrine response to injury.[139] TNF and IL-1 administration led to increased in vitro release of corticotropin-releasing factor and adrenocorticotropic hormone by hypothalamic and pituitary cells.[110,140–142] Interestingly, this effect is experimentally abrogated in vivo through the administration of exogenous glucocorticoids.[143] Similarly, a proinflammatory cytokine blockade leads to diminished glucocorticoid response during severe bacteremia.[144]

Several experimental studies have demonstrated that glucocorticoid administration is protective in septic shock.[11] Dexamethasone also attenuates the release of purported antiinflammatory cytokines (e.g., IL-4 and IL-10) in vitro.[145,146] Glucocorticoid-mediated TNF suppression may be reversed or overcome in vitro by other cytokines, including IFNγ.[136] Finally, in the absence of severe injury, cortisol administration or excess reduces the appearance of TNF during brief human endotoxemia.[147]

Human studies of glucocorticoid administration in the presence of severe SIRS and inflammation have not replicated the more dramatic results of steroid administration in animals. A meta-analysis of nine glucocorticoid therapy clinical trials in septic patients showed no decrease in mortality, and in fact several of the individual studies showed increased mortality.[148]

Like corticosteroids, catecholamines may have potent antiinflammatory effects.[149] For example, norepinephrine has been shown to reduce directly endotoxin-induced TNF and IL-6 in whole blood models.[150] Epinephrine infusion has been shown to reduce the appearance of TNF and IL-1 in dose-dependent fashion after endotoxin administration in human studies; and, importantly, it enhanced IL-10 production.[151–153] This effect was mediated through a combined effect on the α- and β-adrenergic receptors.

Apoptosis

The term apoptosis, or programmed cell death, describes a highly regulated, energy-dependent process by which cellular death and disposal occurs. Though the process is ubiquitous to all cells, the role of programmed cell death in the immune system is of particular importance during states of severe inflammation or infection. Evidence suggests that programmed cell death of immunocytes and perhaps of solid organ parenchymal cells may direct the temporal nature and perhaps the magnitude of the postinjury response. An orderly efficient apoptotic process regulates the systematic deletion of senescent and dysfunctional cells following initial activation or the proliferative response to injury. This process is believed to occur without the release of proinflammatory cytokines or potent chemical mediators, inlcuding toxic granule components and reactive oxygen metabolites.[56,154–157] At sites of inflammation, however, the altered mediator environment may disrupt this process. Several proinflammatory cytokines, including TNF, IL-1, IL-6, IL-8, and granulocyte/macrophage colony-stimulating factor, (GM-CSF), as well as endotoxin, have been shown to reduce or delay immunocyte apoptosis in vitro.[158–161] As a consequence, these cells may predominantly undergo necrosis, with a further release of toxic metabolites into the local environment.[158,162–164] Ultimately, this process may increase the immunocyte half-life and prolong an acute or chronic inflammatory response[165,166] (Fig. 17.1).

Solid organ parenchymal cells have been demonstrated to upregulate proapoptotic pathways in response to local injury.[167–169] Altered solid organ function is influenced by the presence of local inflammatory cells and the ability to maintain their normal metabolic function. It remains to be determined if parenchymal cell apoptosis is increased or decreased in such an inflammatory milieu. Although early death of normally functioning cells is an unwanted consequence of local inflammation, the capacity to delete dysfunctional cells efficiently is critical.

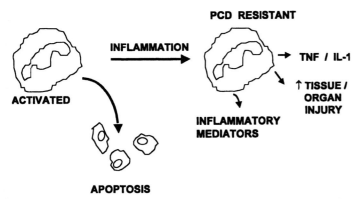

FIGURE 17.1. Programmed cell death (PCD) in immunocyte regulation. Mechanism by which inflammatory states delay immunocyte apoptosis and thus may further direct the temporal nature and perhaps magnitude of the response after injury/sepsis.

Role of Cytokines and Endocrine Hormones in Apoptosis

Proinflammatory Cytokines

Depending on study conditions, TNF may induce, inhibit, or have little influence on neutrophil apoptosis.[154,160,170,171] These effects are also concentration-dependent and vary with cell type and culture conditions in both human and murine cell lines. Neutrophils from healthy subjects suggest that recombinant TNF causes a significant decrease in spontaneous apoptosis, whereas little to no change in the rate of spontaneous apoptosis was observed in neutrophils isolated from septic patients.[154,160]

Specifically, Murray et al. showed that TNF promoted human granulocyte apoptosis within the first 6 hours of culture but had a much more profound inhibitory effect after 12 hours of incubation in vitro.[160] These effects were abolished through co-incubation with anti-TNF antibodies. Watson et al. also demonstrated in a rodent model that granulocytes at sites of inflammation had a varied response to proapoptotic signals compared with circulating neutrophils. Neutrophils obtained by bronchoalveolar lavage in rodents challenged by intratracheal LPS had delayed apoptosis compared to circulating neutrophils challenged with TNF or Fas receptor agonist antibody. The transmigration of neutrophils to sites of inflammation may alter their response to TNF by downregulation of proapoptotic receptors and cellular protein activities.[172,173]

The effect of TNF on macrophage apoptosis is also condition-dependent. TNF has been shown to inhibit spontaneous apoptosis in resting human Langerhans cells.[174] However, during *Mycobacterium tuberculosis* infection, TNF promoted human alveolar macrophage apoptosis.[175] Finally, TNF promotes activated T cell apoptosis in both murine and human lymphocytes.[176–178] This effect is more prominent during the initial postactivation phase (Table 17.1).

The role of IL-1 in immune cell apoptosis is an area of continuing debate. IL-1 has been shown to inhibit neutrophil, monocyte, and lymphocyte cell line apoptosis.[156,179–181] William et al. have shown that not only did IL-1 expression delay neutrophil apoptosis but that this effect was abrogated through the administration of IL-1ra in vitro.[180] However, Friedlander et al. suggested that the IL-1 had divergent effects on cellular apoptosis depending on the timing of administration.[179] They found that IL-1 administered before hypoxia-induced apoptosis led to a delay in apoptosis versus controls, whereas when administered simultaneously with stressor, IL-1 induced apoptosis.[179]

Interleukin-6 is also reported to delay neutrophil and lymphocyte apoptosis while inducing macrophage apoptosis.[188,189,207,209] Biffl et al. showed that IL-6 delayed neutrophil apoptosis in vitro.[164,207]

The role of IL-8 on immune cell apoptosis is currently under investigation. Kettritz et al. found in human in vitro studies that IL-8 inhibited both spontaneous and TNF-mediated neutrophil apoptosis. This effect is dose-dependent.[187]

Antiinflammatory Cytokines

Interleukin-10 may partially reverse the antiapoptotic effect of LPS and TNF in healthy and activated human neutrophils.[191] Cox showed that neutrophils obtained by bronchoalveolar lavage from rats administered LPS and then incubated with IL-10 demonstrated more rapid clearance of inflammation via apoptosis.[191] Similar findings were reported by Keel et al. in human in vitro neutrophil models. Their reported effect was partially mediated through decreased production of TNF and IL-1.[154] Pretreatment of healthy neutrophils with IL-10 followed by proinflammatory cytokine incubation led to preservation of cellular apoptosis. Thus the effect of IL-10 on neutrophil apoptosis is mediated through its inhibition of proinflammatory cytokine production and potentially by interfering with cell responsiveness to apoptotic signals. Interestingly, IL-10

TABLE 17.1. Role of Cytokines and Glucocorticoids in Immune Cell Apoptosis.

Cytokine	Neutrophil	Macrophage	Lymphocyte
TNFα	↑↓[154,160]	↑↓[174,175]	↑[176,177]
IL-1	↑↓[179,180]	↓[156]	↓[181]
IL-4	⇔ ↓[154,174]	↑[182,183]	↓[184–186]
IL-6	↓[187]	↓[188]	⇓[189]
IL-8	↓[187]	?	↑[190]
IL-10	↑[154,191]	↑↓[174,192]	↓[193,194]
IL-12	?	?	↑↓[195,196]
IL-18	?	↑[197]	?
TGFβ	↓[198]	↓[192]	↑[199,200]
IFNγ	↑[154]	⇔[201]	↑[202,203]
Glucocorticoids	↓[204,205]	↑[206]	↑[207,208]

Thin and thick solid arrows, human cells; open arrows, murine cells.

administration alone did not increase or affect the baseline spontaneous rate of neutrophil apoptosis to healthy, unchallenged neutrophils.[154]

Interleukin-10 also been shown to inhibit T cell apoptosis.[193,194] However, the effect of IL-10 on macrophages may be dependent on their state of activation. Ludewig et al. demonstrated that IL-10 induced human Langerhans cell apoptosis.[174] By contrast, Bissinger et al. showed that IL-10 rescued human alveolar macrophages from LPS-induced apoptosis,[192] and Arai et al. demonstrated a similar response to IL-10 administration in infected murine peritoneal macrophages.[210]

Both TNF-induced and Fas-mediated lymphocyte apoptosis is delayed by IL-4.[184–186] Similarly, IL-4 has also been shown to delay or have no effect on neutrophil apoptosis.[154,174] In contrast, IL-4 induces human macrophage apoptosis.[182,183]

Macroendocrine Molecules

The role of glucocorticoids in immunocyte apoptosis is an area of intense research. Steroids appear to have differential effects on various immune cell lines. Glucocorticoids increase lymphocyte and macrophage apoptosis in vitro in both mice and humans,[191,206,208,211–214] whereas they inhibit neutrophil apoptosis in both models.[204,205,215] Kato et al. found this suppressive effect to be dose-dependent for both spontaneous and TNF-mediated neutrophil apoptosis.[205] Their findings were substantiated in that this glucocorticoid effect was reversed by administration of glucocorticoid receptor antagonists in a dose-dependent fashion.[204,205,215]

Conclusions

Despite immense progress in our understanding of the postinjury or infection-induced inflammatory response, no clinical therapeutic intervention dramatically reduces the adverse sequelae of severe inflammation. Although there was early enthusiasm that proinflammatory cytokine blockade would improve such outcomes, current approaches have not proved effective.

The regulation of immune cell apoptosis appears to be an integral aspect of the host's inflammatory response. Dysregulation of normal apoptotic pathways and the inability to delete activated immunocytes from the circulation—and perhaps more importantly from inflamed tissues—may contribute to persistent, potentially morbid inflammatory responses.

Therapy directed at regulating parenchymal and immune cell apoptosis represents an exciting arena for investigation and intervention. Central to such therapy is the avoidance of a profoundly immunocompromised state. Thus determining at what juncture such therapy should be administered may be complex. Understanding the relation between soluble and cell-associated ligands and receptors, and how cellular signaling might be influenced by the degree or stage of the inflammatory response, is essential.

Further study to help identify the markers and signs that predict the clinical appearance of sepsis and multisystem organ failure, as well as large clinical trials, may be the most crucial step in treating this complex condition. Finally, because some inflammation is a necessary adjunct to survival, better understanding of immune cell apoptosis and the development of strategies to control programmed cell death may be a key to maintaining this appropriate immune response.

References

1. Davies M, Hagen P: Systemic inflammatory response syndrome. Br J Surg 1997;84:920–935.
2. Bone R: Toward a theory regarding the pathogenesis of the systemic inflammatory response syndrome: what we do and do not know about cytokine regulation. Crit Care Med 1996;24:163–172.
3. Bone R: Immunologic dissonance: a continuing evolution in our understanding of the systemic inflammatory response and the multiple organ dysfunction syndrome. Ann Intern Med 1996;125:680–687.
4. Nystrom P: The systemic inflammatory response syndrome. J Antimicrob Chemother 1998;41:1–7.
5. Schmand J, Ayala A, Morrison M, et al: Effects of hydroxyethyl starch after trauma hemorrhagic shock: restoration of macrophage integrity and prevention of increased circulating interleukin-6. Crit Care Med 1995;23:806–814.
6. Chaudry I, Ayala A, Ertel W, et al: Hemorrhage and resucitation: immunological aspects. Am J Physiol 1990;259:R663–R678.
7. Meldrum D, Ayala A, Perrin M, et al: Diltiazem restores IL-2, IL-3, IL-6, and IFN-gamma synthesis and decreased host susceptibility to sepsis following hemorrage. J Surg Res 1991;51:158–164.
8. Kunkel S, Remick D, Strieter R, et al: Mechanisms that regulate the production and effects of tumor necrosis factor alpha. Crit Rev Immunol 1989;9:93–117.
9. Michie H, Manogue K, Spriggs D, et al: Detection of circulating tumor necrosis factor after endotoxin administration. N Engl J Med 1988;318:1481–1486.
10. Bauss F, Droge W, Mannel D: Tumor necrosis factor mediates endotoxic effects in mice. Infect Immun 1998;55:1622–1625.
11. Fong Y, Lowry S: Cytokines and the cellular response to injury and infection. In: Care in the ICU, vol 2. New York, Scientific American, 1996.
12. Greenfield LJ, Mulholland M, Oldham K, Zelenock G, Lillemore K. (eds) Surgery: Scientific Principles and Practice, 2nd ed. Philadelphia, Lippincott-Raven 1997;108–131.
13. Moser R, Schleiffenbaum B, Groscurth P, et al: Interleukin 1 and tumor necrosis factor stimulate human vascular endothelial cells to promote transendothelial neutrophil passage. J Clin Invest 1989;83:444–455.
14. Clark R: Basics of cutaneous wound repair. J Dermatol Surg Oncol 1993;19:693–706.
15. Salomon G, Kasid A, Cromack D, et al: The local effects of cachectin/tumor necrosis factor on wound healing. Ann Surg 1991;214:175–180.
16. Girardin E, Grau G, Dayer J, et al: Tumor necrosis factor and interleukin 1 in the serum of children with severe infectious purpura. N Engl J Med 1988;319:397–400.
17. Marks J, Marks C, Luce J, et al: Plasma tumor necrosis factor in patients with septic shock: mortality rate, incidence of adult respiratory distress syndrome. Am Rev Respir Dis 1990;141:94–97.

18. Shalaby M, Halgunset J, Haugen O, et al: Cytokine-associated tissue injury and lethality in mice: a comparative study. Clin Immunol Immunopathol 1991;61:69–82.
19. Waage A, Halstensen A, Espevik T: Association between tumor necrosis factor in serum and fatal outcome in patients with meningococcal disease. Lancet 1987;1:355–357.
20. Mustafa M, Lebel M, Ramilo O, et al: Correlation of interleukin 1 beta and cachectin concentrations in cerebrospinal fluid and outcome from bacterial menigitis. J Pediatr 1989;115:208–213.
21. Tracey K, Beutler B, Lowry S, et al: Shock and tissue injury induced by recombinant human cachectin. Science 1986;234:470–474.
22. Remick D, Kunkel R, Larrick J, et al: Acute in vivo effects of human recombinant tumor necrosis factor. Lab Invest 1987;56:583–590.
23. Bevilacqua M, Pober J, Majeau G, et al: Recombinant tumor necrosis factor induces procoagulant activity in cultured human vascular endothelium: characterization and comparison with the actions of interleukin 1. Proc Natl Acad Sci USA 1986;83:4533–4537.
24. Nawroth P, Stern D: Modulation of endothelial cell hemostatic properties by tumor necrosis factor. J Exp Med 1986;163:740–745.
25. Strieter R, Lynch J III, Basha M, et al: Host responses in mediating sepsis and the adult respiratory distress syndrome. Semin Respir Infect 1990;5:233–247.
26. Tracey K, Lowry S, Cerami A: Cachectin/TNF-alpha in the septic shock and septic adult respiratory distress syndrome. Am Rev Respir Dis 1988;138:1377–1379.
27. Nachman R, Hajjar K, Siverstein R, et al: Interleukin 1 induces endothelial cell synthesis of plasminogen activator inhibitor. J Exp Med 1986;163:1595–1600.
28. Gramse M, Brevario F, Pintucci G, et al: Enhancement by interleukin 1 of plasminogen activator inhibitor activity in cultured human endothelial cells. Biochem Biophys Res Commun 1986;139:720–724.
29. Nawroth P, Handley D, Esmon C, et al: Interleukin 1 induces endothelial cell procoagulant while suppressing cell surface anticoagulant activity. Proc Natl Acad Sci USA 1986;83:3460–3464.
30. Loppnow H, Bil R, Hirt S, et al: Platelet derived interleukin 1 induces cytokine production, but not proliferation of human vascular smooth muscle cells. Blood 1998;91:134–141.
31. Van Dam A, Poole S, Schulzberg M, et al: Effects of peripheral administration of LPS on the expression of immunoreactive interleukin-1 alpha, beta, and receptor antagonist in rat brain. Ann NY Acad Sci 1998;840:128–138.
32. Lang C, Fan J, Wogner M, et al: Role of central IL-1 in regulating peripheral IGF-1 during endotoxemia and sepsis Am J Physiol 1998;274:R956–R962.
33. Fischer E, Marano M, Van Zee K, et al: Interleukin 1 receptor blockade improves survival and hemodynamic performance in Escherichia coli septic shock, but fails to alter host response to sublethal endotoxinemia. J Clin Invest 1992;89:1551–1557.
34. Ohlsson K, Bjork P, Bergenfeldt M, et al: Interleukin 1 receptor antagonist reduces mortality from endotoxin shock. Nature 1990;346:550–552.
35. Alexander H, Doherty G, Buresh C, et al: A recombinant human receptor antagonist interleukin 1 improves survival after lethal endotoxemia in mice. J Exp Med 1991;173:1029–1032.
36. Barriere S, Lowry S: An overview of mortality risk prediction in sepsis. Crit Care Med 1995;23:376–393.
37. Fong Y, Moldawer L, Marano M, et al: Cachectin/TNF or IL-1 alpha induces cachexia with redistribution of body proteins. Am J Physiol 1989;256:R659.
38. Cannon J, Friedberg J, Gelfand J, et al: Circulating interleukin 1B and tumor necrosis concentrations after burn injury in humans. Crit Care Med 1992;20:1414–1419.
39. Mills C, Caldwell M, Gann D: Evidence of plasma-mediated "window" of immunodeficiency in rats following trauma. J Clin Immunol 1989;9:139–150.
40. Browder W, Williams D, Pretus H, et al: Beneficial effect of enhanced macrophage function in the trauma patient. Ann Surg 1990;211:605–612.
41. Akira S, Hirano T, Taga T, et al: Biology of multifunctional cytokines: IL-6 and related molecules (IL-1, and TNF). FASEB, J 1990;4:2860–2867.
42. Kopf M, Baumann H, Freer G, et al: Impaired immune and acute phase responses in interleukin 6 deficient mice. Nature, 1994;368:339–342.
43. Castell J, Gomez-Lechon M, David M, et al: Interleukin-6 is the major regulator of acute phase response protein synthesis in adult human hepatocytes. FEBS, Lett 1989;242:237–239.
44. Gauldie J, Baumann H: Cytokines and acute phase protein expression. In: Kimball E (ed). Cytokines in Inflammation. Toronto, Telford Press, 1991.
45. Heinrich P, Castell J, Andus T: Interleukin 6 and acute phase response. Biochem J 1990;265:621–636.
46. Fong Y, Moldawer L, Marano M, et al: Endotexemia elicits increased circulating b-IFN/IL-6 in man. J Immunol 1989;142:2321–2324.
47. Hack C, DeGroot E, Felt-Bersma R, et al: Increased plasma levels of interleukin 6 in sepsis. Blood 1989;74:1704–1710.
48. Castell J, Gomez-Lechon M, David M, et al: Interleukin-6 is the major regulator of acute phase response protein synthesis in adult human hepatocytes. FEBS Lett 1989;242:237–239.
49. Grzelak I, Olswewski W, Zaleska M, et al: Blood cytokine levels rise even after minor surgical trauma. J Clin Immunol 1996;16:159–163.
50. Calandra T, Gerain J, Heumann D, et al: High circulating levels of IL-6 in patients with septic shock: evolution during sepsis, prognostic value and interplay with other cytokines. Am J Med 1991;91:23–29.
51. Rodriguez J, Miller C, Garner W, et al: Correlation of the local and systemic cytokine response with clinical outcome following thermal injury. J Trauma 1993;34:684–695.
52. Frieling J, van Deuren M, Wijdenes J, et al: Circulating interleukin 6 receptor in patients with sepsis syndrome. J Infect Dis 1995;17:469–472.
53. Martich D, Danner R, Ceska M: Detection of interleukin 8 and tumor necrosis factor in normal humans after intravenous endotoxin: the effect of anti-inflammatory agents. J Exp Med 1991;173:1021–1024.
54. Baggiolini M, Walz A, Kunkel S, et al: Neutrophil-activating peptide-1/interleukin 8, a novel cytokine that activates neutrophils. J Clin Invest 1989;84:1045.
55. Lowry S, Calavano S: Soluble cytokine and hormonal mediators of immunity and inflammation. In: Howard R, Simmons R (eds) Surgical Infectious Diseases. Norwalk, CT, Appleton Lange 1995;313–326.

56. Lin E, Lowry S, Calvano S: The systemic response to injury. In: Schwartz S, Shires T, Spencer F, et al (eds) Principles of Surgery. New York, McGraw-Hill, 1999;3–51.
57. Lampe M, Wilson C, Beva M, et al: Gamma interferon production by cytotoxic T lymphocytes is required for resolution of Chlamydia trachomatis infection. Infect Immun 1998;66: 5457–5461.
58. Cano L, Kashino S, Arruda C, et al: Protective role of gamma interferon in experimental pulmonary paracoccidioidomycosis. Infect Immun 1998;66:800–806.
59. Docke W, Randow F, Syrbe U, et al: Monocyte deactivation in septic patients: restoration by IFN-gamma treatment. Nat Med 1997;3:678–681.
60. Miles R, Paxton T, Dries D, et al: Interferon-gamma increases mortality following cecal ligation and puncture. J Trauma 1994;36:607–611.
61. Wasserman D, Ioannovich J, Hinzmann R, et al: Interferon gamma in the prevention of severe burn-related infections: a European phase III multicenter trail; The Severe Burns Study Group. Crit Care Med 1998;26:419–420.
62. Trincheri G: Proinflammatory and immunoregulatory functions of IL-12. Int Rev Immunol 1998;16:365–396.
63. Gately M, Renzetti L, Magram J, et al: The interleukin 12/interleukin 12 receptor system: role in normal and pathologic immune responses. Annu Rev Immunol 1998;16:495–521.
64. Ertel W, Keel M, Neidhardt R, et al: Inhibition of the defense system stimulating interleukin-12 interferon-γ pathway during critical illness. Blood 1997;89:1612–1620.
65. O'Suilleabhain C, O'Sullivan S, Kelley J, et al: Interleukin-12 treatment restores normal resistance to bacterial challenge after burn injury. Surgery 1996;120:290–296.
66. Kohyama M, Saijyo K, Hayasida M, et al: Direct activation of human $CD8^+$ cytotoxic T lymphocytes by interleukin-18. Jpn J Cancer Res 1988;89:1041–1046.
67. Gillespie M, Horwood N: Interleukin-18: perspectives on the newest interleukin. Cytokine Growth Factor Rev 1998;9:109–116.
68. Tomura M, Maruo S, Mu J, et al: Differential capacities of CD 4^+, CD 8^+, and $CD4^- CD8$ T-cell subsets to express IL-18 receptor and produce IFN-gamma in response to IL-18. J Immunol 1998;160:3759–3765.
69. Stoll S, Jonuleit H, Schmitt E, et al: Production of functional IL-18 by different subtypes of murine and human dendritic cells: DC-derived IL-18 enhances IL-12 dependent Th 1 development. Eur J Immunol 1998;28:3231–3239.
70. Kawakami K, Qureshi M, Zhang T, et al: Il-18 protects mice against pulmonary and disseminated infection with Cryptococcus neoformans by inducing IFN-gamma production. J Immunol 1997;159:5528–5534.
71. Bohn E, Sing A, Zumbihl R, et al: Il-18 regulates early cytokine production in, and promotes resolution of, bacterial infection in mice. J Immunol 1998;160:299–307.
72. Tracey K, Yuman F, Hesse D, et al: Anti-cachectin/TNF monoclonal antibodies prevent septic shock during lethal bacteremia. Nature 1987;330:662–664.
73. Fong Y, Tracey K, Moldawer L, et al: Antibodies to cachectin/tumor necrosis factor reduces interleukin 1 beta and interleukin 6 appearance during lethal bacteremia. J Exp Med 1989; 170: 1627–1633.
74. Hinshaw L, Emerson T, Taylor F, et al: Lethal Staphylococcus aureus-induced shock in primates: prevention of death with anti-TNF antibody. J Trauma 1992;33:568–573.
75. Mohler K, Torrance D, Smith C, et al: Soluble tumor necrosis factor receptors are effective therapeutic agents in lethal endotoxemia and function simultaneously as both carriers and TNF antagonists. J Immunol 1993;151:1548.
76. Vincent J, Bakker J, Marecaux G, et al: Administration of anti-TNF antibody improves left ventricular function in septic shock patients. Chest 1992;101:810–815.
77. Pinsky M: Clinical studies on cytokines in sepsis: role of serum in the development of multiple-systems organ failure. Nephrol Dial Transplant 1994;9:94–98.
78. Eskardri M, Bolgos G, Miller C, et al: Anti-tumor necrosis antibody therapy fails to prevent lethality after cecal ligation and puncture or endotoxinemia. J Immunol 1992;148:2724–2730.
79. Wayte J, Silva A, Krausz T, et al: Observations on the role of tumor necrosis factor in a murine model of shock due to Streptococcus pyogenes. Crit Care Med,1993;21:1207–1212.
80. Sawyer R, Adams R, May A, et al: Anti-tumor necrosis factor antibody reduces mortality in the presence of antibiotic. Arch Surg 1993;128:173–177.
81. Reinhart K, Wiegand-Lohnert C, Grimminger F: Assessment of the safety and efficacy of the monoclonal anti-tumor necrosis factor monoclonal antibody fragment, MAK 195, in patients with sepsis and septic shock: a multicenter, randomized, placebo-controlled, dose ranging study. Crit Care Med 1996;24:733–742.
82. Dhainaut J, Vincent J, Richard C: CDP571, a humanized antibody to human necrosis factor alpha: safety, pharmacokinetics, immune response, and influence of the antibody on the cytokine concentrations in patients with septic shock. Crit Care Med 1995;23:1461–1469.
83. Abraham E, Wunderink R, Silverman H, et al: Efficacy and safety of monoclonal antibody to human tumor necrosis factor alpha in patients with sepsis syndrome: a randomized, controlled, double-blind, multicenter clinical trial; TNF-alpha Mab Sepsis Study Group JAMA 1995;273:934–941.
84. Tartaglia L, Goeddel D: Tumor necrosis factor receptor signaling: a dominant negative mutation suppresses the activation of 55 kDa tumor necrosis factor receptor. J Biol Chem 1992;267:4304–4307.
85. Tartaglia L, Pennica D, Goeddel D: Ligand passing: the 75 kDa tumor necrosis factor receptor recruits TNF signaling by the p55 TNF receptor. J Biol Chem 1993;25:18542–18548.
86. Loetscer H, Stueber D, Banner D, et al: Human tumor necrosis factor alpha mutants with exclusive specificity for the 55 kd or 75 kd TNF receptors. J Biol Chem 1993;268:26350–26357.
87. Engelman H, Aderka A, Rubinstein M, et al: A tumor necrosis factor binding protein purified to homogeneity from human urine protects from tumor necrosis factor toxicity. J Biol Chem 1989;20:11974–11980.
88. Heilig B, Fiehn C, Brockhaus M, et al: Evaluation of soluble tumor necrosis factor receptor antibodies in patients with systemic lupus erythematosus, progressive systemic sclerosis, and mixed connective tissue disease. J Clin Immunol 1993;13:321–328.
89. Neilson D, Kavanagh JP, Rao P: Kinetics of circulating TNF alpha and TNF soluble receptors following surgery in a clinical model of sepsis. Cytokine 1996;8:938–943.
90. Van Zee K, Kohno T, Fischer E, et al: Tumor necrosis factor soluble receptors circulate during experimental and clinical inflammation and can protect against excessive tumor necrosis factor alpha in vitro and in vivo. Proc Natl Acad Sci USA 1992;89:4845–4849.

91. Calvano S, van der Poole T, Coyle S, et al: Monocyte tumor necrosis factor levels as a predictor of risk in human sepsis. Arch Surg 1996;131:434–437.
92. Read R: Experimental therapies for sepsis directed against tumor necrosis factor. J Antimicrob Chemother 1998;41:65–69.
93. Bertini R, Delgado R, Faggioni R, et al: Urinary TNF-binding protein protects mice against the lethal effect of TNF and endotoxin shock. Eur Cytokine Netw 1993;4:39–42.
94. Abraham E, Glauser M, Butler T, et al: P55 tumor necrosis factor fusion protein in the treatment of patients with severe sepsis and septic shock: a randomized controlled multicenter trial; Ro 45-2081 Study Group. JAMA 1997;277:1531–1538.
95. Fisher C, Agosti J, Opal S, et al: Treatment of septic shock with the tumor necrosis factor receptor: Fc fusion protein; the soluble TNF Receptor Sepsis Study Group. N Engl J Med 1996;334:1697–1702.
96. Matsukawa A, Fukumoto T, Maeda T, et al: Detection and characterization of Il-1 receptor antagonist in tissues from healthy rabbits: Il-1 receptor antagonist is probably involved in health. Cytokine 1997;9:307–315.
97. Eisenberg S, Evans R, Arend W, et al: Primary structure and functional expression from complimentary DNA of human interleukin-1 receptor antagonist. Nature 1990;343:341–346.
98. Shimauchi H, Takayama S, Imai-Tanaka T, et al: Balance of interleukin-1 beta and interleukin-1 receptor antagonist in human periapical lesions. J Endod 1998;24:116–119.
99. Dripps D, Brandhuber B, Thompson R, et al: Interleukin -1 (IL-1) receptor antagonist binds to the 80-kDa IL-1 receptor but does not initiate IL-1 signal transduction. J Biol Chem 1991;16:10331–10336.
100. Lumpkin M: The regulation of ACTH secretion by IL-1. Science 1987;238:452–454.
101. Gabay C, Smith M, Eidlen D, et al: Interleukin-1 receptor antagonist is an acute phase protein. J Clin Invest 1997;99:2930–2940.
102. Guirao X, Lowry S. Biologic control of injury and inflammation: much more than too little or too late. World J Surg 1996;20:437–446.
103. Fukomoto T, Matsukawa A, Ohkawara S, et al: Administration of neutralizing antibody against rabbit IL-1 receptor antagonist exacerbates lipopolysaccharide induced arthritis in rabbits. Inflamm Res 1996;45:479–485.
104. Kasai T, Inada K, Takakuwa Y, et al: Anti-inflammatory cytokine levels in patients with septic shock. Res Commun Mol Pathol Pharmacol 1997;98:34–42.
105. Dinarello C, Wolff S: The role of IL-1 in disease. N Engl J Med 1993;328:106–113.
106. Fischer E, Van Zee K, Marano M, et al: Interleukin-1 receptor antagonist circulates in the experimental inflammation and human disease. Blood 1992;79:2196–2200.
107. De Bont E, de Leij L, Okken A, et al: Increased plasma concentrations of interleukin 1 receptor antagonist in neonatal sepsis. Pediatr Res 1995;37:626–629.
108. Endo S, Inada K, Yamada Y, et al: Plasma levels of interleukin 1 receptor antagonist and severity of illness in patients with burns. J Exp Med 1996;27:57–61.
109. Pellicane J, DeMaria E, Abd-Elfattah A, et al: Interleukin-1 receptor antagonist improves survival and preserves organ adenosine-5′-triphosphate after hemorrhagic shock. Surgery 1993;114:278–284.
110. Shito M, Wakabayashi G, Ueda M, et al: Interleukin-1 receptor blockade reduces tumor necrosis factor production, tissue injury, and mortality after hepatic ischemia/reperfusion in the rat. Transplantation 1997;63:143–148.
111. Colagiovanni DB, Shopp GM: Evaluation of interleukin-1 receptor antagonist and tumor necrosis factor binding protein in a rodent abscess model of host resistance. Immunopharmacol Immunotoxicol 1996;18:397–419.
112. Fisher C, Slotman G, Opal S, et al: Initial evaluation of human interleukin-1 receptor antagonist in the treatment of sepsis syndrome: a randomized, open-labeled, placebo-controlled multicenter trial. Crit Care Med 1994;22:12–21.
113. Opal S, Fisher C, Dhainaut J, et al: Confirmatory interleukin 1 receptor antagonist trial in severe sepsis: a phase III, randomized, double-blinded, placebo controlled, multicenter trial. Crit Care Med 1997;25:1115–1124.
114. Mantovani A, Musio M, Ghezzi P, et al: Regulation of inhibitory pathways of the interleukin-1 system: Ann NY Acad Sci 1998;840:338–351.
115. Chomarat P, Banchereau J: An update on interleukin-4 and its receptor. Eur Cytokine Netw 1997;8:33–34.
116. Brown M, Hural J: Functions of IL-4 and control of its expression. Crit Rev Immunol 1997;17:1–32.
117. Banchereau J: Converging and diverging properties of human interleukin-4 and interleukin-10. Behring Inst Mitt 1995;96:58–77.
118. Marie C, Pitton C, Fitting C: IL-10 and IL-4 synergize with TNF alpha to induce IL-1ra production by human neutrophils. Cytokine 1996;8:147–151.
119. Urban J, Maliszewski C, Madden K, et al: IL-4 treatment can cure established gastrointestinal nematode infections in immunocomponent and immunodeficient mice. J Immunol 1995;154:4675–4684.
120. Jain-Vora S, Le Vine A, Chroneos Z, et al: Interleukin 4 enhances pulmonary clearance of *Pseudomonas aeruginosa*. Infect Immun 1998;66:4229–4236.
121. Hultgren O, Kopf M, Tarkowski A, et al: *Staphylococcus aureus*-induced septic arthritis and septic death is decreased in IL-4 deficient mice: role of IL-4 as promoter for bacterial growth. J Immunol 1998;160:5082–5087.
122. Himmelrich H, Parra-Lopez C, Tacchini-Cottier F, et al: The IL-4 rapidly produced in BALB/c mice after infection with Leishmania major down-regulates IL-12 receptor beta 2-chain expression on $CD4^+$ T cells resulting in a state of unresponsiveness to IL-12. J Immunol 1998;161:6156–6163.
123. Tascini C, Baldelli F, Monari C, et al: Inhibition of fungicidal activity of polymorphonuclear leukocytes from HIV-infected patients by interleukin-4 and IL-10. AIDS 1996;10:477–483.
124. Opal S, Wherry J, Grint P: Interleukin-10: potential benefits and possible risks in clinical infectious diseases. Clin Infect Dis 1998;27:1497–1507.
125. De Waal Malefyt R, Abrams J, Bennet B, et al: Interleukin-10 inhibits cytokine synthesis by human monocytes: an autoregulatory role of IL-10 produced by monocytes. J Exp Med 1991;174:1209–1220.
126. Marchant A, Bruyns C, Vandenabelle P, et al: IL-10 controls IFN-gamma and TNF production by activated macrophages. Eur J Immunol 1994;24:1167–1171.
127. Rogy M, Auffenberg T, Espat N, et al: Human tumor necrosis factor receptor and interleukin 10 gene transfer in the mouse

reduces mortality to lethal endotoxemia and also attenuates local inflammatory responses. J Exp Med 1995;181:2289–2293.
128. Marchant A, Vincent J, Goldman M: Interleukin 10 as a protective cytokine produced during sepsis. In: Morrison J, Ryans. (eds) Novel Strategies in the Treatment of Sepsis. 1996; 301–311.
129. Marchant A, Deviere B, Byl B, et al: Interleukin 10 production during septicemia. Lancet 1994;343:707–708.
130. Derkx B, Marchant M, Goldman R, et al: High levels of interleukin 10 during the initial phase of fulminant meningoccal septic shock. J Infect Dis 1995;171:229–232.
131. Parsons P, Moss M, Vannice J, et al: Circulating Il-1ra and IL-10 levels are increased but do not predict the development of acute respiratory distress syndrome in at risk patients. Am J Respir Crit Care Med 1997;155:1469–1473.
132. Han J, Thompson F, Beutler B: Dexamethasone and pentoxifiline inhibit endotoxin induced cachectin tumor necrosis factor synthesis at separate points in the signaling pathway. J Exp Med 1990;172:391–394.
133. Van der Poll T, Jansen P, Montegut, et al: Effects of IL-10 on systemic inflammatory responses during sublethal primate endotoxemia. J Immunol 1997;158:1971–1975.
134. Van der Poll T, de Waal Malefyt R, Coyle S, et al: Antiinflammatory cytokine responses during clinical sepsis and experimental endotoxemia: sequential measurements of plasma soluble interleukin-1 receptor type II, IL-10, and IL-13. J Infect Dis 1997;175:110–122.
135. Zuckerman S, Shellhaas J, Butler L: Differential regulation of lipopolysaccharide induced interleukin-1 and tumor necrosis factor and synthesis: effects of endogenous glucocorticoids and the role of the pituitary-adrenal axis. Eur J Immunol 1989; 19:301–305.
136. Luedke C, Cerami A: Interferon gamma overcomes glucocorticoid suppression of cachectin/tumor necrosis factor biosynthesis by murine macrophages. J Clin Invest 1990;86:1234–1240.
137. Ray A, LaForge K, Sehgal P: On the mechanism for efficient repression of the interleukin-6 promoter by glucocorticoids: enhancer, TATA box, and RNA start site occlusion. Mol Cell Biol 1990;10:5736–5746.
138. Brown E, Dare H, Marsh C, et al: The combination of endotoxin and dexamethasone induces type II interleukin-1 receptor in monocytes: a comparison to interleukin-1 beta and interleukin-1 receptor antagonist. Cytokine 1996;8:828–836.
139. Horai R, Asano M, Sudo K, et al: Production of mice deficient in genes for IL-1 alpha, Il-1 beta, Il-1 alpha/beta, and Il-1 receptor antagonist shows that Il-1 beta is crucial in turpentine induced fever development and glucocortioid secretion. J Exp Med 1988;187:1463–1475.
140. Bernton E, Beach J, Holaday J, et al: Release of multiple hormones by direct action of interleukin 1 on pituitary cells. Science 1997;230:519–521.
141. Berkenbosch F, van Oers J, del Rey A, et al: Corticotropin-releasing factor producing neurons in the rat activated by interleukin 1. Science 1987;238:522–524.
142. Sapolsky R, Rivier C, Yamamot G, et al: Interleukin 1 stimulates the secretion of hypothalamic corticotropin-releasing factor. Science 1987;238:522–524.
143. Bernardini R, Kamilaris T, Calogero A, et al: Interactions between tumor necrosis factor alpha, hypothalamic corticotropin-releasing hormone, and adrenocorticotropin secretion in the rat. Endocrinology 1990;126:2876–2881.
144. Gwosdow A: Mechanisms of interleukin 1 induced hormone secretion from rat adrenal gland. Endocr Res 1995;21:25–37.
145. Joyce DA, Steer J, Kloda A: Dexamethasone antagonizes IL-4 and IL-10 induced release of IL-1ra by monocytes but augments IL-4, Il-10, and TGF beta induced suppression of TNF alpha release. J Interferon Cytokine Res 1996;16:511–517.
146. Sauer J, Castren M, Hopfner U, et al: Inhibition of lipopolysaccharide induced monocyte interleukin-1 receptor antagonist synthesis by cortisol: involvement of mineralocorticoid receptor. J Clin Endocrinol Metab 1996;81:73–79.
147. Barber A, Coyle S, Marano M, et al: Glucocorticoid therapy alters hormonal and cytokine response to endotoxin in man. J Immunol 1993;150:1999–2006.
148. Natanson C: Anti-inflammatory therapies to treat sepsis and septic shock: a reassessment. Crit Care Med 1997;25:1095–1099.
149. Pastores S, Hasko G, Vizi E, et al: Cytokine production and its manipulation by vasoactive drugs. New Horiz 1996;4:252–264.
150. Van der Poll T, Jansen J, Endert E, et al: Noradrenaline inhibits lipopolysaccharide-induced tumor necrosis factor and interleukin 6 production in human whole blood. Infect Immun 1994;62:2046.
151. Van der Poll T, Braxton C, Coyle S, et al: Effect of epinephrine on cytokine release during human endotoxemia. Surg Forum 1995;46:102.
152. Van der Poll T, Coyle S, Barbosa K, et al: Epinephrine inhibits tumor necrosis factor-alpha and potentiates interleukin 10 production during human endotoxemia. J Clin Invest 1996;97:713–719.
153. Van der Poll T, Lowry S: Epinephrine inhibits endotoxin-induced IL-1 beta production: roles of tumor necrosis factor-alpha and IL-10. Am J Physiol 1997;273:1885–1890.
154. Keel M, Ungethum U, Steckholzer U, et al: Interleukin-10 counteregulates proinflammatory cytokine – induced inhibition of neutrophil apoptosis during severe sepsis. Blood 1997;90:3356–3363.
155. Cohen J: Programmed cell death in the immune system. Adv Immunol 1991;50:55.
156. Haslett C, Savill JS, Whyte M, et al: Granulocyte apoptosis and the control of inflammation. Philos Trans R Soc Lond B 1994;345:327.
157. Haslett C: Resolution of acute inflammation and the role of apoptosis in the tissue fate of granulocytes. Clin Sci 1992;83:639.
158. Colotta F, Polentarutti N, Sozzani S, et al: Modulation of granulocyte survival and programmed cell death by cytokines and bacterial products. Blood 1992;80:2012.
159. Lee A, Whyte M, Haslett C: Inhibition of apoptosis and prolongation of neutrophil functional longevity by inflammatory mediators. J Leukoc Biol 1993;54:283.
160. Murray J, Barbara J, Dunkley S, et al: Regulation of neutrophil apoptosis by tumor necrosis factor-alpha: requirement for TNFR 55 and TNFR 75 for induction of apoptosis in vitro. Blood 1997;90:2772–2783.
161. Brach M, de Vos S, Gruss H, et al: Prolongation of survival of human polymorphonuclear neutrophils by granulocyte-macrophage colony-stimulating factor is caused by inhibition of programmed cell death. Blood 1992;80:2920.
162. Chitnis D, Dickerson C, Munster A, et al: Inhibition of apoptosis in polymorphonuclear neutrophils from burn patients. J Leukoc Biol 1996;59:835–839.
163. Ertel W, Keele M, Infanger M, et al: Circulating mediators in serum of injured patients with septic complication inhibit

neutrophil apoptosis through upregulation of protein-tyrosine phosphorylation. J Trauma 1998;44:767–775.
164. Biffl W, Moore E, Moore F, et al: Interleukin 6 delays neutrophil apoptosis. Arch Surg 1996;131:24–30.
165. Saville DJ, Wyllie A, Henson J, et al: Macrophage phagocytosis of aging neutrophils in inflammation: programmed cell death in the neutrophil leads to its recognition by macrophages. J Clin Invest 1989;83:865–875.
166. Whyte EM, Meagher L, MacDermot J, et al: Impairment of function in aging neutrophils is associated with apoptosis. J Immunol 1993;150:5124–5134.
167. Ogasawara J, Watanabe-Funkunaga R, Adachi M, et al: Lethal effect of the anti-Fas antibody in mice. Nature 1993;377;348–351.
168. Galle P, Hofmann W, Walczak H, et al: Involvement of the CD95 receptor and ligand in liver damage. J Exp Med 1995;11:1223–1230.
169. Leist CM, Gatner F, Bohlinger I, et al: Tumor necrosis-induced hepatocyte apoptosis preceeds liver failure in experimental murine shock models. Am J Pathol 1995;146:1220–1234.
170. Hsu H, Xiong I, Goeddel D, et al: The TNF receptor 1-associated protein TRADD signals cell death and NF-κB activation. Cell 1995;81:495–504.
171. Tsuchida H, Tekeda Y, Takei H, et al: In vivo regulation of rat neutrophil apoptosis occurring spontaneously or induced with TNF-α or cyclohexamide. J Immunol 1995;154:2403.
172. Watson W, Rotstein O, Parodo J, et al: Impaired apoptotic death signalling in inflammatory lung neutrophils is associated with decreased expression of interleukin 1 beta converting enzyme family proteases. Surgery 1997;122:163–172.
173. Watson R, Rotstein O, Nathenes A, et al: Neutrophil apoptosis is modulated by endothelial transmigration and adhesion molecule engagement. J Immunol 1997;158:945–953.
174. Ludewig B, Graf D, Gelderblom H, et al: Spontaneous apoptosis of dendritic cells is efficiently inhibited by TRAP and TNF-alpha, but strongly enhanced by interleukin-10. Eur J Immunol 1995;25:1943–1950.
175. Balcewicz-Sablinska M, Keane J, Kornfeld H, et al: Pathogenic Mycobacterium tuberculosis evades apoptosis of host macrophages by release of TNF-R2, resulting in inactivation of TNF-alpha. J Immunol 1998;161:2636–2641.
176. Klein S, Dobmeyer J, Dobmeyer T, et al: TNF alpha mediated apoptosis of CD4 positive T-lymphocytes: a model of T cell depletion in HIV infected individuals. Eur J Med Res 1996;5:249–258.
177. Ware C, Van Arsdale S, Van Arsdale T: Apoptosis mediated by the TNF-related cytokine and receptor families. J Cell Biochem 1996;60:47–55.
178. Zheng L, Fisher G, Miller R, et al: Induction of apoptosis in mature T cells by tumor necrosis factor. Nature 1995;377:348–351.
179. Tatsuta T, Cheng J, Mountz J, et al: Intracellular IL-1 beta is an inhibitor of fas mediated apoptosis. J Immunol 1996;157:3949–3957.
180. William R, Watson G, Rotstein O, et al: The IL-1 beta-converting enzyme inhibits apoptosis of inflammatory neutrophil through activation of IL-1 beta. J Immunol 1998;161:957–962.
181. Furukawa Y, Kikuchi J, Terui Y, et al: Preferential production of interleukin 1 beta over interleukin 1 receptor antagonist contributes to proliferation and suppression of apoptosis in leukemic cells. Jpn J Cancer Res 1995;86:208–216.

182. Yamamoto M, Kawabata K, Fujihashi K, et al: Absence of exogenous interleukin-4-induced apoptosis of gingival macrophages may contribute to chronic inflammation in periodontal diseases. Am J Pathol 1996;148:331–339.
183. Mangan D, Robertson B, Wahl S, et al: IL-4 enhances programmed cell death in stimulated human monocytes. J Immunol 1992;148:1812–1816.
184. Manna S, Aggarwal B: Interleukin-4 down regulates both forms of tumor necrosis factor receptor and receptor-mediated apoptosis, NF-kappaB, AP-1, and c-Jun N-terminal kinase: comparison with interleukin 13. J Biol Chem 1998;273:33333–33341.
185. Foote L, Marshak-Rothstein A, Rothstein T: Tolerant B lymphocytes acquire resistance to Fas-mediated apoptosis after treatment with interleukin 4 but not after treatment with specific antigen unless a surface immunoglobulin threshold is exceeded. J Exp Med 1998;187:847–853.
186. Foote L, Howard R, Marshak-Rothstein A, et al: Il-4 induces Fas resistance in B-cells. J Immunol 1996;157:2749–2753.
187. Kettritz R, Gaido M, Haller H, et al: Interleukin 8 delays spontaneous and tumor necrosis factor alpha–mediated apoptosis of human neutrophils. Kidney Int 1998;53:84–91.
188. Afford S, Pongracz J, Stockley R, et al: The induction by human interleukin-6 of apoptosis in the promonocytic cell lnie U937 and human neutrophils. J Biol Chem 1992;267:21612–21616.
189. Teague T, Marrack P, Kappler J, et al: IL-6 rescues resting mouse T cells from apoptosis. J Immunol 1996;157:3949–3957.
190. Terui Y, Ikeda M, Tomizuka H, et al: Activated endothelial cells induce apoptosis in leukemic cells by endothelial interleukin 8. Blood 1998;92:2672–2680.
191. Cox G: IL-10 enhances resolution of pulmonary inflammation in vivo by prompting apoptosis of neutrophils. Am J Physiol 1996;L566–L570.
192. Bissinger R, Stey C, Weller M, et al: Apoptosis in human alveolar macrophages is induced by endotoxin and is modulated by cytokines. Am J Respir Cell Mol Biol 1996;15:64–70.
193. Cohen B, Crawley J, Kahan M, et al: Interleukin-10 rescues T cells from apoptotic cell death: association with an upregulation of Bcl-2. Immunology 1997;92:1–5.
194. Pawelec G, Hambrecht A, Rehbein A, et al: Interleukin 10 protects activated human T lymphocytes against growth factor withdrawal-induced cell death but only anti-Fas antibody can prevent activation-induced cell death. Cytokine 1996;8:877–881.
195. Radrizzani M, Accornero P, Amidei A, et al: IL-12 inhibits apoptosis induced in a human Th1 clone by gp 120/CD4 crosslinking and CD3/TCR activation or by IL-2 deprivation. Cell Immunol 1995;161:14–21.
196. Marth T, Strober W, Kelsall B, et al: High dose oral tolerance in ovalbulmin TCR-transgenic mice: systemic neutralization of IL-12 augments TGF-beta secretion and T cell apoptosis. J Immunol 1996;157:2348–2357.
197. Ohtsuki T, Micallef M, Kohno K, et al: Interleukin 18 enhances Fas ligand expression and induces apoptosis in Fas-expressing human myelomonocytic KG-1 cells. Anticancer Res 1997;17:3253–3258.
198. Ward C, Hannah S, Chilvers E, et al: Transforming growth factor-beta increases the inhibitory effects of GM-CSF and dexamethasone on neutrophil apoptosis. Biochem Soc Trans 1997;25:244S.
199. Saltzman A, Murro R, Searfoss G, et al: Transforming growth factor-beta-mediated apoptosis in the Ramos B-lymphoma cell

199. line is accompanied by caspase activation and Bcl-XL downregulation. Exp Cell Res 1998;242:244–254.
200. Lomo J, Blomhoff H, Beiske K, et al: TGF-beta 1 and cyclic AMP promote apoptosis in resting human B lymphocytes. J Immunol 1995;154:1634–1643.
201. Ranjan P, Sodhi A, Singh S, et al: Murine peritoneal macrophages treated with cisplatin and interferon-gamma undergo NO-mediated apoptosis via activation of an endonuclease. Anticancer Drugs 1998;9:333–341.
202. Novelli F, Bernabei P, Ozmen L, et al: Swithching on the proliferation or apoptosis of activated human T lymphocytes by IFN-gamma is correlated with differential expression of the alpha- and beta-chains of its receptor. J Immunol 1996;157:1935–1943.
203. Selleri C, Sato T, Anderson S, et al: Interferon-gamma and tumor necrosis factor-alpha suppress both early and late stages of hematopoiesis and induce programmed cell death. J Cell Physiol 1995;165:538–546.
204. Nittoh T, Fujimori H, Kozumi Y, et al: Effects of glucorticoids on apoptosis on infiltrated eosinophils and neutrophils in rats. Eur J Pharmacol 1998;354:73–81.
205. Kato T, Takeda Y, Nakada T, et al: Inhibition by dexamethasone of human neutrophil apoptosis in vitro. Nat Immun 1995;14:198–208.
206. Horigome A, Hirano T, Oka K, et al: Glucocorticoids and cyclosporine induce apoptosis in mitogen-activated human peripheral mononuclear cells. Immunopharmacology 1997;37:87–94.
207. Biffl W, Moore E, Moore F, et al: Interleukin 6 delays neutrophil apoptosis via a mechanism involving platelet activating factor. J Trauma 1996;40:575–577.
208. Schwartzman R, Cidlowski J: Glucocorticoid-induced apoptosis of lymphoid cells. Int Arch Allergy Immunol 1994;105:347–354.
209. Oritani K, Kaisho T, Nakajima, et al: Retinoic acid inhibits interleukin-6-induced macrophage differentiation and apoptosis in a murine hematopoietic cell line, Y6. Blood 1992;80:2298–2305.
210. Arai T, Hiromatsu K, Nishimura H, et al: Endogenous interleukin 10 prevents apoptosis in macrophages during Salmonella infection. Biochem Biophys Res Commun 1995;213:600–607.
211. Meagher L, Cousin J, Seckl J, et al: Opposing effects of glucocorticoids on the rate of apoptosis in neutrophilic and eosinophilic granulocytes. J Immunol 1996;156:4422–4428.
212. Kato Y, Morikawa A, Sugiyama T, et al: Role of tumor necrosis factor alpha and glucocorticoid on lipopolysaccharide induced apoptosis of thymocytes. FEMS Immunol Med Microbiol, 1995;12:195–204.
213. Gruol D, Bourgeois S: Expression of the mdr1 P-glycoprotein gene: a mechanism of escape from glucocorticoid-induced apoptosis. Biochem Cell Biol 1994;72:561–571.
214. Cox G: Glucocorticoid treatment inhibits apoptosis in human neutrophils: separation of survival and activation outcomes. J Immunol 1995;154:4719–4725.
215. Murosaki S, Inagaki-Ohara K, Kusaka H, et al: Apoptosis of intestinal intraepithelial lymphocytes induced by exogenous and endogenous glucocorticoids. Microbiol Immunol 1997;41:139–148.

18
Reactive Oxygen Species in Clinical Practice

Aruna Nathan and Mervyn Singer

Reactive oxygen species (ROSs) are oxidants produced in both health and disease by various processes, for example, from the phagocytic respiratory burst, during mitochondrial aerobic respiration, and as a by-product of both ischemia and reperfusion. In health, ROSs serve a variety of roles, including defense, cell signaling, and as a trigger for inflammation (Fig. 18.1). A number of endogenous mechanisms are in place to protect the body against excessive oxidant effect, including circulating antioxidants (e.g., albumin) intracellular antioxidants (e.g., reduced glutathione), and specific enzymes (e.g., superoxide dismutase) (Table 18.1). When the equilibrium is grossly disrupted by excess production of oxidants or loss of endogenous defenses, widespread damage can ensue to protein, lipid, DNA, and mitochondria. This damage is implicated in various local or systemic clinical syndromes, such as after reperfusion of an ischemic heart, limb, or bowel, or with acute respiratory distress syndrome (ARDS) or sepsis.

Chemistry

Reactive oxygen species may or may not contain one or more unpaired electrons (e). Those that do are termed free radicals. Oxygen exists in air in a molecular form (O_2, dioxygen) that contains two unpaired electrons. In this form, oxygen is not highly reactive, as the electrons have the same spin quantum number (parallel spin). Only when this spin restriction is overcome does oxygen become highly reactive.

Formation of Reactive Oxygen and Nitrogen Species

Reactive oxygen species can be formed in the body via several mechanisms (Fig. 18.2). Aerobic metabolism, the most efficient method of generating energy from metabolic substrate, utilizes O_2 to generate adenosine triphosphate (ATP). During this process, O_2 is reduced via a series of reactions to generate ROSs, including hydroperoxyl and hydroxyl free radicals and hydrogen peroxide. At physiologic pH the hydroperoxyl radical dissociates into the superoxide radical, which can be further converted to other reactive oxygen species.

$$O_2^{\bullet} + e + H^+ \to HO_2^{\bullet} \quad \text{(hydroperoxyl radical)}$$
$$HO_2^{\bullet} \to H^+ + O_2^{\bullet} \quad \text{(superoxide radical)}$$
$$O_2^{\bullet} + 2H^+ + e \to H_2O_2 \quad \text{(hydrogen peroxide)}$$
$$H_2O_2 + e \to {}^{\bullet}OH^- + OH^{\bullet} \quad \text{(hydroxyl radical)}$$
$$OH^{\bullet} + e + H^+ \to H_2O$$

The clinically relevant species are the superoxide radical, hydrogen peroxide, and the highly reactive hydroxyl radicals. Superoxide ($O_2^{\bullet}$) is formed by adding one electron to O_2. Its reactivity is variable. Superoxide is a weak oxidizing agent, though it is a strong reductive agent able to reduce iron-containing complexes such as cytochrome c. Superoxide dismutates into hydrogen peroxide (H_2O_2) and H_2O in solution. This reaction is accelerated by the presence of the enzyme superoxide dismutase (SOD).[1] This enzyme is found in various forms in plant and animal cells and forms an important defense mechanism against oxidative stress. The $HO_2^{\bullet}$ radical is highly reactive but is present only in minute quantities at physiologic pH. H_2O_2 is much less reactive and is stable in the absence of transitional metal ions. It readily diffuses across biologic membranes and can form the highly reactive hydroxyl ($OH^{\bullet}$) radical in the presence of metal ions, especially iron and copper. It is removed by enzymes, including catalase and glutathione peroxidase. The $OH^{\bullet}$ radical is a powerful oxidant that can cause severe tissue damage. The presence of iron accelerates the formation of $OH^{\bullet}$ from H_2O_2, as described by the Fenton reaction.[2]

$$Fe^{2+} + H_2O_2 \to Fe^{3+} + OH^- + OH^{\bullet}$$
$$Fe^{3+} + H_2O_2 \to Fe^{2+} + HO_2^{\bullet} + H^+$$

Ferrous (Fe^{2+}) Hiron is rapidly oxidized to ferric (Fe^{3+}) iron in the presence of phosphate and O_2. $O_2^{\bullet}$ is formed by the addition of one electron to O_2 during this process, as is perferryl iron ($Fe^{2+} O_2$ and $Fe^{3+} O_2^{\bullet}$).

Hypochlorous acid (HOCl), formed by the enzyme myeloperoxidase, catalyzes the formation of HOCl from H_2O_2 and chloride ions in phagocytes. HOCl can itself generate $OH^{\bullet}$.[3,4]

Some of the oxides of nitrogen are free radicals, as they also have unpaired electrons. They include the nitrosyl radical,

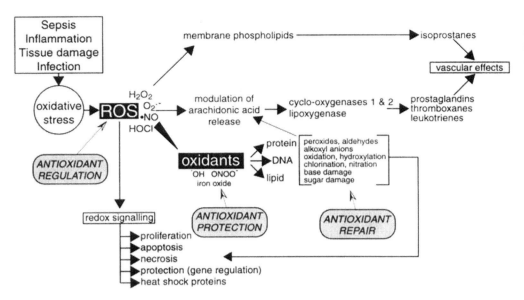

FIGURE 18.1. Putative role of reactive oxygen species in modulating inflammation, cell signaling, and tissue damage.

produced by the one-electron reduction of nitric oxide ($NO^{\bullet}$), and nitrogen dioxide ($NO_2^{\bullet}$). These reactive oxygen species may affect other biological molecules by oxidation, nitration, or nitrosalation.[5,6]

Studies have shown both cytotoxic and cytoprotective roles for NO.[5,7,8] These roles may or may not involve the generation of reactive NO species.[9–11]

In the presence of $O_2^{\bullet}$, RNOSs such as peroxynitrite ($ONOO^-$) and N_2O_3 are formed.[12,13] Concomitant generation of NO and $O_2^{\bullet}$ produces $ONOO^-$, a more highly reactive molecule than either of its congenitors; but it may not be particularly toxic in normal situations.[7] Nitric oxide synthase may also generate $NO^{\bullet}$ directly,[14,15] which can be reduced to NO by electron acceptors such as superoxide dismutase.

$$NO^{\bullet} + SOD\ (Cu^{2+}) \rightarrow NO + SOD\ (Cu^{3+})$$

Nitric oxide may also be generated indirectly through the formation of N-hydroxy-L-arginine (HO-Arg), which generates $NO^{\bullet}$ under conditions of oxidative stress.[16,17] $NO^{\bullet}$ can also be formed during the decomposition of S-nitrosothiols and in conditions of nitrosative stress.[18] The cytotoxic effect of $NO^{\bullet}$ can result in DNA double strand breaks.[19] This effect is enhanced by oxygen, which may continue the process of lipid peroxidation initiated by $NO^{\bullet}$ or can enhance generation of $ONOO^-$. Toxicity might be influenced by low cellular levels of reduced glutathione (GSH). $NO^{\bullet}$ oxidizes thiols including GSH, thereby enhancing the toxicity of RNOSs and ROSs. Co-generation of $NO^{\bullet}$ and ROS may also enhance the toxicity of H_2O_2 owing to reduced levels of intracellular GSH.[5]

TABLE 18.1. Examples of Antioxidants.

Antioxidant	Mode of action
Enzyme antioxidants	
Glutathione peroxidase	Removal of H_2O_2, hydroperoxides
Superoxide dismutase	Catalytic removal of O_2
Catalase	Catalytic reduction of H_2O_2 to H_2O
Non enzymatic antioxidants	
Membrane antioxidants	
Vitamin E	Chain-breaking antioxidant
β-Carotene	Scavenger of ROS
Coenzyme Q	?Antioxidant role
Compounds that reduce availability of transition metals	
Transferrin	Binds ferric iron
Lactoferrin	Binds ferric iron at lower pH
Haptoglobins	Bind hemoglobin
Albumin	Binds heme and copper
Scavengers	
Bilirubin	Scavenges peroxyl radicals
Uric acid	Scavenges FOR (Free Oxygen Radicals)
Ascorbic acid	Scavenges hydroxyl radical
Mucus	Scavenges hydroxyl radicals
Ceruloplasmin	Scavenges $O_2^{\bullet}$, binds copper ions
Thiol group donors	
Reduced glutathione (GSSH)	Binds free radical, SH group oxidized to disulfide group (GSSG)
Synthetic antioxidants	
N-Acetylcysteine	Increases intracellular GSSH
Desferrioxamine	Heavy metal chelator
Allopurinol	Xanthine oxidase inhibitor
Lazaroids	Free radical scavengers; inhibitors of lipid peroxidation
Mannitol	Free radical scavenger

Lipid Peroxidation

Free radicals oxidize lipids, proteins, and DNA. The oxidation of polyunsaturated fatty acids, termed lipid peroxidation, involves a chain reaction that progresses through three stages: initiation, propagation, and termination.[20] When a hydrogen atom is removed by a free radical from a methylene group

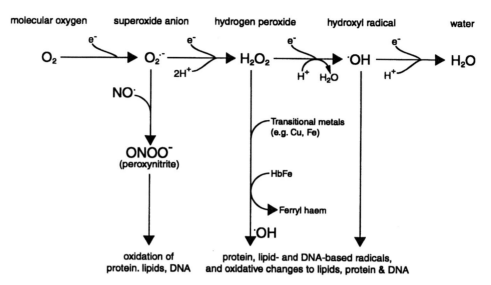

FIGURE 18.2. Derivation of reactive oxygen and nitrogen oxygen species (NO•, nitric oxide; Cu, copper; Fe, iron; e^-, unpaired electron; O_2^-, superoxide; OH•, hydroxyl radical; DNA, deoxyribonucleic acid).

(–CH2–), an unpaired electron is left behind on the carbon atom (–•CH–). This is the process of initiation. Compounds that can initiate lipid peroxidation include OH•, alkoxyl (RO•), and peroxyl (ROO•) radicals. Alkoxyl radicals are formed when reduced or oxidized metal complexes react with lipid peroxides. The radical then undergoes a conformational change to form a conjugated diene, which can directly react with O_2 to form peroxyl radicals (ROO•). The peroxyl radical is a powerful oxidant, and the process is thereby continued.

Lipid peroxides are stable except in the presence of transitional metals or metal complexes. Iron complexes can accelerate lipid peroxide decomposition, as can heme proteins such as hemoglobin and the cytochromes, by releasing chelatable iron.[21] Iron ions are free radicals that play a vital role in lipid peroxidation by catalyzing the formation of the highly reactive OH• from $O_2^{\bullet-}$. This action is probably site-specific, as the iron and copper complexes are normally bound to specific molecules. The peroxidation reaction is usually terminated when it reaches a protein. These damaged proteins are detected in and removed from the cell.[22,23]

Markers of ROS Generation

Electron spin resonance (ESR) spectroscopy is the only technique that measures free radical activity directly. Compounds ("spin traps") that react with the free radicals to form more stable adducts can be added if desired. ESR spectroscopy, however, is both sophisticated and expensive. Indirect markers of ROS generation are used, seeking evidence of damage (e.g., lipid peroxidation) or depletion of endogenous antioxidants. This subject was well reviewed by Gutteridge.[20]

Natural Antioxidant Systems

The body has both enzymatic and nonenzymatic antioxidant defense systems that protect against reactive oxygen species. Nonenzymatic defense systems include vitamins E and C, α-lipoic acid, vitamin A, β-carotene, and the reduced form of glutathione. Enzyme systems include superoxide dismutase (SOD), catalase, and glutathione peroxidase. SOD exists in three forms: cytosolic Cu SOD, mitochondrial Mn SOD, and extracellular Zn SOD. SOD catalyzes the conversion of $O_2^{\bullet-}$ to H_2O and H_2O_2. Catalase is found mainly in peroxisomes and catalyzes the conversion of H_2O_2 to H_2O and O_2. Glutathione peroxidase reduces H_2O_2 to H_2O by oxidizing glutathione (GSH). The oxidized glutathione (GSSG) is reduced back to glutathione by glutathione reductase in the presence of reduced nicotinamide adenine dinucleotide phosphate (NADPH) (Fig. 18.3).

$$H_2O_2 + 2GSH \rightarrow GSSG + 2H_2O$$
$$GSSG + NADPH + H^+ \rightarrow 2GSH + NADP^+$$

All these enzymes require metal cofactors, such as iron for catalase, selenium for glutathione peroxidase, and copper, zinc, or manganese for SOD.

Mechanisms of Damage

Oxidative stress occurs in clinical conditions involving tissue hypoxia, ischemia, and reperfusion. Such conditions include shock of different etiologies; revascularization of ischemic limbs, bowel, or heart; pancreatitis; organ transplantation; and the systemic inflammatory response syndrome (SIRS). ROSs formed in these situations initiate lipid peroxidation and protein and nucleic acid damage, generate chemotactic substances, and induce expression of cell adhesion molecules, resulting in microvascular thrombosis.[24] ROSs are also generated by mitochondrial oxidation, metabolism of arachidonic acid, activation of NADPH oxidase in phagocytes, and activation of xanthine oxidase (Fig. 18.4). Apart from increasing the activity of this enzyme, ischemia and hypoxia also increase its substrate (hypoxanthine/xanthine) via increased ATP hydrolysis and a

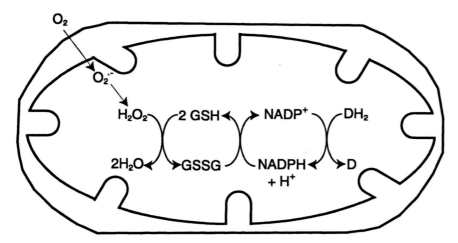

FIGURE 18.3. Protective role of mitochondrial glutathione (GSH reduced form, GSSG oxidized form) against hydrogen peroxide (H_2O_2) and restoration of its reduced form by reactions involving nicotinamide adenine dinucleotide phosphate (NADPH and NADP) and a nonspecificed NADP reducing system (DH_2 and D).

subsequent increase in adenosine monophosphate (AMP) levels. Metabolism of hypoxanthine/xanthine leads to increased generation of $O_2^{\bullet-}$.[25]

$$\text{Xanthine/hypoxanthine} + H_2O + 2O_2$$
$$\rightarrow \text{uric acid} + O_2^{\bullet-} + 2H^+$$

Clinical Overview

Sepsis

Sepsis-related multiple organ failure is the leading cause of death in intensive care units.[26] Infection incites a systemic inflammatory response, with neutrophil infiltration, activation, and phagocytosis. During the "respiratory burst" $O_2^{\bullet-}$ is generated by the NADPH-dependent oxidase present in neutrophils,[27] as is HOCl (generated by myeloperoxidase) and $NO^\bullet$. Nitric oxide further reacts with $O_2^{\bullet-}$ to form $ONOO^\bullet$, ultimately generating the toxic hydroxyl ($OH^\bullet$) radical.

Inflammatory cascade activation results in ongoing generation of proinflammatory mediators plus induction of nitric oxide synthase (iNOS). Increased expression of iNOS has been found in circulating neutrophils of patients with sepsis or SIRS.[28] Endothelial cells have also been shown to produce $O_2^{\bullet-}$ by xanthine oxidase activation induced by activated neutrophils and mediators.[29,30] Increased xanthine oxidase activity plus evidence of ROS-mediated damage was found by Galley et al. in septic patients, although it was lowest in those who died.[31] Studies conducted on whole blood oxidant output and superoxide production in leukocytes of septic patients and controls suggest impaired phagocyte function. Although total oxidant output was increased, the normalized oxidative output for the individual phagocytes was subnormal in response to a variety of stimuli.[32] The apparent increase in total oxidative output may be due to the increased number of leukocytes.

Breakdown products of lipid peroxides have been found in organs and plasma of septic animals.[32-36] Lipid peroxide levels were also found to be elevated in critically ill, ventilated patients.[37]

Cellular antioxidant defense mechanisms limit the damage produced by free radicals. α-Tocopherol (vitamin E) is the major chain-breaking antioxidant found in cells.[38] Ascorbic acid (vitamin C) is a powerful antioxidant that reduces $O_2^{\bullet-}$, H_2O_2, and $OH^\bullet$, forming dehydroascorbic acid (DHA).[39] Glutathione reductase reduces DHA back to ascorbic acid. Another impor-

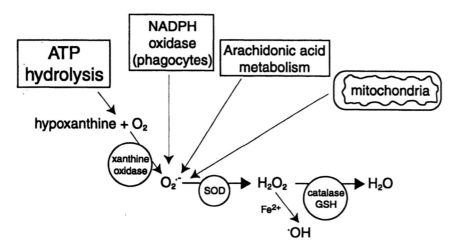

FIGURE 18.4. Sources of intracellular oxidative stress.

tant function of ascorbic acid is regeneration of α-tocopherol from the tocopherol radical. Under certain situations, ascorbic acid is prooxidant, catalyzing the conversion of Fe^{3+} to Fe^{2+} which fuels the Fenton reaction leading to formation of $OH^{\bullet}$.[40] β-Carotene (provitamin A) is also believed to exert an antioxidant function in hypoxic conditions.[41] Trace elements contribute to antioxidant mechanisms as they form the metal centers of enzyme systems.[39]

In those with sepsis the above defense mechanisms may be compromised. Low concentrations of vitamin C[42] and vitamin E[43–46] have been found in septic patients. In the study of Goode et al.[46] low antioxidant vitamin concentrations were associated with increased lipid peroxidation and urinary nitrite excretion. The highest values of lipid peroxidation were found in patients with three or more organ failures, acute inflammation, and altered protein metabolism. Borelli et al.[47] found decreased vitamin C levels and high copper/zinc ratios in patients developing multiple organ failure, in association with increased levels of interleukin-6 (IL-6) and soluble tumor necrosis factor (TNF) receptors. A low total antioxidant capacity has also been shown in the critically ill, in those with uremia, and in renal transplant recipients.[48] Of interest, Pascual et al.[49] found that total antioxidant activity was subnormal in septic patients but elevated in those in septic shock. Fukuyama et al.[50] reported a marked increase in plasma nitrite/nitrate and nitrotyrosine levels in chronic renal failure patients with septic shock, suggesting excessive $ONOO^-$ formation. Hammarqvist et al.[51] found decreased levels of reduced glutathione in skeletal muscle of critically ill patients and a low reduced/total muscle glutathione ratio.

Treatment with antioxidants including SOD, catalase, and N-acetylcysteine (NAC) have produced variable results.[52,53] Their benefits in human sepsis are still unclear. NAC is a low-molecular-weight precursor of glutathione that possibly replenishes intracellular glutathione stores. NAC also has antiinflammatory effects on neutrophils and monocytes. Pretreatment with NAC had a positive effect on myocardial function in a canine model of endotoxic shock.[54] It was attributed to enhanced glutathione peroxidase activity and inhibition of TNF release secondary to a decrease in ROS release. Interestingly, it did not increase plasma total antioxidant potential (TAP) in critically ill patients.[55] Although NAC may restore intracellular glutathione levels, it may not reflect on the TAP. Galley et al.[56] reported an improvement in hemodynamic parameters in septic, critically ill patients treated with intravenous antioxidants. Ascorbate loading in septic patients and healthy controls resulted in increased ascorbyl radical activity in both groups, revealing suboptimal ascorbate levels in the controls and rapid consumption of ascorbate in septic patients.[57]

Specific Infections

Reactive oxygen species and NO mediate pathophysiologic changes in bacterial meningitis-related brain injury.[58] Injury due to cerebral malaria is considered to result in part from free radical-mediated lipid peroxidation of cellular and subcellular structures. Oxidative stress is also involved in the neutrophil-mediated destruction of these parasites.[59] Hemolysis and dyserythropoiesis are common in children with malaria and are associated with increased transferrin saturation. The resultant increase in free iron can fuel formation of free radicals. Gordeuk et al.[60] found that elevated transferrin saturation was associated with delayed recovery in those with cerebral malaria.

Oxidant stress also plays a role in viral illness [e.g., influenza-related cytotoxicity[61] and human immunodeficiency virus (HIV) replication]. Malorni et al. [62] found that an increase in intracellular oxidant stress resulted in activation of latent HIV and that pretreatment with NAC could decrease the degree of virus activation and apoptosis. Diethyldithiocarbamate, which is used for the treatment of acquired immunodeficiency syndrome (AIDS), has powerful antioxidant properties, scavenging HOCl and $OH^{\bullet}$ radicals and inhibiting SOD and cytochrome P450.[63]

Acute Renal Failure

Acute renal failure may result from conditions involving hypoperfusion, hypotension, or tissue hypoxia. Reactive oxygen species are involved in the pathogenesis of both ischemia-mediated and immune complex-mediated renal failure. In vitro experiments have demonstrated the generation of $O_2^{\bullet}$, H_2O_2, and $OH^{\bullet}$ by proximal tubule cells under normoxic conditions.[64] Free radical production was increased, during hypoxia and reoxygenation, as was lipid peroxidation. There was an efflux of adenine metabolites and a decrease in cellular ATP concentration and cell lysis. $O_2^{\bullet}$ is generated by increased expression of xanthine oxidase and by activated neutrophils that adhere to the vascular endothelium in the ischemic kidney.[65]

Drug-Induced Toxicity

Aminoglycoside nephrotoxicity is well recognized. It is of interest that gentamicin has been shown to enhance generation of $O_2^{\bullet}$, H_2O_2, and $OH^{\bullet}$[66,67] and to produce a time- and dose-dependent increase in the release of iron from renal cortical mitochondria.[68] Reactive oxygen species are also involved in cyclosporin A-induced nephrotoxicity. Oxidant mechanisms in toxic acute renal failure have been reviewed by Baliga et al.[69]

Rhabdomyolysis

The acute renal failure secondary to rhabdomyolysis is now considered to be related to iron-catalyzed free radical formation and lipid peroxidation of proximal tubular cell membranes, rather than myoglobin tubular blockage per se. The terminal mitochondrial electron transport chain may be a source of these free radicals.[70] The heme iron from myoglobin might fuel the Haber–Weiss reaction with formation of $OH^{\bullet}$, or it may produce highly reactive iron-based free radicals, namely ferryl or perferryl radicals. Heme oxygenase (HO) seems to play a significant role in this injury by generation of free iron from the heme moiety.[71]

ROSs in Hepatic and Pancreatic Disease

Oxidative damage occurs in the liver, mainly as a consequence of ischemia/reperfusion injury (as in shock states), metabolism of toxic substances (e.g., alcohol), and iron overload. The liver generates up to 80% of total body glutathione, a tripeptide of glutamate, cysteine, and glycine, with the thiol (SH) group of the cysteine moiety conferring significant reducing capacity. The reduced form of glutathione (GSH) can be oxidized to the disulfide (S–S) form. Ninety percent of cellular GSH is cytosolic, the remainder being mitochondrial. During normal aerobic mitochondrial respiration, 1–5% of total oxygen consumption is used to generate superoxide, which is converted by SOD to H_2O_2. Mitochondrial GSH provides the reducing power to inactivate H_2O_2, thereby protecting the mitochondria against this oxidative stress. GSH is also involved in the detoxification of oxidants and electrophilic compounds. Malnutrition reduces GSH levels and is associated with an increased risk of multiple organ dysfunction syndrome (MODS) and death in septic patients.[72] These two effects may be linked. In a rodent model of sepsis, Robinson et al.[73] found that starvation increased ROS generation by 200% following endotoxemia.

Hepatocytes produce a variety of reactive oxygen and nitrogen intermediates in response to cytokines, microbes, or hypoxia.[74] NO seems to exert a protective role on oxidant injury of the liver.[75] Studies by Shu et al.[76] suggested that NO might enhance oxidative stress by modifying the GSH content of hepatocytes. They suggested that during sepsis, especially in the presence of acidosis, it is important to normalize the acidosis prior to inhibition of NO, the rationale being that both $OH^{\bullet}$ and $ONOO^-$ are more stable at acidic pH, and a reduced OH baseline results in increased intracellular GSH. Enhanced ROS production has also been described in patients with cirrhosis and portal hypertension and as part of the reperfusion injury following orthotoptic liver transplantation.[77] Several animal studies also indicate a role for ROSs in the pathogenesis of acute pancreatitis.[78] Allopurinol, a xanthine oxidase inhibitor, had a significant protective effect in a rat model of L-arginine-induced acute pancreatitis.[79]

Acute Lung Injury and Acute Respiratory Distress Syndrome

Acute lung injury (ALI) and the acute respiratory distress syndrome (ARDS) are clinical syndromes that represent increasing severity of lung injury associated with the myriad conditions causing SIRS and multiple organ dysfunction. Although the numbers involved are small, several studies have demonstrated evidence of oxidative stress in ARDS. In a study of eight patients with severe ARDS requiring high-frequency jet ventilation, survivors had higher plasma thiol levels than nonsurvivors; the latter also had rising protein carbonyl levels.[80] A deficiency of glutathione in the alveolar fluid has also been reported in patients with ARDS.[81,82]

Both ROSs and peroxynitrite ($ONOO^-$) are implicated in the injury process.[83] ROSs can cause indirect damage by damaging enzymes and depleting antioxidants. They may also lead to pulmonary endothelial dysfunction, which appears to be associated with impaired NO synthesis and release. These ROSs could be produced by activated neutrophils or endothelial cells. Nitrotyrosine residues, the metabolites of $ONOO^-$, have also been found in the lungs of ARDS patients.[84] Enhanced formation of ROSs has been demonstrated with other pulmonary conditions, as well, such as asthma,[85,86] acid aspiration pneumonitis,[87] and inhalational burns,[88] and in patients undergoing pulmonary resection.[89]

Ischemia/Reperfusion Injury

It is known that ischemia/reperfusion injury lies behind a host of clinical conditions, such as ischemic hepatitis, pancreatitis, brain injury, major vascular surgery, myocardial infarction, and cardiopulmonary bypass. It is also common following global insults such as cardiac arrest and shock states.

Acute coronary syndromes are associated with enhanced generation of ROSs. Reilly et al.[90] have shown that urinary excretion of isoprostanes (a marker of lipid peroxidation) is increased after acute coronary angioplasty. In a study on isolated perfused rat hearts, Samaja et al.[91] found that the severity of the reperfusion injury depended more on the low oxygen supply than on low coronary flow. Preconditioning has a putative protective effect from subsequent ischemic stress on the heart. Upregulation of antioxidant systems is one mechanism by which it occurs.[92] In a small study, pulmonary vascular permeability was found to be increased in patients following cardiopulmonary bypass compared to that in normal subjects.[93] These patients had increased markers of lipid peroxidation products and decreased antioxidant levels. Endothelial cells have been shown to generate ROSs upon reoxygenation following a period of hypoxia.[94] There is evidence that ROSs are involved in cerebral ischemia/reperfusion following carotid endarterectomy.[95] SOD activity seems to be reduced in patients with ischemic strokes.[96] ROSs have also been implicated in the pathophysiology of tissue damage following vascular surgery.[97–99]

Conclusions

There has been an increasing appreciation of the role of reactive oxygen and nitrogen–oxygen species in clinical disease states. However, no antioxidant therapeutic modalities are yet in routine use, except N-acetylcysteine for acetaminophen (paracetamol) poisoning.

References

1. McCord JM, Fridovich I: Superoxide dismutase, an enzymic function of erythrocuprein (hemocuprrein). J Biol Chem 1969;244:6049–6055.
2. Koppenol WH: The centennial of the Fenton reaction. Free Radic Biol Med 1993;15:645–651.
3. Candeias LP, Patel KB, Stratford MRL, Wardman P: Free hydroxyl radicals are formed as reaction between the neutrophil

derived species superoxide and hypochlorous acid. FEBS Lett 1993; 333:151–153.
4. Candeias LP, Stratford MRL, Wardman P: Formation of hydroxyl radicals on reaction of hypochlorous acid with ferrocyanide, a model iron(II) complex. Free Radic Res Commun 1994;20:241–249.
5. Wink DA, Cook J, Pacelli R, et al: The effect of various nitric oxide donors agents on hydrogen peroxide mediated toxicity: a direct correlation between nitric oxide formation and protection. Arch Biochem Biophys 1996;331:241–248.
6. Pryor WA, Squadrito GL: The chemistry of peroxynitrite: a product from the reaction of nitric oxide with superoxide. Am J Physiol 1996;268:L699–L721.
7. Wink DA, Hanbauer I, Krishna MC, DeGraff W, Gamson J, Mitchell JB: Nitric oxide protects against cellular damage and cytotoxicity from reactive oxygen species. Proc Natl Acad Sci USA 1993;90:9813–9817.
8. Wink DA, Cook JA, Krishna MC, et al: Nitric oxide protects against alkyl peroxide mediated cytotoxicity: further insights into the role nitric oxide plays in oxidative stress. Arch Biochem Biophys 1995;319:402–407.
9. Rubbo H, Radi R, Trujillo M, et al: Nitric oxide regulation of superoxide and peroxynitrite-dependent lipid peroxidation. Formation of novel nitrogen-containing oxidized lipid derivatives. J Biol Chem 1994;269:26068–26075.
10. Hogg N, Kalyanaraman B, Joseph J, Struck A, Parthasarathy S: Inhibition of low density lipoprotein oxidation by nitric oxide. potential role in atherogenesis. FEBS Lett 1993;334:170–174.
11. Gorbunov NV, Osipov AN, Day BW, et al: Reduction of ferrylmyoglobin and ferrylhemoglobin by nitric oxide: a protective mechanism against ferryl hemoprotein induced oxidation. Biochemistry 1995;34:6689–6699.
12. Beckman JS, Beckman TW, Chen J, Marshall PA, Freeman BA: Apparent hydroxyl radical formation by peroxynitrite: implications for endothelial injury from nitric oxide and superoxide. Proc Natl Acad Sci USA 1990;87:1620–1624.
13. Saran M, Michel C, Bors W: Reaction of NO with implications for endothelial injury from nitric oxide and superoxide. Free Radic Res Commun 1990;10:221–226.
14. Hobbs AJ, Fukuto JM, Ignarro LJ: Formation of free nitric oxide from L-arginine by nitric oxide synthase: direct enhancement of generation by superoxide dismutase. Proc Natl Acad Sci USA 1994;91:10992–10996.
15. Schmidt HH, Hoffmann H, Schindler U, Shutenko ZS, Cunningham DD, Feelisch M: No •NO from NO synthase. Proc Natl Acad Sci USA 1996;93:14492–14497.
16. Griffith OW, Stuehr DJ: Nitric oxide synthases: properties and catalytic mechanism. Annu Rev Physiol 1995;57:707–736.
17. Pufahl RA, Wishnock JS, Marletta MA: Hydrogen peroxide supported oxidation of N^G-hydroxyl-L-arginine by nitric oxide synthase. Biochemistry 1995;34:1930–1941.
18. Arnelle DR, Stamler JS: NO^+, NO and NO^- donation by S: nitrosothiols: implications for regulation of physiological functions by S-nitrosylation and regulation of disulfide formation. Arch Biochem Biophys 1995;318:279–285.
19. Wink DA, Feelisch M, Fukuto J, et al: The cytotoxicity of nitroxyl: possible implications for the pathophysiological role of NO. Arch Biochem Biophys 1998;351:66–74.
20. Gutteridge JMC: Lipid peroxidation and antioxidants as biomarkers of tissue damage. Clin Chem 1995;41:1819–1828.
21. Gutteridge JMC: Iron promoters of the Fenton reaction and lipid peroxidation can be released from haemoglobin by peroxides. FEBS Lett 1986;20:291–295.
22. Davies KJA: Protein damage and degradation by oxygen radicals. 1. General Aspects. J Biol Chem 1987;262:9895–9901.
23. Wolff S, Dean RT: Fragmentation of proteins by free radicals and its effect on their susceptibility to enzymic hydrolysis. Biochem J 1986;234:399–403.
24. Fraticelli A, Serrano CV, Bochner BS, et al: Hydrogen peroxide and superoxide modulate leukocyte adhesion molecule expression and leukocyte endothelial adhesion. Biochem Biophys Acta 1996;1310:251–259.
25. McCord JM: Oxygen-derived free radicals in postischemic tissue injury. N Engl J Med 1985;312:159–163.
26. Bone RC: The pathogenesis of sepsis. Ann Intern Med 1991; 115:457–469.
27. Klebanoff SL: Oxygen metabolism and the toxic properties of phagocytes. Ann Intern Med 1980;93:480–489.
28. Tsukahara Y, Morisaki T, Horita Y, Torisu M: Tanaka M: Expression of inducible nitric oxide synthase in circulating neutrophils of the systemic inflammatory response syndrome and septic patients. World J Surg 1998;22:771–777.
29. Phan SH, Gannon DE, Varani J, et al: Xanthine oxidase activity in rat pulmonary artery endothelial cells and its modulation by activated neutrophils. Am J Pathol 1989;134:1201–1211.
30. Friedl HP, Till GO, Ryan US: Mediator induced activation of xanthine oxidase in endothelial cells. FASEB J 1989;3:2512–2518.
31. Galley HF, Davies MJ, Webster NR: Xanthine oxidase activity and free radical generation in patients with sepsis syndrome. Crit Care Med 1996;24:1649–1653.
32. Pascual C, Karzai W, Meier-Hellmann A, et al: A controlled study of leukocyte activation in septic patients. Intensive Care Med 1997;23:743–748.
33. Morgan RA, Manning PB, Coran AG, et al: Oxygen free radical activity during live E. coli septic shock in the dog. Circ Shock 1988;25:319–323.
34. Kunimoto F, Morita T, Ogawa R, et al: Inhibition of lipid peroxidation improves survival rate of endotoxemic rats. Circ Shock 1987;21:15–22.
35. Ogawa R, Kunimoto F, Morita T, et al: Changes in hepatic lipid peroxide concentration in endotoxemic rats. Circ Shock 1982;9:369–374.
36. Demling D, LaLonde C, Jin LJ, et al: Endotoxemia causes an increased lung lipid peroxidation in unanesthetised sheep. J Appl Physiol 1986;60:2094–2100.
37. Ben Baquali A, Aube H, Maupoil V, et al: Plasma lipid peroxidation in critically ill patients: importance of mechanical ventilation. Free Radic Biol Med 1994;16:223–227.
38. Burton GW, Joyce A, Ingold KU: First proof that vitamin E remains the major lipid soluble chain-breaking antioxidant in human plasma. Lancet 1982;2:327.
39. Goode HF, Webster NR: Free radicals and trace element metabolism in sepsis and injury. Br J Intensive Care 1992;2: 312–322.
40. Halliwell B, Gutteridge JMC: Oxygen toxicity, oxygen radicals, transition metals and disease. Biochem J 1984;167:92–98.
41. Krinsky NI: Antioxidant functions of carotenoids. Free Radic Biol Med 1989;7:617–635.

42. Cross CE, Forte T, Stocker R, et al: Oxidative stress and abnormal cholesterol metabolism in patients with adult respiratory distress syndrome. J Lab Clin Med 1990;115:396–404.
43. Richard C, Lemmonier F, Thibbault M, et al: Vitamin E deficiency and lipid peroxidation during the adult respiratory distress syndrome. Crit Care Med 1990;18:4–9.
44. Bertrand Y, Pincemail J, Hanique G, et al: Differences in tocopherol-lipid ratios in ARDS and non-ARDS patients. Intensive Care Med 1989;15:87–93.
45. Ogilvie AC, Groenveld ABJ, Straub JP, Thijs LG: Plasma lipid peroxides and antioxidants in human septic shock. Intensive Care Med 1991;17:40–44.
46. Goode HJ, Cowley HC, Walker BE, et al: Decreased antioxidant status and increased lipid peroxidation in patients with septic shock and secondary organ dysfunction. Crit Care Med 1995;23:646–651.
47. Borelli E, Roux-Lombard P, Grau G, et al: Plasma concentrations of cytokines, their soluble receptors, and antioxidant vitamins can predict the development of multiple organ failure in patients at risk. Crit Care Med 1996;24:392–397.
48. Dasgupta A, Malhotra D, Levy H, et al: Decreased total antioxidant capacity but normal lipid hydroperoxide concentrations in sera of critically ill patients. Life Sci 1997;60:335–340.
49. Pascual C, Karzai W, Meier-Hellmann A, et al: Total plasma antioxidant capacity is not always decreased in sepsis. Crit Care Med 1998;26:705–709.
50. Fukuyama N, Takebayashi Y, Hida M, et al: Clinical evidence of peroxynitrite formation in chronic renal failure patients with septic shock. Free Radic Biol Med 1997;22:771–774.
51. Hammarqvist F, Luo Jia-Li, Cotgreave IA, et al: Skeletal muscle glutathione is depleted in critically ill patients. Crit Care Med 1997;25:78–84.
52. Goode HF, Webster N: Antioxidants in intensive care medicine. Clin Intensive Care 1993;4:265–269.
53. Goode HF, Webster NR: Free radicals and antioxidants in sepsis. Crit Care Med 1993;21:1770–1776.
54. Zhang H, Spapen H, Nguyen DN, et al: Protective effects of N-acetyl-L-cysteine in endotoxaemia. Am J Physiol 1994;266:H1746–H1754.
55. Molnar Z, Mackinnon KL, Shearer E, et al: The effect of N-acetylcysteine on total serum antioxidant potential and urinary albumin excretion in critically ill patients. Intensive Care Med 1998;24:230–235.
56. Galley HF, Howdle PD, Wlaker B, Webster N: The effect of intravenous antioxidants in patients with septic shock. Crit Care Med 1997;23:768–774.
57. Galley HF, Davies MJ, Webster N: Ascorbyl radical formation in patients with sepsis: effect of ascorbate loading. Free Radic Biol Med 1996;20:139–143.
58. Koedel U, Bernatowitcz A, Paul R, et al: Experimental pneumococcal meningitis: cerebrovascular alterations, brain oedema, and meningeal inflammation are linked to the production of nitric oxide. Ann Neurol 1995;37:313–323.
59. Golenser J, Kamyl M, Tsafack A, et al: Correlation between destruction of malarial parasites by polymorphonuclear leucocytes and oxidative stress. Free Radic Res Commun 1992;17:249–262.
60. Gordeuk VR, Thuma PE, McLaren C, et al: Transferrin saturation and recovery from coma in cerebral malaria. Blood 1995;85:3297–3301.
61. Knobil K, Choi AMK, Weigand G, Jacoby DB: Role of oxidants in influenza virus-induced gene expression. Am J Physiol 1998;274:L134–L142.
62. Malorni W, Rivabene R, Santini MT, Donelli G: N-Acetylcysteine inhibits apoptosis and decreases viral particles in HIV-chronically infected U937 cells. FEBS Lett 1993;327:75–78.
63. Liu J, Shigenaga MK, Yan L, et al: Antioxidant activity of diethyldithiocarbamate. Free Radic Res 1996; 24:461–472.
64. Paller MS, Neumann TV: Reactive oxygen species and rat renal epithelial cells during hypoxia and reoxygenation. Kidney int 1991;40:1041–1049.
65. Yoshida N, Granger DN, Anderson DC, et al: Anoxia-reoxygenation induced neutrophil adherence to cultured endothelial cells. Am J Physiol 1992;262:H1891–H1898.
66. Walker PD, Shah SV: Gentamycin enhanced production of hydrogen peroxide by renal cortical mitochondria. Am J Physiol 1987;253:C495–C499.
67. Yang CL, Du XH, Han YX: Renal cortical mitochondria are the source of oxygen free radicals enhanced by gentamycin. Ren Fail 1995;17:21–26.
68. Ueda N, Guidet B, Shah SV: Gentamycin induced mobilisation of iron from renal cortical mitochondria. Am J Physiol 1993;265:F435–F439.
69. Baliga R, Ueda N, Walker PD, Shah SV: Oxidant mechanisms in toxic acute renal failure. Am J Kidney Dis 1997;29:465–477.
70. Zager RA: Mitochondrial free radical production induces lipid peroxidation during myohemoglobinuria. Kidney Int 1996;49:741–751.
71. Zager RA, Burkhart K: Myoglobin toxicity in proximal human kidney cells: roles of Fe, Ca, and terminal mitochondrial electron transport. Kidney Int 1997;51:728–738.
72. Pacelli F, Doglietto GB, Alfieri S, et al: Prognosis in intra-abdomianl infections: multivariate analysis on 604 patients. Arch Surg 1996;11:641–646.
73. Robinson MK, Rustum RR, Chambers EA, et al: Starvation enhances hepatic free radical release following endotoxemia. J Surg Res 1997;69:325–330.
74. Arthur MJ: Reactive oxygen intermediates and liver injury. J Hepatol 1988;6:125–131.
75. Kuo PC, Slivka A: Nitric oxide diminishes oxidant-mediated hepatic injury. J Surg Res 1994;56:594–600.
76. Shu Z, Jung M, Beger HG, Marzinzig M, et al: pH dependent changes of nitric oxide, peroxynitrite and reactive oxygen species in hepatocellular damage. Am J Physiol 1997;273:G1118–G1126.
77. Bzeizi KI, Dawkes R, Dodd NJF, et al: Graft dysfunction following liver transplantation: role of free radicals. J Hepatol 1997;26:69–74.
78. Schoenberg MH, Buchler M, Beger HG: The role of oxygen radicals in experimental acute pancreatitis. Free Radic Biol Med 1992;12:515–522.
79. Czako L, Tkacs T, Varga I, et al: Involvement of oxygen derived free radicals in L-arginine induced acute pancreatitis. Dig Dis Sci 1998;43:1770–1777.
80. Quinlan GJ, Evans TW, Gutteridge JMC: Oxidative damage to plasma proteins in adult respiratory distress syndrome. Free Radic Res 1994;20:289–298.
81. Pacht ER, Timerman AP, Lykens MG, Merola AJ: Deficiency of alveolar fluid glutathione in patients with sepsis and the adult respiratory distress syndrome. Chest 1991;100:1397–1403.

82. Bunnell E, Pacht ER: Oxidized glutathione is increased in the alveolar fluid of patients with the adult respiratory distress syndrome. Am Rev Respir Dis 1993;148:1174–1178.
83. Chabot F, Mitchell JA, Gutteridge JMC, Evans TW: Reactive oxygen species in acute lung injury. Eur Respir J 1998;11:745–757.
84. Kooy NW, Royall JA, Ye YZ, et al: Evidence for in vivo peroxynitrite production in human acute lung injury. Am J Respir Crit Care Med 1995;151:1250–1254.
85. Smith LJ, Shamsuddin M, Sporn PHS, et al: Reduced superoxide dismutase in lung cells of patients with asthma. Free Radic Biol Med 1997;22:1301–1307.
86. Vachier I, Chanez P, Doucen CL, et al: Enhancement of reactive oxygen species formation in stable and unstable asthmatic patients. Eur Respir J 1994;7:1585–1592.
87. Nader-Djalal N, Knight PR III, Thusu K, et al: Reactive oxygen species contribute to oxygen related lung injury after acid aspiration. Anesth Analg 1998; 87:127–133.
88. Youn Y-K, Lalonde C, Demling R: Oxidants and the pathophysiology of burn and smoke inhalational injury. Free Radic Biol Med 1992;12:409–415.
89. Williams EA, Quinlan GJ, Goldstraw P, et al: Post operative lung injury and oxidative damage in patients undergoing pulmonary wedge resection. Eur Respir J 1998;11:1028–1034.
90. Reilly MP, Delanty N, Roy I, et al: Evidence for oxidant stress during acute coronary reperfusion in humans. Circulation 1997;96:3314–3320.
91. Samaja M, Motterlini R, Santoro F, et al: Oxidative injury in reoxygenated and reperfused hearts. Free Radic Biol Med 1994;16:255–262.
92. Richard V, Kaeffer N, Thuillez C: Delayed protection of the ischemic heart: from pathophysiology to therapeutic applications. Fundam Clin Pharmacol 1996;10:409–415.
93. Messent M, Sinclair DG, Quinlan GJ, et al: Pulmonary vascular permeability after cardiopulmonary bypass and its relationship to oxidative stress. Crit Care Med 1997;25:425–429.
94. Zweier JL, Kuppusamy P, Thompson-Gorman S, et al: Measurement and characterisation of free radical generation in reoxygenated human endothelial cells. Am J Physiol 1994;266:C700–C708.
95. Bacon PJ, Love SA, Gupta AK: Plasma antioxidant consumption with ischemia/reperfusion during carotidendarterectomy. Stroke 1996;27:1808–1811.
96. Spranger M, Krempien S, Schwab S, et al: Superoxide dismutase activity in serum of patients with acute cerebral ischemic injury: correlation with clinical course and infarct size. Stroke 1997;28: 2425–2428.
97. Thompson MM, Nasim A, Sayers RD, et al: Oxygen free radica and cytokine generation during endovascular and conventional aneurysm repair. Eur J Vasc Endovasc Surg 1996;12: 70–75.
98. Spark JI, Chetter IC, Gallavin L, et al: Reduced total antioxidant capacity predicts ischemia reperfusion injury after femoro-distal bypass. Br J Surg 1998;85:217–220.
99. Kretzschmar M, Klein U, Palutke M, Schirrmeister W: Reduction of ischemia reperfusion syndrome after abdominal aortic aneurysmectomy by N-acetylcysteine but not mannitol. Acta Anaesthesiol Scand 1996;40:657–664.

19
Nitric Oxide as a Modulator of Sepsis: Therapeutic Possibilities

A. Neil Salyapongse and Timothy R. Billiar

The systemic inflammatory response syndrome (SIRS), multiple organ dysfunction syndrome (MODS), and multiple organ failure (MOF) remain the most common causes of death in the intensive care unit. Despite the elucidation of many of the mediators contributing to the physiologic changes observed during these processes, a "magic bullet" capable of treating SIRS and preventing MODS/MOF continues to evade identification. This difficulty rests, at least in part, on the nature of these pathophysiologic states as final common pathways deriving from a variety of insults (e.g., infection, trauma, burns).[1] Interest in nitric oxide (NO) as a potential mediator of SIRS, MODS, and MOF stems from its ability to modulate inflammation, vascular reactivity, and cardiac function, some of the key elements comprising these inflammatory syndromes. This chapter presents the evidence for NO as a key participant in these inflammatory syndromes and reviews the promises and limitations of NO modulation suggested by experimental and clinical trials.

Biochemistry of Nitric Oxide

Generated in nature by elements as diverse as lightning and bacteria[2] and produced as a by-product of technology in electrical power plants and automotive exhaust,[3] NO was identified as a significant mammalian cell secretory product only during the late 1980s. Although the first suggestion that mammals produced nitrogen oxides occurred in 1916,[4] confirmation of mammalian nitrate production,[5–7] its enhancement by endotoxin,[8] and its dependence on L-arginine[9] did not arrive until the 1970s and 1980s. By 1987 Palmer et al.[10] and Ignarro et al.[11] had identified NO as the endothelial-derived relaxing factor originally described by Furchgott and Zawadzki,[12] laying the groundwork for further revelations of NO as a mediator in physiologic processes ranging from vascular tone and microbial killing to neurotransmission and sphincter relaxation.

Composed of one atom each of nitrogen and oxygen, NO is a relatively unstable (half-life 2–30 seconds), uncharged free radical. These properties allow rapid diffusion across cell membranes with activity limited to the local environment. NO may directly interact with molecular targets, such as heavy metals and protein thiol groups, or with superoxide to form other radicals, such as peroxynitrite, nitrogen dioxide, and hydroxyl radicals, which can in turn target other proteins. In the presence of oxygen and hemoglobin, NO rapidly oxidizes, yielding the stable, measurable end-products nitrite and nitrate.

Generation of NO occurs following five-electron oxidation of the guanidino nitrogen of L-arginine to citrulline via one of the family of nitric oxide synthase (NOS) enzymes.[13] Three NOS isoforms exist, each named for the cell type in which it was originally identified (Table 19.1). Neuronal NOS (nNOS, NOS1)[14] and endothelial NOS (ecNOS, NOS3)[15] represent constitutively present enzymes that remain inactive until intracellular calcium levels increase. With the influx of calcium, a calcium–calmodulin complex binds to and activates NOS. These isoforms continue to produce low levels of NO until intracellular calcium levels fall[16] (Fig. 19.1).[17] The dependence of NO generation on calcium flux allows moment-to-moment alterations in NO concentration necessary for homeostatic processes such as regulation of vascular tone and sphincter relaxation. In contrast, inducible NOS (iNOS, NOS2) is not typically present in unstimulated cells and is transcriptionally regulated rather than calcium flux-dependent. Stimuli including endotoxin or inflammatory cytokines, such as interleukin-1 (IL-1), interferon-γ (IFNγ), and tumor necrosis factor-α (TNFα) induce expression of iNOS,[18,19] which, provided adequate substrate is present, leads to sustained production of high levels of NO over the life of the enzyme. Each NOS enzyme is a homodimer that contains a protoporphyrin IX heme group and relies on the presence of nicotinamide adenine dinucleotide phosphate (NADPH), flavin adenine dinucleotide (FAD), flavin mononucleotide (FMN), and tetrahydrobiopterin (H$_4$B) as cofactors. iNOS differs from cNOS (ecNOS and nNOS) in that a calmodulin molecule is permanently bound to each subunit of the homodimer, a property that allows calcium-independent generation of NO by iNOS.[20]

Because tissues at nearly every site in the body contain cells capable of expressing one or more of the NOS isoforms, it is not surprising that NO can participate in a wide variety of

TABLE 19.1. Comparison of NOS Isoforms.

Parameter	nNOS (type 1)	iNOS (type 2)	eNOS (type 3)
Cellular location	Cytosol	Cytosol, vesicles	Cytosol, membrane caveolae
Ca^{2+} dependence	Yes	No	+/−
Primary regulation	Ca^{2+} flux	Transcription	Ca^{2+} flux phosphorylation
NO production	Picomolar	Nanomolar	Picomolar
Duration of activity	Transient	Sustained	Transient

physiologic processes. Preformed and able to respond to intracellular calcium shifts, cNOS can increase local NO concentrations almost immediately, whereas induction and expression of NO from iNOS may require hours. Once formed, however, iNOS may release levels of NO that dwarf the contributions of cNOS. These differences may help explain the challenges inherent in manipulation of NO as a therapeutic intervention in the setting of SIRS, MODS, and MOF.

Molecular Action of Nitric Oxide

Whereas most bioactive signaling molecules, (e.g., growth factors, neurotransmitters, cytokines) transmit their message by binding to specific cell surface or intracellular protein receptors, NO effects its message by interacting with specific elements of target molecules, thereby altering the function of a wide variety of enzymes. NO is lipophilic and readily diffuses from cell to cell through cell membranes.[21] Direct interaction often occurs with protein thiol groups or metals,[1] such as the iron–heme complex.

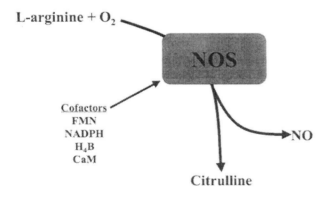

FIGURE 19.1. Generation of nitric oxide (NO) by nitric oxide synthase (NOS). NOS catalyzes the five-electron conversion of L-arginine to citrulline and NO. Cofactors include flavin mononucleotide (FMN), nicotinamide adenine dinucleotide phosphate (NADPH), tetrahydrobiopterin (H_4B), and calmodulin (CaM). iNOS differs from the cNOS isotype in that calmodulin is permanently bound to each subunit of the homodimeric enzyme, allowing iNOS to function independently of calcium flux.

An example of the latter case is activation of soluble guanylate cyclase. NO interacts with the iron–heme component of the enzyme, liberating a histidine and resulting in cyclic guanosine monophosphate (cGMP) synthesis. In the vasculature this increase in cGMP leads to vasorelaxation,[22] and the same signal in smooth muscle may induce relaxation as well.[13] Reaction of NO with iron complexes in other enzymes (e.g., aconitase,[23] nicotinamide adenine dinucleotide:ubiquinone reductase,[23,24] catalase,[25,26] cytochrome P450[27]), however, results in enzyme inactivation. Furthermore, NO can decrease its own biosynthesis by reacting with the iron–heme group in cNOS and iNOS.[8,28] Through a thiol reaction known as S-nitrosylation, NO reactive products that contain the NO^+ moiety (e.g., N_2O_3) can modulate the function of a wide range of proteins. For example, S-nitrosylation of p21 ras activates this regulatory, intracellular signaling molecule; and thiol modulation accounts for the opening of the ryanodine receptor[29] and K^+-regulated Ca^{2+} channel.[30] Evidence also suggests that NO may circulate bound to hemoglobin through a reversible NO–thiol interaction, allowing hemoglobin to act as a NO carrier/donor.[31]

Indirect actions of NO may occur through interaction with superoxide, resulting in generation of other free radicals, including peroxynitrite, nitrogen dioxide, and hydroxyl radicals.[32,33] These radicals may damage cells directly, a process that may be central to the antimicrobial and antitumor properties of NO.[34,35] Either NO or peroxynitrite may directly damage DNA through inducing single-strand breakage.[36] In vascular smooth muscle cells this can result in attempts at DNA repair through the activation of poly-ADP-ribosyl transferase (PARS), thereby consuming ATP and NAD^+ stores, resulting in decreased vascular contractility. Furthermore, peroxynitrite can disrupt the activity of calcium[37] and sodium-potassium[38] membrane pumps, thereby inhibiting the contractility of smooth muscle cells.

Inhibitors of NOS and NO Activity

Regulation of NO activity could conceivably occur at any of three stages: activation of NOS gene expression (perhaps relevant only for iNOS), inhibition of NOS activity, or blockade of NO actions. Prevention of iNOS expression can be accomplished with a variety of agents, including glucocorticoids,[39] nifedipine,[40] and insulin-like growth factor-I (IGF-I).[41] Methylene blue and hemoglobin represent the classic inhibitors of guanylate cyclase activity, but, more specific inhibitors, such as 1-H-[1,2,4] oxadiazolo [4,3,a] quinozalin-1-one (ODQ),[42] are now available. Despite the availability of the above agents, most of those in clinical use today fall in the category of NOS inhibitors (reviewed by Southan and Szabo[43]). The challenge remains to improve isoform selectivity so specific generation of NO during SIRS may be blocked. As discussed later, the available data suggest that it is dangerous to inhibit eNOS during sepsis as it can result in endothelial injury, microvascular thrombosis, and tissue damage. The objective thus becomes suppression or removal of iNOS-generated NO.

TABLE 19.2. Agents that Enhance Expression of NO.

Agent[a]	Mechanism of NO generation	NO production	Limitations
SIN-1	Electron transfer	1 NO/molecule	In vitro may generate superoxide and NO
SNAP	Spontaneous decomposition	1 NO/molecule	Wide variability in rate of NO production based on milieu
NO gas	Direct	1 NO/molecule	Typically inhaled
NG, SNP	Electron transfer, Chemical reduction	1 NO/molecule	SNP by-product, cyanide, inhibits NO activity
NONOates	Spontaneous decomposition	2 NO/molecule	pH, temperature, and nucleophile determine release rate

[a]SIN-1, linsidomine; SNAP, S-nitroso-amino-penicillamine; NG, nitroglycerin; SNP, sodium nitroprusside; NONOates, nucleophile–NO conjugates.

TABLE 19.3. Agents that Limit Expression of NO.

Agent[a]	Mechanism of action	Relative potency (vs. iNOS)[b]	Relative potency (vs. eNOS)[b]
Glucocorticoids	Transcription inhibition	++	–
L-arginine analogues			
L-NA	Competitive inhibition	+	++
L-NMMA	Competitive inhibition	++	++
L-NAME	Competitive inhibition	++	+++
L-NIL	Competitive inhibition	++	+
Isothioureas			
S-MITU	Competitive inhibition	+++	++
S-EITU	Competitive inhibition	+++	++
Other inhibitors			
AG	Competitive inhibition	+	–
1400W	Competitive inhibition	++++	–
ODQ	Guanylate cyclase inhibition	N/A	N/A
NO scavengers			
Hemoglobin	NO–Fe^{2+} interaction	N/A	N/A
Dithiocarbamates[c]	NO–Fe^{2+} interaction	N/A	N/A

[a]L-arginine analogues, see text; S-MITU, S-methyl-isothiourea; S-EITU, S-ethyl-isothiourea; AG, aminoguanidine; 1400W, N-(3-(aminomethyl)benzyl)-acetamidine; ODQ, 1-H-[1,2,4]oxadiazolo[4,3,a]quinozalin-1-one.
[b]Relative effect: minimal (–); increasing relative potency (+, ++, +++, ++++). Compiled and adapted from Southan and Szabo,[43] Garvey et al.,[44,45] and Rees et al.[46]
[c]Reviewed by Pieper et al.[47]

All isoforms of NOS contain a specific binding site for L-arginine, which positions that guanidino group (the ultimate source of NO) adjacent to the heme prosthetic group of the catalytic site. Apart from L-arginine, only a handful of substrates, mostly slight modifications of L-arginine, can be used by NOS to generate NO. This has led to the development of numerous guanidino- or carboxyl-substituted versions of L-arginine as NOS inhibitors (Table 19.2). All of these L-arginine analogues can inhibit each NOS isoform, although slight selectivity may exist. N^G-Nitro-L-arginine (L-NA) and N^ω-Nitro-L-arginine-methyl-ester (L-NAME), for instance, show greater inhibition of eNOS than iNOS (Table 19.3). In contrast, another substituted amino acid, L-N^6-(1-aminoethyl)lysine (L-NIL), demonstrates 30-fold selectivity for iNOS over nNOS.[48]

Nonamino acids, including the isothioureas, such as S-methyl isothiourea (S-MITU) and S-ethyl isothiourea (S-EITU), have been shown to demonstrate anywhere from a 2- to 19-fold selectivity for iNOS over eNOS.[44] Aminoguanidine (AG) represents one of the substituted guanidine family of inhibitors that show slight selectivity for iNOS but demonstrate weaker activity than the L-arginine analogues.[49] Newer agents, including N-[3-(aminomethyl)benzyl]acetamidine (1400W) with an in vivo 50-fold selectivity for iNOS,[45] promise that specific, clinically useful NOS inhibition may soon be available.

NO as Mediator of Vascular Tone

Exogenously supplied nitrates had long been in clinical use; but identification of NO as the "endothelial-derived relaxing factor"[33] provided concrete evidence that this endogenously produced bioactive molecule was key to regulating vascular tone. Investigations over the past decade have revealed that small amounts of endothelial-derived NO (EDNO) function to maintain a basal state of vasodilation. Inhibition of NOS activity in healthy rats,[50–52] dogs,[53,54] and humans[55,56] has resulted variously in significant elevations in systemic, pulmonary, and renal vascular resistances as well as elevations in blood pressure. Examination of flow to specific vascular beds, including the brain,[57,58] heart,[59] and intestine,[60] has further cemented the role of EDNO as an autoregulator of blood flow. Studies of mice in which the eNOS gene has been mutated (eNOS knockouts) have revealed that, in the absence of EDNO, mice become hypertensive.[61]

The importance of not exceeding low basal levels of NO (e.g., those provided by cNOS) became evident as investigators sought to explain the etiology of hypotension associated with immunomodulation therapy for cancer. Endothelial cells cultured with TNF, IL-1, or endotoxin (lipopolysaccharide, or LPS), alone or in combination, accumulated nitrate (a stable end-product of NO generation) in the culture medium.[62] The NO produced by such stimulation exhibited a delay in appearance but was capable of rising to concentrations orders of magnitude (millimolar) above that generated at baseline (micromolar), characteristics that would be ultimately related to iNOS activity. In addition, patients undergoing cytokine therapy with IL-2 demonstrated significant increases in plasma nitrates associated with decreases in both systolic and diastolic blood pressures.[63] Inhibition of NOS activity in the setting of TNF,[64] IL-1,[65] and IL-2[66,67] prevented hypotension in both animals and patients, confirming induced expression of NO as the culprit. The observation that exposure of rat aortic rings to the NOS inhibitor N^G-monomethyl-L-arginine (L-NMMA) restored the contractile response to norepinephrine[68] even in the absence of endothelium eventually led to the confirmation that iNOS expression in vascular smooth muscle[69] was responsible for the demonstrated hyporeactivity.

NO and Inflammation

Although virtually all cell types can generate NO, activated macrophages are capable of expressing some of the highest levels of NOS and therefore producing large amounts of NO. As mentioned above, the free radical NO and the peroxynitrite it engenders can result in cytotoxic effects. The high levels of NO generated by iNOS may contribute to the killing of a wide array of microorganisms including bacteria, fungi, and viruses (reviewed by DeGroote and Fang[70]). Inhibition of NOS activity has been shown to impair macrophage ability to kill both tumor cells and microbes. In addition to direct cytotoxic effects, NO may also upregulate production of inflammatory cytokines such as TNF and IL-8 as well as proinflammatory prostaglandins.[71,72] Specific examples of NO acting as a proinflammatory agent have come from studies in hemorrhagic shock[73] and Leishmania infections.[74] In these examples, the expression of cytokines in tissues was dependent on the expression of iNOS. Of note, NO has also demonstrated antiinflammatory effects by inactivating neutrophil NADPH oxidase. Despite this fact, the high levels of NO generated by iNOS appear primarily proinflammatory.

SIRS and the Culpability of NO

Levels of NO increase during sepsis,[75-77] supporting the next logical hypothesis that NO may be responsible for the vascular hyporeactivity to pressors that leads to hypotension and shock during the inception and progression of SIRS. Our group[75] and others[78] have found, when comparing septic patients with shock to those without shock, that the levels of nitrite and nitrate positively correlated with cardiac output and levels of endotoxin and negatively correlated with systolic blood pressure. Additional evidence for the key role of iNOS in septic shock comes from the demonstration that iNOS knockout mice are at least partially resistant to the effects of endotoxin.[79] Perhaps the most convincing argument for NO as a mediator of SIRS and shock, however, is the multitude of studies of the effects of NOS inhibitors on both experimental and clinical shock.

NOS Inhibition and Vascular Reactivity

Elucidation of the effects of NO on the vasculature derived in large part from experiments with NOS inhibition and isolated aortic rings. Numerous studies have now confirmed that arginine analogues,[46,80-83] aminoguanidine,[84] isothiurea derivatives,[80,85-87] and the PARS inhibitor 3-aminobenzamide[36] are capable of reversing the hypotensive effects of endotoxin across a variety of species. The general response to NOS inhibition in these systems involves vasoconstriction in both arterial and venous circulations with a concomitant increase in blood pressure and decrease in cardiac output. Using the arginine analogues L-NAME, L-NMMA, and L-NA, similar results were found in a few case reports and preliminary clinical studies,[88-92] and were confirmed in more recent phase I and phase II trials.[67,93] Observations of a pressor effect by diaspirin cross-linked hemoglobin (DCLHb), a cell-free oxygen carrier proposed as a resuscitative fluid, in rats[94] and humans[95] led to experiments confirming that elevations in blood pressure were secondary to reduced NO activity.[96] Thus scavenging NO might prove as beneficial for hypotension as preventing NO formation.

Renal Effects of NOS Inhibition

In contrast to the hyporeactivity of the systemic vasculature in sepsis, the renovascular response is characterized by vasoconstriction and decreased glomerular filtration rate (GFR).[97] After administration of endotoxin to rodents, these renal changes occur within the first 1–2 hours, even before systemic hypotension arises.[98] Treatment of endotoxemic rodents with NOS inhibitors resulted in what initially appeared to be conflicting results. Nonselective NOS inhibition worsened the renal vasoconstriction[99] and resulted in glomerular thrombosis.[100] More selective NOS inhibition, however, restored renal medullary blood flow as measured by laser Doppler technique, improved inulin clearance,[102] and improved GFR as manifested by decreased serum creatinine levels.[82,83,86] Clarification of the significance of specific NOS inhibition came with comparison of the effects of the nonspecific NOS inhibitor L-NAME and the more specific iNOS inhibitor L-NIL.[101] After treatment with LPS, rats received one of the two NOS inhibitors. All endotoxemic rats experienced decreased GFR. Those rats receiving L-NAME manifested further decreases in GFR, and the GFR in L-NIL-treated rats returned to baseline. These results suggested that eNOS may play a critical role in maintaining renal perfusion and the GFR, and that the high levels of NO generated by iNOS may play a role in reducing eNOS activity in the renal vasculature. In septic patients, serum nitrate levels have demonstrated both an absence of[75-77] and a positive correlation with[78,102] creatinine levels. Groeneveld et al. proposed an association between high levels of NO and renal insufficiency that cannot be explained simply by decreased excretion of NO.[102] This suggests that high levels of NO during sepsis may play a role in the pathogenesis of renal insufficiency.

Pulmonary Effects of Nitric Oxide

Pulmonary failure, as a component of MODS, represents the constellation of pulmonary arterial hypertension, decreased lung compliance, and ventilation/perfusion (V/Q) mismatch. Most of these changes can be traced to alterations in pulmonary vascular function, including increased microvascular permeability, pulmonary hypertension, and intrapulmonary shunting of venous blood.[103] As an effector of vascular relaxation and a modulator of inflammation, NO has been the focus of seemingly conflicting trials of NOS inhibition, inhaled NO supplementation, and combinations of the two modalities. Combined, these studies have revealed some of the complexity underlying the roles of the NOS isoforms in the acute lung injury (ALI) of SIRS.

ALI one of the earliest manifestations of ALI is the loss of capillary barrier function resulting in increased leakage of protein and fluid into the lung interstitium.[104] This contributes to the impaired gas exchange the decreased lung compliance found in ALI. In the setting of ischemia/reperfusion-, antigen-, or LPS-induced ALI, nonspecific inhibition of NOS with either L-NA[104] or L-NAME[105–107] reduced capillary leak, as measured by pulmonary extravasation of Evan's blue, a vital dye. Antigen-induced leakage was not reversed by administration of the iNOS selective inhibitor aminoguanidine,[106] suggesting that only eNOS participated in the phenomenon of capillary leak; however, one study of endotoxemia in iNOS knockout mice revealed no increase in the wet/dry ratio of LPS-treated mice over controls,[108] suggesting that iNOS plays a role in the increased parenchymal fluid. Thus it remains to be clarified whether capillary leak occurs secondary to NO derived from iNOS, eNOS, or both.

Pulmonary arterial hypertension occurs as a result of vasoconstriction and occlusion of the pulmonary microvasculature.[109] Agents responsible for these changes include thromboxane A_2,[110] neuropeptide Y, and norepinephrine.[111] This hypertension aggravates capillary leak and can contribute to intrapulmonary shunting. Given its vasodilating property and rapid inactivation by hemoglobin, inhaled NO became a prime candidate for selective pulmonary vasodilation. With occasional exceptions,[112] most trials have since proved the efficacy of inhaled NO not only in reversing pulmonary hypertension induced by hypoxia[113] and heparin-protamine[114] but also preexisting pulmonary hypertension.[115] Benefits of inhaled NO in experimental endotoxic shock have also included improved oxygenation,[116,117] decreased intrapulmonary shunting,[117,118] and improved right ventricular function.[119] Given the probable aggravating role of NO in the accumulation of parenchymal water and decreased compliance, it is not surprising that inhaled NO did not improve either condition in experimental animals.[112,120] These findings have led to multiple clinical trials testing the efficacy of inhaled NO for reversing the pulmonary hypertension and hypoxia of acute respiratory distress syndrome (ARDS). An observational trial of seven children with ARDS resulting primarily from sepsis (one patient from near-drowning) revealed improvements in oxygenation with concentrations of inhaled NO ranging from 1 to 4 ppm.[121] Similar improvements were found in adults in a prospective, randomized trial of inhaled NO (0.5–40.0 ppm, daily).[122] The improvements were noted during the first 24 hours of therapy, with no further benefits detected thereafter. Combining inhaled NO with adjunctive therapies such as phenylephrine,[123] almitrine, and prone positioning[124] has succeeded in improving oxygenation, sometimes to a greater extent than that seen with inhaled NO alone. In the largest study published to date, Doering et al. and the Inhaled Nitric Oxide in ARDS Study Group demonstrated acute improvement in oxygenation with inhaled NO (concentration 1.25–80.00 ppm) over the first 4 hours of therapy and sustained improvement, as manifested by the decreased fraction of inspired oxygen and intensity of ventilation, over the ensuing 4 days compared to placebo-treated controls. No difference in adverse effects was noted between the groups.[123]

The finding that systemic, nonspecific NOS inhibition with L-NAME potentiated the pulmonary hypertension induced by LPS administration to swine[125] raised the possibility that combination therapy with inhaled NO could treat not only systemic hypotension but pulmonary hypertension as well. Attempts with combination therapy, however, have met with mixed results. In the porcine model, inhaled NO with L-NA[126] or L-NMMA[127] consistently improved pulmonary hypertension and systemic arterial hypotension. Addition of L-NA resulted in decreased cardiac output, whereas L-NMMA significantly improved cardiac output. Given the relatively nonselective nature of both agents (L-NA has slight eNOS selectivity), this difference is difficult to explain, and further studies with more isoform selective inhibitors are needed to clarify the potential benefits of combination therapy.

Cardiac Function and NOS Inhibition

Myocardial failure has clearly been established as a component of ongoing SIRS. Indeed, normal volunteers who have received endotoxin manifest depressed left ventricular function.[128] With the discovery of increased NO production in SIRS and the finding that L-arginine could decrease contractile force in isolated, electrically stimulated hamster papillary muscles by 80–90%,[129] NO as a mediator of decreased myocardial function came to the fore. Debate has since raged over the cardiac effects of NO both in vitro and in vivo; one study employing NO gas and NO donors (e.g., S-nitroso-amino-penicillamine, or SNAP) found a decrease in papillary muscle contractility only with concomitant β-adrenergic stimulation with norepinephrine.[130] Others have demonstrated decreased myocyte contractility in cells harvested from endotoxin-treated animals[131] and in endothelium/myocyte co-cultures from control animals treated with bradykinin or sodium nitroprusside.[132] In both cases the decreased contractility could be reversed by administering L-NAME. The findings in animal trials have been less homogeneous. Trials of NOS inhibition in dogs rendered septic with endotoxin have revealed aggravation of myocardial depression with both L-NMA[133] and L-NMMA[134,135] and decreased peripheral tissue oxygenation. In contrast, L-NAME administered to septic sheep resulted in normalization of the hyperdynamic state and maintenance of normal tissue oxygenation.[82] The relatively iNOS-selective inhibitor SMT (S-methylisothiourea) has produced improved cardiac output in vivo in septic rats; however, ex vivo preparations of the SMT-treated rat hearts lost this improvement, suggesting that another factor in the septic milieu was essential for the effects of NOS inhibition.[136] Further complicating the cardiac role of NO in SIRS is the finding that blockade of either NO synthesis (L-NA) or NO function (methylene blue) results in local areas of myocardial ischemia as imaged by NADH surface fluorescence.[137] However, there was no correlation between this local ischemia and cardiac function. Clearly, the effects of NOS inhibition in SIRS are mixed and may vary not only with the animal model but also with the specificity of the NOS inhibitor.

Hepatic Effects of NOS Inhibition

Hepatocytes were the first nonmacrophage cell type[138] and first human cell type found to express iNOS.[139] Cytokine combinations, including TNF, IL-1, and IFNγ, as well as LPS[140] have been shown to upregulate expression of iNOS. In addition, inflammatory states such as endotoxemia,[141] hepatitis, liver regeneration, and parasitic infection[142] can stimulate iNOS production. In vitro studies had shown that NO could suppress protein synthesis,[143] impair mitochondrial respiration,[144] and decrease cytochrome P450 activity in hepatocytes.[145] Given the potential for generating high local levels of hepatic NO and the in vitro data demonstrating detrimental effects of NO on hepatocyte function, the discovery that inhibition of NO generation in SIRS results in increased hepatic damage came as somewhat of a surprise. Administration of L-NMMA to mice treated with endotoxin resulted in increased levels of plasma aspartate aminotransferase (AST) and lactate dehydrogenase (LDH)[146] as well as increased hepatocellular necrosis and intrahepatic thrombosis.[147] Conversely, endotoxemic rabbits that received linsidomine (SIN-1), an NO donor, maintained portal venous blood flow and plasma lactate levels comparable to those in nonendotoxemic animals.[148] The hepatic arterial flow in SIN-1-treated animals even increased above control. Recognition that use of nonselective NOS inhibition discriminates the functions of constitutive NOS versus inducible NOS, other investigators have demonstrated a hepatic protective effect of specific iNOS inhibition using SMT,[86] L-canavanine,[149] and AG.[150] In contrast, work in our laboratory has shown that selective iNOS inhibition results in increased hepatic apoptosis.[151] The antiapoptotic effect of NO in the liver has been borne out by several studies showing that NO is a potent inhibitor of hepatocyte[152] and endothelial cell[153] apoptosis. We have postulated that eNOS limits necrosis by protecting the endothelium and that iNOS limits TNFα-induced apoptosis. Furthermore, we have suggested that the protective effects seen by others with iNOS inhibition is a manifestation of improved systemic hemodynamics. This conclusion raises the possibility that complete iNOS inhibition may have untoward effects in the presence of sepsis and that partial iNOS inhibition may be that ultimate goal.

Short, repetitive episodes of ischemia interspersed with reperfusion have been shown to render organs, including the heart and liver, more resistant to subsequent ischemic injury. Attempts to elucidate the protective mechanism underlying preconditioning in hepatic ischemia/reperfusion injury have identified NO as one of the central mediators of this effect. When an NO donor, spermine NONOate (nucleophile–NO conjugate), was infused in rats 5 minutes prior to a 90-minute hepatic ischemic injury, plasma levels of AST, alanine aminotransferase (ALT), and LDH paralleled the improvements seen with ischemic preconditioning.[154] Treatment with L-NAME prior to ischemic preconditioning abolished the protective effect of preconditioning. Exogenous portal administration of L-arginine to rats following hepatic ischemia resulted in increased hepatic NO, increased total hepatic blood flow, and decreased plasma levels of AST and ALT.[155] One potential explanation for the protective effect of NO is the described antagonism of endothelin (ET-1), a possible mediator of the disturbances in hepatic microcirculation. When infused prior to an ischemic insult, spermine NONOate decreases the expression of ET-1.[156]

NOS Inhibition and the Gastrointestinal Tract

One popular theory of the development of SIRS and MODS rests on disruption of the normal barrier function of the gut, which allows translocation of bacteria and endotoxin from the intestinal lumen and worsening systemic inflammation.[157] Underperfusion of the gut mucosa resulting in mucosal hypoxia[158,159] and increased permeability has been postulated as the mechanism of barrier impairment. Despite expression of iNOS in the mesentery of LPS-treated rodents, response of the mesenteric vessels to multiple vasoconstrictors, including ET-1, a thromboxane A₂ mimetic, phenylephrine, and 5-hydroxytryptamine, was unaffected.[160] In the presence of L-NAME, vasoconstrictor effects were potentiated, suggesting that during sepsis mesenteric NO may be essential for counterbalancing some of the effects of endogenous vasoconstrictors. Confirming the importance of NO in the maintenance of intestinal barrier function, rodent models of endotoxemia have demonstrated increased vascular permeability resulting from inhibition of NOS activity.[161–163] As complementary evidence, decreased intestinal mucosal damage and attenuated plasma leakage were noted in rats that received the NO donor SNAP beginning 10 minutes prior to LPS administration.[163] Topical mucosal application of an NO donor has been proposed as a means of augmenting local microcirculatory flow without systemic effects and has shown preliminary success in a rodent model.[164] As in other organ systems, however, evidence exists that selective isoform inhibition may reveal differing roles for NO. Rats receiving AG for 18 hours prior to LPS challenge demonstrated significantly reduced bacterial translocation (22% incidence vs. 100% in control rats) and higher transmembrane potential (as a measure of epithelial viability) than control rats.[165] Furthermore, the timing of NOS inhibition may be critical to the effect on intestinal vascular injury. Concurrent administration of L-NMMA or L-NAME and LPS has resulted in increased vascular injury as measured by intestinal albumin leakage; in contrast, administration of either inhibitor 3 hours following LPS challenge, a time of known expression of iNOS, reduces subsequent damage to the intestinal vasculature.[161]

Evidence continues to accrue implicating NO in the etiology of the intestinal ileus often present in the critically ill. Studies in canine jejunum reveal that NO functions as the neurotransmitter responsible for the nonadrenergic, noncholinergic inhibitory junctional potential (NANC-IJP).[166] NANC-IJP provides one of the major deterrents for progression of the intestine into the migrating motor complex III (MMC III), the key propulsive force in the intestine. Similar results were found in human volunteers receiving infusions of L-NMMA.[167] Data have also implicated iNOS as a major source of NO leading to ileus in endotoxemia.[168] The NO effects of increased transit time plus the increased intestinal permeability could conceivably aggravate bacterial translocation and contribute to the inception/progression of SIRS.

NOS Inhibition and Mortality

Despite the apparently promising effects of NOS inhibition on hypotension, decreased GFR, and impaired cardiac output and intestinal mucosal barrier, the survival benefits of NOS inhibition have been decidedly mixed. Most murine models of endotoxemia exhibit decreased survival following administration of L-NAME[169,170] or L-NMMA.[171] A study of specific NOS inhibition via N^ω-amino-L-arginine in endotoxemic dogs revealed a similar decrease in survival despite improvements in the aforementioned parameters.[172] In contrast, experimental murine sepsis that proved uniformly fatal even with administration of imipenem-cilastatin exhibited 80–100% survivability with co-administration of L-NMMA. Explanation of the difference between the latter study and the former trials may rest in the timing when administering the NOS inhibitor. During each trial demonstrating decreased survival the NOS inhibitor was administered concurrently with the endotoxic challenge; the survivors in the latter experiment received L-NMMA 7 hours following a lethal intraperitoneal injection of *Escherichia coli*. The temptation to attribute success in this experiment to blockade of NO derived from iNOS (as expression by 7 hours after infection should be maximal) must be tempered by the finding that iNOS knockout mice demonstrated no increase in survival over controls following a lethal dose LPS.[173] Finally, Nava et al. demonstrated that whereas high-dose (300 mg/kg) L-NMMA resulted in 100% mortality in endotoxic rats, co-administration of SNAP (300 μg/kg/hr) via continuous infusion afforded reversal of systemic hypotension and 100% survival.[81]

It is interesting to note that the experimental results have been replicated in a recent phase III clinical trial.[174] In this trial involving more than 700 septic patients, administration of the nonspecific NOS inhibitor L-NMMA resulted in increased mortality. When divided into groups based on L-NMMA dose, patients receiving low doses (5 mg/kg/hr or less) had improved survival. This result corresponds to those of experimental studies demonstrating that nonspecific NOS inhibition can be toxic at high doses; and that approaches to suppress, but not completely block, NO production could be beneficial.

Conclusion

As the studies to date have shown, manipulation of the wide-reaching effects of NO during SIRS holds great promise for improving physiologic processes in a variety of organ systems. This spectrum of NO activity also poses the greatest challenge for establishing an intervention that improves both organ protection and survival. When systemic NOS inhibition is employed, techniques aimed at allowing ongoing expression of NO from eNOS and attenuating but not completely blocking the avalanche of NO that arrives with iNOS induction (e.g., delaying administration of the NOS inhibitor or using highly selective iNOS inhibitors) appear to yield the best results. Another, possibly adjunctive approach to achieve this objective is through the use of NO scavengers that remove only excess NO. Such scavengers include hemoglobin and dithiocarbamates. Complementary therapies could include systemic NOS inhibition with concurrent administration of small amounts of NO, either through inhaled NO (as in the ARDS trials) or through low-dose infusion of an NO donor (e.g., SNAP). Ultimately, the goal is to allow generation of just enough NO to exert its benefits without crossing the threshold into detrimental effects.

References

1. Baue AE: Multiple organ failure, multiple organ dysfunction syndrome, and systemic inflammatory response syndrome: why no magic bullets? Arch Surg 1997;132:703–707.
2. Nathan C: Nitric oxide as a secretory product of mammalian cells. FASEB J 1992;6:3051–3064.
3. Lowenstein CJ, Dinerman JL, Snyder SH: Nitric oxide: a physiologic messenger. Ann Intern Med 1994;120:227–237.
4. Mitchell HH, Shonle HA, Grindley HS: The origin of nitrate in the urine. J Biol Chem 1916;24:461.
5. Green LC, Tannenbaum SR, Goldman P: Nitrate synthesis in the germ free and conventional rat. Science 1981;212:56–58.
6. Tannenbaum SR, Fett D, Young VR, Land PD, Bruce WR: Nitrite and nitrate are formed by endogenous synthesis in the human intestine. Science 1978;200:1487–1489.
7. Green LC, Ruiz de Luzuriaga K, Wagner DA: Nitrate biosynthesis in man. Proc Natl Acad Sci USA 1981;78:7764–7768.
8. Wagner DA, Young VR, Tannenbaum SR: Mammalian nitrate biosynthesis: incorporation of $^{15}NH_3$ into nitrate is enhanced by endotoxin treatment. Proc Natl Acad Sci USA 1983;80:4518–4521.
9. Hibbs JBJ, Taintor RR, Vavrin Z: Macrophage cytotoxicity: role for L-arginine deiminase and imino nitrogen oxidation to nitrite. Science 1987;235:473–476.
10. Palmer RM, Ferrige AG, Moncada S: Nitric oxide release accounts for the biological activity of endothelium-derived relaxing factor. Nature 1987;327:524–526.

11. Ignarro LJ, Buga GM, Wood KS, Byrns RE, Chaudhuri G: Endothelium-derived relaxing factor produced and released from artery and vein is nitric oxide. Proc Natl Acad Sci USA 1987;84:9265–9269.
12. Furchgott RF, Zawadzki JV: The obligatory role of endothelial cells in the relaxation of arterial smooth muscle by acetylcholine. Nature 1980;288:373–376.
13. Stuehr DJ, Griffith OW: Mammalian nitric oxide synthases. Adv Enzymol Relat Areas Mol Biol 1992;65:287–346.
14. Bredt DS, Glatt CE, Hwang PM, Fotuhi M, Dawson TM, Snyder SH: Nitric oxide synthase protein and mRNA are discretely localized in neuronal populations of the mammalian CNS together with NADPH diaphorase. Neuron 1991;7:615–624.
15. Marsden PA, Schappert KT, Chen HS, et al: Molecular cloning and characterization of human endothelial nitric oxide synthase. FEBS Lett 1992;307:287–293.
16. Bredt DS, Snyder SH: Isolation of nitric oxide synthetase, a calmodulin-requiring enzyme. Proc Natl Acad Sci USA 1990;87:682–685.
17. Busse R, Mulsch A: Calcium-dependent nitric oxide synthesis in endothelial cytosol is mediated by calmodulin. FEBS Lett 1990;265:133–136.
18. Nathan C, Xie QW: Regulation of biosynthesis of nitric oxide. J Biol Chem 1994;269:13725–13728.
19. Morris SMJ, Billiar TR: New insights into the regulation of inducible nitric oxide synthesis. Am J Physiol 1994;266:E829–E839.
20. Cho HJ, Xie QW, Calaycay J, et al: Calmodulin is a subunit of nitric oxide synthase from macrophages. J Exp Med 1992;176:599–604.
21. Lancaster JRJ: Simulation of the diffusion and reaction of endogenously produced nitric oxide. Proc Natl Acad Sci USA 1994;91:8137–8141.
22. Furchgott RF, Zawadzki JV: The obligatory role of endothelial cells in the relaxation of arterial smooth muscle by acetylcholine. Nature 1980;288:373–376.
23. Lowenstein CJ, Dinerman JL, Snyder SH: Nitric oxide: a physiologic messenger. Ann Intern Med 1994;120:227–237.
24. Nathan C: Nitric oxide as a secretory product of mammalian cells. FASEB J 1992;6:3051–3064.
25. Tannenbaum SR, Fett D, Young VR, Land PD, Bruce WR: Nitrite and nitrate are formed by endogenous synthesis in the human intestine. Science 1978;200:1487–1489.
26. Green LC, Ruiz de Luzuriaga K, Wagner DA: Nitrate biosynthesis in man. Proc Natl Acad Sci USA 1981;78:7764–7768.
27. Green LC, Tannenbaum SR, Goldman P: Nitrate synthesis in the germ free and conventional rat. Science 1981;212:56–58.
28. Hibbs JBJ, Taintor RR, Vavrin Z: Macrophage cytotoxicity: role for L-arginine deiminase and amino nitrogen oxidation to nitrite. Science 1987;235:473–476.
29. Xu L, Eu JP, Meissner G, Stamler JS: Activation of the cardiac calcium release channel (ryanodine receptor) by poly-S-nitrosylation. Science 1998;279:234–237.
30. Mistry DK, Garland CJ: Nitric oxide (NO)-induced activation of large conductance Ca^{2+}-dependent K^+ channels [BK(Ca)] in smooth muscle cells isolated from the rat mesenteric artery. Br J Pharmacol 1998;124:1131–1140.
31. McMahon TJ, Stamler JS: Concerted nitric oxide/oxygen delivery by hemoglobin. Methods Enzymol 1999;301:99–114.
32. Ignarro LJ, Buga GM, Wood KS, Byrns RE, Chaudhuri G: Endothelium-derived relaxing factor produced and released from artery and vein is nitric oxide. Proc Natl Acad Sci USA 1987;84:9265–9269.
33. Palmer RM, Ferrige AG, Moncada S: Nitric oxide release accounts for the biological activity of endothelium-derived relaxing factor. Nature 1987;327:524–526.
34. Marsden PA, Schappert KT, Chen HS, et al: Molecular cloning and characterization of human endothelial nitric oxide synthase. FEBS Lett 1992;307:287–293.
35. Bredt DS, Hwang PM, Glatt CE, Lowenstein C, Reed RR, Snyder SH: Cloned and expressed nitric oxide synthase structurally resembles cytochrome P-450 reductase. Nature 1991;351:714–718.
36. Szabo C, Zingarelli B, O'Connor M, Salzman AL: DNA strand breakage, activation of poly (ADP-ribose) synthetase, and cellular energy depletion are involved in the cytotoxicity of macrophages and smooth muscle cells exposed to peroxynitrite. Proc Natl Acad Sci USA 1996;93:1753–1758.
37. Viner RI, Huhmer AF, Bigelow DJ, Schoneich C: The oxidative inactivation of sarcoplasmic reticulum Ca^{2+}-ATPase by peroxynitrite. Free Radic Res 1996;24:243–259.
38. Szabo C: The pathophysiological role of peroxynitrite in shock, inflammation, and ischemia-reperfusion injury. Shock 1996;6:79–88.
39. Paya D, Gray GA, Fleming I, Stoclet JC: Effect of dexamethasone on the onset and persistence of vascular hyporeactivity induced by E. coli lipopolysaccharide in rats. Circ Shock 1993;41:103–112.
40. Szabo C, Mitchell JA, Gross SS, Thiemermann C, Vane JR: Nifedipine inhibits the induction of nitric oxide synthase by bacterial lipopolysaccharide. J Pharmacol Exp Ther 1993;265:674–680.
41. Schini VB, Catovsky S, Schray-Utz B, Busse R, Vanhoutte PM: Insulin-like growth factor I inhibits induction of nitric oxide synthase in vascular smooth muscle cells. Circ Res 1994;74:24–32.
42. Moro MA, Russel RJ, Cellek S, et al: cGMP mediates the vascular and platelet actions of nitric oxide: confirmation using an inhibitor of the soluble guanylyl cyclase. Proc Natl Acad Sci USA 1996;93:1480–1485.
43. Southan GJ, Szabo C: Selective pharmacological inhibition of distinct nitric oxide synthase isoforms. Biochem Pharmacol 1996;51:383–394.
44. Garvey EP, Oplinger JA, Tanoury GJ, et al: Potent and selective inhibition of human nitric oxide synthases: inhibition by nonamino acid isothioureas. J Biol Chem 1994;269:26669–26676.
45. Garvey EP, Oplinger JA, Furfine ES, et al: 1400W is a slow, tight binding, and highly selective inhibitor of inducible nitric-oxide synthase in vitro and in vivo. J Biol Chem 1997;272:4959–4963.
46. Rees DD, Monkhouse JE, Cambridge D, Moncada S: Nitric oxide and the haemodynamic profile of endotoxin shock in the conscious mouse. Br J Pharmacol 1998;124:540–546.
47. Pieper GM: Review of alterations in endothelial nitric oxide production in diabetes: protective role of orginine on endothelial dysfunction. Hypertension 1998;31:1047–1060.
48. Moore WM, Webber RK, Jerome GM, Tjoeng FS, Misko TP, Currie MG: L-N^6-(1-iminoethyl)lysine: a selective inhibitor of inducible nitric oxide synthase. J Med Chem 1994;37:3886–3888.
49. Corbett JA, Tilton RG, Chang K, et al: Aminoguanidine, a novel inhibitor of nitric oxide formation, prevents diabetic vascular dysfunction. Diabetes 1992;41:552–556.

50. Ikeda K, Gutierrez OGJ, Yamori Y: Dietary N^G-nitro-L-arginine induces sustained hypertension in normotensive Wistar–Kyoto rats. Clin Exp Pharmacol Physiol 1992;19:583–586.
51. Kobayashi Y, Ikeda K, Shinozuka K, Nara Y, Yamori Y, Hattori K: L-Nitroarginine increases blood pressure in the rat. Clin Exp Pharmacol Physiol 1991;18:397–399.
52. Baylis C, Mitruka B, Deng A: Chronic blockade of nitric oxide synthesis in the rat produces systemic hypertension and glomerular damage. J Clin Invest 1992;90:278–281.
53. Perrella MA, Hildebrand FLJ, Margulies KB, Burnett JCJ: Endothelium-derived relaxing factor in regulation of basal cardiopulmonary and renal function. Am J Physiol 1991;261:R323–R328.
54. Persson PB, Baumann JE, Ehmke H, Nafz B, Wittmann U, Kirchheim HR: Phasic and 24-h blood pressure control by endothelium-derived relaxing factor in conscious dogs. Am J Physiol 1992;262:H1395–H1400.
55. Haynes WG, Noon JP, Walker BR, Webb DJ: Inhibition of nitric oxide synthesis increases blood pressure in healthy humans. J Hypertens 1993;11:1375–1380.
56. Vallance P, Collier J, Moncada S: Effects of endothelium-derived nitrix oxide on peripheral arteriolar tone in man. Lancet 1989;2:997–1000.
57. Faraci FM, Breese KR: Nitric oxide mediates vasodilatation in response to activation of N-methyl-D-aspartate receptors in brain. Circ Res 1993;72:476–480.
58. Toda N, Okamura T: Mechanism underlying the response to vasodilator nerve stimulation in isolated dog and monkey cerebral arteries. Am J Physiol 1990;259:H1511–H1517.
59. Broten TP, Miyashiro JK, Moncada S, Feigl EO: Role of endothelium-derived relaxing factor in parasympathetic coronary vasodilation. Am J Physiol 1992;262:H1579–H1584.
60. Iwata F, Joh T, Kawai T, Itoh M: Role of EDRF in splanchnic blood flow of normal and chronic portal hypertensive rats. Am J Physiol 1992;263:G149–G154.
61. Huang PL, Huang Z, Mashimo H, et al: Hypertension in mice lacking the gene for endothelial nitric oxide synthase. Nature 1995;377:239–242.
62. Kilbourn RG, Belloni P: Endothelial cell production of nitrogen oxides in response to interferon gamma in combination with tumor necrosis factor, interleukin-1, or endotoxin. J Natl Cancer Inst 1990;82:772–776.
63. Ochoa JB, Curti B, Peitzman AB, et al: Increased circulating nitrogen oxides after human tumor immunotherapy: correlation with toxic hemodynamic changes. J Natl Cancer Inst 1992;84:864–867. Erratum. J Natl Cancer Inst 1992;84:1291.
64. Kilbourn RG, Gross SS, Jubran A, et al: N^G-Methyl-L-arginine inhibits tumor necrosis factor-induced hypotension: implications for the involvement of nitric oxide. Proc Natl Acad Sci USA 1990;87:3629–3632.
65. Kilbourn RG, Gross SS, Lodato RF, et al: Inhibition of interleukin-1-alpha-induced nitric oxide synthase in vascular smooth muscle and full reversal of interleukin-1-alpha-induced hypotension by N-omega-amino-L-arginie. J Natl Cancer Inst 1992;84:1008–1016.
66. Kilbourn RG, Owen-Schaub LB, Cromeens DM: N^G-Methyl-L-arginine, an inhibitor of nitric oxide formation, reverses IL-2-mediated hypotension in dogs. J Appl Physiol 1994;76:1130–1137.
67. Kilbourn RG, Fonseca GA, Griffith OW, et al: N^G-Methyl-L-arginine, an inhibitor of nitric oxide synthase, reverses interleukin-2-induced hypotension. Crit Care Med 1995;23:1018–1024.
68. Julou-Schaeffer G, Gray GA, Fleming I, Schott C, Parratt JR, Stoclet JC: Loss of vascular responsiveness induced by endotoxin involves L-arginine pathway. Am J Physiol 1990;259:H1038–H1043.
69. Knowles RG, Salter M, Brooks SL, Moncada S: Anti-inflammatory glucocorticoids inhibit the induction by endotoxin of nitric oxide synthase in the lung, liver and aorta of the rat. Biochem Biophys Res Commun 1990;172:1042–1048.
70. De Groote MA, Fang FC: NO inhibitions: antimicrobial properties of nitric oxide. Clin Infect Dis 1995;21(suppl 2):S162–S165.
71. Remick D, Villarete L: Regulation of cytokine expression by reactive oxygen and reactive nitrogen intermediates. J Leukoc Biol 1996;59:471–475.
72. Van Dervort A, Yan L, Madara P, et al: Nitric oxide regulates endotoxin-induced TNF-alpha production by human neutrophils. J Immunol 1994;152:4102–4109.
73. Hierholzer C, Harbrecht B, Menezes JM, et al: Essential role of induced nitric oxide in the initiation of the inflammatory response after hemorrhagic shock. J Exp Med 1998;187:917–928.
74. Diefenbach A, Schindler H, Donhauser N, et al: Type 1 interferon (IFNalpha/beta) and type 2 nitric oxide synthase regulate the innate immune response to a protozoan parasite. Immunity 1998;8:77–87.
75. Ochoa JB, Udekwu AO, Billiar TR, et al: Nitrogen oxide levels in patients after trauma and during sepsis. Ann Surg 1991;214:621–626.
76. Wong HR, Carcillo JA, Burckart G, Shah N, Janosky JE: Increased serum nitrite and nitrate concentrations in children with the sepsis syndrome. Crit Care Med 1995;23:835–842.
77. Evans T, Carpenter A, Kinderman H, Cohen J: Evidence of increased nitric oxide production in patients with the sepsis syndrome. Circ Shock 1993;41:77–81.
78. Gomez-Jimenez J, Salgado A, Mourelle M, et al: L-Arginine: nitric oxide pathway in endotoxemia and human septic shock. Crit Care Med 1995;23:253–258.
79. MacMicking JD, Nathan C, Hom G, et al: Altered responses to bacterial infection and endotoxic shock in mice lacking inducible nitric oxide synthase. Cell 1995;81:641–650. Erratum. Cell 1995;81:following 1170.
80. Thiemermann C, Ruetten H, Wu CC, Vane JR: The multiple organ dysfunction syndrome caused by endotoxin in the rat: attenuation of liver dysfunction by inhibitors of nitric oxide synthase. Br J Pharmacol 1995;116:2845–2851.
81. Nava E, Palmer RM, Moncada S: The role of nitric oxide in endotoxic shock: effects of N^G-monomethyl-L-arginine. J Cardiovasc Pharmacol 1992;20(suppl 12):S132–S134.
82. Meyer J, Lentz CW, Stothert JCJ, Traber LD, Herndon DN, Traber DL: Effects of nitric oxide synthesis inhibition in hyperdynamic endotoxemia. Crit Care Med 1994;22:306–312.
83. Meyer J, Traber LD, Nelson S, et al: Reversal of hyperdynamic response to continuous endotoxin administration by inhibition of NO synthesis. J Appl Physiol 1992;73:324–328.
84. Wu CC, Chen SJ, Szabo C, Thiemermann C, Vane JR: Aminoguanidine attenuates the delayed circulatory failure and improves survival in rodent models of endotoxic shock. Br J Pharmacol 1995;114:1666–1672.
85. Seo HG, Fujiwara N, Kaneto H, Asahi M, Fujii J, Taniguchi N: Effect of a nitric oxide synthase inhibitor, S-ethylisothiourea, on cultured cells and cardiovascular functions of normal and

lipopolysaccharide-treated rabbits. J Biochem (Tokyo) 1996; 119:553-558.
86. Szabo C, Southan GJ, Thiemermann C: Beneficial effects and improved survival in rodent models of septic shock with S-methylisothiourea sulfate, a potent and selective inhibitor of inducible nitric oxide synthase. Proc Natl Acad Sci USA 1994; 91:12472-12476.
87. Vromen A, Szabo C, Southan GJ, Salzman AL: Effects of S-isopropyl isothiourea, a potent inhibitor of nitric oxide synthase, in severe hemorrhagic shock. J Appl Physiol 1996;81: 707-715.
88. Lin PJ, Chang CH, Chang JP: Reversal of refractory hypotension in septic shock by inhibitor of nitric oxide synthase. Chest 1994;106:626-629.
89. Petros A, Bennett D, Vallance P: Effect of nitric oxide synthase inhibitors on hypotension in patients with septic shock. Lancet 1991;338:1557-1558.
90. Petros A, Lamb G, Leone A, Moncada S, Bennett D, Vallance P: Effects of a nitric oxide synthase inhibitor in humans with septic shock. Cardiovasc Res 1994;28:34-39.
91. Lorente JA, Landin L, De Pablo R, Renes E, Liste D: L-Arginine pathway in the sepsis syndrome. Crit Care Med 1993;21: 1287-1295.
92. Avontuur JA, Tutein NR, van Bodegom JW, Bruining HA: Prolonged inhibition of nitric oxide synthesis in severe septic shock: a clinical study. Crit Care Med 1998;26:660-667.
93. Anonymous editor: Nitric oxide synthase inhibition: clinical aspects. Acta Hostichemica 1997;99:127-128.
94. Mourelatos MG, Enzer N, Ferguson JL, Rypins EB, Burhop KE, Law WR: The effects of diaspirin cross-linked hemoglobin in sepsis. Shock 1996;5:141-148.
95. Reah G, Bodenham AR, Mallick A, Daily EK, Przybelski RJ: Initial evaluation of diaspirin cross-linked hemoglobin (DCLHb) as a vasopressor in critically ill patients. Crit Care Med 1997; 25:1480-1488.
96. Moisan S, Drapeau G, Burhop KE, Rioux F: Mechanism of the acute pressor effect and bradycardia elicited by diaspirin cross-linked hemoglobin in anesthetized rats. Can J Physiol Pharmacol 1998;76:434-442.
97. Fink MP, Fiallo V, Stein KL, Gardiner WM: Systemic and regional hemodynamic changes after intraperitoneal endotoxin in rabbits: development of a new model of the clinical syndrome of hyperdynamic sepsis. Circ Shock 1987;22:73-81.
98. Millar CG, Thiemermann C: Intrarenal haemodynamics and renal dysfunction in endotoxemia: effects of nitric oxide synthase inhibition. Br J Pharmacol 1997;121:1824-1830.
99. Spain DA, Wilson MA, Bloom ITM, Garrison RN: Renal microvascular responses to sepsis are dependent on nitric oxide. J Surg Res 1994;56:524-529.
100. Shultz PJ, Raij L: Endogenously synthesized nitric oxide prevents endotoxin-induced glomerular thrombosis. J Clin Invest 1992;90:1718-1725.
101. Schwartz D, Mendonca M, Schwartz I, et al: Inhibition of constitutive nitric oxide synthase (NOS) by nitric oxide generated by inducible NOS after lipopolysaccharide administration provokes renal dysfunction in rats. J Clin Invest 1997;100:439-448.
102. Groeneveld PH, Kwappenberg KM, Langermans JA, Nibbering PH, Curtis L: Nitric oxide (NO) production correlates with renal insufficiency and multiple organ dysfunction syndrome in severe sepsis. Intensive Care Med 1996;22: 1197-1202.
103. Fox GA, McCormack DG: The pulmonary physician and critical care 4. A new look at the pulmonary circulation in acute lung injury. Thorax 1992;47:743-747.
104. Tavaf-Motamen H, Miner TJ, Starnes BW, Shea-Donohue T: Nitric oxide mediates acute lung injury by modulation of inflammation. J Surg Res 1998;78:137-142.
105. Turnage RH, Wright JK, Iglesias J, et al: Intestinal reperfusion-induced pulmonary edema is related to increased pulmonary inducible nitric oxide synthase activity. Surgery 1998;124: 457-462.
106. Mehta S, Boudreau J, Lilly CM, Drazen JM: Endogenous pulmonary nitric oxide in the regulation of airway microvascular leak. Am J Physiol 1998;275:L961-L968.
107. Arkovitz MS, Wispe JR, Garcia VF, Szabo C: Selective inhibition of the inducible isoform of nitric oxide synthase prevents pulmonary transvascular flux during acute endotoxemia. J Pediatr Surg 1996;31:1009-1015.
108. Kristof AS, Goldberg P, Laubach V, Hussain SN: Role of inducible nitric oxide synthase in endotoxin-induced acute lung injury. Am J Respir Crit Care Med 1998;158:1883-1889.
109. Rossaint R, Falke KJ, Lopez F, Slama K, Pison U, Zapol WM: Inhaled nitric oxide for the adult respiratory distress syndrome. N Engl J Med 1993;328:399-405.
110. Demling RH, Smith M, Gunther R, Flynn JT, Gee MH: Pulmonary injury and prostaglandin production during endotoxemia in conscious sheep. Am J Physiol 1981;240:H348-H353.
111. Benedict CR, Grahame-Smith DG: Plasma noradrenaline and adrenaline concentrations and dopamine-beta-hydroxylase activity in patients with shock due to septicaemia, trauma and haemorrhage. Q J Med 1978;47:1-20.
112. Rayhrer CS, Edmisten TD, Cephas GA, Tribble CG, Kron IL, Young JS: Nitric oxide potentiates acute lung injury in an isolated rabbit lung model. Ann Thorac Surg 1998;65:935-938.
113. Frostell C, Fratacci MD, Wain JC, Jones R, Zapol WM: Inhaled nitric oxide: a selective pulmonary vasodilator reversing hypoxic pulmonary vasoconstriction. Circulation 1991;83:2038-2047. Erratum. Circulation 1991;84:2212.
114. Fratacci MD, Frostell CG, Chen TY, Wain JCJ, Robinson DR, Zapol WM: Inhaled nitric oxide: a selective pulmonary vasodilator of heparin-protamine vasoconstriction in sheep. Anesthesiology 1991;75:990-999.
115. Pepke-Zaba J, Higenbottam TW, Dinh-Xuan AT, Stone D, Wallwork J: Inhaled nitric oxide as a cause of selective pulmonary vasodilatation in pulmonary hypertension. Lancet 1991;338: 1173-1174.
116. Weitzberg E, Rudehill A, Lundberg JM: Nitric oxide inhalation attenuates pulmonary hypertension and improves gas exhange in endotoxin shock. Eur J Pharmacol 1993;233:85-94.
117. Dahm PL, Jonson B, De Robertis E, et al: The effects of nitric oxide inhalation on respiratory mechanics and gas exchange during endotoxaemia in the pig. Acta Anaesthesiol Scand 1998; 42:536-544.
118. Ogura H, Offner PJ, Saitoh D, et al: The pulmonary effffect of nitric oxide synthase inhibition following endotoxemia in a swine model. Arch Surg 1994;129:1233-1239.
119. Offner PJ, Ogura H, Jordan BS, Pruitt BAJ, Cioffi WG: Effects of inhaled nitric oxide on right ventricular function in endotoxin shock. J Trauma 1995;39:179-185.
120. Shah NS, Nakayama DK, Jacob TD, et al: Efficacy of inhaled nitric oxide in a porcine model of adult respiratory distress syndrome. Arch Surg 1994;129:158-164.

121. Okamoto K, Hamaguchi M, Kukita I, Kikuta K, Sato T: Efficacy of inhaled nitric oxide in children with ARDS. Chest 1998;114:827–833.
122. Troncy E, Collet JP, Shapiro S, et al: Inhaled nitric oxide in acute respiratory distress syndrome: a pilot randomized controlled study. Am J Respir Crit Care Med 1998;157:1483–1488.
123. Doering EB, Hanson CW, Reily DJ, Marshall C, Marshall BE: Improvement in oxygenation by phenylephrine and nitric oxide in patients with adult respiratory distress syndrome. Anesthesiology 1997;87:18–25.
124. Gillart T, Bazin JE, Cosserant B, et al: Combined nitric oxide inhalation, prone positioning and almitrine infusion improve oxygenation in severe ARDS. Can J Anaesth 1998;45:402–409.
125. Robertson FM, Offner PJ, Ciceri DP, Becker WK, Pruitt BA J: Detrimental hemodynamic effects of nitric oxide synthase inhibition in septic shock. Arch Surg 1994;129:149–155.
126. Weitzberg E, Rudehill A, Modin A, Lundberg JM: Effect of combined nitric oxide inhalation and N^G-nitro-L-arginine infusion in porcine endotoxin shock. Crit Care Med 1995;23:909–918.
127. Klemm P, Thiemermann C, Winklmaier G, Martorana PA, Henning R: Effects of nitric oxide synthase inhibition combined with nitric oxide inhalation in a porcine model of endotoxin shock. Br J Pharmacol 1995;114:363–368.
128. Suffredini AF, Fromm RE, Parker MM, et al: The cardiovascular response of normal humans to the administration of endotoxin. N Engl J Med 1989;321:280–287.
129. Finkel MS, Oddis CV, Jacob TD, Watkins SC, Hattler BG, Simmons RL: Negative inotropic effects of cytokines on the heart mediated by nitric oxide. Science 1992;257:387–389.
130. Weyrich AS, Ma XL, Buerke M, et al: Physiological concentrations of nitric oxide do not elicit an acute negative inotropic effect in unstimulated cardiac muscle. Circ Res 1994;75:692–700.
131. Brady AJ, Poole-Wilson PA, Harding SE, Warren JB: Nitric oxide production within cardiac myocytes reduces their contractility in endotoxemia. Am J Physiol 1992;263:H1963–H1966.
132. Brady AJ, Warren JB, Poole-Wilson PA, Williams TJ, Harding SE: Nitric oxide attenuates cardiac myocyte contraction. Am J Physiol 1993;265:H176–H182.
133. Klabunde RE, Ritger RC: N^G-Monomethyl-L-arginine (NMA) restores arterial blood pressure but reduces cardiac output in a canine model of endotoxic shock. Biochem Biophys Res Commun 1991;178:1135–1140.
134. Statman R, Cheng W, Cunningham JN, et al: Nitric oxide inhibition in the treatment of the sepsis syndrome is detrimental to tissue oxygenation. J Surg Res 1994;57:93–98.
135. Freeman BD, Zeni F, Banks SM, et al: Response of the septic vasculature to prolonged vasopressor therapy with N^ω-monomethyl-L-arginine and epinephrine in canines. Crit Care Med 1998;26:877–886.
136. McDonough KH, Smith T, Patel K, Quinn M: Myocardial dysfunction in the septic rat heart: role of nitric oxide. Shock 1998;10:371–376.
137. Avontuur JA, Bruining HA, Ince C: Inhibition of nitric oxide synthesis causes myocardial ischemia in endotoxemic rats. Circ Res 1995;76:418–425.
138. Curran RD, Billiar TR, Stuehr DJ, Hofmann K, Simmons RL: Hepatocytes produce nitrogen oxides from L-arginine in response to inflammatory products of Kupffer cells. J Exp Med 1989;170:1769–1774.
139. Nussler AK, Di Silvio M, Billiar TR, et al: Stimulation of the nitric oxide synthase pathway in human hepatocytes by cytokines and endotoxin. J Exp Med 1992;176:261–264.
140. Geller DA, Nussler AK, Di Silvio M, et al: Cytokines, endotoxin, and glucocorticoids regulate the expression of inducible nitric oxide synthase in hepatocytes. Proc Natl Acad Sci USA 1993;90:522–526.
141. Geller DA, Di Silvio M, Nussler AK, et al: Nitric oxide synthase expression is induced in hepatocytes in vivo during hepatic inflammation. J Surg Res 1993;55:427–432.
142. Klotz FW, Scheller LF, Seguin MC, et al: Co-localization of inducible-nitric oxide synthase and plasmodium berghei in hepatocytes from rats immunized with irradiated sporozoites. J Immunol 1995;154:3391–3395.
143. Billiar TR, Curran RD, Stuehr DJ, West MA, Bentz BG, Simmons RL: An L-arginine-dependent mechanism mediates Kupffer cell inhibition of hepatocyte protein synthesis in vitro. J Exp Med 1989;169:1467–1472.
144. Stadler J, Billiar TR, Curran RD, Stuehr DJ, Ochoa JB, Simmons RL: Effect of exogenous and endogenous nitric oxide on mitochondrial respiration of rat hepatocytes. Am J Physiol 1991;260:C910–C916.
145. Muller CM, Scierka A, Stiller RL, et al: Nitric oxide mediates hepatic cytochrome P450 dysfunction induced by endotoxin. Anesthesiology 1996;84:1435–1442.
146. Harbrecht BG, Billiar TR, Stadler J, et al: Nitric oxide synthesis serves to reduce hepatic damage during acute murine endotoxemia. Crit Care Med 1992;20:1568–1574.
147. Harbrecht BG, Billiar TR, Stadler J, et al: Inhibition of nitric oxide synthesis during endotoxemia promotes intrahepatic thrombosis and an oxygen radical-mediated hepatic injury. J Leukoc Biol 1992;52:390–394.
148. Pastor CM, Losser MR, Payen D: Nitric oxide donor prevents hepatic and systemic perfusion decrease induced by endotoxin in anesthetized rabbits. Hepatology 1995;22:1547–1553.
149. Liaudet L, Feihl F, Rosselet A, Markert M, Hurni JM, Perret C: Beneficial effects of L-canavanine, a selective inhibitor of inducible nitric oxide synthase, during rodent endotoxaemia. Clin Sci (Colch) 1996;90:369–377.
150. Ruetten H, Southan GJ, Abate A, Thiemermann C: Attenuation of endotoxin-induced multiple organ dysfunction by 1-amino-2-hydroxy-guanidine, a potent inhibitor of inducible nitric oxide synthase. Br J Pharmacol 1996;118:261–270.
151. Ou J, Carlos TM, Watkins SC, et al: Differential effects of nonselective nitric oxide synthase (NOS) and selective inducible NOS inhibition on hepatic necrosis, apoptosis, ICAM-1 expression, and neutrophil accumulation during endotoxemia. Nitric Oxide 1997;1:404–416.
152. Kim YM, de Vera ME, Watkins SC, Billiar TR: Nitric Oxide protects cultured rat hepatocytes from tumor necrosis factor-alpha-induced apoptosis by inducing heat shock protein 70 expression. J Biol Chem 1997;272:1402–1411.
153. Tzeng E, Kim YM, Pitt BR, Lizonova A, Kovesdi I, Billiar TR: Adenoviral transfer of the inducible nitric oxide synthase gene blocks endothelial cell apoptosis. Surgery 1997;122:255–263.
154. Peralta C, Hotter G, Closa D, Gelpi E, Bulbena O, Rosello-Catafau J: Protective effect of preconditioning on the injury associated to hepatic ischemia-reperfusion in the rat: role of nitric oxide and adenosine. Hepatology 1997;25:934–937.
155. Shiraishi M, Kusano T, Aihara T, Ikeda Y, Koyama Y, Muto Y: Protection against hepatic ischemia/reperfusion

injury by exogenous L-arginine. Transplant Proc 1996;28: 1887–1888.
156. Peralta C, Closa D, Hotter G, Gelpi E, Prats N, Rosello-Catafau J:Liver ischemic preconditioning is mediated by the inhibitory action of nitric oxide on endothelin. Biochem Biophys Res Commun 1996;229:264–270.
157. Swank GM, Deitch EA: Role of the gut in multiple organ failure: bacterial translocation and permeability changes. World J Surg 1996;20:411–417.
158. Nelson DP, Samsel RW, Wood LD, Schumacker PT: Pathological supply dependence of systemic and intestinal O_2 uptake during endotoxemia. J Appl Physiol 1988;64:2410–2419.
159. Theuer CJ, Wilson MA, Steeb GD, Garrison RN: Microvascular vasoconstriction and mucosal hypoperfusion of the rat small intestine during bacteremia. Circ Shock 1993;40:61–68.
160. Mitchell JA, Kohlhaas KL, Sorrentino R, Warner TD, Murad F, Vane JR: Induction by endotoxin of nitric oxide synthase in the rat mesentery: lack of effect on action of vasoconstrictors. Br J Pharmacol 1993;109:265–270.
161. Laszlo F, Whittle BJ, Moncada S: Time-dependent enhancement or inhibition of endotoxin-induced vascular injury in rat intestine by nitric oxide synthase inhibitors. Br J Pharmacol 1994; 111:1309–1315.
162. Hutcheson IR, Whittle BJ, Boughton-Smith NK: Role of nitric oxide in maintaining vascular integrity in endotoxin-induced acute intestinal damage in the rat. Br J Pharmacol 1990;101:815–820.
163. Boughton-Smith NK, Hutcheson IR, Deakin AM, Whittle BJ, Moncada S: Protective effect of S-nitroso-N-acetyl-penicillamine in endotoxin-induced acute intestinal damage in the rat. Eur J Pharmacol 1990;191:485–488.
164. Hersch M, Madorin WS, Sibbald WJ, Martin CM: Selective gut microcirculatory control (SGMC) in septic rats: a novel approach with a locally applied vasoactive drug. Shock 1998;10:292–297.
165. Sorrells DL, Friend C, Koltuksuz U, et al: Inhibition of nitric oxide with aminoguanidine reduces bacterial translocation after endotoxin challenge in vivo. Arch Surg 1996;131:1155–1163.
166. Stark ME, Bauer AJ, Szurszewski JH: Effect of nitric oxide on circular muscle of the canine small intestine. J Physiol (Lond) 1991;444:743–761.
167. Russo A, Fraser R, Adachi K, Horowitz M, Boeckxstaens G: Evidence that nitric oxide mechanisms regulate small intestinal motility in humans. Gut 1999;44:72–76.
168. Eskandari MK, Kalff JC, Lee KK, Bauer AJ: Lipopolysaccharide activates jejunal muscularis macrophages and suppresses circular muscularis activity. Transplant Proc 1998;30:2670.
169. Minnard EA, Shou J, Naama H, Cech A, Gallagher H, Daly JM: Inhibition of nitric oxide synthesis is detrimental during endotoxemia. Arch Surg 1994;129:142–147.
170. Fukatsu K, Saito H, Fukushima R, et al: Detrimental effects of a nitric oxide synthase inhibitor (N^{ω}-nitro-L-arginine-methyl-ester) in a murine sepsis model. Arch Surg 1995;130:410–414.
171. Evans T, Carpenter A, Silva A, Cohen J: Inhibition of nitric oxide synthase in experimental gram-negative sepsis. J Infect Dis 1994;169:343–349.
172. Cobb JP, Natanson C, Hoffman WD, et al: N^{ω}-amino-L-arginine, an inhibitor of nitric oxide synthase, raises vascular resistance but increases mortality rates in awake canines challenged with endotoxin. J Exp Med 1992;176:1175–1182.
173. Laubach VE, Shesely EG, Smithies O, Sherman PA: Mice lacking inducible nitric oxide synthase are not resistant to lipopolysaccharide-induced death. Proc Natl Acad Sci USA 1995;92: 10688–10692.
174. Grover R, Lopez A, Lorente J, Steingrub J, Bakker J, Wilatts S: Multi-center, randomized, placebo-controlled, double-blind study of the nitric oxide synthase inhibitor 546V88: effect on survival in patients with septic shock. Crit Care Med 1999;27:A33.

20
Mast Cells

Donald E. Fry

Mast cells are ubiquitously identified cells that have been clearly identified as participants in the human inflammatory response, although since their initial identification by Ehrlich in 1878[1] these cells have generally been viewed as a biologic nemesis. Hypersensitivity reactions and allergic asthma are the most common associations enjoyed by mast cells. Yet the preservation of these cells across the evolutionary process suggests that they have value for the host and that they play an important role in nonspecific host defense. This chapter addresses the mast cell as an important initiator of human inflammation, with potential for both beneficial and destructive roles in the development of systemic inflammatory response syndrome (SIRS) and multiple organ dysfunction syndrome (MODS). Regulation and control of mast cell function and of the numerous secreted products may be yet another potential treatment modality to be considered in the ever-expanding domain of potential therapies.

Cell Biology

The mast cell is rich in cytoplasmic granules and releases the presynthesized contents of these granules when specific stimuli activate the inflammatory response (Fig. 20.1). In addition to this release, mast cells acutely synthesize important active products of human inflammation. Whether degranulation, synthesis of new inflammatory products, or both occur varies depending on the activation stimulus. The mast cell shares many morphologic and functional characteristics with the circulating basophil[2] but resides within the tissues and does not circulate in the blood after full maturation. The mast cell is derived from the pleuripotential hematopoietic cell of the bone marrow,[3] appears to migrate through the circulation to a final tissue residence, and then differentiates to assume specific fundamental characteristics dictated by the hormonal and cytokine milieu of its local environment.[4]

The mast cell is particularly interesting relative to its eccentric tissue locations. It is located in skin, in intestine, around nerves, and around blood and lymph vessels.[5] These locations imply a "first response" role for the mast cell in meeting external transgressions of the host epithelial barrier or vascular tree.

The particularly well known products released from mast cells granules include heparin, histamine, and neutral protease enzymes. The types of neutral proteases present within the cytoplasmic granules have become the principal basis for differentiating populations of mast cells.[5-7] The mucosa-associated mast cell population is found in the intestinal mucosa and within alveolar tissues. The granules of the mucosa-associated cells contain only tryptase as a neutral protease. They are T cell-dependent and have unique morphologic features. The second population of mast cells are found within the skin and the submucosa of the intestinal tract. These cells also have tryptase, but chymase, carboxypeptidase, and cathepsin G reside within their granules as well. This population of mast cells is T cell-independent.

The maturation and maintenance of mast cells require stem cell factor[8,9] and interleukin-3 (IL-3).[10,11] Both stem cell factor and IL-3 are required for the differentiation of connective tissue-type mast cells.[8] Proliferation of mast cells appears to be stimulated by IL-4, IL-10, and other cytokines, but they only proliferate when IL-3 is present as well.[12-14] Under normal conditions, the total number of mast cells appears to be relatively constant.[15] Mast cell viability and maturation require the constant presence of stem cell factor.[16] Deprivation of IL-3 results in mast cell apoptosis, which can be rescued by the presence of stem cell factor.[17] Thus either IL-3 or stem cell factor must be present. Apoptosis appears to be the normal mechanism for regulation of mast cell populations in tissue as clinical conditions change.[5]

Activation of mast cells results in the release of a host of mediators. Activation results from the binding of the mediator signal to specific receptor sites. A large array of mediator signals may activate mast cells (Table 20.1).[18-38] The most extensively studied activation signal for mast cells is the immunoglobulin E (IgE)–allergen complex, which plays an important role in initiating the type I hypersensitivity reaction. The Fc component of the IgE antibody binds to a specific receptor on the plasma membrane of the plasma membrane. Binding of the IgE molecule alone does not activate the cell but does put it in a state of readiness when the appropriate antigen for the antibody is bound. Binding of the allergen on

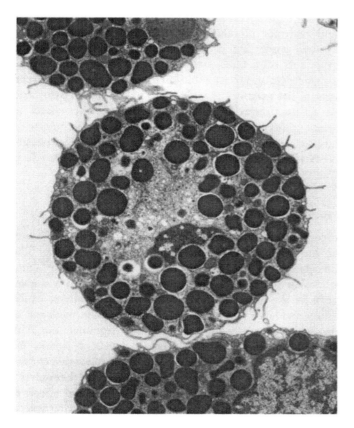

FIGURE 20.1. Electron micrograph of a rat peritoneal mast cell. The cell measures about 10 μm in diameter. The cytoplasm is rich with 0.5- to 1.0-μm cytoplasmic granules, which undergo exocytosis with the appropriate stimulus.

TABLE 20.1. Mediators That Activate Mast Cell.

IgE–antigen complex[5]

Peptides
  Mellitin (Bee vonom peptide)[18]
  Adrenocorticotropic hormone[19]
  Substance P[20]
  Calcitonin gene-related peptide[21]
  Compound 48/80[22]
  Neurotensin[23]

Cytokines
  Interleukin-1, interleukin-3[24,25]
  Platelet factor 4[26]
  Stem cell factor[27,28]
  Macrophage inflammatory protein-1 α[29]

Others
  C3a, C4a, C5a[30,31]
  Dextran[32]
  Lectins[33]
  Fibrin/collagen degradation products[34]
  Morphine[35]
  Bacterial toxins[36]
  Live bacteria[37,38]

the exposed Fab component of the antibody initiates activation of the cell.

A number of biologically relevant activation signals for the mast cell are significant contributors to the acute inflammatory response following tissue injury or infection. IL-1 and several chemokines activate mast cells. Granulocyte/monocyte colony-stimulating factor (GM-CSF) activates mast cells. The cleavage products of complement activation (C3a, C4a, C5a) are the best known activators of mast cell degranulation; and the various mast cell populations appear to have specific activation sensitivity to different activation signals. For example, C5a from the activation of complement activates skin mast cells but does not activate pulmonary mast cells.

Mediator Products

When activated, the mast cell releases a pleiotropic array of varied secretory products. As is commonly the case with all phases of human inflammation, these secreted mediators from the mast cell have redundancy with each other and represent duplicate products or redundant functions with products from other cells. The secreted products may be preformed mediators or enzymes that reside within the abundant granules of the cytoplasm. Other lipid-derived and cytokine signals are generally viewed as requiring synthesis when activation occurs.

Histamine

Among the stored cell products within the cytoplasmic granules, histamine is the most noted.[39] The action of histidine decarboxylase on the amino acid histidine results in synthesis of histamine. The histamine product is ionically bound to proteoglycans within the granule. Activation of the mast cell results in cationic exchange of the histamine product for extracellular sodium and the extracellular release of histamine. Histamine has a short biologic elimination half-life before it is metabolized to several possible end-products. The short half-life (a few minutes) probably means that the effects of this amino acid are paracrine in scope. Systemic measurements of histamine during significant stimulation by activation signals may not be easily identified because of the short half-life, which prevents large accumulation. With episodic release, as may be seen in clinical sepsis secondary to invasive infection, consistent systemic measurements of histamine concentrations have been elusive.[40,41] The absence of measurable histamine from the blood of SIRS patients, as with the numerous other cytokines, does not mean that significant biologic effects from mast cells are not being experienced by the host.

The biologic effects of histamine are numerous. Histamine may act as a vasodilator by stimulating H_2-receptors or as a vasoconstrictor through H_1-receptors.[42] The H_2-receptor-mediated vasodilation is through receptors directly present on the vascular smooth muscle itself. Evidence suggests that some of the vasodilatory effects of histamine may be through nitric oxide (NO)-dependent pathways.[43] The vasodilation effects of histamine similarly result in increased microvascular permeability and edema formation. Gap formation between endothelial cells may be secondary to morphological changes within these cells, which is mediated by histamine.[44] As discussed later, these functions of vasodilation, increased vascular permeability, and edema formation are shared by other mast cell products.

Numerous other effects of histamine are seen. Selectin activation on endothelial cells by histamine facilitates the leukocyte "rolling" phenomenon on the endovascular surface to initiate the process of margination. P-selectin on platelets is expressed by the histamine effect.[45] Histamine may locally inhibit the release of histamine from other populations of cells (i.e., basophils and perivascular mast cells).[46] Mast cell histamine may be taken up by platelets,[47] so mast cell histamine acts as a reservoir for the platelet for a portion of platelet-derived histamine that is not synthesized within the platelet itself. The uptake of histamine by the platelet may constitute a regulatory control mechanism to avoid systemic histamine effects during maximum mast cell activation.

Further evidence of the diverse effects of histamine is seen in cell populations with H_1-receptors. In addition to vasoconstriction effects, H_1-receptor stimulation mediates bronchoconstriction[48] and constriction of gastrointestinal smooth muscle.[49]

Finally, some evidence indicates that histamine from mast cells may have antiinflammatory and immunomodulatory effects that participate in the yin-yang relationship of pro- and counterinflammatory signaling seen in the summed effects of all elements of the human inflammatory response.[50,51] Histamine may have a scavenger function for reactive oxygen intermediates,[52] and it appears to inhibit neutrophil generation of reactive oxygen intermediates.[53]

Neutral Proteases

Neutral proteases are present in the cytoplasmic granules of all mast cells, although the specific proteases present differ among the mast cell populations.[54] Tryptase is the only neutral protease present in most of the resident mast cells of the lung and small intestinal mucosa. The neutral proteases of the predominant mast cells of the skin and the submucosa of the intestinal tract are tryptase, chymase, carboxypeptidase, and cathepsin G.[5] Mixed populations of the two mast cell types are seen in the nasal mucosa and tonsils. This composition of tryptase alone versus the presence of multiple proteases becomes the method for separating the two major phenotypes of mast cells in humans.[6] The different phenotypic composition of neutral proteases speaks to differentiated mast cell functions among the various populations.

Proteolysis appears to be the principal function of the neutral proteases. Digestion of the extracellular matrix as part of the inflammatory response following injury seems to be a nonspecific and salutary effect of mast cells. However, this proteolysis function appears to be injurious to the host when activation is the result of an allergic response.

Specific functions are identified with the various enzymes found in different mast cell populations. Tryptase and chymase have the specific capacity to cleave collagen.[55,56] Thus the capacity to disrupt the basement membrane appears to be a functional capacity of all mast cell populations. Chymase is a potent activator of other mast cells and also mediates the enzymatic production of angiotensin II.[57] Differences in the composition of neutral proteases in rat mast cells can be associated with specificity to degranulation of the proteoglycan matrix of the mast cell granule itself, which is then associated with different rates of histamine release.[58] The effects of different stimuli result in different rates of histamine release as a function of the protease content of the granule. The neutral proteases have extracellular effects as well as intracellular effects within the mast cell granule.

Proteoglycans

Proteoglycans are complex molecules with a central protein core that has multiple side chains of disaccharide units. The proteoglycans of the human mast cell are heparin[59] and chondroitin sulfate E.[60] The proteoglycan serves as a storage matrix for the histamine and neutral protease contents of the granule and may also serve as an extracellular mediator of secondary events following activation and degranulation. With mast cell activation, protease enzyme activation within the granule results in proteoglycan degranulation, histamine release, and subunit release of the proteoglycan molecules themselves.

Heparin is a potent anticoagulant. The potential effects of heparin's anticoagulant effects can be viewed as having several benefits for the host. Heparin maintains a fluid extracellular environment that allows the ready ingress and movement of phagocytic cells through tissues with injury or active infection. Local anticoagulation by heparin may alter excessive activation of the coagulation cascade and platelets. If one views the activation of coagulation and platelets as the primary event in human inflammation, local release of heparin may appropriately be viewed as a modulating effect on inflammation. Heparin suppresses complement activation—yet another potential modulating effect.[61] Heparin interferes with blastogenesis.[62] Heparin may be bound to platelets and may bind to specific phagocytic cell receptor sites.[63] The chondroitin sulfate E and heparin may be internalized by connective tissue cells, fibroblasts,[64] and endothelial cells.[65] Whether proteoglycans that are disposed by internalization in other cells comprise a signaling mechanism or simply a route of elimination is undefined at this time.

Cytokine Production

As another example of the redundancy that exists in the inflammatory cascade, an array of cytokines are produced by mast cells. The proinflammatory cytokines tumor necrosis factor-α (TNFα),[66] IL-1,[67] IL-6,[67] GM-CSF,[68] and interferon-γ (IFNγ)[69] have been shown to be synthesized and released by mast cells following activation. Presynthesized and stored TNFα have been identified within the granules, a unique feature of cytokine biology for the mast cell.[70] IL-3 is produced, which is most interesting given the requirement of this cytokine by mast cells to avoid apoptosis.[71] IL-4[72] and IL-5[73] have also been demonstrated from mast cells. The chemokines of IL-8,[74] [H macrophage chemotactic protein-1, macrophage inflammatory protein-1 (MIP-1α, MIP-1β) I 309, RANTES (Regulated on Activated Normal T-cell expressed and secreted) and others have been documented to be synthesized and released by activated mast cells.[75] The capacity of the mast cell to rapidly produce the numerous proinflammatory, chemotactic, and counterinflammatory signals gives this cell a quick response function in the various elements of inflammation.

Lipid Products

Cyclooxygenase and lipoxygenase products are synthesized and released by mast cells following an activation stimulus. Prostaglandin D is a multifunctional product of activated mast cells that causes vasodilation, inhibits platelet aggregation, and has chemoattractant properties for neutrophils.[76] The lipoxygenase pathway activation in the mast cell produces an array of various leukotriene (LT) molecules including LTB_4, LTC_4, LTD_4, and LTE_4.[77] The lipoxygenase pathway products are chemoattractants, enhance vascular permeability, promote the release of lysosomal enzymes from neutrophils, and stimulate the production of reactive oxygen intermediates.

Platelet activating factor (PAF) is another lipid-based product of the stimulated mast cell.[78] It serves a host of proinflammatory functions, including leukocyte trafficking, activation of platelets, and vasodilation.

Potential Role of Mast Cells in SIRS/MODS

In Chapter 10 mast cells were identified as one of the five initiators of human inflammation. These initiators set into motion phase I (i.e., vasodilation, increased vascular permeability, edema) and phase II (i.e., phagocytosis) of inflammation. The ubiquitous and strategic location of mast cells at epithelial surfaces and around vascular channels means that any major surface injury or systemically disseminated activating event (e.g., endotoxin, bacteremia) can potentially activate their inflammatory response. It is reasonable based on the broadly defined roles of the mast cell to accept their participation in (1) acute vasodilation, (2) chemokine production and leukocyte trafficking, (3) proinflammatory cytokine signaling, (4) degradation of the extracellular matrix, (5) immunomodulatory and counterinflammatory signaling, and 6) angiogenesis and wound healing.

Acute Vasodilation

The potency of histamine in promoting vasodilation in inflammatory events is well recognized. Systemic vasodilation is a clearly identified event in the patient with SIRS/MODS. Systemic histamine release is a response commonly associated with mast cells, but histamine may arise from basophils and platelets. Furthermore, measurable histamine in patients with sepsis has been inconsistently found in blood, although measurability in blood may not be a requirement as evidence of systemic participation of the either histamine or the mast cell. In addition to histamine, the synthesis of prostaglandin D is yet another mast cell product that seems likely to participate in regional and systemic vasodilation when systemic activators of inflammation are present. The separation of mast cell-specific influences versus the contribution of the alternative and additive other vasodilatory effects (e.g., NO) is not defined at this time. It is certainly reasonable to conclude that all of these vasodilatory influences are working in concert in the SIRS/MODS patient.

Chemokine Production and Leukocyte Trafficking

Among mast cell functions, their role in leukocyte mobilization into soft tissues has been studied most extensively. It is the production of chemokines and other chemoattractant signals that are identified with both the positive responses and the damaging effects of mast cells. The summed effects of chemoattractant production leads to expression of P- and E-selectin, which initiates leukocyte "rolling" within the postcapillary venule and slowing of leukocyte movement within the bloodstream in preparation for final margination. The chemokine gradient provides direction for leukocyte diapedesis into an area of acute infection or injury. Unfortunately, with generalized release of chemoattractant signals, margination and activation of the leukocyte occurs without a directional gradient and leads to the microcirculatory and tissue injury of SIRS/MODS.

Experiments with W/W^v mice have most clearly identified the important chemoattractant role of the mast cell. W/W^v mice are genetically deficient in mast cells.[79] They also have a chronic anemia that adds a certain problematic feature to direct interpretation of data used with this experimental animal. With mast cell repletion from tissue culture mast cells, the effects of mast cell deficiency can be interpreted.

Peritonitis created with bacterial and chemical models have produced common results in the W/W^v mouse,[80-85] (Table 20.2). Mobilization of neutrophils into the inflammatory milieu is slower, and there are fewer infiltrating leukocytes. Mortality rates are higher than those of normal mice of the same strain. Restoration of the mast cells with bone marrow culture mast cells restores appropriate responsiveness for the inflammatory response. Similar findings are found when gram-negative bacteria are aerosolized into the lung of the mast cell-deficient animals.[85] Reduced bacterial clearance and impaired neutrophil infiltration are seen. Normal bacterial clearance is restored with reconstitution of the mast cells. It should be emphasized that although the mast cell-deficient mice had reduced infiltration of the inflammatory site with neutrophils, this response was not completely ablated. This again illustrates the redundant mechanisms of the inflammatory response. In another provocative study, the administration of stem cell factor to normal mice appeared to increase total mast cell numbers and improved survival from cecal ligation and puncture (CLP)-induced peritonitis.[86]

These studies also showed the beneficial and potentially negative aspects of the component parts of the inflammatory

TABLE 20.2. Mast Cells in Various Models of Clinically Relevant and Other Types of Peritonitis[a].

Study year	Peritonitis model	Findings
Qureshi[80] 1988	Thioglycollate peritonitis	Delay in neutrophil influx in deficient mice; 75% total reduction in neutrophils at 14 hours, normal neutrophil response 9 days after mast cell transplantation.
Ramos[81] 1990	Egg albumin–antibody complex	Neutrophil influx into peritoneal cavity started later and maximum response had 50% fewer neutrophils than normal littermates. Transplantation of mast cells restored normal response.
Zhang[82] 1992	Egg albumin–antibody complex	Delay in neutrophil influx and maximum response at 8 hours resulted in 45% fewer neutrophils. Immediate TNF response of mast cell-deficient mice was lost. Transplantation of mast cells normalized response.
Rao[83] 1994	Calcium ionophore	Showed reduced enzyme markers for neutrophil-deficient mice. No difference between deficient and normal mice with respect to eicosanoid-derived mediators.
Echtenacher[84] 1996	Cecal ligation and puncture	Mast cell-deficient mice had 100% mortality; controls had only 25% mortality. Improved survival with mast cell-transplanted mice. Anti-TNF antibody eliminated protection of reconstituted mice.
Malaviya[85] 1996	Intraperitoneal *Klebsiella pneumoniae*	Mast cell deficient mice 20-fold less efficient in bacterial clearance from peritoneal cavity. Mortality 80% in mast cell-deficient mice. Bacterial clearance and survival restored with mast cell transplantation.

TNF, tumor necrosis factor.
[a]The findings in these studies comparing the mast cell-deficient W/W^v mouse have been consistent. Most experiments have transplanted mast cells back into the deficient mice to confirm the findings.

response. Although not specifically studied, the peritoneal and pulmonary responses of mast cell activation can similarly be viewed as negative when systemic activation of inflammation occurs. There is an amazing absence of experimental studies that have studied the mast cell consequences of bacteremia, sepsis, endotoxemia, and shock. Some experimental evidence supports a role for mast cells in ischemia/reperfusion injury.[87]

Proinflammatory Cytokine Signaling

Mast cells have been documented to produce TNF, IL-1, IL-6, and other proinflammatory cytokines. Mast cell proinflammatory cytokines must act in concert with cytokine production from other populations of cells to yield both the beneficial and deleterious effects of these signals. Anti-TNF antibody blunts the benefits of mast cell repletion in the models of peritonitis with the W/W^v mast cell-deficient mouse.[84] Mast cell-derived TNF is likely not only to serve a beneficial role in the acute infection but also to initiate the systemic effects of the exaggerated SIRS response.

The observation that mast cells have preformed TNF and perhaps other cytokines within the granule gives these cells a "first responder" role in acute inflammation. The beneficial effects of the preformed TNF may give the mast cell the earliest role in activation of the salutary local events of inflammation. Synthesis of TNF after activation likely gives the mast cell (with other cell populations) a negative role in the excessive production observed in SIRS patients.

Degradation of the Extracellular Matrix

Protease release with degranulation of the mast cell is associated with extracellular proteolysis. In acutely injured or acutely infected tissues, this proteolytic effect permits salutary digestion of the effete self. Digestion of injured and nonviable tissues surely permits more efficient infiltration of the environment by phagocytic cells. With this understanding of the possible benefits of the neutral proteases, excessive release of these enzymes in extreme circumstances of injury or necrotizing infection might well lead to inflammatory damage.

Immunomodulatory and Counterinflammatory Signaling

The mast cell appears to have not only proinflammatory functions but also a role in counterinflammatory effects. Mast cells produce IL-4, IL-13,[88] and transforming growth factor-β (TGFβ).[89] Again, situations of extreme stimulation of the cell may result in the excessive production or dyscoordinated production of these counterinflammatory signals. The mast cell may well participate in the compensatory antagonist response (CARS) (see Chapter 62). Heparin is yet another mast cell product with antiinflammatory effects. The stimuli responsible for the mast cell assuming production of pro- or counterinflammatory signals at any point in the evolution of inflammation remain to be defined.

Angiogenesis and Wound Healing

The mast cell promotes angiogenesis and wound healing. These clearly important functions of the mast cell must be preserved in the SIRS/MODS patient. These positive functions contribute to the paradox of the mast cell having both beneficial and negative effects.

There remain functions of the mast cell that are unclear in terms of benefit or liability for the host. Mast cells degranulate and are activated by neural mediators, suggesting a central neural mechanism that is involved in inflammation. Mast cells exhibit phagocytic activity.[90] Is this a "first responder" role that is beneficial to the host, or does phagocytosis activate the mast cell to an inappropriate level of proinflammatory response? Does phagocytosis result in antigen processing, similar to that seen with the monocyte, as part of the initial phase of specific immunity?

Like other components of the human inflammatory response, the mast cell shares many functions with other cell populations. Mast cells and basophils are distinct cell populations but with numerous common functions. Mast cells have extensive overlap with the monocyte or the fixed tissue macrophage. Although few studies have looked at mast cell responses to systemic events (e.g., bacteremia, shock), the evidence at present supports the idea that when the scope of the mast cell secretory products are autocrine or paracrine with acute injury or infection, the effects can generally be viewed as beneficial. The endocrine domain of its granule and synthetic products, like those of cytokines, and mediator signals from other cell populations are likely to be negative in the context of SIRS, MODS, and CARS.

References

1. Ehrlich P: Beitrage zur theorie und Praxis der histologischer Farbung. PhD thesis, University of Leipzig, 1878.
2. Huntley JF: Mast cells and basophils: a review of their heterogeneity and function. J Comp Pathol 1992;107:349–372.
3. Fodinger M, Fritsch G, Winkler K, et al: Origin of human mast cells: development from transplanted hematopoietic stem cells after allogenic bone marrow transplantation. Blood 1994;84:2954–2959.
4. Agis H, Willheim M, Sperr WR, et al: Monocytes do not make mast cells when cultured in the presence of SCF: characterization of the circulating mast cell progenitor as a c-kit$^+$, CD34$^+$, Ly$^-$, CD14$^-$, CD17$^-$, colony-forming cell. J Immunol 1993;151:4221–4227.
5. Metcalfe DD, Baram D, Mekori YA: Mast cells. Physiol Rev 1997;77:1033–1079.
6. Schwartz LB, Irani AMA, Roller K, et al: Quantitation of histamine, tryptase and chymase in dispersed human T and TC mast cells. J Immunol 1987;138:2611–2615.
7. Weidner N, Austen KF: Evidence for morphologic diversity of human mast cells: an ultrastructural study of mast cells from multiple body sites. Lab Invest 1990;63:63–72.
8. Tsai M, Takashi H, Thompson K, et al: Induction of mast cell proliferation, maturation and heparin synthesis by the rat c-kit ligand, stem cell factor. Proc Natl Acad Sci USA 1991;88:6382–6386.
9. Martin FH, Suggs SV, Langley KE: Primary structure and functional expression of rat human stem cell factor DNAs. Cell 1990;63:203–211.
10. Rottem M, Goff JP, Albert JP, Metcalfe DD: The effects of stem cell factor on the ultrastructure of FcRI$^+$ cells developing in IL-3 dependent murine bone marrow-derived cell cultures. J Immunol 1993;151:4950–4963.
11. Denburg JA: Basophil and mast cell lineages in vitro and in vivo. Blood 1992;79:846–860.
12. Rottem M, Hull G, Metcalfe DD: Demonstration of differential effects of cytokines on mast cells derived from murine bone marrow and peripheral blood mononuclear cells. Exp Hematol 1994;22:1147–1155.
13. Hultner L, Druez C, Moeller J: Mast cell growth enhancement activity (MEA) is structurally related and functionally identical to the novel mouse T cell growth factor P_{40}/TCGFIII. Eur J Immunol 1990;20:1413–1416.
14. Thompson-Nieps L, Dahr V, Bond MW, et al: Interleukin 10: a novel stimulatory factor for mast cells and their progenitors. J Exp Med 1991;173:507–510.
15. Garriga MM, Friedman M, Metcalfe DD: A survey of the number and distribution of mast cells in the skin of patients with mast cell disorders. J Allergy Clin Immunol 1988;82:425–430.
16. Mekori YA, Oh CK, Metcalfe DD: IL-3 dependent mast cells undergo apoptosis on removal of IL-3: prevention of apoptosis by c-kit ligand. J Immunol 1993;151:3775–3784.
17. Iemura A, Tsai M, Ando A, et al: The c-kit ligand, stem cell factor, promotes mast cell survival by suppressing apoptosis. Am J Pathol 1994;144:321–328.
18. Roy PD, Moran DM, Bryant V, et al: Further studies on histamine release from rat mast cells in vitro induced by peptides: characteristics of a synthetic intermediate with potent releasing activity. Biochem J 1980;191:233–237.
19. Hinson JP, Vinson GP, Kopas S, Teja R: The relationship between adrenal vascular events and steroid secretion: the role of mast cells and endothelin. J Steroid Biochem Mol Biol 1991;40:381–389.
20. Johnson AR, Erdos EG: Release of histamine from mast cells by vasoactive peptides. Proc Soc Exp Biol Med 1973;142:1252–1256.
21. Ottosson A, Edvinsson L: Release of histamine from dural mast cells by substance P and calcitonin gene-related peptide. Cephalgia 1997;17:166–174.
22. Lagunoff D, Martin TW, Read G: Agents that release histamine from mast cells. Annu Rev Pharmacol Toxicol 1983;23:331–351.
23. Miller LA, Cochrane DE, Feldberg RS, Carraway RE: Inhibition of neurotensin-stimulated mast cell secretion and carboxypeptidase A activity by the peptide inhibitor of carboxypeptidase A and neurotensin-receptor antagonist SR 48692. Int Arch Allergy Immunol 1998;116:147–153.
24. Subramanian N, Bray MA: Interleukin 1 releases histamine from human basophils and mast cells in vitro. J Immunol 1987;138:271–275.
25. Nitschke M, Sohn K, Dieckmann D, et al: Effects of basophil-priming and stimulatory cytokines in histamine release from isolated human skin mast cells. Arch Dermatol Res 1996;288:463–468.
26. McLaren KM, Holloway L, Pepper DS: Human platelet factor 4 and tissue mast cells. Thromb Res 1980;19:293–297.
27. Klimpel GR, Chopra AK, Langley KE, et al: A role for stem cell factor and c-kit in the murine intestinal tract secretory response to cholera toxin. J Exp Med 1995;182:1931–1942.
28. Taylor AM, Galli SJ, Coleman JW: Stem-cell factor, the kit ligand, induces direct degranulation of rat peritoneal mast cells in vitro and in vivo. Immunology 1995;86:427–433.
29. Alam R, Kumar D, Anderson-Walters D, Forsythe PA: Macrophage inflammatory protein-1 alpha and monocyte chemoattractant peptide-1 elicit immediate and late cutaneous reactions and

activate murine mast cells in vivo. J Immunol 1994;152: 1298–1303.
30. Hugli TE, Muller-Eberhard HJ: Anaphylatoxins: C3A and C5A. Adv Immunol 1978;26:1–53.
31. Johnson AR, Hugli TE, Muller-Eberhard HJ: Release of histamine from rat mast cells by complement peptides C3a and C5a. Immunology 1975;28:1067–1072.
32. Ennis M, Trimble ER: Comparison of histamine release from peritoneal mast cells derived from diabetic and control rats. Agents Actions 1991;33:23–25.
33. Lagunoff D, Martin TW, Read G: Agents that release histamine from mast cells. Annu Rev Pharmacol Toxicol 1983;23:331–351.
34. Wojtecka-Lukasik E, Maslinski S: Fibronectin and fibrinogen degradation products stimulate PMN-leukocyte and mast cell degranulation. J Physiol Pharmacol 1992;43:173–181.
35. DiBello MG, Masini E, Ioannides C, et al: Histamine release from rat mast cells induced by the metabolic activation of drugs of abuse into free radicals. Inflamm Res 1998;47:122–130.
36. Leal-Berumen I, Conlon P, Marshall JS: IL-6 production by rat peritoneal mast cells is not necessarily preceded by histamine release and can be induced by bacterial lipopolysaccharide. J Immunol 1994;152:5468–5476.
37. Malaviya R, Ross E, Jakschik BA, Abraham SN: Mast cell degranulation induced by type 1 fimbriated *Escherichia coli* in mice. J Clin Invest 1994;93:1645–1653.
38. Malaviya R, Ross EA, MacGregor JI, et al: Mast cell phagocytosis of FimH-expressing enterobacteria. J Immunol 1994;152: 1907–1914.
39. White MV, Slater JE, Kaliner MA: Histamine and asthma. Am Rev Respir Dis 1987;135:1165–1176.
40. Neugebauer E, Lorenz W, Beckurts T, et al: Significance of histamine formation and release in the development of endotoxic shock: proof of current concepts by randomized controlled studies in rats. Rev Infect Dis 1987;9(Suppl 5):S585–S593.
41. Neugebauer E, Lorenz W, Rixen D, et al: Histamine release in sepsis: a prospective, controlled, clinical study. Crit Care Med 1996;24:1670–1677.
42. Mannaioni PF, Di Bello MG, Masini E: Platelets and inflammation: role of platelet-derived growth factor, adhesion molecules and histamine. Inflamm Res 1997;46:4–18.
43. Mayhan WG: Nitric oxide accounts for histamine-induced increases in macromolecular extravasation. Am J Physiol 1994;226:H2369–H2373.
44. Majno G, Shea SM, Leventhal M: Endothelial contraction induced by histamine type mediator: an electron microscope study. J Cell Biol 1969;42:647–667.
45. Eppihimer MJ, Wolitzky B, Anderson DC, et al: Heterogeneity of expression of E- and P-selectin in vivo. Circ Res 1996;79:560–569.
46. Lichtenstein LM, Gillespie E: Inhibition of histamine release by histamine controlled by H2 receptor. Nature 1973;244:287–288.
47. Gill DS, Barradas MA, Mikhailidis DP, Dandona P: Histamine uptake by human platelets. Clin Chim Acta 1987;168:177–185.
48. Myers AC, Undem BJ: Antigen depolarizes guinea pig bronchial parasympathetic ganglion neurons by activation of histamine H1 receptors. Am J Physiol 1995;268:L879–L894.
49. Sim SS, Jo YH, Hahn SJ, et al: H1 receptor mediates inositol phosphate response to histamine in gastric smooth muscle of guinea pigs. Scand J Gastroenterol 1993;28:69–72.
50. Al-Imara LJ, Dale MM: The inhibitory effect of histamine on lymphoid tissue the proliferation in mice. Cell Immunol 1985;91:284–288.
51. Carlsson R, Dohlsten M, Sjogren HO: Histamine modulates the production of interferon-gamma and interleukin-2 mitogen-activated human mononuclear blood cells. Cell Immunol 1985;96:104–112.
52. Ching TL, van der Hee RM, Bhoelan NM, et al: Histamine as a marker for hydroxyl radicals. Med Inflamm 1995;4: 339–343.
53. Fantozzi R, Brunelleschi S, Banchelli Soldaini G, et al: N-formylmethionyl-leucyl-phenyl-alanine: different releasing effects on human neutrophils and rat mast cells. Agents Actions 1983;13:218–221.
54. Irani A-MA, Bradford TR, Kepley CL, et al: Detection of MCT and MCTC types of human mast cells by immunohistochemistry using new monoclonal anti-tryptase and anti-chymase antibodies. J Histochem Cytochem 1989;37:1509–1515.
55. Gruber BL, Marchese MJ, Suzuki K, et al: Synovial procollagenase activation by human mast cell tryptase dependence upon matrix metalloproteinase 3 activation J Clin Invest 1989;84: 1657–1662.
56. Saarinen J, Kalkkinen N, Welgus HG, Kovanen PT: Activation of human interstitial procollaginase through direct cleavage of the leu83-thr84 bond by mast cell chymase. J Biol Chem 1994;269:18134–18140.
57. Reilly CF, Tewksbury DA, Schechter NM, Travis J: Rapid conversion of angiotensin I to angiotensin II by neutrophil and mast cell proteinase. J Biol Chem 1982;257:8619–8622.
58. Goldstein SM, Leong J, Schwartz LB, Cooke D: Protease composition of exocytosed human skin mast cell protease-proteoglycan complexes: tryptase resides in a complex distinct from chymase and carboxypeptidase. J Immunol 1992;148:2475–2482.
59. Metcalfe DD, Lewis RA, Silbert JE, et al: Isolation and characterization of heparin from human lung. J Clin Invest 1979;64:1537–1543.
60. Thompson HL, Schulman ES, Metcalfe DD: Identification of chondroitin sulfate E in human lung mast cells. J Immunol 1988;140:2708–2713.
61. Strunk R, Colten HR: Inhibition of the enzymatic activity of the first component of complement by heparin. Clin Immunol Immunopathol 1976;6:248–255.
62. Frieri M, Metcalfe DD: Analysis of the effect of mast cell granules on lymphocyte blastogenesis in the absence and presence of mitogen. J Immunol 1983;131:1942–1948.
63. Leculier C, Benzerara O, Couprie N, et al: Specific binding between human neutrophils and heparin. Br J Haematol 1992;81:81–85.
64. Subba Rao PV, Friedman MM, Atkins FM, Metcalfe DD: Phagocytosis of mast cell granules by cultured fibroblasts. J Immunol 1983;130:341–349.
65. Atkins FM, Friedman MM, Metcalfe DD: Biochemical and microscopic evidence for the internalization and degradation of heparin-containing mast cell granules by bovine endothelial cells. Lab Invest 1985;52:278–286.
66. Okhawara Y, Yamauchi K, Tanno Y: Human lung mast cells and pulmonary macrophages produce tumor necrosis factor-alpha in sensitized lung tissue after IgE receptor triggering. Am J Respir Cell Mol Biol 1992;7:385.
67. Grabbe J, Welker P, Moller A, et al: Comparative cytokine release from human monocytes, monocyte-derived immature mast cells, and a human mast cell line (HMC-1). J Invest Dermatol 1994;103:504–508.

68. Okayama Y, Kobayashi H, Ashman LK, et al: Human lung mast cells are enriched in the capacity to produce granulocyte-macrophage colony-stimulating factor in response to IgE-dependent stimulation. Eur J Immunol 1998;28:708–715.
69. Gupta AA, Leal-Berumen I, Croitoru K, Marshall JS: Rat peritoneal mast cells produce IFN-gamma following IL-12 treatment but not in response to IgE-mediated activation. J Immunol 1996;157:2123–2128.
70. Gordon JR, Galli SJ: Mast cells as a source of both performed and immunologically inducible TNF-alpha/cachectin. Nature 1990;346:274–276.
71. Buckley MG, Williams CM, Thompson J, et al: IL-4 enhances IL-3 and IL-8 gene expression in a human leukemia mast cell line. Immunology 1995;84:410–415.
72. Bradding P, Feather IH, Howarth PH, et al: Interleukin-4 is localized to and released by human mast cells. J Exp Med 1992;1381–1386.
73. Bressler RB, Lesko J, Jones M, et al: Production of IL-5 and granulocyte-macrophage colony-stimulating factor by naive human mast cells activated by high affinity IgE receptor ligation. J Allergy Clin Immunol 1997;99:508–514.
74. Moller A, Pippert U, Lessmann D, et al: Human mast cells produce IL-8. J Immunol 1993;151:3261–3266.
75. Selvan RS, Butterfield JH, Krangel MS: Expression of multiple cytokine genes by a human mast cell leukemia. J Biol Chem 1994;269:13893–13898.
76. Lewis RA, Austen KF: The biologically active leukotrienes: biosynthesis, metabolism, receptors, functions and pharmacology. J Clin Invest 1984;73:889–897.
77. Lewis RA, Austen KF, Soberman RJ: Leukotrienes and other products of the 5-lipoxygenase pathway-biochemistry and relation to pathobiology in human disease. N Engl J Med 1990;323:645–655.
78. Gaboury JP, Johnston B, Niu XF, Kubes P: Mechanisms underlying acute mast cell-induced leukocyte rolling and adhesion in vivo. J Immunol 1995;154:804–813.
79. Kitamura Y, Go S, Hatanaka K: Decrease of mast cells in W/W^v mice and their increase by bone marrow transplantation. Blood 1978;52:447–452.
80. Qureshi R, Jakschik BA: The role of mast cells in thioglycollate-induced inflammation. J Immunol 1988;141:2090–2096.
81. Ramos BF, Qureshi R, Olsen KM, Jakschik BA: The importance of mast cells for the neutrophil influx immune complex-induced peritonitis in mice. J Immunol 1990;145:1868–1873.
82. Zhang Y, Ramos BF, Jakschik BA: Neutrophil recruitment by tumor necrosis factor from mast cells in immune complex peritonitis. Science 1992;258:1957–1959.
83. Rao TS, Shaffer AF, Currie JL, Isakson PC: Role of mast cells in calcium ionophore (A23187)-induced peritoneal inflammation in mice. Inflammation 1994;18:187–192.
84. Echtenacher B, Mannel DN, Hultner L: Critical protective role of mast cells in a model of acute septic peritonitis. Nature 1996;381:75–77.
85. Malaviya R, Iikeda T, Ross E, Abraham SN: Mast cell modulation of neutrophil influx and bacterial clearance at sites of infection through TNF-alpha. Science 1996;381:77–80.
86. Maurer M, Echtenacher B, Hultner L, et al: The c-kit ligand, stem cell factor, can enhance innate immunity through effects on mast cells. J Exp Med 1998;188:2343–2348.
87. Kanwar S, Hickey MJ, Kubes P: Postischemic inflammation: a role for mast cells in intestine but not in skeletal muscle. Am J Physiol 1998;275:G212–G218.
88. Toru H, Pawankar R, Ra C, et al: Human mast cells produce IL-13 by high affinity IgE receptor cross-linking: enhanced IL-13 production by IL-4 primed human mast cells. J. Allergy Clin Immunol 1998;102:491–502.
89. Kendall JC, Li XH, Galli SJ, Gordon JR: Promotion of mouse fibroblast proliferation by IgE-dependent activation of mouse mast cells: role for mast cell tumor necrosis factor-alpha and transforming growth factor-beta 1. J Allergy Clin Immunol 1997;99:113–123.
90. Malaviya R, Ross EA, MacGregor JI, et al: Mast cell phagocytosis of FimH-expressing enterobacteria. J Immunol 1994;152:1907–1914.

21
Eicosanoids

Geoffrey T. Manley, Mary J. Vassar, and James W. Holcroft

Over the past 40 years a number of acute and chronic inflammatory mediators such as bradykinin, histamine, and eicosanoids have been studied. More recently, studies have focused on the pathophysiologic role of cytokines, growth factors, and nitric oxide. Using the powerful techniques of molecular biology, complex and interrelated pathways for these mediators have been established. These methods have also led to the recent discovery of an inducible form of prostaglandin synthase (cyclooxygenase-2, or COX-2) and a number of new phospholipase A_2 family members. These discoveries in turn have led to renewed interest in the role of eicosanoids in acute and chronic inflammation. This is fitting, given that aspirin and other nonsteroidal antiinflammatory drugs (NSAIDs) continue to be the most widely used medications for a variety of disorders. The purpose of this chapter is to review the molecular, pharmacologic, and clinical aspects of eicosanoid biosynthesis with a focus on recent developments in this important pathway.

Overview of Eicosanoid Pathways

The eicosanoids are a family of lipid-based mediators derived from an essential 20-carbon polyunsaturated fatty acid precursor, arachidonic acid (AA). These molecules were identified through their actions on smooth muscle contraction.[1] Unlike classic protein hormones, eicosanoids are not stored or transported in the bloodstream. Instead, they are rapidly synthesized, released, and metabolized in their local environment. Because of these properties they are often referred to as "autocoids." The eicosanoids are produced by nearly all mammalian cells and tissues with the exception of the red blood cell. The first step in eicosanoid synthesis involves the release of AA from membrane phospholipids catalyzed by phospholipases (Fig. 21.1). Free AA is then rapidly converted to intermediates of prostaglandin (PG) synthesis by PG synthase. Depending on the cell type or tissue, AA can also be enzymatically metabolized to precursors of the leukotriene (LT) pathway by several lipoxygenases. In addition to these classic pathways of AA metabolism, an important nonenzymatic pathway has recently been elucidated whereby free radical attack on AA results in the production of isoeicosanoids.

Arachidonic Acid Release

In general, AA release from the phospholipid membrane is the rate-limiting step in eicosanoid production.[2] This reaction is carried out by the phospholipase family of enzymes. These proteins also play a significant role in other signal transduction pathways, cellular membrane restructuring, and general lipid metabolism. The two most important groups in the eicosanoid pathway are phospholipase A_2 and phospholipase C.

Phospholipase A_2 is a rapidly growing family of enzymes that hydrolyze the *sn*-2 ester bond of glycerophospholipids to generate free fatty acids and lysophospholipids. These products can be reesterified or metabolized into downstream bioactive molecules. Lysophospholipids can alter membrane fluidity or be converted to the inflammatory mediators platelet-activating factor[3] and lysophosphatidic acid.[4] Lysophospholipids can also induce expression of vascular adhesion molecules and growth factor receptors, and they can stimulate protein kinase C and cyclic phosphodiesterases. Following a pathologic event such as trauma, the increased activity of phospholipase A_2 favors the production of these lipid mediators as well as the eicosanoids, thereby promoting membrane and cellular dysfunction.

The increased number of phospholipase A_2 enzymes recognized has led to a revised classification system based on substrate and cofactor specificity, molecular weight, and amino acid sequence (Table 21.1).[5] Groups I, II, and III are low-molecular-weight enzymes (13–15 kDa) that require calcium and are secreted. These well characterized phospholipases were first identified in poisonous snake venom. In mammals the group IB phospholipases are primarily secreted by the pancreas for extracellular digestion of lipids.[6] They are also expressed in other organs, suggesting a secondary nondigestive role.[7] The group IIA enzymes are found in the synovial fluid of arthritic joints and in the serum of patients with sepsis, adult respiratory distress syndrome (ARDS), and acute pancreatitis, suggesting a role in inflammation.[8] Group IV phospholipases are larger

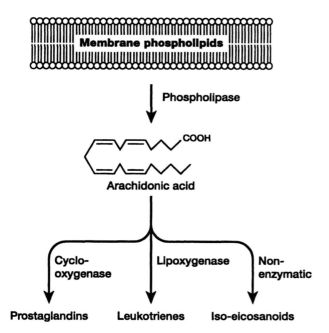

FIGURE 21.1. Overview of eicosanoids pathways. Arachidonic acid released from membrane phospholipids is catalyzed by phospholipases. Arachidonic acid can be enzymatically converted to prostaglandins and leukotrienes. Nonenzymatically, free radicals attach as arachidonic acid leads to isoeicosanoid formation.

(85 kDa) enzymes that have a smaller calcium requirement and are cytosolic. Group IV enzymes can also be regulated by phosphorylation.[9] They have phospholipase A_1, transacylase, and lysophospholipase activity.[10] Group V enzymes are found in heart, lung, and liver and are thought to be an evolutionary precursor of the group I and II proteins.[6] Cytosolic calcium-independent group VI phospholipases are found in ovarian and macrophage cell lines. This enzyme remodels the phospholipid membrane to facilitate esterification of arachidonic acid for subsequent stimulated release.[11] The enzyme that degrades platelet-activating factor (PAF), PAF acetylhydrolase, has recently been cloned and found to be a phospholipase A_2. This group VII enzyme is found in plasma and has antiinflammatory activity.[12] A second intracellular form of PAF acetylhydrolase is placed in the group VIII phospholipases. A number of other biochemically characterized phospholipases have yet to be cloned, so the size and classification scheme of this crucial family of enzymes will certainly continue to expand.

Phospholipase C can also initiate a cascade that results in the release of free AA. This complex pathway was first identified in platelets. The initial step involves release of the phosphatidyl moiety from the third position of the phospholipid molecule, typically phosphatidyl inositol. The free phosphatidyl inositol can then participate in downstream signal transduction pathways. The residual diacylglycerol molecule can activate protein kinase C or be sequentially metabolized by diacylglyceride lipase and monoglyceride lipase to generate AA for eicosanoid synthesis.[13]

It is apparent that phospholipase activity not only results in the release of free AA for eicosanoid synthesis, it can also generate a number of other significant inflammatory mediators. The rate-limiting aspect of these enzymes makes them prime targets for pharmacologic intervention. It was thought for some time that steroids inhibited phospholipase A_2 through an intermediate protein, but no direct inhibition of phospholipase A_2 has yet been demonstrated. Although steroids do have the ability to regulate a number of inflammatory processes, the exact mechanisms of these interactions are still poorly understood. To date, no specific inhibitors have been identified for clinical use. As our knowledge of this complex group of enzymes increases, the future development of clinically important phospholipase inhibitors is likely.

Prostaglandin Biosynthesis

The synthesis of prostaglandins and thromboxanes occurs in a stepwise fashion beginning with the conversion of free AA to an unstable endoperoxide (Fig. 21.2). The enzyme responsible for the first two steps in the pathway is PGH_2 synthase, also known as cyclooxygenase. This protein has two catalytic sites that first oxygenate and cyclize AA to form the cyclic endoperoxide PGG_2 and then reduce PGG_2 to the hydroxyl endoperoxide PGH_2. These endoperoxides are then transformed enzymatically by specific synthases into a variety of prostaglandins such as PGD_2, PGE_2, $PGF_{2\alpha}$, prostacyclin (PGI_2), and thromboxane (TXA_2). Thromboxane and prostacyclin synthase have been purified, cloned, and sequenced; prostaglandin D, E, and F synthase await more extensive characterization.

Prostaglandins play a key role in tissue homeostasis and inflammation.[14] In the stomach prostaglandins such as PGI_2 and PGE_2 have a cytoprotective function due to their ability to

TABLE 21.1. Classification and Characterization of Major Phospholipase A_2 Groups.

Group	Source	Size (kDa)	Location	Ca^{2+} dependency (mM)
IA	Snake venom	13–15	Secreted	Dependent
IB	Pancreas	13–15	Secreted	Dependent
IIA	Synovial fluid, platelets,		Secreted	Dependent
IIB	Snake venom		Secreted	Dependent
IIC	Testes		Secreted	Dependent
III	Bees, lizards		Secreted	Dependent
IV	Platelets, kidney, cell lines (U937, Raw 264.7)		Cytosolic	Dependent (<1)
V	Heart, lung, P338D1 macrophages		Secreted	Dependent
VI	P338D1 macrophages, CHO cells		Cytosolic	Independent
VII	Plasma		Secreted	Independent
VIII	Brain		Cytosolic	Independent
IX	Marine snail		Secreted	Dependent (<1)

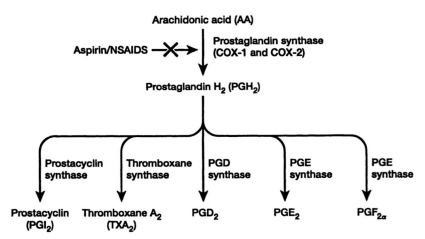

FIGURE 21.2. Biosynthesis of prostaglandins. Free arachidonic acid is converted to unstable prostaglandin endoperoxide (PGH_2) by COX-1 and COX-2. PGH_2 can be converted to a variety of prostaglandins by specific synthases. Aspirin and NSAIDs inhibit COX-1 and COX-2.

enhance mucosal blood flow. Prostaglandins are also important in maintaining renal blood flow in patients with congestive heart failure or adrenal insufficiency. The effect of TXA_2 on platelet aggregation is well characterized and forms the basis of prophylactic cyclooxygenase inhibition for thromboembolic disease. Endothelial cells produce prostacyclin, a potent vasodilator that also serves as an antiaggregatory counterbalance to TXA_2. PGE_2 and PGD_2 are major prostaglandins in the central nervous system. It is believed that fever is a result of PGE_2 produced in the organum vasculosum laminae terminalis, which activates the thermoregulatory center in the anterior hypothalamus.[15] Another nervous system effect of prostaglandins is hyperalgesia. During inflammation prostaglandins are generated near the terminals of peripheral sensory neurons and cause pain.[16] It is clear from this limited review that prostaglandins are ubiquitous with a wide array of important functions.

One of the most exciting events in eicosanoid biology in recent years is the discovery of a second isoform of cyclooxygenase.[17] The original enzyme, now referred to as cyclooxygenase-1 (COX-1), was first purified during the mid-1970s and cloned in 1988. The second enzyme, COX-2, was identified based on its homology to COX-1. Subsequent studies have revealed a number of similarities and clinically important differences in these two isoforms (Table 21.2). They are similar in size (71 kDa) and have 63% amino acid sequence identity. The gene structure and expression, however, are quite different. COX-1 is located on chromosome 9 and constitutively expresses a 2.8-kb mRNA. COX-2 is located on chromosome 1 with inducible expression of a 4.3-kb mRNA that is highly unstable, consistent with its function as an immediate early gene. The catalytic activities of the two isoforms are identical. A comparison of the X-ray crystal structures reveals that the catalytic site, substrate binding channel, and adjacent residues are identical, with divergence at only two sites (positions 434 and 523). Biochemically, there are significant differences in substrate specificity and inhibitor selectivity (see below). COX-2, for example, can accept and transform 18-carbon polyunsaturated fatty acids more readily than COX-1.

There are significant differences in the physiologic roles of the two cyclooxygenase isoforms. COX-1 is expressed on the endoplasmic reticulum of nearly all cells and participates in normal functions.[18] Examples of COX-1 housekeeping functions are consistent with its expression in the stomach, kidney, platelets, endothelium, uterus, and brain. In contrast, COX-2 is rapidly induced in response to a number of inflammatory mediators, growth factors, and tumor promoters and is expressed in the endoplasmic reticulum and nuclear envelope. The brain is one of the few organs that constitutively expresses of COX-2, where it is thought to participate in synaptic transmission. Interestingly, corticosteroids and antiinflammatory cytokines can decrease COX-2 induction.[19] Further exploration of the inhibitory actions of steroids on COX-2 is important to clarify their effect on prostaglandin synthesis, as noted in previous reports.

Both isoforms of cyclooxygenase are inhibited by aspirin and NSAIDs, although, different NSAIDs have differential inhibitory activity on COX-1 and COX-2.[20] Structural studies of cyclooxygenase suggest that the active site of the enzyme is located at the end of a tubular channel.[14] Aspirin irreversibly inhibits COX-1 by acetylating a specific serine residue (Ser^{530}) that blocks AA entry into the channel. Although aspirin also acetylates a comparable amino acid (Ser^{516}) of COX-2, the enzyme retains

TABLE 21.2. Comparison of COX-1 and COX-2.

Parameter	COX-1	COX-2
Gene	Chromosome 9; 22 kb	Chromosome 1; 8 kb
Expression	Constitutive 2.8-kb mRNA	Inducible 4.3-kb mRNA (unstable)
Protein	71-kDa membrane protein	71-kDa membrane protein
Cellular location	Endoplasmic reticulum	Endoplasmic reticulum and nuclear envelope
Tissue distribution	All tissues	Inflammatory tissues
Function	Housekeeping functions in stomach, kidney, platelets, endothelium	Inflammatory response in macrophages, leukocytes, endothelium, fibroblasts
Inhibition	Aspirin, NSAIDs	Aspirin, NSAIDs, glucocorticoids

its oxygenase activity, allowing conversion of AA to 15(R)-hydroxyeicosottetraenoic acid (HETE). It has been postulated that this metabolite may be involved in the protective effects of aspirin on colorectal cancer.[21] A comparison of the inhibitory effects of NSAIDs on COX-1 and COX-2 has demonstrated variable selectivity for these enzymes, which has created an opportunity for the development of specific COX-2 inhibitors. The different biologic effects of the isoforms suggests that a specific COX-2 inhibitor may be effective in preventing inflammation while preserving the housekeeping functions of COX-1. This concept has generated significant pharmaceutical interest, resulting in the development of a number of COX-2-specific drugs. Early reports show that these drugs are effective antiinflammatory agents that appear to have few renal and gastrointestinal side effects. The continued development of new cyclooxygenase inhibitors will likely lead to more effective treatments for a number of acute, chronic, and inherited diseases.

Leukotriene Biosynthesis

The lipoxygenase pathway is another major conduit for eicosanoid production in mammalian cells (Fig. 21.3). These compounds were first identified as active components of the slow-reacting substance of anaphylaxis.[22] The first step in this pathway begins with the introduction of molecular oxygen into AA by a lipoxygenase.[23] The three major lipoxygenases (5-, 12-, and 15-lipoxygenase) differ in their tissue-specific expression and specificity for the substrate placement of the hydroxyperoxy group. All of these enzymes are similar in size and have Fe^{2+} near the active site. These enzymes catalyze a two-step reaction wherein AA is first converted to a hydroperoxy fatty acid. These hydroxyperoxyeicosottetraenoic acids (HPETEs) are highly unstable and rapidly converted to a more stable HETE. In platelets, 12-lipoxygenase converts arachidonic acid to 12-HETE. Leukocytes have both 15- and 5-lipoxygenase. In the 15-lipoxygenase pathway further metabolism generates lipoxins, which are mediators of neutrophil activity.

The 5-lipoxygenase pathway has been studied most extensively, as it leads to the production of leukotrienes. Once 5-lipoxygenase has generated 5-HPETE, LTA_4 synthase, which is part of this enzyme, catalyzes the rearrangement into LTA_4. This second unstable intermediate can then be converted to LTB_4, or it can be conjugated with glutathione to form LTC_4. Subsequent cleavage of the glutamic acid and glycine results in the formation of LTD_4 and LTE_4. The latter three compounds are often referred to as the cysteinyl leukotrienes.

Leukotriene B_4 is a significant inflammatory mediator.[24] It stimulates neutrophil chemotaxis and activation, resulting in the release of additional enzyme mediators and superoxides. LTB_4 also stimulates the production of cytokines in mononuclear cells. It is thought to have a role in pain through its reduction in the nociceptive threshold in inflamed tissue. The cysteinyl leukotrienes (LTC_4, LTD_4, LTE_4) are powerful smooth muscle constrictors in the airway.[25] They also increase vascular permeability, resulting in tissue edema. Because these activities mimic many of the features of asthma, several groups have pursued the development of 5-lipoxygenase and cysteinyl leukotriene receptor antagonists.[26] A number of leukotriene receptor antagonists have been developed using a combination of strategies based on structure–activity relations.[27] Several of these compounds have been introduced for the treatment of asthma. Other leukotriene receptor antagonists will soon become available and will likely extend the range of diseases that can be treated with this approach. The structure–activity paradigm used in the successful development of these drugs serves as a model for future antieicosanoid drug development.

Isoeicosanoids

The isoeicosanoids are a relatively new family of eicosanoid isomers derived from the nonenzymatic oxidative modification of AA.[28] Members of this family include the isoleukotrienes, isoprostaglandins, or isoprostanes of the D_2, E_2, and F_2 series and the isothromboxanes. In contrast to the "classic" leukotriene and prostaglandin enzymatic pathways where free arachidonic acid is used as a substrate, the isoeicosanoid pathway begins with the free radical-catalyzed modification of arachidonic acid while it is still attached to the membrane phospholipids. This conversion may result in alterations in cellular membrane fluidity and function. The release of isoeicosanoids is

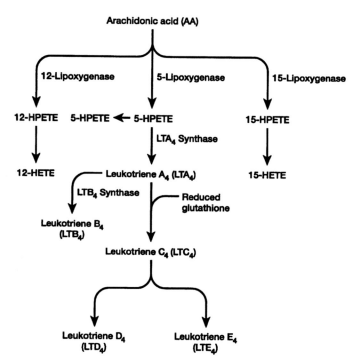

FIGURE 21.3. Biosynthesis of leukotrienes. Arachidonic acid can be converted to 5-, 12-, and 15-hydroxyeicosattetraenoic acid (HETE) by their respective lipoxygenases. 5-HETE can be converted to leukotriene A_4 (LTA_4). LTA_4 can proceed to LTB_4 or, with introduction of reduced glutathione, can be converted to form cysteinyl-leukotrienes (LTC_4, LTD_4, LTE_4).

presumably carried out through a phospholipase-mediated event. Unlike most of the prostaglandins and leukotrienes, the isoeicosanoids are highly stable compounds, which has allowed a number of studies to examine the serum and urinary concentrations in a variety of pathologic conditions.[29,30]

Oxidative damage is thought to play an important role in the pathophysiology of acute ischemia/reperfusion, trauma, hypercholesterolemia, and smoking-related cardiovascular disease. The best studied isoeicosanoid, 8-epi-$PGF_{2\alpha}$, is a potent vasoconstrictor and a vascular smooth muscle mitogen.[28] Exposure of human monocytes to low density lipoprotein (LDL) results in the formation of 8-epi-$PGF_{2\alpha}$ and hydroperoxide.[30,31] This reaction is inhibited by free radical scavengers and superoxide dismutase but not by cyclooxygenase inhibitors. The levels of 8-epi-$PGF_{2\alpha}$ are thought to be a measure of oxidative stress in vivo.[32] Morrow et al. demonstrated increased F_2 isoprostanes in smokers, suggesting increased lipid peroxidation.[33] Increased urinary excretion of 8-epi-$PGF_{2\alpha}$ has also been documented during cardiac reperfusion following successful angioplasty for myocardial infarction.[34] In general, the study of oxidative stress and free radical damage in the clinical arena is difficult. The significant association between isoeicosanoid production and these events may provide a new endpoint for monitoring these pathologic conditions and for their treatment.

Role of Eicosanoids in the Pathogenesis of Pulmonary Failure

In critically ill and injured patients the lungs are typically the first organ clinically to manifest the effects of secondary insults associated with hemorrhage, shock, ischemia, and sepsis. Activation of coagulation and inflammation at the site of tissue injury or infection is critical for wound healing, but difficulties arise when these processes become malignant and pose a significant threat to patient survival. Understanding the triggers and multiple biochemical pathways involved in the pathogenesis of pulmonary failure and the progression to ARDS has demonstrated the significant role of eicosanoids in modulating and mediating neutrophil and platelet interactions. Eicosanoid-mediated microaggregation and adherence of neutrophils and platelets within the pulmonary microvasculature initiates disruption of the endothelium and subsequent production of interstitial and alveolar edema. Substances released by activated neutrophil and platelet microaggregates include toxic oxygen metabolites, cytokines, lysosomal enzymes, prostaglandins, thromboxanes, leukotrienes, and histamine. (The roles of noneicosanoids are discussed in other chapters.)

Understanding the actions of eicosanoids is complicated by the capacity of these substances to enhance or inhibit each other's actions and the actions of other inflammatory mediators. In the lung, the cyclooxygenase products, $PGF_{2\alpha}$, and TXA_2 are potent bronchoconstricting and vasoconstricting agents. In contrast, prostaglandins I_2, E_1, and E_2 have bronchodilating and vasodilating effects. Lipoxygenase products are strong modulators of neutrophil function and interactions with other cells, with some products having proinflammatory actions and others having both pro- and antiinflammatory actions. LTB_4 is a potent chemotactic and chemokinetic agent for neutrophils; it amplifies the process of neutrophil lysosomal enzyme release and superoxide production. LTC_4 and LTD_4 disrupt the endothelium and increase pulmonary microvascular permeability, which leads to exudation of plasma. In critically ill patients with trauma and sepsis the plasma levels of phospholipase A_2, metabolites of TXA_2, and PGI_2 (TXB_2 and 6-keto-$PGF_{1\alpha}$) are uniformly elevated.[35–46] In Fig. 21.4 serial measurements collected from patients with active sepsis and major trauma show significant elevations of 6-keto-$PGF_{1\alpha}$ and TXB_2.[41] Leukotrienes are not substantially elevated in the plasma of ARDS patients, although analysis of bronchoalveolar lavage samples from these patients has shown increased release of leukotrienes from neutrophils, macrophages, and mast cells.[46] The difficulty of interpreting the implications of circulating elevations and local production of these compounds is complicated by their ability to exert their effects in nanomolar concentrations, the lack of organ specificity, and opposing effects of products from different pathways. Because the pathways use the same substrate, AA, selective inhibition of one pathway may enhance the activity of the other pathway above and beyond a mere reduction in production of the competing product. The ability to selectively control either pathway could theoretically result in either enhancement or inhibition of the repair/fibrotic process.

Successful therapy for pulmonary failure requires a drug that can be safely administered for several days and that inhibits

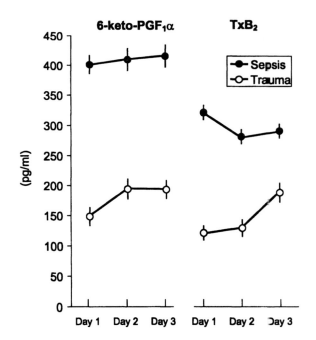

FIGURE 21.4. Serial measurements of 6-keto-prostaglandin $F_{1\alpha}$ ($PGF_{1\alpha}$) and thromboxane B_2 (TxB_2) levels (mean ± standard error) in 35 septic surgical patients and 16 major trauma patients. (From Vassar et al.,[41] with permission).

coagulation and inflammation in the lungs but not in the injured or infected peripheral tissues where wound healing or recovery from infection is in progress. Accordingly, inhibition of AA metabolism with thromboxane synthetase inhibitors, corticosteroid therapy, or NSAIDs seemed promising for treatment of ARDS, but they have not been successful. There has been recent interest in the benefits of nutritional formulations containing antiinflammatory fatty acids to reduce the intrapulmonary synthesis of proinflammatory eicosanoids.[47] Animal studies have demonstrated that the administration of PGE_1 and PGI_2 significantly reduces lung microvascular permeability and improves survival of shock due to hemorrhage and endotoxin.[48-50] Prostaglandins of the E series have also been safely used for a variety of clinical disorders. In addition to its vasodilating effects and antiplatelet aggregating properties, PGE_1 is a potent modulator of neutrophil function. The manner in which PGE_1 regulates these effects appears to be dose-dependent. In micromolar concentrations PGE_1 reduces in vitro neutrophil oxygen radical production, LTB_4 production, lysosomal enzyme release, chemotaxis, and membrane depolarization.[51-56] In nanomolar concentrations PGE_1 enhances the chemotactic response of neutrophils[57,58] promotes healing of duodenal ulcers, and stimulates DNA synthesis in cultured cells.[59-62] When administered to patients with ARDS, on average two-thirds of PGE_1 is metabolized during a single passage through the lungs.[63] Thus high concentrations of PGE_1 in the lungs may suppress the inflammatory insult, and lower concentrations in the periphery may augment the inflammatory response needed to recovery from infection and heal wounds.

Administration of PGE_1 has been under investigation since the early 1980s as a means of preventing and treating the acute inflammatory response associated with ARDS. A 7-day infusion of PGE_1 versus placebo for treatment of surgical patients with ARDS due to trauma and sepsis showed significant improvement in survival, with 71% of the PGE_1-treated patients alive at 30 days versus 35% survival in the placebo group.[64] A subsequent multicenter study in medical and surgical patients with advanced ARDS did not confirm these findings.[65] In the former study, the most benefit was found in patients with multiple trauma without sepsis or other organ failure at the time of entry into the protocol, with survival of 90% in the PGE_1 group versus 44% in the placebo group. This prompted a trial designed to evaluate the efficacy of early administration of PGE_1 for prevention of ARDS in high risk trauma patients and monitor the correlation with plasma suppressive factors for neutrophil activation.[66] The incidence of ARDS in the PGE_1-treated patients was 13% versus 32% in the placebo-treated patients; however, 48 patients were not sufficient to demonstrate statistical significance. Interestingly, the infusion of PGE_1 produced significant reversal of the baseline posttraumatic plasma suppressive activity upon normal neutrophil N-formyl-methionyl-leucyl-phenylalanine (FMLP)-stimulated superoxide production 24 hours after the start of the infusion (Fig. 21.5) and that persisted after 7 full days of infusion. In vitro addition of PGE_1 to the placebo-patient plasma did not result in enhancement of normal polymorphonuclear neutrophil (PMN) superoxide release. The PGE_1-treated patients were also found to have significant loss of neutrophil lysozyme content on day 1 of the infusion in association with the reduction of the plasma suppressive activity upon PMN superoxide production (Fig. 21.4). Neutrophil primary granule contents (β-glucoronidase and elastase) were unchanged from baseline to day 1, strongly suggesting that the loss of lysozyme content was a consequence of selective degranulation of secondary granule contents during PGE_1 administration. Secondary granules are not classic lysosomes; and unlike primary granules, they do not contain acid hydrolases capable of inducing tissue damage. The loss of PMN secondary granules may in fact reflect other aspects of PMN activation, such as the upregulation of adherence proteins, oxidative burst, and actin polymerization.[67,68] PMN secondary granules may contribute to the normal events involved in localization of the acute inflammatory response by interacting with the complement system to enhance chemotactic and microbicidal activity. While these experiments do not exclude the possibility of a direct in vivo action of PGE_1 on PMNs, a more likely explanation is an indirect action of PGE_1 on pulmonary and peripheral vascular flow in combination with alterations in mediator release from sites of tissue injury and inflammation that contribute to activation of PMNs.

Interest in the potential therapeutic benefits of PGE_1 has been renewed, with benefit shown in the prevention of postoperative thrombocytopenia, ARDS, and morbidity associated with liver transplantation.[69-71] New prostaglandin analogues that reduce the incidence of side effects and have longer half-lives are now

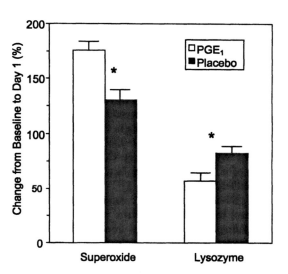

FIGURE 21.5. Relationship between loss of in vitro suppressive activity of plasma measured by N-formyl-methionyl-leucyl-phenylalanine (FMLP)-stimulated polymorphonuclear neutrophil (PMN) superoxide production (nanomoles cytochrome C reduced/10^6 PMNs/15 min) and in vivo PMN degranulation determined by PMN lysozyme content (μg/5 × 10^6 PMNs). Data are shown as the percent change from baseline (preinfusion) to 24 hours of infusion of PGE_1 versus placebo. *Significant differences between the two groups for superoxide ($p < 0.04$) and lysozyme ($p < 0.001$). (From Vassar et al.,[41] with permission).

available along with liposomal carriers that solve the problem of rapid degradation. How the pro- and antiinflammatory eicosanoids exert their effects is still not clear because of their ubiquitous nature and diverse range of physiologic and pathologic actions. The events related to pulmonary and other organ failure are multifactorial; and when the processes of coagulation and inflammation are fully understood, it will have important implications for the development of selective therapies to prevent organ failure.

References

1. Abrahamson S, Bergstrom S, Sameulsson B: The absolute configuration of PG F2-1. J Chem Soc 1962;332.
2. Dennis E, Rhee S, Billah M, et al: Role of phospholipases in generating lipid second messengers in signal transduction. FASEB J 1991;5:2068–2077.
3. Chao W, Olson M: Platelet-activating factor: receptors and signal transduction. Biochem J 1993;292:617–629.
4. Moolenaar W: Lysophosphatidic acid, a multifunctional phospholipid messenger. J Biol Chem 1995;270:12949–12952.
5. Dennis E: The growing phospholipase A_2 superfamily of signal transduction enzymes. Trends Biochem Sci 1997;22:1–2.
6. Tischfield J: A reassessment of the low molecular weight phospholipase A_2 gene family in mammals. J Biol Chem 1997;272:17247–17250.
7. Sakata T, Nakamura E, Tsuruta Y, et al: Presence of pancreatic-type phospholipase A_2 mRNA in rat gastric mucosa and lung. Biochim Biophys Acta 1989;1007:124–126.
8. Nevalainen T: Serum phospholipases A_2 in inflammatory diseases. Clin Chem 1993;39:2453–2459.
9. Beorsch-Haubold A: Regulation of cytosolic phospholipase A_2 by phosphorylation. Biochem Soc Trans 1998;26:350–345.
10. Reynolds L, Hughes L, Louis A, et al: Metal ion and salt effects on the phospholipase A_2, lysophospholipase, and transacylase activities of human cytosolic phospholipase A_2. Biochim Biophys Acta 1993;1167:272–280.
11. Balsinde J, Bianco I, Ackermann E, et al: Inhibition of calcium-independent phospholipase A_2 prevents arachidonic acid incorporation and phospholipid remodeling in P388D1 macrophages. Proc Natl Acad Sci USA 1995;92:8527–8531.
12. Tjoelker L, Wilder C, Eberhardt C, et al: Anti-inflammatory properties of a platelet-activating factor acetylhydrolase. Nature 1995;374:549–553.
13. Balsinde J, Diez E, Mollinedo F: Arachidonic acid release from diacylglycerol in human neutrophils: translocation of diacylglycerol-deacylating enzyme activities from an intracellular pool to plasma membrane upon cell activation. J Biol Chem 1991;266:15638–15643.
14. Vane J, Botting R: Biological properties of cyclooxygenase products. In: F Cunningham (ed) Lipid Mediators. London, Academic, 1994;61–97.
15. Blatties C, Sehic E: Fever: how many circulating pyrogens signal the brain? News Physiol Sci 1997;12:1–8.
16. Ferreira S: Prostaglandins, aspirin-like drugs and analgesia. Nature [New Biol] 1972;240:200–203.
17. Smith W, Garavito R, DeWitt D: Prostaglandin endoperoxide H synthases cyclooxygenases-1 and -2. J Biol Chem 1996;271:33157–33160.
18. Morita I, Schindler M, Regie M, et al: Different intracellular locations for prostaglandin endoperoxide H synthase-1 and -2. J Biol Chem 1995;270:10902–10908.
19. Bakhle Y, Botting R: Cyclo-oxygenase-2 and its regulation in inflammation. Mediat Inflamm 1996;5:305–323.
20. Meade E, Smith W, DeWitt D: Differential inhibition of prostaglandin endoperoxide synthase cyclooxygenase isozymes by aspirin and other non-steroidal anti-inflammatory drugs. J Biol Chem 1993;268:6610–6614.
21. Claria J, Serhan C: Aspirin triggers previously undescribed bioactive eicosanoids by human endothelial cells-leukocyte interactions. Proc Natl Acad Sci USA 1995;92:9475–9479.
22. Samuelsson B: Leukotrienes: mediators of immediate hypersensitivity reactions and inflammation. Science 1983;220:568–575.
23. Samuelsson B, Dahlaen S, Lindgren J, et al: Leukotrienes and lipoxins: structures, biosynthesis, and biological effects. Science 1987;237:1171–1176.
24. Ford-Hutchinson A: Leukotriene B_4 in inflammation. Crit Rev Immunol 1990;10:1–12.
25. Dahlaen S, Hansson G, Hedqvist P, et al: Allergen challenge of lung tissue from asthmatics elicits bronchial contraction that correlates with the release of leukotrienes C_4, D_4, and E_4. Proc Natl Acad Sci USA 1983;80:1712–1716.
26. Drazen JM: Pharmacology of leukotriene receptor antagonists and 5-lipoxygenase inhibitors in the management of asthma. Pharmacotherapy 1997;17:22S–30S.
27. Bernstein P: Chemistry and structure-activity relationships of leukotriene receptor antagonists. Am J Respir Crit Care Med 1998;157:S220–S226.
28. Patrono C, FitzGerald G: Isoprostanes: potential markers of oxidant stress in atherothrombotic disease. Arterioscler Thromb Vasc Biol 1997;17:2309–2315.
29. Morrow J, Hill K, Burk R, et al: A series of prostaglandin F_2-like compounds are produced in vivo in humans by a non-cyclooxygenase, free radical-catalyzed mechanism. Proc Natl Acad Sci USA 1990;87:9383–9387.
30. Lynch S, Morrow J, Roberts L, et al: Formation of non-cyclooxygenase-derived prostanoids F_2-isoprostanes in plasma and low density lipoprotein exposed to oxidative stress in vitro. J Clin Invest 1994;93:998–1004.
31. Praticao D, FitzGerald G: Generation of 8-epiprostaglandin $F_{2\alpha}$ by human monocytes: discriminate production by reactive oxygen species and prostaglandin endoperoxide synthase-2. J Biol Chem 1996;271:8919–8924.
32. Praticao D, Iuliano L, Mauriello A, et al: Localization of distinct F_2-isoprostanes in human atherosclerotic lesions. J Clin Invest 1997;100:2028–2034.
33. Morrow J, Frei B, Longmire A, et al: Increase in circulating products of lipid peroxidation F_2-isoprostanes in smokers: smoking as a cause of oxidative damage. N Engl J Med 1995;332:1198–1203.
34. Reilly M, Lawson J, FitzGerald G: Eicosanoids and isoeicosanoids: indices of cellular function and oxidant stress. J Nutr 1998;128:434S–438S.
35. Uhl W, Büchler M, Nevalainen T, et al: Serum phospholipase A_2 in patients with multiple injuries. J Trauma 1990;31:1285–1290.
36. Green J, Smith G, Buchta R, et al: Circulating phospholipase A_2 activity associated with sepsis and septic shock is indistinguishable from that associated with rheumatoid arthritis. Inflammation 1991;15:355–367.

37. Vadas P, Scott K, Smith G, et al: Serum phospholipase A_2 enzyme activity and immunoreactivity in a prospective analysis of patients with septic shock. Life Sci 1992;50:807–811.
38. Anderson B, Moore E, Banerjee A: Phospholipase A_2 regulates critical inflammatory mediators of multiple organ failure. J Surg Res 1994;56:199–205.
39. Nyman K, Waldemar U, Forsström J, et al: Serum phospholipase A_2 in patients with multiple organ failure. J Surg Res 1996;60:7–14.
40. Reines H, Haluska P, Cook J, et al: Plasma thromboxane concentrations are raised in patients dying with septic shock. Lancet 1982;24:174–175.
41. Vassar M, Weber C, Holcroft J: Measurement of 6-keto-$PGF_{1\alpha}$ and thromboxane B_2 levels in critically ill surgical patients. Prostaglandins Leukot Essent Fatty Acids 1988;33:129–135.
42. Carmona R, Tsao T, Trunkey D: The role of prostacyclin and thromboxane in sepsis and septic shock. Arch Surg 1984;119:189–192.
43. Yellin S, Nguyen D, Quinn J, et al: Prostacyclin and thromboxane A_2 in septic shock: species differences. Circ Shock 1986;20:291–297.
44. Webb P, Westwick J, Scully M, et al: Do prostacyclin and thromboxane play a role in endotoxic shock? Br J Surg 1981;68:720–724.
45. Deby-Dupont G, Braum M, Lamy M, et al: Thromboxane and prostacyclin release in adult respiratory distress syndrome. Intensive Care Med 1987;13:167–164.
46. Stephenson A, Lonigro A, Hyers T, et al: Increased concentration of leukotrienes in bronchoalveolar lavage fluid of patients with ARDS or at risk for ARDS. Am Rev Respir Dis 1988;138:714–719.
47. Mancuso P, Whelan J, DeMichele S, et al: Dietary fish oil and fish and borage oil suppress intrapulmonary proinflammatory eicosanoid biosynthesis and attenuate pulmonary neutrophil accumulation in endotoxic rats. Crit Care Med 1997;25:1198–1206.
48. Bolliger C, Fourie P, Coetzee A: The effect of prostaglandin E_1 on acute pulmonary artery hypertension during oleic acid-induced respiratory dysfunction. Chest 1991;99:1501–1506.
49. Lefer A, Sollott S, Galvin M: Beneficial actions of prostacyclin in traumatic shock. Prostaglandins 1979;17:761–767.
50. Raflo G, Wangensteen S, Glenn T, et al: Mechanism of the protective effects of prostaglandins E_1 and $F_{2\alpha}$ in canine endotoxin shock. Eur J Pharmacol 1973;24:86–95.
51. Fantone J, Kinnes D: Prostaglandin E_1 and prostaglandin I_2 modulation of superoxide production by human neutrophils. Biochem Biophys Res Commun 1983;113:506–512.
52. Fantone J, Kunkel S, Ward P, et al: Suppression by prostaglandin E_1 of vascular permeability induced by vasoactive inflammatory mediators. J Immunol 1980;125:2591–2596.
53. Fantone J, Marasco W, Elgas L, et al: Stimulus specificity of prostaglandin inhibition of rabbit polymorphonuclear leukocyte lysosomal enzyme release and superoxide anion production. Am J Physiol 1984;115:9–16.
54. Kunkel S, Thrall R, Kunkel R, et al: Suppression of immune complex vasculitis in rats by prostaglandin. J Clin Invest 1979;64:1525–1529.
55. Fletcher M: Prostaglandin E_1 inhibits N-formyl-methionyl-leucyl-phenylalanine — mediated depolarization responses by decreasing the proportion of responsive cells without affecting chemotaxin-induced forward light scatter changes. J Immunol 1987;139:4167–4173.
56. Ham E, Soderman D, Saneti M, et al: Inhibition by prostaglandins of leukotriene B_4 release from activated neutrophils. Proc Natl Acad Sci USA 1984;80:4349–4353.
57. Van Epps D, Wiik A, Garcia M, et al: Enhancement of human neutrophil migration by prostaglandin E_2. Cell Immunol 1978;37:142–150.
58. Downey G, Gumbay D, Doherty J, et al: Enhancement of pulmonary inflammation by PGE_2: evidence for a vasodilator effect. J Appl Physiol 1988;64:728–741.
59. Whittle B, Steel G: Evaluation of the protection of rat gastric mucosa by prostaglandin analogue using cellular enzyme marker and histologic technique. Gastroenterology 1985;88:315–327.
60. Owen N: Effect of prostaglandin E_1 on DNA synthesis I vascular smooth muscle cells. Am J Physiol 1986;250:C584–C488.
61. Pentland A, Needleman P: Modulation of keratinocyte proliferation in vitro by endogenous prostaglandin synthesis. J Clin Invest 1986;77:246–251.
62. Rozengurt E, Collins M, Keehan M: Mitogenic effect of prostaglandin E_1 in Swiss 3T3 cells: role of cyclic AMP. J Cell Physiol 1983;116:379–384.
63. Cox J, Andreadis N, Vassar M, et al: Pulmonary extraction and pharmacokinetics of prostaglandin E_1 during continuous intravenous infusion in patients with adult respiratory distress syndrome. Am Rev Respir Dis 1988;137:5–12.
64. Holcroft J, Vassar M, Weber C: Prostaglandin E_1 and survival in patients with the adult respiratory distress syndrome. Ann Surg 1986;203:371–378.
65. Bone R, Slotman G, Maunder R, et al: Randomized double-blind, multicenter study of prostaglandin E_1 in patients with the adult respiratory distress syndrome. Chest 1989;96:114–119.
66. Vassar M, Fletcher M, Perry C, et al: Evaluation of prostaglandin E_1 for prevention of respiratory failure in high risk trauma patients: a prospective clinical trial and correlation with plasma suppressive factors for neutrophil activation. Prostaglandins Leukot Essent Fatty Acids 1991;44:223–231.
67. Wright D, Malawista S: The mobilization and extracellular release of granular enzymes from human leukocytes during phagocytosis. J Cell Biol 1972;53:788–797.
68. Goldstein I, Weissmann G: Generation of C5-derived lysosomal enzyme releasing activity (C_5a) by lysates of leukocyte lysosomes. J Immunol 1974;113:1583–1588.
69. Locker G, Staudinger T, Knapp S, et al: Prostaglandin E_1 inhibits platelet decrease after massive blood transfusions during major surgery: influence on coagulation cascade? J Trauma 1997;42:525–531.
70. Abraham E, Park Y, Covington P, et al: Liposomal prostaglandin E_1 in acute respiratory distress syndrome: a placebo-controlled, randomized, double-blind, multicenter clinical trial. Crit Care Med 1996;24:10–15.
71. Henley K, Lucey M, Normolle D, et al: A double-blind, randomized, placebo-controlled trial of prostaglandin E_1 in liver transplantation. Hepatology 1995;21:366–372.

22
Platelet-Activating Factor

M. Poeze, W.A. Buurman, G. Ramsay, and J.W.M. Greve

Research leading to the discovery of platelet-activating factor (PAF) came from studying a reaction that triggered platelets to release histamine. It was attributed to a factor actively released from leukocytes. Platelet-activating factor was first identified by Benveniste et al. in 1972.[1] Later it was recognized that this phospholipid mediator is also released from a number of other cell types, such as macrophages, basophils, and mast cells and that it displayed diverse immunomodulatory actions. The role PAF plays in the process leading to sepsis has especially attracted attention. PAF was identified as an important factor in sepsis leading to the release of many other inflammatory mediators.[2]

Since 1972 a large number of studies have provided insight to the mechanisms by which PAF is synthesized and metabolized. This chapter summarizes recent knowledge on the mechanisms by which PAF exhibits its actions and the advances made in the use of various PAF antagonists, with emphasis on the research performed regarding sepsis.

Basic Biology of PAF

Chemical Structure

Platelet-activating factor is a chiral phosphorylcholine derivate (1-O-alkyl-2-acetyl-sn-glycero-3-phosphocholine) (Fig. 22.1). It is generally regarded as a single moiety, but a variety of structurally related molecules have been identified with the same pathophysiologic effects, including PAF-acether (*ace* for acetate and *ether* for the alkyl bond), acetyl glycerol ether phosphorylcholine (alkyl-PAF; AGEPC), and acyl-PAF (AGPC).[3] The PAF structure consists of four parts: a glycerol backbone with sn-2-acetate, sn-1-O-alkyl ether, and sn-3-phosphocholine side chains attached. When synthesizing PAF, it is generally preferred to introduce the C_2-O-acetyl group to the glycerol chain after the C_1-alkoxy-side chain and the C_3-phosphorylcholine moiety to avoid acetyl migration.[4] These complex interactions lead to yields of only 5–25%. Attempts to form PAF from synthetic starting products have failed to improve these results.

Biochemistry

In vitro and in vivo data showed that PAF is synthesized by cells through two pathways. In the first pathway, called the remodeling pathway, PAF-acether is formed from the precursor lyso-PAF, as shown by Wykle's group,[5] and catalyzed by acetyltransferase (Fig. 22.2), which is the rate-limiting step in the formation of PAF. This lyso-PAF is formed from alkyl-acyl-glycero-phosphocholine (GPC) with phospholipase A_2 as catalyst. The lyso-PAF can be transformed again into this alkylacyl-GPC by an acyl-transferase.[5] Intracellularly, PAF-acether is rapidly broken down by acetylhydrolase into acetate and lyso-PAF. The deacylation–reacylation cycle constitutes the primary pathway of PAF biosynthesis and degradation in leukocytes, macrophages, and endothelial cells. The biosynthesis part of the pathway can be triggered by numerous agents and particles, such as endotoxins, opsonized particles, and granulocyte/macrophage colony-stimulating factor (GM-CSF)[6–8] (Fig. 22.3). The inactivation and conversion of PAF to lyso-PAF is not dependent on cell stimulation. Depending on the cell type from which PAF is secreted, PAF is either retained in the plasma membrane or rapidly released into the extracellular space.[9] The endothelial cell-associated PAF synthesis was shown to be related to cell-to-cell signal transduction after injury.[10] The difference in localization seems to be related to the difference in the paracrine and endocrine function of PAF in the inflammatory response. In plasma secreted PAF-acether can be degraded to lyso-PAF by circulating PAF-acetylhydrolase. This PAF-acetylhydrolase, mainly secreted by liver cells and monocytes/macrophages,[11–13] has been used as a marker for PAF levels in the circulation.[14] Decreased PAF-acetylhydrolase is correlated with an increased mortality rate, which may indicate high plasma levels of PAF.[15]

The second pathway for the synthesis of PAF seems to be restricted mainly to brain and kidney tissue.[16] The formation of PAF by this de novo pathway maintains physiologic PAF levels in resting cells and functions without the need for specific stimulation. These data suggest that this pathway may be involved in controlling blood flow in these organs.[17,18] Acetyl-coenzyme-A acetyltransferase catalyzes conversion of the sn-2 hydroxyl group

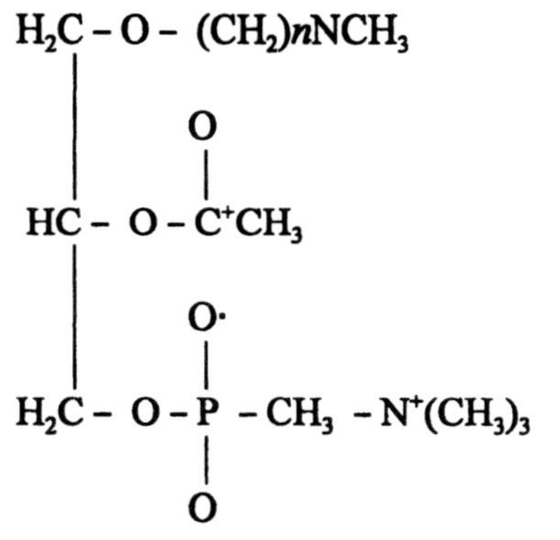

22. Platelet-Activating Factor

FIGURE 22.1. Structure of platelet-activating factor, a chiral phosphorylcholine derivative (1-O-alkyl-2-acetyl-sn-glycero-3-phosphocholine).

of the 1-O-alkyl-sn-glycero-3-phosphate to an acetyl group[9] (Fig. 22.2). This compound is further processed by phosphohydrolase and by a specific CDP-cholinephosphotransferase to form PAF.[3] Alternatively, the sn-2 hydroxy group is converted to an acyl group. The latter can be further processed to alkylacyl-GPC, which forms the start of the "remodeling pathway."[19] Alkylacyl-GPC is the biologically inactive precursor of PAF, which is stored linked to cellular membranes.[20]

In addition to this specific, direct mechanism for the production of PAF, an alternative nonenzymatic pathway for the production of PAF-like phospholipids constitutes the third pathway for the formation of PAF during injury. In the presence of sepsis and trauma the formation of oxidative radicals has been shown to oxidize phospholipids to form PAF-like oxidized phospholipids, which can be degraded to a phosphocholine moiety by PAF-acetylhydrolase. The bioactivity of these PAF-like phospholipids is less than the PAF formed by the other two pathways.[21]

Irrespective of the pathway used or the tissue involved, PAF mediates its effects via a receptor-mediated interaction[22] (Fig. 22.4). PAF receptors are found in virtually all tissues in the body. The primary biologic signal induced by PAF after binding to the receptor is an increase in phosphatidylinositol (PI) and diacylglycerol (DAG), mediated by G-proteins.[9] The receptor has been identified as a guanosine 5'-triphosphate-

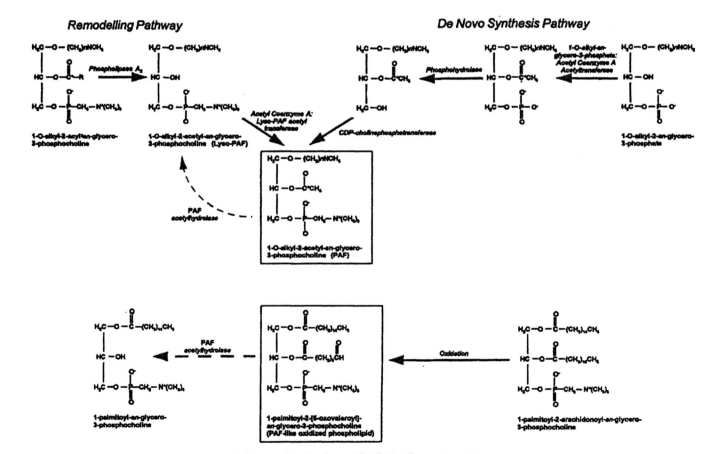

FIGURE 22.2. Platelet-activating factor (PAF) in shock and sepsis. PAF is synthesized by cells via two pathways: the remodeling pathway and the de novo synthesis pathway. (From Ayala and Chaudry,[9] with permission.)

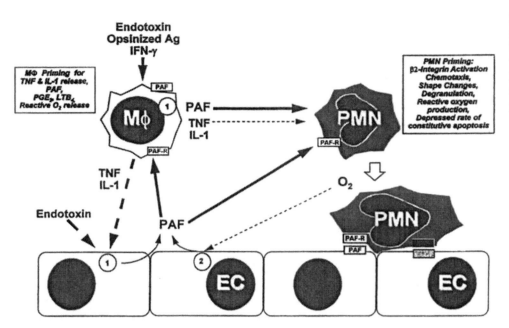

FIGURE 22.3. Biosynthesis portion of the deacylation-reacylation cycle is triggered by agents and particles such as endotoxins, opsonized particles, and granulocyte/macrophage colony-stimulating factor. (From Ayala and Chaudry,[9] with permission.)

binding protein-linked acetylcholine-like receptor complex,[22] sharing its structure with receptors of chemotactic substances, such as C5a, leukotriene-B_4, interleukin-8 (IL-8), and macrophage inflammatory protein (MIP-1).[9] DAG is a potent activator of protein kinase C (PKC), and breakdown of PI forms inositol triphosphate (IP_3), which results in an increase in intracellular free calcium concentration by increased cellular influx. The increased calcium influx and activation of PKC act synergistically to enhance the biologic actions of PAF.

Pharmacology and Pharmacobiology

The PAF is rapidly broken down with a half-life ($t_{1/2}$) of 1–3 minutes in plasma and a $t_{1/2}$ of 5–15 minutes in cell supernatants.[15] This has made measurement of PAF difficult. The bioassay used to measure PAF levels is based on the ability of PAF to aggregate platelets. Difficulties with the accuracy of this measurement has led to a search for alternative methods. One such method is mass spectrometry, which can accurately distinguish between the levels of PAF and the levels of PAF-like phospholipids,[23] but it is not easy to perform and is usually not readily available. Measurement of substrates with a longer half-life, which can be indicative of PAF-levels (e.g., the lyso-PAF[9]), could provide an alternative. PAF-acetylhydrolase was also shown to be indicative of PAF levels.[14,15]

Several PAF analogues have been synthesized in search of antagonists and has led to an increased understanding of the structure-related activity of PAF. A large number of PAF analogues have been made by varying the glyceryl backbone structure. These variations made it clear that the length of the backbone is essential for appropriate PAF function. In general it can be stated that the chemical structure of PAF cannot be changed substantially without loss of biologic activity, indicating that the effects of PAF are mediated through binding to a

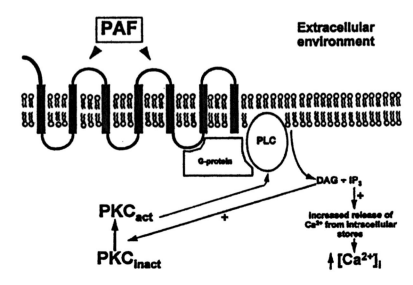

FIGURE 22.4. Platelet-activating factor (PAF) mediates its effects via a receptor-mediated interaction. (From Ayala and Chaudry,[9] with permission.)

receptor. Saturation of the carbon–carbon bonds in the sn-1 alkyl groups[3] and hydrolysis of the acetyl group at the sn-2 acetyl group reduce the potency of PAF.[24] PAF can be found in both dextro- and levo-isomers but is active only in the levo-isomer.[25] Changes in function by the above-mentioned structural changes are not equal for all properties of PAF; for example, a large increase in hypotensive property was accompanied by a much smaller increase in the ability to activate neutrophils.[26]

In vitro data suggest that many cells produce PAF. In addition to the kidney glomerular cells and brain tissue cells already mentioned,[16,27] gastrointestinal endothelium and lung endothelial cells, neutrophils, pneumocytes, and macrophages are capable of producing PAF,[3,28–31] as are granulocytes, monocytes, mast cells, and platelets in the circulation. The production of PAF in these cells can be stimulated in vitro by many inflammatory mediators, such as tumor necrosis factor (TNF), IL-1, and PAF, thereby creating a positive feedback loop.[29,32]

Compared to other stimuli, PAF is a weak inducer of neutrophil activation. Only with relatively high concentrations of PAF can a low, short-lived respiratory burst be measured in neutrophils.[33] However, low concentrations of PAF "prime" inflammatory cells. In contrast to the high concentrations of PAF needed to activate resting neutrophils, low concentrations (10^{-12} M) are needed to increase the TNF-induced respiratory burst effectively.[34] Evidence for involvement of endogenous PAF in the activation of neutrophils suggests that PAF might have a regulatory role in many pathophysiologic conditions.[34] Activation of leukocytes causes rigidification and adhesion of the leukocytes to the endothelium. This adhesion and the subsequent occurrence of migration of leukocytes into the tissues inhibit vascular flow. Such changes in adhesive properties tend to remain after reperfusion has occurred. This reperfusion can subsequently direct new leukocytes to the inflammatory process, after which they can be activated by the circulating mediators. These effects contribute to enhancement of the local defense against an infectious agent.

Other cells such as macrophages and platelets are activated by PAF to release TNF, IL-1, eicosanoids, histamine, and serotonin.[16,29] Endothelial cells were shown to produce PAF both early (after 2–40 minutes) through activation of the remodeling pathway and late (after 4–8 hours) through activation of the de novo pathway, depending on the stimulus involved.[35] In vitro data showed that the delayed reaction is stimulated by cytokines, such as TNF and IL-1.[29] The microvascular injury induced by PAF is related to the induction of direct damage to the endothelial cells.[36]

In vivo data suggest that PAF is released during several pathologic conditions, such as ischemia/reperfusion, peritonitis, and endotoxemia.[37–39] The heart and gut were shown to release PAF after ischemia/reperfusion injury.[37] The importance of the role of PAF in these conditions was confirmed by reducing the effects of ischemia/reperfusion with a PAF antagonist.[39] In rats, intraperitoneal injection of *Escherichia coli* was followed by production of PAF in the peritoneal cells;[38] and in pigs, intravenous infusion of endotoxin was followed after 20–30 minutes by an increase in systemic levels of PAF.[40] On the other hand, in vivo data showed that intravenous injection of PAF results in a condition characterized by hypotension,[41] pulmonary hypertension,[42] bronchoconstriction,[43] increased vascular permeability, thrombocytopenia,[36] neutropenia,[44] and increased mortality.[41,42] These effects of PAF are highly species-dependent and also depend on the route of administration.[3]

In humans, septic patients had decreased levels of PAF-acetylhydrolase, indicating increased levels of PAF in their circulation.[15] This finding was confirmed by Patrick et al. in trauma patients developing multiple organ failure (MOF).[14] In another study by Botha et al. in patients with postinjury MOF, superoxide release of primed neutrophils was reduced using a PAF antagonist.[45] Bussolino et al. showed that elevated levels of PAF were present in children with sepsis and bacterial meningitis.[46]

In summary, there appears to be strong evidence that PAF plays an important role during the inflammatory response that accompanies infection and ischemia/reperfusion. Most of the other data indicating that PAF is pathophysiologically important in sepsis and ischemia/reperfusion are drawn from studies using PAF antagonists.

PAF Antagonists

The inhibitors of PAF can be divided into two main groups: those specifically inhibiting PAF and the more nonspecific inhibitors. The specific PAF antagonists can be divided into two subgroups (1) synthetic PAF antagonists and (2) natural products. The number of PAF antagonists discovered or synthesized is large, but only a few can be discussed here. The natural compounds include the PAF antagonists FR 900452, PCA 4248, SCH 37370, the ginkgolides, kadsurenone, chantancin, phomactin, swietemohonin A, prehispalone, THC-7-oic acid, and aglafoline. The synthetic compounds include CV-3988, CV-6209, TCV-309, Ono 6420, Ro 19-3704, Ro 24-4736, Ro 24-0238, SRI 63-119, SRI 63-072, SRI 63-441, UR-10324, UR-11353, E-5880, CL 184005, 6-mono and bis-aryl phosphate antagonists, Ro-74719, WEB 2086, Y 24180, BN 50726, BN 50727, BN 50730, BN 50739, RP 55778, RP 59227, RP 66681, YM 264, YM 461, SM 10661, SR 27417, UK 74505, BB 182, BB 823, BB 654, BB 882, SDZ 64-412, SDZ 65-123, L 652731, L 659898, L 668750, L 671284, L 680573, L 680574, CIS 19, ABT-299, and pinusolide.

Specific Inhibition

PAF-Related Antagonists

The nonconstrained backbone PAF antagonists are directly derived from the chemical structure of the PAF molecule.[3] The first compound in this group was developed by Takeda Chemical Industries and called CV 3988.[47] In this compound the three sites of the glyceryl backbone of PAF were changed, but it had antagonist activity only when it was used in high concentrations. An analogue of CV 3988, named CV 6209, was 80 times as potent as CV 3988.[48] The newest analogue of CV

6209 is TCV-309, which is 260–444 times as potent as CV 3988 in terms of inhibiting platelet aggregation.[49] The IC_{50} value for PAF-induced platelet aggregation of rabbit and human platelets by TCV-309 were 3.0×10^{-8} and 3.6×10^{-8} M, respectively. ONO 6240 and related antagonists were formed by placing a heptamethylene thiazolium on position 3 in the glyceryl backbone.[50] ONO 6240 is the most potent antagonist among this group as measured with PAF-induced platelet aggregation in the guinea pig. Burri et al. synthesized several PAF antagonists by chemically altering PAF-acether[51] stereospecifically from (R)glycerol acetonide, such as Ro 19-3704 with an IC_{50} of 10^{-6} M. Investigators at Sandoz formed SRI 63-119 and SRI 63-072 with IC_{50} values of 3.8×10^{-6} and 2.23×10^{-5} M, respectively.[52] Two other compounds formed by this group were SaRI 62586 and SaRI 62436, which have only moderate antagonistic activity.[53] Wichrowski et al. reported formation of a PAF antagonist, RU-45703,[54] by placing an ester linkage in place of the phosphoryl group[3] with an IC_{50} of 8×10^{-6} M. In summary, several synthetic, nonconstrained PAF antagonists have been formed by modifying the glyceryl backbone, of which TCV-309 is the most potent. TCV-309 has been carried forward for use in clinical trials in patients with septic shock.

The process of cyclization of the PAF structure yielded another group of PAF antagonists, the constrained backbone antagonists. Two of these PAF antagonists have been reported: the PAF antagonist related to piperidine, SRI 63-073,[55] and the PAF antagonist related to dioxanone. Inhibition of platelet aggregation of human platelets by this substance had an IC_{50} of 3.77×10^{-5} M. The last subgroup of PAF-related antagonists are the tetrahydrofuran derivatives. SRI 63-441 is the most potent antagonist derived from tetrahydrofuran, with an IC_{50} of 3.3×10^{-3} M.[56]

Natural Products

Several natural products, derived from plants (terpenes and lignans) and bacteria (gliotoxines), were found to have PAF antagonistic properties. Of the terpenes the ginkgolide BN 52021 is the most well known, it has been used in clinical trials and is more efficient than BN 52020, BN 52023, BN 52024, or BN 52063, with an IC_{50} of 10^{-7} M.[57–59]

The lignan antagonists can be divided into several subgroups: benzofuranoid neolignans, substituted furanoid lignans, butanolide lignans, substituted furofuranoid lignans, and other lignans. Of the benzofuranoid neolignans, kadsurenone, one the first natural products, was shown specifically to inhibit platelet aggregation with an IC_{50} of 9.9×10^{-7} M. Another PAF antagonist, L-652,731, belongs to a subgroup of the substituted furanoid lignans (synthetic PAF antagonist); and is orally active.[60] The lignans from the other three groups are weak to moderately active PAF antagonists.

Fermentation of several fungi and microorganisms yielded another group of PAF antagonists, the gliotoxins. Two products, FR 900452 and FR 49175, have been tested for their anti-PAF action but have given variable results, with strong inhibition of bronchoconstriction and thrombocytopenia, but not PAF-induced hypotension.[61,62]

Nonspecific Inhibition

Triazolobenzodiazepines

The PAF antagonists triazolobenzodiazepines belong to the group of psychotropic substances. In addition to the classic drugs triazolam and alprazolam, which have specific PAF antagonistic actions, the PAF antagonist WEB 2086 was synthesized as a derivate of triazolobenzodiazepine. WEB 2086 has been widely used in experimental studies.[63–65]

Calcium Channel Blocking Agents

Nonspecific inhibitors such as verapamil or diltiazim, which are calcium channel blocking agents, act through competitive and noncompetitive antagonistic mechanisms. Few trials have been reported using this group of drugs. Most of them are under development, and only a few have undergone clinical trials.

PAF Antagonists: Putative Therapeutic Effects and Experimental Evidence

General Information

Most of the attention to the potential effects of treatment with PAF antagonists has been focused on the clear role of PAF in gram-negative sepsis. It was shown that pretreatment with a PAF antagonist could effectively reduce not only lipopolysaccharide (LPS)-induced TNF release but also LPS-induced mortality.[66–68] However, the effect is highly dependent on the antagonist used and on which species the experiment is performed.[69] This illustrates the complexity of the problem. Even a well controlled (experimental) environment with comparable subgroups, exact timing of the (pre)treatment with PAF antagonist, and controlled induction of the septic insult (e.g., LPS or bacteria) does not guarantee consistent results when the experiments are performed in different species. When compared with the clinical situation—with a diverse group of patients in whom the moment of treatment is always long after the first septic insult, and the start of treatment different in all patients within the different treatment arms—the experimental setting can be considered ideal, although these experimental studies certainly provide results that overestimate the true clinical relevance. Nevertheless, there are indications that PAF antagonists might positively affect the course of events in critically ill patients.

Sepsis and PAF Antagonist Treatment

The effects of PAF inhibition have been studied in several settings. Most of these studies are based on endotoxin-induced or gram-negative bacteria-induced inflammatory responses with either pretreatment (i.e., prevention of the release of inflammatory mediators) or true treatment, where the PAF antagonist was applied minutes to hours after the septic insult.

Kuipers et al. showed in a experimental primate model that the PAF antagonist TCV-309 could significantly reduce the

LPS-induced release of TNF-α, TNF-r, IL-6, and IL-8.[68] These results were comparable to those of Ogata et al.,[66] who showed that TCV-309 could reduce TNFα release in endotoxin-treated mice and also reduced mortality. In a model with rabbits the PAF antagonist E5880 significantly reduced MOF and disseminated intravascular coagulation (DIC) in a biliary sepsis model.[70] Murakami et al. found similar results in septic rats: decreased DIC and acute respiratory distress syndrome (ARDS); in their study TNF levels were also reduced by PAF antagonist treatment.[71] However in all these experiments the PAF antagonists were given as prevention (i.e., before inflammation was induced).

In contrast, Spapen et al. did not find a significant effect of treatment with the PAF antagonist BB-882 when it was given 1 hour after endotoxin administration, with respect to the hemodynamic status in fluid-resuscitated dogs.[72] In a similar experiment they found that global oxygen extraction was not improved, although cardiac performance appeared to be improved at low filling pressures.[69] The number of studies in which PAF antagonists were given as treatment (i.e., after induction of an inflammatory response) is limited. In an overview on PAF and sepsis, Mathiak et al. could identify only 7 (of 50) experimental studies in which treatment was used.[73] It should be stressed that the treatment was applied relatively soon (minutes to hours) after the induction of inflammation, which is far from the clinical reality.

The experiments with systemic inflammation induced by endotoxins, bacteria, or other agents mainly focus on the effects ascribed to the PAF released in the circulation. However, PAF could be more important on a local level in the various organ systems. It is therefore interesting to summarize some studies that specifically focus on organ systems such as the lung, heart, or kidney, which are "key figures" in the complex play of the systemic inflammatory response syndrome (SIRS).

Important effects of experimental PAF infusion are hemoconcentration and vascular leakage, indicating an effect on the endothelial cells in the capillaries of various tissues. It results, for example, in pulmonary edema. In several models of lung injury induced with local infusion of endotoxins or gram-negative bacteria, pretreatment with PAF antagonists inhibited leukocyte sequestration and microvascular damage,[28] reduced pulmonary vasoconstriction and edema,[74,75] and blocked increased capillary leakage.[76] Not only are the local effects reduced, treatment with PAF antagonists improves survival after endotoxin- or bacteria-induced lung injury.[76,77]

With respect to cardiac function, PAF infusion causes a decreased cardiac index, lower left ventricle stroke work index, and reduced contractility of the muscle fibers. All these effects can be blocked efficiently with a PAF receptor antagonist.[78] However, Spapen et al. found that the beneficial effect of a PAF antagonist on cardiac function was time-dependent and that it did not improve global oxygen extraction, indicating that its usefulness for treatment of septic shock may be limited.[69]

Another important effect of PAF is the enhanced adhesion of neutrophils or leukocytes to endothelium, which can result in an enhanced local inflammatory response.[79–81] This could be a contributing factor to the development of SIRS, which is considered to be an "overshoot" of a normally effective defense mechanism resulting in systemic release of inflammatory mediators. The adhesion of neutrophils can be blocked with PAF receptor antagonists,[79,80] which reduces the inflammatory response; however, it also reduces the local defense against infection or ischemia/reperfusion damage, which could be a drawback for this treatment strategy.

The kidney, another organ at risk in critically ill patients, was also studied with respect to treatment with PAF antagonists. It was shown that PAF antagonists could reduce the alterations in tissue perfusion after LPS injection, reducing impairment of renal function.[73] In a different line of research (transplantation) it was shown that PAF antagonists such as TCV-309 could significantly reduce tissue damage in the kidney after ischemia/reperfusion.[82] The latter may play a role in protecting the kidney from ischemic damage in low-flow situations such as septic shock.

Finally, research has focused on the effect of PAF on the digestive tract. In septic patients the integrity of the gastrointestinal wall is often impaired, resulting for example in ulcerations and hemorrhage from the stomach. Experimentally it was shown that PAF plays an important role in derangement of the gut barrier.[83,84] Furthermore, it was shown that PAF is involved in ischemia/reperfusion damage of the gut, which in turn results in MOF.[85] Several PAF antagonists were shown to protect against endotoxin- or PAF-induced gastrointestinal damage.[86] In other inflammatory processes in the gut, such as experimentally induced colitis, PAF appeared to play a pivotal role in the resulting damage.[87] Interesting results were also found in studies that focused on the treatment of severe acute pancreatitis. Acute pancreatitis in itself is not a major component of the sepsis syndrome; but on the other hand, patients with severe acute pancreatitis often develop severe sepsis. Several experimental studies have shown that PAF antagonists and lexipafant in particular can prevent and even be used to treat animals with experimental pancreatitis.[88,89] It was also shown that a PAF antagonist could preserve bowel wall integrity, thereby preventing translocation of bacteria and toxins in the acute pancreatitis model.[90] Hypothetically, the latter could explain the putative beneficial effect of PAF antagonists in patients with ongoing sepsis. When endotoxins translocating from the gut cause the secondary phase of sepsis, PAF antagonists preventing gut barrier dysfunction (thus preventing further stimulation of the inflammatory cascade) may be beneficial even during a late phase of the disease.

Clinical Studies: PAF as an Important Inflammatory Mediator in Trauma and Sepsis

Only limited data are available on PAF levels in septic patients. One of the main reasons is the difficult or unreliable assay. The short half-life of PAF in plasma is another obstacle to reliable determination of PAF levels in vivo. Evidence of increased PAF levels in plasma and bronchoalveolar lavage fluid was reported in a study with only eight patients and from a single measurement within 24 hours after admission on an intensive care unit (ICU).[91] In this study the PAF levels were related to survival of the patient. Another four studies reported increased PAF levels in septic patients, but only a limited number of patients were subjected to measurements, and the results are difficult to interpret.[92-95] On the other hand, at least as many studies did not show that PAF levels were higher in septic patients than in controls.[15,96] That PAF plays a role in patients with endotoxemia can be concluded from a study in healthy volunteers. In this study the PAF antagonist Ro 24-4736, given orally 18 hours before endotoxin infusion, significantly reduced such symptoms as rigor and myalgia.[97] However, in contrast to previous studies in primates,[68] the release of inflammatory mediators was not influenced.

PAF Antagonists as a Therapeutic Option in Septic Patients

A number of clinical studies in septic patients have been reported. The first phase II study with the PAF antagonist BN 52021 was published in 1994.[98] The results were promising to the extent that the antagonist appeared to be safe and that a survival benefit was found in a subgroup of patients (post hoc analysis) with severe gram-negative sepsis. However, in a phase III study done by the same group, it was proven again that retrospective analysis is dangerous. In the second study, which comprised 609 patients with severe gram-negative sepsis studied in a multicenter, randomized, placebo-controlled, double-blind fashion, the PAF antagonist BN 52021 did not improve overall mortality.[58] It was shown, though, that BN 52021 could be given safely to the patient, and there was a slight tendency toward improved organ function (reduced hepatic dysfunction) in the treated group.

A second series of clinical studies was performed with the PAF antagonist TCV-309. The first study (multicenter, phase II, double-blind, placebo-controlled) included 29 patients with severe sepsis, of whom 28 could be evaluated.[99] Overall mortality was not different, and again treatment with the PAF antagonist did not cause adverse events; furthermore, levels of the measured inflammatory parameters (TNF, IL-6, IL-8, soluble E-selectin) were not different between the placebo- and TCV-309-treated patients. Comparable to the study with BN 52021, a difference was found in the level of organ dysfunction in favor of the TCV-309-treated patients. In a second randomized multicenter study in which 97 patients were included, organ dysfunction was one of the primary endpoints.[100] In this study the patients were treated for a prolonged period (2 weeks) with a twice-daily dosage of TCV-309. Again there was no difference in overall mortality (50%); there was, however, a significant reduction in organ dysfunction (cardiovascular, pulmonary, renal, hepatic, and hematologic systems) in the TCV-309-treated group.

Interesting results were also reported from studies in patients with severe acute pancreatitis. In the phase II study with lexipafant as the PAF antagonist, organ dysfunction improved significantly in the treated patients.[101] In yet another study of severe acute pancreatitis a significant survival benefit was found in patients treated with lexipafant within 48 hours of onset of the pancreatitis.[102] It was only after post hoc analysis, however, that this benefit became obvious. The results of a large phase III study, in which the preset goal of treatment is within 48 hours of onset of the pancreatitis, must be awaited before final conclusions can be drawn. Theoretically (if this positive survival benefit is confirmed), patients with severe acute pancreatitis may represent a group of patients in whom the disease is detected before the onset of sepsis and therefore who can undergo preventive treatment with a PAF antagonist. This in turn could explain why this selected group of severely ill patients may benefit from treatment with PAF antagonists.

Conclusions

Results from clinical studies of treatment with a PAF antagonist in septic patients are so far disappointing. However, it is an illusion to believe that a complex mechanism as is seen with severe SIRS and sepsis, in which numerous inflammatory mediators have been identified and many are still to be found, can be treated by a single, even though potent, agent. Not only the complexity of the inflammatory response and the many organs involved in an organ-specific way, but also the time of detection, make medical treatment of the underlying cause of sepsis a difficult if not impossible task.

Hypothetically, PAF antagonists could play a role in the treatment of septic patients in the future. It may be in a selected group of patients, such as those with severe acute pancreatitis; but it could also be part of a multimodality treatment in which a combination of agents, each with a separate target, may be applied in a balanced way to improve the outcome of severely ill septic patients. A major benefit of PAF antagonists in this setting is the absence of adverse effects during treatment.

References

1. Benveniste J, Henson PM, Cochrane CG: Leukocyte-dependent histamine release from rabbit platelets: the role of IgE, basophils, and a platelet-activating factor. J Exp Med 1972;136:1356-1377.
2. Braquet P, Paubert-Braquet M, Bourgain RH, Bussolino F, Hosford D: PAF/cytokine auto-generated feedback networks in microvascular immune injury: consequences in shock, ischemia and graft rejection. J Lipid Med 1989;1:75-112.
3. Braquet P, Touqui L, Shen TY, Vargaftig BB: Perspectives in platelet-activating factor research. Pharmacol Rev 1987;39:97-145.
4. Heymans F, Michel E, Borrel MC, et al: New total synthesis and high resolution 1H NMR spectrum of platelet-activating factor, its enantiomer and racemic mixtures. Biochim Biophys Acta 1981;666:230-237.
5. Venable ME, Olson SC, Nieto ML, Wykle RL: Enzymatic studies of lyso platelet-activating factor acylation in human

neutrophils and changes upon stimulation. J Biol Chem 1993;268:7965–7975.
6. Hanahan DJ: The continuing biochemical challenge of PAF and closely related lipid mediators. Adv Exp Med Biol 1996;416:1–3.
7. Gomez-Cambronero J, Durstin M, Molski TF: Calcium is necessary but not sufficient for the platelet-activating factor release in human neutrophils stimulated by physiological stimuli: role of G-proteins. J Biol Chem 1989;264:12699–12704.
8. Marquis O, Robaut C, Cavero I: Evidence for the existence and ionic modulation of platelet-activating factor receptors mediating degranulatory responses in human polymorphonuclear leukocytes. J Pharmacol Exp Ther 1989;250:293–300.
9. Ayala A, Chaudry IH: Platelet activating factor and its role in trauma, shock, and sepsis. New Horiz 1996;4:265–275.
10. Zimmerman GA, Lorant DE, McIntyre TM, Prescott SM: Juxtacrine intercellular signaling: another way to do it. Am J Respir Cell Mol Biol 1993;9:573–577.
11. Stafforini DM, McIntyre TM, Carter ME, Prescott SM: Human plasma platelet-activating factor acetylhydrolase: association with lipoprotein particle and role in the degradation of platelet-activating factor. J Biol Chem 1987;162:4214–4222.
12. Elstad MR, Stafforini DM, McIntyre TM, Prescott SM, Zimmerman GA: Platelet-activating factor acetylhydrolase increases during macrophage differentiation: a novel mechanism that regulates accumulation of platelet-activating factor. J Biol Chem 1989;264:8467–8470.
13. Satoh K, Imaizumi T, Kawamura Y, et al: Platelet-activating factor (PAF) stimulates the production of PAF acetylhydrolase by the human hepatoma cell line, HepG2. J Clin Invest 1991;87:476–481.
14. Patrick DA, Moore EE, Moore FA, Biffl WL, Barnett CC: Reduced PAF-acetylhydrolase activity is associated with postinjury multiple organ failure. Shock 1997;7:170–174.
15. Graham RM, Stephens CJ, Silvester W, Leong LL, Sturm MJ, Taylor RR: Plasma degradation of platelet-activating factor in severely ill patients with clinical sepsis. Crit Care Med, 1994;22:204–212.
16. Prescott SM, Zimmerman GA, McIntyre TM: Platelet-activating factor. J Biol Chem 1990;265:17381–17384.
17. Satoh K, Imaizumi T, Yoshida H, Hiramoto M, Takamatsu S: Increased levels of blood platelet-activating factor (PAF) and PAF-like lipids in patients with ischemic stroke. Acta Neurol Scand 1992;85:122–127.
18. Domingo MT, Spinnewyn B, Chabrier PE, Braquet P: Presence of specific binding sites for platelet activating factor (PAF) in brain. Biochem Biophys Res Commun 1988;151:730–736.
19. Anderson BO, Bensard DD, Harken AH: The role of platelet activating factor and its antagonists in shock, sepsis and multiple organ failure. Surg Gynecol Obstet 1991;172:415–424.
20. Touqui L, Jacquemin C, Dumarey C, Vargaftig BB: 1-O-Alkyl-2-alkyl-2-acyl-sn-glycero-3-phosphocholine is the precursor of platelet-activating factor in stimulated rabbit platelets: evidence for an alkylacetyl-glycero-phosphocholine cycle. Biochim Biophys Acta 1985;833:111–118.
21. Smiley PL, Stremler KE, Prescott SM, Zimmerman GA, McIntyre TM: Oxidatively fragmented phosphatidylcholines activate human neutrophils through the receptor for platelet-activating factor. J Biol Chem 1991;266:11104–11110.
22. Kunz D, Gerard NP, Gerard C: The human leukocyte platelet-activating factor receptor: cDNA cloning, cell surface expression, and construction of a novel epitope-bearing analog. J Biol Chem 1992;267:9101–9106.
23. Polonsky J, Tence M, Varenne P, Das BC, Lunel J, Benveniste J: Release of 1-O-alkylglyceryl 3-phosphorylcholine, O-deacetyl platelet-activating factor, from leukocytes: chemical ionization mass spectrometry of phospholipids. Proc Natl Acad Sci USA 1980;77:7019–7023.
24. Anderson BO, Bensard DD, Harken AH: The role of platelet activating factor and its antagonists in shock, sepsis and multiple organ failure. Surg Gynecol Obstet 1991;172:415–424.
25. Wykle RL, Miller CH, Lewis JC, et al: Strereospecific activity of 1-O-alkyl-2-O-acetyl-sn-glycero-3-phosphocholine and comparison of analogs in the degranulation of platelets and neutrophils. Biochem Biophys Res Commun 1981;100:1651–1658.
26. Ohno M, Fujita K, Shiraiwa M, et al: Molecular design toward biologically significant compounds based on platelet activating factor: a highly selective agonist as a potential antihypertensive agent. J Med Chem 1986;29:1812–1814.
27. Hanahan DJ: Platelet-activating factor: a biologically active phosphoglyceride. Annu Rev Biochem 1986;55:483–509.
28. Anderson BO, Poggetti RS, Shanley PF, et al: Primed neutrophils injure rat lung through a platelet-activating factor-dependent mechanism. Surgery 1991;109:51–61.
29. Camussi G, Tetta C, Bussolino F, Baglioni C: Tumor necrosis factor stimulates human neutrophils to release leukotriene B$_4$ and platelet-activating factor: induction of phospholipase A$_2$ and acetyl-CoA:1-alkyl-sn-glycero-3-phosphocholine O$_2$-acetyltransferase activity and inhibition by antiproteinase. J Exp Med 1987;166:1390–1404.
30. Whatley RE, Zimmerman GA, McIntyre TM, Prescott SM: Endothelium from diverse vascular sources synthesizes platelet-activating factor. Arteriosclerosis 1988;8:321–331.
31. Whittle BJ, Boughton-Smith NK, Hutcheson IR, Esplugues JV, Wallace JL: Increased intestinal formation of PAF in endotoxin-induced damage in the rat. Br J Pharmacol 1991;92:3–4.
32. Doebber TW, Wu MS: Platelet-activating factor (PAF) stimulates the PAF synthesizing enzyme acetyl-CoA:1-alkyl-sn-glycero-3-phosphocholine O$_2$-acetyltransferase and PAF synthesis in neutrophils. Proc Natl Acad Sci USA 1987;84:7557–7561.
33. Ingraham LM, Coates TD, Allen JM, Higgins CP, Baehner RL, Boxer LA: Metabolic, membrane, and functional responses of human polymorphonuclear leukocytes to platelet-activating factor. Blood 1982;59:1259–1266.
34. Braquet P, Hosford D, Koltz P, Guilbaud J, Paubert-Braquet M: Effect of platelet-activating factor on tumor necrosis factor-induced superoxide generation from human neutrophils: possible involvement of G proteins. Lipids 1991;26:1071–1075.
35. Nakamura M, Honda Z, Izumi T, et al: Molecular cloning and expression of platelet-activating factor receptor from human leukocytes. J Biol Chem 1991;266:20400–20405.
36. Bussolino F, Camussi G, Aglietta M, et al: Human endothelial cells are target for platelet-activating factor. I. Platelet-activating factor induces changes in cytoskeleton structures. J Immunol 1987;139:2439–2446.
37. Montrucchio G, Alloatti G, Tetta C, et al: Release of platelet-activating factor from ischemic-reperfused rabbit heart. Am J Physiol 1989;256:H1236–H1246.
38. Inarrea P, Gomez-Cambronero J, Pascual J, Ponte MC, Hernando L, Sanchez-Crespo M: Synthesis of PAF-acether and blood volume changes in gram-negative sepsis. Immunopharmacology 1985;9:45–52.

39. Doebber TW, Wu MS, Robbins JC, Choy BM, Chang MN, Shen TY: Platelet activating factor (PAF) involvement in endotoxin-induced hypotension in rats: studies with PAF-receptor antagonist kadsurenone. Biochem Biophys Res Commun 1985;127: 799-808.
40. Dobrowsky RT, Voyksner RD, Olson NC: Effect of SRI 63-675 on hemodynamics and blood PAF levels during porcine endotoxemia. Am J Physiol 1991;260:H1455-H1465.
41. Bessin P, Bonnet J, Apffel D, et al: Acute circulatory collapse caused by platelet-activating factor (PAF-acether) in dogs. Eur J Pharmacol 1983;86:403-413.
42. Argiolas L, Fabi F, del BP: Mechanisms of pulmonary vasoconstriction and bronchoconstriction produced by PAF in the guinea-pig: role of platelets and cyclo-oxygenase metabolites. Br J Pharmacol 1995;114:203-209.
43. Touvay C, Vilain B, Taylor JE, Etienne A, Braquet P: Proof of the involvement of platelet activating factor (PAF-acether) in pulmonary complex immune systems using a specific PAF-acether receptor antagonist: BN 52021. Prog Lipid Res 1985;25: 277-288.
44. Smallbone BW, Taylor NE, McDonald JW: Effects of L-652,731, a platelet-activating factor (PAF) receptor antagonist, on PAF- and complement-induced pulmonary hypertension in sheep. J Pharmacol Exp Ther 1987;242:1035-1040.
45. Botha AJ, Moore FA, Moore EE, Peterson VM, Silliman CC, Goode AW: Sequential systemic platelet-activating factor and interleukin 8 primes neutrophils in patients at risk of multiple organ failure. Br J Surg 1996;83:1407-1412.
46. Bussolino F, Porcellini MG, Varese L, Bosia A: Intravascular release of platelet activating factor in children with sepsis. Thromb Res 1987;48:619-620.
47. Terashita Z, Tsushima S, Yoshioka Y, Nomura H, Inada Y, Nishikawa K: CV-3988: a specific antagonist of platelet activating factor (PAF). Life Sci 1983;32:1975-1982.
48. Terashita Z, Takatani M, Tsushima S, Nishikawa K: CV-6209: a highly potent platelet-activating factor (PAF) antagonist [abstract]. Presented at the Second International Congress on Platelet-Activating Factor and Structurally Related Alkyl Ether Lipids 1986;29.
49. Terashita Z, Kawamura M, Takatani M, Tsushima S, Imura Y, Nishikawa K: Beneficial effects of TCV-309, a novel potent and selective platelet activating factor antagonist in endotoxin and anaphylactic shock in rodents. J Pharmacol Exp Ther 1992; 260:748-755.
50. Miyamoto T, Ohno M, Yano T, Okada T, Hamanaka N, Kawasaki A: ONO-6420: a new potent antagonist of platelet-activating factor [abstract]. Adv Prostaglandin Thromboxane Leukotriene Res 1985;15:719-720.
51. Burri K, Barner R, Cassal J-M, Hadvary P, Hirth G, Müller K: PAF: from agonists to antagonists by synthesis. Prostaglandins 1985;30:691.
52. Handley DA, Anderson RC, Saunders RN: Inhibition by SRI 63-072 and SRI 63-119 of PAF-acether and immune complex effects in the guinea pig. Eur J Pharmacol 1987;141:409-416.
53. Winslow CM, Vallespir SR, Frisch GE, et al: A novel platelet activating factor receptor antagonist. Prostaglandins 1985;30:697.
54. Wichrowski B, Jouquey S, Heymans F, et al: Platelet activating factor analogs from agonists to antagonists by synthesis by carboxylate isosters [abstract]. Presented at the Sixth International Conference on Prostaglandins and Related Compounds 1986;309.
55. Patterson R, Harris KE, Lee ML, Houlihan WJ: Inhibition of rhesus monkey airway and cutaneous responses to platelet-activating factor (PAF) (AGEPC) with the anti-PAF agent SRI 63-072 [abstract]. Int Arch Allergy Immunol 1986;81:265-268.
56. Handley DA, Tomesch JC, Saunders RN: Inhibition of PAF-induced systemic responses in the rat, guinea pig, dog and primate by the receptor antagonist SRI 63-441. Thromb Haemost 1986;56:40-44.
57. Sanchez CM, Fernandez GS, Nieto ML, Baranes J, Braquet P: Inhibition of the vascular actions of IgG aggregates by BN 52021, a highly specific antagonist of PAF-acether. Immunopharmacology 1985;10:67-75.
58. Dhainaut JF, Tenaillon A, Hemmer M, et al: Confirmatory platelet-activating factor receptor antagonist trial in patients with severe gram-negative bacterial sepsis: a phase III, randomized, double-blind, placebo-controlled, multicenter trial: BN 52021 Sepsis Investigator Group. Crit Care Med 1998;26:1963-1971.
59. Lachachi H, Plantavid M, Simon MF, Chap H, Braquet P, Douste BL: Inhibition of transmembrane movement and metabolism of platelet activating factor (PAF-acether) by a specific antagonist, BN 52021. Biochem Biophys Res Commun 1985;132:460-466.
60. Wu MS, Biftu T, Doebber TW: Inhibition of the platelet activating factor (PAF)-induced in vivo responses in rats by trans-2,5-(3,4,5-trimethoxyphenyl) tetrahydrofuran (L-652,731), a PAF receptor antagonist. J Pharmacol Exp Ther 1986;239:841-845.
61. Okamoto M, Yoshida K, Nishikawa M, Kohsaka M, Aoki H: Platelet activating factor (PAF) involvement in endotoxin-induced thrombocytopenia in rabbits: studies with FR-900452, a specific inhibitor of PAF. Thromb Res 1986;42:661-671.
62. Okamoto M, Yoshida K, Uchida I, Kohsaka M, Aoki H: Studies of platelet activating factor (PAF) antagonists from microbial products. II. Pharmacological studies of FR-49175 in animal models. Chem Pharm Bull Tokyo 1986;34:345-348.
63. Casals SJ, Muacevic G, Weber KH: Pharmacological actions of WEB 2086, a new specific antagonist of platelet activating factor. J Pharmacol Exp Ther 1987;241:974-981.
64. Brambilla A, Ghiorzi A, Giachetti A: WEB 2086: a potent PAF antagonist exerts protective effect toward PAF-induced gastric damage. Pharmacol Res Commun 1987;19:147-151.
65. Casals SJ: Protective effect of WEB 2086, a novel antagonist of platelet activating factor, in endotoxin shock. Eur J Pharmacol 1987;135:117-122.
66. Ogata M, Matsumoto T, Koga K, et al: An antagonist of platelet-activating factor suppresses endotoxin-induced tumor necrosis factor and mortality in mice pretreated with carrageenan. Infect Immun 1993;61:699-704.
67. Yue TL, Farhat M, Rabinovici R, Perera PY, Vogel SN, Feuerstein G: Protective effect of BN 50739, a new platelet-activating factor antagonist, in endotoxin-treated rabbits. J Pharmacol Exp Ther 1990;254:976-981.
68. Kuipers B, van der Poll T, Levi M, et al: Platelet-activating factor antagonist TCV-309 attenuates the induction of the cytokine network in experimental endotoxemia in chimpanzees. J Immunol 1994;152:2438-2446.
69. Spapen H, Zhang H, Verhaeghe V, Smail N, Vincent JL: The platelet-activating factor antagonist BB-882 does not improve tissue oxygen extraction in endotoxic shock. J Crit Care 1998; 13:81-90.
70. Ou MC, Kambayashi J, Kawasaki T, et al: Potential etiologic role of PAF in two major septic complications; disseminated intravas-

cular coagulation and multiple organ failure. Thromb Res 1994;73:227–238.
71. Murakami K, Okajima K, Uchiba M, Johno M, Okabe H, Takatsuki K: A novel platelet activating factor antagonist, SM-12502, attenuates endotoxin-induced disseminated intravascular coagulation and acute pulmonary vascular injury by inhibiting TNF production in rats. Thromb Haemost 1996;75:965–970.
72. Spapen H, Zhang H, Verhaeghe V, Rogiers P, Cabral A, Vincent JL: Treatment with a platelet-activating factor antagonist has little protective effects during endotoxic shock in the dog. Shock 1997;8:200–206.
73. Mathiak G, Szewczyk D, Abdullah F, Ovadia P, Rabinovici R: Platelet-activating factor (PAF) in experimental and clinical sepsis. Shock 1997;7:391–404.
74. Olson NC, Joyce PB, Fleisher LN: Role of platelet-activating factor and eicosanoids during endotoxin-induced lung injury in pigs. Am J Physiol 1990;258:H1674–H186.
75. Siebeck M, Weipert J, Keser C, et al: A triazolodiazepine platelet activating factor receptor antagonist (WEB 2086) reduces pulmonary dysfunction during endotoxin shock in swine. J Trauma 1991;31:942–949.
76. Chang SW, Fernyak S, Voelkel NF: Beneficial effect of a platelet-activating factor antagonist, WEB 2086, on endotoxin-induced lung injury. Am J Physiol 1990;258:H153–H158.
77. Makristathis A, Stauffer F, Feistauer SM, Georgopoulos A: Bacteria induce release of platelet-activating factor (PAF) from polymorphonuclear neutrophil granulocytes: possible role for PAF in pathogenesis of experimentally induced bacterial pneumonia. Infect Immun 1993;61:1996–2002.
78. Gupta JB, Prasad M, Kalra J, Prasad K: Platelet-activating-factor-induced changes in cardiovascular function and oxyradical status of myocardium in presence of the PAF antagonist CV-6209. Angiology 1994;45:25–36.
79. Adams DH, Nash GB: Disturbances of leucocyte circulation and adhesion to the endothelium as factors in circulatory pathology. Br J Anaesth 1996;77:17–31.
80. Coughlan AF, Hau H, Dunlop LC, Berndt MC, Hancock WW: P-selectin and platelet-activating factor mediate initial endotoxin-induced neutropenia. J Exp Med 1994;179:329–334.
81. Kubes P, Ibbotson G, Russell J, Wallace JL, Granger DN: Role of platelet-activating factor in ischemia/reperfusion- induced leukocyte adherence. Am J Physiol 1990;259:G300–G305.
82. Yin M, Kurvers HAJM, Buurman WA, et al: Beneficial effect of platelet-activating factor antagonist TCV-309 on renal ischemia-reperfusion injury. Transplant Proc 1995;27:774–776.
83. Wallace JL, Hogaboam CM, McKnight GW: Platelet-activating factor mediates gastric damage induced by hemorrhagic shock. Am J Physiol 1990;259:G140–G146.
84. Fink MP: Gastrointestinal mucosal injury in experimental models of shock, trauma, and sepsis. Crit Care Med 1991;19:627–641.
85. Biffl WL, Moore EE: Splanchnic ischaemia/reperfusion and multiple organ failure. Br J Anaesth 1996;77:59–70.
86. Wallace JL, Steel G, Whittle BJR, Lagente V, Vargaftig B: Evidence for platelet-activating factor as a mediator of endotoxin-induced gastrointestinal damage in the rat: effects of three platelet-activating factor antagonists. Gastroenterology 1987;93:765–773.
87. Meenan J, Grool TA, Hommes DW, et al: Lexipafant (BB-882), a platelet activating factor receptor antagonist, ameliorates mucosal inflammation in an animal model of colitis. Eur J Gastroenterol Hepatol 1996;8:569–573.
88. Hofbauer B, Saluja AK, Bhatia M, et al: Effect of recombinant platelet-activating factor acetylhydrolase on two models of experimental acute pancreatitis. Gastroenterology 1998;115:1238–1247.
89. Yamano M, Umeda M, Miyata K, Yamada T: Protective effects of a PAF receptor antagonist and a neutrophil elastase inhibitor on multiple organ failure induced by cerulein plus lipopolysaccharide in rats. Naunyn Schmiedebergs Arch Pharmacol 1998;358:253–263.
90. Andersson R, Wang XD, Sun ZW, Deng XM, Soltesz V, Ihse I: Effect of a platelet-activating factor antagonist on pancreatitis-associated gut barrier dysfunction in rats. Pancreas 1998;17:107–119.
91. Sorensen J, Kald B, Tagesson C, Lindahl M: Platelet-activating factor and phospholipase A$_2$ in patients with septic shock and trauma. Intensive Care Med 1994;20:555–561.
92. Ono S, Tamakuma S, Mochizuki H, et al: Clinical and experimental studies on the role of platelet-activating factor (PAF) in the pathogenesis of septic DIC. Surg Today 1993;23:228–233.
93. Heuer HO, Darius H, Lohmann HF, Meyer J, Schierenberg M, Treese N: Platelet-activating factor type activity in plasma from patients with septicemia and other diseases. Lipids 1991;26:1381–1385.
94. Lopez DF, Nieto ML, Fernandez-Gallardo S, Gijon MA, Sanchez CM: Occupancy of platelet receptors for platelet-activating factor in patients with septicemia. J Clin Invest 1989;83:1733–1740.
95. Bussolino F, Porcellini MG, Varese L, Bosia A: Intravascular release of platelet activating factor in children with sepsis [letter]. Thromb Res 1987;48:619–620.
96. Shinozaki K, Kawasaki T, Kambayashi J, et al: A new method of purification and sensitive bioassay of platelet-activating factor (PAF) in human whole blood. Life Sci 1994;54:429–437.
97. Thompson WA, Coyle S, Van Zee K, et al: The metabolic effects of platelet-activating factor antagonism in endotoxemic man. Arch Surg 1994;129:72–79.
98. Dhainaut J-F, Mira J-P, Brunet F: Platelet-activating factor antagonists as therapeutic strategy in sepsis. In: Anonymous Bacterial Endotoxins: Basic Science to Anti-sepsis Strategies, 1st ed. New York, Wiley-Liss 1994;277–293.
99. Froon AM, Greve JW, Buurman WA, et al: Treatment with the platelet-activating factor antagonist TCV-309 in patients with severe systemic inflammatory response syndrome: a prospective, multi-center, double-blind, randomized phase II trial. Shock 1996;5:313–319.
100. Poeze M, Froon AHM, Ramsay G, Buurman WA, Greve JW: Organ failure and MOF-related death is reduced in patients with septic shock treated with the PAF-antagonist TCV-309. Intensive Care Med 1998;24(Suppl 1):S69.
101. Kingsnorth AN, Galloway SW, Formela LJ: Randomized, double-blind phase II trial of lexipafant, a platelet-activating factor antagonist, in human acute pancreatitis. Br J Surg 1995;82:1414–1420.
102. Kingsnorth AN, British Acute Pancreatitis Study Group: Early treatment with lexipafant, a platelet activating factor antagonist reduces mortality in acute pancreatitis: a double blind, randomized, placebo controlled study [abstract]. Gastroenterology 1997;112:A453.

23
Therapeutic Complement Inhibition

Katrin Jurianz and Michael Kirschfink

Excessive complement activation significantly contributes to the pathogenesis of a large number of inflammatory diseases, including ischemia/reperfusion injury, sepsis, and multiple organ failure syndrome. Current strategies to interfere with the deleterious action of complement include the application of endogenous soluble complement inhibitors (C1 inhibitor, recombinant soluble complement receptor 1-rsCR1), administration of antibodies, blocking key proteins of the cascade reaction (e.g., C5), neutralizing the action of the complement-derived anaphylatoxin C5a, or interfering with complement receptor 3 (CR3, CD18/11b)-mediated adhesion of inflammatory cells to the vascular endothelium. Incorporation of membrane-bound complement regulators (DAF-CD55, MCP-CD46, CD59) has provided a major step forward in protecting xenografts from hyperacute rejection. Numerous animal studies and first clinical trials strongly suggest that complement inhibition is a suitable novel therapeutic approach to preventing inflammatory disorders.

Introduction

Complement as a vital part of the body's immune system provides a highly effective means for the destruction of invading microorganisms and for immune complex elimination.[1,2] However, as a key mediator of inflammation, complement also significantly contributes to tissue damage in various clinical disorders.

The complement system comprises a group of at least 30 proteins, which act within a cascade-like reaction sequence or serve as control proteins or cellular receptors (Fig. 23.1). The activation of any of the three pathways—the antibody-dependent classic pathway, the alternative pathway, or the recently discovered lectin pathway[3]—leads to the formation of the cytolytic membrane attack complex, C5b-9. Following complement activation, biologically active peptides are generated that transfer most effector functions of an activated complement system to inflammatory cells. These proinflammatory peptides, especially the anaphylatoxins C5a and C3a, elicit a number of biologic effects: chemotaxis of leukocytes; degranulation of phagocytic cells, mast cells, and basophils; smooth muscle contraction; and increased vascular permeability.[4] The complement-mediated inflammatory response is further amplified by subsequent generation of toxic oxygen radicals and the induction of synthesis and release of arachidonic acid metabolites and cytokines. Consequently, an (over)activated complement system presents a considerable risk of harming the host by directly and indirectly mediating inflammatory tissue destruction.

Under physiologic conditions, uncontrolled activation of complement is prevented by the coordinated action of soluble and membrane-associated regulatory proteins[5] (Fig. 23.1). Our own cells are protected against the detrimental attack of homologous complement by surface proteins, such as the complement receptor 1 (CR1, CD35), the membrane cofactor protein (MCP, CD46), and the glycosylphosphatidylinositol (GPI)-anchored proteins, decay-accelerating factor (DAF, CD55), C8-binding protein/homologous restriction factor (C8bp/HRF), and CD59. In body fluids, soluble complement regulators such as C1 inhibitor, C4-binding protein (C4bp), factors H and I, clusterin, and S-protein (vitronectin) restrict the action of complement at several sites of the cascade reaction.

A large body of clinical and experimental evidence has accumulated to underline the decisive role of complement in the pathogenesis of numerous inflammatory diseases[6–8] (Table 23.1). These diseases include not only immune complex and autoimmune disorders but also organ failure subsequent to ischemia/reperfusion injury, sepsis, multiple trauma, and burns. Complement activation after polytrauma substantially contributes to development of the systemic inflammatory reaction syndrome (SIRS) and multiple organ failure.[9,10] Reperfusion injury, at least in part mediated by complement activation, is of great pathophysiologic relevance to the development of stroke, myocardial infarction, and graft failure.[11] Insufficient tissue perfusion and oxygenation are also hallmarks of endotoxinemia and sepsis. Activation of complement is a critical event in the pathogenesis of sepsis and septic shock.[12–14] Complement activation has been correlated with severity and clinical outcome in patients with meningococcal sepsis.[15] In acute pancreatitis, complement activation products, in part directly generated by

FIGURE 23.1. Complement activation pathways. During the course of the reaction sequence, proinflammatory peptides are generated and the membrane attack complex is formed. Under physiologic conditions the complement cascade reaction is controlled by the fluid phase and membrane-associated (boldface letters) regulatory proteins. MBL, mannan-binding ligand; MASP, mannan-binding ligand-associated serine protease; DAF, decay accelerating factor; MCP, membrane cofactor protein; C4bp, C4-binding protein.

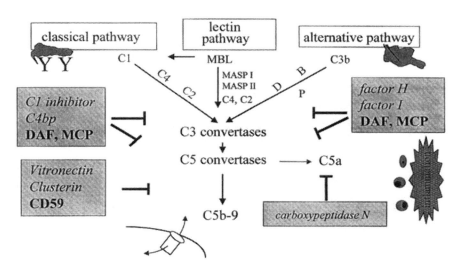

trypsin-mediated cleavage, have been associated with priming and entrapment of neutrophils in the lung vasculature, a first step in the development of lung injury.[16]

The inflammatory response induced by artificial surfaces in hemodialysis and extracorporeal circuits may lead to organ dysfunction. Complement activation has been shown to be associated with transient neutropenia, pulmonary vascular leukostasis, and occasionally anaphylactic shock of variable severity in patients undergoing hemodialysis[17] or cardiopulmonary bypass (CPB).[18] Biomedical polymers differ considerably in their capacity to activate complement.[19] It is therefore generally accepted that evaluation of the biocompatibility of artificial surfaces must include analysis of the activation of both the coagulation and complement systems.[20–22]

Great progress has been made in complement analysis to better define disease severity, evolution, and response to therapy. Modern diagnostic technologies that focus on the quantification of complement-derived split products or protein-protein complexes now provide a comprehensive insight into the activation state of the system.[23,24] Complement analysis has been shown to be of prognostic value in early recognition of, for example, patients at risk to develop acute respiratory distress syndrome (ARDS),[25,26] multiple organ failure after trauma,[9] or individuals with impending graft rejection following renal transplantation.[27] Developments in complement diagnosis focus on a combination of affinity chromatography with immunoassay procedures. This protocol allows us to assess plasma concentrations within 20–30 minutes, thereby meeting an essential prerequisite for the introduction of complement analysis in intensive care units.[28] Applying this novel assay to a recent polytrauma study[26] and in patients with sepsis or SIRS,[29] it was demonstrated that C3a plasma levels correlated with the clinical outcome and helped to distinguish between patients with sepsis and those with SIRS. Thus focusing on complement inhibition appears to be a logical approach to arresting the process of inflammatory disorders.[30–33]

Strategies of Complement Inhibition

Application of Complement Regulatory Proteins

Control of complement activation (Fig. 23.2) is most effectively provided by the system's physiologic regulators (Fig. 23.1). The specificity and the absence of toxic side effects of endogenous complement inhibitors provides an excellent prerequisite for their therapeutic application.

C1 Inhibitor

C1 inhibitor, a member of the serpin superfamily of protease inhibitors,[34] is the only known plasma inhibitor of C1r and C1s.[35] Later studies defined the spectrum of proteases inactivated by C1 inhibitor to include activated factors XI and XII of the contact phase,[36] kallikrein, plasmin,[37] and tissue-type plasminogen activator (tPA),[38] thus controlling the generation of various kinin-like molecules. C1 inhibitor reacts with susceptible proteases at their substrate binding site and is subsequently cleaved by its enzyme ligands; C1 inhibitor–protease complexes are rapidly removed from the circulation after binding to serpin–enzyme complex receptors on monocytes and hepatocytes.[39] Additional proteolytic inactivation of C1 inhibitor by neutrophil elastase is presumed to contribute to the deregulation of plasma cascade systems in severe inflammation.[40]

TABLE 23.1. Inflammatory Disorders Associated with Complement Activation.

Severe trauma, burn, sepsis
Systemic inflammatory reaction syndrome
Multiple organ dysfunction syndrome
Ischemia/reperfusion injury
Angioedema, capillary leak syndrome
Hyperacute graft rejection
Vasculitis, nephritis
Autoimmune disorders: systemic lupus erythematosus, rheumatoid arthritis, multiple sclerosis
Alzheimer's disease
Dialysis, cardiopulmonary bypass

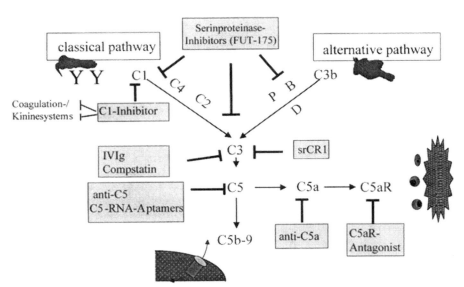

FIGURE 23.2. Complement activation, potentially leading to severe inflammation, can be blocked by administration of physiologic regulatory proteins, blocking antibodies, receptor antagonists, RNA aptamers, or serine proteinase inhibitors or by intravenous application of high-dose immunoglobulins (IVIg).

C1 inhibitor-deficient individuals suffer from recurrent attacks of partly life-threatening mucosal edema, called hereditary angioedema or Quincke edema.[41] Replacement of the regulator by plasma-derived C1 inhibitor concentrates (Behring/Centeon, Marburg, Germany; Immuno, Vienna, Austria) has for many years proved beneficial in the acute treatment of hereditary or acquired angioedema.

A secondary deficiency of C1 inhibitor, resulting from excessive complement activation, subsequently leads to disturbance of the protease–antiprotease balance. Diminished plasma levels of functional active C1 inhibitor have been observed in various states of severe inflammation, such as sepsis,[13] severe burn,[42] polytrauma,[9] capillary leak syndrome after bone marrow transplantation,[43] pancreatitis,[44] urticarial reactions to contrast medium,[45] and in ARDS patients connected to an extracorporeal circuit.[46]

Despite the availability of the purified regulator and more than 30 years' experience in its application to angioedema patients, further indications for C1 inhibitor treatment are still not established by large-scale multicenter trials. In recent years, however, reports have accumulated describing the benefit of C1 inhibitor treatment in various experimental and clinical settings.[47]

C1 inhibitor has been shown to prevent endotoxin-induced pulmonary dysfunction in dogs.[48] In a rabbit model of endotoxin-induced hypercoagulability, Scherer et al.[49] showed the benefit of C1 inhibitor treatment on early disseminated intravascular coagulation. Although the impact of C1 inhibitor on complement is restricted to the classic pathway, its additional regulatory function in the coagulation system appears to be of importance in situations such as septic shock, where activation of either system is associated with a poor clinical outcome. This is supported by findings in C3- and C4-deficient mice, where administration of purified mouse C1 inhibitor was effective in preventing lethal endotoxic shock,[50] pointing to the pathophysiologic contribution of other C1 inhibitor-regulated kinins. A beneficial but modest effect of C1 inhibitor treatment on the clinical course and outcome of severe sepsis in nonhuman primates was observed by Jansen et al.[51] In an early clinical study, application of high doses of a C1 inhibitor concentrate led to an improved clinical outcome in four of five patients suffering from septic shock.[52] Walger et al.[53] reported five cases of streptococcal toxic shock syndrome, where administration of C1 inhibitor concentrate was followed by a rapidly decreasing need for adrenergic agents and a marked fluid shift from the extravasal to the intravasal space.

Acute pancreatitis is associated with systemic activation of protein cascade systems and a dysbalance of antiprotease capacity.[54,55] In an early study of experimental pancreatitis, Ruud et al.[56] had shown that C1 inhibitor substitution reduces mortality and ameliorates the course of disease. These results have been supported by Yamaguchi et al.,[57] who demonstrated that regardless of whether the regulators were given prophylactically or therapeutically the combined application of C1 inhibitor and antithrombin III improved survival after severe hemorrhagic pancreatitis. In an early clinical trial in patients undergoing endoscopic sphincterotomy, infusion of the regulator prevented hyperamylasemia, thereby reducing the risk of inducing acute pancreatitis.[58] In contrast, C1 inhibitor failed to exert a major beneficial effect in three models of experimental pancreatitis in mice or rats and, more importantly, in patients, suffering from acute pancreatitis.[59] In a rat model of traumatic shock, C1 inhibitor administration (15 minutes after trauma) preserved endothelial function and diminished neutrophil accumulation, thereby reducing mortality and prolonging the survival time.[60]

Due to proteolytic degradation, plasma levels of functional C1 inhibitor are often reduced in burned patients.[42] We investigated the possible protective effect of C1 inhibitor in an animal model of thermal trauma. Scalded pigs treated with C1 inhibitor presented with reduced edema formation, diminished bacterial translocation, and a reduction of inflammatory tissue damage.[61,62] Jostkleigrewe et al.[63] described a pilot study with 15 severely burned patients, where C1 inhibitor treatment substantially improved long-term survival and clinical outcome compared to that in a historic control group.

Capillary (or vascular) leak(age) syndrome (CLS), characterized by vascular leakage and hypotension, is a well known complication following bone marrow transplantation and systemic cytokine therapy. The administration of high doses of interleukin-2 (IL-2) to cancer patients often induces life-threatening capillary leakage.[64] Here, activation of complement is reflected by increased plasma levels of C5a, which precede edema formation.[65] In a clinical trial, Ogilvie et al.[66] were able to demonstrate that treatment of patients with C1 inhibitor concentrate not only led to a greater tolerance of high doses of IL-2 but also to a reduced incidence of therapy-associated capillary leak. Systemic complement activation and reduced C1 inhibitor function is also commonly observed in patients with CLS after bone marrow transplantation.[43] In these patients replacement therapy with high doses of C1 inhibitor, leading to supranormal plasma levels of the regulator, suppressed classic pathway activation and substantially improved the clinical outcome.[67] Administration of C1 inhibitor to children with congenital heart disease was effective in terminating bypass-induced capillary leak.[68]

A cardioprotective effect of C1 inhibitor was observed in a cat model of myocardial ischemia and reperfusion[69] and was confirmed in an animal study, where intracoronary application of the human regulator significantly reduced reperfusion injury in pigs.[70] After successful treatment of three patients undergoing emergency surgical revascularization in whom postoperative hemodynamic stabilization could otherwise not be achieved, Bauernschmitt et al.[71] suggested C1 inhibitor administration as rescue therapy in cases of postoperative myocardial dysfunction due to reperfusion injury.

Effective protection from reperfusion injury is also required for successful transplantation. In dogs undergoing lung transplantation, pretreatment with C1 inhibitor prevented early pulmonary dysfunction.[72] In a sheep lung transplant model, reperfusion organ damage was reduced upon C1 inhibitor administration prior to and during initial reperfusion, as reflected by improved oxygenation and pulmonary vascular resistance.[73] In our own experiments in a rat model of transplantation-related liver ischemia/reperfusion injury, we observed by in vivo microscopy reduced cell adherence and tissue infiltration upon C1 inhibitor pretreatment.[74] In patients, a stable C1 inhibitor level of more than 110–130% of normal appears to be favorable for an uneventful outcome after lung transplantation. Patients who developed symptoms of reperfusion injury after lung transplantation received high doses of C1 inhibitor concentrate and recovered completely.[75]

Soluble Complement Receptor 1 (sCR1, CD35)

Complement receptor 1 (CR1, CD35), a single-chain membrane-bound glycoprotein, mediates phagocytosis of C3b-opsonized targets and serves as a potent regulator of C3 and C5 activation.[76] CR1 binds C3b and C4b, exerts cofactor activity for factor I-mediated proteolytic degradation of these molecules, and accelerates the decay of both the classic and alternative C3/C5 convertases. The extramembranous part of CR1, which retains full regulatory activity, can be isolated from plasma. A truncated soluble molecule, lacking the transmembrane and cytoplasmic domains, was then prepared from Chinese hamster ovarian cells transfected with a modified CR1 cDNA.[77] The recombinant soluble complement receptor-1 (sCR1) was found to be more effective than the endogenous soluble C3/C5 convertase inhibitors C4bp and factor H.[78] In addition, the recombinant inhibitor reacted with its target molecules in serum of various other species, a prerequisite for in vivo testing in appropriate animal models of inflammatory disease.

In a rat model of myocardial ischemia/reperfusion injury, treatment of animals with sCR1 reduced the myocardial infarction size by 44% along with an absence of C5b-9 tissue deposition and decreased accumulation of leukocytes within the infarction zone.[79] Administration of sCR1 to rats with intestinal ischemia/reperfusion injury resulted in reduced intestinal mycloperoxide (MPO) activity, mucosal injury, and decreased lung permeability.[80] sCR1 was also shown to exert protective effects in various models of hepatic ischemia/reperfusion injury. Jaeschke et al.[81] found that sCR1 treatment was more protective than systemic complement depletion with cobra venom factor (CVF) (see below), as demonstrated by reduced hepatic necrosis and attenuated neutrophil infiltration in the postischemic liver. In vivo microscopic analysis in rats revealed that after ischemia reperfusion sCR1 significantly diminishes leukocyte rolling and sticking in hepatic vessels, thereby reducing tissue damage.[82] In addition, complement-induced Kupffer cell activation leading to release of reactive oxygen can be diminished by sCR1 treatment.[81-83]

In rats undergoing immune complex-induced alveolitis, sCR1 reduced vascular permeability and hemorrhage by more than 70%.[84] In a rat model of ARDS, Rabinovici et al.[85] demonstrated that sCR1 pretreatment prevented pulmonary edema and polymorphonuclear neutrophil (PMN) infiltration and attenuated complement deposition to lung vessels.

Beneficial effects of sCR1 treatment were also reported for reverse passive Arthus reaction, complement-mediated experimental glomerulonephritis,[86] demyelinating experimental allergic encephalitis,[87] and allogeneic lung transplantation in the rat[88] and pig.[89] Local therapy with sCR1 was shown to be effective in a rat arthritis model.[90]

Initial human trials indicate that sCR1 (TP10; T Cell Sciences/Avantimmune, Boston, MA, USA) is well tolerated, effectively inhibits complement activation, and reduces the need for mechanical ventilation.[91] Phase II clinical trials are in progress to evaluate the regulator's therapeutic potential in patients with ARDS or myocardial infarction and to establish its efficacy in reperfusion injury subsequent to lung transplantation. The problem of rapid clearance of therapeutic reagents such as sCR1 from the blood may be solved by creating chimeric proteins of the inhibitory molecules and other proteins with longer half-lives, such as immunoglobulins[92] or albumin-binding receptor.[93] Further developments include the generation of sCR1 molecules with a selective inhibitory profile by reducing the number of complement control protein repeat (CCP) molecules. A truncated version [sCR1(desLHR-A)] has been created that lacks the C4b-binding long homologous repeat sequence-A and thereby selectively inhibits the alternative pathway.[94,95] Incorporation into sCR1 of the seLe^x oligosaccharide, the common carbohydrate ligand for the P-, E-, and L-selectin adhesion molecules, allows combined inhibition of complement activation and selectin-mediated cellular interaction.[96,97]

Blocking Complement Components

Inhibition of the complement cascade reaction at the level of C5 prevents formation of the membrane attack complex and generation of the anaphylatoxin C5a while maintaining important complement functions such as opsonization and immune complex clearance. C5-deficient mice are, at least to a certain degree, protected against the consequences of fulminant complement activation, as observed in septic shock.[98] Anti-C5 therapy was shown to inhibit significantly cell apoptosis, necrosis, and PMN infiltration in rat myocardial ischemia/reperfusion, despite the reduction of C3 tissue deposition.[99] In two murine preclinical models of systemic lupus erythematosus (SLE)[100] and rheumatoid arthritis,[101] respectively, treatment with monoclonal anti-C5 antibodies led to marked amelioration of the course of renal disease and joint inflammation, respectively. For clinical application, in addition to a humanized monoclonal anti-C5 antibody (h5G.1.1-Mab), a single-chain anti-C5 antibody (h5G1.1-scFv) is now available (Alexion Pharmaceutical, New Haven, CT, USA) that has been shown to be a potent inhibitor of complement as well as of platelet and leukocyte activation in an in vitro model of extracorporeal circulation relevant to cardiopulmonary bypass.[102] Pharmacokinetic and pharmacodynamic data from a phase I clinical trial indicate that a single bolus of the humanized anti-C5 scFv may sufficiently block complement activation during CPB.[103] In addition, CPB-induced myocardial damage, as measured by cardiac-specific creatine phosphokinase, could be significantly reduced.[104] At present, phase I/II trials are performed to test the efficacy of h5G.1.1-Mab in rheumatoid arthritis and SLE and of h5G1.1-scFv in CPB (phase II) and acute myocardial infarction (phase I), respectively.

A C3-binding 13-residue cyclic peptide called compstatin has been identified and shown to inhibit C3 activation in primates.[105] Compstatin inhibited complement and cellular activation in an in vitro model of extracorporeal circulation[106] and prolonged survival of ex vivo-perfused pig xenografts.[107]

Short RNA strings, termed aptamers, specifically binding to C1q and C5, respectively, have been created, employing the SELEX (systematic evolution of ligands and exponential enrichment) methodology. They were shown to bind with high affinity and to inhibit effectively the respective complement proteins in vitro. Human and rat aptamer inhibitors of C5 (Nexstar Pharmaceuticals, Boulder, CO, USA) are currently being evaluated for treatment of human disease.[108] Selective inhibition of C1s or factor D by specific serine protease inhibitors, potentially arising from a structure-based drug design, represents another attractive strategy for focusing on the control of one complement pathway recognized to be primarily involved in inflammatory tissue destruction.

Inhibition of the Anaphylatoxin C5a

The complement-derived anaphylatoxin C5a is considered to be one of the most potent phlogistic peptides.[4] Inflammatory cells react to nanomolar concentrations of C5a with chemotaxis, upregulation of adhesion molecules, and the release of destructive oxygen radicals and lysosomal proteases. Prophylactic administration of anti-C5a antibodies in two models of septic shock caused the mortality rate to be significantly reduced, and the animals showed considerably improved hemodynamic conditions.[109,110] Anti-rat C5a also efficiently blocked complement (C5a)-mediated upregulation of lung vascular intercellular adhesion molecule-1 (ICAM-1) and P-selectin[111] and lung vascular permeability in two rat models of thermal trauma and ischemia/reperfusion injury. Reperfusion injury during myocardial infarction was also markedly reduced in pigs pretreated with monoclonal anti-C5a immunoglobulin G (IgG).[112] The antibody was shown to inhibit C5a generation selectively without attenuating formation of the membrane attack complex C5b-9.[113] In contrast, monoclonal antibodies directed against a porcine C5a/C5adesArg neoepitope failed to exert a beneficial effect on mortality and organ function in a pig septic model. However, improved oxygen use was observed in treated animals, and significantly less IL-6 was generated, supporting the notion of an immunoregulatory role of C5a.[114,115] It therefore appears that certain therapeutic effects observed in previous experiments applying polyclonal anti-C5a (which usually cross-reacts with native C5) may, rather, be due to C5 inhibition and the inability of the animals to generate cytolytic C5b-9 molecules. This observation is in line with those described for C5 inhibition using anti-C5 antibodies (see above). Neutralizing anti-C5a antibodies have also been generated from phage display libraries[116,117] but await testing in vivo.

Synthetic C5a analogues are considered valuable tools for analyzing C5a-mediated biologic functions. However, the design of low-molecular-weight antagonists aimed at interfering with the high-affinity binding of C5a to its receptor is still a challenging problem.[117] C5a receptor antagonists inhibited C5a-induced dermal edema in rabbits and neutropenia in minipigs.[118] In three models of reverse Arthus reaction (skin, lung, peritoneum) a C5a receptor antagonist selected from a phage display library was shown to attenuate PMN influx.[119] In a mouse model of intestinal reperfusion injury, the same antagonist tissue injury significantly reduced lung vascular permeability (J. Koehl, Hannover, Germany, personal communication). Anti-C5a receptor antibodies[120] or inhibitors of C5a receptor binding, such as substituted 4,6-diaminoquinolines,[121] may provide further avenues for reducing anaphylatoxin-mediated inflammation.

Multiple Target Inhibition

A variety of synthetic compounds have been tested for their impact on the complement system, but most are toxic, are not complement-specific, or require unrealistically high concentrations to inhibit complement in vivo.[30] The synthetic serine proteinase inhibitor 6-amidino-2-naphthyl-4-guanidinobenzoate (nafamstat mesilate, or *FUT-175*), is a potent inhibitor of C1s, factor D, and C3/C5-convertase activity.[122] FUT-175 was successfully tested in animal experiments on acute experimental pancreatitis[123] and myocardial ischemia/reperfusion injury.[124] FUT-175 also significantly reduced the incidence of cerebral infarction in a clinical trial on subarachnoid hemorrhage. In a comparative study of FUT-175 and K76-COOH, both molecules inhibited deposition of C5b-9 in the lung, but, neither drug was useful as a single agent to prolong survival in a pig-to-human lung xenograft model if given at nontoxic doses.[125]

Heparin, known for its anticoagulation effect, is considered a potent inhibitor of the complement system, especially if it is bound to the activating surface.[126] A substantial improvement of biocompatibility of CPB devices could be achieved by endpoint attachment of heparin to the surfaces of a extracorporeal circuit as tested in animal experiments and in vitro with human blood in closed circuits.[21,22] One clinical study with patients randomized to operation with uncoated or heparin-coated surfaces demonstrated a significant reduction of complement activation accompanied by attenuation of the leukocyte integrin and selectin response.[127] Schreurs et al.[128] reported reduced release of inflammatory mediators and a clinical benefit in patients with heparin-coated CPB in pediatric cardiac operations.

Supraphysiologic doses of intravenous *immunoglobulin* (IVIg), currently used in a number of inflammatory and autoimmune diseases, probably exert some of their therapeutic effect by acting as a scavenger for activated C3 and C4, thereby preventing the cascade reaction from taking place on the patient's tissue.[129] The inhibitory activity appears to be most pronounced in a mixture of immunoglobulins of different isotypes and may also be due to the ability of IgG to augment factor H- and I-dependent inactivation of C3b-containing complexes.[130] IVIg treatment was beneficial in patients suffering from dermatomyositis and correlated with significantly reduced deposition of C3b and C5b-9 in endomysial capillaries.[131]

Complement Depletion by Cobra Venom Factor

Cobra venom factor (CVF), a nontoxic protein in cobra venom, forms (like C3b) together with factor B and factor D a stable bimolecular C3/C5 convertase,[132] which subsequently leads to unrestricted complement consumption. For many years complement depletion by CVF provided the only experimental means by which to analyze the significance of complement to inflammation.[133] As a "gold standard," CVF is still used to compare the efficacy of most inhibitory molecules described in this overview. Despite its capacity to exert significant protection in complement-mediated pulmonary injury,[134,135] demyelinating experimental allergic neuritis,[136] vasculitis,[137] and hyperacute xenograft rejection,[138–140] the strong immunogenicity of purified CVF has hitherto precluded its clinical application. After cloning the molecule[132] a new generation of modified recombinant forms of CVF may become available for medical therapy.

Complement Inhibition During Xenotransplantation by Gene Transfer

Despite its rare occurrence, hyperacute graft rejection, mediated by the action of natural antibodies and complement, is a significant problem after transplantation surgery. In addition, it represents the major barrier to xenotransplantation, which is frequently discussed as a potential solution to the shortage of human donor organs.[141]

To overcome complement-mediated hyperacute rejection of discordant xenografts,[142,143] human membrane-associated regulatory proteins have been transferred to xenogeneic tissue. Dalmasso et al.[144] demonstrated that human DAF can be directly inserted by its GPI anchor into porcine endothelial cell membranes, thereby preventing lysis of the cells by human complement. Subsequently, protection of xenogeneic cells was achieved by transfection with cDNA of human MCP, DAF, or CD59. In a recent series of experiments we demonstrated that expression on porcine endothelial cells of human CD59 by itself or in combination with soluble regulators effectively inhibited cell destruction by human serum complement.[145] Kooyman et al.[146] showed that GPI-linked complement regulatory proteins expressed on the surface of transgenic mouse or pig erythrocytes can be transferred in a functional, active form to vascular endothelium in vivo.

A major step toward clinical application of xenotransplantation was generation of transgenic donor animals that express human complement inhibitor proteins on their tissue.[147,148] Quantitative analysis of the human regulator DAF in various pig organs displayed an expression level comparable or even higher than that on normal human endothelium. Morphologic and functional analysis revealed that in xenoperfused huDAF or huCD59 transgenic pig hearts and kidneys the human regulators were expressed sufficiently to inhibit complement activation and to reduce significantly the morphologic alterations indicative of hyperacute graft rejection.

Conclusions

With the availability of recombinant complement regulatory molecules, monoclonal antibodies to key complement components and genetically engineered pigs, carrying protecting human complement control proteins, the prospects are favorable for the development of a new strategy to prevent inflammatory tissue destruction by specific complement targeting. However, only convincing results from ongoing and future clinical trials will finally decide the fate of this exciting new avenue in antiphlogistic therapy.

References

1. Müller-Eberhard HJ: Molecular organization and function of the complement system. Annu Rev Biochem 1988;57:321–347.
2. Rother K, Till GO, Hänsch GM: The Complement System, 2nd rev ed., New York, Springer, 1998.
3. Turner MW: Mannose-binding lectin: the pluripotent molecule of the innate immune system. Immunol Today 1996;17:532–540.
4. Hugli TE: Biochemistry and biology of anaphylatoxins. Complement 1986;3:111–127.
5. Morgan BP, Harris CL: Complement Regulatory Proteins. San Diego, Academic, 1999.
6. Dalmasso AP: Complement in the pathophysiology and diagnosis of human diseases. Crit Rev Clin Lab 1986;24:123–183.
7. Morgan BP: Complement: Clinical Aspects and Relevance to Disease. New York, Harcourt Brace Jovanovich, 1990.
8. Volanakis JE, Frank MM: The Human Complement System in Health and Disease. New York, Marcel Dekker, 1998.
9. Zilow G, Sturm JA, Rother U, et al: Complement activation and the prognostic value of C3a in patients at risk of adult respiratory distress syndrome. Clin Exp Immunol 1990;79:151–157.
10. Mollnes TE, Fosse E: The complement system in trauma-related and ischemic tissue damage: a brief review. Shock 1994;2:301–310.
11. Lucchesi BR, Kilgore KS: Complement inhibitors in myocardial ischemia/reperfusion injury. Immunopharmacology 1997;38:27–42.
12. De Boer JP, Creasey AA, Chang A, et al: Activation of the complement system in baboons challenged with live *Escherichia coli*: correlation with mortality and evidence for a biphasic activation pattern. Infect Immun 1993;61:4293–4301.
13. Hack CE, Nuijens JH, Felt-Bersma RJ, et al: Elevated plasma levels of the anaphylatoxins C3a and C4a are associated with a fatal outcome in sepsis. Am J Med 1989;86:20–26.
14. Colman RW: The role of plasma proteases in septic shock. N Engl J Med 1989;320:1207–1209.
15. Hazelzet JA, de Groot R, van Mierlo G, et al: Complement activation in relation to capillary leakage in children with septic shock and purpura. Infect Immun 1998;66:5350–5356.
16. Acioli JM, Isobe M, Kawasaki S: Early complement system activation and neutrophil priming in acute pancreatitis: participation of trypsin. Surgery 1997;122:909–917.
17. Johnson RJ: Complement activation during extracorporeal therapy: biochemistry, cell biology and clinical relevance. Nephrol Dial Transplant 1994;9(Suppl 2):36–45.
18. Gardinali M, Circardi M, Agostoni A, et al: Complement activation in extracorporeal circulation: physiological and pathological implications. Pathol Immunopathol Res 1986;5:352–370.
19. Janatova J, Cheung AK, Parker CJ: Biomedical polymers differ in their capacity to activate complement. Complement Inflamm 1991;8:61–69.
20. Cheung AK, Parker CJ, Hohnholt M: Soluble complement receptor type 1 inhibits complement activation induced by hemodialysis membranes in vitro. Kidney Int 1994;46:1680–1687.
21. Kirschfink M, Kovacs B, Mottaghy K: Extracorporeal circulation: in vivo and in vitro analysis of complement activation by heparin-bonded surfaces. Circ Shock 1993;40:221–226.
22. Mollnes TE: Biocompatibility: complement as mediator of tissue damage and as indicator of incompatibility. Exp Clin Immunogenet 1997;14:24–29.
23. Cooper NR, Nemerow GR, Mayes JT: Methods to detect and quantitate complement activation. Springer Semin Immunopathol 1983;6:195–212.
24. Kirschfink M: The clinical laboratory: testing the complement system. In: Rother K, Till GO, Hänsch GM (eds) The Complement System, 2nd rev ed. New York, Springer, 1998;522–547.
25. Gama de Abreu M, Kirschfink M, Quintel M, et al: White blood cell counts and plasma C3a have synergistic predictive value in patients at risk for acute respiratory distress syndrome. Crit Care Med 1998;26:1040–1048.
26. Hecke F, Schmidt U, Kola A, et al: Circulating complement proteins in multiple trauma patients: correlation with injury severity, development of sepsis, and outcome. Crit Care Med 1997;25:2015–2024.
27. Kirschfink M, Wienert K, Rother K, et al: Complement activation in renal allograft recipients. Transplant Proc 1992;24:2556–2557.
28. Hartmann H, Lubbers B, Casaretto M, et al: Rapid quantification of C3a and C5a using a combination of chromatographic and immunoassay procedures. J Immunol Methods 1993;166:35–44.
29. Stove S, Welte T, Wagner TO, et al: Circulating complement proteins in patients with sepsis or systemic inflammatory response syndrome. Clin Diagn Lab Immunol 1996;3:175–183.
30. Asghar SS: Pharmacological manipulation of complement system. Pharmacol Rev 1984;36:223–244.
31. Kirschfink M: Controlling the complement system in inflammation. Immunopharmacology 1997;38:51–62.
32. Liszewski M-K, Atkinson JP: Novel complement inhibitors. Exp Opin Invest Drugs 1998;7:323–332.
33. Makrides SC: Therapeutic inhibition of the complement system. Pharmacol Rev 1998;50:59–87.
34. Tosi M, Duponchel C, Bourgarel P, et al: Molecular cloning of human C1 inhibitor: sequence homologies with alpha 1-antitrypsin and other members of the serpins superfamily. Gene 1986;42:265–272.
35. Sim RB, Reboul A, Arlaud GJ, et al: Interaction of ^{125}I-labelled complement subcomponents C-1r and C-1s with protease inhibitors in plasma. FEBS Lett 1979;97:111–115.
36. Forbes CD, Pensky J, Ratnoff OD: Inhibition of activated Hageman factor and activated plasma thromboplastin antecedent by purified serum C1 inactivator. J Lab Clin Med 1970;76:809–815.
37. Ratnoff OD, Pensky J, Ogston D, et al: The inhibition of plasmin, plasma kallikrein, plasma permeability factor, and the C'1r subcomponent of the first component of complement by serum C'1 esterase inhibitor. J Exp Med 1969;129:315–331.
38. Ranby M, Bergsdorf N, Nilsson T: Enzymatic properties of the one- and two-chain form of tissue plasminogen activator. Thromb Res 1982;27:175–183.
39. Perlmutter DH, Glover GI, Rivetna M, et al: Identification of a serpin-enzyme complex receptor on human hepatoma cells and human monocytes. Proc Natl Acad Sci USA 1990;87:3753–3757.
40. Brower MS, Harpel PC: Proteolytic cleavage and inactivation of alpha 2-plasmin inhibitor and C1 inactivator by human polymorphonuclear leukocyte elastase. J Biol Chem 1982;257:9849–9854.
41. Davis AE III: C1 inhibitor and hereditary angioneurotic edema. Annu Rev Immunol 1988;6:595–628.
42. Faymonville ME, Micheels J, Bodson L, et al: Biochemical investigations after burning injury: complement system, protease–antiprotease balance and acute-phase reactants. Burns 1987;13:26–33.

43. Nürnberger W, Michelmann I, Petrik K, et al: Activity of C1 esterase inhibitor in patients with vascular leak syndrome after bone marrow transplantation. Ann Hematol 1993;67:17–21.
44. Berling R, Ohlsson K: Effects of high-dose intraperitoneal aprotinin treatment on complement activation and acute phase response in acute severe pancreatitis. J Gastroenterol 1996;31:702–709.
45. Mikkonen R, Aronen HJ, Kivisaari L, et al: Plasma levels of prekallikrein, alpha-2-macroglobulin and C1-esterase inhibitor in patients with urticarial reaction to contrast media. Acta Radiol 1997;38:466–473.
46. Gerlach M, Fohre B, Keh D, et al: Global and extended coagulation monitoring during extracorporeal lung assist with heparin-coated systems in ARDS patients. Int J Artif Organs 1997;20:29–36.
47. Kirschfink M, Nürnberger W: C1 inhibitor in anti-inflammatory therapy: from animal experiment to clinical application. Mol Immunol 1999; 36:225–232.
48. Guerrero R, Velasco F, Rodriguez M, et al: Endotoxin-induced pulmonary dysfunction is prevented by C1-esterase inhibitor. J Clin Invest 1993;91:2754–2760.
49. Scherer RU, Giebler RM, Schmidt U, et al: The influence of C1-esterase inhibitor substitution on coagulation and cardiorespiratory parameters in an endotoxin-induced rabbit model of hypercoagulability. Semin Thromb Hemost 1996;22:357–366.
50. Fischer MB, Prodeus AP, Nicholson-Weller A, et al: Increased susceptibility to endotoxin shock in complement C3- and C4-deficient mice is corrected by C1 inhibitor replacement. J Immunol 1997;159:976–982.
51. Jansen PM, Eisele B, de Jong IW, et al: Effect of C1 inhibitor on inflammatory and physiologic response patterns in primates suffering from lethal septic shock. J Immunol 1998; 160:475–484.
52. Hack CE, Voerman HJ, Eisele B, et al: C1-esterase inhibitor substitution in sepsis [letter]. Lancet 1992;339:378.
53. Walger P, Fronhoffs S, Steuer K, et al: The effect of C1-esterase inhibitor in five patients with streptococcal toxic syndrome. Ann Hematol 1997;74(Suppl III):A160.
54. Goodman AJ, Bird NC, Johnson AG: Antiprotease capacity in acute pancreatitis. Br J Surg 1986;73:796–798.
55. Yamaguchi H, Kimura T, Mimura K, et al: Activation of proteases in cerulein-induced pancreatitis. Pancreas 1989;4: 565–571.
56. Ruud TE, Aasen AO, Stadaas JO, et al: Effects on peritoneal proteolysis and hemodynamics of prophylactic and therapeutic infusions of high doses of aprotinin in experimental acute pancreatitis. Scand J Gastroenterol 1986;21:1011–1017.
57. Yamaguchi H, Weidenbach H, Luhrs H, et al: Combined treatment with C1 esterase inhibitor and antithrombin III improves survival in severe acute experimental pancreatitis. Gut 1997;40:531–535.
58. Testoni PA, Cicardi M, Bergamaschini L, et al: Infusion of C1-inhibitor plasma concentrate prevents hyperamylasemia induced by endoscopic sphincterotomy. Gastrointest Endosc 1995; 42:301–305.
59. Niederau C, Brinsa R, Niederau M, et al: Effects of C1-esterase inhibitor in three models of acute pancreatitis. Int J Pancreatol 1995;17:189–196.
60. Kochilas L, Campbell B, Scalia R, et al: Beneficial effects of C1 esterase inhibitor in murine traumatic shock. Shock 1997;8: 165–169.
61. Radke A, Mottaghy K, Goldmann Ch, et al: C1-Inhibitor prevents capillary leakage after thermal trauma. Crit Care Med 2000 (in press).
62. Khorram-Sefat R, Goldmann C, Radke A, et al: The therapeutic effect of C1-inhibitor on gut-derived bacterial translocation after thermal injury. Shock 1998;9:101–108.
63. Jostkleigrewe F, Brandt KA, Janssen AC: C1-esterase inhibitor (C1-INH) as adjuvant therapy for septic shock following severe thermal trauma. Ann Hematol 1997;74(Suppl III):A159.
64. Rosenstein M, Ettinghausen SE, Rosenberg SA: Extravasation of intravascular fluid mediated by the systemic administration of recombinant interleukin 2. J Immunol 1986;137:1735–1742.
65. Thijs LG, Hack CE, Strack van Schijndel RJ, et al. Activation of the complement system during immunotherapy with recombinant IL-2: relation to the development of side effects. J Immunol 1990;144:2419–2424.
66. Ogilvie AC, Baars JW, Eerenberg AJ, et al: A pilot study to evaluate the effects of C1 esterase inhibitor on the toxicity of high-dose interleukin 2. Br J Cancer 1994;69:596–598.
67. Nürnberger W, Heying R, Burdach S, et al: C1 esterase inhibitor concentrate for capillary leakage syndrome following bone marrow transplantation. Ann Hematol 1997;75:95–101.
68. Stieh J, Harding P, Scheewe J, et al: Capillary leak syndrom after open heart surgery for congenital heart defects: therapy with C1-inhibitor. Biomed Progr 1996;9:13–16.
69. Buerke M, Murohara T, Lefer AM: Cardioprotective effects of a C1 esterase inhibitor in myocardial ischemia and reperfusion. Circulation 1995;91:393–402.
70. Horstick G, Heimann A, Götze O, et al: Intracoronary application of C1 esterase inhibitor improves cardiac function and reduces myocardial necrosis in an experimental model of ischemia and reperfusion. Circulation 1997;95:701–708.
71. Bauernschmitt R, Bohrer H, Hagl S: Rescue therapy with C1-esterase inhibitor concentrate after emergency coronary surgery for failed PTCA. Intensive Care Med 1998;24:635–638.
72. Salvatierra A, Velasco F, Rodriguez M, et al: C1-esterase inhibitor prevents early pulmonary dysfunction after lung transplantation in the dog. Am J Respir Crit Care Med 1997; 155:1147–1154.
73. Graeter T, Demertzis S, Scherer M, et al: Amelioration of ischemia/reperfusion injury with C1-esterase inhibitor in a sheep lung transplant model. Ann Hematol 1997;74(Suppl III):A156.
74. Lehmann TG, Heger M, Münch S, et al: Complement inhibition by C1-esterase inhibitor reduces microvascular disturbance after warm hepatic ischemia. Langenbecks Arch Chir 1999 (in press).
75. Hentjes B, Jankowski M, Vangerow B, et al: C1-esterase-inhibitor levels in patients with and without reperfusion injury following lung transplantation (LTx). Ann Hematol 1997;74(Suppl III):A157.
76. Fearon DT: Regulation of the amplification C3 convertase of human complement by an inhibitory protein isolated from human erythrocyte membrane. Proc Natl Acad Sci USA 1979;76: 5867–5871.
77. Weisman HF, Bartow T, Leppo MK, et al: Recombinant soluble CR1 suppressed complement activation, inflammation, and necrosis associated with reperfusion of ischemic myocardium. Trans Assoc Am Physicians 1990;103:64–72.
78. Fearon DT: Anti-inflammatory and immunosuppressive effects of recombinant soluble complement receptors. Clin Exp Immunol 1991;86(Suppl 1):43–46.

79. Weisman HF, Bartow T, Leppo MK, et al: Soluble human complement receptor type 1: in vivo inhibitor of complement suppressing post-ischemic myocardial inflammation and necrosis. Science 1990;249:146–151.
80. Hill J, Lindsay TF, Ortiz F, et al: Soluble complement receptor type 1 ameliorates the local and remote organ injury after intestinal ischemia/reperfusion in the rat. J Immunol 1992;149:1723–1728.
81. Jaeschke H, Farhood A, Bautista AP, et al: Complement activates Kupffer cells and neutrophils during reperfusion after hepatic ischemia. Am J Physiol 1993;264:801–809.
82. Lehmann TG, Koeppel TA, Kirschfink M, et al: Complement inhibition by soluble complement receptor type 1 improves microcirculation after rat liver transplantation. Transplantation 1998;66:717–722.
83. Chavez-Cartaya RE, DeSola GP, Wright L, Jamieson NV, White DJ: Regulation of the complement cascade by soluble complement receptor type 1: protective effect in experimental liver ischemia and reperfusion. Transplantation 1995;59: 1047–1052.
84. Mulligan MS, Yeh GC, Rudolph AR, Ward PA: Protective effects of soluble CR1 in complement- and neutrophil-mediated tissue injury. J Immunol 1992;148:1479–1485.
85. Rabinovici R, Yeh CG, Hillegass LM, et al: Role of complement in endotoxin/platelet-activating factor-induced lung injury. J Immunol 1992;149:1744–1750.
86. Couser WG, Johnson RJ, Young BA, Yeh CG, Toth CA, Rudolph AR: The effects of soluble recombinant complement receptor 1 on complement-mediated experimental glomerulonephritis. J Am Soc Nephrol 1995;5:1888–1894.
87. Piddlesden SJ, Storch MK, Hibbs M, et al: Soluble recombinant complement receptor 1 inhibits inflammation and demyelination in antibody-mediated demyelinating experimental allergic encephalomyelitis. J Immunol 1994;152:5477–5484.
88. Naka Y, Marsh HC, Scesney SM, et al: Complement activation as a cause for primary graft failure in an isogeneic rat model of hypothermic lung preservation and transplantation. Transplantation 1997;64:1248–1255.
89. Pierre AF, Xavier AM, Liu M, et al: Effect of complement inhibition with soluble complement receptor 1 on pig allotransplant lung function. Transplantation 1998;66:723–732.
90. Goodfellow RM, Williams AS, Levin JL, et al: Local therapy with soluble complement receptor 1 (sCR1) suppresses inflammation in rat mono-articular arthritis. Clin Exp Immunol 1997;110:45–52.
91. Keshavjee RD, Zamora MR, Schulman L, et al: Inhibition of complement in human lung transplant reperfusion injury: a multicenter clinical trial. J Heart Lung Transplant 1998;17:43A.
92. Kalli KR, Hsu PH, Bartow TJ, et al: Mapping of the C3b-binding site of CR1 and construction of a (CR1)2-F(ab)2 chimeric complement inhibitor. J Exp Med 1991;174:1451–1460.
93. Makrides SC, Nygren PA, Andrews B, et al: Extended in vivo half-life of human soluble complement receptor type 1 fused to a serum albumin-binding receptor. J Pharmacol Exp Ther 1996;277:534–542.
94. Scesney SM, Makrides SC, Gosselin ML, et al: A soluble deletion mutant of the human complement receptor type 1, which lacks the C4b binding site, is a selective inhibitor of the alternative complement pathway. Eur J Immunol 1996;26:1729–1735.
95. Gralinski MR, Wiater BC, Assenmacher AN, et al: Selective inhibition of the alternative complement pathway by sCR1[des-LHR-A] protects the rabbit isolated heart from human complement-mediated damage. Immunopharmacology 1996;34:79–88.

96. Akahori T, Yuzawa Y, Nishikawa K, et al: Role of a sialyl Lewis(x)-like epitope selectively expressed on vascular endothelial cells in local skin inflammation of the rat. J Immunol 1997;158:5384–5392.
97. Lowe JB, Ward PA: Therapeutic inhibition of carbohydrate-protein interactions in vivo. J Clin Invest 1997;100:S47–S51.
98. Hsueh W, Sun X, Rioja LN, et al: The role of the complement system in shock and tissue injury induced by tumour necrosis factor and endotoxin. Immunology 1990;70:309–314.
99. Vakeva AP, Agah A, Rollins SA, et al: Myocardial infarction and apoptosis after myocardial ischemia and reperfusion: role of the terminal complement components and inhibition by anti-C5 therapy. Circulation 1998;97:2259–2267.
100. Wang Y, Hu Q, Madri JA, et al: Amelioration of lupus-like autoimmune disease in NZB/WF1 mice after treatment with a blocking monoclonal antibody specific for complement component C5. Proc Natl Acad Sci USA 1996;93: 8563–8568.
101. Wang Y, Rollins SA, Madri JA, et al: Anti-C5 monoclonal antibody therapy prevents collagen-induced arthritis and ameliorates established disease. Proc Natl Acad Sci USA 1995;92: 8955–8959.
102. Thomas TC, Rollins SA, Rother RP, et al: Inhibition of complement activity by humanized anti-C5 antibody and single-chain Fv. Mol Immunol 1996;33:1389–1401.
103. Rollins SA, Rinder HM, Rinder CS, et al: A humanized anti-C5 scFv blocks platelet and leukocyte activation and exhibits prolonged pharmacokinetics and pharmacodynamics in human. Exp Clin Immunogent 1997;14:36A.
104. Rollins SA, Fitch JCK, Sherman S, et al: Anti-C5 single chain antibody therapy blocks complement and leukocyte activation and reduces myocardial tissue damage in CBP patients. Mol Immunol 1998;35:397A.
105. Morikis D, Assa-Munt N, Sahu A, et al: Solution structure of Compstatin, a potent complement inhibitor. Protein Sci 1998;7:619–627.
106. Nilsson B, Larsson R, Hong J, et al: Compstatin inhibits complement and cellular activation in whole blood in two models of extracorporeal circulation. Blood 1998;92:1661–1667.
107. Fiane AE, Mollnes TE, Videm V, et al: Prolongation of ex vivo-perfused pig xenograft survival by the complement inhibitor compstatin. Transplant Proc 1999;31:934–935.
108. Biesecker G, Dihel L, Enney K, et al: Derivation of RNA aptamer inhibitors of human C5. Mol Immunol 1998;35:371A.
109. Stevens JH, O'Hanley P, Shapiro JM, et al: Effects of anti-C5a antibodies on the adult respiratory distress syndrome in septic primates. J Clin Invest 1986;77:1812–1816.
110. Smedegard G, Cui LX, Hugli TE: Endotoxin-induced shock in the rat: a role for C5a. Am J Pathol 1989;135:489–497.
111. Schmid E, Piccolo MT, Friedl HP, et al: Requirement for C5a in lung vascular injury following thermal trauma to rat skin. Shock 1997;8:119–124.
112. Bless NM, Warner RL, Padgaonkar VA, et al: Roles of C-X-C chemokines and C5a in lung injury after hindlimb ischemia/reperfusion. Am J Physiol 1999;276:57–63.
113. Amsterdam EA, Stahl GL, Pan HL, et al: Limitation of reperfusion injury by a monoclonal antibody to C5a during myocardial infarction in pigs. Am J Physiol 1995;268:448–457.
114. Höpken U, Mohr M, Strüber A, et al: Inhibition of interleukin-6 synthesis in an animal model of septic shock by anti-C5a monoclonal antibodies. Eur J Immunol 1996;26:1103–1109.

115. Mohr M, Höpken U, Oppermann M, et al: Effects of anti-C5a monoclonal antibodies on oxygen use in a porcine model of severe sepsis. Eur J Clin Invest 1998;28:227–234.
116. Ames RS, Tornetta MA, Jones CS, et al: Isolation of neutralizing anti-C5a monoclonal antibodies from a filamentous phage monovalent Fab display library. J Immunol 1994;153:910.
117. Kola A, Baensch M, Bautsch W, et al: Epitope mapping of a C5a neutralizing mAb using a combined approach of phage display, synthetic peptides and site-directed mutagenesis. Immunotechnology 1996;2:115–126.
118. Pellas TC, Boyar W, van Oostrum J, et al: Novel C5a receptor antagonists regulate neutrophil functions in vitro and in vivo. J. Immunol 1998;160:5616–5621.
119. Heller T, Hennecke M, Baensch M, et al: A C5a mutant selected from a phage library is a potent C5a-receptor antagonist in vitro and in vivo. Mol Immunol 1998;35:365A.
120. Morgan EL, Ember JA, Sanderson SD, et al: Anti-C5a receptor antibodies: characterization of neutralizing antibodies specific for a peptide, C5aR-(9–29), derived from the predicted amino-terminal sequence of the human C5a receptor. J Immunol 1993;151:377–388.
121. Lanza TJ, Durette PL, Rollins T, et al: Substituted 4, 6-diaminoquinolines as inhibitors of C5a receptor binding. J Med Chem 1992;35:252–258.
122. Inagi R, Miyata T, Maeda K, et al: FUT-175 as a potent inhibitor of C5/C3 convertase activity for production of C5a and C3a. Immunol Lett 1991;27:49–52.
123. Araida T, Frey CF, Ruebner B, et al: Therapeutic regimens in acute experimental pancreatitis in rats: effects of a protease inhibitor, a beta-agonist, and antibiotics. Pancreas 1995;11:132–140.
124. Homeister JW, Satoh P, Lucchesi BR: Effects of complement activation in the isolated heart: role of the terminal complement components. Circ Res 1992;71:303–319.
125. Blum MG, Collins BJ, Chang AC, et al: Complement inhibition by FUT-175 and K76-COOH in a pig-to-human lung xenotransplant model. Xenotransplantation 1998;5:35–43.
126. Cheung AK, Parker CJ, Janatova J, et al: Modulation of complement activation on hemodialysis membranes by immobilized heparin. J Am Soc Nephrol 1992;2:1328–1337.
127. Moen O, Hogasen K, Fosse E, et al: Attenuation of changes in leukocyte surface markers and complement activation with heparin-coated cardiopulmonary bypass. Ann Thorac Surg 1997;63:105–111.
128. Schreurs HH, Wijers MJ, Gu YJ, et al: Heparin-coated bypass circuits: effects on inflammatory response in pediatric cardiac operations. Ann Thorac Surg 1998;66:166–171.
129. Miletic VD, Hester CG, Frank MM: Regulation of complement activity by immunoglobulin. I. Effect of immunoglobulin isotype on C4 uptake on antibody-sensitized sheep erythrocytes and solid phase immune complexes. J Immunol 1996;156:749–757.
130. Lutz HU, Stammler P, Jelezarova E, et al: High doses of immunoglobulin G attenuate immune aggregate-mediated complement activation by enhancing physiologic cleavage of C3b in C3bn–IgG complexes. Blood 1996;88:184–193.
131. Basta M, Dalakas MC: High-dose intravenous immunoglobulin exerts its beneficial effect in patients with dermatomyositis by blocking endomysial deposition of activated complement fragments. J Clin Invest 1994;94:1729–1735.
132. Fritzinger DC, Bredehorst R, Vogel CW: Molecular cloning and derived primary structure of cobra venom factor. Proc Natl Acad Sci USA 1994;91:12775–12779.
133. Cochrane CG, Müller-Eberhard HJ, Aikin BS: Depletion of plasma complement in vivo by a protein of cobra venom: its effect on various immunologic reactions. J Immunol 1970;105:55–69.
134. Ren XD, Huang SJ, Sun JJ, et al: Protective effect of cobra venom factor on pulmonary injury induced by oleic acid. Int J Immunopharmacol 1994;16:969–975.
135. Dehring DJ, Steinberg SM, Wismar BL, et al: Complement depletion in a porcine model of septic acute respiratory disease. J Trauma 1987;27:615–625.
136. Vriesendorp FJ, Flynn RE, Pappolla MA, et al: Complement depletion affects demyelination and inflammation in experimental allergic neuritis. J Neuroimmunol 1995;58:157–165.
137. Mathieson PW, Qasim FJ, Thiru S, et al: Effects of decomplementation with cobra venom factor on experimental vasculitis. Clin Exp Immunol 1994;97:474–477.
138. Gewurz H, Clark DS, Cooper MD, et al: Effect of cobra venom-induced inhibition of complement activity on allograft and xenograft rejection reactions. Transplantation 1967;5:1296–1303.
139. Chrupcalla M, Pomer S, Staehler G, et al: Prolongation of discordant renal xenograft survival by depletion of complement: comparative effects of systematically administered cobra venom factor and soluble complement receptor type 1 in a guinea pig-to-rat model. Transplant Int 1994;7:650–653.
140. Azimzadeh A, Wolf P, Dalmasso AP, et al: Assessment of hyperacute rejection in a rat-to-primate cardiac xenograft model. Transplantation 1996;61:1305–1313.
141. Platt JL, Bach FH: The barrier to xenotransplantation. Transplantation 1991;52:937–947.
142. Dalmasso AP: The complement system in xenotransplantation. Immunopharmacology 1992;24:149–160.
143. Kirschfink M, Haferkamp A, Pomer S, et al: Significance of the complement system for xenotransplantation: strategies for therapeutic intervention. Zentralbl Chir 1998;123:793–797.
144. Dalmasso AP, Vercellotti GM, Platt JL, et al: Inhibition of complement-mediated endothelial cell cytotoxicity by decay-accelerating factor: potential for prevention of xenograft hyperacute rejection. Transplantation 1991;52:530–533.
145. Heckl-Östreicher B, Wosnik A, Kirschfink M: Protection of porcine endothelial cells from complement-mediated cytotoxicity by the human complement regulators CD59, C1 inhibitor, and soluble complement receptor type 1: analysis in a pig-to-human in vitro model relevant to hyperacute xenograft rejection. Transplantation 1996;62:1693–1696.
146. Kooyman DL, Byrne GW, McClellan S, et al: In vivo transfer of GPI-linked complement restriction factor from erythrocytes to the endothelium. Science 1995;269:89–92.
147. Cozzi E, White DJ: The generation of transgenic pigs as potential organ donors for humans. Nat Med 1995;1:964–966.
148. Kroshus TJ, Bolman RM III, Dalmasso AP: Studies on transfer of primate membrane-associated complement inhibitors from recipient blood to porcine donor organs. Transplant Proc 1996;28:601–602.

24
Leukocyte–Endothelial Cell Interactions: Review of Adhesion Molecules and Their Role in Organ Injury

Milind S. Shrotri, James C. Peyton, and William G. Cheadle

The causes of multiple organ injury, which are likely multifactorial, include microcirculatory vasoconstriction, local organ inflammatory mediator production, endothelial activation, and inappropriate polymorphonuclear neutrophil (PMN) sequestration and activation. This review focuses on leukocyte–endothelial interactions involving neutrophils and leading to tissue injury.

The role of neutrophils in tissue injury was first postulated by Metchnikoff in 1887.[1] Inflammatory mediators form an important component of the systemic inflammatory response; and the resultant sequestration of neutrophils (PMNs) into vital organs (e.g., lungs, liver) leads to amplification of the local release of such mediators. Reactive oxygen radicals (O_2^-, H_2O_2), myeloperoxidase, hypochlorous acid (HOCl), and proteases such as elastase, collagenase, and cathepsins, are some of these important early mediators released by activated PMNs. Thus PMNs play a key role in tissue injury. Experimental evidence suggests that activated neutrophils, once firmly adherent to the endothelium, can cause endothelial injury.[2] In some pathologic states (e.g., sepsis, ischemia/reperfusion), functional alterations of neutrophil and endothelium precede undirected, inappropriate, widespread neutrophil–endothelial adhesion throughout the organism.[3,4] The result can be neutrophil-mediated tissue injury in susceptible organs (e.g., liver, lung) that may evolve into organ dysfunction. After an acute inflammatory insult, large number of PMNs, which reside in the marginated pool (mainly lungs and spleen) in "standby mode," are actively released (demargination) into the general circulation under the influence of epinephrine. The release of newly formed PMNs from the bone marrow is probably more important in later persistent inflammatory states.

Leukocyte–endothelial interaction and its regulation are therefore of considerable importance. Leukocyte migration across the endothelial layer into tissues has been shown to involve several steps[5] that require specific adhesion molecule binding between leukocytes and the endothelium (Fig. 24.1). These studies have been mainly performed in exteriorized mesenteric or skeletal muscle vasculature, which is more accessible to study than solid organs such as lungs or liver. Selectins and integrins are responsible for leukocyte rolling and sticking to the endothelium of the postcapillary venules, which is then followed by diapedesis along a chemotactic gradient. The importance of these adhesion molecules is revealed in nature in two syndromes: leukocyte adhesion deficiency I and II.

Neutrophil–Endothelial Interaction and Neutrophil-Mediated Tissue Injury

Rapid mobilization of PMNs occurs at the focus of a tissue infection; it is a key host response that constitutes an essential part of the process of inflammation (Fig. 24.2). Margination is defined as a natural event in which PMNs reside normally in the vascular compartment by loosely tethering to the endothelium.[6] In contrast, sequestration is a process by which PMNs are localized in tissues or organs with strong adhesion to endothelium, mediated specifically by surface glycoprotein receptor complexes, immunoglobulins binding to their ligands, or both.[7] This strong adhesion may or may not culminate into transendothelial migration depending on the site of adhesion and the focus of inflammation.

Activated neutrophils demonstrate a respiratory or oxidative burst, rapidly resulting in reactive oxygen metabolites (ROMs), phagocytosis, or degranulation, with release of digestive cytotoxic enzymes. ROMs cause bacterial destruction by protein oxidation and cell membrane lipid peroxidation. Conversely, granular enzymes generally work through oxygen-independent mechanisms, allowing direct digestion of bacteria, with the exception of myeloperoxidase, which converts H_2O_2 to more destructive ROMs.[8] Activation is also involved in adhesive interaction with the endothelium but is not necessarily followed by phagocytic and cytotoxic activities. Neutrophil-mediated tissue injury, as occurs in multiple organ failure after sepsis or hypovolemic shock, is characterized by increased microvascular permeability.

Neutrophil-Endothelial Cell Adherence/Interaction

The marginated pool of PMNs constitutes two to three times the circulating pool of PMNs. The natural tendency of PMNs to

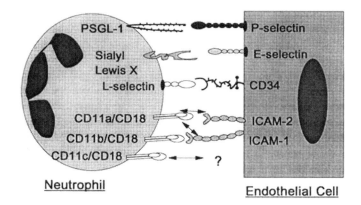

FIGURE 24.1. Various adhesion molecules present or upregulated on neutrophil and endothelial cell surfaces. PSGL-1, P-selectin glycoprotein-1; ICAM, intercellular adhesion molecule.

marginate can be related to their attraction to endothelium by a divalent cation-dependent process. The physics of particulate flow also favors the retardation of PMNs, with the red blood cells moving faster. This is reversed when the blood flow is increased, with the sluggishly moving PMNs pushed back into the circulation, and evident during release of catecholamines and exercise.[9] Compared to spontaneous adherence, stimulated PMN adherence to endothelium is a much stronger adhesive interaction and, unlike the former, is governed by adhesion molecule upregulation/expression and chemical gradients generated at the focus of tissue perturbation.

There are essentially two parts to the individual neutrophil–endothelial interaction: (1) stimulation and alteration of the endothelium to present a sticky surface for capturing the moving PMNs and a chemical gradient for directing the neutrophil transmigration; and (2) stimulation of the PMNs (through selectins and integrins) to become sticky and the subsequent activation necessary for transendothelial migration. The endothelial stimulants include thrombin, leukotrienes, and cytokines such as tumor necrosis factor-α (TNFα) and interleukin-1 (IL-1). Leukotrienes (e.g., leukotriene B_4) and cytokines are produced by local tissue cells, such as mast cells and macrophages, which in turn stimulate the endothelial cells to produce more cytokines and chemoattractants. Chemoattractants released systemically (activated complement, formyl peptides FMLP and FNLP) and factors such as mast cell-derived histamine are also involved in selectin upregulation and other glycoprotein expression on PMNs. These sticky cells are then captured by the sticky endothelium and exposed to the localized chemical gradient. Factors such as CXC chemokines (PMN-specific chemoattractant cytokines) form a chemical gradient and induce shedding of L-selectin and Mac-1 (CD11b/CD18) upregulation, converting

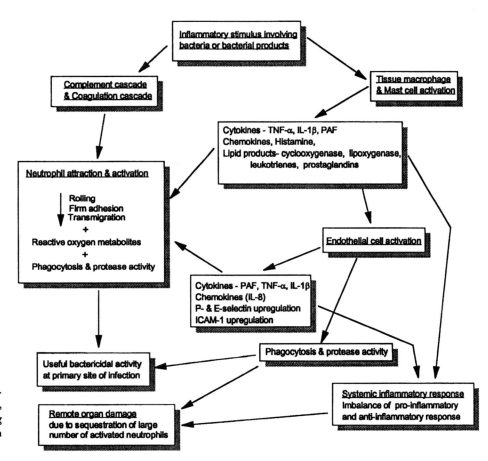

FIGURE 24.2. Inflammatory cascade. TNF-α, tumor necrosis factor-α; IL-1β, interleukin-1β; PAF, platelet-activating factor; ICAM, intercellular adhesion molecule.

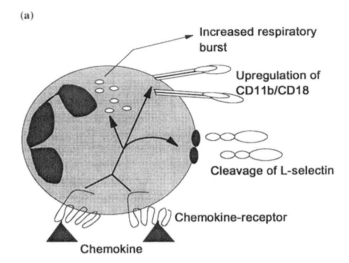

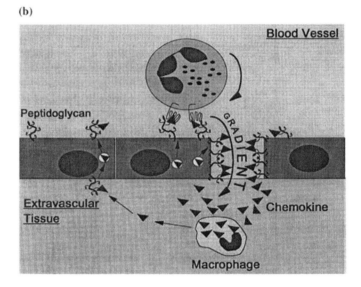

FIGURE 24.3. (a) Role of CXC chemokines on neutrophil activation. (b) Neutrophils follow the chemokine gradient, digesting their way through intercellular junctions.

Paradoxically, endothelial cells can also participate in tissue destruction by producing ROMs, proteases, and phagocytosis.[11-13] Endothelial-derived xanthine oxidase in ischemia/reperfusion injury is responsible for producing ROMs, whereas human PMNs do not have xanthine oxidase.[14] ROMs and proteases are responsible for the process of tissue damage. Tissue injury is best documented by histology, although quantitation is less objective. Morphologic changes of injury can occur late, and nonspecific changes are likely to be mistaken for tissue injury.[15] In the mouse model of cecal ligation and puncture (CLP),[16] we demonstrated that with use of anti-PMN antibody lung PMN sequestration can be reduced with

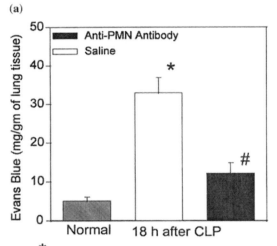

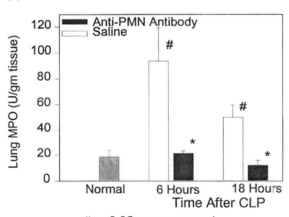

FIGURE 24.4. Effect of anti-PMN antibody on lung injury (a) as measured by Evans blue and on lung neutrophil sequestration (b) measured as tissue myeloperoxidase (MPO). (From Wickel et al.,[16] with permission.)

the transient stickiness of rolling to firm adhesion (Fig. 24.3a). CXC chemokines also cause the activation of PMNs, resulting in increased respiratory burst and perhaps localized degranulation, enabling the cells to digest their way through the intercellular junctions following the chemical gradient (Fig. 24.3b).

Neutrophil activation involves a spectrum of events, including the sequentially occurring adherence and chemotaxis, followed by phagocytosis and degranulation. Various mediators are involved in the initiation of one or more of these functions and may do so in an overlapping fashion, indicating the physiologic backup mechanisms that are involved in the inflammatory cascade of events. Although adherence can occur independent of phagocytosis and degranulation, the latter can be prevented by blocking adhesion.[10]

concomitant reduction in the lung injury, as measured by leakage of Evans blue dye (Fig. 24.4).

Leukocyte Migration: Multistep Paradigm

Once it is clear how PMN-mediated tissue injury occurs, the next important aspect is to understand the process of PMN migration from the vascular space into tissues. This has been categorized into various overlapping steps for most leukocytes, with some differences for individual leukocytic subpopulations. PMN migration is governed by various cells and their mediator products, with adhesion molecules playing the most important part (Fig. 24.5). Intravital microscopy has demonstrated that PMN migration begins with loose tethering or rolling along the endothelium in vessels with high velocity.[17] This initial phase of adhesion is mediated by adhesion molecules of the selectin family, which includes P-selectin, L-selectin, and E-selectin. After a period of rolling, PMNs firmly adhere to the endothelial cell surface and assume a flattened shape.[17] This firm adhesion is regulated by the interaction between the β_2-integrin adhesion molecule (CD11b/CD18) present on PMNs and its endothelial ligand, the intercellular adhesion molecule ICAM-1.[18,19] Transmigration across the endothelial monolayer requires a chemotactic gradient and interactions with another adhesion molecule, the platelet–endothelial cell adhesion molecule PECAM-1.[20] Complements C3a and C5a, peptides such as FMLP, and chemokines play important roles in establishing a chemotactic gradient. Endothelial expression of CXC chemokines is induced by TNFα or IL-1.[21] An overlap of steps may be involved in the process of PMN migration, and the regulation of PMN influx may vary among tissue beds and with different animal models.

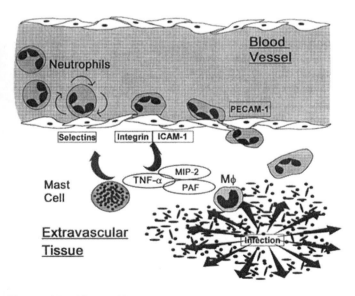

FIGURE 24.5. Neutrophil migration process in response to an infective stimulus. PECAM-1, platelet-endothelial cell adhesion molecule-1; ICAM, intercellular adhesion molecule; MIP-2, macrophage inflammatory protein-2; TNF-α, tumor necrosis factor-α; PAF, platelet-activating factor; Mϕ, macrophage.

Factors Regulating PMN Sequestration

Acute PMN infiltration into the perturbed tissues, with subsequent sequestration in remote organs, is a central event in the process of PMN-mediated tissue injury. The necessity or redundancy of the steps of PMN sequestration is dependent mainly on the following: (1) shear rates in the local vascular bed; (2) site of PMN migration; and (3) the nature of the inflammogen (or type of infective organism, in case of sepsis).

1. *Shear rates in the local vascular bed.* PMN migration into the peritoneal cavity[22] has been shown to occur in the postcapillary venules, whereas in lungs it occurs in the capillary beds.[23] Rolling is perhaps an unnecessary event in the latter situation because of the smaller diameter of the capillary bed;[24] the role of selectins therefore may be limited. Similarly, in the liver PMN migration has been shown to occur in the sinusoids, where the blood flow is again sluggish.

2. *Site of PMN migration.* The local tissue response to inflammation or circulating mediators significantly influences PMN influx. It is known that local mast cells release certain products in response to inflammatory stimuli that cause PMN infiltration.[25] Histamine, for example, causes P-selectin expression or release, and platelet-activating factor (PAF) increases β_2-integrin expression. TNFα (preformed/synthesized) up-regulates E- and P-selectins and β_2 integrin expression, and it may be responsible for the amplified and sustained PMN response.

3. *Nature of the inflammogen.* It has been shown that various infective microorganisms or inflammatory stimuli may induce PMN infiltration by invoking different mechanisms in different tissues. This is exemplified by studies showing that the peritoneal PMN response to experimental *Salmonella typhimurium* peritonitis is abolished by CD11b or CD18 blockade, whereas a similar blockade is ineffective in experimental *Listeria monocytogenes*-induced peritonitis.[26] Similarly, CD18 blockade reduces PMN emigration (and consequent bacterial clearance) in response to pulmonary *Escherichia coli* inoculation but not after *Staphylococcus aureus*.[27] It is important therefore to study a particular model that most closely mimics the clinical scenario.

Endothelial and Leukocytic Adhesion Molecules

Leukocytes, PMNs, and endothelial cells express a variety of adhesion molecules; some are constitutively expressed, whereas others are inducible on cytokine or chemotactic stimulation. There are many adhesion molecules; the three broad categories are the selectins, the integrins, and the immunoglobulin superfamily (Table 24.1). The differential heterophilic and homophilic interactions between these adhesion molecules are responsible for the variable leukocytic response observed under different inflammatory conditions, in different tissues, and in different experimental models.

TABLE 24.1. Adhesion Molecules: Their Ligands, Distribution, and Functions.

Adhesion molecule	Ligand	Distribution	Function
Selections			
L-selectin, CD61L, LAM-1	PSGL-1, CD34, GlyCAM-1, MAdCAM-1	Leukocytes	Lymphocyte homing, leukocyte–endothelial adhesion (rolling)
P-selectin, CD61P	As above	Platelets, endothelial cells	Platelet–leukocyte adhesion, leukocyte–endothelial adhesion (rolling)
E-selectin, CD61E, ELAM-1	PSGL-1	Endothelial cells	Leukocyte–endothelial adhesion (rolling)
Integrins			
LFA-1, CD11a/CD18	ICAM-1,2,3	Leukocytes	Adhesion to endothelial cells
Mac-1, CD11b/CD18	iC3b, CD54, fibrinogen, factor X	Monocytes, macrophages, granulocytes	Adhesion to endothelial cells
gp 150, 95, CD11c/CD18	iC3b	Monocytes, macrophages, granulocytes	Adhesion to endothelial cells
Immunoglobulins			
ICAM-1, CD54	LFA-1, Mac-1	Monocytes, epithelial cells, fibroblasts	Cell–cell adhesion
ICAM-2, CD102	CD11a	Endothelial cells, leukocytes	Leukocyte–endothelial cell adhesion
ICAM-3, CD50	CD11a	Endothelial cells, leukocytes	Leukocyte–endothelial cell adhesion
PECAM-1, CD31	CD31 (homotypic binding)	Endothelial cells, leukocytes	Initiation of endothelial cell–cell adhesion, platelet–monocyte or PMN–endothelial cell adhesion

LAM, lymphocyte adhesion molecule; PSGL, P-selectin glycoprotein ligand; GlyCAM, glycoprotein cell adhesion molecule; MAdCAM, mucosal addressin cell adhesion molecule; ELAM, endothelial–lymphocyte adhesion molecule; LFA, lymphocyte function antigen; ICAM, intercellular adhesion molecule; iC3b, activated complement 3b; gp, glycoprotein; PECAM, platelet–endothelial cell adhesion molecule; PMN, polymorphonuclear leukocyte (neutrophil).

Selectins (Rolling)

The P-, E-, and L-selectins are members of a family of adhesion molecules discovered between 1983 and 1987 by independent groups using monoclonal antibodies.[28-31]

Structure of Selectins and Their Counterreceptors

Selectins are a family of transmembrane glycoproteins.[32] The common structure of all the selectins consists of a lectin-type domain (N-terminal Ca^{2+}-dependent), an epidermal growth factor (EGF)-like domain, multiple short consensus repeats as in complementary regulatory proteins, a transmembrane region, and a short cytoplasmic C-terminal domain. This arrangement results in a structure that is elongated and projects from the cell surface, ideal for interaction between circulating cells and endothelial cells. The lectin and EGF domains mediate ligand binding, as the ligands for the selectins are the fucosylated, sialylated, and usually sulfated glycans, such as sialyl-Lewis X. A peptide backbone of the carbohydrate ligands introduces high affinity and a level of specificity. The ligands for L-selectin have been speculated as glycoprotein cell adhesion molecule (GlyCAM)-1, CD34, and mucosal addressin cell adhesion molecule (MAdCAM)-1 (in mice). P-selectin glycoprotein ligand (PSGL)-1 is a counterreceptor for P-selectin and is present on all leukocytes.[33] It also binds E- and L-selectins with lower affinity and may be responsible in part for neutrophil aggregation.

L-Selectin

An inducible cell adhesion molecule, L-selectin is constitutively expressed on the surface of all leukocytes and is shed (Fig. 24.6a) after cell activation.[28,34] It has been postulated that L-selectin may serve to provide a sialyl-Lewis X molecule to which either E- or P-selectin may bind.[35,36] L-selectin plays a role in trafficking of all leukocytes. Upon activation, L-selectin is rapidly cleaved and shed by the action of a membrane-bound protease. Cleaved L-selectin may reach high levels in blood and may act as a negative feedback inhibitor of leukocyte five migration.[37]

P-Selectin

P-selectin is present in Weibel-Palade bodies in endothelial cells and preformed α-granules in platelets. It is quickly mobilized to the cell surface within minutes of stimulation (Fig. 24.6a) by histamine, thrombin, bradykinin, IL-1, or leukotriene C_4.[35] P-selectin transcription has also been shown to be upregulated in endothelial cells activated by cytokines.[38,39] A role in chronic inflammation has been suggested by the constitutive expression observed in the vessels of rheumatoid synovium.[40]

E-Selectin

E-selectin is expressed by endothelial cells only in response to cytokine stimulus and is neither constitutively expressed nor stored in the cells. In vitro studies have shown that the production of E-selectin is induced by activation of endothelial cells via stimulants such as TNFα, IL-1, and endotoxin,[41,42] with the protein synthesis-dependent expression (Fig. 24.6b) occurring after 4–6 hours of stimulation.[31] In vitro studies have suggested that CD18-independent transendothelial migration may involve E-selectin.[43]

Effect of Selectin Blockade at Primary Site of Infection

We used the CLP model of peritonitis in P-selectin-deficient mice and in mice treated with P-selectin antibody.[44] PMN influx

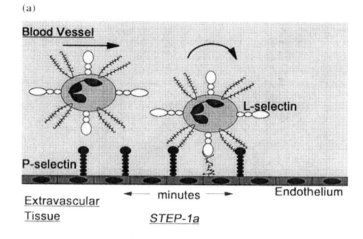

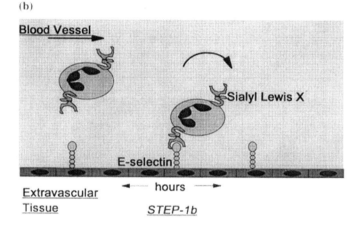

FIGURE 24.6. (a) Rolling of neutrophils (STEP-1a) occurring within minutes of L- and P-selectin upregulation. (b) Neutrophil rolling (STEP-1b) occurring over hours under the influence of E-selectin.

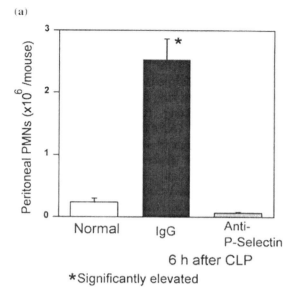

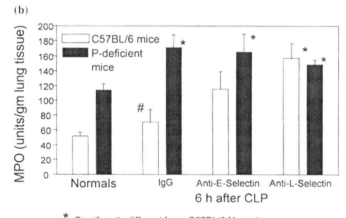

FIGURE 24.7. (a) Effect of blocking P-selectin with a monoclonal antibody on peritoneal neutrophil migration 6 hours after cecal ligation and puncture CLP. (b) Effect on lung neutrophil sequestration 6 hours after CLP in P-selectin-deficient mice and the effect of blocking E- and L-selectins in both normal and P-selectin-deficient mice. (From Wickel et al.,[44] with permission.)

into the peritoneum was shown to be markedly reduced at 6 hours after CLP (Fig. 24.7a). Others have used a different model of peritonitis to show that this attenuation is restored at later time points.[45] The restoration may be related to E-selectin expression, which takes about 6 hours after an inflammatory stimulus for maximal surface expression to occur.[32] Anti-E- and anti-L-selectin antibody treatments alone did not significantly reduce early peritoneal PMN migration. In response to TNFα, P-selectin-deficient animals exhibit significant leukocyte rolling in vivo, which is completely blocked by the anti-E-selectin antibodies, indicating substitution by the E-selectin pathway in the absence of P-selectin.[46] A P-selectin- and E-selectin-deficient double mutant model has been shown to have complete blockade of early PMN migration into the peritoneal cavity in response to *Streptococcus pneumoniae* peritonitis.[47] This also occurs in a thioglycollate model of peritonitis.[48] Therefore although P- and E-selectins both function in the process of PMN adhesion and emigration, it is likely that they do not function completely independently. Because maximal surface expression of E-selectin develops later, in contrast to the rapid expression of P-selectin, it is possible that the relative contribution of

E-selectin is important for continued PMN influx. Studies have demonstrated a role for L-selectin in peritoneal PMN migration in thioglycollate-induced peritonitis.[49,50] This was not evident in our CLP model.[44] Furthermore, selectin blockade did not increase bacteremia, unlike after CD18 blockade in our model (vide infra).

Effect of Selectin Blockade Away from Primary Site of Infection

We have observed that PMN sequestration in lungs after CLP does not decrease in P-selectin-deficient mice (Fig. 24.7b).[44] PMN rolling most likely does not occur in the lung,[24] and therefore selectin expression may be unnecessary. Acute lung injury in experimental models, on the other hand, has been shown to be selectin-dependent. Blockade of P-selectin decreased acute lung injury in a model of experimental ischemia/reperfusion.[51] Blockade of P-selectin[52] or L-selectin[50] has been shown to reduce cobra venom factor-induced pulmonary injury, and immune complex-mediated lung injury has been shown to be E-selectin-dependent.[53] Lung PMN sequestration observed after administration of TNFα is significantly influenced by E-selectin ligands,[54] although in an *S. pneumoniae* model of peritonitis no difference was observed in lung PMNs in E-selectin "knockout" mice when compared with controls.[49] These studies support the postulation that the nature of the inflammogen may influence the mechanisms of PMN infiltration in various tissues

Integrins (Firm Adhesion)

Integrins comprise a large family of glycoproteins involved in cell–cell and cell–matrix interactions. They play a key role in diverse physiologic and pathologic conditions such as embryogenesis, wound healing, inflammatory responses, and tumor immunology.

Structure and Types of Integrin

Integrins consist of two subunits: α and β chains. The 15 α and 8 β subunits identified are known to form at least 19 functionally active integrins.[55] Current subclassification into eight subfamilies is based on structurally distinct β chains. The most important integrin group mediating firm adhesion of PMNs with the endothelium utilizes the β_2 subunit of CD18. Although upregulation of this integrin is necessary for the occurrence of firm adhesion, there is evidence that this adhesion can be mediated through some molecular modulation of preexisting surface integrin without overall receptor expression.[10]

β_2 Integrin

Four β_2 integrins are described: CD11a/CD18 (leukocyte function antigen, or LFA-1, $\alpha_L\beta_2$), CD11b/CD18 (Mac-1, $\alpha_M\beta_2$), CD11c/CD18 (p150, $\alpha_X\beta_2$), and CD11d/CD18 ($\alpha_D\beta_2$). Leukocyte integrins are not constitutively active but need activation to become adhesive. CD11a/CD18 is primarily expressed on leukocytes of lymphoid origin but is present to some extent on all leukocytes. CD11b/CD18 is present mainly on leukocytes of myeloid origin, whereas CD11c/CD18 and CD11d/CD18 are strongly expressed on monocytes and macrophages. Most leukocytes express more than one integrin; therefore α-chain deficiency disease has not been described. Following selectin interaction with their respective ligands, integrin upregulation occurs under chemokine influence (Fig. 24.8). The subsequent firm adhesion accomplished by β_2-integrin binding to ICAM-1 is important for two reasons. First, a firmly adherent neutrophil can form a protected microenvironment next to the endothelium (Fig. 24.9). If it degranulates within this microenvironment, serum antiproteases and free radical scavengers are unable to neutralize the injurious contents.[56] Second, adherence by a CD18-mediated mechanism is known to potentiate the effect of TNFα on neutrophil cytotoxicity, making neutrophils even more capable of injuring the endothelium.[57] Thus inhibition of CD18 may reduce endothelial injury without affecting tissue neutrophil sequestration if neutrophil adhesion is occurring by CD18-independent mechanisms.[4]

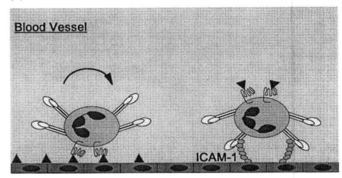

FIGURE 24.8. (a) Chemokine influence on expression of CD11b/CD18, with shedding of L-selectin (STEP-2). (b) Firm adhesion (STEP-3) brought about by CD/11b/CD18 interacting with its ligand intercellular adhesion molecule (ICAM-1).

Effect of Integrin Blockade at Primary Site of Infection

Our own data demonstrated that peritoneal neutrophil migration in response to an endogenous fecal challenge is CD11b/CD18-dependent (Fig. 24.10a).[58] More significantly, inhibition of early peritoneal neutrophil migration resulted in increases in bacteremia, neutrophil sequestration in the liver and lung, and liver injury. CD18-dependent peritoneal neutrophil migration was also reported in a rabbit peritonitis model using intraperi-

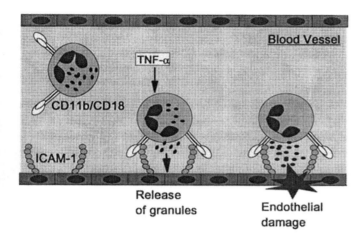

FIGURE 24.9. Tumor necrosis factor (TNFα)-activated neutrophils adhere to endothelial cells and release granular contents to initiate endothelial cell damage.

toneal *Escherichia coli*.[59] This dependence was proven only during the early time periods, as the effect of antibody blockade diminished with time despite repeated dosing with the anti-CD18 antibody.[60] In mice, peritoneal neutrophil migration in response to peritoneal inoculation with *Salmonella typhimurium* was blocked by CD18 antibodies, whereas inoculation with *Listeria monocytogenes* was not, suggesting that the mechanism of peritoneal neutrophil recruitment depended on the inciting organism.[25] Our results[58] show nearly complete dependence on the common CD18 portion of β_2 integrin for early peritoneal neutrophil migration in response to an endogenous polymicrobial challenge, although CD18-independent mechanisms appear increasingly important at 18 hours.

Effect of Integrin Blockade Away from Primary Site of Infection

CD18 blockade after gram-negative bacterial or endotoxin challenges reduces liver and lung neutrophil sequestration. In contrast, inhibition of CD18 in the CLP model causes a paradoxical increase in both liver and lung neutrophil sequestration (Fig. 24.10b).[58] It may be attributed to the observed increase in bacteremia, but more probably it is secondary to increased circulating neutrophils that are prevented from migrating into the peritoneal cavity. Even if firm adhesion was reduced by blocking CD18, it is apparent from our results that in both liver and lung other factors assume greater importance in determining overall organ neutrophil sequestration when the flux of neutrophils between body compartments is altered. The mechanism of neutrophil emigration depends on both the anatomic site and the nature of the inflammatory stimulus. In the systemic circulation, neutralizing antibodies to CD18 inhibited neutrophil migration to abdominal wall-implanted sponges impregnated with either *Escherichia coli* endotoxin, *S. pneumoniae*, phorbol myristate acetate (PMA), or hydrochloric acid. However, when the same challenges were given intratracheally, anti-CD18 antibodies failed to inhibit alveolar neutrophil migration.[61]

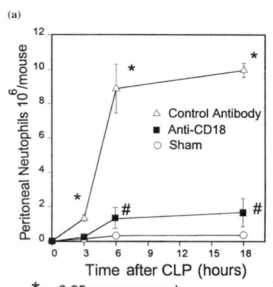

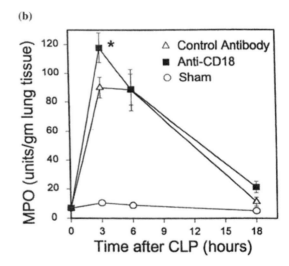

FIGURE 24.10. Effect of blocking CD18 on peritoneal neutrophil migration (a) and lung neutrophil sequestration (b) after CLP in Swiss Webster mice. (Modified from Mercer-Jones et al.,[58] with permission.)

Immunoglobulin Superfamily

The immunoglobulin superfamily consists of glycoproteins with immunoglobulin domains that have evolved to serve different functions, such as receptors for growth factors, receptors for the Fc region of immunoglobulins, and most commonly adhesion molecules.[62] More than 50% of leukocyte surface glycoproteins include various members of this superfamily, such as ICAMs, PECAM-1s, vascular cell adhesion molecules (VCAMs), and mucosal addressin cell adhesion molecule-1 (MAdCAM-1).

Intercellular Adhesion Molecules

Intercellular adhesion molecules are the ligands for integrins[63] and are present on leukocytes, endothelial cells, and many other cell types. Leukocyte rolling mediated by selectins does not progress to firm adhesion unless the immunoglobulin molecules are upregulated. The most important members of this family are ICAM-1, ICAM-2, and ICAM-3. ICAM-1 (CD54) has binding sites for both CD11a/CD18 (LFA-1) and CD11b/CD18; and it is expressed weakly on leukocytes, epithelial cells, and resting endothelial cells. Lipopolysaccharide (LPS) and proinflammatory cytokines [e.g., TNFα, IL-1β, interferon-γ (IFNγ)] can stimulate the expression of ICAM-1.[64] ICAM-2 (CD102) has only the LFA-1 binding domain and is mainly found at a high level on resting endothelial cells. It is also expressed by most leukocytes and plays a key role in initial localization of PMNs to sites of tissue injury. ICAM-3 (CD50) is constitutively expressed at high levels by all resting leukocytes and is a dominant ligand for LFA-1. ICAM-3 appears to play a key role in cell adhesion, initiating immune responses, signal transduction, and T cell antigen stimulation during skin immune reactions.[64] The highest ICAM-3 expression is observed on monocytes/macrophages and B cells. The differential intensity of ligand binding of the various ICAMs is probably responsible for selective recruitment of leukocytes in various pathologic situations.

Involvement of ICAM-1, the endothelial ligand for CD18, is necessary for peritoneal neutrophil migration. ICAM-1-deficient "knockout" mice showed a 70% reduction in peritoneal neutrophil migration in response to intraperitoneal injection of *S. pneumoniae* compared with matched controls.[65] Similarly, P-selectin and ICAM-1 double mutant knockout mice showed complete loss of neutrophil migration in response to intraperitoneally injected *S. pneumoniae*; but as with our observations of isolated P-selectin or CD18 blockade, there was no blockade of alveolar neutrophil migration.[65] In a murine model of endotoxic shock and liver failure, PMN sequestration was unaffected when ICAM-1 was blocked.[66] These results indicate that ICAM blockade does not affect remote organ PMN sequestration, whereas it can have a serious negative impact on host defense at the primary site of infection.

Platelet–Endothelial Cell Adhesion Molecule-1 (Transmigration)

Platelet–endothelial cell adhesion molecule-1 (PECAM-1), or CD31, is a 130-kDa transmembrane immunoglobulin that is expressed on PMNs, monocytes, select T cell subsets, and platelets; it is also a major constituent of endothelial intercellular junctions.[67–69] PECAM-1 is a key mediator in leukocyte–endothelial interactions and is considered to be responsible for transmigration across the endothelial layer. Homophilic engagement of PECAM-1 is postulated to upregulate integrin function, which in turn, through further cell signaling, can upregulate PECAM-1 function and enable transendothelial migration.[70] Antibodies to PECAM-1 inhibited in vitro and in vivo transmigration of PMNs and monocytes across endothelium.[71,72] PECAM-1 blockade has shown to be beneficial in animal models of ischemia/reperfusion.[73,74]

Vascular Cell Adhesion Molecule-1

Vascular cell adhesion molecule-1 (VCAM-1), a 90- to 110-kDa glycoprotein, is the immunoglobulin ligand for the very late antigen (VLA)-4 ($\alpha_4\beta_1$), which is present on eosinophils, basophils, and monocytes, and for $\alpha_4\beta_7$ on activated peripheral T cells. Proinflammatory cytokines upregulate VCAM-1 expression on activated endothelium.[75,76] VCAM-1 appears to be important in acute graft-versus-host disease and various inflammatory conditions such as rheumatoid arthritis and encephalitis due to simian immunodeficiency virus.[77–79]

Role of Adhesion Molecules in Cellular Activation (Nonadhesive Interaction of Adhesion Molecules)

Selectins

L-selectin-deficient mice were shown to be resistant to the lethal effects of high doses of endotoxin (LPS).[80] In addition to decreased leukocyte migration, this benefit may be related to decreased PMN activation, affecting LPS-induced superoxide production and TNFα release in the L-selectin-deficient mice.[81] Thus L-selectin, in addition to being an adhesion molecule, is postulated to act as a signaling receptor for LPS and lipoteichoic acid.[82] E-selectin has been suggested to have a cell-signaling role with a nonadhesive downstream effect, resulting in blockade of PMN migration in the inflamed peritoneal cavity of Balb/c mice.[83]

Integrins

Various integrins are involved in cell signaling pathways and are particularly important in tumor immunology. One example is the specific cooperation of $\alpha_v\beta_3$ integrin with the insulin receptor substrate-1 and the subsequent interaction enhancing the growth-stimulating effects of insulin and insulin-like growth factor. Another important example is the ability of $\alpha_5\beta_1$ integrin to protect cells against apoptosis under certain culture conditions.[84] Only those Chinese hamster ovarian (CHO) cells that attached through this integrin survived in serum-free culture, and this phenomenon was associated with an elevated expression of the antiapoptotic protein Bcl-2. Protease activation has also been shown through the action of specific integrin $\alpha_v\beta_3$.[85] It is postulated that selective interaction prevents cells from attaching to inappropriate sites within an organism, as attachment through an incorrect integrin induces apoptosis.[86] It is likely that similar factors may affect leukocyte trafficking during inflammation.

Immunoglobulins

Platelet–endothelial cell adhesion molecule-1 may play a role in activation of T cells in a mixed lymphocyte reaction.[87] It may also be involved in the process of acute graft-versus-host disease during bone marrow transplantation.[88]

Chemokine Interaction with Adhesion Molecules

The CXC chemokines are peptides with a conserved cysteine residue near the amino-terminus.[89] CXC chemokines identified in humans include IL-8 and GRO-α, GRO-β, GRO-γ.[90] The protein IL-8 is not found in rodents, and the identified CXC chemokines are functional homologues of human GRO proteins. Macrophage inflammatory protein (MIP)-2[91,92] mouse granulocyte chemotactic protein-2 (a recently described CXC chemokine), and KC in mice are the GRO homologues.[93] Murine KC was one of the first platelet-derived growth factor-inducible competence genes to be identified and described.[92] In rats, the functional homologues are the cytokine-induced neutrophil chemotactic proteins (CINC-1, CINC-2α, CINC-2β, CINC-3).[94]

Through a heparin-binding domain, chemokines are able to bind to endothelial cell proteoglycans and are presented to neutrophils rolling along the endothelium.[95] The subsequent activation of the chemokine transmembrane receptor through a juxtacrine mechanism causes upregulation of CD11b/CD18 on the neutrophil and increases respiratory burst.[96] Thereafter, activated PMNs can cause tissue injury through the release of proteases and reactive oxygen species.[97,98] We have shown that concurrent with peritoneal, liver, and lung increases in neutrophil sequestration, the CXC chemokine MIP-2 is induced within the peritoneal cavity (Fig. 24.11a), liver, and lung.[99] We have also shown that MIP-2 increases the peritoneal TNFα content (Fig. 24.11b).[100] Consistent with local upregulation of neutrophil CD18, Zhang et al.[101] showed in a rat CLP model an increase in CD11b/CD18 expression in isolated liver neutrophils compared to that in circulating neutrophils.

Mast Cell Interaction with Adhesion Molecules

Mast cells and CXC chemokines play an important role in the early peritoneal neutrophil response during experimental peritonitis. In humans, the CXC chemokine IL-8 has been shown to cause histamine release from the basophil, a cell closely related to the mast cell.[102] Mast cell-derived histamine has been shown to upregulate endothelial cell P-selectin; and blocking either histamine or P-selectin after mast cell activation inhibited endothelial leukocyte capture and rolling.[25]

Mast cells uniquely contain preformed, releasable TNFα that upregulates P- and E-selectins.[38] We showed a requirement of P-selectin for PMN migration in response to intraperitoneally injected MIP-2.[100] Mast cell-deficient mice had an attenuated peritoneal PMN influx in response to intraperitoneal injection of MIP-2 when compared with mast cell-normal mice, suggesting a co-requirement for mast cells in the chemotactic action of MIP-2. Intraperitoneal MIP-2 injection in Swiss Webster mice

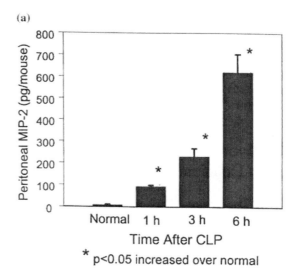

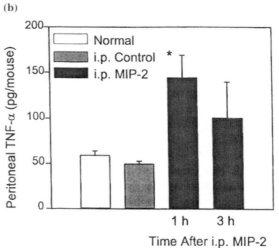

FIGURE 24.11. (a) Peritoneal macrophage inflammatory protein (MIP-2) levels after CLP. (b) Effect of intraperitoneal (i.p.) injection of macrophage inflammatory protein (MIP-2) on peritoneal TNFα. (From Mercer-Jones et al.,[100] with permission.)

resulted in early increases in peritoneal TNFα, paralleling peritoneal PMN sequestration, whereas peritoneal histamine did not increase.[100] This finding suggests that MIP-2 may stimulate mast cells to release TNFα selectively and result in endothelial P-selectin upregulation. This postulation was supported by Malaviya et al.,[103] who reported that after intraperitoneal injection of *Enterobacter* in mast cell-deficient and normal mice there was a significant reduction in PMN migration in the deficient mice, with a corresponding reduction in detectable peritoneal TNFα levels. A similar reduction in PMN migration was observed when reconstituted mast cell-deficient mice were injected intraperitoneally with *Enterobacter* and anti-TNFα antibodies. We showed a reduction in peritoneal PMN migration 6 hours after CLP in mast cell-deficient mice compared to that in normal mice (Fig. 24.12a).[100] A similar dependence was not observed in the lungs (Fig. 24.12b). Mast cells thus play an important role in the early PMN–endothelial interaction after fecal peritonitis. This is further confirmed in other models such as immune complex-mediated inflammation and ischemia/reperfusion injury in the heart.[104,105]

Clinical Syndromes of Adhesion Molecule Deficiency

The clinical importance of adhesion molecules is revealed in nature in two syndromes: leukocyte adhesion deficiency (LAD) I and II.[106–108] LAD was first defined as an autosomal recessive trait characterized by recurrent bacterial infections, impaired pus formation, and wound healing, as well as abnormalities in adherence-dependent function of leukocytes.[109] There is some evidence of a defective response to viral infections as well.[110] With LAD I the abnormality is attributed to impaired synthesis of the β_2 chain of the integrins[111] and exhibits a severe deficiency in leukocyte adhesion. LAD II, discovered later, is a result of deficiency of sialyl-Lewis X, the ligand for selectins, and results in a lesser degree of deficient leukocyte adhesion. The classic form of LAD I is a more severe condition with a high mortality in early childhood, whereas the clinical picture is less severe in LAD II.

Crowley et al.[112] were the first to suggest that defects in neutrophil chemotaxis and phagocytosis were secondary to defects in adhesion seen in LAD I. Mac-1 (CD11b/CD18) is also a complement receptor (CR3); it binds the activated complement 3b (iC3b) ligand[113] and thus helps in the phagocytosis of iC3b opsonized particles. Similarly, LFA-1 (CD11a/CD18) is involved in lymphocyte and monocyte functions such as natural killing and antibody-dependent killing by K cells (and granulocytes), as well as T-helper cell interactions.[114]

Clinical Applications for Reducing Systemic Inflammatory Response and Multiple Organ Injury

Cytokine and Receptor Antagonism

When the complex cascade of inflammation is considered, which is partly sequential and partly simultaneous, it would be simplistic to assume that blockade of a single mediator would significantly alter the host response. This is especially significant when the overlapping nature of the action of the numerous cytokines, chemokines, and adhesion molecules is considered. It is essential to realize that not all results from animal models can be extrapolated to clinical circumstances. This is evident through the numerous failed clinical trials that have used antagonists to endotoxin, TNF, or IL-1 receptor.[115–117] In fact,

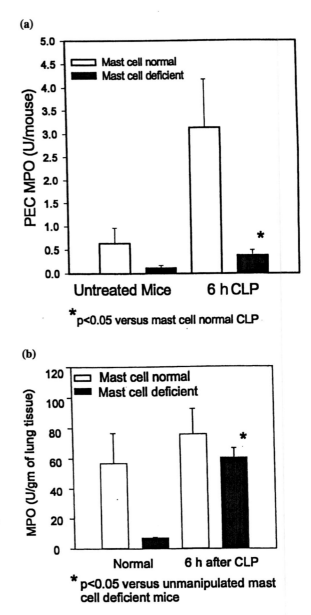

FIGURE 24.12. Peritoneal neutrophil migration (a) and lung neutrophil sequestration (b) 6 hours after CLP in mast cell-deficient and normal mice.

in a study using recombinant human TNF receptor in patients with sepsis syndrome,[118] the mortality rate was higher in the treatment group than in the placebo group. Furthermore, proinflammatory cytokines are part of the natural host defense mechanisms to mount an inflammatory response against microorganisms and events such as trauma or hemorrhage. It is the excessive response that is deleterious to the host. There is evidence of suppression of the normal inflammatory response under certain circumstances,[119–121] and that in these situations immune enhancement may in fact be beneficial.[122,123] Critically ill patients have shown no correlation of mortality with serum TNF levels.[124,125] The latter finding underscores the fact that in animal models a detailed study of local paracrine cytokine

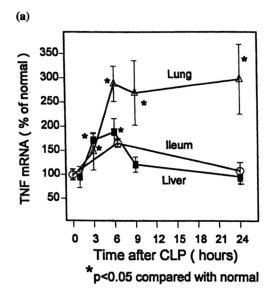

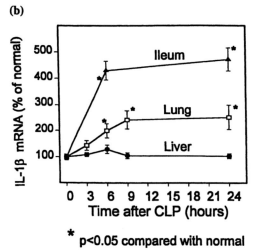

FIGURE 24.13. (a) Tumor necrosis factor-α (TNF) mRNA expression. (b) Interleukin-1β (IL-1β) mRNA expression in various tissues after CLP. (a: Modified from Hadjiminas et al.,[126] with permission.)

responses necessary for inflammation in various tissues is possible (Fig. 24.13),[126] whereas in a clinical scenario a similar study of responses is restricted mostly to peripheral blood. Blockade of other mediators such as platelet-activating factor (PAF)[127] and bradykinin[128] have shown no overall treatment benefits so far.

Adhesion Molecule Blockade for Prevention of PMN-Mediated Tissue Injury

It is most logical to consider blockade of PMN adhesion to reduce tissue injury because PMN-mediated tissue toxicity can occur only after adhesion to endothelium. Adhesion molecule blockade has been used extensively in experimental models, but there are no clinical trials to validate these results. Adhesion blockade appears to be useful when PMN sequestration in organs (lungs, liver, gastrointestinal tract, heart) is reduced in situations such as hemorrhagic shock or ischemia/reperfusion injury.[129-131] Strategies directed more downstream involve the blockade of specific adhesion molecules that regulate the leukocyte-endothelial interaction. This point is of particular relevance, as the final tissue injury is a result of this interaction. Ever since the discovery and elucidation of leukocyte adhesion molecule function in the regulation of leukocyte trafficking during inflammation, many potential applications of antiadhesion molecule therapies have been investigated. Neutrophil adhesion and injury that occurs in the lung and liver after endotoxemia or gram-negative bacterial challenge have been of particular interest.[132-134] Neutrophil-mediated tissue injury is perhaps the most important contributory factor in multiple organ dysfunction. Therefore it is logical to focus on strategies aimed at reducing tissue neutrophil influx or sequestration.

Selectin Blockade

Selectins and their ligands appear to be attractive targets for intervention in pathologic states because of their early role in tissue neutrophil sequestration. The clinical picture presented in the rare human LAD II of recurrent bacterial infection due to selectin dysfunction[32,108] lends support to this speculation. There is evidence from animal models that antiselectin therapy may be protective in ischemia/reperfusion injury. However, there is little evidence that blocking selectins (individually or together) can prevent early neutrophil sequestration in lungs, for example, during peritonitis.[44] The role for intervention in multiple organ injury during peritoneal sepsis is therefore doubtful. Such a treatment approach may in fact attenuate the peritoneal neutrophil influx and worsen the infective complications.

Integrin Blockade

Numerous groups have reported a reduction in liver and lung neutrophil sequestration or injury using antibodies inhibiting neutrophil CD11/CD18.[132,133,135] However, inhibiting neutrophil trafficking and phagocytic function with anti-CD11/CD18 antibodies could be potentially disastrous in the face of a persistent, localized infectious challenge.[136,137] Eichacker et al.[138] showed worsening of endotoxemia and cardiovascular injury in a gram-negative bacterial peritonitis study in dogs. Our own study indicated that blockade of CD18 during experimental fecal peritonitis worsens bacteremia and paradoxically increases remote organ PMN sequestration.[57] Antiadhesion therapies targeted at neutrophils therefore may worsen outcome if provided during an ongoing, localized infection. The precise regulation of neutrophil sequestration in the peritoneal cavity, lung, or liver during prolonged endogenous and polymicrobial peritonitis needs precise defining, which may ultimately allow fine-tuning of the PMN response and reduce organ dysfunction remote from the focus of infection.

Conclusions

Leukocyte–endothelial interactions are complex events that involve adherence of stimulated leukocytes to activated endothelium, which chiefly culminates in transendothelial leukocyte migration. Under certain circumstances, an inappropriately excessive interaction results in tissue injury mostly mediated by neutrophils. Leukocyte migration in various tissues is differentially regulated, and a multistep paradigm has been accepted for this process. If rolling mediated by selectins (P-selectin during the early time period) or firm adhesion mediated by CD11b/CD18 is blocked, the peritoneal response is abrogated in experimental peritonitis. On the other hand, remote organ PMN sequestration is unaffected and may even increase as seen after CD18 blockade.

It is also essential to study the selectin- and CD18-independent mechanisms of PMN infiltration or sequestration in remote organs after bacterial peritonitis, as the results of selectin and integrin blockade are model-dependent. Identification of these factors may play a key role in attempts to modulate PMN trafficking away from these organs and into the peritoneal cavity.

Extrapolation of data from various experimental models to clinical situations has resulted in failed clinical trials in the past. It is therefore essential to work with experimental models that closely represent a clinical scenario to ensure the best opportunity to translate experimental results into appropriate clinical therapy.

Finally, the usefulness of adhesion molecule blockade in clinical trials remains an unanswered question. It is possible that, as with the anticytokine trials, there may be a subset of clinical scenarios in which this treatment protocol is beneficial.

References

1. Metchnikoff E: Sur la lutte des cellules de l'organisme contre l'invasion des microbes. Ann Inst Pasteur 1887;1:321–336.
2. Harlan JM, Schwartz BR, Reidy MA, et al: Activated neutrophils disrupt endothelial monolayer integrity by oxygen radical-dependent mechanism. Lab Invest 1985;52:141–150.
3. Williams JH Jr, Patel SK, Hatakeyama D, et al: Activated pulmonary vascular neutrophils as early mediators of endotoxin-induced lung inflammation. Am J Respir Cell Mol Biol 1993;8:134–144.
4. Hill J, Lindsay T, Rusche J, et al: A Mac-1 antibody reduces liver and lung injury but not neutrophil sequestration after intestinal ischemia-reperfusion. Surgery 1992;112:166–172.
5. Springer TA: Traffic signals for lymphocyte recirculation and leukocyte emigration: the multistep paradigm. Cell 1994;76:301–304.
6. Anderson BO, Brown JM, Shanley PF, et al: Marginating neutrophils are reversibly adherent to normal lung endothelium. Surgery 1991;109:51–61.
7. Worthen GS, Tonnesen MG, Lien DC, et al: Interactions of leukocytes with pulmonary endothelium. In: Ryan US (ed) Pulmonary Endothelium in Health and Disease. New York, Marcel Dekker, 1987;123–160.
8. Wiernik PH: Neutrophil functions in infection. In: Andriole VT (ed) Mediguide to Infectious Diseases, vol 9. New York, Lawrence DellaCorte Publications, 1989;1–8.
9. Muir AL, Cruz M, Martin BA, et al: Leukocyte kinetics in the human lung: role of exercise and catecholamines. J Appl Physiol 1984;57:711–719.
10. Schleiffenbaum B, Moser R, Patarroyo M, et al: The cell surface glycoprotein Mac-1 (CD11b/CD18) mediates neutrophil adhesion and modulates degranulation independently of its quantitative cell surface expression. J Immunol 1989;142:3537–3545.
11. Ryan US: Activation of endothelial cells. Ann NY Acad Sci 1987;516:22–38.
12. Matsubara T, Ziff M: Superoxide anion release by human endothelial cells: synergism between a phorbol ester and a calcium ionophore. J Cell Physiol 1986;127:207–210.
13. Gross JL, Moscatelli D, Rifkin DB: Increased capillary endothelial cell protease activity in response to antigenic stimuli in vitro. Proc Natl Acad Sci USA 1983;80:2623–2627.
14. Linas SL, Whittenburg D, Repine JE: Role of xanthine oxidase in ischemia/reperfusion injury. Am J Physiol 1990;258:F711–F716.
15. Shaw JO, Henson PM: Pulmonary intravascular sequestration of activated neutrophils: failure to induce light-microscopic evidence of lung injury in rabbits. Am J Pathol 1982;108:17–23.
16. Wickel DJ, Cheadle WG, Mercer-Jones MA, Garrison RN: Poor outcome from peritonitis is caused by disease acuity and organ failure, not recurrent peritoneal infection. Ann Surg 1997;225:744–756.
17. Harlan JM, Winn RK, Vedder NB, et al: In vivo models of leukocyte adherence to endothelium. In: Harlan JM, Lui DY (eds) Adhesion: Its Role in Inflammatory Disease. New York, Freeman, 1992;117–150.
18. Wright SD, Lo SL, Detmers PA: Specificity and regulation of CD18-dependent adhesions. In: Springer TA, Anderson DC, Rosenthal AS, Rothlein R (eds) Leukocyte Adhesion Molecules: Structure, Function, and Regulation. New York, Springer, 1990;190–207.
19. Pober JS, Cotran RS: The role of endothelial cells in inflammation. Transplantation 1990;50:537–544.
20. Muller WA: The role of PECAM-1 (CD31) in leukocyte emigration: studies in vitro and in vivo. J Leukoc Biol 1995;57:523–528.
21. Huber AR, Kunkel SL, Todd RF, et al: Regulation of transendothelial neutrophil migration by endogenous interleukin-8. Science 1991;253:1–4.
22. Ley K, Gaehtgens P: Endothelial, not hemodynamic, differences are responsible for preferential leukocyte rolling in rat mesenteric venules. Circ Res 1991;69:1034–1039.
23. Downey GP, Worthen GS, Henson PM, et al: Neutrophil sequestration and migration in localized pulmonary inflammation. Ann Rev Respir Dis 1993;147:168–176.
24. Doerschuk CM, Beyers N, Coxson HO, et al: Comparison of neutrophil and capillary diameters and their relation to neutrophil sequestration in the lung. J Appl Physiol 1993;74:3040–3045.
25. Gaboury JP, Johnston B, Niu X-F, et al: Mechanisms underlying acute mast cell-induced leukocyte rolling and adhesion in vivo. J Immunol 1995;154:804–813.
26. Conlan JW, North R: *Listeria monocytogenes*, but not *Salmonella typhimurium*, elicits a CD18-independent mechanism of neutrophil extravasation into the murine peritoneal cavity. Infect Immun 1994;62:2702–2706.

27. Ramamoorthy C, Sasaki SS, Su DL, et al: CD18 adhesion blockade decreases bacterial clearance and neutrophil recruitment after intrapulmonary *E. coli*, but not after *S. aureus*. J Leukoc Biol 1997;61:167–172.
28. Gallatin WM, Weissman IL, Butcher EC: A cell-surface molecule involved in organ-specific homing of lymphocytes. Nature 1983;304:30–34.
29. Hsu-Lin SC, Berman CL, Furie BC, et al: A platelet membrane protein expressed during platelet activation and secretion. J Biol Chem 1984;259:9121–9126.
30. McEver RP, Martin MN: A monoclonal antibody to a membrane glycoprotein binds only to activated platelets. J Biol Chem 1984;259:9799–9804.
31. Bevilacqua MP, Pober JS, Mendrick DL, et al: Identification of an inducible endothelial-leukocyte adhesion molecule. Proc Natl Acad Sci USA 1987;84:9238–9242.
32. Tedder TF, Steeber DA, Chen A, et al: The selectins: vascular adhesion molecules. FASEB J 1995;9:866–873.
33. Sako D, Chang XJ, Barone KM, et al: Expression cloning of a functional glycoprotein ligand for P-selectin. Cell 1993;75:1179–1186.
34. Kishimoto TK, Jutila MA, Berg EL, et al: Neutrophil Mac-1 and MEL-14 adhesion proteins inversely regulated by chemotactic factors. Science 1989;245:1238–1241.
35. Albelda SM, Smith CW, Ward PA: Adhesion molecules inflammatory injury. FASEB J 1994;8:504–512.
36. Von Andrian UH, Chambers JD, Berger EM, et al: L-selectin mediates neutrophil rolling in inflamed venules through sialyl Lewis X-dependent and independent recognition pathways. Blood 1993;82:182–191.
37. Gearing AJ, Newman W: Circulating adhesion molecules in disease. Immunol Today 1993;14:506–512.
38. Weller A, Isnemann S, Vestweber D: Cloning of the mouse endothelial selectins: expression of both E- and P-selectin is inducible by tumor necrosis factor α. J Biol Chem 1992;267:15176–15183.
39. Gotsch U, Jager U, Dominis M, et al: Expression of P-selectin on endothelial cells is upregulated by LPS and TNF-alpha in vivo. Cell Adhes Commun 1994;2:7–14.
40. Symon FA, Walsh GM, Watson S, et al: Eosinophil adhesion to nasal polyp endothelium is P-selectin dependent. J Exp Med 1994;180:371–376.
41. Keelan ETM, Licence ST, Peters AM, et al: Characterization of E-selectin expression in vivo with use of a radio labeled monoclonal antibody. Am J Physiol 1994;266:H279–H290.
42. Bevilacqua MP, Stengelin S, Gimbrone MA, et al: Endothelial leukocyte adhesion molecule. 1. An inducible receptor for neutrophils related to complement regulatory proteins and lectins. Science 1989;243:1160–1164.
43. Issekutz AC, Chuluyan HE, Lopes N: CD11/CD18-independent transendothelial migration of human polymorphonuclear leukocytes and monocytes: involvement of distinct and unique mechanisms. J Leukoc Biol 1995;57:553–561.
44. Wickel DJ, Mercer-Jones M, Peyton JC, et al: Neutrophil sequestration during early fecal peritonitis is P-selectin dependent in peritoneum but selectin independent in lung. Shock 1998;10:265–269.
45. Mayadas TN, Johnson RC, Rayburn H, et al: Leukocyte rolling and extravasation are severely compromised in P-selectin deficient mice. Cell 1993;74:541–554.
46. Kunkel EJ, Jung U, Bullard DC, et al: Absence of trauma-induced leukocyte rolling in mice deficient in both P-selectin and intercellular adhesion molecule-1. J Exp Med 1996;183:57–65.
47. Bullard DC, Kunkel EJ, Kubo H, et al: Infectious susceptibility and severe deficiency of leukocyte rolling and recruitment in E-selectin and P-selectin double mutant mice. J Exp Med 1996;183:2326–2336.
48. Ley K, Tedder TF: Leukocyte interactions with vascular endothelium. J Immunol 1995;155:525–528.
49. Arbones ML, Ord DC, Ley K, et al: Lymphocyte homing and leukocyte rolling and migration are impaired in L-selectin-deficient mice. Immunity 1994;1:247–260.
50. Mulligan MS, Miyasaka M, Tamatani T, et al: Requirement for L-selectin in neutrophil-mediated lung injury in rats. J Immunol 1994;152:832–840.
51. Carden DL, Young JA, Granger DN: Pulmonary microvascular injury after intestinal ischemia-reperfusion: role of P-selectin. J Appl Physiol 1993;75:2529–2534.
52. Mulligan MS, Polley MJ, Bayer RJ, et al: Neutrophil-dependent acute lung injury. J Clin Invest 1992;90:1600–1607.
53. Mulligan MS, Lowe JB, Larsen RD, et al: Protective effects of sialylated oligosaccharides in immune complex-induced acute lung injury. J Exp Med 1993;178:623–631.
54. Lo SK, Bevilacqua MB, Mali AB: E-selectin ligand mediate tumor necrosis factor induced neutrophil sequestration and pulmonary edema in guinea pig lungs. Circ Res 1994;75:955–960.
55. Ruoslahti E, Noble NA, Kagami S, Border WA: Integrins. Kidney Int 1994;45:17–22.
56. Windsor ACJ, Mullen PG, Fowler AA, et al: Role of the neutrophil in adult respiratory distress syndrome. Br J Surg 1993;80:10–17.
57. Nathan C, Srimal S, Farber C, et al: Cytokine-induced respiratory burst of human neutrophils: dependence on extracellular matrix proteins and CD11/CD18 integrins. J Cell Biol 1989;109:1341–1349.
58. Mercer-Jones MA, Heinzelmann M, Peyton JC, et al: Inhibition of neutrophil migration at the site of infection increases remote organ neutrophil sequestration and injury. Shock 1997;8:193–199.
59. Mileski W, Harlan J, Rice C, Winn R: Streptococcus pneumoniae-stimulated macrophages induce neutrophils to emigrate by a CD18-independent mechanism of adherence. Circ Shock 1990;31:259–267.
60. Winn RK, Harlan JM: CD18-independent neutrophil and mononuclear leukocyte emigration into the peritoneum of rabbits. J Clin Invest 1993;92:1168–1173.
61. Doerschuk CM, Winn RK, Coxson HO, et al: CD18-dependent and independent mechanisms of neutrophil emigration in the pulmonary and systemic microcirculation of rabbits. J Immunol 1990;144:2327–2333.
62. Holness C, Simmons DL: Structural motifs for recognition and adhesion in members of the immunoglobulin superfamily. J Cell Sci 1994;107:2065–2070.
63. Breider MA: Endothelium and inflammation. J Am Vet Med Assoc 1993;203:300–306.
64. Acevedo A, del Pazo MA, Arrayo AG, et al: Distribution of ICAM-3 bearing cells in normal human tissues: expression of a novel counter-receptor for LFA-1 in epidermal Langerhans cells. Am J Pathol 1993;143:774–783.
65. Bullard DC, Qin L, Lorenzo I, et al: P-selectin/ICAM-1 double mutant mice: acute emigration of neutrophils into the peritoneum

is completely absent but is normal into pulmonary alveoli. J Clin Invest 1995;95:1782–1788.
66. Essani NA, Fisher MA, Farhood A, et al: Cytokine-induced hepatic intercellular adhesion molecule-1 (ICAM-1) mRNA expression and its role in the pathophysiology of murine endotoxin shock and acute liver failure. Hepatology 1995;21:1632–1639.
67. Van Mourik JA, Leeksma OC, Reinders JH, et al: Vascular endothelial cells synthesize a plasma membrane protein indistinguishable from platelet membrane glycoprotein IIa. J Biol Chem 1985;260:11300–11306.
68. Albelda SM, Oliver PD, Romer LH, et al: EndoCAM: a novel endothelial cell–cell adhesion molecule. J Cell Biol 1990;110:1227–1237.
69. Newman PJ: The role of PECAM-1 in vascular cell biology. In: Fitzgerald GA, Jennings LK, Patrono C (ed) Platelet-Dependent Vascular Occlusion. New York, New York Academy of Sciences 1994;165–174.
70. Newman PJ: The biology of PECAM-1. J Clin Invest 1997;99:3–8.
71. Muller WA, Weigl SA, Deng X, et al: PECAM-1 is required for transendothelial migration of leukocytes. J Exp Med 1993;178:449–460.
72. Vaporciyan AA, DeLisser HM, Yan H, et al: Involvement of platelet endothelial cell adhesion molecule-1 in neutrophil recruitment in vivo. Science 1993;262:1580–1582.
73. Murohara T, Delyani SM, Albelda SM, et al: Blockade of platelet endothelial cell adhesion molecule-1 protects against myocardial ischemia reperfusion injury in cats. J Immunol 1996;156:3550–3557.
74. Gumina RJ, Schultz J, Yao Z, et al: Antibody to platelet-endothelial cell adhesion molecule-1 reduces myocardial infarct size in a rat model of ischemia-reperfusion injury. Circulation 1996;94:3327–3333.
75. Ruegg C, Postigo AA, Sikorski EE, et al: Role of integrin $\alpha_4\beta_7$/$\alpha_4\beta_p$ in lymphocyte adherence to fibronectin and VCAM-1 and in homotypic cell clustering. J Cell Biol 1992;117:179–189.
76. Zimmerman GA, Prescott SM, McIntyre TM: Endothelial cell interactions with granulocytes: tethering and signaling molecules. Immunol Today 1992;13:93–100.
77. Steinhoff G, Behrend M, Schrader B, et al: Expression patterns of leukocyte adhesion ligand molecules on human liver endothelia. Am J Pathol 1993;42:481–488.
78. Kreigsmann J, Keyszer GM, Geiler TG, et al: Expression of vascular cell adhesion molecule-1 mRNA and protein in rheumatoid synovium demonstrated by in situ hybridization and immunohistochemistry. Lab Invest 1995;72:209–214.
79. Sasseville VG, Newman WA, Lackner AA, et al: Elevated vascular cell adhesion molecule-1 in AIDS encephalitis induced by simian immunodeficiency virus. Am J Pathol 1992;141:1021–1030.
80. Tedder TF, Steeper DA, Pizcueta P: L-selectin deficient mice have impaired leukocyte recruitment into inflammatory sites. J Exp Med 1995;181:2259–2264.
81. Malhotra R, Priest R, Bird MI: Role of L-selectin in lipopolysaccharide-induced activation of neutrophils. Biochem J 1996;320:589–593.
82. Malhotra R, Bird MI: L-selectin: a novel receptor for lipopolysaccharide and its potential role in bacterial sepsis. Bioessays 1997;19:919–923.
83. Ramos CL, Kunkel EJ, Lawrence MB, et al: Differential effect of E-selectin antibodies on neutrophil rolling and recruitment to inflammatory sites. Blood 1997;89:3009–3018.
84. Zhang Z, Vuori K, Reed JC, et al: The $\alpha_5\beta_1$ integrin supports survival of cells on fibronectin and upregulates Bcl-2 expression. Proc Natl Acad Sci USA 1995;92:6161–6165.
85. Seftor REB, Seftor EA, Gehlsen KR, et al: Role of the $\alpha_v\beta_3$ integrin in human melanoma cell invasion. Proc Natl Acad Sci USA 1992;89:1557–1561.
86. Ruoslahti E: Integrins as signaling molecules and targets for tumor therapy. Kidney Int 1997;51:1413–1417.
87. Zehnder JL, Shatsky M, Leung LLK, et al: Involvement of CD31 in lymphocyte-mediated immune responses: importance of the membrane-proximal immunoglobulin domain and identification of an inhibiting CD31 peptide. Blood 1995;85:1282–1288.
88. Behar E, Chao NJ, Hirake DD, et al: Polymorphism of adhesion molecule CD31 and its role in acute graft-versus-host disease. N Engl J Med 1996;334:286–291.
89. Baggiolini M: Chemotactic and inflammatory cytokines -C-X-C and CC proteins. In: Lindley IJD, Westwick J, Kunkel S (eds) The Chemokines: Biology of the Inflammatory Peptide Supergene Family II, New York, Plenum, 1993;1–18.
90. Haskill S, Peace A, Morris J, et al: Identification of three related human GRO genes encoding cytokine functions. Proc Natl Acad Sci USA 1990;87:7732–7736.
91. Wolpe SD, Sherry B, Juers D, et al: Identification and characterization of macrophage inflammatory protein 2. Proc Natl Acad Sci USA 1989;86:612–616.
92. Cochran BH, Reffel AC, Stiles CD: Molecular cloning of gene sequences regulated by platelet-derived growth factor. Cell 1983;33:939–947.
93. Wuyts A, Haelens A, Proost P, et al: Identification of mouse granulocyte chemotactic protein-2 from fibroblasts and epithelial cells. J Immunol 1996;157:1736–1743.
94. Shibata F, Kato H, Konishi K, et al: Differential changes in the concentrations of cytokine-induced neutrophil chemoattractant (CINC)-1 and CINC-2 in exudate during lipopolysaccharide-induced inflammation. Cytokine 1996;8:222–226.
95. Tanaka Y, Adams DH, Shaw S: Proteoglycans on endothelial cells present adhesion-inducing cytokines to leukocytes. Immunol Today 1993;14:111–115.
96. Fevert CW, Huang S, Danaee H, et al: Functional characterization of the rat chemokine KC and its importance in neutrophil recruitment in a rat model of pulmonary inflammation. J Immunol 1995;154:335–344.
97. Jaeschke H: Reactive oxygen and ischaemia-reperfusion injury of the liver. Chem Biol Interact 1991;79:115–136.
98. Mavier P, Preaux AM, Guigui B, et al: In vitro toxicity of polymorphonuclear neutrophils to rat hepatocytes evidence for a proteinase-mediated mechanism. Hepatology 1988;8:254–258.
99. Mercer-Jones MA, Shrotri MS, Peyton JC, et al: Neutrophil sequestration in liver and lung is differentially regulated by C-X-C chemokines during experimental peritonitis. Inflammation 1999;23:305–319.
100. Mercer-Jones MA, Shrotri MS, Heinzelmann M, et al: Regulation of peritoneal neutrophil migration by macrophage inflammatory protein-2 and mast cells in experimental peritonitis. J Leukoc Biol 1999;65:249–255.

101. Zhang P, Xie M, Spitzer JA: Hepatic neutrophil sequestration in early sepsis: enhanced expression of adhesion molecules and phagocytic activity. Shock 1994;2:133–140.
102. Dahinden CA, Kurimoto Y, De Weck AL, et al: The neutrophil-activating peptide NAF/NAP-1 induces histamine and leukotriene release by interleukin 3-primed basophils. J Exp Med 1989;170:1787–1792.
103. Malaviya R, Ikeda T, Ross E, et al: Mast cell modulation of neutrophil influx and bacterial clearance at sites of infection through TNF-α. Nature 1996;381:77–80.
104. Zhang Y, Ramos BF, Jakshick BA: Neutrophil recruitment by tumor necrosis factor from mast cells in immune complex peritonitis. Science 1992;258:1957–1959.
105. Parenteau GL, Clark RE: Prevention of ischemia-reperfusion injury by the allergy drug lodoxamide tromethamine. Ann Thorac Surg 1992;52:832–838.
106. Harlan JM: Leukocyte adhesion deficiency syndrome: insight into the molecular basis of leukocyte emigration. Clin Immunol Immunopathol 1993;69:S16–S24.
107. Etzioni A, Frydman M, Pollack S, et al: Severe recurrent chest infections due to a novel adhesion molecule defect. N Engl J Med 1992;327:1789–1792.
108. Etzioni A, Phillips LM, Paulson JC, et al: Leukocyte adhesion deficiency (LAD) II. Ciba Found Symp 1995;189:51–62.
109. Dana N, Todd RF III, Pitt J, et al: Deficiency of a surface membrane glycoprotein (Mo1) in man. J Clin Invest 1984;73:153–159.
110. Anderson DC, Schmalstieg FC, Finegold MJ, et al: The severe and moderate phenotypes of heritable Mac-1, LFA-1 deficiency: their quantitative definition and relation to leukocyte dysfunction and clinical features. J Infect Dis 1985;152:668–689.
111. Anderson DC, Springer TA: Leukocyte adhesion deficiency: an inherited defect in the Mac-1, LFA-1, and p150,95 glycoproteins. Annu Rev Med 1987;38:175–194.
112. Crowley CA, Curnutte JT, Rosin RE, et al: An inherited abnormality of neutrophil adhesion: its genetic transmission and its association with a missing protein. N Engl J Med 1980;302:1163–1168.
113. Beller DI, Springer TA, Schreiber RD: Anti-Mac-1 selectively inhibits the mouse and human type three complement receptor. J Exp Med 1982;156:1000–1009.
114. Springer TA, Dustin ML, Kishimoto TK, et al: The lymphocyte function-associated LFA-1, CD2, and LFA-3 molecules: cell adhesion receptors of the immune system. Annu Rev Immunol 1987;5:223–252.
115. Fisher CJ, Opal SM, Dhainaut JF, et al: Influence of an anti-tumor necrosis factor monoclonal antibody on cytokine levels in patients with sepsis. Crit Care Med 1993;21:318–327.
116. Abraham E, Wunderink R, Silverman H, et al: Efficacy and safety of monoclonal antibody to human tumor necrosis factor alpha in patients with sepsis syndrome: a randomized, controlled, double blind multicentric clinical trial. JAMA 1995;273:934–941.
117. Fisher CJ, Dhainaut JF, Opal SM, et al: Recombinant human interleukin 1 receptor antagonist in the treatment of patients with sepsis syndrome. JAMA 1994;271:1836–1843.
118. Denz H: Soluble TNF receptors. In: Faist E, Baue AE, Schildberg FW (eds) The Immune Consequences of Trauma, Shock and Sepsis: Mechanisms and Therapeutic Approaches, vol II. Berlin, Pabst Science, 1996;155–157.
119. Chaudry IH, Ayala A, Ertel W, et al: Hemorrhage and resuscitation: immunological aspects. Am J Physiol 1990;259:R663–R678.
120. Schmand JF, Ayala A, Morrison MH, et al: Effects of hydroxyethyl starch after trauma hemorrhagic shock: restoration of macrophage integrity and prevention of increased circulating interleukin-6 levels. Crit Care Med 1995;23:806–814.
121. Fabian TC, Croce MA, Fabian MJ, et al: Reduced tumor necrosis factor production in endotoxin-spiked whole blood after trauma: experimental results and clinical correlation. Surgery 1995;118:63–72.
122. Faist E, Kupper TS, Baker CC, et al: Depression of cellular immunity after major injury: its association with posttraumatic complications and its reversal with immunomodulation. Arch Surg 1986;121:1000–1005.
123. Polk HC Jr, Cheadle WG, Livingston DH, et al: A randomized prospective clinical trial to determine the efficacy of interferon-gamma in severely injured patients. Am J Surg 1992;163:191–196.
124. Debets JM, Kampmeijer R, van der Linden MP, et al: Plasma tumor necrosis factor and mortality in critically ill septic patients. Crit Care Med 1989;17:489–494.
125. Rogy MA, Coyle SM, Oldenburg HS, et al: Persistently elevated soluble tumor necrosis factor receptor and interleukin-1 receptor antagonist levels in critically ill patients. J Am Coll Surg 1994;178:132–138.
126. Hadjiminas DJ, McMasters KM, Peyton JC, Cheadle WG: Tissue tumor necrosis factor mRNA expression following cecal ligation and puncture or intraperitoneal injection of endotoxin. J Surg Res 1994;56:549–555.
127. Dhainaut JF, Tenaillon A, Le Tulzo Y, et al: Platelet-activation factor receptor antagonist BN52021 in the treatment of severe sepsis: a randomized, double-blinded, placebo-controlled, multicenter clinical trial. Crit Care Med 1994;22:1720–1728.
128. Cortech News Release: Phase II Bradycor Trial Does Not Show Clinically Meaningful Reduction of 28-Day Mortality in Sepsis. Denver, Cortech, 1994.
129. Ismail G, Morganroth ML, Todd RF, et al: Prevention of pulmonary injury in isolated perfused rat lungs by activated human neutrophils preincubated with anti-Mo1 monoclonal antibody. Blood 1987;69:1167–1174.
130. Vedder NB, Fouty BW, Winn RK, et al: Role of neutrophils in generalized reperfusion injury associated with resuscitation from shock. Surgery 1989;106:509–516.
131. Mileski WJ, Winn RK, Vedder NB, et al: Inhibition of CD18-dependent neutrophil adherence reduces organ injury after hemorrhagic shock in primates. Surgery 1990;108:206–212.
132. McCandless BK, Kaufman RP, Cooper JA, et al: Mediation of lung neutrophil uptake after endotoxin by CD18-integrin-dependent and -independent mechanisms. Am J Physiol 1994;266:H1451–H1456.
133. Morisaki T, Goya T, Toh H, et al: The anti Mac-1 monoclonal antibody inhibits neutrophil sequestration in lung and liver in a septic murine model. Clin Immunol Immunopathol 1991;61:365–375.
134. Ridings PC, Windsor ACJ, Jutila MA, et al: A dual-binding antibody to E- and L-selectin attenuates sepsis-induced lung injury. Am J Respir Crit Care Med 1995;152:247–253.

135. Walsh CJ, Carey PD, Cook DJ, et al: Anti-CD18 antibody attenuates neutropenia and alveolar capillary-membrane injury during gram-negative sepsis. Surgery 1991;110:205–212.
136. Sharar SR, Winn RK, Murry CE, et al: A CD18 monoclonal antibody increases the incidence and severity of subcutaneous abscess formation after high-dose *Staphylococcus aureus* injection in rabbits. Surgery 1991;110:213–220.
137. Garcia N, Mileski WJ, Lipsky P: Differential effects of monoclonal antibody blockade of adhesion molecules on in vivo susceptibility to soft tissue infection. Infect Immun 1995;63:3816–3819.
138. Eichacker PQ, Hoffman WD, Farese A, et al: Leukocyte CD18 monoclonal antibody worsens endotoxemia and cardiovascular injury in canines with septic shock. J Appl Physiol 1993;74:1885–1892.

Part IV
Prevention and General Therapy

25
Care of Injured Patients in the Field, During Transport, and in the Emergency Department

Steffen Ruchholtz, Christian Waydhas, and Dieter Nast-Kolb

Multiple organ failure in the severely injured patient is caused by direct trauma to one or more organs or secondary impairment of organ function from tissue hypoperfusion and shock (i.e., hypoxia, reduced perfusion, reperfusion) or from mediator-associated inflammation and immune reactions. The early treatment of severely injured patients focuses on rapid, comprehensive treatment of the possible causes of secondary organ injury, such as hypoxia and hypotension, and on avoiding additional stress due to surgical trauma and infection.

To what extent and by which measures these goals can be reached for during prehospital care or only later in the clinic is a matter of discussion. Such discussions are characterized by the lack of controlled trials for most questions, the problem of comparability of the cohorts studied, and the different prehospital health care policies and systems in the individual regions and countries.

In this chapter we present concepts of prehospital and emergency department (ED) therapy of severe trauma based on the relevant literature. Technical advice on medical procedures is not given. For such issues there is an excellent, extensive body of literature (i.e., ATLS[1]).

Resuscitation in the Field

Endotracheal Intubation and Ventilation

Treatment of severely injured patients aims at supporting vital functions, thereby ensuring sufficient oxygen supply to the organism. Causes of primary hypoxia are (1) central asphyxia due to severe brain injury (sTBI) or severe hemorrhagic shock; (2) obstruction of the airway; and (3) massive chest trauma. Patients suffering apnea or severe respiratory dysfunction (e.g., respiratory rate less than 10 or more than 35–40 breaths per minute) must be intubated immediately.

Endotracheal intubation on the scene for patients without or with moderate respiratory disorder is still a matter of discussion in terms of preventing later complications. Conclusions are impeded mainly by the lack of evidence from controlled clinical trials and sociopolitical differences in emergency systems, such as prehospital treatment (e.g., by paramedical personnel in the United States versus physicians in Germany). Which patients profit from prehospital intubation? The focus here is on patients with (1) severe chest trauma, (2) sTBI [Glasow Coma Score (GCS) < 9], and (3) high injury severity.

Severe Chest Trauma

Direct blunt chest trauma results in parenchymal pulmonary lesions, intrapulmonary hemorrhage, and alveolar collapse. Additional negative factors are continuous supine positioning of the patient, reduced tidal volume because of dyspnea or pain (or both), increased respiratory effort by diminished pulmonary compliance, and an impaired ventilation/perfusion ratio.[2–5] Most of these conditions result in an inadequate ability to supply the work of breathing required. This is also true for conditions with hypoperfusion of the respiratory muscles during circulatory shock.

On the capillary side, pulmonary contusion may lead to interstitial edema, interstitial and alveolar hemorrhage, or even large perivascular hematomas. Subsequent mediator effects generate interstitial edema also in the nontraumatized lung regions by impairing capillary permeability and altering alveolar surfactant.[5,6] Depending on the injury severity, early respiratory insufficiency can be expected in 50–70% of patients with severe chest trauma.[2–5]

The positive effects of early ventilation after severe chest trauma with pulmonary contusion are ascribed to intermittent or continuous (positive end-expiratory pressure, or PEEP) inflation, which prevents alveolar collapse and improves access for bronchial suctioning.[6–8] In a study of multiply-injured patients with thoracic trauma, delayed intubation (compared to early intubation within 2 hours after trauma) resulted in a higher incidence of respiratory failure (55% vs. 48%), a similar rate of organ failure (55% vs. 58%), and a higher mortality rate (16% vs. 2%), despite a significantly lower Injury Severity Score (ISS: 26 vs. 36; $p < 0.001$).[6]

Severe Brain Injury

An important task when treating patients with sTBI is minimizing secondary brain damage, which may further influence the prognosis negatively. Factors that may substantially aggravate the primary damage and prevent recovery of not definitively destroyed brain areas are hypoxia, hypotension, anemia, and hypovolemia.[9-11] Chesnut et al.[9] found an increase in mortality rate from 17% to 33% after sTBI if only one additional prehospital hypoxic period was present.

A number of airway and respiratory disturbances may be observed following severe head injury. Hypoxia, hypercapnia, and aspiration may result from upper airway obstruction (i.e., relaxed tongue), depressed or absent protective airway reflexes, abnormal breathing patterns due to irritation of vegetative centers in the brain stem, and associated injuries (chest trauma, hypovolemic shock).[10-12]

Winchell and Hoyt[11] reported on 1092 patients regarding the impact of preclinical intubation on prognosis. Mortality in the nonintubated group of sTBI patients (GCS < 9) was 57% compared to 36% for intubated patients with comparable injury severity. For patients with isolated sTBI there was an even larger difference in mortality (50% vs. 23%).

High Injury Severity

The risk to trauma patients of developing lethal multiorgan failure rises with the grade of injury severity.[6,13] Impaired pulmonary gas exchange and circulatory shock results in decreased oxygen delivery to injured organs, which aggravates hypoxic tissue damage, inducing the release of cytokines with subsequent activation of macrophages and neutrophils. These changes, in turn, precipitate pulmonary and systemic microvascular alterations and lead to the multiple organ dysfunction syndrome (MODS). The acute respiratory distress syndrome (ARDS) is frequently a precursor of MODS, suggesting that altered pulmonary function plays a key role in subsequent organ failure.[14,15]

The prognostic value of early intubation (within 2 hours after trauma) was analyzed in a study of 40 patients with severe skeletal injuries and without severe chest or head trauma. Early intubation of patients with high overall injury severity. (ISS 33) resulted in a significantly lower rate of organ failure (60%) than that of (80%) in patients with comparable injury severity (ISS 32) who were intubated later in the course. The mortality rate for intubated patients was 14% versus 30% for controls.[5,6]

Prehospital intubation plays an important role in aggressive early therapy for severe trauma. Several studies analyzing this issue retrospectively,[16] by international comparison (Germany vs. United States[17]), or in differently treated cohorts[6,11,18-20] were able to provide evidence for the positive effect of prehospital intubation on outcome.

Accordingly, urgent endotracheal intubation is recommended for:

- Upper airway obstruction that cannot be cleared with simple maneuvers
- Cardiopulmonary resuscitation (CPR) or profound circulatory shock states
- Severe head injury with GCS < 9
- Respiratory failure

There is also strong evidence that prophylactic early endotracheal intubation in polytraumatized patients without signs of circulatory or respiratory dysfunction may reduce the incidence of posttraumatic (multiple) organ failure and hereby improve outcome in the following situations:[5]

- Multiply injured patients with major chest trauma [Abbreviated Injury Score (AIS) > 3]
- High injury severity (ISS > 24)
- Two or more major fractures combined with extensive soft tissue and skeletal injury (crush injury) and a high risk of posttraumatic organ failure due to overwhelming mediator release and cellular activation

Fluid Resuscitation

Inadequate cellular perfusion in trauma victims can be attributed to hypovolemia due to blood loss (hemorrhage), increased microvascular permeability, or redistribution of intravascular volume to the capacitance vessels.[21] The end result is a vicious cycle of oxygen debt leading to metabolic acidosis, cellular dysfunction, and ultimately cell death. The goal of resuscitation during traumatic shock is to correct this deficit in plasma volume and restore oxygen delivery to the tissues.

Therapy of mild shock seems not to influence the patients' prognosis greatly.[22] Treatment of severe shock [≥40% blood volume loss = systolic blood pressure (BP) of 80–90 mmHg], particularly the timing of volume therapy (in the field, ED, or operating room), is a matter of controversy. The benefit of early fluid resuscitation after severe trauma has been repeatedly challenged.[23-25] The main reason for postponing volume replacement until after major bleeding sites are surgically controlled is the concern that aggressive fluid resuscitation may disturb natural hemostatic mechanisms by preventing the formation of (or disrupting) clots in injured blood vessels, leading to increased or recurrent hemorrhage and decreased survival. A rise in blood pressure may augment blood loss. A controlled trial from the early 1990s revealed impaired outcome for patients with penetrating trunk injuries if they were treated by volume replacement during the prehospital period.[24]

Delay of definitive surgical treatment and bleeding control by attempts to puncture the collapsed veins of a trauma victim in shock will lead to loss of time, particularly when the trauma center is close-by.[26] Although this practice appears reasonable for patients with penetrating injuries (stab and gunshot wounds), it may not be generalizable to patients with blunt trauma.

A number of problems remain unresolved.

1. What should be done for blunt trauma? There is evidence that in sTBI patients (GCS < 9) hypotonic states (systolic BP < 90 mmHg) lead to secondary brain damage, worsening the prognosis.[9,10]
2. How do we treat patients with profound circulatory shock?
3. How do we resuscitate patients in shock with transport times longer than the usual 10–20 minutes to the nearest clinic?

There is evidence that the key to treating hemorrhagic shock after blunt trauma is moderate fluid replacement during the prehospital phase. Three animal studies showed that subjects treated with delayed fluid resuscitation (depending on the time of the clinical shock control) and those treated early and aggressively (with an increase of blood loss) had the highest mortality rate. The animals treated by moderate shock/fluid therapy [i.e., stabilization of the mean arterial pressure (MAP) up to 40 mmHg in the rat] had the highest survival rate.[27-29]

Prehospital Fluid Resuscitation by Crystalloids and Colloids

Crystalloid solutions, such as Ringer's lactate or sodium chloride 0.9%, and colloidal solutions, such as hydroxyethyl starch, are available for prehospital volume therapy. In the United States only electrolyte solutions are used, whereas other countries such as Germany use a combination of crystalloid and colloidal solutions (mostly at 2:1). Both strategies were compared in a large number of studies during the 1980s but with equivocal results. Two meta-analyses of controlled trials have evaluated the evidence on volume replacement.[30,31] Both found a tendency (4%) toward increased mortality in trauma patients treated with colloids. Because there is no significant mortality-rate advantage to using colloids, and because the cost-effectiveness ratio for crystalloids is much lower than that for colloids, electrolyte therapy seems to be the prehospital fluid treatment of choice.[32]

Hypertonic Solutions and Small-Volume Resuscitation

As an alternative concept for prehospital and clinical volume therapy, hypertonic solutions have been subjected to meticulous analysis since the beginning of the 1990s.[33] Those most often used are pure saline solutions, such as sodium chloride 7.5%, and combined hypertonic saline and hyperoncotic solutions (6–10% dextran 60/70 in sodium chloride 7.5%) administered in cases of imminent or manifest shock by way of a single 250-ml application.[34] Adding a hyperoncotic solution (dextran) prolonged the volume effect for up to 3 hours.[35]

The administration of hypertonic or hypertonic/hyperoncotic solutions takes into consideration the shock-related alterations at the microcirculatory and cellular levels. The immediate, strong circulatory effect is based on a prompt increase of plasmatic osmolarity building up an osmotic gradient between the intravascular and extravascular compartments and between the two sides of the cell membrane.[36,37] Therefore rapid infusion (taking no longer than 2–5 minutes) is of maximum importance. A new osmotic balance between the intra- and extracellular compartments is quickly established, followed by a volume shift from the intra-cellular to the extracellular space. In animal studies the administration of 7.5% NaCl/6% dextran 70 (4 ml/kg) brought about plasma volume expansion of approximately 10–12 ml/kg.[35] On the basis of their clinical experience, Vassar and Holcroft[38] estimated the increase in plasma volume after a bolus infusion of 250 ml of 7.5% sodium chloride/6% dextran in a patient weighing 79 kg with a blood loss of 2 liters as at least 700 ml (small-volume resuscitation). To achieve a similar volume increase with Ringer's solution, no less than 2.8 liters are needed.

Another effect of small-volume resuscitation is based on the mobilization of endogenous fluids from the vessel endothelium, which is swollen owing to shock and hypoxia. The results are increased vascular diameter, decreased hydrostatic resistance (particularly in the postcapillary venules), and restitution of microvascular perfusion.[36,37]

In addition to the mobilization of endogenous fluids, the following mechanisms are thought to add to the circulatory effects of hypertonic/hyperoncotic solutions: peripheral (precapillary) vasodilatation, hemodilution with improved blood fluidity, restitution or an increase in physiologic vasomotion (microangiodynamics),[33] and reduction of postischemic leukocyte adherence to the endothelium of postcapillary venules.[39] The direct influence of hyperosmolar solutions on myocardial contractility is controversial.[40]

Superiority of this technique to the conventional method of volume replacement must still be proven, although a positive influence on prognosis was found by Vassar et al.[41] when patients with sTBI were treated with hypertonic/hyperosmolar solutions. In a meta-analysis of 11 controlled trials, volume substitution by hypertonic solutions was found not to be superior to the conventional treatment. On the other hand, administration of hypertonic/hyperoncotic solutions resulted in a tendency toward improved survival (3.5%) compared to controls treated by isotonic fluids.[34]

Artificial Oxygen Carriers

Intense interest continues in developing a clinically useful artificial oxygen carrier to serve as a substitute for blood.[42] Such a resuscitative fluid should provide simultaneous volume expansion and oxygen-carrying capacity; moreover, it should be universally compatible, immediately available, free of vasoactive properties, free of disease transmission, and capable of long-term storage. An alternative to human blood would be particularly desirable with acute, unplanned blood loss and would simplify the approach to resuscitation.[43]

Despite intensive research efforts, a substance applicable during routine emergency therapy has not yet been identified. The main principles of alternative oxygen carriers studied are (1) perfluorocarbons, (2) liposome-encapsulated hemoglobin, and (3) stroma-free hemoglobin.

Perfluorocarbons

Perfluorocarbons are not dilutable in water and remain relatively inert during metabolism. Oxygen dissolves much better in many fluorocarbons than in water.[44] To use fluorocarbons for oxygen transport in blood they must be prepared by further chemical processing.[44,45]

Problems with the use of perfluorocarbon erythrocyte substitutes are based on the fact that oxygen is dissolved only physically in fluorocarbons. Neither a sigmoidal attachment curve nor oxygen saturation results, requiring ventilation with a high partial pressure of oxygen. In contrast to the carbon dioxide transport capacity of hemoglobin, perfluorocarbons have no such ability.

Furthermore, perfluorocarbons have a relatively short half-life; they are removed by ventilation or stored in the reticuloendothelial system (RES). There is no renal excretion due to their insolubility in water.[45] Further research on the long-term implications of perfluorocarbon storage in the RES organs is needed before clinical application.[44,45]

Liposome-Encapsulated Hemoglobin

The basic idea of liposome-encapsulated hemoglobin is to coat the hemoglobin in lipid membranes. The advantage of such artificial erythrocytes (<1 μm in diameter) is similar to the effect of encapsulated 2,3-diphosphoglycerate, allowing normal hemoglobin function in contrast to freely diluted hemoglobin.[46] The effectiveness of liposome-encapsulated hemoglobin, in terms of sufficient oxygen transport and delivery to the tissue, was proven in an animal shock model.[47] Up to 90% of erythrocytes were substituted successfully in rats.[44] The main problems are due to the short half-life caused by rapid take-up of the artificial particles by the RES.[44]

Stroma-free Hemoglobin

A so-called stroma-free hemoglobin is produced by lysis and separation of the remaining parts (especially membrane remnants). Human and animal (i.e., bovine) erythrocytes may be used.[48] There is also a possibility of genetically engineering human hemoglobin.[49]

The first clinical trials with dissociable tetrameric hemoglobin solutions had unacceptable adverse effects.[50,51] These trials consistently demonstrated adverse effects on renal function and vasoconstriction. The early explanations for these complications emphasized residual stromal contamination, but several notable advances have been made in recent years. The most important advance was recognition of the key role of nitric oxide (NO), or endothelial-derived relaxing factor, in the regulation of vascular tone.[52] NO produced by the vascular endothelial cell is present on both sides of the vascular conduit. The tetramer readily binds NO within the lumen, but it also extravasates through the endothelial cell wall to the vascular muscle layer, binding abluminal NO and resulting in vasoconstriction. Renal dysfunction, probably because of a combination of monomer and dimer filtration in the glomeruli with secondary mechanical tubular damage, may be worsened by renal vasoconstriction.[43]

By polymerization of the hemoglobin and separation of the tetramers from the solution, the hazardous affinity of free hemoglobin to NO and the passage through the endothelium seem to be preventable. In a clinical trial after administration of polymerized hemoglobin there was no vasoconstriction with increased systemic or pulmonary vascular resistance.[53] The first randomized trial on 44 trauma patients (ISS 21) by Gould et al.[43] proves the effectiveness of polymerized hemoglobin. The study group received an average of 4.4 units of polymerized hemoglobin, accounting for approximately 40% of the circulating volume. The use of allogenic blood could be reduced by 3.6 units compared to that in the controls. Side effects were not described. Despite these promising results, the method of applying polymerized hemoglobin must still be analyzed in trials with larger cohorts.

Thoracic Tube Insertion

Thoracic tube (TT) insertion is the definitive procedure for treating pneumothoraces and hematothoraces. The use of prehospital TT insertion for the treatment of patients with thoracic trauma is controversial because of its potential hazards.

Complication rates after TT insertion in trauma patients in the literature vary from 5%[54] to 36%,[55] with large differences in severity. Severe complications are recurrent pneumothoraces (about 10%[56], malpositioning (i.e., intraparenchymal insertion, about 10%[56], and empyemas in 2%[56] to 3%.[55,57] Thoracotomy for decortication in empyema or clotted hemothorax was necessary in 2–3%.[55,56] Barton et al.[58] and Schmidt et al.,[54] who analyzed prehospital TT insertion by experienced helicopter emergency physicians, found a much lower rate of complications.

The experience of the physician on the scene may partly explain the different complication rates. Etoch et al.[56] found considerable differences in complication rates when comparing TT insertion performed by ED physicians (complications in 13%) and surgeons (complications in 4%). None of the authors found lethal complications after TT insertion.

According to most authors, blunt dissection and tube insertion without a trocar in the fourth or fifth intercostal space anterior to the midaxillary line is associated with the fewest complications.[54,55,59] Insertion in the second to third intercostal space in the midclavicular line appears to be comparably safe, with easier access to the chest wall. Controlled comparisons of these two insertion sites are lacking, however.

To date there are no controlled trials on the implications of prehospital TT insertion. Barton et al.[58] showed that respiratory improvement resulted in 61% of cases with prehospital TT insertion.

Prehospital TT insertion is an essential element of the aggressive therapeutic strategy for the severely injured. Several trials[11,16–20] showed a significant improvement in prognosis after intensified prehospital management, including a high rate of TT insertion. Tension pneumothorax is the main indication for immediate TT insertion according to most of the authors.[5,54,56,59]

For ventilated patients with accompanying thoracic trauma, the possibility of developing tension pneumothorax must be considered.[5] Therefore in these patients prophylactic TT insertion should be performed before helicopter transport. TT insertion should also be considered for ground transport of ventilated patients with thoracic trauma, particularly if decreased breath sounds, subcutaneous emphysema, elevated peak airway pressure, or penetrating chest wounds are present.[5,54]

Helicopter Transport

Helicopter transport ensures rapid transport directly from the scene or during secondary transport from a primary hospital to a trauma center. For rural areas with large distances between the scene and a hospital, helicopter transport has had a positive influence on outcome.[18,60]

Aggressive prehospital management by the helicopter teams seems to have a beneficial influence on outcome. Helicopter transport with its reduced diagnostic and therapeutic possibilities during flight requires maximum caution (i.e., securing airways by intubation for manifest or imminent respiratory distress and prophylactic TT insertion for ventilated patients with severe thoracic injury). Patients transported by helicopter are more often intubated,[18,60,61] given more fluids,[18,60,61] and treated more often with TT insertion.[54] Accordingly, several authors have ascribed a better prognosis to the intensified prehospital treatment for helicopter transport particularly when prehospital times were not shorter than those for ground transport.[17-19,60,61]

Important disadvantages are the high cost of helicopter transport (about $7000 per patient[60,61]) and lack of time savings compared to ground transport for many cases in large cities.[62-64] The problem of unnecessary helicopter use can be solved by guidelines for the prehospital transport of severely injured patients.[62,65] These guidelines should consider the resources of a region, the average distance between the scene of an accident and the receiving hospital or trauma center, and the injury severity and prognosis of the patient. An overall concept for prehospital and clinical treatment for a city or a region integrating ground and airbone transport and primary hospitals and trauma centers is recommended.[65]

Resuscitation in the Emergency Department

The early treatment of severely injured patients is based on up-to-date diagnostic and therapeutic methods and a multidisciplinary approach of several medical professionals. The aim is to identify vital threats rapidly, diagnose the causes, and treat them immediately according to priority. In later therapy, all injuries must be diagnosed and treated.

The main prerequisites for coordinated, effective management are the clear distribution of duties and treatment based on clinical guidelines.[66-69] For treatment and coordination of diagnostic and therapeutic procedures in the ED, Nast-Kolb and colleagues[66] developed a priority-based algorithm comprising complete ED management with all parallel diagnostic and therapeutic procedures. The algorithm[70] helps with clinical decisions and formulates guidelines for the ED management of severe trauma. The clinical use of such an algorithm requires continuous critical reevaluation of its practicality and scientific evidence. The impact of the algorithm was analyzed in a prospective study and resulted in acceleration of important treatment phases and improvement of treatment quality.[70] The important steps and decision criteria during treatment of severe trauma are outlined below.

Indications for ED Treatment

Severely injured patients should be treated in the ED of a trauma center or be transferred as soon as possible from a

TABLE 25.1. Indications for Trauma Center Emergency Department Treatment.

Parameter	Indication
Mechanism of injury	Fall from a height of 3 m
	Ejection from a vehicle
	Passenger compartment intrusion (45 cm on patient side, 60 cm on opposite side)
	Death of a passenger
	Pedestrian or bike rider in an automotive accident
	Explosion injury
	Wedging/burying
Pattern of injury	Unstable chest wall
	Open thoracic injury
	Unstable pelvic fracture
	Fracture of more than one major bone of the lower extremity
	Proximal amputation
Vital parameters	Glasgow Coma Scale < 10
	Systolic blood pressure < 80 mmHg
	Respiratory rate < 10 > 35–40 breaths/min
	Oxygen saturation < 90%

primary hospital. The structural and personnel requirements of a trauma center are clearly defined.[1,71] The criteria for ED admission of trauma patients are based on injury severity, trauma mechanism, and the state of vital functions (Table 25.1).[1,66,72]

First Phase of Clinical Therapy of Severe Trauma

The first phase of clinical treatment of severe trauma is in the first 30 minutes for all patients with suspected severe trauma (Table 25.1). Because an accurate assessment of the extent of injury severity anatomically and physiologically is impossible during this early phase, treatment follows a basic diagnostic and therapeutic strategy. The main task is to ensure that vital functions are stabilized and potentially life-threatening lesions are diagnosed simultaneously. In patients with suspected lesions of more than one body region (i.e., penetrating injury) the complete basic diagnostic and therapeutic program should be applied (see below).

Also when sTBI (GCS < 9) is suspected, this basic program should proceed with cranial computed tomography (CT) to identify potential causes for imminent or manifest circulatory instability because of the negative influence of shock (systolic BP < 90 mmHg) and hypoxia (oxygen saturation < 90 mmHg) on the outcome after sTBI[73] and the frequent combination with life-threatening lesions in other body regions. With road accidents, sTBI is associated with severe multiple trauma in 40–70% of cases.[9,74,75] The chance of an unconscious, hypotensive patient requiring emergency laparotomy or thoracotomy is 8.5 times higher than the need for craniotomy.[75]

Patient Admission and ED Team

To ensure optimal management the complete team involved in treatment must be present in the ED before patient arrival. The team leader should be competent in the management of severe trauma and know all relevant aspects of trauma. Surgeons take the responsibility for decision making and the performance of emergency surgical interventions during the early treatment of the trauma victim. Initially a detailed prehospital history is given orally to the physician in charge to ensure complete information (i.e., initial GCS) and to prevent treatment delay.

Stabilizing Vital Parameters and Life-saving Emergency Interventions

The initial phase of ED treatment includes support and stabilization of respiration circulation and establishment of relevant monitoring. Early endotracheal intubation should be performed within 10 minutes for the above guidelines (see Endotracheal Intubation and Ventilation). If necessary, the indications for tracheostomy, bronchoscopy, and TT insertion are considered at this stage.

For circulatory stabilization at least two adequate peripheral venous catheters or a central catheter (i.e., Sheldon catheter) with a diameter large enough for high-speed blood transfusion are required. Invasive blood pressure monitoring is not mandatory during the initial phase.

In the presence of hypotension caused by hemorrhage (systolic BP < 80–90 mmHg) rapid substitution of oxygen carriers is needed. The use of unmatched O-negative blood must be considered.

Several authors have found blood transfusion to be an independent risk for later infection and multiorgan failure (MOF).[13,76,77] An explanation could be that stored blood primes neutrophils (i.e., polymorphonuclear leukocytes, or PMNs) for enhanced cytotoxicity, presumably via platelet-activating factor and possibly amplified by interleukin-6 and interleukin-8.[78,79] Most injured patients at risk for MOF, however, require moderate to high hemoglobin loading to meet oxygen transport demands before surgical bleeding control can be achieved. Current early therapy of severe traumatic shock is based on the administration of allogenic blood, as substitutes are not yet available for routine clinical use (see Artificial Oxygen Carriers, above). Alternative strategies include using only blood products stored for a short time, more extensive washing of blood before infusion, and simultaneously administering antagonists to pro-inflammatory mediators (e.g., recombinant platelet-activating factor acetylhydrolase) with stored-blood transfusion.[13,78]

Tension pneumothorax and pericardial tamponade must be considered if typical signs are present or circulatory stabilization is not achieved. For suspected massive abdominal, thoracic, or pelvic hemorrhage, an emergency intervention (emergency laparotomy, thoracotomy, or pelvic stabilization) should be performed (see Urgent Surgical Interventions, below). All fractures and subluxations of the spine must be addressed.

The initial procedure should include determination of the patient's blood group, continuous electrocardiograms (ECGs), BP, and pulse oximetry. Urine excretion is measured every 15 minutes, hemoglobin and blood gas levels every 30 minutes, and abdominal ultrasonography is repeated every 30 minutes. Blood loss by TT should be examined every 15 minutes.

Basic Diagnostics

The first diagnostic phase serves to identify life-threatening injuries. It provides a basis by which to make decisions about further therapeutic and diagnostic procedures. The surgeon in charge performs a complete physical examination (Advanced Trauma Life Support, or (ATLS). In cases of suspected sTBI the neurosurgeon is informed.

Initially, radiography of the chest (AP), cervical spine (cross-table), and pelvis (AP) is required. Radiography of the thoracic and lumbar spine and possibly fractured major bones may be postponed in favor of urgent cranial CT or emergency operations, but they must be performed before admission to the intensive care unit (ICU).

Ultrasound examination of the abdomen, pericardium, and pleural space is standard procedure for basic diagnostics of trauma in many European trauma centers because of its high precision, the possibility of quantitative evaluation of intracavitary fluid, infinite repeatability, and lack of complications.[80–82] Diagnostic peritoneal lavage has been replaced by ultrasonography. In patients with unclear ultrasound findings (i.e., presence of subcutaneous emphysema) and a stable circulatory condition, contrast-enhanced CT of the chest and abdomen is performed.

Second Phase of Clinical Emergency Therapy of Severe Trauma

The second phase of emergency treatment is determined by the gradual revelation of the underlying anatomic and physiologic injury severity. Important steps of the priority oriented procedure are outlined.

Urgent Surgical Interventions

If, despite initial volume and blood replacement, circulatory instability or a need for continuous substitution persists or if the source of severe hemorrhage is identified, the patient should be operated (for indications see Table 25.2).

Severe Brain Injury

Traumatic intracranial bleeding leads to brain compression, with the risk of hypoperfusion of intact areas and wedging of the brain stem, sTBI patients require rapid decompression of space-occupying hemorrhage. Emergency trephination is performed most frequently for acute subdural (aSDH) and acute epidural (aEDH) hematomas. According to the findings of several authors, delayed trephination, (2–4 hours after trauma) leads to a significantly worse outcome.[83–85]

Considering the average prehospital time of up to 1 hour[16,17,19,86] for severe blunt trauma (ISS > 15), trephination should be performed no later than 60 minutes after admission to

TABLE 25.2. Indications for Early Surgical Intervention (Within 60 Minutes).

Site	Indication
Head	More than 1 cm of maximum diameter of acute subdural or epidural hematoma on CT-scan or intracerebral bleeding of >30 ml with suspected elevated intracranial pressure on CT
Chest	Initial blood loss through thoracic tube of >2000 ml or persistent bleeding through thoracic tube Pericardial tamponade
Abdomen	Intraabdominal hemorrhage
Extremities	Severe dorsal pelvic fractures with bleeding with circulatory effect (systolic blood pressure < 80 mmHg or substitution needed)

respect the 2-hour limit for cranial decompression after trauma. Therefore cranial CT must be carried out within 30 minutes after admission for sTBI when the basic diagnostic tests are completed.

Cranial CT and trephination should be performed under stable circulatory conditions. Severe hemorrhage must be controlled surgically (i.e., emergency laparotomy) before or simultaneously. All other operations (i.e., fracture reduction or soft tissue reconstructions) take place simultaneously or after trephination. Because of the negative influence of additional intraoperative blood loss on sTBI outcome,[87] less invasive procedures (i.e., external fixation) should be chosen.

If trephination is not necessary, continuous intracranial pressure (ICP) monitoring may be indicated.[73,88] Ventilated patients with sTBI and lesions that do not require surgical treatment (i.e., small contusions) may profit from ICP monitoring because of their high risk of developing increased ICP. ICP monitoring is standard procedure during ICU treatment of ventilated patients with sTBI and intracranial lesions. This is supported by a reduction in mortality from 50–54% to 12–36% when ICU treatment is directed by ICP monitoring.[73]

Additional Diagnostic Procedures

After examining the need for urgent intervention and stabilization of vital signs, additional diagnostic procedures should be performed. Radiographic diagnosis of fractures and luxations of small bones and joints should be completed in the ED. If the patient is already in the CT room, the necessary CT scans graphics are obtained first (Table 25.3). For ED management, helical CT is of utmost value owing to its high resolution, rapid performance (i.e., chest CT in 20 seconds vs. 10 minutes with the conventional technique) and its capacity in representing large vessels dynamically.

Computed tomography may add important information, with thoracic trauma suspected by physical examination or chest radiography. A study at our institution[89] on 103 patients revealed an additional lesion (i.e., occult pneumothorax, hemothorax, pulmonary contusion) on CT in 65% of cases. In 41% of cases the CT findings led to therapeutic interventions (i.e., TT insertion). Possible indications for CT are summarized in Table 25.3. Further diagnostic procedures used in the ED are bronchoscopy, selective angiography, transesophageal echography, and retrograde cystoscopy.

TABLE 25.3. Indications for Emergency Computed Tomography.

Parameter	Indication
Absolute indications	Cranium: TBI and Glasgow Coma Score < 9 Cervical spine: if not clearly represented during radiography Chest: clinical and radiologic suspicion of thoracic trauma; suspected dissection of the thoracic aorta
Relative indications	Abdomen: abdominal trauma and sonography not possible; suspect lesion in parenchymal organ Pelvis: acetabular or complex fracture if simultaneous CT of other body region is performed

TBI, traumatic brain injury.

Life-saving and Organ-saving Early Operations

After completion of the ED treatment or urgent surgical intervention, early operations are performed. They should start as soon as possible after stabilization of vital functions. Possible indications for early surgery are outlined in Table 25.4.

Considering the good results of intermittent prone positioning for traumatic respiratory failure, sufficient stabilization of fractures for turning the patient seems beneficial.[90–92] Additional interventions are required for unstable pelvic and femoral fractures. All other fractures may be treated by splints or casts to avoid unnecessary long operations and added surgical trauma.[93,94] The least damaging methods should be chosen for pelvic and femoral interventions in the trauma patient. Primary intramedullary nailing, particularly with thoracic trauma, presents an additive secondary trauma.[93–96] In many institutions a femoral fracture is often stabilized by external fixation because of the minimal surgical trauma and the short operating time. For lesions of the pelvic ring, primary stabilization by external fixation with subsequent definitive care or

TABLE 25.4. Indications for Early Surgical Intervention Within 120 Minutes.

Site	
Head	Penetrating eye injury Open skull and facial bone injuries
Chest	Lesions of bronchus or trachea Covered aortic rupture
Abdomen	Lesions of cavernous organs High retroperitoneal bleeding Peritoneal bladder rupture
Extremities	Fractures with vessel lesion Fractures with severe soft tissue damage and/or compartment syndrome Open joint fractures Fractures leading to necrosis Spinal injuries with secondary paraplegia

secondary dorsal stabilization after primary ventral osteosynthesis (i.e., open reduction of the symphysis in open-book lesions) can be used. Complex and dorsal stabilization of the acetabulum should be postponed and performed secondarily, if possible during the first week.

Quality Management

Despite a significant reduction in mortality after trauma during the last two decades, there are still deviations from treatment guidelines with a negative influence on outcome noted in European and North American trauma centers.[97–103] The principles of quality management (QM),[104,105] already proven successful in industry, offer improved methods for implementation in the treatment of severe trauma. QM requires relevant feedback loops for process and outcome data to optimize the procedural organization and structural resources.

In a prospective study, a clinical QM system for severely injured patients was developed at the Surgical Clinic, Klinikum Innenstadt, of the Ludwig-Maximilians-University (LMU) Munich, Germany, and later validated at the Department for Trauma Surgery of the University Hospital, Essen, Germany.[106] The following parameters were necessary before implementation of the QM system.

1. *Data assessment*: Based on an analysis of the documented data of 126 severely injured patients treated before the study in the Surgical Clinic of the LMU, Munich, an adequate protocol for documentation containing more than 80 parameters was developed.[107]
2. *Assessment criteria*: To guarantee objective analysis of the process and to measure the influence of the QM system continuously, assessment criteria (19 criteria in Munich, 21 in Essen) were defined following the audit filters of the American College of Surgeon (ACS).[1] Patient data were consecutively saved in a database and revised before each meeting of the quality circle.
3. *Quality circle*: Based on the multidisciplinary approach, the ED courses were assessed by a quality circle consisting of the relevant professionals from trauma surgery, general and neuro-surgery, anesthesiology, radiology, and laboratory and transfusion medicine, including both physicians and technical staff.

The quality circle compiled and implemented measures for therapy improvement. The impact of the measures was studied directly based on the online documented data.

Validation of the QM system at the Department for Trauma Surgery of the University Hospital, Essen revealed significantly improved treatment quality 1 year (5/1998–4/1999) after implementation. Altogether 325 severely injured patients (ISS 22 ± 18) treated consecutively in the ED were included in the study; and 14 long-term improvement measures (4 structural, 10 organizational) were implemented during the course of eight quality circle meetings.

Improvement in the treatment course was reflected in 15 (71%) of the assessment criteria comparing the first (5/1998–8/1998) with the last 4-month (third) period (1/1999–4/1999). Improvements were, for example, increased punctuality of the ED team: the team leader appearance was delayed 23% of the time during the first period versus 4% of the time during the third period. ($p < 0.05$); reduced time for radiologic-sonographic basic diagnostics (from 24 ± 12 minutes to 13 ± 5 minutes) ($p < 0.05$); and the time until the performance of a cranial CT in sTBI patients with GCS < 9 from 45 ± 22 minutes to 30 ± 5 minutes ($p < 0.05$). Further improvements were found in the therapeutic sector, such as reduced time to blood substitution in patients with shock (from 35 ± 20 minutes to 18 ± 13 minutes), time to emergency operation in those with shock (from 67 ± 41 minutes to 45 ± 21 minutes) and time elapsed until trephination was performed (from 77 ± 41 minutes to 68 ± 24 minutes). In addition to these important accelerations of treatment the rate of delayed diagnosis of lesions was diminished from 4% to 2%. After assessing the deaths, none could be classified as "preventable death."

Conclusions

Severely injured patients should be admitted as soon as possible to a trauma center. Nevertheless, any important impairment of vital functions must be treated immediately to prevent or at least limit the extent of impending secondary organ damage. Early airway management (endotracheal intubation, thoracic tube insertion) along with a short time at the scene of the injury correlates with better outcome.

The quantity and type of solution used for fluid resuscitation for treatment of hemorrhagic shock is still a matter of discussion. Aggressive prehospital volume therapy may not be beneficial in patients with penetrating injuries. Sound clinical data for the fluid management of patients with blunt trauma is lacking, but experimental studies indicate a need for moderate fluid resuscitation before bleeding can be controlled surgically.

Early clinical treatment of severely injured patients implies the need for concomitant diagnostics and therapy. Medical decision making should follow the relevant priority-oriented guidelines. Blood replacement and surgical hemorrhage control in patients with hemorrhagic shock as well as rapid decompression for space-occupying intracerebral bleeding are first-line measures. The quality of care for the severely injured patient can be improved significantly with respect to treatment by implementing a QM system for the clinical routine of a trauma center.

References

1. American College of Surgeons Committee on Trauma: Resources for Optimal Care of the Injured Patient. Library of Congress, Chicago, 1993.
2. Barone JE, Pizzi WF, Nealon TF, Richman H: Indications for intubation in blunt chest trauma. J Trauma 1986;26:334–337.
3. Pepe PE: Acute posttraumatic respiratory physiology and insufficiency. Surg Clin North Am 1989;69:157–173.

4. Putensen C, Waibel U, Koller W, Putensen-Himmer G, Beck R, Benzer H: Das akute Lungenversagen nach Thoraxtrauma. Anaesthesist 1990;39:530–534.
5. Nast-Kolb D, Trupka A, Waydhas C: Early intubation in trauma patients. In: Goris RJA, Trentz O (eds) The Integrated Approach to Trauma Care. Springer, New York, 1995.
6. Trupka A, Waydhas C, Nast-Kolb D, Schweiberer L: Early intubation in severely injured patients. Eur J Emerg Med 1994; 1:1–8.
7. Pepe PE, Hudson LD, Carrico CJ: Early application of positive end exspiratory pressure in patients at risk for the adult respiratory distress syndrome. N Engl J Med 1984;311:281–286.
8. Bailen-Ruiz M, Fernandez-Mondejar E, Hurtado-Ruiz B, et al: Immediate application of positive-end expiratory pressure is more effective than delayed positive-end expiratory pressure to reduce extravascular lung water. Crit Care Med 1999;27:380–384.
9. Chesnut RM, Klarshall LF, Klauber MR: The role of secondary brain injury in determining outcome from severe head injury. J Trauma 1993;34:216–222.
10. Wald SL, Shackford SR, Fenwick J: The effect of secondary insults on mortality and long-term disability after severe head injury in a rural region without a trauma system. J Trauma 1993;34:377–382.
11. Winchell RJ. Hoyt DB: Endotracheal intubation in the fields improves survival in patients with severe head injury. Arch Surg 1997;132:592–597.
12. Erhard J, Waydhas C, Lackner CK, Kanz KG, Ruchholtz S, Schweiberer L: Präklinische Diagnostik und Versorgung beim schweren SHT. Unfallchirurg 1996;99:534–540.
13. Moore FA, Moore EE, Sauaia A: Blood transfusion: and independent risk factor for postinjury multiple organ failure. Arch Surg 1997;132:620–625.
14. Meade P, Shoemaker WC, Donnelly TJ, Abraham E: Temporal patterns of hemodynamics, oxygen transport, cytokine activity and complement acitivity in the development of adult respiratory distress syndrome after severe injury. J Trauma 1994;36:651–657.
15. Gosling P, Path MR, Sanghera K, Dickson G: Generalized vascular permeability and pulmonary function in patients following serious trauma. J Trauma 1994;36:447–481.
16. Regal G, Lobenhoffer P, Grotz M, Pape HC, Lehmann U, Tscherne H: Treatment results of patients with multiple trauma: an analysis of 3406 cases treated between 1972 and 1991 at a German level I trauma center. J Trauma 1993;38:70–78.
17. Schmidt U, Frame SB, Nerlich M, et al: On-scene helicopter transport of patients with multiple injuries: comparison of a German and an American system. J Trauma 1992;33:548–555.
18. Moylan JA, Fitzpatrick KT, Beyer J, Georgiade GS: Factors improving survival in multisystem trauma patients. Ann Surg 1988;207:679–685.
19. Lehman U, Grotz M, Regel G, Rudolph S, Tscherne H: Hat die Initialversorgung des polytraumatisierten Patienten Einfluß auf die Ausbildung eines multiplen Organversagens? Unfallchirurg 1995;98:442–446.
20. Frankel H, Rozycki G, Champion H, Harviel JD, Bass R: The use of TRISS methodology to validate prehospital intubation by urban EMS providers. Am J Emerg Med 1997;15:630–632.
21. Falk JL, O'Brien JF, Kerr R: Fluid resuscitation in traumatic hemorrhagic shock. Crit Care Clin 1992;8:323–340.
22. Mondy JS III, Blaisdell W: Volume infusion in traumatic shock. In: Goris RJA, Trentz O (eds) The Integrated Approach to Trauma Care. Springer, New York, 1995.
23. Kaweski SM, Sise MJ, Virgilio RW: The effect of prehospital fluids on survival in trauma patients. J Trauma 1990;30:1215–1220.
24. Bickell WH, Wall MJ, Pepe PE, et al: Immediate versus delayed fluid resuscitation for hypotensive patients with penetrating torso injuries. N Engl J Med 1994;331:1105–1109.
25. Sakles JC, Sena MJ, Knight DA, Davis JM: Effect of immediate fluid resuscitation on the rate, volume, and duration of pulmonary vascular hemorrhage in a sheep model of penetrating thoracic trauma. Ann Emerg Med 1997;29:392–399.
26. Sampalis JS, Tamin H, Denis R, et al: Ineffectiveness of on-site intravenous lines: is prehospital time the culprit. J Trauma 1997;43:608–617.
27. Burris D, Rhee P, Kaufmann C, et al: Controlled resuscitation for uncontrolled hemorrhagic shock. J Trauma 1999;46:216–223.
28. Leppaniemi A, Solterro R, Burris D, et al: Fluid resuscitation in a model of uncontrolled hemorrhage: too much too early, or too little too late. J Surg Res 1996;63:413–418.
29. Capone AC, Safar P, Stezoski W, Tisherman S, Peitzman AB: Improved outcome with fluid restriction in treatment of uncontrolled hemorrhagic shock. J Am Coll Surg 1995;180:49–56.
30. Schierhout G, Roberts I: Fluid resuscitation with colloid or crystalloid solutions in critically ill patients: a systematic review of randomised trials. BMJ 1998;316:961–964.
31. Choi PT, Yip G, Quinonez LG, Cook DJ: Crystalloids vs. colloids in fluid resuscitation: a systematic review. Crit Care Med 1999;27:200–210.
32. Bisonni RS, Holtgrave DR, Lawler F, Marley DS: Colloids versus crystalloids in fluid resuscitation: an analysis of randomized trials. J Fam Pract 1991;32:387–390.
33. Kreimeier U, Christ F, Frey L, et al: Small-volume resuscitation beim hypovolämischen Schock. Anaesthesist 1997;46:309–328.
34. Wade CE, Kramer GC, Grady JJ, Fabrian TC, Younes RN: Efficacy of hypertonic 7.5% saline and 6% dextran-70 in treating trauma: a meta-analysis of controlled clinical studies. Surgery 1997;122:609–616.
35. Smith GJ, Kramer GC, Perron P, Nakayama SI, Gunther RA, Holcroft JW: A comparison of several hypertonic solutions for resuscitation of bled sheep. J Surg Res 1985;39:517–528.
36. Marshall RJ, Shephard JT: Effect of injections of hypertonic solutions on blood flow through the femoral artery of the dog. Am J Physiol 1959;197:951–954.
37. Mazzoni MC, Lundgren E, Arfors KE: Volume changes of an endothelial cell monolayer on exposure to anisotonic media. J Cell Physiol 1989;140:272–280.
38. Vassar MJ, Holcroft JW: Use of hypertonic/hyperoncotic fluids for resuscitations of trauma patients. J Intensive Care Med 1992;7:189–198.
39. Rizoli SB, Kapus A, Fan J, Li YH, Marshall JC, Rotstein OD: Immunomodulatory effects of hypertonic resuscitation on the development of lung inflammation following hemorrhagic shock. J Immunol 1998;161:6288–6296.
40. Ogino R, Suzuki K, Kohno M, Nishina M, Kohama A: Effects of hypertonic saline and dextran 70 on cardiac contractility after hemorrhagic shock. J Trauma 1998;44:59–69.
41. Vassar MJ, Perry CA, Gannaway WL, Holcroft JW: 7.5% Sodium chloride/dextran for resuscitation of trauma patients undergoing helicopter transport. Arch Surg 1991;126:1065–1072.
42. Gould SA, Moss GS: The clinical development of human polymerized hemoglobin as a blood substitute. World J Surg 1996;20:1200–1207.

43. Gould SA, Moore EE, Hoyt DB, et al: The first randomized trail of human polymerized hemoglobin as a blood substitute in acute trauma and emergency sugery. J Am Coll Surg 1998;187:113–122.
44. Förster H: Künstlicher Blutersatz. Chirurg 1994;65:1085–1094
45. Ravis WR, Hoke JF, Parsons DL: Perfluorochemical erythrocyte substitutes: disposition and effects on drug distribution and elimination. Drug Metab Rev 1991;23:375–380.
46. Chang TMS: The use of modified hemoglobin as an oxygen carrying blood substitute. Transfus Med Rev 1989;3:312–320.
47. Usaba A, Osaka F, Kinura T, et al: Liposome encapsulated hemoglobin as a resuscitation fluid for hemorrhagic shock. Artif Organs 1998;22:116–122.
48. Waschke KF: Haemoglobinmodifikationen als sauerstofftransportierende Blutersatzmittel. Anaetheisist 1995;44:1–12.
49. Loeb AL, McIntosh LJ, Raj NR, Longnecker DE: Resuscitation after hemorrhage using recombinant human hemoglobin (rHb1,1) in rats: effects on nitric oxide and prostanoid systems. Crit Care Med 1998;26:1071–1080.
50. Savitsky JP, Doczi J, Black J, Arnold JD: A clinical safety trial of stoma-free hemoglobin. Clin Pharmacol Ther 1978;23:73–80.
51. Brandt JL, Frank R, Lichtman HC: The effect of hemoglobin solutions on renal functions in man. Blood 1951;6:1152–1159.
52. Moncada S, Palmer RMJ, Higgs EA: Nitric oxide: physiology, pathophysiology, and pharmacology. Pharmacol Rev 1991;43:109–142.
53. Johnson JL, Moore EE, Offner PJ, Haenel JBB, Hides GA, Tamura DY: Resuscitation of the injured patient with polymerized stoma-free hemoglobin does not produce systemic hypertension. Am J Surg 1998;176:612–617.
54. Schmidt U, Stalp M, Gerich T, Blauth M, Maull KI, Tscherne H: Chest tube decompression of blunt chest injuries by physicians in the field: effectiveness and complications. J Trauma 1998;44:98–101.
55. Helling TS, Gyles NR III, Eisenstein CL, Soracco CA: Complications following blunt and penetrating injuries in 216 victims of chest trauma requiring tube thoracostomy. J Trauma 1989;9:1367–1370.
56. Etoch SW, Bar-Natan MF, Miller FB, Richardson JD: Tube thoracostomy: factors related to complications. Arch Surg 1955;130:521–526.
57. Millikan JS, Moore EE, Steiner E, Argaon GE, Van Way CW III: Complications of tube thoracostomy for acute truama. Am J Surg 1980;140:738–741.
58. Barton ED, Epperson M, Hoyt DB, Forlage D, Rosen P: Prehospital needle aspiration and tube thoracotomy in trauma victims: a six year experience with aeromedical crews. J Emerg Med 1995;13:155–163.
59. Deakin CD, Davies G, Wilson A: Simple thoracostomy avoids chest drain insertion in prehospital trauma. J Trauma 1995;39:373–374.
60. Baxt WGT, Moody P: The impact of advanced prehospital emergency care on the mortality of severely brain injured patients. J Trauma 1987;27:365–370.
61. Fischer RP, Flynn TC, Miller PW, Duke JH: Urban helicopter response to the scene of injury. J Trauma 1984;24:946–951.
62. Cocanour CS, Fischer RP, Caesar MU: Are scene flights for penetrating trauma justified? J Trauma 1997;43:83–88.
63. Schiller WR, Knox R, Zinnecker H: Effect of helicopter transport of trauma victims on survival in an urban trauma center. J Trauma 1988;28:1127–1132.
64. MacKenzie CF, Shin B, Fischer R: Two year mortality in 760 patients transported by helicopter direct from the road accident scene. Am Surg 1979;45:101–108.
65. Burney RE, Fischer RP: Ground versus air transport of trauma victims: medical and logistical considerations. Ann Emerg Med 1986;15:1491–1495.
66. Nast-Kolb D, Waydhas C, Kanz KG, Schweiberer L: Algorithmus für das Schockraummanagement beim Polytrauma. Unfallchirurg 1994;97:292–302.
67. Shoemaker WC, Corley RD, Liu M, et al: Development and testing of a decision tree for blunt trauma. Crit Care Med 1988;1199–1123.
68. Mancini ME, Klein J: Decision Making in Trauma Management: A Multidisciplinary Approach. Decker, Philadelphia, 1991.
69. Waydhas C, Nast-Kolb D, Kanz KG: Schockraum-Algorithmus. Langenbecks Arch Chir Suppl 1994;379:1140–1148.
70. Ruchholtz S, Zintl B, Nast-Kolb D, et al: Improvement in the therapy of polytraumatized patients by introduction of clinical management guidelines. Injury 1998;29:115–129.
71. Haas NP: Empfehlungen zur Struktur, Organisation und Ausstattung der präklinischen und klinischen Patientenversorgung an Unfallchirurgischen Abteilungen in Kranken häusern der Bundesrepublik Deutschland. Unfallchirurg 1997;100:2–7.
72. Esposito TJ, Offner PJ, Jurkovich GJ, Griffith J, Maier RV: Do prehospital trauma center triage criteria identify major trauma victims? Arch Surg 1995;130:171–176.
73. Bullock R, Chesnut RM, Clifton G, et al: Guidelines for the management of severe head injury. J Neurosurg 1996;13:639–734.
74. Ruchholtz S, Nast-Kolb D, Waydhas C, Schweiberer L: Das Verletzungsmuster beim Polytrauma: Stellenwert der Information über den Unfallhergang zum Zeitpunkt der klinischen Akutversorgung. Unfallchirurg 1996;99:633–641.
75. Thomasen M, Messik J, Rutledge R, et al: Head CT scanning versus urgent exploration in the hypotensive blunt trauma patient. J Trauma 1993;34:40–45.
76. Agarwal N, Murphy JG, Cayten CG, Stahl WM: Blood transfusion increases the risk of infection after trauma. Arch Surg 1993;128:171–177.
77. Edna TH, Bjerkeset T: Association between blood transfusion and infection in injured patients. J Trauma 1992;33:659–661.
78. Patrick DA, Moore EE, Barnett CC: Human polymerized hemoglobin as a blood substitute avoids transfusion induced neutrophil priming. Surg Forum 1996;47:36–38.
79. Silliman CC, Clay KL, Thurman GW, Johnson CA, Ambruso DR: Partial characterization of lipids that develop during the routine storage of blood and prime neutrophil NADPH oxidase. J Lab Clin Med 1994;124:684–694.
80. Waydhas C, Nast-Kolb D, Blahs U, Schweiberer L: Abdominelle Sonographie versus Peritoneallavage in der Schockraumdiagnostik beim Polytrauma. Chirurg 1991;62:789–793.
81. Glaser K, Tschmelitsch J, Klingler A, Wetscher G: The role of ultrasound in the management of blunt abdominal trauma. In: Goris RJA, Trentz O (eds) The Integrated Approach to Trauma Care Springer, New York, 1995.
82. Boulanger BR, McLellan BA, Brenneman FD, et al: Emergency abdominal sonography as a screening test in a new diagnostic algorithm for blunt trauma. J Trauma 1996;40:867–874.
83. Cohen JE, Montero A, Israel Z: Prognosis and clinicl relevance of anisocoriacraniotomy latency for epidural hematoma in comatose patients. J Trauma 1996;41:120–122.

84. Haselsberger K, Pucher R, Auer LM: Prognosis after acute subdural or epidural hemorrhage. Acta Neurochir (Wien) 1988;90:111–116.
85. Seelig JM, Becker DP, Miller JD, et al: Traumatic acute subdural hematoma: major mortality reduction in comatose patients treated within four hours. N Engl J Med 1981;304:1511–1518.
86. Ruchholtz S: Arbeitsgemeinschaft-Polytrauma: Das Traumaregister der Deutschen Gesellschaft für Unfallchirurgie als Grundlage des interklinischen Qualitätsmanagements in der Schwerverletztenversorgung. Unfallchirurg (in press).
87. Russel RJ, Cohn SM, Moller BA: Early fracture fixation may be deleterious after head injury. J Trauma 1997;42:1–6.
88. Ruchholtz S, Waydhas C, Müller A, et al: Percutaneous computer tomography controlled ventriculostomy in severe traumatic brain injury. J Trauma 1998;45:505–511.
89. Trupka A, Waydhas C, Hallfeldt KK, Nast-Kolb D, Pfeifer KJ, Schweiberer L: Value of thoracic computed tomography in the first assessment of severely injured patients with blunt chest trauma: results of a prospective study. J Trauma 1997;43:405–415.
90. Voggenreiter G, Neudeck F, Obertacke U: Die dorsoventrale Wechsellagerung in der Therapie der schweren posttraumatischen Lungenfunktionsstörung. Unfallchirurg 1995;98:72–78.
91. Walz M, Muhr G: Die kontinuierlich wechselnde Bauch- und Rückenlagerung beim akuten Lungenversagen. Chirurg 1992;63:931–937.
92. Erhard J, Waydhas C, Ruchholtz S, et al: Einfluß der kinetischen Therapie auf den Behandlungsablauf bei ptienten mit posttraumatischem Lungenversagen. Unfallchirurg 1998;101:928–934.
93. Nast-Kolb D, Waydhas C, Jochum M, Duswald KH, Schweiberer L: Günstiger Operationszeitpunkt für die Versorgung von Femurschaftfrakturen beim Polytrauma. Chirurg 1990;61:259–265.
94. Waydhas C, Nast-Kolb D, Trupka A, et al: Posttraumatic inflammatory response, secondary operations and latent multiple organ failure. J Trauma 1996;40:624–631.
95. Neudeck F, Wozsasek G, Obertacke U, Turnher M, Schlag G: Nailing versus plating in thoracic trauma: an experimental study in sheep. J Trauma 1996;40:980–984.
96. Pape HC, Aufmkolk M, Paffrath T, Regel G, Sturm JA, Tscherne H: Primary intramedullary femur fixation in multiple trauma patients with associated lung contusion: a cause of posttraumatic ARDS? J Trauma 1993;34:540–548.
97. Ruchholtz S, Nast-Kolb D, Waydhas C, Betz P, Schweiberer L: Frühletalität beim Polytrauma: eine kritische Analyse vermeidbarer Fehler. Unfallchirurg 1994;97:285–291.
98. Draaisma JMT, de Haan AFJ, Goris RJA: Preventable deaths in The Netherlands: a prospective multicenter study. J Trauma 1987;29:1552–1557.
99. Yates DW, Woodford M, Hollis S: Preliminary report of the care of injured patients in 33 British hospitals: first report of the U.K. Mayor Trauma Outcome Study. BMJ 1992;305:737–740.
100. Acosta JA, Yang JC, Winchell RJ, et al.: Lethal injuries and time to death in a level I trauma center. J Am Coll Surg 1998;186:528–533.
101. Cayten GC, Stahl WM, Agarwal N, Murphy JG: Analysis of preventable deaths by mechanism of injury among 13.500 trauma admissions. Ann Surg 1991;214:510–521.
102. Davis JW, Hoyt DB, McArdle MS, et al: An analysis of errors causing morbidity and mortality in a trauma system: a guide for quality improvement. J Trauma 1992;32:660–667.
103. Hoyt DB, Hollingsworth-Fridlund P, Winchell RJ, Simons RK, Holbrook T, Fortlage D: Analysis of recurrent process errors leading to provider-related complications on an organized trauma service: directions for care improvement. J Trauma 1994;36:377–384.
104. Ishikawa K: What Is Total Quality Control? Englewood Cliffs, NJ, Prentice-Hall, 1985.
105. Deming WE: Out of the Crisis. Cambridge, Ma, MIT-CAES, 1985.
106. Nast-Kolb D, Ruchholtz S: Qualitätsmanagement der frühen klinischen Behandlung schwerverletzter Patienten. Unfallchirurg 1999;102:338–346.
107. Zintl B, Ruchholtz S, Nast-Kolb D, Waydhas C, Schweiberer L: I. Qualitätsmanagement in der frühen klinischen Polytraumaversorgung. I. Dokumentation der Behandlung und Beurteilung der Versorgungsqualität. Unfallchirurg 1997;100:811–819.

26
Intensive Care Monitoring

Orlando C. Kirton and Joseph M. Civetta

Intensive care medicine, as a discipline to treat the most critically ill patients, had its beginnings during the last quarter of the twentieth century. From the beginning, hemodynamic monitoring needs evolved as physicians sought to optimize their patients' hemodynamic status, provide early intervention, and establish a warning system of impending cardiovascular deterioration. A perennial concern of the intensivist is the adequacy of the systemic circulation.

The purpose of hemodynamic monitoring in the intensive care unit (ICU) is to ensure that adequate amounts of oxygen (and substrate nutrients) are delivered to all the body's cells to support aerobic metabolism and cellular function. Achieving adequate oxygen delivery to meet the metabolic needs of the tissues and cells requires in-depth understanding of: (1) cardiopulmonary physiology; (2) the pathophysiology underlying cardiovascular decompensation; and of equal importance (3) the available physiologic monitoring systems and their indications, physics, and potential limitations. Furthermore, the intensivist must be able to ensure the quality of the measurements obtained from these monitoring methods and be able to interpret and correctly apply the obtained numbers to guide therapy.

There is ample evidence that unmet needs of oxygen demand are associated with progressive oxygen debt at the cellular, tissue, and subsequent organ levels, resulting in multiple organ system failure and increased mortality.[1-4] Not infrequently, measurements of total body oxygen delivery/demand, mixed venous oxygen saturation, and blood lactate concentrations fail to reflect adequately regionally ischemic tissue.[5-10] Hemodynamic monitoring has now shifted toward assessment of tissue oxygenation by less invasive and more continuous real-time techniques.[5,10-12] There has been substantial interest in developing methods to guide resuscitation using organ- and tissue-specific, rather than global monitoring, measurements.

Gastric intramucosal tonometry with resuscitation aimed at normalizing calculated intramucosal pH or reducing measured mucosal carbon dioxide (PCO_2) generated by neutralization of hydrogen ions is a by-product of this emerging monitoring approach.[9,13-15] Tissue PO_2 probes, near-infrared spectroscopy, and phosphorus magnetic resonance spectroscopy are other emerging technologies that may offer clinicians the ability to monitor specific tissues and organs during resuscitation.[11,12,16-19] Invasive and noninvasive global monitoring systems continue to be used extensively in ICUs. Enhanced right heart pulmonary artery catheters (e.g., right heart ejection fraction, continuous cardiac output, dual oximetry catheters) are available.[20-28] Minimally invasive and noninvasive global monitoring systems (thoracic bioelectric impedance, echocardiography, Doppler cardiography) have gained increasing attention.[29-37] The later noninvasive systems may be used as screening instruments to select patients for subsequent invasive monitoring, providing early data for corrective action before the patient's hemodynamic alterations deteriorate significantly.[33-35]

In this chapter we discuss the most common invasive, minimally invasive, and noninvasive hemodynamic monitoring techniques (intermittent and continuous approaches) in the ICU setting. In addition, emerging monitoring technology (e.g., near-infrared spectroscopy, phosphorus magnetic resonance spectroscopy, fiberoptic oxygen probes) are introduced.

Principles of Hemodynamic Optimization

Resuscitation of patients in shock due to inflammatory disorders such as sepsis, acute respiratory distress syndrome (ARDS), or hemorrhagic shock is a common clinical scenario in critical care units. The appropriate goal for shock resuscitation is an ongoing source of controversy. The mainstay of treatment in the hypovolemic victim remains aggressive fluid resuscitation.[38] The rationale behind this approach is that the noncompromised cardiovascular system predictably responds to volume infusion with increased stroke volume and peripheral oxygen delivery. Fluid resuscitation therefore can be guided by readily available bedside clinical parameters of systemic blood pressure, heart rate, and urine output. Correction of base deficit and blood lactate concentrations confirms the restoration of aerobic metabolism at the tissue and cellular levels. In the critically ill, severely injured patient cardiopulmonary dynamics change quickly, often with grave consequences. In this clinical scenario, it is often difficult for the clinician to determine the appropriate balance between the restoration of adequate tissue perfusion and maximization of systemic oxygen delivery (DO_2). Invasive hemodynamic monitoring has become a standard for monitoring these patients.

Cardiac output is determined by multiplying the heart rate by the stroke volume. If the heart rate increases, the diastolic filling time decreases, which may then decrease stroke volume. Increasing the heart rate is therefore not considered to be a viable mechanism for increasing cardiac output, except in the case of severe bradycardia. Augmentation of stroke volume is the primary mechanism by which cardiac function is optimized. There are three primary determinants of stroke volume: (1) filling of the ventricle during diastole (i.e., preload); (2) the resistance against which the ventricle must empty (afterload); and (3) the force of contraction of the ventricle (contractility). During shock resuscitation, each of these goals is optimized by administering a combination of fluids, vasopressors, vasodilators, and inotropes to improve cardiac output and global oxygen delivery.

Current thinking defines oxygen transport as the overall balance between oxygen supply and demand for oxygen at the cellular level. The oxygen extraction ratio looks at the oxygen consumption/oxygen delivery balance; it can be isolated by factoring the Fick equation. If oxygen demand exceeds consumption, anaerobic metabolism occurs with progressive lactic acidosis. Mixed venous saturation is a measure of the balance between delivery and demand and can be dissected by solving the Fick equation. There are four primary determinants of mixed venous oxygen saturation: (1) cardiac output; (2) hemoglobin concentration; (3) arterial oxyhemoglobin saturation; and (4) oxygen consumption. Low mixed venous oxygen saturation suggests that lactic acidosis is caused by ongoing oxygen consumption/delivery imbalance, rather than reperfusion and delayed peripheral washout or decreased metabolism of lactate.

The relation between myocardial fiber stretch and force of ventricular systolic contraction is curvilinear and is described by Starling's law.[39] Clinically, this principle describes the relation between end-diastolic volume and cardiac output during volume loading. In patients with normally compliant hearts there is a linear relation between pressure and volume within the left ventricle, and intraventricular volume is inferred from pressure. The measurement of left ventricle end-diastolic pressure (EDP) allows the clinician to construct a therapeutic goal to optimize cardiac output based on the response to changes in end-diastolic pressure. This conceptualization forms the backbone of resuscitative strategies for many types of shock.[23,40] The first step in resuscitation for any type of shock (hypovolemic, neurogenic, septic, cardiogenic) is to maximize the preload (with crystalloid and colloids) to optimize ventricular stretch, therapy augmenting cardiac output. With a right heart pulmonary artery catheter in place, measurement of pulmonary artery occlusion pressure and the response of cardiac output to changes in filling pressure can be used to develop a Starling response curve. However, the clinician must be aware that the relation between filling pressure and cardiac output can be acutely and dramatically altered in the presence of ischemia, inotropes, cardiomyopathy, ventricular hypertrophy, pericardial disease, and positive end-expiratory pressure (PEEP), all of which affect the compliance of the left ventricle—and potentially this relation.[15,21,23,40] As ventricular compliance changes, the relation between pressure and volume within the ventricle is altered and the same filling pressure may result in different end-diastolic volumes.

The published report of the right heart/pulmonary artery catheter by Ganz, Swan, and Forrester in 1970 revolutionized our understanding of the relation of oxygen delivery and the determinants of cardiac output.[41] During the 1980s and 1990s a new generation of enhanced right heart catheters were introduced for use when therapeutic benefits were anticipated from the information based on knowledge of oxygen transport endpoints and mixed venous saturation (continuous venous oximeteric catheter), ventricular preload (right ventricular function/ejection fraction catheter), or when knowledge of the continuous display of variables was important to titration of therapy (continuous cardiac output monitor).[10,20] Unfortunately, there are no clinical studies using continuous mixed venous oximetry, right heart function (right ventricular ejection fraction) catheters, or continuous cardiac output measurements that demonstrate improved outcome compared to standard right heart pulmonary artery catheters. Future research must focus on the value of the data for clinical decision making and its ability to improve the efficiency of patient care and overall patient outcome.

Several clinical studies have suggested that failure to achieve supranormal circulatory parameters and utilize supranormal levels of oxygen during the acute phase of injury are associated with increased mortality and shock-related complications, including multiple organ system failure.[2–4,14,42,43] The presumption is that with inflammatory disorders (e.g., sepsis, major trauma, shock, ARDS) occult hypoxia or hypoperfusion of regional tissue beds can exacerbate the inflammatory process. Therapeutic goals such as supranormal values of oxygen delivery and oxygen consumption have been tested prospectively in randomized controlled trials, with varying conclusions, exemplified by the reports by Durham et al.[44] and Gattinoni and colleagues.[24] They demonstrated that optimizing oxygen delivery to supranormal levels or normalizing mixed venous oxygen content does not change mortality. The preceding observations have led investigators to search for other means of monitoring regional tissue perfusion, such as gastric intramucosal tonometry, near-infrared spectroscopy, base deficit, and plasma lactate concentration and to look for therapeutic goals during resuscitation that may prevent occult tissue hypoxemia.[10,11,44–47]

Central Venous Catheter

The most common indications for central venous catheter placement include (1) reliable central venous access for massive fluid therapy, vasoactive drug infusions, and total parenteral nutrition; and (2) monitoring the central venous pressure (CVP).[48] There are no absolute contraindications for CVP catheter placement, but conditions that place the patient at increased risk of bleeding (e.g., acquired coagulopathy, thrombocytopenia, specific coagulation factor deficiency), the presence of vessel thrombosis, local infection or inflammation, or anatomic distortion due to trauma or previous surgery may be considered relative contraindications to a specific site of catheterization. When monitoring CVP, the catheter should be attached to a pressure transducer for electronic measurement. The CVP is often helpful in the hypotensive patient to differentiate among cardiogenic insufficiency, conditions of hypervolemia associated with hypotension (i.e., pericardial tamponade), and absolute hypovolemia. Analysis of the CVP tracing may also be helpful for diagnosing certain cardiac arrhythmias (e.g., atrial fibrillation: absent a-waves) and valvular dysfunction (tricuspid insufficiency: prominent v-waves).

Pulmonary Artery Catheter

Physician prediction of hemodynamic status is typically inaccurate in critically ill patients, regardless of whether the patient has cardiac disease. Among patients considered for right heart catheterization, appropriate interpretation of data obtained from pulmonary artery catheterization results in a change of therapy in 40–60% of patients. However, survival ultimately depends on the patient's underlying disorder, co-morbidities, and overall response to appropriate therapy. For example, in trauma patients hemodynamic data obtained from the right heart pulmonary artery catheter appear to be beneficial for the following indications: (1) to ascertain the status of underlying cardiovascular performance or the need for improvement; (2) to direct therapy when less invasive monitoring appears inadequate or misleading, or the endpoints of resuscitation are difficult to define; (3) to assess response to resuscitation; (4) potentially to decrease secondary injury when severe head or spinal cord injuries are components of multisystem trauma; (5) to augment clinical decision making when major trauma is complicated by severe ARDS, progressive oliguria/anuria, myocardial ischemia, congestive heart failure, or major thermal injury.[38] In general, there are not enough carefully designed studies (i.e., level I evidence) to define and establish definitively the benefit of global invasive hemodynamic monitoring in the individual patient.[20,49,50] It is reasonable to assume that more precise bedside knowledge of fundamental cardiovascular parameters would facilitate early diagnosis and guide therapy. It is accepted practice that pulmonary artery catheters are indicated whenever the data obtained can facilitate therapeutic decision making without unnecessary risks (Table 26.1).

From the perspective of the clinician at the bedside, the pulmonary artery catheter has provided a quantum leap in the physiologic information available for management of critically ill patients. Information that can be obtained include the CVP, pulmonary artery diastolic pressure (PADP), pulmonary artery systolic pressure, mean pulmonary artery pressure, pulmonary artery occlusion pressure ("wedge") pressure (PAOP), cardiac output by thermodilution, and mixed venous saturation by intermittent sampling or continuous mixed venous oximetry. The pulmonary artery occlusion pressure represents the left atrial pressure (LAP) so long as the column of blood distal to the pulmonary artery tip is uninterrupted to the left atrium. Pulmonary artery occlusion pressure reflects the thoracic alveolar pressure if the catheter tip is situated predominantly in West's zones 1 and 2, where pulmonary airway or arterial pressure exceeds pulmonary venous pressure, respectively. The proportion of the lung in these zones is exaggerated in states of low pulmonary vascular perfusion (e.g., cardiogenic insufficiency, hypovolemia) or if the patient is being exposed to high levels of PEEP. Fortunately, most inserted pulmonary artery catheters float into the dependent regions of the lung where pulmonary blood flow is high and pulmonary venous pressure exceeds alveolar pressure (West's zone 3). In this location a continuous column of blood exists between the distal tip of the catheter and the left atrium. Another factor favoring appropriate catheter position is supine positioning of the patient.

Right Heart Function Monitoring Catheter

The advent of rapid response thermisters have made possible bedside calculations of right ventricular volume. The right heart

TABLE 26.1. Clinical Situations for Which Pulmonary Artery Catheterization Can Be of Diagnostic Value.

General
  Shock despite perceived adequate fluid therapy
  Oliguria that persists despite perceived adequate fluid therapy
  To assess the effect of intravascular volume expansion on cardiac function
  To delineate the cardiovascular component of multiple organ system dysfunction.

Surgical
  Preoperative assessment and perioperative management of high risk surgical patients.
  Patients who need cardiac or major vascular surgery
  Postoperative cardiovascular complications

Trauma
  Ascertain the status of underlying cardiovascular performance and the need for improvement
  Direct therapy when noninvasive monitoring may be inadequate, misleading, or the endpoints of resuscitation difficult to define
  Potentially decrease secondary injury when severe closed-head or acute spinal cord injuries are components of multisystem trauma
  Augment clinical decision-making when major trauma is complicated by severe adult respiratory distress syndrome (ARDS), progression oliguria/anuria/myocardial ischemia/congestive heart failure or major thermal injury

Pulmonary
  Differentiate noncardiogenic (ARDS) from cardiogenic pulmonary edema
  Assess effects of high levels of ventilatory support on cardiovascular status

Cardiac
  Myocardial infarction complicated by pump failure or pulmonary edema
  Treatment of unstable angina with intravenous nitroglycerin therapy
  Congestive heart failure unresponsive to simple therapy (to guide preload and vasodilator therapy)
  Pulmonary hypertension: for diagnosis and to monitor drug therapy

pulmonary artery catheter is modified to disburse more uniformly the thermal indicator bolus. The rapid response feature of this thermister allows beat-to-beat changes in electrical resistance to be correlated with the electrocardiogram (ECG), allowing precise R-R interval timing. The computer is therefore able to calculate the residual temperature and convert this measure to the right ventricular ejection fraction by accurately measuring the temperature change between consecutive heartbeats during the logarithmic portion of the temperature decay curve.[51,52] The stroke volume index (calculated by dividing the cardiac index by the heart rate) is divided by the ejection fraction to yield right ventricular end-diastolic volume (RVEDV). Abnormalities of heart rate and rhythm may cause erroneous readings because of the inability to capture the R-wave and determine the appropriate R-R interval. Heart rates higher than 150 beats/min, atrial fibrillation/supraventricular tachycardia with frequent ectopic beats, or frequent ventricular ectopy can render the signal uninterpretable. The right ventricular ejection fraction and calculation is highly dependent on right ventricular afterload; therefore an increase in pulmonary vascular resistance affects the ejection fraction and hence calculation of the end-diastolic volume and cardiac index. Although the right ventricular ejection fraction may not consistently reflect right ventricular contractility, it has been shown to be a predictor of survival in patients with trauma[23] and coronary artery disease.[24] Ventricular end-diastolic volume is a significantly better predictor of what several authors have termed preload recruitable end-diastolic volume as it relates to increases in cardiac index following fluid challenge.[6,40] This is particularly true in situations where there is an increase in pleural pressure (i.e., high positive airway and mean airway pressures), significant minute ventilation rates, or intraabdominal hypertension.[15,21,23]

Although preload status is a fundamental, important aspect of resuscitation, other variables reflecting acid-base status, regional perfusion, and oxygen utilization should be considered. Therefore it may be wrong to consider RVEDV a resuscitation endpoint of any sort. It is simply an indicator of preload and should be used in conjunction with afterload and contractility, the other independent determinants of ventricular function. Kraut and associates[22] made concurrent measurements of RVEDV and the left ventricular end-diastolic volume (LVEDV). The RVEDV was measured using a residual fraction right heart function catheter, and the LVEDV was measured using transesophageal echocardiography with acoustic amplification. They found that the RVEDV overestimated left ventricular preload. Measuring the RVEDV and intramucosal pH (pHi) and performing pulse oximetry simultaneously showed that higher preloads are associated with improved intestinal perfusion and important outcomes in critically injured patients.[53] Preload may be better defined in terms of optimal systemic and regional perfusion beyond minimum levels that result in an adequate cardiac index. Furthermore, the ability to measure end-diastolic and end-systolic volumes with the volumetric pulmonary artery catheter enables clinicians to assess contractility and afterload in conjunction with preload in a unified methodologic framework. This technique has allowed identification of patterns of preload, contractility, and afterload associated with high levels of ventricular stroke work in survivors after traumatic shock.[54]

Continuous Mixed Venous Oximetric Catheter

The continuous mixed venous oximetric catheter is an enhanced right heart catheter. With it, mixed venous oxygen saturation can be monitored continuously using fiberoptic cables in the thermodilution catheter.[20,24,27] With this technology, narrow wave bands of light are selected for their reflectance characteristics for both total hemoglobin and oxyhemoglobin. These reflectance signals are transmitted and received by two fiberoptic bundles within the catheter. As red blood cells flow past the fiberoptic catheter tip, light is reflected back to an optical transducer and the mixed venous oxygen saturation calculated.[55] Calibration errors can lead to a fixed error in the mixed venous oxygen saturation value, and malposition of the catheter can cause sporadic errors. Therefore these enhanced catheters require routine calibration and ascertainment of a nonwedge position of the catheter tip. Current monitoring systems sense pulsatile flow to warn of deterioration in signal quality. When mixed venous oxygen saturation falls to less than 0.65, further information must be obtained to understand which of the four determinants of oxygen transport and consumption must be addressed.

Continuous Cardiac Output Catheter

New technology, the continuous cardiac output catheter measures temperature change as blood flows past the catheter tip. It uses a thermal pulse generated by the heating filament on the catheter.[25-28] The cardiac output computer senses temperature changes in pulmonary artery blood distal to the heating filament. Cardiac output is calculated by correlating the amount of energy imparted to the heating filament and the temperature change produced in the blood distal to this filament. The cardiac output is displayed and updated every 30 seconds, with the display representing the averaged cardiac output for the previous 3-6 minutes. The derived continual data allow titration of vasoactive agents based on trends in cardiac output.

Continuous cardiac output monitors have been demonstrated to provide clinically acceptable measurements in the hemodynamically stable patient.[25-28] However, at high cardiac outputs the difference with other methods increases, and the results should be interpreted cautiously.[28] The continuous method for measuring cardiac output allows recognition (within the time frame chosen to average the cardiac output) of hemodynamic changes so therapeutic interventions can be initiated rapidly. The measurement influences patient care only when the data are used in a comprehensive, dynamic patient care plan.

Gastrointestinal Tonometry

Gastrointestinal tonometry is a relatively noninvasive technique that measures stomach mucosal PCO_2, allowing equilibration of CO_2 partial pressure between an intragastric balloon and the gastric mucosal layers. The physiologic basis of gastrointestinal tonometry as a monitor of inadequate tissue oxygen supply is tissue hypercarbic acidosis due to increases in tissue CO_2 production consequent to liberated hydrogen protons [secondary to anaerobic metabolism, unreversed adenosine triphosphate (ATP) hydrolysis, radical–radical interaction during ischemia reperfusion] buffered by tissue bicarbonate. Gastric tonometry measures the partial pressure of CO_2 in the lumen of the stomach.

Several clinical studies have validated the use of gastric tonometry to predict mortality, multiple organ dysfunction system, and length of stay in the ICU.[1,5,56] Furthermore, several, clinical reports suggest that gastric tonometry is a more accurate endpoint of resuscitation from traumatic hypovolemic shock, associated with improved outcome when intestinal tonometry is the selected endpoint of resuscitation.[10,12,13,57] Calculated intramucosal pH (using arterial bicarbonate as an estimate of intramucosal bicarbonate concentration in the Henderson-Hasselbach equation) has been validated against measured mucosal pH (pHi) with implanted microprobes. In cases of diminished or absent flow, the pHi has been shown to decrease in parallel with the pHa (measured by microprobes) but tends to underestimate slightly the degree of intramucosal acidosis. At least four studies in the literature have tested the efficacy of using changes in pHi to guide therapy in critically ill patients.[13,14,58]

Two advances have improved the original method of gastric tonometry. The first is continuous air tonometry. In laboratory models this fluidless gas system demonstrated greater sensitivity in detecting tissue hypoxia than standard saline tonometry, probably because the gas is in constant equilibrium with the tissue. A new method of placing a fiberoptic CO_2 sensor directly in the stomach is being tested in animal models.[12] Sublingual and esophageal tonometry have also emerged as promising less-invasive options. One perceived concern about adopting gastrointestinal tonometry to guide resuscitation has been the inability to improve selectively (gut-directed resuscitation) intestinal perfusion in the setting of otherwise adequate systemic perfusion. Most studies to date direct therapy toward improving the pHi solely by improving cardiac index and systemic acid-base status, providing little information about improving intramucosal pH in patients with adequate systemic parameters but persistently decreased intestinal blood flow.[15] Although some preliminary data suggest that it may be possible, no one has yet conclusively demonstrated the ability to improve gut hypoperfusion selectively as evidenced by pHi or intramucosal PCO_2 production on demand in patients who are otherwise well perfused. Furthermore, until recently, threshold values of the pHi and mucosal-arterial PCO_2 gap for specific subgroups of critically ill patients have never been specifically identified.[57]

TABLE 26.2. Frequency of Administered Agents and Survival.

Agent	Patients	% Total	% Lived
None	4	12	100
Blood	28	83	83
Isoproterenol	22	65	77
Dobutamine	19	56	69
Nitroglycerine	6	18	67
Nitroprusside	5	5	100
Epinephrine	4	12	25

In critically ill trauma patients the arterial-to-mucosal PCO_2 gap may be a more sensitive measure of intramucosal acidosis than gastric intramucosal pH (pHi). Chang and associates[53,54] identified a gap value of 18 mmHg as an important endpoint of inadequate tissue perfusion. At Jackson Memorial Hospital in Miami, Florida, we evaluated a hemodynamic resuscitation protocol based on achieving a pHi of 7.25 or higher that incorporated antioxidants and splanchnic circulation-sparing vasoactive agents in consecutive critically injured blunt and penetrating trauma patients admitted to our level I trauma ICU. On admission, all patients received intravenous doses of mannitol, folate, lidocaine, vitamin C, selenium, polymyxin B, and hydrocortisone in addition to crystalloid and colloid resuscitation. Oxygen-carrying capacity was adjusted to achieve a hemoglobin level of at least 11 g/dl and an SaO_2 of at least 92%. If the pHi remained at less than 7.25, splanchnic circulation-sparing vasopressors and vasodilators (when appropriate) were administered under right heart pulmonary artery catheter guidance. Vasoactive agents that cause splanchnic vasoconstriction (e.g., epinephrine, Neo-Synephrine, norepinephrine) were used only to treat refractory systemic hypotension (mean arterial pressure <55 mmHg). Of 92 patients, 58 (63%) achieved a pHi of at least 7.25 on admission to the ICU with volume resuscitation and the antioxidant regimen, associated with 100% survival; the other 34 patients had a pHi of less than 7.25 and were placed on a splanchnic circulation-sparing vasoactive regimen (Tables 26.2, 26.3). Of these 34 patients, 29 were normalized with this regimen, associated with a survival of 90%. The five patients who did not normalize experienced 60% mortality.

TABLE 26.3. Interventions per Patient and Survival.

No. of interventions	Patients	% Total	% Lived
0	4	12	100
1	4	12	100
2	8	23	100
3	8	24	75
4	5	15	80
5	4	12	25
6	1	2	100
Total	34	100	90

Thoracic Bioelectric Impedance Cardiography

Thoracic bioelectric impedance cardiographic instruments pass a low-energy high-frequency alternating electrical current through the thorax. A pair of detecting electrodes, located within the path, measure changes in tissue impedance (resistance to current flow). Blood, being the most electrically conductive substance in the thorax, shifts the electrical impedance as the intravascular volume changes within the thorax. These phasic changes in thoracic bioelectrical impedance reflect the aortic flow and through a transformation equation can be computed into an estimate of cardiac output.[37] A regression equation calculates an estimate of ejection fraction from the systolic time intervals. The systolic ejection fraction is incorporated into a formula using stroke volume to calculate the LVEDV.

In general, the ratio of the potential differences measured between a pair of electrodes on the body surface to the current passing between another pair of electrodes on the same surface (the impedance) is a function of the size and position of the electrodes, the size and shape of the body, and the resistivity of blood and distribution of other resistances within the body. Stroke volume can be determined by several bioimpedance systems capable of detecting the impedance change in the heart between ventricular systole and diastole and relating this measurement directly to the volume of blood ejected.[59]

Bioelectrical impedance cardiographic devices can theoretically determine left ventricular preload, cardiac output, and contractility. Modern bioelectric impedance devices incorporate microprocessors that allow for state-of-the-art data acquisition and signal processing, and these devices can then generate real-time, continuous hemodynamic data.[33–35,37,59,60] Many studies have compared cardiac output obtained by bioelectric impedance with that obtained by thermodilution; and the results are largely inconclusive.

Marik and colleagues[37] compared hemodynamic parameters derived from transthoracic electrical bioimpedance with those obtained with thermodilution right heart catheters and contrast ventriculography in the stable environment of the cardiac catheterization laboratory. Their study found poor agreement between the cardiac output, systolic ejection fraction, LVEDV estimated by bioimpedance with those values obtained simultaneously by thermodilution or ventriculography, underscored by wide confidence intervals, reflecting the great variation between the techniques. Marik et al. concluded that the considerable discrepancies between bioelectric impedance and traditional methods made the technology clinically unacceptable,[37] potentially leading to inappropriate clinical interventions.

Others have reported good correlation and agreement in critically ill and emergency room patients.[35,36] In separate multicenter trials, thoracic electrical bioimpedance devices were documented to provide accurate, reliable cardiac output estimations compared to simultaneous cardiac output measurements obtained by thermodilution. Thangathurai and colleagues compared a noninvasive thoracic bioimpedance device with the standard thermodilution method during the intraoperative period of high risk patients undergoing oncologic surgery.[36] They concluded that the device was a safe, reliable, clinically acceptable alternative to the invasive thermodilution method in the operating room environment. In critically ill patients, however, the data obtained from thoracic electrical bioimpedance devises can be compromised owing to the presence of central catheters, bulky dressings, and other invasive and noninvasive devices. In addition, these patients tend to be hemodynamically labile. In contradistinction to these observations, Shoemaker et al. reported reliable measurements in this population of patients.[33–35] At this time thoracic bioelectric impedance cardiography should not replace traditional invasive hemodynamic monitoring.[60]

Transesophageal Echocardiography

Minimally invasive transesophageal cardiography can be used for intermittent real-time evaluation of right ventricular filling (i.e., image-acquired adequacy of RVEDV) or continuous monitoring of cardiac output by either multiplane or Doppler modes. Intermittent transesophageal determination of ventricular end-diastolic volume may be especially useful in situations when there is uncertainty regarding right ventricular filling (e.g., high levels of PEEP, inadequate peripheral perfusion in the presence of right heart catheter evidence of adequate left-sided ventricular filling pressures, or uninterpretable or insufficient responses to volume loading).[32] Limitations of this technique include the need for a skilled operator and limited feasibility in hemodynamically unstable patients. Multiple approaches to continuous, real-time cardiac output monitoring by echocardiography or flow Doppler technique have been explored, but, they have not been accepted into general clinical practice because of many shortcomings associated with adequate, reliable measurement of the aortic blood flow velocity and the cross-sectional area of the aorta. The need for a trained operator and maintaining stable probe positions are also problematic with the continuous technology modes.

Current transesophageal echocardiography (TEE) devices provide high-fidelity two-dimensional imaging and greater stability in probe position, thereby minimizing the errors observed with Doppler cardiac output monitoring. Traditional TEE continues to be hampered by limitations in image viewing due to the restricted confines of the esophagus and stomach. Recent multiplane technology has greatly expanded the imaging capability of TEE. It allows the operator to steer the imaging plane, providing multiple perspectives for visualizing the aortic valve and for determining aortic blood flow velocity. Cardiac output can be calculated by combining continuous Doppler waveforms with the imaging capabilities of two-dimensional multiplane TEE.

Perrino and others compared multiplane TEE-determined cardiac output to that obtained by thermodilution in patients scheduled for cardiac or noncardiac surgery necessitating pulmonary artery catheter monitoring. They found multiplane TEE to be an acceptable alternative method for cardiac output determination.[31] The transesophageal probe was positioned in the midesophagus to obtain short-axis views of the aortic valve. The multiple imaging angles were adjusted to align the imaging plane with the cross-sectional plane of the aortic valve, facilitating measurement of aortic blood flow velocity. They found good agreement of this method with thermodilution-derived cardiac output, with a correlation of $R = 0.98$ and $p < 0.001$. The Doppler method was in accord with continuous thermodilution cardiac output results regarding the direction of change in cardiac output in 97% of instances. Unfortunately, even though the Doppler technique tracked the direction of serial changes in cardiac output on a percentage basis, serial changes in Doppler-derived cardiac output averaged 86% of the magnitude of the matched change of thermodilution-derived cardiac output.[31]

Krishnamurthy et al. compared a Doppler esophageal probe placed through the nasopharynx with continuous thermodilution cardiac output monitoring in patients undergoing coronary revascularization.[30] The esophageal Doppler probe was found to be a reliable minimally invasive device that allowed continuous observation of the trend of cardiac output, compared to thermodilution methodology. However, during the postoperative period the continuous cardiac output monitor provided more stable results, and the esophageal Doppler probe required the continuous presence of an experienced anesthetist to obtain comparable cardiac output estimations. They found that the esophageal probe lost its signal during patient turning, tracheal suctioning, and radiologic examinations, in contrast to traditional right heart catheters, which continued to work without the need for adjustment.

Doppler flow measurements are susceptible to underestimation of blood velocities caused by misalignment of the Doppler beam. Sclerosis of the aortic valve leaflets and conditions that restrict their motion can result in an irregularly shaped valve orifice.[31] Greim and associates examined the usefulness of TEE and automated endocardium detection for online calculation of left ventricular stroke volume.[29] They found that signal instability, lack of accuracy, and restricted trend capability limited the intraoperative usefulness of this technique for continuous estimation of stroke volume.

Capnography

Capnography is the graphic display of CO_2 concentrations as a waveform. It should not be confused with capnometry, which refers only to the numerical presentation of the concentration, without a waveform. Capnography includes capnometry when the capnographic display is calibrated. With most stand-alone capnographs, the CO_2 concentration is measured by infrared spectroscopy. The capnograph compares the amount of infrared light absorbed by the patient's gas in a sample cell with the amount absorbed either by gas in a reference cell or by the sample cell during a time of known zero-gas concentration.[48] The capnograph then displays the instantaneous CO_2 concentration.

Normally, there is a fairly predictable relation between the peak exhaled or end-tidal CO_2 ($PETCO_2$) and the $PaCO_2$. In healthy subjects with normal lungs, the $PaCO_2$ is 4–6 mmHg higher than the $PETCO_2$. Patients with chronic obstructive lung disease and other derangements associated with increased deadspace manifest an increased arterial/end-tidal CO_2 gradient ($Pa-ETCO_2$). Measurement of $PETCO_2$ is perhaps one of the most reliable means of determining proper endotracheal tube placement. Esophageal intubations are associated with a rapid fall in $PETCO_2$ to zero. The end-tidal partial pressure CO_2 has been found to correlate with cardiac output and coronary perfusion pressure during cardiopulmonary resuscitation and with successful resuscitation and survival because circulatory arrest creates total deadspace with rapid disappearance of $PETCO_2$. An increase in $PETCO_2$ provides an immediate bedside validation of the efficacy of cardiopulmonary resuscitation (CPR).

In the ICU environment the use of $PETCO_2$ to monitor resuscitation and cardiac output is predicated on maintaining a constant minute ventilation and consistent V/Q matching so changes in $PETCO_2$ result from changes in lung perfusion (and therefore cardiac output) and not ventilation. $PETCO_2$ can be used as a ventilator disconnect alarm as well as a system to determine ventilator malfunction. Measurement of $PETCO_2$ has been proposed as a substitute for arterial blood gas sampling during mechanical ventilation and a stand-alone monitor of the adequacy of cardiac output in critically ill patients, thereby obviating the need to measure arterial blood gases and for thermodilution cardiac output measurements. Unfortunately, $PETCO_2$ trends in critically ill patients are often misleading because the $Pa-ETCO_2$ varies greatly in these individuals, and the V/Q mismatch in supine, intubated ICU patients with acute lung injury or ARDS is commonly characterized by changing physiologic deadspace. Therefore CO_2 monitoring may not adequately represent the alveolar CO_2 and so may inaccurately represent the adequacy of cardiac performance and the adequacy of the cardiovascular circulation.

Pulse Oximetry

Pulse oximetry provides a reliable real-time estimation of arterial hemoglobin oxygen saturation. This noninvasive monitoring technique has gained clinical acceptance in the operating room, recovery room, and ICU. Continuous arterial blood gas monitoring is another alternative.[48,61,62] Pulse oximetry estimates arterial hemoglobin saturation by measuring the absorbance of light transmitted through well perfused tissue, such as the finger or ear. Light absorption is measured at two wavelengths, 600 nm (red) and 900 nm (infrared), to distinguish between two species of hemoglobin: oxyhemoglobin and deoxyhemoglobin. (Pulse oximetry distinguishes only oxyhemoglobin and deoxyhemoglobin.) Oxyhemoglobin absorbs less red light than deoxyhemoglobin. If other hemoglobin species are present, an error is introduced. Laboratory co-oximeters, on the other hand, generally use more than two wavelengths and can quantify other hemoglobin species directly. When abnormal hemoglobins such as carboxyhemoglobin and methemoglobin can be measured, it becomes meaningful to distinguish between functional saturation (100 × oxyhemoglobin + oxyhemoglobin + deoxyhemoglobin) and fractional saturation (100 × oxyhemoglobin/oxyhemoglobin + deoxyhemoglobin + carboxyhemoglobin + methemoglobin). Intravenously administered dyes, particularly methylene blue and indocyanine green, can temporarily induce artificially low saturation readings. Despite its limitations, pulse oximetry is generally acknowledged as one of the most significant advances in clinical monitoring.

Near-Infrared Spectroscopy

Cytochrome A,A_3 is a terminal receptor for oxygen in the electron transport chain. When oxygen supply is inadequate, the rate of electron transport is reduced and oxidative phosphorylation decreases, leading ultimately to anaerobic metabolism.[11,44] Optical devices utilizing near-infrared wavelengths can determine the redox potential of copper atoms on cytochrome A,A_3 and has been used to study intracellular oxidated processes noninvasively. Technologic advances have led to the development of compact, portable spectroscopic devices; and improvements in optical techniques have reduced distortion, scattering, and interference from other biologic tissues. Near-infrared (NIR) wavelengths pass relatively easy through skin and bone and thus have the potential to provide transcutaneous, noninvasive monitoring of tissue oxygen saturation.

Transcranial NIR spectroscopy has been used to monitor cerebral oxygenation in newborns, patients undergoing hypothermic cardiopulmonary bypass, and brain-injured patients. Current trials are investigating the incorporation of NIR probes into nasogastric tubes to measure gastric mucosal oxygen saturation as an end-point of resuscitation. Currently, NIR spectroscopy is also being tested as a means of detecting lower extremity compartment syndrome in critically injured patients and to monitor the viability of tissue flaps and revascularize extremities.[44] NIR can also be used to assess the redox states of chromophores other than the copper ion. Patients who are septic or have ARDS or multiple organ failure often demonstrate impaired ability to consume oxygen.[11] An early reduction of cytochrome A,A_3, despite normal oxygen delivery, has been demonstrated in trauma patients who go on to develop multiple organ failure and in those with endotoxemia.[11]

Fiberoptic Oxygen Probes

Monitoring tissue oxygen partial pressures (PO_2) has appeared to be a relatively noninvasive means of detecting hypoxia. However, changes in skin temperature and the level of adrenergic stimulation can make it difficult to sustain a quantitative relation between oxygen delivery and subcutaneous oxygen tension.

Several studies have utilized tissue PO_2 probes to monitor resuscitation.[17,18] During an oxygen challenge with breathing 100% oxygen, most patients demonstrate a rapid increase in tissue PO_2. That some patients fail to demonstrate this response until provided with additional fluid suggests inadequate peripheral perfusion due to unrecognized hypovolemia. Placement of tissue PO_2 electrodes over skeletal muscle have been described, and an increasing oxygen tension gradient between arterial blood and PO_2 electrodes can be taken as evidence of circulatory compensation. The improvements in design to eliminate drift and calibration problems may enable tissue PO_2 probes to be incorporated into intracranial pressure monitoring devices.

Transcutaneous Oxygen Tension Monitoring

Hypoxemia, frequent during the second to fourth postoperative days after major upper abdominal and thoracic surgery, may be related to the development of cardiac complications. Postoperative or episodic hypoxemia has been verified previously by pulse oximetry. Measurements of transcutaneous oxygen tension is a suitable reference point for validating pulse oximetry monitoring and hypoxemia. Stausholm and colleagues, in a study comparing pulse oximetry with transcutaneous oxygen tension, found that episodic oxygen desaturation was reflected in transcutaneous oxygen tension measurements. In 95% of cases the episodes lasted 1 minute or more.[61] The relation between transcutaneous and arterial oxygen tension, however, is not dependent on skin temperature, skin thickness, the site of the measurement, or correct preparation of the skin.

Phosphorus Magnetic Resonance Spectroscopy

The physics principle underlying the methodology of phosphorus magnetic resonance spectroscopy is based on the observation that when atoms with an odd number of protons or neutrons are placed in a magnetic field they align in a specific orientation. When allowed to return to their original random configuration, energy is released as a weak radiofrequency signal. The energy signal generated can be analyzed to provide information about the chemical composition of tissue.

Phosphorus 31 can be measured to provide information about the relative concentrations of ATP, phosphocreatine (Pcr, the main energy store of the cell), and inorganic phosphate (Pi).[8,14] During periods of reduced oxygen supply cytochrome oxidation decreases, but ATP generation is initially maintained by depletion of Pcr stores. Ischemia is characterized by a fall in high-energy Pcr and an increase in the Pi breakdown products, which can be displayed as a decrease in the Pcr/Pi ratio. The measurement of cellular energy stores, as evidenced by a decrease in Pcr and parallel increase in Pi, is likely to be the most sensitive indicator of the adequacy of tissue metabolism and the irreversibility of ischemic damage. Application of this technology in the ICU has been limited by the size of the currently available systems and the risk of electronic interference due to magnetic fields. However, this technology may enable clinicians to determine if cellular anoxia is corrected during hemodynamic resuscitation.

Conclusions

Flow-directed catheters have been around since the mid-1970s. Technologic innovations have modified these catheters to meet new demands for patient care. Although right heart pulmonary artery catheters have not been demonstrated to improve survival in critically ill patients,[50] they do provide information that cannot be obtained reliably by physical examination at the bedside. Clinical misinterpretation and misapplication of the data appear to be the greatest impediment to using pulmonary catheters to alter the pathophysiologic processes and consistently improve outcome in critically ill patients. Advances in invasive and noninvasive monitoring techniques provide the opportunity to improve our ability to ensure adequate oxygen delivery with restoration of the circulation at the end-organ and cellular level. In general, carefully designed clinical trials are essential to establish the benefit of all global and organ-specific invasive and noninvasive monitoring systems.

References

1. Kirton OC, Windsor J, Wedderburn R, et al: Failure of splanchnic resuscitation in the acutely injured trauma patient correlation with multiple organ system failure and length of stay in the ICU. Chest 1998;113:1064–1069.
2. Moore F, Haenel J, Moore E, et al: Incommensurate oxygen consumption in response to maximal oxygen availability predicts post injury multiple organ failure. J Trauma 1992;3:58–67.
3. Tuchschmidt J, Fried J, Astiz M, et al: Elevation of cardiac output and oxygen delivery improves outcome in septic shock. Chest 1992;102:216–220.
4. Yu M, Levy MM, Smith P, et al: Effect of maximizing oxygen delivery on morbidity and mortality rates in critically ill patients: a prospective, randomized, controlled study. Crit Care Med 1993;21:830–832.
5. Maynard N, Bihari D, Beale R, et al: Assessment of splanchnic oxygenation by gastric tonometry in patients with acute circulatory failure. JAMA 1993;270:1203–1210.
6. Chang MC, Cheatham ML, Nelson LD, et al: Gastric tonometry supplements information provided by systemic indicators of oxygen transport. J Trauma 1994;27:488–494.
7. Landow L, Phillip DA, Heard SO, et al: Gastric tonometry and venous oximetry in cardiac surgery patients. Crit Care Med 1991;19:1226–1233.
8. Gutierrez G: Cellular energy metabolism during hypoxia. Crit Care Med 1991;19:619–626.
9. Ivatury RR, Simon RJ, Havriliak D, et al: Gastric mucosal pH and organ delivery and oxygen consumption indices in the assessment of adequacy of resuscitation after trauma: a prospective randomized study. J Trauma 1995;39:128–134.
10. Porter JM, Ivatury RR: In search of the optimal endpoints of resuscitation in trauma patients: a review. J Trauma 1998;44:908–914.
11. Carins CB, Moore FA, Haenel JB, et al: Evidence for early supply independent mitochondrial dysfunction in patients developing multiple organ failure after trauma. J Trauma 1997;42:532–536.
12. Soto Y, Weil MH, Tang W: Tissue hypercarbic acidosis as a marker of acute circulatory failure (shock). Chest 1998;114:263–274.
13. Mythen MO, Webb AR: The role of gut mucosal hypoperfusion in the pathogenesis of post-operative organ dysfunction. Intensive Care Med 1994;20:203–209.
14. Kirton OC, Civetta JM: Splanchnic flow and resuscitation. In: Civetta JM, Taylor RW, Kirby RR (eds) Critical Care, 3rd ed. Philadelphia, Lippincott-Raven.
15. Barquist E, Kirton OC, Windsor J, et al: The impact of antioxidant and splanchnic-directed therapy on persistent uncorrected gastric mucosal pH in the critically injured trauma patient. J Trauma 1998;14:355–359.
16. Gutierrez G, Andry JM: Nuclear magnetic resonance measurements: clinical applications. Crit Care Med 1989;17:73–82.
17. Knudson MM, Bermudez KM, Doyle CA, et al: Use of tissue oxygen tension measurements during resuscitation from hemorrhagic shock. J Trauma 1997;42:608–614.
18. Waxman K, Annas C, Daughters K, et al: A method to determine the adequacy of resuscitation using tissue oxygen monitoring. J Trauma 1994;36:852–858.
19. Lee P, Langdale L, Mock C, et al: Near-infrared spectroscopy: continuous measurement of cytochrome oxidation during hemorrhagic shock. Crit Care Med 1997;25:166–170.
20. Nelson L: The new pulmonary artery catheters: continuous venous oximetry, right ventricular ejection fraction and continuous cardiac output. New Horiz 1997;5:251–258.
21. Diebel LN, Meyers T, Dulchausky S: Effects of increasing airway pressure and PEEP on the assessment of cardiac preload. J Trauma 1997;42:585–591.
22. Kraut EJ, Owings JT, Anderson JT, et al: Right ventricular volumes over estimate left ventricular preload in critically ill patients. J Trauma 1997;42:839–846.
23. Chang MC, Blinman TA, Rutherford EJ, et al: Preload assessment in trauma patients during large-volume shock resuscitation. Arch Surg 1996;131:728–731.
24. Gattinoni L, Brazzi L, Pelosi P, et al: A trial of goal-oriented hemodynamic therapy in critically ill patients. N Engl J Med 1995;333:1025–1032.
25. Boldt J, Menges T, Wollbruk M, et al: Is continuous cardiac output measurement using thermodilution reliable in the critically ill patient? Crit Care Med 1994;22:1913–1918.
26. Mihm FG, Gettinger A, Hanson W, et al: A multicenter evaluation of a new continuous cardiac output pulmonary artery catheter system. Crit Care Med 1998;26:1346–1350.
27. Burchell SA, Yu M, Takiguchi SA, et al: Evaluation of a continuous cardiac output and mixed venous oxygen saturation catheter in critically ill surgical patients. Crit Care Med 1997;25:388–391.
28. Jacquet L, Hanique G, Glorieux D, et al: Analysis of the accuracy of continuous thermodilution cardiac output measurements. Intensive Care Med 1996;22:1125–1129.

29. Greim CA, Roewer N, Lavx G, et al: On-line estimation of left ventricular stroke volume using transesophageal echocardiography and acoustic quantification. Br J Anesth 1996;77:365–369.
30. Krishnamurthy B, McMurray TJ, McClean E: The perioperative use of the esophageal Doppler monitor in patients undergoing coronary artery revascularization. Anesthesia 1997;52:624–629.
31. Perrino AC, Harris SN, Luther MA: Intraoperative determination of cardiac output using multiplane transesophageal echocardiography. Anesthesiology 1998;89:350–357.
32. Greim CA, Roewer N, Apfel C, et al: Relation of echocardiographic preload indices to stroke volume in critically ill patients with normal and low cardiac index. Intensive Care Med 1997;23:411–416.
33. Shoemaker WC, Wo CCJ, Bishop MH, et al: Noninvasive physiologic monitoring of high-risk surgical patients. Arch Surg 1996;131:732–737.
34. Shoemaker WC, Wo CCJ, Bishop MH, et al: Multicenter trial of a new thoracic electrical bioimpedance device for cardiac output estimation. Crit Care Med 1994;22:1907–1912.
35. Shoemaker WC, Belzberg H, Wo CCJ, et al: Multicenter study of noninvasive monitoring systems as alternatives to invasive monitoring of acutely ill emergency patients. Chest 1998;114:1643–1652.
36. Thangathurai D, Charbonnet C, Roessler P, et al: Continuous intraoperative noninvasive cardiac output monitoring using a new thoracic bioimpedance device. J Cardiothorac Vasc Anesth 1997;11:440–444.
37. Marik PE, Pendelton JE, Smith R: A comparison of hemodynamic parameters derived from transthoracic electrical bioimpedance with those parameters obtained by thermodilution and ventricular angiography. Crit Care Med 1997;25:1545–1550.
38. Kirton OC, Civetta JM: Do pulmonary artery catheters alter outcome in trauma patients? New Horiz 1997;5:222–227.
39. Levy M: Pulmonary capillary pressure and tissue perfusion: clinical implications during resuscitation from shock. New Horiz 1996;4:504–518.
40. Deibel LN, Wilson RF, Tagett MG, et al: End-diastolic volume; a better indicator of preload in the critically ill. Arch Surg 1992;127:817–821.
41. Swan HJC, Ganz W, Forrester JS, et al: Catheterization of the heart and pulmonary artery was accomplished by floating a flow-directed balloon-tipped catheter. N Engl J Med 1970;283:447–451.
42. Bishop MH, Shoemaker WC, Appel PL, et al: Relationship between supranormal circulatory values, time delays, and outcome in severely traumatized patients. Crit Care Med 1993:21:51–63.
43. Abou-Khalil B, Scalea TM, Trooskin SZ, et al: Hemodynamic responses to shock in young trauma patients: need for invasive monitoring. Crit Care Med 1994;22:633–639.
44. Durham RM, Neunaber K, Mazuski JE, et al: The use of oxygen consumption and delivery as endpoints for resuscitation in critically ill patients. J Trauma 1996;41:32–40.
45. Davis JW, Kaups KL: Base deficit in the elderly: a marker of severe injury and deaths. J Trauma 1998;45:873–877.
46. Abramson D, Scalea TM, Hitchcock R, et al: Lactate clearance and survival following injury. J Trauma 1993;35:585–589.
47. Rhee P, Langdale L, Mock C, et al: Near-infrared spectroscopy: continuous measurement of cytochrome oxidation during hemorrhagic shock. Crit Care Med 1997;25:166–170.
48. Varon AJ, Kirton OC, Civetta JM: Physiologic monitoring of the surgical patient. In: Schwartz SI (ed) Principles of Surgery, vol 12. 1999;485–509.
49. Robin ED: Death by pulmonary artery flow-directed catheter: time for a moratorium? Chest 1987;92:727–731.
50. Connors AF, Speroff T, Dawson NV, et al: The effectiveness of right heart catheterization in the initial care of critically ill patients. JAMA 1996;276:889–897.
51. Urban P, Scheidegger D, Gabathuler J, et al: Thermodilution measurement of right ventricular volume and ejection fraction: a comparison with biplane angiography. Crit Care Med 1987;15:652–655.
52. Ferris S, Konno M: In vivo validation of a thermodilution right ventricular ejection fraction method. J Clin Monit 1992;8:74–79.
53. Chang MC, Meredith JW: Cardiac preload, splanchnic perfusion, and their relationship during resuscitation in trauma patients. J Trauma 1997;42:577–584.
54. Chang MC, Mondy JS, Meredith JW, et al: Redefining cardiovascular performance during shock resuscitation: ventricular stroke work, power, and the pressure–volume diagram. J Trauma 1998;45:470–478.
55. Beele PL, McMichan JC, Marsh HM, et al: Continuous monitoring of mixed venous oxygen saturation in critically ill patients. Anesth Analg 1982;61:513–517.
56. Doglio GR, Pusajo JF, Equrrola MA, et al: Gastric mucosal pH as a prognostic index of mortality in critically ill patients. Crit Care Med 1991;19:1037–1040.
57. Miller PR, Kincaid EH, Meredith JW, et al: Threshold values of pH and mucosal-arterial CO_2 gap during resuscitation. J Trauma 1998;45:868–872.
58. Ivatury R, Simon R, Havriliak D, et al: Gastric mucosal pH and oxygen delivery and oxygen consumption indices in the assessment of adequacy of resuscitation after trauma: a prospective randomized study. J Trauma 1995;39:128–134.
59. Smith DN: Bioimpedance measurement of cardiac output [letter to the editor]. Crit Care Med 1994;22:1513–1514.
60. Weil MH: Electrical bioimpedance for noninvasive measurement of cardiac output [letter to the editor]. Crit Care Med 1997;25:1455.
61. Stausholm K, Rosenberg-Adamson S, Edvardsen L, et al: Validation of pulse oximetry for monitoring of hypoxemic episodes in the late postoperative period. Br J Anaesth 1997;78:86–87.
62. Larson CP: Continuous arterial blood gas monitoring: a technology in transition. Intensive Care Med 1996;22:1141–1143.

27
Peritonitis: Management of the Patient with SIRS and MODS

Donald E. Fry

Peritonitis continues to be a complex illness that requires the coordinated efforts of timely surgical intervention, systemic antibiotic therapy, and supportive critical care management. Peritonitis and its accompanying sequela of intraabdominal abscess are frequently associated with activation of the systemic inflammatory response syndrome (SIRS) and is commonly associated with the development of the multiple organ dysfunction syndrome (MODS). Many authors consider peritonitis to be the prototypical infection associated with MODS, although there is general consensus at the present time that any infectious source could potentially activate SIRS and lead to MODS.[1] The general perception is that effective intervention in the initial management of patients with peritonitis can avoid subsequent evolution of the multiple organ failure cascade. Some have reported reversal of organ failure with surgical intervention in intraabdominal infection.[2-4] This chapter summarizes the significant aspects of the treatment of the complex constellation of diseases called peritonitis.

Pathophysiology and Microbiology

Effective treatment of peritonitis requires a clear understanding of the pathophysiology and microbiology of this disease entity. Peritonitis can be identified as being primary, secondary, or tertiary (Table 27.1). Tertiary peritonitis is addressed at the end of the chapter. Primary peritonitis implies that the microbial pathogen has gained access to the peritoneal cavity by a hematogenous or lymphatic route.[5] Primary peritonitis means that the patient does not have a fundamental disease process within the abdomen that is responsible for the developing infection. The most common current clinical scenario for primary peritonitis is the patient with hepatic cirrhosis and ascites. Excessive quantities of free intraperitoneal fluid appear to render the peritoneal cavity vulnerable to lymphatic or hematogenously disseminated microorganisms. Although commonly discussed in the medical literature, primary peritonitis is uncommon and constitutes fewer than 1% of the total number of peritonitis patients customarily treated.

Secondary bacterial peritonitis is clearly the disease entity that is of greatest concern to the physician. Secondary peritonitis occurs when patients have a primary biliary or enteric disease that results in transmural tissue necrosis and perforation, followed by secondary contamination of the peritoneal sac. Common diseases that result in secondary peritonitis include perforated appendix, perforated gastrointestinal track malignancies (e.g., colon cancer) perforated diverticular disease, and perforated peptic ulcer.[6] Occasionally, perforations of the biliary track are responsible for peritonitis, and complex complicated cases of pancreatitis may lead to peritonitis as well.

The process begins with perforation of the viscus as the primary event, followed by secondary contamination of the peritoneal cavity. The magnitude of microbial contamination with the perforation can be highly variable. Patients with a perforated peptic ulcer ordinarily have few microorganisms in the peritoneal cavity, as normal gastric acid production limits microbial colonization within the stomach. On the other hand, perforation of obstructed bowel or perforations from the distal colon may have high densities of microorganisms, which may approach 10^{10} or even more per gram of intraluminal content. In these circumstances the perforative event of the colon represents a catastrophic insult to the peritoneal cavity by virtue of the large number of microbial organisms. When one compares the consequences of a perforated peptic ulcer with that of a perforated diverticulum, it is apparent that the disease entities covered under the umbrella of peritonitis are a diverse group of illnesses, and their therapy is different as well.

With contamination of the peritoneal cavity there is prompt dissemination of the microbial pathogens.[7] The peritoneal cavity ordinarily has a small amount of peritoneal fluid, which is the consequence of increased hydrostatic pressure within the mesenteric circulation. This peritoneal fluid customarily moves toward the diaphragm as a function of the patient's normal breathing patterns while lying in a recumbent position. Each time the patient exhales peritoneal fluid moves toward the area of reduced pressure; the movement of peritoneal fluid toward the diaphragmatic surface serves the biologic purpose of allowing peritoneal fluid to be cleared through the normal lymphatic fenestrations on the abdominal surface of the

TABLE 27.1. Salient Features of the Various Phases of Peritonitis.

Type of peritonitis	Source of bacteria	Pathogens	Treatment and comments
Primary	Hematogenous or lymphatic "seeding" of peritoneal cavity	*Escherichia coli*, *Klebsiella* sp., pneumococci	Antibiotics alone; must be sure of the diagnosis; no anaerobes and not a polymicrobial infection
Secondary	Perforation of viscous or biliary tract	Enteric gram-negatives and obligate anaerobes	Surgical source control; drainage and débridement of peritoneal cavity; antibiotics against pathogens
Tertiary	Environment of ICU or resistant colonization from the host	Resistant gram-negatives (e.g., *Pseudomonas* sp.), enterococci, *Candida* sp.	Mechanical débridement; frequent reoperations; meticulous wound care; antimicrobial therapy

diaphragm.[8,9] These lymphatic fenestrations communicate directly with the thoracic duct. This process of normal peritoneal fluid formation and clearance through the lymphatic system underscores the fact that the peritoneal cavity is a giant lymphocele in direct communication with the lymphatic system.

As the microbe disseminates and adheres to the surface of the peritoneal cavity, the process of human inflammation is activated. The activation of the process is similar to that described for other areas of the body (see Chapter 9). The fact that the peritoneal surface represents in an adult the equivalent of approximately 40% of the total body surface area reflects the enormous interface that exists between the host inflammatory response and the disseminated pathogens within the abdominal cavity. This vast mesothelial surface becomes a potentially large surface for the access of microbes, microbial cell products, and proinflammatory cytokines into the systemic circulation of the host.

As with infection at other sites, the severity of infection in the peritoneal cavity relates to the number of microbes released and to the presence of adjuvant factors that enhance microbial virulence. Hemoglobin, dead tissue, and foreign bodies are the most relevant. Hemoglobin is a potent adjuvant because of the availability of ferric iron, which enhances microbial proliferation;[10] but it may also have an adjuvant effect because of a metabolic end-product of microbial action on hemoglobin that is toxic to host phagocytic cells.[11] Foreign bodies become particularly significant in peritonitis, as the nonbacterial components of human fecal material and food products within the gastrointestinal tract serve to enhance microbial virulence and to inhibit host responsiveness. When peritonitis is the consequence of abdominal trauma, there may also be dead tissue, free hemoglobin, and other foreign bodies to enhance microbial virulence.

Host response to the proliferating microorganisms is through the human inflammatory response (see Chapter 9). The primary phase of vasodilation, increased microcirculatory flow, and local tissue edema lead to the secondary phase of phagocytic cell delivery to the inflamed peritoneal tissues. A second mechanism for microbial removal from the peritoneal cavity is the clearance of bacteria through the lymphatic fenestrations as part of the normal clearance of bacterial fluid (described above). Thus microbial invaders within the abdominal cavity are eradicated by phagocytic cell activity or by clearance through the lymphatic system of the diaphragm.

When the density of microbes within the abdominal cavity is in excess of those that can be eradicated by normal physiologic forces, the "court of last resort" of the peritoneal cavity is to loculate, or wall off, the pathogen. The inflammatory process creates a fibrin perimeter about these dense collections of microbes, and the loculation process results in an abscess. The process of having an abscess in the abdominal cavity means that dense collections of microbes are contained. The abscess cavity then may serve as a repository for a dense collection of pus, from which microbes, cellular products of the bacteria, or inflammatory mediators can gain access to the systemic circulation. The patient continues to have systemic sequela from the abscess even though the microbes are contained within a localized area. These abscess collections characteristically occur in dependent portions of the abdominal cavity,[12] characteristically in the subphrenic space, pericolic gutters, and pelvis. When patients have had prior abdominal operations, false dependencies within the peritoneal cavity may be created by adhesions between loops of intestine or between adhesions from the bowel to the abdominal wall. These false dependencies can create unusual sites for abscesses in the subfascial space or even in the interloop areas.

An abscess usually is associated with continued spiking fevers in the patient and clinical evidence systemically that infection is an active process. Thus it can be safely said that although inflammation and its associated processes may be effective in containing the dense microbes within the abscess cavity, the continued dynamic process of host-pathogen interaction continues, and the patients usually have systemic consequences from an abscess. Commonly, the successful or unsuccessful management of an abscess dictates the ultimate outcome of the patient with an intraabdominal infection. Furthermore, a persistent abscess and sustained SIRS become the clinical setting leading to MODS.

The microbiology of peritonitis deserves special consideration. When perforations due to a peptic ulcer occur, most of the cultures are negative; positive cultures usually are due to mouth flora that were present within the upper gastrointestinal tract at the time of the perforation. Perforations of the biliary tract are associated with the customary biliary microorganisms: *Escherichia coli*, *Klebsiella* sp., and *Enterococcus* sp.[13] Distal small

TABLE 27.2. Bacterial Isolates Commonly Cultured in Patients with Acute Secondary Bacterial Peritonitis.[a]

Cultured organism	Percent of patients with positive cultures
Aerobes	
Escherichia coli	57–83
Streptococcus sp.	26–63
Enterococcus sp.	11–28
Proteus sp.	3–11
Klebsiella sp.	4–20
Pseudomonas sp.	3–19
Anaerobes	
Bacteroides sp.	61–323[b]
Bacteroides fragilis	31–76
Peptostreptococcus sp.	6–68
Peptococcus sp.	1–28
Fusobacterium sp.	3–33
Eubacterium sp.	2–33
Clostridium sp.	6–40

(Data were derived from four major publications).
[a] Note the highly variable probabilities of recovering even the most common pathogens that are recognized in patients with peritonitis.
[b] More than 100% indicates multiple isolates per patient.

bowel and colonic perforations represent the most complex microflora and customarily have both enteric gram-negative rods (e.g., *E. coli*) and obligate anaerobes (e.g., *Bacteroides fragilis*). It is generally thought that *E. coli* and *B. fragilis* in community-acquired bacterial peritonitis represent the prototypical microorganisms. These aerobic and anaerobic bacteria appear to have a synergistic relationship.[14] The results of cultures of the peritoneal cavity are highly variable (Table 27.2)[6,15–17] and may not be of any clinical value,[6] although this opinion has been disputed.[17]

Diagnosis

The diagnosis of acute bacterial peritonitis is primarily based on clinical findings and does not require sophisticated methodology. The diagnosis is somewhat more difficult in the elderly patient, where the prompt, vigorous inflammatory response appears to be blunted by the aging process. In general, the history of a patient with peritonitis begins with the precipitous onset of acute abdominal pain. Patients who have acute peptic ulcer disease, acute cholecystitis, or diverticulitis may have had antecedent periods of pain caused by the primary disease process that preceded the perforation. In patients with acute appendicitis the pain commonly begins in the periumbilical area and then localizes to the right lower quadrant; perforation customarily follows within 24–36 hours of untreated localized right lower quadrant pain. Patients with acute peritonitis customarily have attendant nausea and vomiting, but the remaining historical symptoms are usually specific for the underlying disease, not for the peritonitis.

The fundamental and most important aspect of establishing the diagnosis of acute bacterial peritonitis is the physical examination. The palpatory examination of the abdomen characteristically identifies severe tenderness that may be quite diffuse depending on the duration of the infectious process. Rebound tenderness reflects severe inflammation of the parietal peritoneum and is the sine qua non for establishing the diagnosis of acute bacterial peritonitis. An appropriate history and the physical finding of rebound tenderness fulfill the necessary criteria for establishing the diagnosis.

Laboratory studies are commonly performed and are extraordinarily nonspecific in establishing the diagnosis of peritonitis. Leukocytosis may be present, but this measurement can be treacherous in the elderly and is frequently not impressive in patients who have had a recent onset of perforated appendix. With severe peritonitis plus SIRS and evolving MODS, the leukocyte count may be high or low. In general, an elevated white blood cell (WBC) count and a shift of the count to premature forms is collaborative but nonspecific evidence; it is seldom a major determinant in establishing the diagnosis of peritonitis.

Conventional abdominal roentgenographic studies continue to be done for diagnosing peritonitis. The "three-way" abdomen series includes a supine roentgenogram of the abdomen, an upright chest roentgenogram, and a lateral decubitus film. Free air can be identified on the upright chest roentgenogram usually underneath the left hemidiaphragm (Fig. 27.1) but is common only with perforated peptic ulcers; it is highly unusual with other perforative events. Other nonspecific findings of perforation can be identified but are usually not helpful (Fig. 27.2). In general, the findings of the three-way abdomen series are of so little value that its continued use in the evaluation of these patients is viewed as a waste of resources and

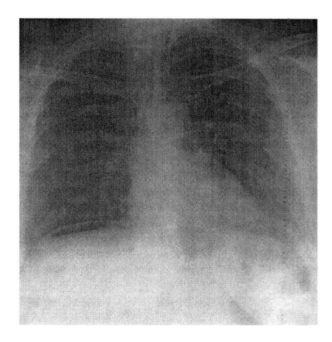

FIGURE 27.1. Upright chest roentgenogram with free air under the right hemidiaphragm.

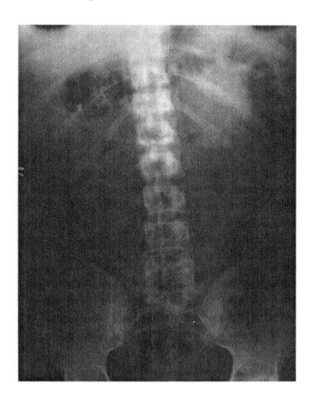

FIGURE 27.2. Obligatory abdominal "flat plate" obtained on virtually every patient with a suspected diagnosis of peritonitis. As seen here, such radiographs are rarely of any value.

does not to have any relevance in establishing the diagnosis for most of these patients.

More sophisticated imaging studies with acute peritonitis are of limited value. Computed tomography (CT) and abdominal ultrasonography can identify free fluid within the peritoneal cavity and occasionally visualizes acute appendicitis. Imaging studies are not of value for most patients with acute bacterial peritonitis and are generally used for evaluating of patients with suspected abscess within the peritoneal cavity.

The diagnosis of primary peritonitis is a highly specialized situation. Patients with primary peritonitis commonly have cirrhosis and ascites. They have severe, diffuse abdominal pain, usually with rebound tenderness in all quadrants of the abdomen. The treacherous part of establishing the diagnosis of primary peritonitis is that the patient with primary peritonitis commonly has multiple risk factors for secondary peritonitis as well. Thus when evaluating the patient with cirrhosis and ascites and a presumed diagnosis of primary peritonitis, one should bear in mind that a perforated viscus is still more likely in that patient than is primary peritonitis. The diagnosis of primary peritonitis is best achieved by paracentesis and examining the peritoneal fluid. If the peritoneal fluid demonstrates a high leukocyte count and gram-positive organisms (e.g., *Streptococcus pneumoniae*), one can be confident that primary peritonitis is the correct diagnosis and so proceed with antibiotic therapy alone. When gram-negative bacteria are identified, caution must be exercised and a careful assessment of the patient undertaken to ensure that secondary peritonitis is not present. Failure of the patient to respond to antibiotic therapy may be the basis for promptly proceeding with abdominal exploration of the patient with secondary peritonitis.

Our group has applied the use of diagnostic laparoscopy to patients with gram-negative primary peritonitis to eliminate a perforated viscus as being the cause of the peritonitis in the presence of ascites and clinical peritonitis. It must be emphasized that ascitic fluid with polymicrobial microflora or that is culture-positive for an anaerobe is likely to indicate a perforated viscus, and abdominal exploration is necessary. Anaerobes are not recognized pathogens of primary peritonitis.[18]

Treatment

The principal treatment for acute bacterial peritonitis is abdominal exploration. Findings of rebound tenderness with a history consistent with perforated appendix, perforated diverticular disease, or perforated ulcer should lead promptly to surgical exploration. Some presentations have suggested that selected patients with perforated peptic ulcer can be treated with conservative nonsurgical methods.[19] Even patients with a perforated appendix that presents with an abscessed mass can be successfully treated without operation.[20] However, the diagnosis of diffuse peritonitis is commonly a diagnosis of uncertain intraabdominal pathology. The surgeon must be cautious about making assumptions as to which viscus is perforated, and validation of that perforation through operation is important.

The standard treatment of acute bacterial peritonitis has four basic components. First and foremost is source control. The perforation within the abdominal cavity must be contained. Second is drainage and débridement of exudate, pus, and dead tissue from within the abdominal cavity. Third, antibiotics are addressed to the expected pathogens within the infectious process. Finally, appropriate systemic supportive care of the patient must be supplied by vigorous administration of intravenous fluids and other measures.

Source Control

Source control begins with selection of the abdominal incision. When there is a high degree of confidence that the perforative event is from the appendix, a transverse incision in the right lower quadrant is selected. This incision is chosen, rather than the traditional McBurney incision, so that if unexpected pathology is encountered the incision can be extended medially and across into the left lower quadrant as a low transverse incision. This flexibility obviously allows comprehensive exploration of the abdomen by using the original transverse right lower quadrant approach. When other sources of intraabdominal infection are anticipated or the source of infection is unclear, the safest surgical incision approach is generally through the midline. Extension of the midline incision in a superior or inferior direction gives the surgeon maximum flexibility when approaching pathology at any location within the abdominal cavity.

Once the abdominal cavity is open, the surgeon searches for the quadrant in which exudative material appears to be in greatest density. Tracing the exudate within the peritoneal cavity with an acute perforation generally is the fastest route for identifying the primary source. If patients have had a delay in having their operation for whatever cause, the inflammation and exudate can be diffuse within the peritoneal cavity, and one must then systematically go through all of the possible sites of perforation to identify the offending source.

Source management is always an important issue for discussion. Traditionally, for acute perforated peptic ulcers most surgeons opted for acute vagotomy and pyloroplasty as treatment, given a limited amount of contamination within the abdomen. When patients are unstable and contamination is severe, a traditional plication procedure may be chosen. Uncommonly, one may be confronted with a giant perforation (>2 cm in diameter). The perforation and local inflammation are so severe and the adjacent tissues so friable that plication may serve to obstruct the outlet of the stomach, or it cannot be safely done. In such unusual circumstances the surgeon may be forced to pursue gastrectomy. In general, gastrectomy as an alternative for acute management of perforated peptic ulcer is not encouraged. Source control for the perforated appendix is customarily appendectomy alone. Again in highly unusual circumstances one may find necrosis of the cecal wall when the inflammatory process has existed for a long time. In unusual circumstances an emergency right hemicolectomy may be chosen. In such circumstances it is my preference to perform a primary ileotransverse colostomy as a primary anastomosis rather than doing a cutaneous ileostomy procedure. Perforated sigmoid diverticular disease requires resection of the involved segment and customarily a colostomy. A Hartmann pouch may be necessary; or if the segment of rectosigmoid colon distal to the area of resection is long enough, a mucous fistula may be created. Perforations of colon cancers require resection of the disease, not diversion alone. A perforated colonic cecum from distal obstruction in the colon is a difficult management problem and is commonly attended by massive contamination within the peritoneal cavity. Under these circumstances the extent of inflammation and the severity of peritonitis may make ileostomy an appropriate temporizing measure for these patients. However, every general surgeon knows that ileostomy is attended by problems of stomal morbidity (e.g., necrosis, stricture) and the longer-term problems of fluid and electrolyte losses, especially in the elderly. The magnitude of contamination and the severity of the inflammation of the cecal wall commonly make cecostomy somewhat undesirable.

The method of source control is important and is commonly not standardized in clinical trials of peritonitis. The problem of standardization is that judgment at the time of the procedure commonly dictates the treatment options. Variation in methods of source control may be a significant variable in the evaluation of outcomes reported in the literature for management of complex cases of acute bacterial peritonitis.

Débridement and Drainage

Following source control, the surgeon is confronted with managing copious amounts of exudate and pus in the peritoneal cavity due to the inflammatory response. The fibrin within the peritoneal cavity is laden with large numbers of microbes, and it is desirable to try to remove that which is readily available. All loose debris and pus are evacuated with suction. Irrigation may be employed to facilitate removal of debris, but it should be emphasized that the conventional irrigation strategy (pouring warm saline into the peritoneal cavity) does little to reduce the bacterial load adherent to the peritoneal surface in the abdomen. This irrigation strategy is useful for removing loose devitalized debris and fibrin but probably does not materially reduce bacterial counts. In recent years our group has employed pulsed lavage, commonly used to manage open fractures,[21] as it provides higher-velocity irrigation. We have found that it effectively separates much of the debris on the peritoneal surface on both the parietal peritoneum and the visceral peritoneum overlying the intestine itself; and it may be more effective in reducing the bacterial density. It clearly does not remove all of the densely adherent fibrin sometimes encountered, but this method does not risk injury to the wall of the intestine, which would be an issue if sharp dissection were used to remove this adherent fibrin.

Efforts to remove all debris within the peritoneal cavity have resulted in attempts to use radical peritoneal débridement.[22] The concept here is to sharply dissect all of the fibrin from the surface of the peritoneum. This process is fraught with considerable blood loss given the acute inflammation that exists. Furthermore, it is attended by complications when the patient subsequently develops an enterocutaneous fistula. A prospective randomized trial of radical peritoneal débridement failed to show an improvement in outcome in the patients who underwent that therapy when compared to more conventional strategies.[23]

Drains are commonly employed within the peritoneal cavity by some surgeons but serve no value in the patient with diffuse bacterial peritonitis. The entire peritoneal cavity cannot be drained; and, in fact, the patient with severe bacterial peritonitis has microorganisms disseminated throughout the abdominal compartment. Prospective studies have failed to show any benefit of intraabdominal drains in patients with peritonitis;[24] nevertheless, many types of drain are available, and the practice continues. It is unlikely that any drainage system can be of value.

A variation on the theme of using irrigation and drainage systems is the use of continuous peritoneal lavage with or without antibiotic solutions in the irrigant solution. Some reports have identified improved results with this treatment in patients with complex peritonitis.[25-29] Irrigation catheters are placed anteriorly at the time of the operation, and bilateral drainage catheters are placed in the paracolic gutters. Hourly introduction of irrigation solution is employed, with sequential drainage. These hourly exchanges are used for about 72 hours. This strategy is labor-intensive and has not gained acceptance. Systemic absorption of antibiotics does occur when antibiotics are introduced into the irrigant solution,[30] but antibiotics in the irrigation solution are of uncertain value when appropriate systemic antibiotics are being employed.

A final aspect when completing the surgical part of the procedure is wound closure. Debate continues over the merits of delayed primary closure versus primary closure of the surgical wound.[31] When contamination is massive and the patient is clearly seriously ill, wound management is hardly an issue in the overall length of stay in hospital; accordingly, delayed primary closure or even secondary closure may be preferable to the risks of an attempt at primary closure of the wound and the morbidity of a necrotizing infection of the abdominal wall. This point is of special concern when one is confronted with colonic perforations and sizable contamination. Postoperative management is best achieved with saline moist dressings. In general, topical antiseptics are toxic to the open wound and are not employed.

Antibiotics

Antibiotic therapy for patients with acute bacterial peritonitis customarily is oriented toward covering enteric gram-negative rods and obligate anaerobes. Table 27.3 defines a number of acceptable antibiotic combinations that have been shown in prospective randomized trials to be effective for treatment of patients with acute bacterial peritonitis.[32-42] It subscribes, with few exceptions, to the general recommendations of the Surgical Infection Society [43] but is certainly not all-inclusive of the potential choices studied in prospective randomized trials. Antibiotic strategies for the treatment of patients with intraabdominal infection can be classified into three general groups.

First, a popular antibiotic strategy is to use triple-drug therapy. This strategy uses an aminoglycoside (e.g., gentamicin) to cover the enteric gram-negative rods, metronidazole or clindamycin to cover the obligate anaerobes, and ampicillin directed against the enterococci. (Enterococcal coverage has not been proven to add measurably to the patient's outcome and generally is discouraged.) Metronidazole is generally chosen over clindamycin in that it has been shown to be clinically equivalent, and it is less expensive.[44]

An alternative double-drug combination of antibiotics is generally identified as the "gold standard" of antibiotic therapy for peritonitis. Probably the most data have been collected on the use of an aminoglycoside plus either clindamycin or metronidazole to treat patients with peritonitis. This strategy covers the likely pathogens of peritonitis and has consistently given good results. Aminoglycoside dosing can be precarious in the septic patient.[45] It is fraught with the potential risk of undosing when the patient has an expanded volume of distribution and exhibits the hyperdynamic septic response. Aggressive antibiotic dosing with aminoglycosides is generally encouraged during the initial phases of management in young patients with normal renal function. Dosing requirements diminish as the hyperdynamic response to SIRS declines.

Finally, considerable evidence supports use of a single antibiotic preparation that covers both aerobes and anaerobes. These strategies are usually with drugs that have a more favorable therapeutic ratio than do the aminoglycosides;

TABLE 27.3. Antibiotic Choices for Treatment of Acute Bacterial Peritonitis Supported by Randomized Clinical Trials.

Therapy	Dosage	Comments
Single agent		
Cefoxitin[32]	1–2 g q4–6h	Short half-life (45 min); low toxicity
Cefotetan[33]	1–2 g q12h	Longer half-life (3.5 hr); low toxicity
Ceftizoxime[34]	2 g q8–12h	Excellent gram-negative coverage; controversial anaerobic coverage
Ampicillin/sulbactam[35]	3 g q6h	Short half-life (1 hr); some gram-negative resistance
Ticarcillin/clavulanate[36]	3.1 g q4–6h	Short half-life (1 hr)
Piperacillin/tazobactam[37]	3.375 g q6h	Short half-life (1 hr); excellent comprehensive coverage
Imipenem/cilastatin[38]	0.5 g q6h	Short half-life (1 hr); excellent coverage
Meropenem[39]	1 g q8h	Short half-life (1 hr); excellent coverage
Combinations (one aerobic drug with one anaerobic drug)		
Aerobic choices		
Gentamicin	1–2 mg/kg q8h	Nephrotoxicity; unpredictable pharmacology; excellent gram-negative coverage
Tobramycin	1–2 mg/kg q8h	Same as gentamicin
Amikacin	5 mg/kg q8h	Same as gentamicin
Aztreonam[41]	2 g q8–12 h	Low toxicity; gram-negative coverage suspect
Ciprofloxacin[42]	750 mg q12h	Low toxicity
Anaerobic choices		
Clindamycin	600–900 mg q6h	Expensive; adds gram-positive coverage
Metronidazole	500 mg q6h	Inexpensive; strictly anaerobic coverage

prospective randomized trials of these agents compared to combination therapy have consistently demonstrated equivalent responses. Again there are few data that clearly define the unique features of dosing strategies for these agents in the patient with severe peritonitis. Generally it is desirable to use aggressive dosing strategies when confronted with patients who have severe bacterial peritonitis, particularly when the agent employed has a favorable therapeutic ratio.

The general supportive care of the patient with peritonitis is covered in numerous other chapters in this text. Briefly, the critical elements of managing these patients includes maximizing tissue perfusion, adequate oxygen delivery, and nutritional support. Optimum support assists appropriate management of the infection by minimizing the risks of the transition from SIRS to MODS.

Indications for Reoperation

A more extensive discussion of reoperation appears in Chapter 30. Generally, reoperation for patients with peritonitis must to be considered for two basic reasons. First, the patient may have had failure of a repair or failure of source control after the initial procedure. The characteristic feature of a patient with failed source control is severe decompensation, which can be identified during the first couple of days after the initial operation for peritonitis. Patients pursuing a rapid, fulminant septic course (e.g., severe SIRS) with rapid evolution of organ failure (MODS) after an operation where the source was presumably controlled probably justifies urgent, immediate reoperation. Any questions the surgeon may have had about potentially nonviable intestine from the original procedure may also warrant reexploration.

The judgment to pursue reoperation under these circumstances is purely empiric. No specific diagnostic study is of any value when trying to discern whether emergent reoperation is necessary. Furthermore, when patients have had an abdominal incision and abdominal exploration during the preceding 48–72 hours, physical examination of the abdomen is of limited value. Abdominal distension, spiking fever and leukocytosis, reduced urine output, increase volumes of fluid resuscitation, deteriorating pulmonary function, and overall evidence of end-organ failure within the first 2–3 days after abdominal exploration represent findings that necessitate reoperation.

The more common scenario for reoperation is the development of an abdominal abscess. Abdominal abscess is identified in approximately 10% of patients who have had operations for acute peritonitis.[6] Patients who have had a reoperation for abdominal infection may require a second.[12] Reoperation for abscess must be evaluated with less-invasive methods to drain pus. Accordingly, abdominal CT scanning becomes the diagnostic modality of choice for evaluating the patient with abscess; one should be prepared when doing an abdominal CT scan to have the radiologist perform percutaneous drainage if selected and specific conditions are met (Fig. 27.3). It is important to understand that patients who have undergone major abdominal operations for trauma or peritonitis as their first procedure can have a CT scan too soon after their original procedure. In general, diagnostic CT studies for abscess should not be done before the 7 days after the abdominal exploration. Anatomic landmarks are obscure, and commonly residual irrigation fluid may give false-positive results relative to the abscess. CT scans should not be performed during the first few days following exploration.

The CT scan can identify abscesses in the physiologic drainage basins of the abdomen. Many of these abscessed cavities are approachable by direct CT percutaneous drainage. If the patient is tolerating the septic process well and the CT catheter can gain access to the abscess cavity without traversing another hollow viscus within the abdomen, percutaneous drainage must be used. However, the patient with severe sepsis characterized by bacteremia and emerging organ failure should undergo formal abdominal exploration (see Chapter 30).

The reoperated patient poses formidable problems relative to the issue of wound management. The reoperated wound commonly has evidence of necrosis when there is a deep-seeded septic event. The multiply-operated abdominal wound commonly develops friable edges, and abdominal distension makes closure of the abdominal cavity extraordinarily difficult, running the risk of creating an abdominal compartment syndrome. Fascial margins become necrotic, and adequate débridement may simply make wound closure not feasible. Commonly these wounds must be left open and managed in an open fashion with or without the use of synthetic mesh (see Chapter 30).

Tertiary Peritonitis

Occasionally patients have such catastrophic situations in terms of the massive degree of peritoneal contamination that multiple sequential operations are necessary to achieve mechanical control of the infectious process. Furthermore, the magnitude and severity of the exudative response is such that effective drainage cannot be achieved closing the abdomen, which necessitates leaving the entire abdominal cavity open for frequent if not daily local explorations and irrigation of the peritoneal cavity. This circumstance of having a chronic fibrinopurulent peel and exudate across the surface of the visceral and parietal peritoneum in a patient with an open wound is termed *tertiary peritonitis*. These patients have this chronic exudative peritonitis usually with hospital-acquired gram-negative organisms.

Although antibiotics are inevitably used for these patients, this disease process requires meticulous, daily mechanical management. It is the overall systemic support of the patient and the local mechanical management of the open wound that ultimately results in survival. Extreme care when managing the tertiary peritonitis patient to avoid injuring the intestine with the daily débridement process is essential so fistula formation is avoided. Creation of a fistula in the middle of this open tertiary peritonitis wound is commonly a fatal complication. Thus, technical precision in irrigating and managing the open wound and in the day-to-day management of the dressings used for managing this wound are essential to avoid this complication.

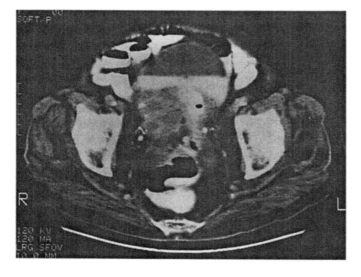

FIGURE 27.3. Abdominal/pelvic CT scan showing air bubbles within a pelvic abscess from a prior perforated appendix.

Conclusions

Peritonitis represents a complex disease process that requires precise judgment as to when operation is to be performed and what operative procedure is undertaken. The fundamental application of source control with drainage and dèbridement are paramount for patient recovery. Administration of systemic antibiotics against enteric gram-negative rods and the obligate anaerobes of the human colon is generally thought to be an important adjunctive measure in the management of these patients. Antibiotic therapy is probably best executed with aggressive dosing and at the earliest possible time in the patient's course. When an abscess and tertiary peritonitis evolve, it is unlikely that systemic antibiotic therapy is of primary value; rather, mechanical elimination of pus and exudate are the major features of successful management. Reoperation is always a difficult undertaking, but the precise use of clinical judgment and abdominal imaging techniques can allow either reoperation or percutaneous drainage methods to be employed to the patient's advantage. Hopefully, future developments that aid in augmenting the host responsiveness in the setting of acute peritonitis will add to the established armamentarium already employed in the management of these patients.

References

1. Deutschman CS, Konstantinides FN, Tsai M, et al: Physiology and metabolism in isolated viral septicemia: further evidence of an organism-independent, host-dependent response. Arch Surg 1987;122:21.
2. Eiseman B, Beart R, Norton L: Multiple organ failure. Surg Gynecol Obstet 1977;144:323–326.
3. Polk HC Jr, Shields CL: Remote organ failure: a valid sign of occult intra-abdominal infection. Surgery 1977;81:310–313.
4. Hinsdale JG, Jaffe BM: Reoperation for intraabdominal sepsis: indications and results in modern critical care setting. Ann Surg 1984;199:31–36.
5. Hoefs JC, Runyon BA: Spontaneous bacterial peritonitis. Dis Mon 1985;31:1.
6. Mosdell DM, Morris DM, Voltura A, et al: Antibiotic treatment for surgical peritonitis. Ann Surg 1991;214:543–549.
7. Autio V: The spread of intraperitoneal infection: studies with roentgen contrast medium. Acta Chir Scand Suppl 1964;321:5
8. Allen L, Weatherford T: Role of fenestrated basement membrane in lymphatic absorption from the peritoneal cavity. Am J Physiol 1956;197:551–554.
9. Tsilibary EC, Wissig SL: Absorption from the peritoneal cavity: SEM study of the mesothelium covering the peritoneal surface of the muscular portion of the diaphragm. Am J Anat 1977;149:127–132.
10. Polk HC Jr, Miles AA: Enhancement of bacterial infection by ferric iron: kinetics, mechanisms, and surgical significance. Surgery 1971;70:71–77.
11. Pruett TL, Rotstein OD, Fiegel VD, et al: Mechanisms of the adjuvant effect of hemoglobin in experimental peritonitis. VII. A leukotoxin is produced by *Escherichia coli* metabolism in hemoglobin. Surgery 1984;96:375–383.
12. Fry DE, Garrison RN, Heitsch RC, et al: Determinants of death in patients with intraabdominal abscess. Surgery 1980;89:517–523.
13. Chetlin SH, Elliott DW: Biliary bacteremia. Arch Surg 1971;102:303–307.
14. Onderdonk AB, Bartlett JC, Louie T, et al: Microbial synergy in experimental intraabdominal abscess. Infect Immun 1976;13:22–26.
15. Lorber B, Swenson RM: The bacteriology of intraabdominal infections. Surg Clin North Am 1975;55:1349–1358.
16. Bennion RS, Baron EJ, Thompson Jr JE, et al: The bacteriology of gangrenous and perforated appendicitis-revisited. Ann Surg 1990;211:165.
17. Christou NV, Turgeon P, Wassef R, et al: Management of intra-abdominal infections: the case for intraoperative cultures and comprehensive broad-spectrum antibiotic coverage. Arch Surg 1996;131:1193–1201.
18. Sheckman P, Onderdonk AB, Bartlett JG: Anaerobes in spontaneous peritonitis. Lancet 1977;2:1223.
19. Donovan AJ, Berne TV, Donovan JA: Perforated duodenal ulcer: an alternative plan. Arch Surg 1998;133:1166–1171.
20. Hurme T, Nylano E: Conservative versus operative treatment of appendicular abscess: experience of 147 consecutive patients. Ann Chir Gynecol 1995;84:33–36.
21. Rodeheaver GT, Pettry D, Thacker JG, et al: Wound cleansing by high pressure irrigation. Surg Gynecol Obstet 1975;141:357.
22. Hudspeth AS: Radical surgical debridement in the treatment of advanced generalized bacterial peritonitis. Arch Surg 1975;110:1233–1236.
23. Polk HC Jr, Fry DE: Radical peritoneal dèbridement for established peritonitis. Ann Surg 1980;192:350–355.
24. Stone HH, Hooper CA, Millikan WJ Jr: Abdominal drainage following appendectomy and cholecystectomy. Ann Surg 1978;187:606–612.
25. Atkins RC, Scott DF, Holdsworth SR, et al: Prolonged antibiotic peritoneal lavage in the management of gross generalized peritonitis. Med J Aust 1976;1:954.
26. Stephen M, Loewenthal J: Continuing peritoneal lavage in high-risk peritonitis. Surgery 1979;85:604–606.
27. Uden P, Eskilsson P, Brunes L, et al: A clinical evaluation of postoperative peritoneal lavage in the treatment of perforated appendicitis. Br J Surg 1983;70:348–349.
28. Leiboff AR, Soroff HS: The treatment of generalized peritonitis by closed postoperative peritoneal lavage. Arch Surg 1987;122:1005–1010.
29. Dobrin PB, O'Keefe P, Tatarowicz W, et al: The value of continuous 72-hour peritoneal lavage for peritonitis. Am J Surg 1989;157:368–371.
30. Fry DE, Trachtenburg L, Polk HC Jr: Serum kinetics of intraperitoneal moxalactam. Arch Surg 1986;121:282–284.
31. Brasel KJ, Borgstrom DC, Weigelt JA: Cost-utility analysis of contaminated appendectomy wounds. J Am Coll Surg 1997;184:23–30.
32. Malangoni MA, Condon RE, Spiegel CA: Treatment of intra-abdominal infections is appropriate with single-agent or combination antibiotic therapy. Surgery 1985;98:648–655.
33. Huizinga WK, Baker LW, Kadwa H, et al: Management of severe intra-abdominal sepsis: single agent antibiotic therapy with cefotetan versus combination therapy with ampicillin, gentamicin, and metronidazole. Br J Surg 1988;75:1134–1138.
34. Harding G, Vincelette J, Rachlis A, et al: A preliminary report on the use of ceftizoxime versus clindamycin-tobramycin for the therapy of intraabdominal and pelvic infections. J Antimicrob Chemother 1982;10(Suppl C):191–192.

35. Walker AP, Nichols RL, Wilson RF, et al: Efficacy of a beta-lactam inhibitor combination for serious intraabdominal infections. Ann Surg 1993;217:115–121.
36. Dougherty SH, Sirinik KR, Schauer PB, et al: Ticarcillin/clavulanate compared with clindamycin/gentamicin (with or without ampicillin) for the treatment of intraabdominal infection in pediatric and adult patients. Am Surg 1995;61:297–303.
37. Arguedas A, Sifuentes-Osornis J, Loaiza C, et al: An open, multicenter clinical trial of piperacillin/tazobactum in the treatment of pediatric patients with intraabdominal infections. J Chemother 1996;8:130–136.
38. Solomkin JS, Dellinger EP, Christou NV, Busuttil RW: Results of a multicenter trial comparing imipenem/cilastatin to tobramycin/clindamycin for intraabdominal infections. Ann Surg 1990;212:581–591.
39. Geroulanos SJ: Meropenem versus imipenem/cilastatin in intraabdominal infections requiring surgery. J Antimicrob Chemother 1995;36(Suppl A):191–205.
40. Donahue PE, Smith DL, Yellin AE, et al: Trovafloxacin in the treatment of intraabdominal infections: results of a double-blind, multicenter comparison with imipenem/cilastatin. Am J Surg 1998;176(Suppl 6A):53S–61S.
41. Barboza E, del Castillo M, Yi A, Gotuzzo E: Clindamycin plus amikacin versus clindamycin plus aztreonam in established intraabdominal infection. Surgery, 1994;116:28–35.
42. Solomkin JS, Reinhardt HH, Dellinger EP, et al: Results of a randomized trial comparing sequential intravenous/oral treatment with ciprofloxacin plus metronidazole to imipenem/cilastatin for intraabdominal infection. Ann Surg 1996;223:303–315.
43. Bohnen JMA, Solomkin JS, Dellinger EP, et al: Guidelines for clinical care: anti-infective agents for intra-abdominal infection. Arch Surg 1992;127:83–92.
44. Anonymous: Prospective, randomized comparison of metronidazole and clindamycin, each with gentamicin for the treatment of serious intra-abdominal infection. Surgery 1983;93:221–229.
45. Niemiec PW, Allo MD, Miller CF: Effect of altered volume of distribution on aminoglycoside levels in patients in surgical intensive care. Arch Surg 1987;122:207.

28
Hypothermia-Coagulopathy-Acidosis Syndrome: When to Operate/When to Stop Operating

Asher Hirshberg and Kenneth L. Mattox

Determining when to operate has traditionally been the most problematic decision when managing critically injured patients. Today the advent of aggressive trauma management algorithms now makes the decision to operate relatively straightforward. With few exceptions, the trauma patient in hemorrhagic shock is taken to the operating room within minutes of arrival at the hospital. Point of service adjuncts, including focused abdominal sonography, assist in the decision to operate.

Paradoxically, the most difficult decision trauma surgeons of the 1990s face is not when to operate but when to *stop* operating. This shift is a result of a major change in civilian wounding patterns characterized by an increased incidence of multivisceral, high-energy transfers (from automatic weapons and fast motor vehicles). Rapid access, control of hemorrhage, and reconstruction—the traditional operative sequence for trauma—are clearly inappropriate for the exsanguinating patient with extensive damage to multiple organs. Definitive repairs require lengthy, complex procedures that result in a lethal triad of hypothermia, coagulopathy, and acidosis.[1]

These observations led to the evolution of a revised operative sequence whereby only immediately life-threatening visceral damage is addressed using rapid temporary control measures. The operation is then stopped and the patient transferred to the intensive care unit (ICU) for resuscitation and stabilization. Definitive anatomic repair of the injuries is undertaken at a later date, when the patient is more hemodynamically stable and warmed. This staged repair is called "damage control".[2] Damage control represents a major paradigm shift in trauma surgery and is a revolutionary change in the way trauma surgeons view their role in the operating room. The center of attention has shifted from anatomic reconstruction to restitution of physiologic reserves. Anatomic integrity is temporarily sacrificed so the physiologic insult can be addressed before it becomes irreversible.[1,3] Herein lies the fundamental difference between the traditional operative approach to severe trauma, which views the operation as a single definitive event, and the damage control concept of staged repair.

"Physiologic Envelope"

The concept of the "physiologic envelope" is central to understanding the rationale behind the damage control approach. Despite technologic advances, the operating room remains a physiologically unfavorable and outright hostile environment for the severely wounded patient. The extensive peritoneal exposure during a laparotomy after trauma results in accelerated heat loss, which is further aggravated by massive transfusion. Hypothermia, in turn, contributes to coagulopathy and subsequently to shock, metabolic acidosis, and the need for further transfusion.[3]

This triad—hypothermia, coagulopathy, acidosis (HCA)—is a self-propagating vicious circle that eventually leads to an irreversible physiologic insult. It may present in the operating room as diffuse bleeding that cannot be controlled surgically, followed by refractory ventricular arrhythmias and intraoperative death.[4] More frequently, the operation is rapidly terminated and the irreversible insult manifests as ongoing postoperative oozing and rapidly evolving multisystem organ failure. In the surgical ICU, the trauma team attempts to contend with a refractory systolic blood pressure of 60–80 mmHg, oliguria, peripheral vasoconstriction, progressive hypoxemia, and troublesome oozing from every incision or vascular access site in addition to massive fluid accumulation in the face, tongue, and subcutaneous tissue. Death almost invariably occurs within the first few postoperative hours. Thus the HCA syndrome defines the patient's "physiologic envelope," a set of physiologic parameters that together mark the boundary between a survivable physiologic insult and an irreversible derangement. Termination of the operation before the "physiologic envelope" is breached is the essence of damage control strategy. Current understanding of the significance of the three components of this lethal syndrome and their interactions is partial at best. Other chapters in this book discuss the contribution of inflammatory mediators to the preservation or destruction of this physiologic envelope. It is important to examine these pathophysiologic mechanisms in some detail, as they are the most obvious cues the conditioned trauma surgeon looks for to support the decision to terminate the operation abruptly.

Coagulopathy

Diffuse "nonsurgical" bleeding is the most apparent clinical manifestation of the HCA syndrome. Although hemodilution and hypotension are contributing factors,[5] hypothermia is clearly the major cause of coagulopathy in the critically injured patient. Hypothermia affects clotting primarily through alteration of platelet function.[6] In the hypothermic patient, platelets are sequestered in the liver and spleen and exhibit marked morphologic changes.[7-9] Platelet activation is inhibited in vivo during hypothermia,[10] and thromboelastogram studies of hypothermic patients reveal altered platelet function.[11]

Additionally, because the enzymes of the clotting cascade are temperature-sensitive, the cascade is strongly inhibited during hypothermia.[3,12] Fibrinolysis, once presumed to play a key role in hypothermia-induced coagulopathy, is probably a lesser contributor. Nevertheless, consumption of clotting factors undoubtedly occurs late in the HCA syndrome and may well be considered a preterminal signal. Late-appearing consumption coagulopathy is indicative of multiorgan failure, systemic inflammatory response syndrome (SIRS), or infection. Coagulopathy in the critically injured patient is a clinical, not a laboratory, diagnosis. Standard coagulation tests often fail to reflect the full magnitude of the clotting disorder in these patients because they are routinely performed at 37°C.[13]

Acidosis

Lactic acidosis is the result of anaerobic glycolysis, reflecting inadequate tissue perfusion. It has been shown to affect myocardial contractility and cardiac output adversely in animal models,[14,15] but the precise physiologic and metabolic effects of acidosis in humans remain unclear. Acidosis is a closely monitored parameter in trauma patients because it is a useful measure of the severity of shock and a reliable predictor of survival. Serum lactate levels, base deficit, and the time interval to normalization of serum lactate have all been shown to correlate closely with mortality due to severe trauma in both animal models and clinical studies.[16] However, no well defined cutoff value is universally accepted as indicating irreversible shock. Furthermore, numerous extraneous factors, such as the presence of cocaine, may contribute to abnormal serum lactate and base deficit levels.

Hypothermia

Of the three components of the HCA syndrome, hypothermia is emerging as the central pathophysiologic event. Patients in shock secondary to penetrating torso injuries have a mean temperature of 34.5°C by the time they reach the operating room.[17] Most adult resuscitation and operating rooms are at temperatures approaching 22°C, as are the solutions stored in these rooms. Banked blood is stored at 4°C. When rapidly infused without warming devices, these cold solutions contribute to hypothermia. The open peritoneal cavity is another dominant source of accelerated intraoperative heat loss.[18]

The HCA syndrome is not always present in hypothermic syndromes, even with some element of trauma superimposed. Thus the mere presence of hypothermia (especially in the absence of coagulopathy) is not a predictor of death. However, hypothermia is harmful and adversely affects survival independently of other variables, such as injury severity.[19,20]

The full spectrum of the physiologic and metabolic effects of hypothermia remains ill-defined, but it has been associated with increased systemic vascular resistance, decreased cardiac output, cardiac arrhythmias, and a leftward shift in the oxyhemoglobin dissociation curve.[21,22] In the context of severe trauma, the adverse effect of hypothermia on coagulation is the most important one because coagulopathy sets in motion the self-propagating vicious circle of the HCA syndrome.

Of the three components of the "physiologic envelope," hypothermia is the only one for which there is a well defined endpoint. In 1987 Jurkovich et al.[20] convincingly demonstrated that in severely wounded patients undergoing laparotomy a core temperature below 32°C is associated with 100% mortality.

Damage Control Strategy

Damage control for severe trauma consists of: (1) initial operation; (2) surgical ICU resuscitation; and (3) planned reoperation.[1,23] The initial operation is a rapid "bail-out" procedure where sometimes unorthodox and temporary techniques are used to control bleeding, prevent spillage of intestinal content or urine, restore blood flow to vital vascular beds, and effect rapid closure of the abdomen or chest.[24] In other words, the surgeon does only the absolute minimum necessary to save the patient's life, deliberately avoiding formal resections and reconstructions or definitive closure of the visceral cavities.

The timing and technique of abdominal damage control tactics are the keys to success. Recognition that a patient potentially has exsanguinating hemorrhage and enteral spillage that must be rapidly controlled is one of the most difficult lessons to learn. Control should be accomplished literally within a few minutes of entering the abdomen. A hand is swept over the liver and spleen, seeking the presence of a large injury; if present, numerous laparotomy packs are placed preparatory to further exploration. Contained right-sided suprarenal hematomas are *not* opened and explored. Contained nonexpanding pelvic hematomas are *not* opened and explored. The retroperitoneum at the areas of the aorta, inferior vena cava, portal vein, and mesenteric vessels is examined.

In patients for whom the damage control approach has been chosen, uncontrolled bleeding sites or expanding hematomas are exposed and control attempted, reserving reconstruction for later staged operations. Considerations for temporary intravascular stents in the portal vein, inferior vena cava, or abdominal aorta are part of the damage control tactics. The packs in the area of the spleen and liver are examined and replaced with fresh laparotomy pads, ensuring that the vena cava is not compressed. Laparotomy and instrument counts are unnecessarily time-consuming, as exploration and radiographs are part of subsequent operations to ensure removal of all foreign bodies. Use of umbilical tapes, gross sutures, or intestinal staples are rapidly applied to control enteric spillage, even if temporary blind loops are created. Only the skin is closed, with application of skin towel clips (20–35 clips) or a large running synthetic suture. Should an abdominal compartment be created by the closure, a "Bogota bag" plastic sheet is applied, even at the original operation, suturing the bag to the skin.

The patient is then transferred to the surgical ICU for aggressive resuscitation, hemodynamic stabilization, and correction of hypothermia. Reoperation is undertaken in a stable patient, usually within 24–48 hours of the initial operation. It includes definitive repair of injuries and formal closure of the operated cavity.

The traditional single definitive operation is appropriate for most wounded patients. The damage control approach is indicated in the few trauma patients who sustain multivisceral injuries requiring complex repairs or those who are exsanguinating. The price of a staged repair is a high incidence of major complications related mainly to intraabdominal infection, fistula formation, and problems with delayed abdominal closure.[1,4,23] One of the most difficult aspects of this surgical strategy is determining when to abandon the traditional operative sequence and embark on an approach that may give the patient a better chance of survival but is also associated with much higher morbidity if used unnecessarily.[24]

Neural Network Model

We attempted to analyze the decision to "bail out" by means of an artificial neural network model. The underlying hypothesis was that a neutral network could be built and trained to predict early postoperative death (within 12 hours of the operation) using a limited set of injury severity and physiologic data. The neural network was constructed using a commercial software package (Brainmaker Pro; California Scientific Software, Nevada City, CA, USA). The input layer of the network consisted of six nodes representing parameters available to the surgeon during the first hour of the operation (patient's age, lowest intraoperative systolic blood pressure, lowest pH of arterial blood, lowest core temperature, volume of transfused blood, and the Abdominal Trauma Index). There was one node in the output layer predicting survival or death. A back-propagation algorithm was used to train the network on clinical data sets from 117 injured patients in shock who underwent emergency laparotomy. Despite repeated runs using various configuration of hidden layers, the neural network could be trained to predict the patient's outcome only with an error rate of 15%, well above the desired rate of less than 5%. This failure of the neural network to predict imminent death reliably in critically injured patients based on physiologic and injury severity parameters shows that the decision to "bail out" cannot be made on the basis of objective quantifiable data alone. The decision must incorporate other factors, such as precise circumstances in the operating room, human factors, and subjective surgical judgment. Thus the decision to stop operating is a complex, multifaceted one that is difficult to analyze and teach.

Experienced trauma surgeons tend to make the critical decision to "bail out" early in the course of the operation, as supported by data from two retrospective studies. In one series of 56 trauma patients whose operations were abruptly terminated, 37 patients had intraoperative evidence of diffuse coagulopathic bleeding, and 19 patients did not.[23] Of the 37 patients, 16 died. Among the 19 patients without a clinical coagulopathy, only 3 died. In another series of 70 patients[25] early decision to employ temporary hemostasis by packing was a key determinant of survival after severe abdominal trauma.

Instead of relying on physiologic parameters, experienced trauma surgeons use injury pattern recognition on which to base the decision to "bail out." Major abdominal vascular injury combined with hollow or solid visceral damage, destruction of the pancreaticoduodenal complex, highgrade liver injury, and open pelvic fracture are examples of injury patterns where an early decision to employ damage control is indicated.[24]

Quantitative Analysis of the Physiologic Envelope

Attempts to define quantitatively the physiologic envelope in the severely injured patient are currently the focus of much attention. Burch et al.[4] first attempted to predict physiologic irreversibility by regression analysis of intraoperative pH and transfusion requirement data from a series of 200 patients undergoing damage control laparotomy at the Ben Taub General Hospital in Houston, Texas. However, this analysis, based on incomplete retrospective data, failed to yield useful guidelines that can be applied in practice.

More recently, Cosgriff et al.[26] tried to predict the onset of coagulopathy by prospectively analyzing data from 58 injured patients who received massive transfusions. Multiple logistic regression identified four significant risk factors that predict onset of coagulopathy: (1) pH < 7.10; (2) temperature < 34°C; (3) Injury Severity Score > 25; and (4) systolic blood pressure < 70 mmHg. Approximately one-fourth of these 58 patients developed a coagulopathy; but when all four conditions were present, the probability of developing a coagulopathy was 98%. The diagnosis of coagulopathy in this study was based on prolongation of prothrombin and partial thromboplastin times and carried a mortality rate of only 43%.

In another study with a similar aim, Cushman et al.[27] evaluated a series of 53 patients with iliac vascular injuries. The study showed significant differences between the initial and final operating room temperature and the acid-base status of survivors compared to that of nonsurvivors. An initial pH of <7.1 and a final operating room temperature of <35°C were the best predictors of imminent death in these patients.

Although these studies represent important attempts to quantify the "physiologic envelope," their practical usefulness

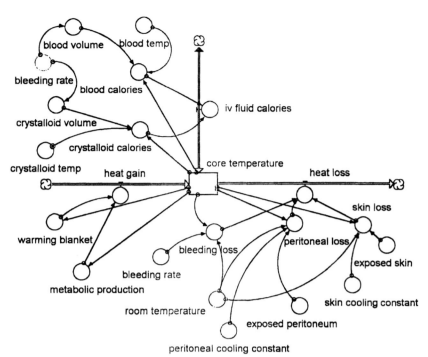

FIGURE 28.1. Single compartment STELLA model of intraopertaive heat loss during laparotomy for exsanguinating hemorrhage in an operating room with an ambient temperature of 21°C. It represents a set of difference equations that are solved numerically. The only accumulation is core temperature, marked by a rectangle. Heat gain and loss are control variables that update the accumulation every 6 minutes. Factors affecting flow are marked by circles. The model equations and parameters were described by Hirshberg et al.[29]

to the operating surgeon is limited. The surgeon may know that pH < 7.1 or a core temperature < 34°C is associated with an increased risk of coagulopathy and death, but the surgeon does not know how quickly or slowly these values will be reached. The extreme clinical circumstances of laparotomy for exsanguinating hemorrhage preclude controlled clinical trials and make it difficult to use animal models to answer this central question. A different approach is clearly needed to define the time frame from beginning of operation to onset of physiologic irreversibility.

Computer Simulation of Intraoperative Heat Loss

Heat loss in the operating room is not only the key element of the physiologic envelope but a continually monitored well defined physical phenomenon that can be described in mathematic terms. Burch et al.[28] calculated heat loss during surgery for severe trauma and were able to quantify the rapid development of hypothermia using a simple mathematic model. Because hypothermia has a well defined endpoint of 32°C, beyond which mortality in trauma patients is 100%,[20] the time interval from the beginning of operation until the core temperature reaches 32°C represents the window of opportunity to salvage the patient.

Using these basic assumptions, a single-compartment dynamic computer model of heat loss during laparotomy for exsanguinating hemorrhage was developed and implemented.[29] The graphic modeling language STELLA 5.0 (High Performance Systems, Hanover, NH, USA) was employed to describe all heat flows into and from a 70-kg patient undergoing laparotomy for exsanguinating hemorrhage (Fig. 28.1). Because a patient in hemorrhagic shock is maximally vasoconstricted, internal redistribution of heat from the core to the periphery is minimal.[30] Thus from the modeling viewpoint, the body can be treated as a single thermal compartment.[31] Heat gain and loss calculations were based on experimental[18] and clinical[32] data in the literature. The time interval from beginning of laparotomy until the patient had reached the critical core temperature of 32°C was computed in successive simulation runs under varying intraoperative conditions. The model predicted an exponential decline in body temperature with time, so that with an initial core temperature of 36°C the time interval to 32°C is only 66 minutes. The patient's thermal balance is dominated by heat loss from the exposed peritoneal surfaces, which cannot be offset by a warming blanket or warmed intravenous fluids. So long as blood and fluid replacement remain in a roughly normothermic range (35°–38°C), the patient's heat loss curve is only moderately affected even by extreme changes in the bleeding rate. Elevating the operating room ambient temperature can buy the surgeon valuable time, but rapid closure of the open peritoneal cavity is the only way to correct from a negative to a positive balance (Fig. 28.2).

This computer model shows that the window of opportunity before physiologic irreversibility sets in cannot be longer than 60–90 minutes, even under the most favorable circumstances; and it is often shorter. For example, if the patient's core temperature at the beginning of the operation is below 35°C, the model predicts that the time frame to irreversibility is about half an hour, too short a time for effective surgical intervention.

This computer model is the first attempt to define the boundaries of the "physiologic envelope" quantitatively, not in terms of target values of selected parameters but as a dynamic

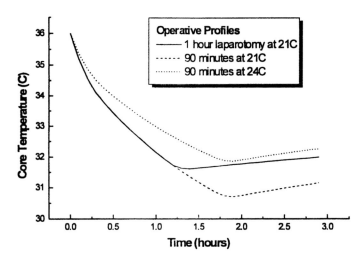

FIGURE 28.2. Simulation of heat loss during "damage control" laparotomy using a typical operative profile. Temporary control of bleeding at 15 minutes reduces blood loss from 100 ml/min to 50 ml/min. Definitive control of bleeding occurs at 30 minutes. Peritoneal exposure is adjusted from 50% to 25% according to the operative steps. Four liters of normothermic blood are administered through a rapid-infusion device (36°C) with 4 liters of crystalloids, only half of which are normothermic; the rest are at room temperature.[29] Heat loss is simulated for a 1-hour "damage control" laparotomy, for a longer peritoneal exposure (90 minutes), and for an elevated ambient temperature.

time frame which, albeit short, can be modified by intraoperative conditions and the surgeon's actions.

Decision to Reoperate

Formal completion of the "damage control" sequence is a planned reoperation on a rewarmed, stable patient in whom the HCA syndrome has been successfully treated. Yet the optimal timing of reoperation remains controversial. Although it is generally believed that longer delays between the original damage control procedure and the planned reoperation increase the risk of infection, good supporting evidence has only recently been published.[33] The surgeon must also be concerned about returning to the operating room "too early," thus setting the stage for a second HCA syndrome. Tissue edema, surgical bleeding, early inflammation, erosions, and even infections are encountered at reoperation; but for a patient with a normal temperature, pH > 7.2, and normal coagulation profile, recurrence of the HCA syndrome is rare, unless the original syndrome is still present.

Clinical circumstances such as a severely ischemic limb, bowel interrupted at several sites (creating a closed loop), and suboptimal control of spillage (e.g., a packed nonrepaired renal or duodenal disruption)[34] occasionally leads to an early reoperation before the "physiologic envelope" is completely restituted. Continued bleeding or progressive intraabdominal hypertension may dictate an urgent (unplanned) reoperation. The decision to reoperate may be difficult in these patients because during the first few hours in the surgical ICU they are cold and coagulopathic and therefore continue to bleed. The key factors are not whether the patient is bleeding but whether the amount and rate of blood loss exceed what is expected in the specific patient and whether bleeding is from a controllable surgical source or due to diffuse coagulopathic oozing.[35] This complex decision relies heavily on impressions gained at the original operative procedures and should therefore be made by the same surgeon.

The need for urgent decompression is obvious in most patients with abdominal compartment syndrome, defined as organ failure secondary to increased intraabdominal pressure[36] and typically presenting with hypotension, oliguria, and grossly impaired ventilatory mechanics. The abdominal compartment syndrome, with a mortality rate of more than 70%, is a dramatic, rapidly lethal complication of damage control surgery. It is not an isolated, unpredictable clinical occurrence but, rather, the result of untreated progressive intraabdominal hypertension.[37] Intraabdominal pressure can easily be monitored in the ICU, and levels above 20–25 cm H_2O are generally considered an indication for decompression. Occasionally, a slowly progressive rise in intraabdominal pressure is observed in a patient who has not yet fully recovered from the HCA syndrome and is still hypothermic and coagulopathic. These patients who have not yet developed the clinical signs of the abdominal compartment syndrome but are prone to do so present some of the most difficult decision dilemmas faced by trauma surgeons.

Conclusions

The "damage control" approach has significantly changed the concept of trauma resuscitation, which begins in the field, continues in the emergency room and operating room, and ends only upon reaching a supported stable state in the surgical ICU. Thus for the exsanguinating trauma patient, the initial surgical procedure is merely one of four links in the "resuscitation chain," not to be used alone for definitive visceral repair.

The critical decisions in "damage control" surgery revolve around the HCA syndrome. In fact, the ultimate purpose of this strategy is to avoid the syndrome. Although fewer than 6% of severely injured patients presenting to a trauma center develop the HCA syndrome, the surgeon must be aware of it and of the ways and means to anticipate and avoid it. The decision to stop operating and to "bail out" should be made 5–10 minutes into the procedure, long before the first clinical signs of the HCA syndrome.

The HCA syndrome following major trauma is a teleologic aberration. Prior to development of advanced prehospital transportation and current management of critically injured patients in trauma centers, this syndrome was not encountered. Patients with the potential for developing the syndrome died before arrival at the trauma center or in the operating room. That this syndrome exists is credit to significant advances in all four links of the "resuscitation chain" for critically injured patients. Further study and better understanding of this syndrome will allow continued advances in the care of this challenging group of trauma patients.

References

1. Hirshberg A, Mattox KL: Planned reoperation for severe trauma. Ann Surg 1995;222:3–8.
2. Rotondo MF, Schwab CW, McGonigal MD, et al: "Damage control": an approach for improved survival in exsanguinating penetrating abdominal injury. J Trauma 1993;35:375–382.
3. Rotondo MF, Zonies DH: The damage control sequence and underlying logic. Surg Clin North Am 1997;77:761–777.
4. Burch JM, Ortiz VB, Richardson RJ, Martin RR, Mattox KL, Jordan GL Jr: Abbreviated laparotomy and planned reoperation for critically injured patients. Ann Surg 1992;215:476–482.
5. Hewson JR, Neame PB, Kumar N, et al: Coagulopathy related to dilution and hypotension during massive transfusion. Crit Care Med 1985;13:387–391.
6. Patt A, McCroskey BL, Moore E: Hypothermia-induced coagulopathies in trauma. Surg Clin North Am 1988;68:775–785.
7. Villalobos T, Adelson E, Barilia T: Hematolytic changes in hypothermic dogs. Proc Soc Exp Biol Med 1955;89:192–196.
8. Hessel E, Schmer G, Dillard D: Platelet kinetics during deep hypothermia. J Surg Res 1980;28:23–27.
9. White T, Krivit W: An ultrastructural basis for the shape changes induced in platelets by chilling blood. Blood 1967;30:635–675.
10. Michelson AD, MacGregor H, Barnard MR, Kestin AS, Rohrer MJ, Valeri CR: Reversible inhibition of human platelet activation by hypothermia in vivo and in vitro. Thromb Haemost 1994;71:633–640.
11. Watts DD, Trask A, Soeken K, Perdue P, Dols S, Kaufmann C: Hypothermic coagulopathy in trauma: effect of varying levels of hypothermia on enzyme speed, platelet function, and fibrinolytic activity. J Trauma 1998;44:846–854.
12. Rohrer MJ, Natale AM: Effects of hypothermia on the coagulation cascade. Crit Care Med 1992;20:1402–1405.
13. Reed RL II, Johnson TD, Hudson JD, Fischer RP: The disparity between hypothermic coagulopathy and clotting studies. J Trauma 1992;33:465–470.
14. Wildenthal K, Mierzwiak DS, Myers RW: Effects of acute lactic acidosis on left ventricular performance. Am J Physiol 1968;214:1352–1359.
15. Yudkin J, Cohen RD, Slack B: The haemodynamic effects of metabolic acidosis in the rat. Clin Sci Mol Med 1976;50:177–184.
16. Porter JM, Ivatury RR: In search of the optimal end points of resuscitation in trauma patients: a review. J Trauma 1998;44:908–914.
17. Bickell WH, Wall MJ Jr, Pepe PE, et al: Immediate versus delayed fluid resuscitation for hypotensive patients with penetrating torso injuries. N Engl J Med 1994;331:1105–1109.
18. English MJM, Papenberg R, Farias E, Scott WAC, Hinchey J: Heat loss in an animal experimental model. J Trauma 1991;31:36–38.
19. Gentilello LM, Jurkovich GJ, Stark MS, Hassantash SA, O'Keefe GE: Is hypothermia in the victim of major trauma protective or harmful? A randomized, prospective study. Ann Surg 1997;226:439–447.
20. Jurkovich GJ, Greiser WB, Luterman A, Curreri PW: Hypothermia in trauma victims: an ominous predictor of survival. J Trauma 1987;27:1019–1022.
21. Michenfelder JD, Uihlein A, Saw EF, Theye RA: Moderate hypothermia in man: hemodynamic and metabolic effects. Br J Anaesth 1965;37:738–745.
22. Coniam SW: Accidental hypothermia. Anesthesia 1979;34:250–256.
23. Hirshberg A, Wall MJ Jr, Mattox KL: Planned reoperation for trauma: a two year experience with 124 consecutive patients. J Trauma 1994;37:365–369.
24. Hirshberg A, Walden R: "Damage control" for abdominal trauma. Surg Clin North Am 1997;77:813–820.
25. Garrison JR, Richardson JD, Hilakos AS, et al: Predicting the need to pack early for severe intra-abdominal hemorrhage. J Trauma 1996;40:923–927.
26. Cosgriff N, Moore EE, Sauaia A, Kenny-Moynihan M, Burch J, Galloway B: Predicting life threatening coagulopathy in the massively transfused trauma patient: hypothermia and acidoses revisited. J Trauma 1997;42:857–862.
27. Cushman JG, Feliciano DV, Renz BM, et al: Iliac vessel injury: operative physiology related to outcome. J Trauma 1997;42:1033–1040.
28. Burch JM, Denton JR, Noble RD: Physiologic rationale for abbreviated laparotomy. Surg Clin North Am 1997;77:779–782.
29. Hirshberg A, Stein M, Walden R: A computer simulation of hypothermia during "damage control" laparotomy. World J Surg 1999;23:960–963.
30. Forstot RM: The etiology and management of inadvertent perioperative hypothermia. J Clin Anesth 1995;7:657–674.
31. Ereth MH, Lennon RL, Sessler DI: Limited heat transfer between thermal compartments during rewarming in vasoconstricted patients. Aviat Space Environ Med 1992;63:1065–1069.
32. Little RA, Stoner HB: Body temperature after accidental injury. Br J Surg 1981;68:221–224.
33. Abikhaled JA, Granchi TS, Wall MJ, Hirshberg A, Mattox KL: Prolonged abdominal packing for trauma is associated with increased morbidity and mortality. Am Surg 1997;63:1109–1112.
34. Hirshberg A, Stein M, Adar R: Reoperation: planned and unplanned. Surg Clin North Am 1997;77:897–907.
35. Hirshberg A, Wall MJ Jr, Ramchandani MK, Mattox KL: Reoperation for bleeding in trauma. Arch Surg 1993;128:1163–1167.
36. Saggi BH, Sugerman HJ, Ivatury RR, Bloomfield GL: Abdominal compartment syndrome. J Trauma 1998;45:597–609.
37. Ivatury RR, Porter JM, Simon RJ, Islam S, John R, Stahl WM: Intraabdominal hypertension after life-threatening penetrating abdominal trauma: prophylaxis, incidence, and clinical relevance to gastric mucosal pH and abdominal compartment syndrome. J Trauma 1998;44:1016–1021.

29
Early Definitive Fracture Fixation with Polytrauma: Advantages Versus Systemic/Pulmonary Consequences

Hans-Christoph Pape and Harald Tscherne

A considerable change in the treatment of fractures in patients with blunt multiple injuries has occurred during the last decades. During the 1950s and 1960s a high mortality rate in multiply-injured patients appeared to be inevitable. The major issue was the rate of fracture healing. Better union of femoral fractures was believed to occur in patients with delayed operative stabilization (more than 6 days after trauma). It was argued that the operation itself represented a major insult, with considerable blood loss. Initial surgical stabilization was allowed only if the patient was in a clinically excellent condition.[1] Some authors even recommended delaying surgery until 10–14 days after the injury.[2] In his book on fracture treatment, Küntscher's recommendations for intramedullary stabilization of major fractures included the following.[3]

1. Do not nail as long as symptoms of fat embolization are present. Take special precautions in cases of multiple fractures ... and extensive injuries to soft tissues.
2. Do not nail immediately, but wait a few days.

The major fear of surgeons treating these patients was the fat embolism syndrome.[4] Pulmonary dysfunction, the hallmark of this problem, develops several days after trauma. Once the fat embolism syndrome becomes full-blown, therapy was often in vain or only postpones death; mortality rates of around 50% were reported.[4] This syndrome was believed due to fat and intramedullary contents liberated in an unstabilized fracture. Consequently it was deduced that stabilization of major fractures can prevent this complication.[5–7]

During the 1970s and 1980s, along with improved intraoperative monitoring, postoperative care, and intensive care, a more aggressive surgical approach for fracture treatment began. The definition of early operative treatment implied stabilization within 24 h.[6] Retrospective analyses reported improved survival and fewer pulmonary complications such as pneumonia and fat embolism syndrome. Seibel et al., in 56 trauma patients with femoral or acetabular fractures, compared the clinical course according to the time of surgical stabilization and found that delayed stabilization was associated with a longer hospital and intensive care unit (ICU) stay.[7] The benefit from early operative treatment was described as directly proportional to the injury severity. A group of 132 trauma patients with ISS > 18 points and primary stabilization (operative intervention within 24 hours) were reviewed. The type of operation was not specified. A severely traumatized group with an ISS > 40 was investigated separately. In this subgroup the incidence of ARDS was 17% if surgery on the femur was done within 24 hours it was 75% in patients with later stabilization. The authors concluded that with more severe injuries a better outcome was provided by early operation.[8] A prospective clinical trial investigated the difference between early (<24 hours) and late (>24 hours after injury) femoral stabilization in 178 patients. One group of 95 patients had minor associated injuries (mean ISS 11.4 points). The other group of 83 multiply-injured patients had an average HTI/ISS of 31.5 points. In the latter group only 1 of 46 patients with early femoral osteosynthesis developed acute respiratory distress syndrome (ARDS) in contrast to 6 of 37 patients following delayed osteosynthesis (type of surgery not specified).[9]

During this time, a stepwise approach was used in other centers that included stabilization of major fractures within 24 hours. Several time intervals are differentiated: The first operative period includes emergency life-saving procedures performed within 1–2 hours ("acute period"). This is followed by the "primary period" (day 1 surgery) for limb-preserving procedures, open fractures, open joints, closed limb fractures, and compartment syndromes. The "secondary" period, defined as 48–72 hours after trauma, serves for reconstructive procedures requiring prolonged operation, such as for severe intraarticular fractures. During the "tertiary" period, defined as >72 hours after injury, more prolonged joint reconstructions, such as for acetabular fractures, may be performed, as may secondary wound closure and bone grafting.[10]

In contrast, at the beginning of the 1990s the dogma of "early total care" (fracture stabilization) in all multiple-trauma patients was reviewed because of a European multicenter study. Among 1127 patients with femoral fractures a remarkably high rate of pulmonary complications was found after primary (<24 hours) stabilization, which was mainly performed by reamed nailing. These problems were particularly noticeable in the young age group, 20–30 years old, with no risk of pulmonary complications due to preexistent disease. Almost no patient had suffered thoracic trauma. Therefore the timing and the type of surgical stabilization were believed to play the major role.[11] This observation was supported by other retrospective reports.[12,13]

Studies that previously advocated primary stabilization in all trauma patients were criticized for the study design (e.g., inclusion of patients who died from hemorrhagic shock and head trauma, inclusion of patients undergoing no fracture reduction in the late operation group, their definition of ARDS.[12-15] It was confirmed that, in general, primary stabilization continues to be the method of choice for major fractures in patients with severe blunt trauma.[12-15] However, it was doubtful that this concept was applicable to all patients. The surgical procedures performed might cause an additional burden for the patient. Questions remain about the relevance of other factors, such as severity of injury, associated chest trauma, the patient's preoperative condition, and the type of the surgical procedure (e.g., reamed versus unreamed nails). The following sections summarize these studies and their clinical significance.

Fracture Treatment in the Polytrauma Patient

Gold Standard: Early Definitive Stabilization of Major Fractures

A major aim of treating the multiple-trauma patient with fractures is rapid stabilization of their extremity injuries. Intramedullary nailing (IMN) is the method of choice for long bone fractures. The biomechanical properties, including a higher bending strength, are more favorable if the implant is inside the medullary canal.[16] Nailing causes less soft tissue injury and less blood loss. Most centers reported more rapid mobilization after IMN.[17] Rogers et al. categorized 67 patients with isolated femur fractures into three groups retrospectively according to immediate (<24 hours), early (24–72 hours), or late (>72 hours) surgical fixation of a femoral shaft fracture. Patients undergoing fracture fixation at 24–72 hours had complication rates similar to those who underwent immediate (<24 hours) fixation. The longest operating time was found in patients stabilized as an emergency. The authors concluded that extending the time for early fixation permitted the patient to be put into the elective operation schedule, allowing more optimal utilization of resources. They stated that "this approach might be more appealing to busy orthopedic surgeons and to the hospital administration since this would reduce the emergency use of the operating room during the evening and night shifts."[18]

A retrospective study used the statewide hospital discharge base in North Carolina and categorized 2805 adults over 16 years of age into two groups according to the ISS (ISS < 15 or ISS > 15). Four groups were identified: group 1, nonsurgical; group 2, surgery < 1 day; group 3, surgery 2–4 days; and group 4, surgery > 4 days. There was a high mortality rate among patients treated nonsurgically regardless of the severity of injury.

However, in the patient groups with ISS > 15, surgery within 1 day was associated with a higher mortality rate (3.8%) than in patients operated at 2–4 days (1.8%) or after 4 days (1.5%); this difference was statistically significant. There was a progressive increase in length of hospitalization with delayed operative intervention. The authors concluded that a patient should undergo "initial stabilization and management of life-threatening interventions followed by repair of the femoral shaft fracture within 4 days after injury."[19]

Reynolds et al. summarized 105 patients with femoral shaft fractures treated by reamed IMN over an 11-year period. Patients were categorized based on immediate nailing (IMN < 24 hours), early treatment (IMN 24–48 hours), and late treatment (IMN > 48 hours). With low injury severity (ISS < 18) there was a tendency toward fewer pulmonary complications in the immediate operation group. No relation between timing and outcome was seen in multiple-trauma patients (ISS > 18). The authors criticized all previous authors stating that "none of these studies have proven that the improvements in outcome were an isolated effect of improved treatment of the femur fracture."[14]

Bosse et al. undertook a retrospective study of patients submitted to either reamed femoral nailing or plate osteosynthesis. No difference in the incidence of ARDS was found.[20] The study design may be criticized because (1) the two patient groups were treated in different hospitals; and (2) patients with both proximal and distal femoral fractures were included, even though the major effect of fat embolization is known to occur with proximal fractures.

We studied pulmonary complications (ARDS) in multiple-trauma patients submitted to reamed IMN. In these patients, early IMN was associated with a significantly lower ventilation time and total ICU stay compared to patients undergoing secondary stabilization. In addition, a higher rate of infectious pulmonary complications was observed in the group with no thoracic trauma and delayed treatment. This finding emphasized a positive effect of primary stabilization in these patients.[15]

In summary, most studies during the 1980s agreed that primary fracture stabilization is advantageous when compared with primary traction of the injured extremity. This concept was also accepted for the multiple-trauma situation. No study has compared the effects of different stabilization procedures or special cases such as additional chest trauma. Reports on this topic are discussed below.

Lung as a Target Organ After Severe Blunt Trauma

Recent emphasis on the pulmonary complications of nonthoracic trauma has increased usage of the term "shock lung" and given the implication that the lung is a target organ in instances of shock.
—Joel H. Horovitz, 1974[21]

Following blunt trauma, debris from open wounds and from the fracture site enters the venous circulation and the lungs. Some authors called the lung a "filter," preventing these

29. Early Definitive Fracture Fixation with Polytrauma

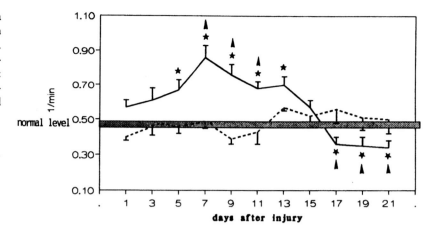

FIGURE 29.1. Changes in reticuloendothelial system function (K_2 value) in blunt multiple trauma patients. In 20 healthy volunteers the normal range was 0.47 ± 0.06. In nonsurvivors (group N; solid line) an increase developed within the first week after injury: group N: 0.86 ± 0.10 on day 7 ($p = 0.003$) compared with survivors (group S; broken line) (0.48 ± 0.08 on day 7) and controls. (From Pape et al.,[35] with permission.)

substances from entering the arterial bloodstream.[22] Trauma-induced hemorrhage causes an increase in microvascular permeability, which occurs in all organs including the lung.[23,24] The lung has an extraordinary ability to clear interstitial fluid via the lymphatic systems.[25] Because the lung has the largest microvascular bed in the body, an increase in interstitial edema and a reduction of oxygenation capacity may occur.[26]

Unreduced and unstabilized fractures are source of intramedullary contents entering the bloodstream,[27] which may induce the formation of thrombi due to a high thromboplastin content.[28] With unreduced fractures care in bed produces additional local soft tissue trauma, muscle necrosis, and pain. These mechanisms alter the systemic immunologic response that may secondarily affect the lung.[7,27,29]

The effects of blunt trauma on the hemostatic response are well known and range from blockage of the pulmonary microvasculature[30] to disseminated intravascular coagulation.[31] Impaired host defense plays a major role, and the increased adhesiveness of inflammatory cells inside the lung is well known.[32,33] External pathogens may enter the bloodstream in shock states[34] and are usually inactivated by the reticuloendothelial system (RES). Nonsurviving trauma patients showed inadequate RES function,[35] which may enable these pathogens to cause adverse effects in the lung (Fig. 29.1).

Pathogenetic Consequences of Intramedullary Fixation of Long Bones

Systemic Mechanisms Induced by Intramedullary Instrumentation

Primary Mechanisms

In uninjured long bone the normal intramedullary pressure ranges between 15 and 30 mmHg.[36,37] Intramedullary instrumentation (IMN) creates a piston-like effect that causes intravasation of bone marrow contents.[38,39] The volume of fat intravasated during insertion of an intramedullary femoral nail was estimated to be 20–80 cc.[40,41] A transient increase in pulmonary arterial pressure occurs, which was up to 10 mmHg in humans and even more in experimental models[42–44] within the first minutes after reaming (Fig. 29.2).

The question is whether intramedullary fat is the only cause of this pressure increase, as fat is able to pass arteriovenous shunting systems in the lung, followed by systemic spread.[45]

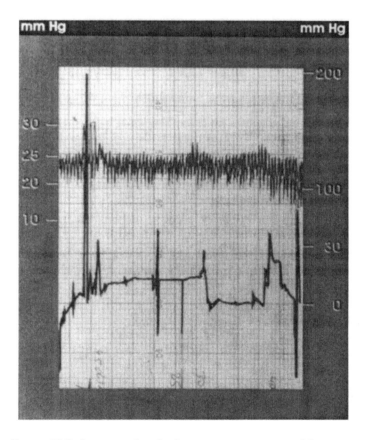

FIGURE 29.2. Intraoperative simultaneous measurements of intramedullary (right x-axis) and pulmonary arterial pressures (left x-axis) in a patient undergoing reamed femoral nailing. A significant transient increase in pulmonary arterial pressure occurred in association with reaming of the femoral canal. After maximum pulmonary artery (PA) pressures had normalized within minutes, an increased amplitude of PA pressure recordings was seen.

Pulmonary capillaries (total length about 3 mm) are much shorter than the capillaries in the general circulation, and the pressure gradient between arterioles and capillaries in the lung is only 5 mmHg. Hence the pulmonary resistance (11 Pa/ml/s) is small compared to that of other systems (vascular resistance of the kidney 740 Pa/ml/s).[46] If pure mechanical occlusion was the cause of a pulmonary artery pressure increase, a huge amount of material would be necessary, and mechanical occlusion alone does not adequately explain the rise of pulmonary artery pressure and functional disturbances associated with IMN.

Secondary Mechanisms

Reactions of the Pulmonary Vasculature

If acute embolization is severe enough to cause local hypoxia, the Cournand–Euler mechanism may be activated, a reflex vasoconstriction teleologically designed to reduce unnecessary perfusion in nonventilated pulmonary segments.[47] This mechanism can augment the pathologic pulmonary arterial pressure increase. Thromboxane, an arachidonic acid derivative, induces vasoconstriction and is released acutely from platelets and endothelial cells in response to various stimuli.[48] Elevated systemic concentrations of thromboxane have been found after reamed IMN in sheep[42] and in a clinical study.[49] This mechanism may contribute to the rise of pulmonary arterial pressure.

Metabolic Effects After Fat Intravasation

A breakdown of neutral fat to free fatty acids inside the lung has been considered.[50,51] Free fatty acids are known to cause pulmonary functional disturbance.[52] An accumulation of free fatty acids occurs after embolization of neutral fat.[53] Baker et al. explained pulmonary dysfunction in patients with fat embolism syndrome with similar effects.[54]

Coagulation Response After Fat Intravasation

The contents of the intramedullary canal have hemostatic properties. Histologic investigations revealed large clusters of platelets around fat droplets exuding from the femoral vein[55] that may be induced by thromboplastin in bone marrow.[56] Injections of bone marrow result in increased pulmonary permeability as well.[57] Tissue disruption by reaming of the medullary canal may cause activation of the intrinsic pathway of the coagulation cascade;[58] increased activation of the coagulation system was seen in sheep that underwent reamed femoral nailing.[59] In a severe trauma setting, consumption of fibrinogen and reduction of the central venous levels of antithrombin III was significantly worse after reamed nailing than after unreamed nailing or plate osteosynthesis[60] (Fig. 29.3). In addition to these effects, tissue trauma may have similar consequences.[61] Activated thrombin induces aggregation and chemotaxis of leukocytes,[62] increases lung permeability,[63,64] and causes other cross reactions between the hemostatic and inflammatory pathways.[65,66]

Inflammatory Response After Fat Intravasation

Monocytes produce thromboplastin if activated by inflammation.[67] Intramedullary contents and neutral fat have the ability to activate inflammatory cells independent of hemostatic reactions.[43,44,68] Polymorphonuclear neutrophil (PMN) activation plays a role in patients with ARDS and has also been demonstrated after IMN.[58] Experimental infusion of neutral fat induces stimulation of PMNs.[69] This inflammatory response appears to be one of the mechanisms responsible for the pulmonary alterations of reamed femoral nailing.

Influence of Cofactors: Inflammatory Stimuli, Hemorrhagic Shock, Thoracic Trauma

In our experience, adverse effects of primary intramedullary stabilization mainly occurred in the presence of additional systemic damage. Inflammatory stimuli such as endotoxin represent some of the most important cofactors.[70–75]

There is a long history of experimental studies regarding *hemorrhagic shock*. However, as an isolated insult, its effects are short-lasting.[76,77] This effect parallels the effects of endotoxin,

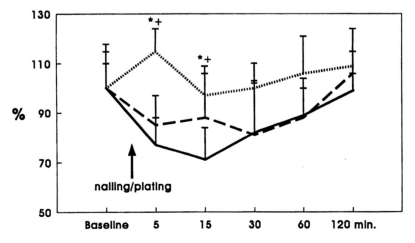

FIGURE 29.3. Central venous fibrinogen levels in sheep submitted to different types of femoral instrumentation (reamed nailing, RFN, solid line; unreamed nailing, UFN, broken line; plate osteosynthesis P, dotted line) after hemorrhagic shock (2 hours, 50 mmHg) and lung contusion. In the P group there were no statistically significant changes during or after femoral instrumentation. In the animals of the UFN group, there was a mild decrease in the plasma fibrinogen levels after femoral instrumentation, but there was no statistically significant change when compared to the baseline values or to P group fibrinogen levels. In contrast, the fibrinogen levels in animals that underwent RFN showed a significant decrease at 5 and 15 minutes after intramedullary reaming and rodding. (From Pape et al.,[60] with permission.)

which also, as an isolated stimulus, does not cause long-lasting adverse effects on organ function. In contrast, hemorrhagic shock plus surgical trauma induced by laparotomy, a combined insult, produces weight loss, dysfunction of several organ systems, and late mortality 3–5 days after resuscitation.[78]

Lung contusion represents a severe injury.[79] The acute functional disturbances after lung contusion depend on the impact velocity.[80] Low impact velocity mainly causes bronchial injury, whereas high energy impact leads to alveolar injury.[81] With lung contusion (1) the disturbance of oxygenation increases with time, and (2) even with unilateral lung injury there is a generalized disturbance in oxygenation. Worsening of hypoxemia was explained by intrabronchial bleeding and flooding of air spaces with blood and plasma.[82] A progressive decrease of pulmonary blood flow and an increase of pulmonary vascular resistance and pulmonary edema were observed,[83–86] mediated by inflammatory cells.[87] This "progressive nature of pulmonary contusion"[88] causes sustained problems during the clinical course. The true severity of pulmonary damage can rarely be fully appreciated early after injury. Blood gas parameters may still be within normal limits, and the chest radiograph may be falsely negative. Only computed tomography (CT) has been claimed to reveal the overall degree of destruction adequately.[89] The mechanisms initiated by pulmonary contusion are comparable to those seen after severe injury, especially in terms of the immune response.[90,91] Even though activated by a different mechanism, the host response to pulmonary contusion is similar to that seen with nonpulmonary injury, resulting in an increased risk of ARDS.

A variety of experimental studies have shown that a combination of stimuli may augment the systemic damage. The combination of hemorrhagic shock and local injury caused a overadditive release of triglycerides and free fatty acids.[92] A transient pulmonary permeability increase caused by endotoxin injection was potentiated by the addition of a bone marrow fat infusion.[69] Pulmonary microvascular damage caused by fat intravasation via intramedullary reaming of the femur was stronger if hemorrhagic shock and unilateral lung contusion had been present previously.[15,42–44] The addition of several stimuli after IMN converted reversible changes[73] to irreversible organ failure.[93–95]

Clinical Consequences of Primary Definitive Fixation: Additional Systemic Burden or Beneficial Treatment?

Systemic Burden of Operative Procedures: Clinical Studies

Attempts have been made to determine the impact of an operation on the patient's general condition by measuring several biochemical mediators.[96–98] Lumbar spine stabilization was associated with considerable activation of several immunologic pathways.[99] Reports dealing with the systemic sequelae of fracture stabilization are limited. Pelvic, femoral, and spinal fractures have been investigated.[100–103] We have measured the inflammatory response in patients submitted to different types of femoral instrumentation (Fig. 29.4). The principal results demonstrated that the systemic impact of intramedullary instrumentation can be measured by biochemical parameters and should not be underestimated.

Current Discussion

The ongoing controversy focuses on two questions: Are the systemic sequelae of reamed femoral nailing worse than those of unreamed femoral nailing? If the combination of chest trauma and femoral shaft fracture occurs, does the intramedullary instrumentation cause significant side effects?

Effect of Reamed Versus Unreamed Nailing

One argument against the reamed procedure is destruction of the intramedullary blood supply.[103] After new implants became available, the unreamed procedure was used for comparison.

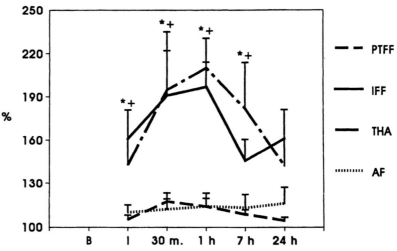

FIGURE 29.4. Clinical measurements of interleukin-6 serum concentrations (percent of baseline levels) in patients submitted to intramedullary instrumentation. Group PTFF: polytrauma patients who had a femoral shaft fracture stabilized with an unreamed femoral nail. Group IFF: patients suffering from a isolated femoral shaft fracture treated by an unreamed femoral nail. Group THA: patients with osteoarthritis of the hip treated with total hip arthroplasty (THA) with the uncemented technique. Group AF: patients with an isolated closed ankle fracture stabilized surgically.

With tibial shaft fractures there was a 70% reduction of blood supply with reamed nailing versus only 30% reduction with unreamed nailing.[104] Also, several cases of heat necrosis were described after reamed nailing of the tibia, and intraoperative temperature increases of more than 50°C were measured.[105] In a sheep tibia model, cortical revascularization occurred by 6 weeks in the unreamed group but not until 12 weeks in the reamed group.[106] The advocates of reamed nailing cite a higher incidence of bolt breakage upon weight-bearing, which they attributed to the fact that less contact surface between nail and the inner cortex is available with the unreamed nailings. So far only one prospective study is available,[107] and this study was criticized because (1) juxtametaphyseal fractures were included, (2) only one locking screw was used, and (3) immediate full weight-bearing was allowed for all fracture types.[108]

The piston-like effect of intramedullary instrumentation is also well known. In the tibia an increased risk of compartment syndrome has been described for reamed nailing.[109] With unreamed nailing only mild, transient pressure increases were measured during reduction and nail passage (maximum 35 mmHg) and were not considered clinically relevant.[110] In the femur, intramedullary pressures were increased up to 1000 mmHg during reamed nailing of the femur, whereas unreamed nailing was associated with pressure increases of only 40–70 mmHg.[39,41] Most authors have described pressure increases between 100 and 1200 mmHg, as summarized previously.[111] Systemic embolization has been extensively documented[112] and includes case reports of fatal outcome.[113]

Wenda separated the appearance of emboli into either a "snowstorm appearance" or "configured" emboli representing solid material. Among 20 nailing procedures no configured emboli in the unreamed group were found, whereas with reamed femoral nailing 8 of 20 femurs developed configured emboli, seen on echocardiography. Reaming was judged to cause a "cumulative effect" owing to repeated instrumentation of the canal. The repetitive maneuvers were thought to allow blood and further intramedullary contents to collect and then to be intravasated into the venous system during the next reaming process.[41]

In a clinical study, we compared the effects of reamed (group R) versus unreamed (group U) femoral nailing on pulmonary hemodynamics. Reamed nailing of closed femoral fractures was associated with a transient, significant increase in pulmonary arterial pressure, whereas unreamed nailing was not (Fig. 29.5).[43] In addition to the primary and secondary effects described earlier in this chapter, pulmonary permeability, determined by bronchoalveolar lavage, was pathologically elevated after reamed nailing of the femur.[114] Some authors wondered whether the reamer design or the degree of predamage may play a role.[44,110,115,116]

Two recent experimental studies doubted the clinical relevance of the negative effects of reamed nailing,[117,118] but several inconsistencies of the study design were criticized.[60] Kröpfl et al. presented the first clinical study of patients with unreamed nailing; 36% of their patients had a thoracic abbreviated injury score (AIS^{thorax}) of more than 2 points, and no patient developed ARDS. They concluded that unreamed femur nailing was a safe method even in the presence of severe thoracic trauma.[119] Moed and Watson suggested retrograde nailing without reaming for femoral shaft fractures in the multiply-injured patient. A transarticular approach was used in 20 patients. The authors stressed the advantage of a short operating time and little blood loss (<100 ml in all patients). A possible drawback appeared to be an unexplained high number of delayed unions that could not be readily explained.[120] A multicenter study from The Netherlands looked at 122 patients with 129 fractures treated with an unreamed nail. In their experience there were no clear-cut advantages regarding handling or fracture healing. No effect was found on pulmonary complications, but there were only 58 patients with multiple injuries.[121]

In summary, the negative effects of reamed nailing (impaired blood supply and the severity of fat embolism) are reduced to a significant extent by the unreamed procedure. Even though to date not all clinicians agree that bone marrow embolism is a clinically relevant entity, almost all researchers have found less damage if the unreamed procedure was chosen. The question "to ream or not to ream" has been addressed at orthopedic trauma meetings, in publications, and in commentary.[84]

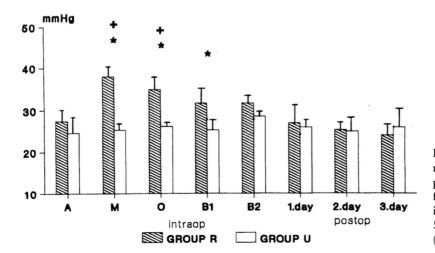

FIGURE 29.5. Intraoperative and postoperative measurements of pulmonary artery pressure in patients submitted to primary reamed (group R) versus unreamed (group U) femoral nailing. A, preoperative values; M, reaming/nail insertion; O, completion of nailing (end of interlocking); B1, 5–15 minutes after nailing; B2, 60 minutes after nailing. (From Pape et al.,[43] with permission.)

Management of the Multiply-Injured Patient with Chest Trauma

Blunt thoracic trauma is accepted as a predisposing factor for the development of pulmonary complications.[85,86] However, fracture management in patients with thoracic injuries remains controversial. In the retrospective report cited above by Fakhry et al., a subgroup of patients who had associated severe chest injuries (AIS > 3 points) demonstrated a mortality rate of 4.6% in patients operated at day 1; no patients died even in the presence of severe chest injury when they were operated on days 2–4 or after day 4. The authors concluded that "the presence of severe chest injury may be an indication to delay the femoral repair for 24–48 hours until these injuries have been stabilized."[19]

In our previously cited report[15] we found that patients with severe thoracic trauma had a worse outcome with primary reamed intramedullary femur stabilization. Selection of the inclusion criteria may play a role. We excluded all patients who died early from head injury or shock and included only those with midshaft fractures treated with a reamed nail. Therefore the patient number dropped from 766 to 106 and represented a well defined group.

Furthermore, strict criteria for the definition of ARDS were used to exclude patients with short, non-life-threatening perioperative deterioration of lung function. In the severely injured groups with thoracic trauma the ISS (52.2 and 55.2) was higher than in other studies (ISS 31.8 and 31.3[9] or 38.0 and 38.2[8]). In our study an alarmingly high ARDS incidence was found among patients with chest trauma submitted to primary reamed IMN. ARDS could not be attributed to thoracic injury severity, as in patients with a comparable thoracic injury and secondary stabilization the ARDS incidence was low. We concluded that the combination of multiple trauma, thoracic trauma, and early operative fracture fixation by reamed IMN is associated with an increased risk of ARDS.[15] The study was criticized because of the inclusion criteria, the number of patients included, and the lack of a statistically significant difference between the groups with severe thoracic trauma.[20,117,121–123]

Other authors have reported inconclusive results. Pelias et al. investigated 130 consecutive patients with blunt chest injury, 85 of whom had rib fractures and 11 a flail chest; they analyzed the outcome of patients with and without a long bone fracture. Even though the two patient groups had comparable injury severity, the authors found a significantly higher rate of pulmonary complications (28%) and death (17%) among patients with long bone fractures compared to those without (pulmonary complications 10.4%, death 8.3%). In another comparison between early and late fixation of long bone fractures, there was no difference in pulmonary complications (early operation 27.6%, late operation 29.4%) or mortality (early operation 16.9%, late operation 17.6%). The authors concluded that: (1) early operative fixation of femoral fractures does not improve the incidence of pulmonary complications, and (2) the incidence of ARDS in these patients is due to chest trauma complicated by the fracture.[124] This study was also criticized because the severity of thoracic injury was not graded. Therefore the thoracic trauma may not have been comparable in the different groups.[125]

In contrast, other groups of authors described no side effects if additional thoracic injuries were present. Van Os et al. compared 30 patients who had chest injuries but no major fractures with 27 patients who had major fractures including fractures of the humerus, forearm, femur (9/14 treated by intramedullary nailing), tibia, pelvis, and vertebrae. They found no statistical difference in the incidence of ARDS and concluded that severe thoracic trauma is not a contraindication for early osteosynthesis.[126]

Bone et al. reported a retrospective study addressing the effect of femoral canal reaming in the polytraumatized patient with associated chest injury. They included patients with an AIS/ISS > 18 points and an AIS > 3 points, and, they differentiated a group submitted to primary (<24 hours) reamed nailing, one with primary (<24 hours) plate osteosynthesis, and patients without femoral fractures. They found no ARDS in the reamed group, 33% ARDS in the plated group, and 27% in the group without femoral fractures. They concluded that the degree of pulmonary injury, rather than the type of instrumentation of the femur, had an impact on pulmonary function and therefore regarded primary reaming of the femur a safe procedure.[127] Several aspects are unclear in this study. Patient groups were not comparable, as the plated group was about 20 years older than the reamed group. The fracture pattern and the degree of soft tissue trauma were different between the groups because the indication for plating included proximal and distal fractures. Likewise, the authors failed to explain why the incidence of ARDS was so low only in the reamed group. It is unclear whether the severity of thoracic trauma was comparable in all groups because the numbers are not given in the paper. Two other retrospective studies concluded that even though fat embolization occurs its effect would be mild and transient and therefore of negligible clinical relevance.[126,127] Boulanger et al.'s study demonstrated only 40–55% admittance to the ICU. Therefore it appears that the degree of severity of the associated injuries was rather low. Patients previously noted to be at special risk of ARDS (i.e., critically injured patient's) appear to have been included.[122] The study was therefore criticized as follows: "the groups were as well matched as possible ...but the Tables 29.1 clearly indicate considerable differences among the groups." In addition, "the other important point is that although we know the average ISS, we do not know how many patients presented with very high scores."[128]

Summary

The data concerning the effect of primary stabilization of major fractures in the patient with associated chest injury remain controversial. The increasing numbers of reports published since the beginning of the 1990s agree with the following statements: In general, primary fracture stabilization in multiple-trauma patients is recommended. With femoral shaft fractures, embolization to the lung can take place if intramedullary reaming is performed. However, two major differences of opinion must be distinguished: (1) Some authors argue that this factor is of little relevance for the future clinical course of the patient. They believe that the benefits of early definitive stabilization outweigh the possible risks induced by embolization of the bone marrow, and ARDS in these patients is a sequela of chest injury. They recommended reamed IMN without exception, even though this opinion lately has been revised in part by stating that in patients with chest injury "overagressive" reaming should be avoided.[127] (2) In the other opinion, early stabilization, irrespective of the method used in a given institution, is generally recommended with the exception of patients with severe chest injury or those admitted in a critical condition or in an uncertain clinical state (borderline patients). In a "borderline situation" there is a predisposition for pulmonary deterioration due to thoracic trauma or previous severe shock, and additional reamed nailing in these patients is regarded as possibly detrimental.[12,15,28,39,111,115,119] These authors question whether it is preferable to stabilize all fractures using definitive stabilization methods, or if temporary stabilization using external fixation is advantageous. Recently, closer attention has been drawn to this option.[129]

Future Perspectives and Treatment Protocol

Treatment protocols of fracture management must consider that operative fracture treatment has developed a great deal, with a variety of technical achievements. A comparison of two decades revealed a reduction of mortality from 40% for 1972–1981 to 22% for 1982–1991.[130] A combination of factors most likely is responsible for this improvement. It is difficult to isolate a single factor, such as *musculoskeletal management*. Studies investigating the impact of fracture management should focus on (1) distinct inclusion criteria, (2) a sufficient number of patients to ensure statistical significance, (3) treatment in the same department, and (4) the same treatment protocols during the study period, and they should be as short as possible. It is difficult to achieve all these criteria: In a recent invited commentary, Court-Brown criticized methodologic problems of retrospective studies and experiments. He stated that "methodological criticism is easy, but we must realize that conventional prospective, comparative studies will be impossible for ethical reasons."[128]

Two studies compared the effects of reamed versus unreamed femoral nailing. Anwar et al. looked at 82 patients with femoral fractures without chest trauma and found a mean Aa gradient of 1.7 after reamed and 1.4 after unreamed fracture treatment. Patients with reamed nailing had a 21.4% incidence of pulmonary complications compared to 12.5% in patients with unreamed nailing. They concluded that reamed nailing of the femur causes no harm.[131] In a prospective multicenter study from Canada, a lower incidence of ARDS was found for unreamed cases (15% reamed, 2.6% unreamed). This study included 235 patients so far and is still ongoing. The authors concluded that there is a tendency toward a lower pulmonary complication rate after unreamed femoral nailing.[132] Müller et al. summarized the relevance of intramedullary pressure increases investigated in relevant publications of recent years.

TABLE 29.1. Criteria to Increase Awareness of the "Borderline Patient" and for the Development of Pulmonary Problems.

Polytrauma + ISS > 20 and additional thoracic trauma (AIS > 2)
Polytrauma with abdominal/pelvic trauma (> Moore 3) and hemorrhagic shock (initial RR < 90 mmHg)
ISS 40 or more in the absence of additional thoracic injury
Radiographic findings of bilateral lung contusion
Initial mean pulmonary arterial pressure > 24 mmHg[134]
Pulmonary artery pressure increase during intramedullery nailing > 6 mmHg

ISS, Injury Severity Score; AIS, Abbreviated Injury Score; RR, Respiratory Rate.

Based on their own and other authors' results, they concluded that "the relevance of pressure differences and the type of nailing procedure is controversial. Intramedullary pressure increases are an important factor in embolization with consequent pulmonary dysfunction and in necrosis of the medullary cortex. Consequently, every possible effort should be made to develop reaming procedures and instruments that maintain low pressures."[133]

Based on our experience, we have developed a stepwise evaluation of the clinical status of severely traumatized patients to distinguish patients at risk (borderline situation). Evaluation of a borderline situation includes the criteria listed in Table 29.1 and distinguishes three patient groups (Table 29.2). If there is doubt about the true pulmonary status (group II), a pulmonary artery (PA) catheter should be inserted and the PA pressure monitored. Early elevated PA pressures document patients at high risk of ARDS.[134] During intramedullary stabilization of the long bone fracture the catheter may indicate embolic events. If evidence of pulmonary injury with an AIS of 2–4 in association with several other injuries is present, we believe that fracture stabilization should be done using an unreamed procedure; that is, reaming should be avoided. The concept of intraoperative patient monitoring has been supported. Patton et al. proposed measuring the alveolar deadspace as a tool to determine whether intensive postoperative monitoring is necessary. A positive predictive value of 76% was found if the index was

TABLE 29.2. Staged Protocol for Treatment of Femoral Shaft Fractures in Hannover.

Group	Injury severity and Injury distribution	Recommendation for treatment
I	Isolated femoral shaft fractures and polytrauma without thoracic trauma	Treatment according to locally preferred method (RFN/UFN/plate)
II	Polytrauma with thoracic trauma (AIS 2–4 points); borderline patient (criteria: see Table 29.1)	UFN + intraop. PA catheter monitoring (intraop. PA pressure increase > 6 mmHg: modification of ventilatory support
III	Polytrauma with severe thoracic trauma (AIS > 4 points) or in critical condition (in extremis)	No intramedullary instrumentation: temporary external fixation or distraction

The protocol was modified according to Pape et al.[111] AIS, Abbreviated Injury Score; RFN/UFN, Reamed/Unreamed Nailing; PA, Pulmonary Artery.

TABLE 29.3. Recommendations Regarding Intraoperative Monitoring During Intramedullary Femoral Nailing.

At 30 minutes after femoral instrumentation: Vd/Vt > 20%	postoperative monitoring required (ventilation)
At 30 minutes after femoral instrumentation: Vd/Vt < 20%	no monitoring required

From Patton et al.,[135] with permission.
The authors described a positive predictive value of 76% if the alveolar deadspace (Vd/Vt) was measured 30 minutes after instrumentation.

TABLE 29.4. Indicators for Patients At Risk of MOF.

Currently used clinical indicators for increased risk of developing organ dysfunction
    Initial thrombocyte count < 95,000/μl
    Input/output ratio > 5 1/6 hr after the initial injury
Potentially useful future indicators for patients at high risk of organ failure
    Increased interleukin levels (Il-1, Il-6)
    Increased serum elastase levels
    Pathologic initial chest CT findings

measured 30 minutes after instrumentation of the medullary canal. This recommendation (Table 29.3) has been reported and may be an additional tool for clinical evaluation.[135] If group III criteria are present and resuscitation does not improve the patient's condition, instrumentation of the femoral canal should be avoided. An external fixation device is placed in the operating room or even in the Surgical ICU. Definitive fixation is delayed until the patient has stabilized. Clinical studies have documented that conversion of external fixation to intramedullary nailing for femoral shaft fractures is a safe method.[136] We have avoided conversion to internal stabilization between days 2 and 4. In contrast, it appears to be safe following post-injury day 4.[136,137] Using this stepwise patient evaluation, separation of borderline patients, and selection of surgical procedures adapted to the clinical status of the patient, we have not observed unexpected deterioration after femoral instrumentation. We are aware that additional factors (Table 29.4) may be useful currently or in the future. We believe that this protocol respects the principle of primary fracture fixation and maintains the advantages of primary definitive stabilization, if possible, considering patient safety.

Acknowledgment. The authors thank Dr. J.D. Wyrick, Department of Orthopedics, University of Cincinnati, for thorough revision of the manuscript.

References

1. Wickstrom J, Corban MS: Intramedullary fixation of fractures of the femoral shaft. J Trauma 1967;7:551–583.
2. Smith JEM: The results of early and delayed internal fixation of fractures of the shaft of the femur. J Bone Joint Surg Br 1964;46: 28–32.
3. Küntscher G: Dangers of intramedullary nailing: fat embolism. In: Küntscher G (ed) Practice of Intramedullary Nailing. Springfield, IL, Charles C Thomas, 1962;36–51.
4. Nöller F: Traumatischer Schock und Fettembolie. Zentralbl Chir 1965;90:1060–1067.
5. Beck JP, Colins JA: Theoretical and clinical aspects of post traumatic fat embolism syndrome. AAOS Instr Course Lett 1973;22:38–44.
6. Riska EB, von Bonsdorff H, Hakkinen S: Primary operative fixation of long bone fractures in patients with multiple injuries. J Trauma 1977;17:111–121.
7. Seibel R, LaDuca J, Hassett JM, et al: Blunt multiple trauma (ISS 36), femur traction and the pulmonary failure septic state. Ann Surg 1985;202:283.
8. Johnson KD, Cadambi A, Seibert B: Incidence of adult respiratory distress syndrome in patients with multiple musculoskeletal injuries: effect of early operative stabilization of fractures. J Trauma 1985;25:375–381.
9. Bone LB, Johnson KD, Weigelt J, et al: Early versus delayed stabilization of fractures. J Bone Joint Surg Am 1989;71: 336–339.
10. Tscherne H: Osteosynthesis of major fractures in polytrauma. World J Surg 1983;7:80–89.
11. Ecke H, Faupel L, Quoika P: Gedanken zum Zeitpunkt der Operation bei Frakturen des Oberschenkelknochens. Unfallchirurgie 1985;11:89–93.
12. Nast Kolb D, Waydhas C, Jochum M, Spannagel M, Duswald KH, Schweiberer L: Günstigster Operationszeitpunkt für die Versorgung von Femurschaftfrakturen beim Polytrauma. Chirurg 1990;61:259–265.
13. Schüller W. Gaudernack T: Lungenkomplikationen nach Oberschenkelmarknagelung Hefte Unfallheilkd 1986;182:273–278.
14. Reynolds MA, Richardson JD, Spain DA, et al: Is timing of fracture fixation important for the patient with multiple trauma? Ann Surg 1995;222:470–481.
15. Pape H-C, Auf m'Kolk MD, Paffrath T, et al: Primary intramedullary fixation in polytrauma patients with associated lung contusion: a cause of posttraumatic ARDS? J Trauma 1993; 34:540–48.
16. Laurence M, Freeman MAR, Swanson SAV: Engineering considerations in the internal fixation of fractures of the tibial shaft. J Bone Joint Surg Br 1969;75:4–9.
17. Winquist RA, Hansen ST, Clawson DK: Closed intramedullary nailing of femoral fractures. J Bone Joint Surg Am 1984;660: 529–539.
18. Rogers FB, Shackford SR, Vane DW, Kaups KL, Harris F: Prompt fixation of isolated femur fractures in a rural trauma center: a study examining the timing of fixation and resource allocation. J Trauma 1994;36:774–777.
19. Fakhry SM, Rutledge R, Dahners LE, Kessler D: Incidence, management and outcome of femoral shaft fracture: a state wide population based analysis of 2805 adult patients in a rural state. J Trauma 1994;37:255–261.
20. Bosse MJ, MacKenzie E, Riemer BL, et al: Adult respiratory distress syndrome, pneumonia, and mortality following thoracic injury and a femoral fracture treated either with intramedullary nailing with reaming or with a plate. J Bone Joint Surg 1997;79:799–809.
21. Horovitz JH, Carrico CH, Shires T: Pulmonary response to major injury. Arch Surg 1974;108:349.

22. Meek RN, Woodruff B, Allardyce DB: Source of fat macroglobules in fractures of the lower extremity. J Trauma 1972;12:432–434.
23. Nuytinck JKS, Offermans XJM, Kubat K, Goris RJA: Whole body inflammation in trauma patients: an autopsy study. Arch Surg 1988;123:1519–1524.
24. Pape H-C, Remmers D, Kleemann W, Goris RJA, Tscherne H: Posttraumatic multiple organ failure: a report on clinical and autopsy findings. Shock 1994;1:228–234.
25. Staub NC: Pulmonary edema. Physiol Rev 1974;54:678.
26. Sturm JA, Wisner D, Oestern HJ: Increased lung permeability after severe trauma: a prospective clinical study. J Trauma 1986;26:409–419.
27. Gossling HR, Pellegrini VD: Fat embolism syndrome: a review of the pathophysiology and physiological basis of treatment. Clin Orthop 1982;165:68–72.
28. Wenda K, Ritter G, Degreif J: Zur Genese pulmonaler Komplikationen nach Marknagelosteosynthesen. Unfallchirurg 1988;91:432–435.
29. Hausberger FX, Whitenack SH: Effect of pressure on intravasation of fat from the bone marrow cavity. Surg Gynecol Obstet 1972;134:931–936.
30. Saldeen T: Intravascular coagulation in the lungs in experimental fat embolism. Acta Chir Scand 1970;135:653–657.
31. Barthels M: Veränderungen der Gerinnung beim Polytrauma. In: Barthels M, Poliwoda M (eds) Gerinnungsanalysen. New York, Thieme Verlag, 1993;83–101.
32. Redl H, Schlag G, Kneidinger R, Dinges HP, Davies J: Activation phenomena of leukocytes and endothelial cells in trauma and sepsis. In: Schlag G, Redl H (eds) Pathophysiology of Shock, Sepsis and Organ Failure. Springer, New York, 1993;549–559.
33. Stephan R, Ayala A, Chaudry IH: Monocyte and lymphocyte responses following trauma. In: Schlag G, Redl H (eds) Pathophysiology of Shock, Sepsis and Organ Failure. Springer, New York, 1993;131–139.
34. Deitch EA, Winterton J, Li M, Berg A: The gut as a portal entry for bacteria. Ann Surg 1987;205:681–685.
35. Pape H-C, Remmers D, Gortz M, et al: Reticuloendothelial system activity and organ failure in multiply injured patients. Arch Surg 1999;134:421–427.
36. Shaw NE: Observations on the physiology of the circulation in bones. Ann Coll Surg Engl 1964;34:214–233.
37. Rehm J: Druckmessungen im Knochenmarksraum und Bestimmung des Gesamtfettgehaltes in den abführenden Venen bei Küntschernagelung. Langebecks Arch Klin Chir 1956;283:452–455.
38. Müller C, McIff T, Rahn BA, et al: Influence of the compression force on the intramedullary pressure development in reaming of the femoral medullary cacity. Injury 1993;24:36–39.
39. Wenda K, Runkel M, Degreif J, Ritter G: Pathogenesis and clinical relevance of bone marrow embolism in medullary nailing demonstrated by intraoperative echocardiography. Injury 1993;24:73–81.
40. Watson AJ: Genesis of fat emboli. J Clin Pathol 1970;23:132–142.
41. Wenda K: Untersuchungen zur Genese und Prophylaxe von Kreislaufkomplikationen bei Operationen im Bereich der Markhöhle der Oberschenkels. Thesis, Johannes Gutenberg University, Mainz, Germany, 1988.
42. Pape H-C, Dwenger A, Grotz M, et al: Does the reamer type influence the degree of lung dysfunction after femoral nailing following severe trauma? J Orthop Trauma 1994;8:300–309.
43. Pape H-C, Regel G, Dwenger A, et al: Influences of different methods of intramedullary femoral nailing on lung function in patients with multiple trauma. J Trauma 1993;35:709–715.
44. Pape H-C, Dwenger A, Regel G, et al: Pulmonary damage after intramedullary femoral nailing in sheep: is there an effect of different nailing methods? J Trauma 1992;33:574–581.
45. Collard M: Pulmonale Reaktionen nach Embolisierungen. In: Fettembolie Baden-Baden, Verlag G Witzstrock, 1973; 2–51.
46. Schmidt RF, Thews G: Physiologie des Menschen, 20th ed. Springer, Berlin, 1980.
47. Wehner W: Ablauf der experimentellen Fettembolie. In: Die Fettembolie. VEB Verlag Volk & Gesundheit, Berlin, 1968.
48. Moncada S, Vane JR: Prostacyclin in the cardiovascular system. Adv Prostaglandin Thromboxane Res 1980;6:43–60.
49. Oettinger W, Bach A: Thromboxanfreisetzung während intramedullärer Nagelung von Femurschaftfrakturen bei Patienten. Chir Forum 1984;15:233–241.
50. Jacks ML, Ashcraft W, Reed WA: Alterations in plasma free fatty acids during extracorporeal circulation. Surg Forum 1964;15:279–281.
51. Clowes GHA, Suschneid W, Dragacevic S: The nonspecific pulmonary inflammatory reactions leading to respiratory failure after shock, gangrene and sepsis. J Trauma 1968;8:899–914.
52. McKay DG, Whitaker AN, Cruise V: Studies of catecholamine shock. Am J Pathol 1969;5:177–200.
53. Fonte DD: Free fatty acid content and histopathology of lungs after experimental fat embolism. Thesis, Department of Anatomy, The Jefferson Medical College of Philadelphia, 1968.
54. Baker PL, Kuenzig MC, Peltier LF: Experimental fat embolism in dogs. J Trauma 1969;9:577–584.
55. Wenda K, Ritter G, Degreif J: Zur Genese pulmonaler Komplikationen nach Marknagelostheosynthesen. Unfallchirurg 1988;91:432–435.
56. Wenda K, Degreif J, Runkel M, Ritter G: Pathogenesis and prophylaxis of circulatory reactions during total hip replacement. Arch Orthop Trauma Surg 1993;112:260–265.
57. Barie PS, Minnear FL, Malik AB: Increase of pulmonary vascular permeablity after bone marrow injection in sheep. Am Rev Respir Dis 1981;123:648–655.
58. Saldeen T: Intravascular coagulation in the lungs in experimental fat embolism. Acta Chir Scand 1970;135:635–658.
59. Heim D, Regazzoni P, Tsakiris DA, et al: Intramedullary nailing and pulmonary embolism: does unreamed nailing prevent embolization? An in vivo study in rabbits. J Trauma 1995;38:899–904.
60. Pape H-C, Bartels M, Pohlemann T, et al: Coagulatory response after femoral instrumentation following severe trauma in sheep. J Trauma 1998;45:720–728.
61. Jacobs RR, Wheeler Ej, Jelenko C, McDonald TF, Bliven FE: Fat embolism: a microscopic and ultrastructure evaluation of two animals models. J Trauma 1973;13:980–993.
62. Bizios R, Lai L, Fenton JW, Malik AB: Thrombin-induced chemotaxis and aggregation of neutrophils. J Cell Physiol 1986;128:485–490.
63. Belloni PN, Carney DH, Nicholson GL: Organ-derived microvessel endothelial cells exhibit differential responsiveness to thrombin and other growth factors. Microvasc Res 1992;43:20–45.
64. De Michele MAA, Minnear FL: Modulation of vascular endothelium permeability by thrombin. Semin Thromb Hemost 1992;18:287–295.

65. Esmon CT: The roles of protein C and thrombomodulin in the regulation of blood coagulation. J Biol Chem 1989;264:4743–4746.
66. Prydz H, Allison AC, Schorlemmer HU: Further link between complement activation and coagulation. Nature 1977;270:173–174.
67. Dean RT, Prydz H: Inflammatory particles stimulate thromboplastin production by human monocytes. Thromb Res 1983;30:357–362.
68. Jacobovitz-Derks D, Derks CM: Pulmonary neutral fat embolism in dogs. Am J Pathol 1979;95:29–37.
69. Regel G, Nerlich ML, Dwenger A, Seidel J, Schmidt C, Sturm JA: Induction of pulmonary injury by polymorphonuclear leucocytes after bone marrow fat injection and endotoxemia: a sheep model. Thor Surg 1989;4:22–30.
70. Demling RH, Proctor R, Grossman J: Lung injury and lung lysosomal enzyme release during endotoxemia. J Surg Res 1981;30:135–141.
71. Lang CH, Spitzer JA: Glucose kinetics and development of endotoxin tolerance during long term endotoxin infusion. Metabolism 1987;36:469–474
72. Egan TM, Saunders NR, Luk SC, Cooper JD: Complement mediated pulmonary edema in sheep. J Surg Res 1988;45:204–214.
73. Pape H-C, Dwenger A, Regel G, et al: Pulmonary damage after recurrent administration of endotoxin and zymosan activated plasma: a sheep model. Thor Surg 1994;9:82–89.
74. Nuytinck JK, Goris RJA, Weerts JG, Schillings PH, Stekhoven JH: Acute generalized microvascular injury by activated complement and hypoxia: the basis of the adult respiratory distress syndrome and multiple organ failure? Br J Exp Pathol 1984;67:548–554.
75. Deitch EA, Berg RD: Endotoxin but not malnutrition promotes bacterial translocation of the gut flora in burned mice. J Trauma 1987;27:161–166.
76. Pretorius JP, Schlag G, Redl H: The 'lung in shock' as a result of hypovolemic-traumatic shock. J Trauma 1987;27:1344–1352.
77. Chaudry IH, Wang P, Singh G, Hauptman JG, Ayla A: Rat and mouse models hypovolemic traumatic shock. In: G Schlag, Redl H (eds) Pathophysiology of Shock, Sepsis and Organ Failure New York, Springer, 1993;371–392.
78. Chaudry IH, Blasko KA, Wagner PA: A clinically relevant model of hemorrhagic shock and resuscitation in the rat. Circ Shock 1989;27:318–319.
79. Stellin G: Survival in trauma victims with pulmonary contusion. Am Surg 1991;57:780.
80. Viano DC: Evaluation of biomechanical response and the potential injury from thoracic impact. Aviat Space Environ Med 1978;49:125.
81. Lau VK, Viano DC: Influence of impact velocity and chest compression on experimental pulmonary injury severity in rabbits. J Trauma 1981;21:1022.
82. Oppenheimer L, Craven KD, Forkert L, et al: Pathophysiology of pulmonary contusion in dogs. J Appl Physiol 1979;47:718.
83. Hellinger A, Konerding MA, Malkush W, et al: Does lung contusion affect both the traumatized and the noninjured lung parenchyma? A morphological and morphometric study in the pig. J Trauma 1995;39:712.
84. Trafton P: ARDS and IM nailing: to ream or not to ream? Complications Orthop 1995;10:5–10.
85. Stellin G: Survival in trauma victims with pulmonary contusion. Am Surg 1991;57:780
86. Pinilla JC: Acute respiratory failure in severe blunt chest trauma. J Trauma 1982;22:221–226.
87. Regel G, Dwenger A, Seidel J, Nerlich ML, Tscherene H: Die Bedeutung der neutrophilen Granulozyten bei der Enstehung des posttraumatischen Lungenversagens. Unfallchirurg 1987;90:99–105.
88. Fulton RL, Peter ET: The progressive nature of pulmonary contusion. Surgery 1970;67:499.
89. Schild HH, Strunk H, Weber W et al: Pulmonary contusion: CT vs plain radiograms. J Comp Assist Tomogr 1989;13:417.
90. Tate RM, Repine JE: Neutrophils and the adult respiratory distress syndrome. Am Rev Resp Dis 1983;128:552.
91. Weiland JE, Davis B, Holter JF, et al: Lung neutrophils in the adult respiratory distress syndrome. Am Rev Respir Dis 1986;133:218–225.
92. Kox W, Schindler HG, Burg E: Biochemische und histologische Veränderungen nach Trauma und Schock: Tierexperimentelle Untersuchungen zur Pathogenese des akuten Lungenversagens und der sogenannten Fettembolie. Hefte Unfallheilkd 1979;138:272–275.
93. Pape H-C, Grotz M, Remmers D, et al: Multiple organ failure after severe trauma: a standardized sheep model. Intensive Care Med 1998;24:590–598.
94. Dwenger A, Remmers D, Grotz M, et al: Aprotinin prevents the development of trauma induced MOF in a chronic sheep model. Eur J Clin Chem Clin Biochem 1996;34:207–214.
95. Remmers D, Dwenger A, Grotz M, Pape H-C, Gruner A, Regel G: Attenuation of multiple organ dysfunction in a chronic sheep model by the 21-aminosteroid U74389 G. J Surg Res 1996;62:278–283.
96. Roumen R, Hendrijks T, ven der Ven-Jongekrijk, Nieuwenhuizen G, Sauerwein R, Goris RJA: Cytokine patterns in patients after major vascular surgery, hemorrhagic shock, and severe blunt trauma. Ann Surg 218;6:769–776.
97. Nast-Kolb D, Waydhas C, Gippner-Steppert C, et al: Indicators of the posttraumatic inflammatory response correlate with organ failure in patients with multiple injuries. J Trauma 1997;42:446–455.
98. Neithardt R, keel M, Steckholzer U, et al: Relationship of interleukin-10 plasma levels to severity of injury and clinical outcome in injured patients. J Trauma 1997;42:863–871.
99. Waydhas C, Nast Kolb D, Kick M, et al: Operationstruama Wirbelsäule in der Behandlung polytraumatisierter Patienten. Unfallchirurg 1993;96:62–65.
100. Goris RJA, Gimbrere JSF, van Niekerk JLM, Schoots FJ, Booy HD: Early osteosynthesis and prophylactic mechanical ventilation in the multitrauma patient. J Trauma 1982;22:895–903.
101. Waydhas C, Nast Kolb D, Kick M, Ritcher-Turnur M, Schweiberer L: Operations-planung von sekundären Eingriffen nach Polytrauma. Unfallchirurg 1994;97:244.
102. Pohlemann T, Gänsslen A, Tscherne H: The technique of packing for control of hemorrhage in complex pelvic fractures. Tech Orthop 1995;9:267–270.
103. Danckwardt-Liljestrom G: Reaming of the medullary canal and its effect on diaphyseal bone. Acta Orthop Scand Suppl 1969;128.
104. Klein MPM, Rahn BA, Frigg R, Kessler S, Perren SM: Reaming versus non-reaming in medullary nailing: interference with

cortical circulation of the canine tibia. Arch Orthop Trauma Surg 1990;109:314–316.
105. Stürmer KM, Schuchardt W: Neue Aspekte der gedeckten Marknagelung und des Aufbohrens der Markhöhle im Tierexperiment. I. Die Tibia als Tiermodell für die Marknagelung. Unfallheikunde 1980;83:341–345.
106. Schemitsch E, Kowalski MJ, Swiontkowski MF, Senft D: Cortical bone blood flow in reamed and unreamed locked intramedullary nailing: a fractured tibia model in sheep. J Orthop Trauma 1994;8:373–382.
107. Court-Brown Cm, Christie J: Reamed or unreamed nailing for tibial fractures. 1996;78:584–587.
108. Tennent, J Bone Joint Surg Br 1997;171.
109. Koval KJ, Clapper MF, Brumback RJ, et al: Complications of reamed intramedullary nailing of the tibia. J Orthop Trauma 1991;5:184–189.
110. Tornetta P, French BG: Compartment pressures during nonreamed nailing without traction. J Orthop Trauma 1997;11:24–27.
111. Pape H-C, Regel G, Tscherne H: Local and systemic effects of fat embolization after intramedullary reaming and its influence by cofactors. Tech Orthop 1996;11:2–13.
112. Pell A, Christie J, Keating JF, Sutherland GR: The detection of fat embolism by transoesophageal echocardiography during reamed intramedullary nailing. J Bone Joint Surg Br 1993;75 921–925.
113. Pape H.-C. Krettek C, Maschek HJ, Regel G, Tscherne H: Fatal pulmonary embolization after reaming of the femoral medullary cavity in sclerosing osteomyelitis. J Orthop Trauma 1996;10:429–432.
114. Obertacke U, Kleinschmidt C, Dresing K, Bardenheuer M, Bruch J: Wiederholbare Routinebestimmung der pulmonalmikrovaskulären Permeabilität nach Polytrauma. Unfallchirurg 1993;96:142–149.
115. Müller C, Frigg G, Perren SM, et al: Effects of flexible drive diameter and reamer design on the increase of pressure in the medullary cavity during reaming. Injury 1993;24(Suppl 3):40–46.
116. Pape H-C, Dwenger A, Regel G, Remmers D, Tscherne H: Intramedullary femoral nailing in sheep: does severe injury predispose to pulmonary dysfunction? Eur J Surg 1995;151:163–171.
117. Schemitsch E. Jain R, Turchin DC, et al: Pulmonary effects of fixation of a fracture with a plate compared with intramedullary nailing. J Bone Joint Surg Am 1997;79:984–996.
118. Duwelius Pj, Huckfeldt R, Mullins R, et al: The effects of femoral intramedullary reaming on pulmonary function in a sheep lung model. J Bone Joint Surg Am 1997;79:194–202.
119. Kröpfl A, Naglik H, Primavesi C, Hertz H: Unreamed intramedullary nailing of femoral fractures. J Trauma 1995:38:717–726.
120. Moed B, Watson T: Retrograde intramedullary nailing, without reaming, of fractures of the femoral shaft in multiply injured patients. J Bone Joint Surg Am 1995;77:1520–1527.
121. Hammacher ER, van Meeteren MC, van der Werken C: Improved results in treatment of femoral shaft fractures with the unreamed femoral nail? A multicenter experience. J Trauma 1998;45:517–521.
122. Boulanger BR, Stephen D, Brennemann FD: Thoracic trauma and early intramedullary nailing of femur fractures: are we doing harm? J Trauma 1997;43:24–29.
123. Carlson DA, Rodman GH, kaehr D, Hage J, Misinski M Femur fractures in chest-injured patients: is reaming contraindicated? J Orthop Trauma 1998;12:164–168.
124. Pelias ME, Townsend MC, Flancbaum L: Long bone fractures predispose to pulmonary dysfunction in blunt chest trauma despite early operative fixation. Surgery 1992;111:576–579.
125. Wagner RB, Schimpf PB: Letter to the editor. Surgery 1993;114:129.
126. Van Os JP, Roumen R, Schoots F, Heystraaten FJ, Goris RJA: Is early osteosynthesis safe in multiple trauma patients with severe thoracic trauma and pulmonary contusion? J Trauma 1994;36:495–498.
127. Bone LB, Babikian G, Stegemann P: Femoral canal reaming in the polytrauma patient with chest injury. Clin Orthop 1995;318:91–94.
128. Court-Brown CM: Invited commentary. J Orthop Trauma 1998;12:175–176.
129. Nowotarski PJ, Turen CH, Brumback RJ, Scaraboro JM: Conversion of external fixation to intramedullary nailing for shaft fractures in polytrauma patients. Presented at the annual meeting, Orthopaedic Trauma Association, Vancouver, Canada, 1998.
130. Regel G, Lobenhoffer P, Lehmann U, et al: Treatment results of patients with multiple trauma: an analysis of 3406 cases treated between 1972 and 1991 at a German level I trauma center. J Trauma 1995;38:70–78.
131. Anwar IA, Olson SA, Battistella FD: Pulmonary consequences of reamed versus unreamed intramedullary femur fixation: a prospective randomized study. Presented to the AAST, 1997.
132. De Groote R, Powell J, Buckley R, et al: A prospective randomized clinical trial comparing reamed versus unreamed intramedullary femoral nailing of femoral shaft fractures: assessment of pulmonary dysfunction. Presented at the annual meeting, Orthopaedic Trauma Association, Vancouver, Canada, 1998.
133. Müller CA, Schavan R, Frigg R, Perren S, Pfister U: Intramedullary pressure increase for different commercial and experimental reaming systems: an experimental investigation. J Orthop Trauma 1998;12:540–546.
134. Sturm JA, Lewis FR, Trentz O, Tscherne H: Cardiopulmonary parameters and prognosis after severe multiple trauma. J Trauma 1979;19:409–418.
135. Patton WC, Rudd JN, Crosby L, Kline J, Norris B: The alveolar dead space fraction predicts respiratory distress after intramedullary fixation of femoral shaft fractures. Annual meeting, Orthopaedic Trauma Association, Vanvouver, Canada, 1998.
136. Strum JA: Introduction. In: Sturm JA (ed) Adult Respiratory Distress Syndrome, Heidelberg, Springer, 1991;1–4.
137. Nerlich ML: Progressive organ failure. In: Sturm JA (ed) Adult Respiratory Distress Syndrome, Heidelberg, Springer, 1991;45–56.

30
Abdominal Compartment Syndrome

Eduardo Bumaschny and Alejandro Rodríguez

Intraabdominal pressure (IAP) is one of the physical constants that can be modified with great ease at an early time in the presence of severe cavity alterations. An increase in IAP produces a hypertensive state (intraabdominal hypertension, or IAH) that is both the result and an indicator of underlying pathophysiologic alterations. IAH has marked effects, both local and systemic, that are liable to lead to multiorgan dysfunction and the full picture of the abdominal compartment syndrome (ACS).[1]

Definition and Incidence

Abdominal compartment syndrome is characterized by massive abdominal distension and multiorgan system dysfunction, with involvement of the cardiovascular, respiratory, renal, and central nervous systems. It is induced by an acute, marked, progressive, sustained, and uncontrolled increase in IAP.[2-5] The clinical course can be managed only by decompressive laparotomy, which if done early enough is able to reverse the dysfunctions. Some authors believe that an IAP higher than 15–20 mmHg is required to validate the presence of ACS,[6] whereas others base the diagnosis on the clinical aspects of the syndrome alone.[7] We agree with Ivatury et al.[1] in that IAH per se is not synonymous with ACS but certainly is one of its components.

Chronic ACS can be present in morbidly obese patients, in whom the IAP is high and predisposes to secondary effects in several systems and organs (venous stasis and endocranial hypertension, among others).[8,9]

The incidence of IAH in critically ill patients is high, with an IAP value that exceeds 20 mmHg in about 30% of patients undergoing scheduled operations. After emergency operations the incidence is even higher. The incidence of ACS is most likely underreported given the diverse criteria used to define the syndrome. Throughout the 12 years' existence of the Vanderbilt Trauma Center, with approximately 2900 annual admissions, Eddy et al. identified ACS in only 34 patients.[10] Meldrum et al. observed ACS in 21 of 145 (14%) patients with trauma and an injury severity score (ISS) higher than 15 subjected to laparotomy.[11]

Historical Background

Wendt first observed the appearance of anuria secondary to renal compression in 1876.[12] In 1911 Emerson measured IAP and the consequences of its increase in small animals in an attempt to discern its mechanism.[13] In 1923 Thorington and Schmidt demonstrated a decrease in urinary flow in dogs with experimentally induced ascites.[13] Salkin in 1924 and Waggoner in 1926 measured IAP in healthy individuals, recording pressures ranging from zero to less than 30 mmH$_2$O, and similar results were obtained by Overholt in 1931 in dogs.[14,15] In 1947 Bradley and Bradley demonstrated alterations in renal function in healthy youths by applying external pressure to the abdomen.[16] Gross in 1948 confirmed the complications produced by attempting to reduce congenital omphalocele and proposed making silos or abdominal chimneys.[17] In 1976 Richardson and Trinkle showed experimentally that elevated IAP leads to high end-inspiratory pressures and decreased cardiac output.[18] Harman et al.[14] in 1982 demonstrated a deterioration in renal function in dogs subjected to increased IAP, and the following year Richards et al.[19] reported four patients with anuric renal failure due to extreme abdominal distension secondary to postoperative hemorrhage. Kron et al. in 1984 indicated that IAP higher than 30 mmHg causes renal failure and proposed a standardized method for IAP measurement; they were the first to suggest decompression in the presence of pressures exceeding 25 mmHg accompanied by oliguria.[20] Lastly, Fietsam et al. in 1989 were the first to indicate that in surgical patients the increase in IAP produces a defined pattern of organic dysfunction, coining the term ACS.[21]

Biophysical Features

The abdomen and its contents may be compared to a relatively incompressible fluid that behaves as a unit according to Pascal's law. Any change in the volume of the contents affects the pressure in its interior.[22-24] This happens with slow, progressive increases where the compliance of the abdominal wall allows it to respond to large variations in volume with mild modifications in pressure, as in cirrhotic patients.[8,25] Some general or local conditions modify this compliance and influence the IAP: surgical incisions, muscular relaxants, sedatives, large soft tissue losses. The application of external pressure and the increase in IAP are transmitted to the retroperitoneal area, as was shown by Shenasky and Gillenwater in dogs.[22] Conversely, an increase in retroperitoneal volume (hemorrhage, edema, pancreatitis) is transferred to the IAP.[8]

Etiology and Pathogenesis of IAH

There is no agreement on the IAP that constitutes IAH, but most accept IAPs ranging from 15 to 25 mmHg as being high. However, upon analyzing IAP in 21 consecutive patients admitted for abdominal operations, our team documented a worse postoperative course in patients with IAP exceeding 10 mmHg than in those who had control levels lower than or equal to that value (Fig. 30.1).[26]

Etiology

Intraabdominal hypertension appears in a great variety of clinical situations in both adults and pediatric patients.[27-32] Often it is attributable to the anatomic or physiologic impact of a traumatic or noxious circumstance combined with operation. As indicated by Schein et al.,[24] its causes may be acute or chronic (Table 30.1). Those most prone to develop an ACS are trauma patients, as they require a large quantity of fluids for resuscitation with hypothermia, clotting disorders, and postoperative hemorrhage, as well as those who for any reason undergo massive volume resuscitation (burns, severe pancreatitis, and shock, among others). In this setting the bowel becomes extremely edematous, preventing abdominal closure if a laparotomy is performed. Should closure be forced, ACS may be

TABLE 30.1. Etiologic Factors for Acute and Chronic Intraabdominal Hypertension.

Condition	Factors
Acute	
Spontaneous	Peritonitis; intraabdominal abscess; ileus; intestinal obstruction; colonic pseudoobstruction; ruptured abdominal aortic aneurysm; hypertensive pneumoperitoneum; severe acute pancreatitis; mesenteric venous or arterial obstruction; bladder distension
Postoperative	Postoperative peritonitis; intraabdominal abscess; ileus; acute gastric dilatation; intraperitoneal hemorrhage; massive gut, retroperitoneum, or solid viscera edema (long operations, prolonged viscera exposure)
Postresuscitation after trauma	Profound hypothermia; large volume infusion; septic shock; cardiac arrest
Posttraumatic	Intraperitoneal, retroperitoneal, or pelvic hemorrhage; postresuscitation visceral edema
Iatrogenic	Laparoscopic procedures using pneumoperitoneum; pneumatic antishock garment; damage control operation; abdominal packing; abdominal tamponade with balloon catheters; parietal, ventral, or diaphragmatic massive hernia reduction with lost domain; abdominal closure under excessive tension; intestinal swelling due to massive volume resuscitation
Chronic	Massive ascites; large abdominal tumor; chronic ambulatory peritoneal dialysis; pregnancy; morbid obesity

From Bumaschny,[5] with permission.

triggered.[13] In the absence of trauma, increased IAP strongly suggests the existence of severe intraabdominal sepsis, particularly in patients who had previously had a laparotomy.[26]

Pathogenesis

Increased IAP is due to the simultaneous or successive changes that (1) increase the volume of the organs contained in the abdomen, (2) incorporate extraanatomic components in the cavity or the retroperitoneum, (3) apply external pressures, or (4) alter the anterior abdominal wall. Some of these factors act progressively, but others may happen quickly and produce dramatic effects.

Increased Volume of Anatomic Abdominal Contents

An increased volume of abdominal contents may be due to visceral edema or intestinal distension. Massive resuscitation with fluids and blood exposes the patient to the effects of hypervolemia at the same time altered distribution of corporeal fluids and hemodilution lead to a decrease in colloidal osmotic pressure.[23] The consequences are aggravated by increased capillary permeability and by inflammation produced by shock. These conditions cause an increase in interstitial fluid that promotes edema of the intestine, mesentery, solid viscera, and

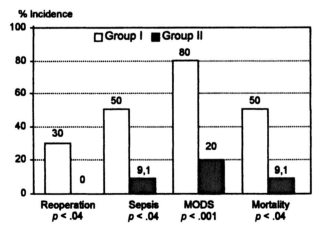

FIGURE 30.1. Incidence of reoperation, sepsis, multiorgan dysfunction syndrome (MODS), and mortality in two patient groups. Group I: one or more intraabdominal pressure measurements >10 mmHg. Group II: all intraabdominal pressure measurements ≤10 mmHg. (From Pusajó et al.,[26] with permission.)

retroperitoneum.[3,12,23,33] Ischemia and reperfusion, the release of vasoactive mediators and free oxygen radicals, and hypothermia due to exposure of the body cavities to ambient temperature also contribute to visceral edema, ileus, and intestinal distension, which in turn increases the IAP.[8,28]

Occupation of the Cavity or Retroperitoneum by Extraanatomic Components

Extraanatomic components in the cavity or retroperitoneum may be collections or packing with laparotomy pads. Severe intraabdominal infection, compression of the systemic venous or portal regions, hemorrhage, ischemia, and reperfusion may produce free fluid or clots whose volume may reach 8–10 liters, surpassing the compliance of the abdominal wall. When packing is used, the effect is more complex as venous compression is added to the volume occupied by the foreign body introduced. At the time of operation for trauma, a paradox arises with a damage control operation by packing in an attempt to interrupt the "bloody vicious cycle" of coagulopathy, hypothermia, and acidosis: IAH may help arrest hemorrhage, but excessive IAP promotes clotting disorders by way of cellular hypoxia.[11]

Application of External Pressures

External pressure by a pneumatic antishock garment reduces the capacity of the abdomen[34] in a setting of traumatic or hypovolemic shock and visceral ischemia. Its pathogenic effects are then compounded.

Alteration of the Abdominal Wall

The loss of soft tissue due to necrosis, severe infection, or defective scars, excessive tension on the abdominal incision, or swelling of the wall in response to intraabdominal alterations leads to loss of compliance, preventing conventional surgical closure.[28] If closure is forced, more pressure is added to the already present internal pressure. Ivatury et al.[1] documented a 100% incidence of IAH in patients in whom the fascia was conventionally closed primarily versus 38% for those in whom large mesh was used.

Consequences of IAH and Adverse Physiologic Effects

The physiologic alterations induced by the increase in IAP are mainly found in the circulatory system, kidneys, and gastrointestinal tract. As summarized by Baue,[35] IAH alters general hemodynamics and blood supply to the gut at the same time it interferes with renal function. No less important are its effects on the abdominal wall, respiratory system, and cellular respiration as well as on the central nervous system, lymphatic system, and endocrine system[36] (Fig. 30.2 and Table 30.2). It is not unlikely that these pathophysiologic changes begin before IAP and may have reached the threshold considered to be hypertension even before clinical manifestations are evident.[1]

Circulatory System

Cardiac Output and Arterial Blood Pressure

The consequences of IAH depend on the status of the blood volume and the magnitude of the IAP. With normovolemia, cardiac output is maintained initially at the expense of an increase in heart rate[22,24] and is reduced when the IAP reaches 40 mmHg.[12] In the presence of hypovolemia, cardiac output falls quickly with an increase in systemic vascular resistance.[37] In hypervolemic dogs cardiac output increases up to 50% when the IAP starts to increase,[27] but falls significantly when the latter reaches 40 mmHg. During certain clinical procedures (e.g., laparoscopic cholecystectomy) the changes occur at much lower IAP levels.[12,22,25,37]

The decrease in cardiac output is attributed to various factors, such as a fall in preload,[4,25] a decrease in ventricular compliance, and an increase in afterload. Ventricular compliance seems to be affected by passive upward displacement of the diaphragm and transmission of abdominal pressure toward the heart and large vessels.[3] However, Marathe et al.[38] failed to observe any modification in contractility of the left ventricle in rats with 25 mmHg IAP and ascribed the fall in cardiac output to preload alterations. Bloomfield et al.[25] and Ali and Qi[34] attributed it to an increase in afterload and a systemic vascular resistance increase due to compression of the abdominal aorta and arterial bed.

An initial increase in mean arterial blood pressure is due to the increase in peripheral resistance. With an IAH higher than 30 mmHg the blood pressure decreases, though peripheral resistance continues to rise.

Central Venous Pressure and Pulmonary Capillary Pressure

Both the central venous pressure and the pulmonary capillary pressure are increased initially, though recordings may be spurious owing to increased pleural pressure or to the application of positive end-expiratory pressure (PEEP). With increased IAP there is inevitably a fall in both central venous pressure and pulmonary capillary pressure. If the transmural pressure is calculated (pulmonary capillary pressure or venous pressure minus pleural pressure), more exact values are obtained.[4] The right ventricular end-diastolic volume seems a better indicator of preload than pulmonary capillary pressure to guide volume resuscitation in these patients.[39]

Alterations in Macrocirculation and Microcirculation

Although pressure is increased in some vessels, such as the hepatic artery, perfusion of abdominal viscera is uniformly reduced with the sole exception of the adrenal glands, as demonstrated by the use of radiolabeled microshperes.[13,29]

Pressure in the inferior vena cava equals the IAP, so venous return decreases owing to (1) the venous resistance being higher than the capillary pressure and (2) functional venous narrowing at the diaphragm. These vary in conditions of hypervolemia, as the larger circulating flow decreases venous compression.[27]

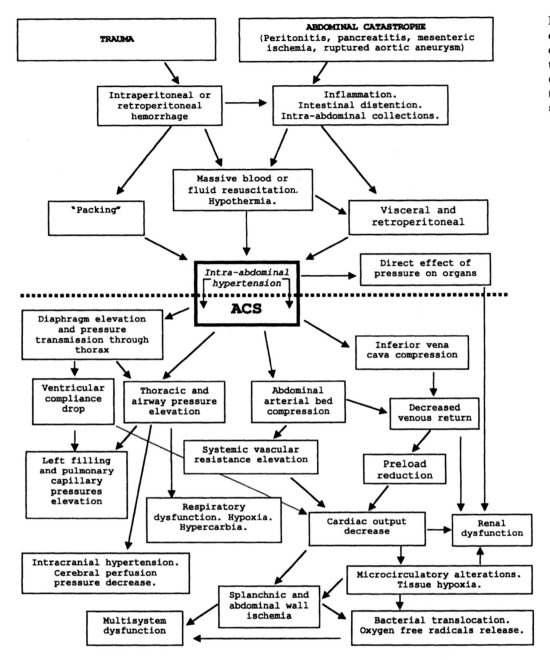

FIGURE 30.2. Causes of intraabdominal hypertension and induced physiologic alterations that give rise to the abdominal compartment syndrome (ACS). (From Bumaschny,[5] with permission.)

Another consequence of IAH is partial obstruction of the femoral veins and generalized edema due to fluid leakage to the extravascular compartment.[22] High venous pressure exerts mechanical stress on the vessels, causing endothelial microlesions and increasing the risk of thrombosis. In the renal veins pressure exceeds that of the vena cava by 1–2 mmHg, and renal vascular resistance increases so it is 15 times higher than the total vascular resistance.[25]

Kidneys

With an IAP of 20 mmHg, oliguria occurs, and renal blood flow and the glomerular filtration rate decrease to 25% normal. With 40 mmHg IAP, anuria occurs, though it may appear earlier in critically ill patients. At 25 mmHg IAP, antidiuretic hormone, renin-angiotensin, and aldosterone levels increase.[22,24,25] During laparoscopic surgery it has been shown that with IAPs of up to 15 mmHg good urinary flow is maintained. If the pressure rises beyond 15 mmHg oliguria appears, and if it exceeds 30 mmHg there is anuria.[40]

Four mechanisms have been identified that interfere with renal function in ACS.

1. *Vascular*: reduction in renal plasma flow due to the drop in cardiac output;[25] difficult venous drainage due to hypertension in the inferior vena cava;[7] compression of cortical arterioles and blood shunting from the cortex toward the medulla.[1,8]

TABLE 30.2. Changes in Physiologic Parameters Induced by Intraabdominal Hypertension.

Parameter	Modification	
Cardiovascular	IAP 10–19 mmHg	IAP ≥ 20 mmHg
Heart rate	↑	↑
Cardiac output	NC	↓
Mean arterial blood pressure	↑	↓
Preload	↑	↓
Systemic vascular resistance (afterload)	↑	↑
Stroke volume and left ventricular work	↓	↓
Cardiac compliance	↓	↓
Pulmonary vascular resistance	NC	↑
Pulmonary artery mean pressure and wedge pressure	↑	↑
Central venous pressure	↑	NC or ↓
Inferior vena cava pressure	↑	↑
Venous return	NC or ↑	↓
Arterial and microvascular hepatic flow	↓	↓
Portal flow	NC or ↓	↓
Mesenteric circulation	↓	↓↓
Renal	IAP 20–39 mmHg	IAP ≥ 40 mmHg
Urine output	Oliguria	Anuria
Renal blood flow	↓	↓↓
Glomerular filtration rate	↓	↓↓
H$_2$O reabsorption	↑	↑
Renal venous pressure	↑	↑↑
ADH-aldosterone	NC	↑
Peripheral edema	No	Yes
Respiratory	IAP ≥ 20 mmHg	
Breath rate	↑	
Airway pressure and peak airway pressure	↑	
PaO$_2$; PaO$_2$/FiO$_2$	↓	
PaCO$_2$	↑	
Ventilation/perfusion index	Mismatch	
Dynamic and static thoracic compliance; pulmonary expansion	↓	
Vital capacity; thoracic volume; diaphragmatic excursion	↓	
Deadspace	↑	
Intrathoracic and pleural pressure	↑	
Gastrointestinal tract and abdomen		
Gastroesophagic reflux	↑	
Splanchnic perfusion; arterial and mucous mesenteric flow	↓	
Gastric intramucosal pH	↓	
Bacterial translocation; oxygen free radical release	Yes	
Abdominal wall compliance; abdominal parietal blood flow	↓	
Diaphragm elevation	Yes	
Central nervous system		
Intracranial pressure	↑	
Cerebral perfusion pressure	↓	

From Bumaschny,[5] with permission.
ADH, antidiuretic hormone; IAP, intraabdominal pressure; NC, no changes; ↑, increase; ↓, decrease; ↑↑, significant increase; ↓↓, significant decrease.

2. *Nephron-related*: reduced glomerular filtration rate and tubular function;[16] increased water reabsorption.
3. *Compressive*: local vascular or endocrine phenomenon caused by direct compression of the kidneys ("renal compartment syndrome").[14,25] Direct action of increased pressure on the ureters or on the bladder is ruled out, as placing stents in the ureteral lumen fails to prevent oliguria.[14]
4. *Endocrine*: increased production of aldosterone due to, among other causes, redistribution of the blood flow from the abdomen to the thorax.[33]

Acute tubular necrosis (ATN) can develop. If it does, it is irreversible without going through a period of anuria. Hopefully there is eventual recovery of renal function.

Gastrointestinal Tract

Intraabdominal hypertension, which gives rise to the ACS, produces ischemia of all the abdominal viscera. The small bowel is probably the most sensitive organ and has subclinical damage before the classic renal, pulmonary, or cardiovascular signs are evident.[8,31] Overt effects are splanchnic hypoperfusion, intestinal mucosa acidosis, local fall in oxygen partial pressure, and failure of mucosal barrier function, events that are independent of the modifications in cardiac output[1] but are proportional to the IAP increase. When the IAP exceeds 20 mmHg, gastric intramucosal pH decreases. The drop in this parameter could be associated with an increase in lactate due to anaerobic glycolysis,[12] and it indicates severe mucosal ischemia and failure of the intestine to use available oxygen, with possible effects on bacterial translocation, nosocomial pneumonia, myocardial depression, and sepsis.[41] Paul et al.,[29] reported intestinal ischemia secondary to laparoscopic surgery.

We found (by gastric tonometry) significant alterations of splanchnic microperfusion during the immediate postoperative period, when the IAP surpassed 10 mmHg (Fig. 30.3). In support, Sugrue et al.[6] have assigned a prognostic value to gastric intramucosal pH: Abnormal results (intramucosal pH ≤ 7.32) are associated with an 11.3 times greater probability of high IAP, hypotension, renal dysfunction, relaparotomy, and death. These observations agree with those in experimental models, as reported by Eleftheriadis et al.,[31] who also demonstrated free oxygen radical production and bacterial translocation. Such findings are similar to those of Diebel et al., who confirmed that although the mesenteric and intestinal mucosal flow reduction occurs when IAP reaches 20 mmHg the hepatic and portal flows are altered from 10 mmHg.[12,42] These data suggest that pathophysiologic alterations begin early, with even mild increases in IAP, and that the appearance of clinical manifestations is delayed and may not present simultaneously in all organs. In contrast, Thaler et al.[41] observed that with an IAP up to 15 mmHg patients who presented neither prior cardiovascular nor humoral alterations preserved their visceral microperfusion within the normal range during the short time it takes to perform a laparoscopic procedure.

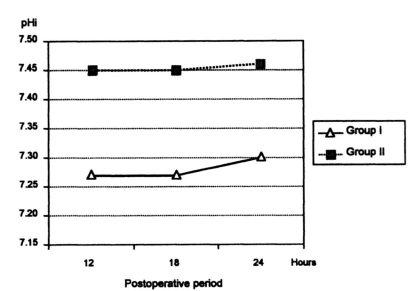

FIGURE 30.3. Gastric intramucosal pH (pHi) at 12, 18, and 24 hours after operation in two patient groups. Group I: one or more intraabdominal pressure measurements >10 mmHg. Group II: all intraabdominal pressure measurements ≤ 10 mmHg. (From Pusajó et al.,[26] with permission.)

Respiratory System

The first consequence of IAH on the respiratory system is failure to ventilate. Pulmonary dysfunction is due to a number of causes: mechanical difficulties for diaphragmatic excursion with increased airway pressure;[7] increased pleural pressure;[2] activation of polymorphonuclear leukocytes (PMNs), leading to endothelial alterations;[43] compression of basal pulmonary segments; and decreased residual functional capacity with increased deadspace.[37] Hemorrhage and subsequent massive resuscitation with fluids may exacerbate the effect of IAH with mechanical ventilation, inducing increased intrathoracic pressure, particularly with PEEP.[43]

The decrease in PaO_2 and the increase in $PaCO_2$ are impossible to correct by a ventilator,[7] as high pressures are required to maintain tidal volume.[13,24,25] The PaO_2/FiO_2 ratio drops[12,33] and respiratory frequency is increased in response to the decrease in compliance and in vital capacity. In a clinical study on 26 patients subjected to laparoscopic cholecystectomy, Obeid et al.[30] confirmed that the increase in IAP (up to 16 mmHg) influenced pulmonary compliance by reducing it to 50%. A ventilation/perfusion imbalance and moderate distress occurred. Ranieri et al.[44] concluded that an increase in IAP also affects thoracic wall mechanics due to configuration changes resulting from abdominal distension. Similar observations were reported by Fok et al.[45] in infants.

Oxygen Transport, Delivery, and Usage: Acid—Base Status

The slowing-down of venous outflow interferes with oxygen availability.[1] Hypoxemia, hypercarbia, and acidosis reflect the difficulties in oxygen transport, delivery, and usage and indicate respiratory chain disorder even in extraabdominal territory. In an animal model an increase in IAP and its combination with PEEP produced respiratory acidosis[22] and increased serum lactate levels, attributable to anaerobic glycolysis or to inhibition of hepatic lactate metabolism due to hypoperfusion. Severe lung changes caused by IAH produce gas-exchange alterations and respiratory acidosis, characterized by a significant decrease in PaO_2 and a small increase in $PaCO_2$.

Central Nervous System

An increase in intracranial pressure is a component of the ACS; its effects are more evident with a more rapid increase in IAP.[2,46] In an animal model, an increase in IAP to 25 mmHg significantly elevated the intracranial pressure and reduced cerebral perfusion pressure.[36] According to Bloomfield et al.,[2,36] it is attributable to increased intrathoracic pressure, which hinders cerebral venous drainage. It is possible that a similar mechanism is operative in preeclampsia and morbid obesity. Elevated IAP has been emphasized in the latter condition. Sugerman et al.[47] demonstrated the existence of IAH and increased intrathoracic pressures in obese patients with "pseudotumor cerebri." Cerebral perfusion pressure can be improved by increasing the cardiac output via volume expansion.[36]

Abdominal Wall Compliance and Circulation

With an IAP of 40 mmHg, a drop in blood flow of the rectus sheath of 20% of normal was observed.[1,48] Extreme parietal expansion leads to a reduction in compliance, which may cause fascial necrosis, wound infection, dehiscence, and evisceration, as resistance to infection and collagen deposition are directly related to tissue perfusion.[49]

Lymphatic System

Lymphatic flow along the thoracic duct ceases when abdominal pressure exceeds 30 cmH_2O.[50] Reduction in abdominal lymphatic drainage and peritoneal fluid transport to thoracic lymphatic vessels is caused by: (1) direct compression of the thoracic duct;[24,50] and (2) diaphragm stretching and decrease in lymphatic lacunare volume.

In experimental studies and in patients with tensely distended abdomens, lymph flow through the cannulated thoracic duct is decreased.[50] Lymphatic drainage increases promptly after abdominal decompression.[24]

Neurohormonal and Humoral Alterations

Certain effects of an elevated IAP, such as alterations of hepatic perfusion and of renal function, are attributable to humoral mechanisms.[22,23,25,42] A similar picture is observed in patients with morbid obesity and preeclampsia. Bloomfield et al.[25] concluded that IAH upregulates the hormonal output of the renin-angiotensin-aldosterone system, probably by increasing renal venous pressure. Hirvonen et al.[51] demonstrated an increase in plasma epinephrine.

Measurement of IAP

Measurement of IAP may be made directly or indirectly. Indirect methods are based on measurement of the pressure in the stomach,[3] rectum, or bladder: When these organs are partially full, they act as extensible and compressible intraabdominal bags. The simplest recording technique, currently considered the gold standard, consists in measurements through a vesical tube (a technique described by Kron et al.,[20]) as described in Table 30.3. Our findings (unpublished data) in patients with extraabdominal disease revealed a mean IAP value of 1.10 ± 0.92 cmH$_2$O.

The intragastric route must be used in the presence of a neurogenic bladder, bladder trauma, or a pelvic hematoma.[9] Measurement is performed through a nasogastric indwelling tube (or through a gastrostomy tube if present) similar to the transvesical method. Even though several animal studies have demonstrated a better correspondence between the true pressure and measurement through the bladder, rather than the stomach or the rectum,[4,30] in our experience[52] and in agreement with other authors[53] there is a good correlation between gastric and bladder pressure.

Clinical Considerations

The clinical course starts with abdominal distension, increased peak airway pressure (exceeding 80 cmH$_2$O), and increased PaCO$_2$. The arterial blood pressure remains stable, the cardiac index falls, and the systemic vascular resistance increases. Urine output decreases gradually, with more concentrated urine; the lower limbs are much colder than the upper limbs. At that time the patient generally receives a fluid challenge, inotropic agents, and diuretics without achieving a significant increase in diuresis despite improvement in the cardiovascular variables. The clinical features of ACS are summarized in Table 30.4.

With early abdominal decompression adequate ventilation is promptly reestablished, the inspiratory pressure drops, urinary flow increases, distal pulses become palpable, and the patient's hemodynamics become normal. The severity of the picture is directly proportional to the degree of IAH. Meldrum et al.[11] classified ACS in four stages: I (IAP 10–15 mmHg), for which it is advised to maintain normovolemia; II (16–25 mmHg), for which hypervolemic resuscitation should be initiated; III (26–35 mmHg), for which decompression should be performed; and IV (>35 mmHg), for which the abdomen should be decompressed and reexplored. In our experience there was a significant correlation between increased postoperative IAP and a reduction in gastrointestinal tract microperfusion, the presence of sepsis and multiple organ dysfunction syndrome (MODS), the need to reoperate, and the mortality rate (Fig. 30.1).[26] Table 30.5 summarizes the papers cited in this review.

Aggravating Clinical Circumstances

The clinical setting in which ACS develops decisively affects outcome. Simon et al.[43] have shown in an experimental model that in the presence of hemorrhage and subsequent resuscitation [a frequent condition in intensive care unit (ICU) patients] the effects of IAH are more severe and have their onset with lower IAP values (10 mmHg). In this setting significant deterioration of cardiac output takes place at an IAP exceeding 10 mmHg. At 20 mmHg the PCO$_2$ increases and the PaO$_2$/FiO$_2$ ratio falls. Oxygenation drops at 30–40 mmHg IAP. Therefore with hemorrhagic shock and resuscitation even moderate IAP elevation should be avoided.

TABLE 30.3. Measurement of Intraabdominal Hypertension.

Transvesical method: Foley catheter connected to a venous pressure manometer or to a transducer

Procedure
- Place patient in supine position
- Empty the bladder
- Instill 75–100 ml of normal saline
- Measure during expiration
- Pubic symphysis is taken as point zero
- Normal pressure is ≤ 0
- Hypertension is reported at 15–25 mmHg

TABLE 30.4. Clinical Features of Abdominal Compartment Syndrome.

Tense, distended abdomen

Hemodynamic instability

Progressive oliguria

Decreased cardiac output with high left filling pressures; increased vascular systemic resistance

Respiratory alterations
- Improper ventilation
- Hypoxemia
- Hypercarbia
- Increased airway pressure
- Decreased pulmonary compliance

TABLE 30.5. Clinical Experience Reported in Literature.

Etiology	No.	Died
Bumaschny (review) [5]		
Aortic aneurysm	9	
Trauma	72	
Trauma (outcome unknown)	21	
Pancreatitis	2	
Hepatic trauma	2	
Abdominal infection	1	
Gastric	2	
Pelvic tumor	2	
Liver transplant	4	
Abdominal closure under tension	1	
Spleen trauma	1	
Hepatic, intestinal trauma	2	
Mesenteric artery thrombosis	1	
Sigmoid colon necrosis[a]	1	
Ischemic postoperative colitis[a]	1	
Total	122	53/101
Chang et al. [54]		
Trauma	11	7/11
Overall total	133	60/112

[a]Postaortic aneurysm operation.

Multiple trauma with craniocephalic involvement and a traumatic diaphragm hernia (singly or together) increase the severity of the picture. Both problems should be kept in mind with multiple trauma. Diagnostic laparoscopy with pneumoperitoneum should be avoided because it may increase neurologic damage or induce sudden cardiorespiratory deterioration, leading to death, as was observed by Ali and Qi[34] in an experimental model.

Diagnosis

The diagnosis of the ACS is based on the clinical history and pathophysiologic responses. These measures should be supplemented by an IAP measurement higher than 15 mmHg, as clinical appraisal alone may prove fallacious.[41] Patients at risk of developing the syndrome should be identified, as ACS is often disregarded owing to the fact that critically ill patients have multiple reasons for a distended abdomen, pulmonary dysfunction, and oliguria.

Characteristic features of ACS include (1) low cardiac output with elevated filling pressures even in the presence of hypovolemia; (2) tachycardia; (3) oliguria; (4) requirement for massive volumes of intravenous fluids; and (5) variations in arterial blood pressure linked to assisted ventilation. Chest radiographs, show raised hemidiaphragms and normal or small ventricles. Dynamic compliance is markedly decreased.[3] In eight ACS patients with mean IAP values of 38 ± 17 mmHg Cullen et al.[3] found high peak airway pressures, markedly decreased dynamic compliance, normal PaO_2 and $PaCO_2$, low urinary flow, tachycardia, reduced systolic volume, and metabolic acidosis.

In a review of 16 cases, Morris et al. diagnosed ACS indirectly by an elevated inspiratory pressure (>85 cmH$_2$O), CO_2 retention, and oliguria. ACS was recognized preoperatively in 83% of their patients; in their experience, IAP measurement through the bladder did not give consistent results.[7] Meldrum et al.[11] defined the syndrome as IAP exceeding 20 mmHg accompanied by one or more of the following signs: peak airway pressure > 40 cmH$_2$O, oxygen availability < 600 ml O$_2$/min/m^2, or diuresis < 0.5 ml/kg/hr. In agreement with Morris et al., most surgeons use clinical signs;[28] we and Schein et al.[24] contend that diagnostic suspicion must be confirmed by objective measurements of IAP. This practice allows earlier, more reliable selection of patients who require decompression.

Treatment

The aims of treatment are correction of hemodynamic, renal, respiratory, and metabolic abnormalities and correction of all reversible causes of IAH.[9,50] Medical treatment can provide only supportive measures: volume expansion to maintain adequate preload, increased heart rate, and optimization of renal flow with dopamine.[3] Abdominal decompression (reopening the incision in a recently operated case or opening the abdominal cavity through a midline incision if the abdomen was not previously opened) is the only procedure that can reverse the picture. This should be done even if the patient's condition is not good and whenever ACS is suspected—or, better still, in anticipation of the syndrome.[7,8,12] It is important to avoid delay. Decompression of the abdominal cavity and reduction in PEEP may prevent a fatal outcome even though the cause of ACS is not or cannot be corrected.[29]

Morris et al.[7] found that the most frequent surgical indication was an abrupt increase in PaCO$_2$ along with the impossibility of ventilating due to high peak airway pressures. Kron et al.[20] preferred not to wait for respiratory complications and postulated that an IAP value higher than 25 mmHg, accompanied by acute oliguria that fails to respond to fluids, is a strong indication of the need for a decompressive laparotomy. Eddy et al.[10] assigned value to worsening hypercarbia and compliance deterioration; they refrained from decompressing without the presence of pulmonary, renal, or cardiovascular compromise. They observed no oliguria in the absence of ventilatory failure. Chang et al.[54] recommended abdominal decompression with oliguria or progressive acidosis despite aggressive resuscitation and with IAP exceeding 25 mmHg. In our experience[26] the association of IAH (IAP > 20 mmHg) with an acidotic gastric intramucosal pH requires prompt decompression to prevent MODS and death. If the patient proceeds from oliguria to anuria without undergoing decompression, ATN may have developed; and with eventual decompression, there is no diuresis.

During the immediate preoperative period patients with elevated IAP should undergo fluid expansion if mixed-venous oxygen saturation is low, even though pulmonary capillary pressure remains high. Adverse effects and IAP or pleural pressure increases were not observed when necessary intravascular volumes were provided.[4] Lack or delay in adequate volume replacement, based on fallacious increases in central venous pressure or pulmonary capillary pressure, may severely decrease splanchnic perfusion.[4]

The goals of intervention are to decompress the abdomen, contain the viscera, reduce abdominal wall tension, preserve the fascia until visceral edema abates, and finally minimize the risks of wound infection and abdominal wall necrosis. Trained medical and ancillary staff are essential, with an ICU team for ventilation and volume management. Morris et al. used an intravenous solution to decrease reperfusion washout of harmful by-products of anaerobic metabolism; it contained 1 liter of normal saline solution plus 50 g mannitol and 50 mEq sodium bicarbonate.[7] Adequate and prompt volume expansion with normal saline or lactated Ringer's solution before abdominal decompression may be satisfactory. Although mannitol is useful as a reactive oxygen species scavenger, it could exacerbate hypovolemia by incurring osmotic diuresis. Monitoring during decompression must include the mean arterial blood pressure, pulse oximetry, pulmonary artery pressures, arterial and mixed-venous oxygen saturation, and core temperature. Restored intravascular volume should maximize oxygen availability and transport and combat the circulating reperfusion metabolites.[24]

The operation should control hemorrhage, evacuate collections, remove necrotic tissue, resect ischemic organs, and close, intubate, or exteriorize digestive tract discontinuities (whatever can be done in the least time). If packing had been placed, it should be partially or totally removed.[11] An important precaution is to avoid hypothermia.[33]

Abdominal wall closure is not possible. Temporary closure, leaving a wide margin between the borders of the fascia, is required with the use of mesh or other prostheses (semiopen technique).[9] This strategy and others, such as open management, planned relaparotomy, and staged abdominal repair, all reverse the negative effects of increased IAP.

Open and semiopen management facilitates reexploration, achieves better diaphragmatic excursion, improves renal perfusion, and reduces absorption of bacterial products by diaphragmatic stomas.[55] However, according to Schein et al.[56] the advantages assigned to open management have not yet been demonstrated, its sole virtue being to avoid repeated reopening and closure, which may damage the abdominal wall.

Prostheses to decompress include meshes composed of polypropylene (Prolene; Ethicon Division of Johnson and Johnson, New Brunswick, NJ, USA); polypropylene monofilament tissue (Bard Marlex Mesh; Davol, Craston, RI, USA); polyglactin 910 reabsorbable (Vicryl; Ethicon); expanded polytetrafluoroethyl (PTFE, Gore-Tex soft tissue patch; W.L. Gore, Flagstaff, AZ, USA); a silicone rubber sheet; or an open 3-L polyvinyl intravenous infusion bag. The material is fixed with a running suture of polypropylene-0. The entire prosthesis may be used without shortening but rolled in the center of the wound without tension, as suggested by Ivatury et al. This method allows it to be loosened as required, without needing to be changed.[1] Another available material is the Velcro-like "artificial burr-like device" (HIDIH Surgical, Doerrebach, Germany), which may be used in the same way.[57] Whenever possible, the omentum is placed on top of the viscera.

With massive intestinal or retroperitoneal edema, which prevents visceral reduction through a flat prosthesis, a silo with a rubber or plastic membrane is used, such as with gastroschisis and omphalocele in newborns. This membrane is cut to cover the gap, taking into account the volume of exteriorized intestine. It is then sutured or stapled to the cutaneous borders. The most popular material and the one preferred by us is an open 3-L intravenous fluid bag previously sterilized (Bogotá bag).[13]

The proper place to perform the decompressive laparotomy is the operating room; but given the transportation difficulties or limitation of ventilator support, the abdomen can be decompressed in the ICU, provided there is no active hemorrhage and the possibility of severe hypotension and asystole due to reperfusion damage is anticipated.[28]

Complications of Operations

Intraoperative Complications

Decompression is hemodynamically safe in patients who are not markedly hypovolemic.[24] When hypovolemia is present cardiovascular collapse may occur, which is attributable to the release of acidotic and vasoactive substances by the intestine and ischemic lower limbs [3] and to the abrupt fall in systemic vascular resistance due to splanchnic vasodilatation.[24] Morris et al.[7] found that 4 of 15 patients with ACS developed asystole when the abdomen was opened, and none survived (lethal reperfusion syndrome). To prevent neurologic damage, volume expansion is required to maintain cardiac output and brain perfusion pressure at normal levels before performing sudden abdominal decompression.[36] The other severe intraoperative complication is hypothermia, which may also lead to death.

Postoperative Complications

Postoperative complications may involve the abdomen or be extraabdominal. With open management evisceration, massive fluid loss, spontaneous fistulas in exposed bowel, and wound contamination may occur. The semiopen technique has a lower complication rate.[55] Other complications depend on the underlying disease. There is a high incidence of dehiscence, acute incisional hernia, and necrotizing infection, as well as skin and subcutaneous tissue necrosis. Burch et al. found complications in 20% of patients in which a silo was used.[33]

With multiple trauma and brain injury, laparoscopic exploration entails the risk of further brain damage due to increased IAP. MacDonnell et al.[58] reported extensive distal venous thrombosis in a patient with a pulmonary embolism after decompression. Simon et al.[43] found that patients with deferred closure had a much lower incidence of pulmonary or renal dysfunction and a better survival rate.

A staged repair strategy requires repeated operations. For patients in whom the systemic inflammatory response is not yet controlled, such a strategy may act as a "second hit" and trigger MODS.[55]

Late Complications

With the use of a silo, a large ventral hernia is present whose treatment may be complex.[33] However, the incidence of parietal sepsis and of incisional hernia upon performing definitive closure is low.

Postoperative Course

During the immediate postoperative period aggressive treatment restores perfusion and normalizes coagulation factors, platelets, and body temperature; prophylactic antibiotic therapy is used for a short period.[13,28] Most patients show immediate improvement after decompression, with prompt recovery of respiratory and renal function.[43] Chang et al.[54] studied the effects of decompression in 11 patients and found improved preload, pulmonary function, and visceral perfusion. Once hemorrhage is controlled, necrotic tissue eliminated, and oxygenation restored, parietal and visceral edema starts to be reabsorbed, depending on the status of cellular repair and the integrity of the endothelial membrane. The result is a brisk diuresis and the possibility of restoring the bowel into the peritoneal cavity.

The wound gap is decreased progressively with control of IAP, reducing the surface of the silo and awaiting the best time for definitive closure. General improvement, satisfactory hemodynamics, diuresis, increased body temperature, normal coagulation tests, and clinical evidence of decreased abdominal wall tension usually occurs between the third and fifth postoperative days.[28] If direct closure is not feasible after 2 weeks, the granulation tissue may be covered with a split-thickness skin graft so long as infection is under control, leaving a large ventral hernia to be repaired 6–12 months later.

Mortality associated with ACS is high.[28,36] Morris et al. reported a mortality rate of 62.5%[7] and Schein et al. 42%;[24] and in the reviewed reports it reached 53.6% (Table 30.5). According to Burch et al.,[13] patients not undergoing decompression failed to survive. Recently we found that the 12-hour postoperative IAP value proved to be a predictive factor for mortality on applying multiple logistic regression to 109 determinations. It had high sensitivity (90.7%), low specificity (27.3%), and a correct classification rate of 65.14%. The goodness-of-fit test was 7.1552 ($p = 0.5200$), demonstrating adequate calibration between predicted and true mortality. According to the odds ratio value obtained, the mean increase in the risk of death is 7% for each point of IAP increase exceeding 20 mmHg. On the basis of logistic regression data and through application of the probability-of-death formula, a curve was plotted relating the latter to IAP value (Fig. 30.4).

Prevention

There are no reports of prospective studies evaluating the application of objective methods to help with the decision for a given surgical strategy or time for managing patients prone to develop ACS. Mayberry et al.[59] retrospectively analyzed the results of abdominal closure with meshes compared with closed management. They found that when a prosthesis was placed during the first laparotomy for prevention there was no postoperative ACS, though the mortality rate remained unchanged. Ivatury et al. confirmed that the incidence of IAH after open abdominal trauma was greater with primary closure of the fascia (52% of cases) than with prophylactic employment of a mesh (22.2%).[60] Oelschlager et al.[32] found a trend toward better survival in patients with ruptured abdominal aortic aneurysms when open management was used; they attributed it to a lower incidence of ACS.

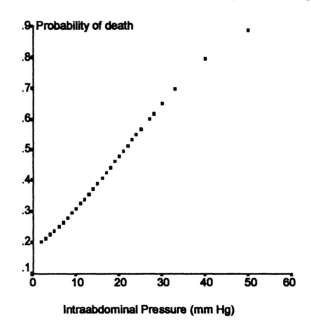

FIGURE 30.4. Correlation between intraabdominal pressure and the likelihood of death.

TABLE 30.6. Prevention of Abdominal Compartment Syndrome.

Identify patients
  Severe abdominal disease
  Ruptured aortic aneurysm
  Peritoneal sepsis
  Pancreatitis
  Severe trauma

Recommendations
  Close the abdomen with a prosthesis if the abdominal wall does not come together easily
  Resort to semiopen or open abdomen and contain viscera with a silo when containment cannot be flat
  Monitor gastric intramucosal pH and check intraabdominal pressure every 4–6 hours
  Decompress when intraabdominal pressure increases pathologically: 20–25 mmHg or 15 mmHg with head trauma
  Do not perform gas laparoscopy after severe abdominal trauma or head trauma owing to possible aggravation of splanchnic and neurologic ischemic conditions, or in the presence of MODS or sepsis, given its potential for a "second hit" effect

Prevention of ACS is based on the control and decrease of IAP; the incidence may be considerably lower with prophylactic measures. Prevention of ACS is summarized in Table 30.6.

Conclusions

Abdominal compartment syndrome is an infrequently reported entity. It may lead to death not only because of its etiology but also because of the pathophysiologic alterations triggered by IAH. It is important to act preventively by timely decompression of the abdomen. IAP and gastric intramucosal pH should be assessed in every critically ill patient prone to this complication. Data obtained by these measurements provide criteria for reexploring the abdomen before cardiorespiratory or renal signs appear. In the presence of elevated IAP accompanied by oliguria and increased central venous and pulmonary capillary pressures, operation must be done promptly to reduce IAP and PEEP before resorting to diuretics or inotropic agents. Use of an abdominal silo can provide the time required for recovery of altered physiologic variables. Although mortality remains high, careful monitoring provides a valuable tool to guide decision making.

References

1. Ivatury RR, Diebel L, Porter JM, Simon RJ: Intra-abdominal hypertension and the abdominal compartment syndrome. Surg Clin North Am 1997;77:783–812.
2. Bloomfield GL, Ridings PC, Blocher CR, Marmarou A, Sugerman HJ: A proposed relationship between increased intra-abdominal, intrathoracic, and intracranial pressure. Crit Care Med 1997;25:496–503.
3. Cullen DJ, Coyle JP, Teplick R, Long MC: Cardiovascular, pulmonary, and renal effects of massively increased intra-abdominal pressure in critically ill patients. Crit Care Med 1989;17:118–121.
4. Ridings PC, Bloomfield GL, Blocher CR, Sugerman HJ: Cardiopulmonary effects of raised intra-abdominal pressure before and after intravascular volume expansion. J Trauma 1995;39:1071–1075.
5. Bumaschny E: The abdominal compartment syndrome. Curr Opin Crit Care 1998;4:236–244.
6. Sugrue M, Jones F, Lee A, et al: Intraabdominal pressure and gastric intramucosal pH: is there an association? World J Surg 1996;20:988–991.
7. Morris JA Jr, Eddy VA, Blinman TA, Rutherford EJ, Sharp KW: Staged celiotomy for trauma: issues in unpacking and reconstruction. Ann Surg 1993;217:576–586.
8. Saggi BH, Sugerman HJ, Ivatury RR, Bloomfield GL: Abdominal compartment syndrome. J Trauma 1998;45:597–609.
9. Sugrue M, Hillman KM: Intra-abdominal hypertension and intensive care. In: Vincent JL (ed) Yearbook of Intensive Care and Emergency Medicine. Berlin, Springer 1998;667–676.
10. Eddy V, Nunn C, Morris JA: Abdominal compartment syndrome: the Nashville experience. Surg Clin North Am 1997;77:801–812.
11. Meldrum DR, Moore FA, Moore EE, Franciose RJ, Sauaia A, Burch JM: Prospective characterization and selective management of the abdominal compartment syndrome. Am J Surg 1997;174:667–673.
12. Diebel LN, Dulchavsky SA, Wilson RF: Effect of increased intraabdominal pressure on mesenteric arterial and intestinal mucosal blood flow. J Trauma 1992;33:45–49.
13. Burch JM, Moore EE, Moore FA, Franciose R: The abdominal compartment syndrome. Surg Clin North Am 1996;76:833–842.
14. Harman PK, Kron IL, McLachlan HD, Freedlender AE, Nolan SP: Elevated intra-abdominal pressure and renal function. Ann Surg 1982;196:594–947.
15. Overholt RH: Intraperitoneal pressure. Arch Surg 1931;22:691–703.
16. Bradley SE, Bradley GP: The effect of increased intra-abdominal pressure on renal function in man. J Clin Invest 1947;26:1010–1022.
17. Gross R: A new method for surgical treatment of large omphaloceles. Surgery 1948;24:277–292.
18. Richardson JD, Trinkle JK: Hemodynamic and respiratory alterations with increased intra-abdominal pressure. J Surg Res 1976;20:401–404.
19. Richards WO, Scovill W, Shin B, Reed W: Acute renal failure associated with increased intra-abdominal pressure. Ann Surg 1983;197:183–187.
20. Kron IL, Harman PK, Nolan SP: Measurement of intra-abdominal pressure as a criterion for abdominal re-exploration. Ann Surg 1984;199:28–30.
21. Fietsam R Jr, Villalba M, Glover JL, Clark K: Intra-abdominal compartment syndrome as a complication of ruptured abdominal aortic aneurysm repair. Am Surg 1989;55:396–402.
22. Shenasky JH, Gillenwater JY: The renal hemodynamic and functional effects of external counterpressure. Surg Gynecol Obstet 1972;134:253–258.
23. Diebel LN, Wilson RF, Dulchavsky SA, Saxe J: Effect of increased intra-abdominal pressure on hepatic arterial, portal venous, and hepatic microcirculatory blood flow. J Trauma 1992;33:279–283.
24. Schein M, Wittmann DH, Aprahamian CC, Condon RE: The abdominal compartment syndrome: the physiological and clinical consequences of elevated intra-abdominal pressure. J Am Coll Surg 1995;180:745–753.
25. Bloomfield GL, Blocher CR, Fakhry BS, Sica DA, Sugerman HJ: Elevated intra-abdominal pressure increases plasma renin activity and aldosterone levels. J Trauma 1997;42:997–1005.
26. Pusajó JF, Bumaschny E, Egurrola MA, et al: Intra-abdominal pressure: its relation to splanchnic perfusion, sepsis, multiple organ failure and surgical reintervention. Intensive Crit Care Dig 1994;13:2–4.
27. Kashtan J, Green JF, Parsons EQ, Holcroft JW: Hemodynamic effects of increased abdominal pressure. J Surg Res 1981;30:249–225.
28. Hirshberg A, Mattox KL: Planned reoperation for severe trauma. Ann Surg 1995;222:3–8.
29. Paul A, Troidl H, Peters S, Stuttmann R: Fatal intestinal ischaemia following laparoscopic cholecystectomy. Br J Surg 1994;81:1207.
30. Obeid F, Saba A, Fath J, et al: Increases in intra-abdominal pressure affect pulmonary compliance. Arch Surg 1995;130:544–548.
31. Eleftheriadis E, Kotzampassi K, Papanotas K, Heliadis N, Sarris K: Gut ischemia, oxidative stress, and bacterial translocation in elevated abdominal pressure in rats. World J Surg 1996;20:11–16.
32. Oelschlager BK, Boyle EM Jr, Johansen K, Meissner MH: Delayed abdominal closure in the management of ruptured abdominal aortic aneurysms. Am J Surg 1997;173:411–415.

33. Burch JM, Ortiz VB, Richardson RJ, Martin RR, Mattox KL, Jordan GL Jr: Abbreviated laparotomy and planned reoperation for critically injured patients. Ann Surg 1992;215:476–484.
34. Ali J, Qi W: The cardiorespiratory effects of increased intra-abdominal pressure in diaphragmatic rupture. J Trauma 1992;33:233–239.
35. Baue AE: The particular problem of peritonitis and increased abdominal pressure. In: Baue AE (ed) Multiple Organ Failure. Patients Care and Prevention. St Louis, Mosby Year Book, 1990;466–470.
36. Bloomfield GL, Ridings PC, Blocher CR, Marmarou A, Sugerman HJ: Effects of increased intra-abdominal pressure upon intracranial and cerebral perfusion pressure before and after volume expansion. J Trauma 1996;40:936–943.
37. Safran DS, Orlando R III: Physiologic effects of pneumoperitoneum. Am J Surg 1994;167:281–286.
38. Marathe US, Lilly RE, Silvestry SC, et al: Alterations in hemodynamics and left ventricular contractility during carbon dioxide pneumoperitoneum. Surg Endosc 1996;10:974–978.
39. Durham R, Neunaber K, Vogler G, Shapiro M, Mazuski J: Right ventricular end-diastolic volume as a measure of preload. J Trauma 1995;39:218–224.
40. O'Leary E, Hbbard K, Torney W, Cunningham AJ: Laparoscopic cholecystectomy: haemodynamic and neuroendocrine responses after pneumoperitoneum and changes in position. Br J Anaesth 1996;75:640–644.
41. Thaler W, Frey L, Marzoli P, Messmer K: Assessment of splanchnic tissue oxygenation by gastric tonometry in patients undergoing laparoscopic and open cholecystectomy. Br J Surg 1996;83:620–624.
42. Diebel LN, Dulchavsky SA, Brown WJ: Splanchnic ischemia and bacterial translocation in the abdominal compartment syndrome. J Trauma 1997;43:852–855.
43. Simon RJ, Friedlander MH, Ivatury RR, DiRaimo R, Machiedo GW: Hemorrhage lowers the threshold for intra-abdominal hypertension-induced pulmonary dysfunction. J Trauma 1997;42:398–405.
44. Ranieri VM, Brienza A, Santostasi S, et al: Impairment of lung and chest wall mechanics in patients with acute respiratory distress syndrome: role of abdominal distension. Am J Respir Crit Care Med 1997;156:1082–1091.
45. Fok TF, Ng PC, Wong W, Lee CH, So KW: High frequency oscillatory ventilation in infants with increased intra-abdominal pressure. Arch Dis Child 1997;76:F123–F125.
46. Irgau I, Koyfman Y, Tikellis JI: Elective intraoperative intracranial pressure monitoring during laparoscopic cholecystectomy. Arch Surg 1995;130:1011–1013.
47. Sugerman HJ, DeMaria EJ, Felton WL, Nakatsuka M, Sismanis A: Increased intra-abdominal pressure and cardiac filling pressures in obesity-associated pseudotumor cerebri. Neurology 1997;49:507–511.
48. Diebel L, Saxe J, Dulchavsky S: Effect of intra-abdominal pressure on abdominal wall blood flow. Am Surg 1992;58:573–576.
49. Nathens A, Boulanger BR: The abdominal compartment syndrome. Curr Opin Crit Care 1998;4:118–120.
50. Savino JA, Cerabona T, Agarwal N, Byrne D: Manipulation of ascitic pressure in cirrhotics to optimize hemodynamic and renal function [discussion]. Ann Surg 1988;208:504–511.
51. Hirvonen EA, Nuutinen LS, Vuolteenaho O: Hormonal responses and cardiac filling pressures in head-up or head-down position and pneumoperitoneum in patients undergoing operative laparoscopy. Br J Anaesth 1997;78:128–133.
52. Rodríguez A, Egurrola A, Chiacchiara D, et al: Presión intra-abdominal en pacientes críticos. Comparación de dos métodos. Medi Intens (Argentina) 1995;12:51–55.
53. Sugrue M, Buist MD, Lee A, Sanchez DJ, Hillman KM: Intra-abdominal pressure measurement using a modified nasogastric tube: description and validation of new technique. Intensive Care Med 1994;20:588–590.
54. Chang MC, Miller PR, D'Agostino R Jr, Meredith W: Effects of abdominal decompression on cardiopulmonary function and visceral perfusion in patients with intra-abdominal hypertension. J Trauma 1998;44:440–445.
55. Wittmann DH, Schein M, Condon RE: Management of secondary peritonitis. Ann Surg 1996;224:10–18.
56. Schein M, Hirshberg A, Hashmonai M: Current surgical management of severe intraabdominal infection. Surgery 1992;112:489–496.
57. Wittmann DH, Aprahamian C, Bergstein JM, et al: A burr-like device to facilitate temporary abdominal closure in planned multiple laparotomies. Eur J Surg 1993;159:75–79.
58. MacDonnell SP, Lalude OA, Davidson AC: The abdominal compartment syndrome: the physiological and clinical consequences of elevated intraabdominal pressure [letter]. J Am Coll Surg 1996;184:419–420.
59. Mayberry JC, Mullins RJ, Crass RA, Trunkey DD: Prevention of abdominal compartment syndrome by absorbable mesh prosthesis closure. Arch Surg 1997;132:957–962.
60. Ivatury RR, Porter JM, Simon RJ, Islam S, John R, Stahl WM: Intraabdominal hypertension after life-threatening penetrating abdominal trauma: prophylaxis, incidence, and clinical relevance to gastric mucosal pH and abdominal compartment syndrome. J Trauma 1998;44:1016–1023.

31
SIRS and MODS: Indications for Surgical Intervention?

Donald E. Fry

Management of the patient with the systemic inflammatory response syndrome (SIRS) and evolving multiple organ dysfunction syndrome (MODS) continues to be a formidable challenge. Although SIRS as a clinical syndrome is usually readily identified and organ failure is ordinarily evident (depending on the definition employed), uncertainty about the specific stimulus that has activated the systemic inflammation commonly exists. Many of these patients are in the intensive care unit (ICU), and any number of apparent or subtle activators of inflammation may be present.

Among the activators of inflammation (discussed in Chapter 9), infection remains the most common cause of SIRS leading to MODS. Surgical patients have numerous potential portals for invasive infection that may be driving the systemic activation of inflammation. Infection at a prior surgical site or at the site of trauma injury must always be considered. In the ICU specific nosocomial infections are possible. Among these nosocomial infections, pneumonia, urinary tract infection, and intravascular device infections are the most common. Infection at the surgical/trauma site or infection where invasive monitoring or support has been employed (e.g., endotracheal tube, Foley catheter, indwelling intravascular catheter) is responsible for clinical infection in 95% of episodes. However, candidemia and bacteremia of unknown origin are increasing in frequency, especially in the patient with a protracted ICU stay and in the patient who has received a lengthy course or multiple courses of antibiotic therapy. Better prevention of infection is thought to reduce the incidence of SIRS, and the hope of clinicians is that better management and control of established infection can reverse the natural history of activated systemic inflammation.

In one of the original treatises on multiple organ failure (MOF), Eiseman et al.[1] identified surgically correctable sources of infection as being major associated events for the organ failure patient. They presented an argument for better surgical management of the primary infection as a strategy to both prevent and reverse organ failure. Polk and Shields[2] reported a small number of patients in whom organ failure complexes were identified, and surgical intervention and drainage of suppurative collections of pus from the intraabdominal cavity resulted in resolution of the organ failure. Similarly, Hinsdale and Jaffe[3] reported successful reversal of organ failure when selected empiric reoperation was pursued in patients with subsequently proven abdominal abscess.

In a series of reports, our group identified surgically manageable sources of infection as a commonly associated clinical event in patients with MODS.[4–7] Among emergency surgical patients, about 50% had uncontrolled intraabdominal infection as the presumed infection "activator" of organ failure.[4] Of note, nearly 50% of patients had pleuropulmonary sources of infection as the identified stimulus for clinical sepsis and MODS. Intraabdominal abscess[5] and anaerobic bacteremia with the enteric pathogen *Bacteroides fragilis*[6] represented specific illnesses associated with SIRS and MODS and commonly required surgical intervention for successful management. However, clear relations between surgical drainage of pyogenic infection and the reversal of established MOF was more implied than proven in these studies.

The microcirculatory hypothesis of MOF was presented in Chapter 9. It is hypothesized that the global activation and progression of systemic inflammation may result in sufficient damage (e.g., necrosis) to the failed organs that even complete control of the inciting event cannot change the natural history of the progressive organ dysfunction and ultimate death of the patient. A point is reached where ischemic damage and end-organ cellular injury itself may serve as the continued stimulus to activation of the inflammatory response. Most surgeons have had patients in whom organ failure pursued a relentless, fatal course even in the face of appropriate, timely surgical intervention for a pyogenic infection. Norton best expressed the ennui of the clinical conundrum of severe organ failure in a report in which it was stated that drainage of an abscess did not improve the outcome of patients with advanced organ failure.[8] Thus the question is whether patients with established organ failure should undergo aggressive surgical intervention in an effort to reverse the process. What are the clinical criteria that should guide such decisions?

Clinical Dilemma

Infection from any anatomic site or from any microbial type of clinical infection can be responsible for activating systemic inflammation. Are there special or specific features of inflammation that are unique to these clinical scenarios where pus within the abdominal cavity may trigger the inflammatory response? SIRS is a nonspecific response of the host to infective and noninfective activation. The clinician must systematically identify the infectious and noninfectious variables that may be relevant in a specific patient and then search for clinical clues to assist in the decision making process.

The patient with severe acute pancreatitis is illustrative of the many faces of SIRS that can be expressed in a given patient across the longitudinal course of time. At presentation, patients with severe acute pancreatitis have evidence of SIRS and evolving MODS by virtue of all the criteria identified by Ranson et al.[9] The patients have fever and leukocytosis. Fluid administration must be given in large quantities to meet (1) extracellular losses into the retroperitoneal inflammation, (2) the requirements of expanded capacitance due to systemic vasodilation, and (3) systemic edema formation in all soft tissues secondary to increased capillary permeability. Early MODS is commonly seen in these patients, who require ventilator support because of arterial desaturation. (Fig. 31.1). Mild elevations of bilirubin and other liver enzymes may be seen, and creatinine elevations may be identified in especially severe cases. The process may abate within 48–72 hours of aggressive, appropriate management, and SIRS then recedes. The patients are weaned from ventilator support, and liver enzyme profiles return to normal.

At 5–7 days following the onset of the disease process and admission to the hospital, these patients commonly have a secondary SIRS event, with a return of fever and leukocytosis. A hyperdynamic response with an increase in cardiac output and reduction of peripheral vascular resistance is identified. The patient again may require ventilator support, and liver enzyme abnormalities may return. This clinical scenario heralds the onset of peripancreatic infection or may be caused by pancreatic necrosis but without infection—yet. Complex clinical decisions are required that commonly lead to multiple operations and débridement/drainage of the lesser sac and pancreatic tissue bed. Management may be complicated by nosocomial infection, with the patient having a ventilation-associated pneumonia with a gram-negative organism (e.g., *Pseudomonas aeruginosa*) or a central line septic event with *Staphylococcus aureus*. Reoperations for abdominal sepsis are frequent, but nosocomial infections at other anatomic sites make the frequency and necessity of these multiple reoperative procedures of uncertain value.

The transition to a third phase of SIRS for these patients occurs in the wake of resolution of the abdominal infection. The patients may have tertiary peritonitis or multiple, resistant gram-negative nosocomial infections at remote sites. These nosocomial infections are usually with highly resistant, hospital-acquired gram-negative bacteria. Blood cultures may be positive for *Candida* sp.[10] or *Enterococcus* sp.[11] as evidence that continued SIRS and evolving MODS may be driven at this time by microbial translocation.

With such a prototypical case one can identify distinct phases where different activation stimuli are initiating the SIRS process. In the reality of a clinical scenario, multiple stimuli may be active in concert or in sequence. The decision to reoperate in these complex clinical situations requires the use of all objective diagnostic tools together with keen clinical judgment.

Patient Selection for Reoperation

Which patients should be considered for abdominal exploration with the hope of reversing SIRS and early MODS? A primary consideration must identify whether an abdominal source of sepsis is a realistic concern. In an open-heart postoperative patient who has a difficult, protracted period of cardiopulmonary bypass and is demonstrating pulmonary failure and jaundice on the third day following the procedure, it is unlikely that an abdominal event is activating SIRS. On the other hand, SIRS in a patient 6–7 days following sigmoid colectomy with colostomy for a perforated diverticulum or in a postoperative abdominal gunshot wound patient with multiple initial injuries represents a setting where the presence of SIRS should stimulate a high index of suspicion that abdominal infection is the clinical event responsible for activating the process.

Early postoperative deterioration (1–3 days postoperatively) with early SIRS and MODS in the abdominal surgical patient

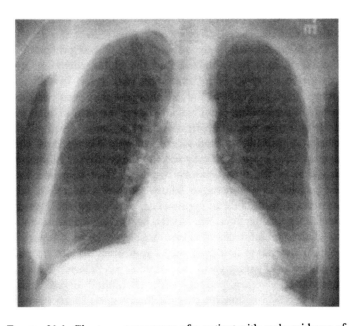

FIGURE 31.1. Chest roentgenogram of a patient with early evidence of adult respiratory distress syndrome (ARDS) on the fifth day following abdominal operation for acute peritonitis. ARDS at this point of the patient's course must give strong consideration to SIRS from an abdominal abscess.

must provoke strong consideration for early reoperation. Such decompensations are associated with catastrophic complications, such as intestinal suture line dehiscence. Ischemic infarctions following abdominal aneurysm or other abdominal aortic procedure are similarly the types of case when reoperation must be entertained to reverse abrupt clinical deterioration. In trauma patients, early SIRS and MODS may be an indication of a missed injury during the initial evaluation or initial abdominal exploration. Because computed tomography (CT) scans within the initial 7 days after celiotomy for trauma are inaccurate because of inflammatory changes or "casual" water from inflammatory fluids or retained irrigation,[12,13] the decision to pursue reoperation may need to be made on clinical grounds alone.

The decision for reoperation must take into consideration whether the patient has obvious, nonabdominal sources for SIRS and MODS. The presence of rapidly evolving pneumonia or infection at another site should diminish the inclination to conclude immediately that SIRS and MODS are arising the consequence of an intraabdominal infection. However, left lower lobe pneumonia or left lower lobe pulmonary effusion may support the presence of a left subphrenic abscess. Even the diagnosis of pneumonia can be tenuous, as rapidly evolving adult respiratory distress syndrome (ARDS) with diffuse pulmonary infiltration may be the consequence of SIRS. Infiltration of the lung secondary to ARDS is in reality an expression of MODS and not due to pneumonia per se. Pneumonia is a common complication of intraabdominal abscess, and its presence appears to increase the mortality rates of abdominal abscess patients.[14] (Figs. 31.2, 31.3). Furthermore, the need for ventilatory support of the patient with SIRS and MODS due to an intraabdominal infection frequently results in pulmonary infection, which may ultimately be the most important variable in the recovery of the patient.

The most important tool when making a decision for reoperation has been the abdominal CT scan, which provides excellent diagnostic accuracy for determining if an abscess is present. The CT scan also affords the opportunity to drain the abscess collection percutaneously and obviates the need for reoperation. Avoiding additional general anesthesia, wound morbidity at the abdominal incision, and the risks of enterocutaneous fistulas from repeated intraabdominal procedures are potentially achieved with percutaneous draining under CT direction. The diagnostic accuracy of the currently available, late-generation CT units makes this diagnostic scan of considerable value. When feasible, intravenous and intraluminal contrast is used to enhance the accuracy of the abdominal CT scan. The confidence of the radiologist and the surgeon in the CT findings can be an important issue when determining whether the abdomen should be reexplored. Determining that a given CT evaluation has equivocal findings that cannot be clearly stated to be pus or inflammatory changes may help select a patient for reoperation. The decision requires correlation of the severity of the patient's clinical condition with the conviction that CT abnormalities may in fact represent a surgically correctable problem. Continued improvement in the diagnostic accuracy of postoperative abdominal CT scanning has resulted in overall improvement for making the decision to reoperate.

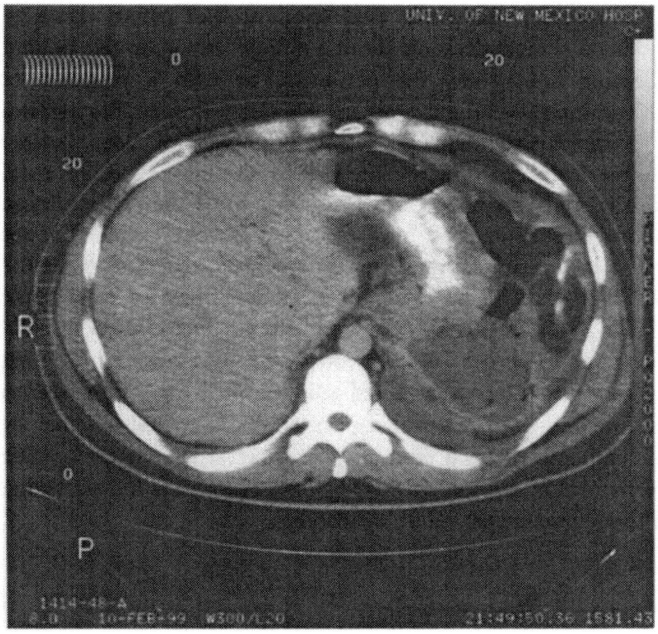

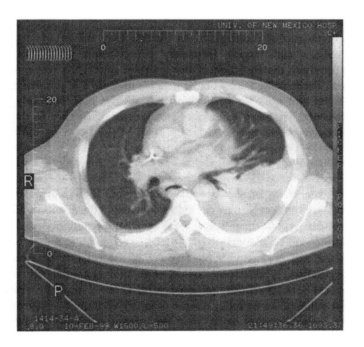

FIGURE 31.2. Computed tomography (CT) scan of the abdomen illustrates a large left upper quadrant abdominal abscess. It was successfully managed by percutaneous drainage.

FIGURE 31.3. Chest CT scan from the same patient in Fig. 31.2. The patient was treated for pneumonia, which failed to resolve on antibiotic therapy. The pulmonary infiltrate did not resolve until the subdiaphragmatic abscess was managed successfully.

When an abscess is identified by CT scan, percutaneous drainage is the first consideration for management.[15-18] When an abscess is accurately defined, it can be drained with minimum morbidity. The pathway of catheter placement for percutaneous drainage should not traverse another hollow viscus in the abdomen as injury to the intestine combined with the local inflammation from an adjacent abscess may be responsible for the development of an enterocutaneous fistula or yet other abscesses. In general, patients with fulminant SIRS and rapidly evolving MODS are not best managed by percutaneous drainage. The extremely ill patient may require other surgical manipulations (e.g., repair, resection, exterioration) in addition to drainage of the abscess collection. The critically ill surgical patient in the ICU with multiple monitors and intravascular access lines and on ventilator support represents a major logistic risk for movement and is not well managed or monitored in the radiology department.

Selected types of abscess may not be well defined by CT-directed, percutaneous drainage methods. The pancreatic abscess is commonly multiloculated, is accompanied by unusually turbid suppuration, and often has sloughed, necrotic tissue debris from the primary process. Effective drainage of these pancreatic abscess collections is associated with a high probability of failure from percutaneous drainage, attempts. In contrast, patients with infected pancreatic pseudocyst collections are amenable to percutaneous drainage as the pseudocyst collection represents contained pancreatic secretions and not necrotic tissue. Percutaneous drainage of an abscess in the subphrenic spaces and pericolic gutters is usually effective using CT-assisted methods. A deep pelvic abscess or interloop abscess is less effectively drained because of the risk of injury to adjacent structures.

Percutaneous drainage of an abscess may fail in selected situations and require secondary percutaneous procedures, appropriate manipulation of the drainage system, or reoperation. Technically, it may not be possible to drain a multilocated abscess and multiple separate abscess cavities percutaneously. However, improved techniques and greater persistence in the pursuit of percutaneous drainage have allowed two or three separate drainage catheters to be placed, with successful resolution of multifocal abdominal abscess. An abscess with excessive tissue debris and necrosis can occlude the small drainage ports of the percutaneous drain. Replacement of drainage catheters over a guidewire may afford successful percutaneous drainage when a catheter has become occluded. Nondependent placement of the catheter can be a source of failure and may require replacement of the catheter or even reoperation. When source control of abdominal contamination has not been successfully achieved owing to failed suture lines or disruption of the bowel by disease or injury, continued soilage of the intraabdominal cavity may not permit resolution of the SIRS and early MODS process. Continued SIRS and progression of MODS after percutaneous drainage efforts is an indication to strongly consider open surgical intervention.

Patients with major abdominal wound morbidity are usually best managed by reoperation and their abdominal compartment reexamined for abscess at the time of this procedure. Wound dehiscence or evisceration usually is the consequence of severe invasive infection of the abdominal wall fascia. If bacterial contamination at the original procedure was sufficiently severe to result in a complex abdominal wall invasive infection, the clinician must be concerned that deeper infection may similarly be present.

Patients with positive blood cultures for enteric microorganisms are commonly in need of drainage and perhaps reoperation. The bacteremic patient obviously has a primary source responsible for dissemination of the microorganism, and a systemic search and evaluation of all probable sites may lead to the conclusion that the abdominal compartment is the likely source. This is particularly true when the bacteremia is due to *Bacteroides fragilis*, and the patient is in a postoperative phase after a complex colon operation or after a procedure for acute bacterial peritonitis due to colonic contamination. A positive blood culture for an obligate enteric anaerobe is certainly presumptive evidence that an anaerobic environment is the source of infection. It is reasonable to assume that the environment is composed of pus from a colonic source of contamination, and that the source needs to be drained. Whereas multiple sites may be implicated by positive cultures for *Escherichia coli*, *Klebsiella* sp., and *Enterobacter* sp. (e.g., urinary tract infection), a blood culture positive for enteric aerobic species must arouse suspicion of an abdominal abscess. In positive blood cultures *Candida* sp., *Staphylococcus epidermidis*, *Enterococcus* sp., and *Pseudomonas* sp. are organisms that remain in the aftermath of extended antibiotic therapy. They are more reflective of a failed host response and do not ordinarily constitute markers of abscess or indicate the need for surgical intervention.

Commonly, the whole evaluation process comes down to making a clinical decision about a difficult postoperative patient following laparotomy for peritonitis or with a complex or difficult intraabdominal problem. Unique postoperative features of inappropriate and persistent postoperative ileus, severe glucose intolerance, acute atrial arrhythmias (especially atrial fibrillation),[19] polyuric syndromes, and acute mental confusion in elderly patients have been identified as "soft" signs of septic events in the surgical patient and require a decision about the likelihood that an intraabdominal process may be responsible (Table 31.1). Early postoperative arterial desaturation or mild elevations in serum bilirubin concentrations may be the first indication that organ dysfunction is looming. Early intervention with definitive mechanical control of the infection, whether by percutaneous or open methods, has a better chance of aborting the natural history of SIRS than when one awaits full activation of the severe organ failure syndromes.

Planned Reoperation

The initial laparotomy in selected patients can provide a clear picture of where there is a high probability of impending uncontrolled postoperative infection or abscess. High velocity

TABLE 31.1. Soft Signs of SIRS.

Clinical event[a]	Comments
Sustained gastrointestinal (GI) ileus	Successful surgical management of acute peritonitis results in an orderly resolution of GI ileus. Ileus beyond the fourth postoperative day suggests that inflammation persists in the abdomen.
Hyperglycemia	Insulin resistance is a consistent feature of the septic state. In the patient without excessive exogenous glucose administration or without latent/established diabetes, postoperative hyperglycemia reflects a possible persistent septic state.
Anaerobic/gram-negative bacteremia	Bacteremia in a postoperative peritonitis patient must have the source defined. A positive blood culture for *Bacteroides fragilis* means an anaerobic environment of infection exists. This usually means pus. *Escherichia coli* or other enteric gram-negative bacteria can come from other sources (e.g., urinary tract), but the abdominal compartment must be considered.
Acute arterial desaturation	In patients without underlying lung disease or early evidence of pneumonia, this may be the first "domino" of MODS.
Chemical hyperbilirubinemia	Early increases in postoperative serum bilirubin in peritonitis patients are commonly ascribed to absorption of hematoma or lysis of old red blood cells. A normal liver can handle a normal bilirubin load. Hyperbilirubinemia in the postoperative peritonitis patient may be heralding MODS.
Acute atrial fibrillation	This may reflect acute increases in cardiac output in the patient with preexistent heart disease. Acute atrial tachyarrhythmias commonly means SIRS and may mean that an intraabdominal focus of residual pus is present in the postoperative peritonitis patient.
Polyuria	Patients with SIRS due to infection may experience corticomedullary redistribution of blood flow and loss of renal concentrating ability. Undrained infection in the postoperative peritonitis patient may be responsible.
Acute mental confusion	Most often seen in older patients, acute mental changes may reflect acute hypoxemia or inadequate cerebral perfusion. Persistent suppuration must be a concern in the postoperative peritonitis patient.
Unilateral pleural effusion/lower lobe pneumonia	This may represent subdiaphragmatic inflammation.
Wound infection/fascial necrosis	If contamination was sufficiently severe to cause a major wound complication, the same magnitude of contamination may have resulted in an abdominal abscess.

[a] These acute clinical events in the postoperative peritonitis patient may reflect ongoing, uncontrolled infection possibly requiring reoperation. Identification of one or more of these clinical events adds to the presumption that reoperation may be necessary.

gunshot wounds of the abdomen with massive tissue destruction and massive contamination from gut contents is one such scenario. Patients with massive contamination from large perforations of the gut or patients with a temporal delay in the source control and management of peritonitis represent other situations. When operation is undertaken in the patient with pancreatic necrosis or pancreatic abscess, it is usually clear at the initial procedure that the complexity of the infectious problem requires one or more reoperative procedures. Finally, every surgeon has encountered the situation where the trauma patient or laparotomy patient has an intestine that does not meet the criteria for being nonviable but arouses suspicion that delayed ischemic death could be a consequence. In these situations a planned reoperation may be the most important strategy to ensure an optimal outcome for the patient.

Planned reoperation has the advantage that the surgeon is not waiting for SIRS and MODS to be fully identified but, rather, is responding to a situation where these outcomes are virtually certain. At the completion of the initial procedure, reoperation is scheduled for a second look 24–48 hours later. When the decision is made to pursue a planned reoperation, the surgeon should not be dissuaded from the task because the patient appears to have done unexpectedly well during the immediate postoperative period. Unfortunately, patients commonly look remarkably well during that initial period, but those with catastrophic abdominal events seldom proceed to an uneventful recovery with antibiotics and divine supplication alone. The earlier intervention makes technical manipulation of the intestine easier than reoperation 6–10 days after the original procedure. The full ravages of the local inflammatory response are not as severe within 48 hours of the original procedure. There are fewer adhesions between loops of bowel, and blood loss is much less than during later interventions, after evidence of SIRS and MODS is present. In pancreatic abscess patients, reoperation may have to be planned on a daily or every-other-day basis for several sessions to ensure adequate local débridement and control of the infectious process.

The results of planned reoperation of the patient with complex peritonitis have been reported by numerous authors. Reported results have indicated that vigorous strategies of timed reexploration may vary from being harmful to patients to being life-saving.[20–24] As suggested by Bohnen and Mustard,[25] a large multicenter prospective trial is necessary to identify the merits and liabilities of this aggressive strategy.

Selected situations may be so severe the surgeon is required to leave the fascia of the entire abdominal wound open. This open abdominal management heralds "tertiary peritonitis," where a chronic fibrinopurulent peel of chronic infection develops across the somatic and parietal surface of the abdominal cavity.[26,27] Open wound management is required to afford complete drainage. The bacteriology of these infections assumes the character of the ICU nosocomial microbes. *Pseudomonas* sp., *Enterobacter* sp., resistant *Enterobacter* sp., and *Candida* sp. are commonly cultured from the abdominal cavity at this point. It is open mechanical management that makes a difference for survival of these patients, not systemic antibiotics. In a patient with an open abdominal wound careful, meticulous wound management is important to avoid catastrophic, commonly fatal complications of fistula within the open wound. Various mesh materials have been used, some with zippers[28-30] and others with Velcro,[31-32] to afford easy access back into the abdomen. We have had a favorable experience using a lubricated gauze (Xeroform) over the surface of the wound, covered by moist saline gauze and then an adhesive plastic drape over the whole wound. Maintaining the moisture of the wound is important to avoid the consequence of wound or serosal desiccation. Delayed abdominal reconstruction is then finished with a nonabsorbable synthetic mesh at a clinically appropriate time.[33]

Conclusions

Selected patients with SIRS and early MODS have a high index of suspicion for uncontrolled infection from the intraabdominal compartment as the activating event for their clinical condition. Conventional wisdom dictates that control of this infection can reverse the natural history of SIRS, which is provoked by invasive infection. Aggressive diagnostic strategies with the use of CT imaging and prudent application of open surgical methods provide the best outcome for most patients.

References

1. Eiseman B, Beart R, Norton L: Multiple organ failure. Surg Gynecol Obstet 1977;144:323-326.
2. Polk HC Jr, Shields CL: Remote organ failure: a valid sign of occult intraabdominal infection. Surgery 1977;81:310.
3. Hinsdale JG, Jaffe BM: Reoperation for intraabdominal sepsis: indications and results in modern critical care setting. Ann Surg 1984;199:31-36.
4. Fry DE, Pearlstein L, Fulton RL, Polk HC Jr: Multiple system organ failure: the role of uncontrolled infection. Arch Surg 1980;115:136-140.
5. Fry DE, Garrison RN, Heitch RC, et al: Determinants of death in patients with intraabdominal abscess. Surgery 1980;89:517-523.
6. Fry DE, Garrison RN, Williams HC: Patterns of morbidity and mortality in splenectomy for trauma. Am Surg 1980;46: 28-32.
7. Fry DE, Garrison RN, Polk HC Jr: Clinical implications in bacteroides bacteremia. Surg Gynecol Obstet 1979;149:189-192.
8. Norton LW: Does drainage of intra-abdominal pus reverse multiple organ failure? Am J Surg 1985;149:347-349.
9. Ranson JHC, Rifkind KM, Roses DF, et al: Prognostic signs and the role of operative management in acute pancreatitis. Ann Surg 1974;139:69.
10. Dyess DL, Garrison RN, Fry DE: Candida sepsis: implications of polymicrobial blood-borne infection. Arch Surg 1985;120: 345-348.
11. Garrison RN, Fry DE, Berberich S, Polk HC Jr: Enterococcal bacteremia: clinical implications and determinants of death. Ann Surg 1982;196:43-47.
12. Neff CC, Simeone JF, Ferrucci JT Jr, et al: The occurrence of fluid collections following routine abdominal surgical procedures: sonographic survey in asymptomatic post operative patients. Radiology 1983;146:463-466.
13. Norwood SH, Civetta JM: Abdominal CT: scanning in critically ill surgical patients. Ann Surg 1985;202:166-175.
14. Richardson JD, DeCamp MM, Garrison RN, Fry DE: Pulmonary infection complicating intra-abdominal sepsis: clinical and experimental observations. Ann Surg 1982;195:732-738.
15. Montgomery RS, Wilson SE: Intraabdominal abscesses: image-guided diagnosis and therapy. Clin Infect Dis 1996;23:28-36.
16. Shuler FW, Newman CN, Angood PB, et al: Non-operative management for intra-abdominal abscesses. Am Surg 1996; 62:218-222.
17. Haaga JR: Imaging intraabdominal abscesses and non-operative drainage procedures. World J Surg 1990;14:204-209.
18. Gerzof SG, Johnson WC, Robbins AH, Nabseth DC: Expanded criteria for percutaneous drainage. Arch Surg 1985;120 227-232.
19. Bender JS: Supraventricular tachyarrhythmias in the surgical intensive care unit: an under-recognized event. Am Surg 1996;62:73-75.
20. Sautner T, Gotzinger P, Redl-Wenzl EM, et al: Does reoperation for abdominal sepsis enhance the inflammatory host response? Arch Surg 1997;132:250-255.
21. Van Goor H, Hulsebos RG, Bleichrodt RP: Complications of planned relaparotomy in patients with severe general peritonitis. Eur J Surg 1997;163:61-66.
22. Schein M: Planned reoperations and open management in critical intra-abdominal infections: prospective experience in 52 cases. World J Surg 1991;15:537-545.
23. Penninckx F, Kerremans R, Filez L, et al: Planned relaparotomies for advanced, established peritonitis from colonic origin. Acta Chir Belg 1990;90:269-274.
24. Schein M, Saadia R, Freinkel Z, Decker GA: Aggressive treatment of severe diffuse peritonitis: a prospective study. Br J Surg 1988;75: 173-176.
25. Bohnen JM, Mustard RA: A critical look at scheduled relaparotomy for secondary bacterial peritonitis. Surg Gynecol Obstet 1991;172(suppl):25-29.
26. Nathans AB, Rotstein OD, Marshall JC: Tertiary peritonitis: clinical features of a complex nosocomial infection. World J Surg 1998;22:158-163.
27. Reemst, PHM, van Goor H, Goris RJA: SIRS, MODS, and tertiary peritonitis. Eur J Surg 1996;576(Suppl):47-49.
28. Sleeman D, Sosa JL, Gonzalez A, et al: Reclosure of the open abdomen. J Am Coll Surg 1995;180:200-204.
29. Hakkiluoto A, Hannukainen J: Open management with mesh and zipper of patients with intraabdominal abscesses or diffuse peritonitis. Eur J Surg 1992;158:403-405.
30. Stone HH, Strom PR, Mullins JR: Pancreatic abscess management by subtotal resection and packing. World J Surg 1984;8: 340-345.
31. Wittman DH, Aprahamian C, Bergstein JM: Etappenlavage: advanced diffuse peritonitis managed by planned multiple laparotomies utilizing zippers, slide fasteners, and velcro analogue for temporary abdominal closure. World J Surg 1990;14:218-226.
32. Wittman DH: Operative and nonoperative therapy of intraabdominal infection. Infection 1998;26:335-341.
33. Fry DE, Osler T: Abdominal wall considerations and complications in reoperative surgery. Surg Clin North Am 1991;71:1-11.

32
Nosocomial Infections in the ICU

Gina Quaid and Joseph S. Solomkin

Although intensive care units (ICUs) have improved the outcome of patients with various shock states and other life-threatening conditions, they are still associated with a high incidence of nosocomial infection.[1-7] Nosocomial infections in the ICU account for 25% of all such infections, and rates of infection are five to ten times higher in the ICU than on general wards. They are endemic and epidemic in ICUs and represent a significant source of morbidity, mortality, and cost.

There are several risk factors that leave the ICU patient susceptible to nosocomial infection. First, the invasive nature of critical care medicine (mechanical ventilatory support, hemodynamic monitoring, total parenteral nutrition, hemodialysis, intracranial pressure monitoring, innovative forms of surgery, and a vast variety of drugs, especially antiinfective agents) breaks down barriers to infection. Second, the severity of illness, preexisting diseases, and immune status are known to contribute to the risk of infection. Finally, health care providers act as carriers of infectious disease. Infection control policies and procedures enforcement and the microbiologic milieu (bacteria, fungus, viruses) of the ICU play a major role in the development and prevention of nosocomial infections.[8,9]

The most common nosocomial infections that occur in the ICU are pneumonia, intravascular catheter-related infections, urinary tract infections (UTIs), invasive fungal infections, sinusitis, antibiotic-associated colitis, and ventriculitis or meningitis from intracranial pressure monitors.[10] This chapter is designed to help in the diagnosis, treatment, and prevention of these infections as they occur within the ICU.

Pneumonia

Fifteen percent of all hospital-acquired infections are pneumonia, and they are the primary cause of deaths due to a nosocomial infection.[10-13] Depending on the severity of acute and underlying diseases of the patient population, mortality rates of 20–50% have been reported.[12,14-19] Several risk factors have been suspected or identified to increase the risk of pneumonia in the ICU, including those identified in the subset of mechanically ventilated patients listed in Table 32.1.

Pathogens/Pathophysiology

Gram-negative bacterial adherence to epithelial cells is important in the pathogenesis of oropharyngeal colonization. Gram-positive organisms normally colonize the oropharynx and help prevent adherence and colonization by gram-negative bacilli. In theory, gram-positive cocci have a greater ability to bind to cells rich in fibronectin than do gram-negative bacilli.[21,22] Patients who have become colonized with gram-negative bacteria have fewer gram-positive cocci per epithelial cell, leaving the way clear for gram-negative organisms to invade and multiply in the lower respiratory tract, eventually resulting in pneumonia.

Gram-negative oropharyngeal colonization takes place within 48 hours after intubation. Organisms responsible for nosocomial pneumonia may originate in the oropharynx and intestinal tract.[23,24] Gastric alkalization secondary to stress ulcer prophylaxis contributes to upper gastrointestinal (GI) tract colonization and creates a source of organisms that may be silently aspirated into the respiratory tract.[25,26] In fact, altering the bacterial flora of the oropharynx and GI tract may be the most important factor contributing to the increased incidence of pneumonia in critically ill patients.

Gram-negative bacilli are responsible for most nosocomial pneumonias (75–90%), and isolates are typically multidrug-resistant. Bacillary pneumonias carry the highest mortality rate in critically ill patients. Multiple studies have reported mortality rates from 56% to 87%.[11,14,16,27-31] *Pseudomonas aeruginosa*, *Acinetobacter* spp., *Stenotrophomonas maltophilia*, and methicillin-resistant *Staphylococcus aureus* are associated with a particularly high risk of mortality.

The onset of nosocomial pneumonia may facilitate predicting the causative organisms. Early infections occur within 4 days of intubation, and late infections occur after 4 days. They are different in regard to severity and types of pathogen encountered. For example, *Haemophilus* spp. and pneumococci are most likely to be found in patients with early-onset pneumonia, trauma victims, and patients who have not received antimicrobial agents. This invasion is thought to be secondary to introduction of oropharyngeal bacteria into the lower airways after intubation or after an aspiration event that may have

TABLE 32.1. Risk Factors Associated with Nosocomial Pneumonia in the ICU.

Ventilator-associated pneumonia
    Age ≥ 60 years
    COPD, PEEP, pulmonary disease
    Coma, impaired consciousness
    Therapeutic intervention
    Organ failure
    Large-volume gastric aspiration
    Prior antibiotics
    H_2-blocker with or without antacids
    Gastric colonization and pH
    Season: winter or fall
    Ventilator circuit changes at 24 hours vs. 48 hours
    Reintubation
    Tracheostomy
    Supine head position
Ventilated and nonventilated patients
    Age > 60 years
    APACHE I > 16, APACHE II score
    Trauma, head injury
    Coma
    Bronchoscopy
    Nasogastric tube
    Endotracheal intubation
    Upper abdominal/thoracic surgery
    Low serum albumin
    Neuromuscular disease
    H_2-blockers

Modified from Hall JB, Schmidt GA, Wood LDH: Principles of Critical Care Medicine, 2nd ed., McGraw-Hill, 1998, with permission of The McGraw-Hill Companies. COPD, chronic obstructive pulmonary disease; PEEP, positive end-expiratory pressure; APACHE, Acute Physiology and Chronic Health Evaluation.

occurred prior to intubation.[10] Gram-negative bacteria, such as *Pseudomonas aeruginosa*, are more common in pneumonias that occur after 4 days of intubation.

Diagnosis

Diagnosis of nosocomial pneumonia is particularly difficult in the ICU patient. Clinical diagnosis in the past has depended on the findings of fever, leukocytosis, purulent secretions, new or progressive chest radiograph infiltrates, and pathogenic bacteria in tracheobronchial secretions. Within 48 hours of intubation, most patients who are mechanically ventilated for respiratory failure develop these same features. The presence of fever and leukocytosis are a result of inflammation due to intubation or other pathologic states. Tracheal secretions may be due to the intubation itself, repeated suctioning, or a tracheobronchitis. A variety of inflammatory conditions that are not infectious in nature can cause infiltrates on chest radiographs: pulmonary edema, atelectasis due to variety of causes, tumors, pulmonary contusions, and acute respiratory distress syndrome (ARDS). These clinical signs did not accurately predict the presence of pneumonia in autopsy studies of patients with ARDS.[32,33] Clinical studies also showed that fewer than 50% of intubated patients who develop these clinical signs have significant infections, as indicated by their clinical improvement without antibiotics.[34,35]

Because of colonization of lower airways secondary to intubation, sputum cultures and tracheal aspirates are unreliable indicators of pneumonia. The standard diagnostic tools for identifying the pathogens are bronchoalveolar lavage (BAL) and protected specimen brushing (PSB). BAL samples a large area of lung parenchyma, whereas PSB samples a segment of the area of interest directly without contamination from the upper airways.[36,37] A positive diagnosis for pneumonia with BAL is a quantitative culture with $≥10^4$ colony-forming units per milliliter (CFU/ml) in combination with Giemsa stains and Gram stains. In a PSB specimen quantitative cultures with $≥10^3$ CFU/ml is considered diagnostic for pneumonia.

Bronchoscopic techniques are currently the standard of care for diagnosing ventilatory-associated pneumonia (VAP). However, the cost and invasive nature of bronchoscopic methods precludes their use as first-line techniques in patients with VAP. Blind catheter techniques are less expensive, safer, and more widely available alternatives to fiberoptic bronchoscopy techniques and have comparable accuracy. Repeated protected specimens obtained blindly provide a useful means for predicting infection and therefore allow early antimicrobial therapy in high risk patients with diffuse lung injury.[38]

Treatment

Empiric antibiotic therapy should be initiated in patients who show clinical signs of sepsis, hemodynamic instability, or persistent acidosis. There is compelling evidence that uncontrolled use of inappropriate antibiotics increases the risk of the patient to become infected with highly resistant organisms. If antibiotic therapy must be instituted prior to obtaining culture results, the onset of pneumonia and microbial profile of the individual ICUs should direct treatment.

In a nonneutropenic patient, culture-directed monotherapy is highly effective as a first line of defense. Several prospective studies comparing monotherapy to combination therapy in nosocomial pneumonia of ICU patients have shown that a response rate of 60% is achievable, which is comparable to historic rates for combination-therapy regimens. Only infections induced by *P. aeruginosa*, *S. aureus*, or other highly resistant pathogens (e.g., *Acinetobacter*, *S. maltophilia*) should be treated with well defined antibiotic combinations.[39]

Immune and biochemical techniques are being developed to treat pneumonia as well. Monoclonal antibodies that bind endotoxin and tumor necrosis factor-α (TNFα) are under investigation, as are interleukin-1 (IL-1) receptor blockers and prostaglandin E_1 (PGE_1). Scavengers for free radicals such as *N*-acetylcysteine and ibuprofen may also be helpful.[40] In the future, immune enhancers may help fight infections such as nosocomial pneumonia.[41]

Prevention

The incidence of nosocomial pneumonias can be greatly reduced by several interventions. The most effective intervention is hand washing along with enforcement of infection control protocols by hospital personnel. Changing the patient's position may also decrease the infection rate. For example, placing a stable patient in a semirecumbent position can decrease aspiration of gastric contents.[42] Oscillating and rotating beds also help minimize complete immobilization, which facilitates atelectasis, alters drainage secretions, and potentially predisposes to pulmonary complications including pneumonia.[43–47] Reduction of infections in clinical studies has not been shown with this technique, but there has been a significant decrease in the length of stay. Aspiration of oropharyngeal secretions continuously or intermittently has been proposed to reduce the chronic aspiration of secretions around the tracheal cuff in intubated patients. There have been no changes in mortality or the incidence of late-onset pathogens; but with early-onset pneumonia there has been a reduction in pathogens.[48,49]

Prophylaxis antibiotics and selective decontamination have been studied aggressively as means to preventing nosocomial pneumonia.[42,44,50–68] At this time, these methods have generated multiresistant bacteria and increased the cost of ICU stays without a significant reduction in the incidence of disease or mortality. Further studies are needed to explore these modalities as possible solutions to preventing nosocomial pneumonia.

Another alternative to preventing nosocomial pneumonia is modifying the approach to alkalinizing gastric secretions. One solution is to utilize sulcrafate, which limits the amount of gastric colonization by coating the lining of the stomach without altering the pH. Antiulcer prophylaxis itself has been questioned in patients who do not have a history of peptic ulcer disease or upper GI bleeding. Studies have shown that the risk of GI bleeding is no different between treated patients and controls.

Chest physiotherapy and incentive spirometry are very helpful in preventing nosocomial pneumonia. This point is important in patients who have undergone any type of surgery, and even more so in patients who have had thoracic surgery. Patients who smoke or have chronic obstructive lung disease are at particular risk for pneumonia, and these patients should have rigorous pulmonary toilette postoperatively.

Catheter-Related Nosocomial Infections

Catheter-related infections (CRIs) leading to bacteremia or fungemia occur in fewer than 1% of hospitalized patients, and most of these infections occur in ICU patients. Ten percent of patients who have been hospitalized for more than 72 hours in surgical ICUs develop nosocomial bacteremia, and many of these bacteremias develop secondary to a CRI. Most nosocomial bloodstream infection epidemics derive from vascular access in some form.[69,70] Definitions of CRIs are presented in Table 32.2.

Risk factors for developing CRIs are dependent on the patient population and the device type and use. Multiple studies have shown that heavy cutaneous colonization of the insertion site is the single most important predictor of CRI with all types of noncuffed catheters.[71,72] Central venous catheters exposed to bacteremia or candidemia from a remote source and catheterizations exceeding 4 days were also shown to be risk factors.[70] Insertion into an internal jugular vein rather than the subclavian vein, catheterization exceeding 3 days, and insertion using less stringent barrier precautions were each associated with significantly increased risk of catheter-related infection with Swan-Ganz catheters.[73] Active UTIs or lower respiratory tract colonization or infection may also increase the risk of central venous catheter-related bloodstream infections.

Pathogenesis/Pathogens

Four major mechanisms cause colonization and subsequent infections of catheters: (1) Bacterial colonization and subsequent infection begins at the interface of the catheter and the skin at the insertion site. (2) Excessive manipulation of the catheter hub may act to inoculate the lumen of the catheter. (3) Hematogenous spread of remote infections in the host produce bacteremia and subsequent catheter seeding. (4) Contamination

TABLE 32.2. Catheter-Related Nosocomial Infection: Definitions.

Local infections
1. Purulent discharge at the exit site, either spontaneous or expressed upon palpation of the site, regardless of whether an organism is cultured from the site
2. Erythema, tenderness, induration (any two of the three) at the exit site with serous or serosanguineous discharge, either spontaneous or expressed upon palpation, in the presence of a positive exit-site culture (moderate to heavy growth of a single or predominant organism)

Definite infection
1. Single positive peripheral blood culture from a patient with clinical and microbiologic data disclosing no other source of the bacteremia in the presence of a semiquantitative or quantitative culture of a catheter segment (proximal or distal from which the same organism (species, antibiogram) was isolated
2. Differential quantitative blood cultures with a ≥10-fold colony count difference between specimens drawn from the catheter and simultaneously from a peripheral venous blood specimen
3. Single positive peripheral blood culture from a patient, with isolation of the same organism (species, antibiogram) from purulent, serous, or serosanguineous discharge from the catheter exit site or along the path of subcutaneously tunneled catheter or from the subcutaneous pocket containing a reservoir of a totally implantable device

Probable infection
1. Two or more positive blood cultures for the same organism (species, antibiogram) from any source (peripheral or retrograde intravascular device cultures) from a patient with clinical and microbiologic data disclosing no other source for the bacteremia except the intravascular device
2. One positive blood culture for *Staphylococcus aureus* or *Candida* species from any source (peripheral or retrograde intravascular device culture) in a patient with clinical and microbiologic data disclosing no other source for the bacteremia except the intravascular device
3. One positive blood culture for any organism commonly associated with intravascular device-related infection (coagulase-negative *Staphylococcus*, *Bacillus* species, *Corynebacterium* species, *Malassezia furfur*) from only one source (peripheral or retrograde culture) in an immunocompromised patient or a neutropenic patient (neutrophils < 500 cells/μl) with clinical and microbiologic data disclosing no other source for the bacteremia except a centrally placed catheter

From Hall JB, Schmidt GA, Wood LDH: Principles of Critical Care Medicine, 2nd ed., McGraw-Hill, 1998, with permission of The McGraw-Hill Companies.

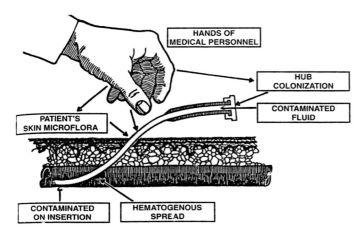

FIGURE 32.1. Sources of catheter-related infections. (From Hall JB, Schmidt GA, Wood LDH: Principles of Critical Care Medicine, 2nd ed., McGraw-Hill, 1998, with permission of The McGraw-Hill Companies.)

of infusate, pressure monitor devices, or line tubing may play a role. Fig. 32.1 represents these various scenarios.

The largest proportion of CRIs evolves from cutaneous microflora at the insertion site.[74] After insertion into a vein, the catheter develops an external fibrin seal, and bacteria travelling down the external surface of the catheter infect this covering. Coagulase-negative staphylococci, which are the predominant organism colonizing skin, cause more than one-half of all CRIs. Furthermore, there is strong concordance between organisms colonizing skin about the catheter and organisms recovered from central venous catheters that have produced bloodstream infection.[75–80] Heavy colonization of the insertion site has a strong predictive value for the occurrence of catheter-related bloodstream infections.[70,79,81,82] The role of cutaneous colonization is further elucidated from surgically implanted Broviac or Hickman catheters, which have a subcutaneous Dacron cuff that becomes ingrown with tissue and poses a mechanical barrier against invasion of the tract by skin organisms. The incidence of CRIs is lower (approximately 0.20 cases per catheter-days) than that with short-term noncuffed central venous catheters (approximately 0.6–1.0 per 100 catheter-days).

Frequent manipulations of the catheter hub are also a source of CRIs. The contamination occurs because of tubing replacements, improper connections, or handling of the hub, which introduces bacteria into the lumen that then migrate down the inner luminal surface to the venous circulation.[83,84] These organisms originate from the hands of the personnel manipulating the catheter. A small percentage of CRIs develop secondary to this scenario.

The third possible source of contamination of catheters is by hematogenous spread from remote areas. This situation especially occurs in patients who have abscesses, drains, or infected wounds.[85] *Enterococcus*, *Klebsiella*, *Escherichia coli*, and fungi are the most common organisms in CRIs caused by hematogenous spread.[86,87] Many factors contribute to the seeding of catheters by hematogenous spread: type of organism, degree and duration of bacteremia, patient's clinical status, and the time of catheter use.[85]

Infusates can be contaminated by intrinsic or extrinsic mechanisms that can cause CRIs. Intrinsic contamination is caused by bacterial inoculation during the processing of infusate fluids. *Klebsiella*, *Enterobacter*, and *Serratia* are specific pathogens responsible for this type of contamination and subsequent infections.[73,88] Extrinsic contamination occurs after manipulation of the tubing, causing breaks in aseptic technique, or when the tubing itself is contaminated, which can innoculate both the catheter and the infusate. This modality of contamination is rare owing to the strict infectious disease control standards required in hospitals today. The estimated incidence as type of contamination is about 1/1000 cannula-related septicemias.

The most common pathogens associated with bacteremia from an intravascular device are *Staphylococcus epidermidis* and *Staphylococcus aureus*. Fifty percent of all catheter-related bacteremias are caused by these organisms. They, especially *S. epidermidis*, are thought to adhere to plastic catheters, which results in a selective advantage for these organisms in causing device-associated infections.[89] Enteric gram-negative bacilli are the next most common, followed by *Candida albicans*, *Pseudomonas*, *Corynebacterium jeikeium*, and *Malassezia furfur*.

Diagnosis

Several laboratory techniques have been developed to assist in the diagnosis of CRIs. Qualitative culture of vascular catheters in broth, semiquantitative culture of catheters on solid media, and quantitative culture of catheters in broth, removing organisms by flush or sonication, are the most common methods used to culture catheters. Semiquantitative cultures are the simplest, most reliable, and most widely used method in hospitals today. The catheter tips are rolled on a plate as described by Maki and colleagues.[90] A positive culture is defined as ≥ 15 CFUs. This method has a specificity of 76–96% and a positive predictive value of 16–31%. There are methods that are more sensitive and more specific, but they have proven to be too time-consuming and expensive to be used on a routine basis in most hospitals.

When a catheter is not removed, catheter blood "draws" (CBDs) may be done. A study investigating the sensitivity and specificity of CBDs found that cultures taken by arterial, pulmonary artery, and central venous catheters found concordant bacteremia with a sensitivity and specificity of 96% and 98%, respectively, compared to cultures obtained simultaneously by peripheral venipuncture.[91] Contamination is a concern with this technique and has limited its usefulness, although CBD is recommended when peripheral culture material is difficult to obtain. Endoluminal brushes can also be used to obtain culture specimens from the intraluminal surface of intravascular catheters. This technique is in the early development phases and may be used as a diagnostic tool in the future.[4]

Clinical diagnosis alone can be difficult with CRIs. Patients with signs of inflammation at the catheter insertion site have a 50% chance of having associated bacteremia. Clinical indicators of a possible catheter-related infection are (1) absence of an alternative source for bacteremia; (2) a septic situation refractory to antimicrobial therapy; (3) the presence of local purulence at the catheter exit site; (4) bacteremia caused by staphylococci or *Candida* species; and (5) concurrent clusters of bacteremia due to *Enterobacter* species, suggesting a common source of contamination of intravenous fluids.

Treatment

Treatment is dependent on several variables, including the type of infection (Fig. 32.1), the microorganisms involved, the type of device (peripheral or central catheter, totally implanted device), and the severity of the illness. Local infections may be treated with catheter removal, local care, and topical or systemic antimicrobial agents (or both). If there is an associated lymphangitis or cellulitis, systemic antibiotic treatment should be instituted.

In bacteremic patients without other sources of infection, the catheter should be removed and sent for culture. A second catheter can be placed at a new site if continued invasive monitoring is necessary. If the catheter is left in place during therapy, septic thrombophlebitis or thrombosis can develop and therefore is not recommended. Antimicrobial therapy should be directed by blood cultures and semiquantitative cultures.

Patients who have long-term indwelling catheters, such as a Hickman, Broviacs, or Cook catheter or a Portocath, can be treated with antimicrobial therapy alone if there is no accompanying tunnel-associated cellulitis, septic thrombophlebitis, tricuspid valve endocarditis, or a persisting bacteremia. *Candida albicans* and *Staphylococcus aureus* cause higher relapse rates of bacteremia and have a higher sepsis-related mortality. Catheter-related infections due to these organisms should be removed early in the treatment.[92]

Local microbiologic patterns and susceptibilities should direct empiric treatment. In most cases a combination of intravenous antistaphylococcal penicillin (vancomycin if methicillin-resistant *S. aureus* is prevalent) and an aminoglycoside or a third-generation cephalosporin provides coverage for most gram-positive and gram-negative microorganisms. Catheter-related bacteremic infections caused by *S. aureus* should be treated for 14 days with parenteral therapy and 2–4 weeks of oral therapy to avoid metastatic infectious complications. The optimal duration of therapy for infections caused by organisms other than *S. aureus* is about 5–10 days. Candidemia may be treated with a short course of amphotericin B (3–7 mg/kg total dose) or fluconazole (400–800 mg/day for 7–10 days). If brief treatment is used, the patient should be recultured at 72 hours to ensure adequate treatment or should be examined for endophthalmitis. For patients at risk for metastatic candidal infections or who continue to have positive cultures, prolonged therapy and further investigations may be warranted.

Prevention

Site care is the most important factor in preventing of catheter-related septicemia. The best method has been shown to be with the use of polymyxin-neomycin-bacitracin ointment for peripheral catheters and iodophor ointment for central and arterial catheters, with dressing changes every 48 hours.

Guidewire exchanges (GWXs) have proven beneficial in decreasing the incidence of catheter-related infections and prolonging catheter site use.[60,61,93] GWXs prevent infection by removing externally and internally adherent bacteria before a "critical mass" develops that may cause bacteremia. A line change via GWX can be done when a new catheter is needed.

Catheter choice and placement can also reduce the risk of infection. Peripheral catheters, such as a peripherally inserted central catheter (PICC) line, may be a better choice in patients who need a long-term central site. Minimizing the number of lumens has been suggested as a preventive measure. Studies have not demonstrated that there is an increased risk of infection with multiple lumens, but they have shown that patients with these catheters are severely ill, requiring numerous infusions, which leads to more handling of the catheter. It is more likely that manipulation of the catheter, rather than the number of lumens, generates the infections. Finally, the use of antiseptic/antimicrobial-bonded devices or subcutaneous cuffs impregnated with antimicrobial agents may be considered. There is a significant decrease in the infection rates (50–80%) with the use of chlorhexidine silver-bonded catheters, silver-impregnated cuffs, and antibiotic-coated catheters.

Hospital-Acquired Urinary Tract Infections

The most common site of nosocomial infection is the urinary tract. UTIs account for 30–40% of all nosocomial infections, and 80% follow urinary tract catheterization.[19,94–96] UTIs are the most common sequelae of ICU admission. Bacteremia arises in 1–3% of patients with UTIs, and the attributable mortality is 13%. These infections are responsible for 2.4–4.5 days of extra hospitalization.[97,98]

The risk of developing a UTI increases with the duration of catheterization, and the risk of developing bacteriuria increases 5–10% for each day of catheterization. Patients at risk of a UTI are pregnant women, elderly or debilitated patients, and those with urologic abnormalities. Other risk factors include diabetes mellitus, use of immunosuppressive agents, parenteral nutrition, disturbances causing decreased urine flow, and radiation therapy.[62] Exposure to broad-spectrum antibiotics increases the risk of a patient having a fungal UTI.

Pathogenesis/Pathogens

Three main pathways allow microorganisms to enter the urinary tract: introduction of bacteria into the bladder by instrumentation; contamination of the catheter lumen by refluxing urine from the collection container; migration of bacteria from the perineum or catheter manipulation to the urethral meatus on a thin film of fluid between the urethral mucosa and external catheter surface.[99]

Bladder catheterization inhibits the ability of the bladder to empty completely. Because there is retained fluid within the bladder, microorganisms can proliferate to high concentrations.[99] Contributing to this situation are the number of catheter manipulations (bladder lavage, catheter exchanges, pulled-out catheter by the patient, blocked catheters); such manipulations cause bladder distension and excessive mucosal damage, promoting bacterial adherence and invasive infections.[100]

Contamination of the collection vessel and retrograde flow of urine also cause UTIs. Urine that has been sitting in the collection bag on or near the floor notoriously becomes contaminated. If urine from the bag is allowed to flow back into the bladder, the bladder can become inoculated with organisms that then generate infection. Irrigation of the bladder via the catheter can introduce organisms into the bladder in a similar manner.

Enteric organisms are the most common pathogens of UTIs. *Escherichia coli*, *Klebsiella*, *Enterobacter*, *Proteus*, enterococci, *Pseudomonas*, and Candida are most often cultured. Because of the close approximation of the urethra and anus, contamination of the nearby skin by fecal organisms explicate the high frequency of infection with fecal flora.

Diagnosis

Diagnosis of UTIs is classically obtained by urinalysis and urine culture. Bacteriuria and pyuria in the ICU are most likely signs of a UTI but may not be the true source of infection, especially if antibiotics have already been administered. Epidemiologic studies show that catheter-acquired bacteriuria is more common in orthopedic and urologic patients, in patients catheterized after 6 days in the hospital, and patients who require catheterization for more than 7 days.[101]

Urinary tract infection is associated with a colony count of $>10^5$ CFU/ml of a predominant species or a mixed culture of 10^5 CFU/ml or more. A colony count of 100 bacteria per milliliter from a suprapubic bladder puncture is considered a UTI, as is the presence of large numbers of bacteria and neutrophils on microscopic examination of urinary sediment. Some have advocated culturing the tip of urinary catheters, but positive catheter-tip cultures have not significantly correlated with bacteriuria.

Treatment

Removing the catheter is the best treatment for UTIs, but often it is not possible in critically ill patients. For patients whose UTI has been identified early, in whom there are no signs of sepsis, and in whom the catheter can be removed, culture-directed single-agent therapy may be warranted.[102] When the catheter cannot be removed, it should be changed and culture-directed antimicrobial therapy instituted. Seven to ten days of treatment with follow-up cultures is recommended. A lower urinary tract infection can be complicated by upper urinary tract contamination, progressing to pyelonephritis or relapse of bacteriuria after short-course therapy. In these cases, 2 weeks of culture-directed therapy is required. Further relapse of these types of infection requires prolonged therapy, in some cases up to 6 weeks.[103,104]

A UTI caused by yeast is not uncommon. Many patients are colonized, especially after prolonged hospitalization and catheterization. In these cases therapy directed toward eradicating fungal colonization with intravenous therapy is appropriate.[105] Irrigation of the bladder is highly controversial and should be avoided in most patients.[106] When a UTI is associated with disseminated candidiasis, prolonged intravenous therapy is recommended with amphotericin B or fluconazole.[107]

Prevention

Use of condom or suprapubic catheters is helpful for reducing the incidence of UTIs. These types of drainage can be used for surgical and general medical patients who may require long-term bladder catheterization. A condom catheter and its attached collection tube are easily managed and should be changed daily to prevent the penis from becoming macerated. Because suprapubic drainage does not obstruct the urethral glands, it has become popular. Preliminary results have shown a delayed onset and reduced incidence of infection in patients with suprapubic urinary catheters. Antibiotic or silver-coated urinary catheters have not been shown to decrease the incidence of UTIs.[108,109]

Fungal Infections

Fungal infections, particularly those caused by *Candida* species, are now so common in many ICUs they approach their bacterial counterparts in terms of being major problems in the care of critically ill patients. Forty-two percent of patients with nosocomial infections have fungi isolated concomitantly.[110] As the magnitude of this problem has increased, there has been considerable effort expended to better understand the epidemiology of fungal infection in the ICU and thereby to define indications for treatment of early infection, prior to candidemia.

The patients at risk for *Candida* infection are those with prolonged ICU stays. The average hospital stay for patients developing candidemia is 18 days.[111] Other risk factors for developing invasive fungal infections are prior antibiotic administration, parenteral nutrition, steroids, burns, granulocytopenia, chemotherapy, irradiation with damaged mucosal barriers, central vascular catheters, and organ transplant.[112,113]

Pathogens/Pathogenesis

Normally, *Candida* organisms live in equilibrium with the host and do not cause disease. When patients have received a multitude of antibiotics, competing bacterial flora are annihilated and there is local overgrowth with *Candida*. This overgrowth can deeply penetrate tissues, with intermittent seeding of organisms into the bloodstream. Microabscesses may form in solid organ structures after hematogenous spread of the organisms.

Candida albicans is the most common yeast to be pathogenic. Other recognized pathogens are *C. Krusei, C. parapsilosis, C. guilliermondi, C. lusitaniae,* and *C. glabrata*.

Diagnosis

Candidiasis that has disseminated is difficult to diagnoses. The most common dilemma is suspicion of fungal infection in patients without positive blood cultures or histologic evidence of tissue invasion. At-risk patients typically manifest fever, leukocytosis, and other potential indicators of infection because of noninfectious inflammatory disease; and they are often under treatment for bacterial infection without resolution of the signs of infection. The criteria for diagnosis and systemic treatment include positive blood cultures after removal of intravascular catheters, culture of *Candida* from three or more sites, or endophthalmitis.[93,114] Currently there are no other reliable diagnostic tests for detecting invasive fungal infections. The polymerase chain reaction (PCR) is being used to determine dissemination of *Candida* after UTIs with good sensitivity and specificity.[115]

Isolation of *Candida* from certain sites merits special attention. The risk of subsequent infection increases as more sites become positive. This is particularly true for patients found to have *Candida* in the peritoneal cavity of either recurrent intraabdominal infection or following elective operation.[114] Growth of *Candida* from bronchoalveolar lavage cultures is likely indicative of a *Candida* pneumonia, although this disease entity requires further definition and investigation. The significance of urine cultures, especially if persistently positive after catheter removal or exchange, may be indicative of a significant systemic infection.[116]

Treatment

The indications for treatment have recently been expanded as more experience has accumulated. Candidemia, defined as one or more positive blood cultures for any *Candida* species, is now viewed as a clear indication for antifungal therapy. There is strong evidence that patients colonized with *Candida*, that is, who grow the same species from the same site (urine, sputum, surgical drain sites) on two or more occasions, are at an approximately 30–50% risk of progressing to candidemia.[117]

In the past, because of the toxicity associated with amphotericin B, therapy for fungal infections was generally withheld until there was overwhelming evidence of systemic infection. A more aggressive approach to treatment has been made possible by the relative safety of fluconazole. Fluconazole has been shown to be suitable as a replacement for amphotericin B in many clinical settings. It is a water-soluble triazole agent with good activity against many *Candida* species. Its minimal toxicity compared to that of amphotericin B has clearly broadened the indications for treatment.

It is now well established that the minimum adult dosage of fluconazole is 400 mg/day. Because of an increase in the incidence of non-*C. albicans* species, with lessened susceptibility to fluconazole, dosages of 600–800 mg may be useful if the particular ICU has a high incidence of such organisms.[118-120] Various studies have demonstrated the excellent absorption of fluconazole in enterally fed ICU patients, and this is therefore the preferred route.

Prevention

To reduce the risk of developing invasive *Candida* infections, intravascular and Foley catheters are removed as early as possible, and long-term or multiple regimens of antibiotics are avoided. High dose oral nystatin can be useful in reducing the number of *Candida* in the intestine and can reduce the incidence of fungemia in various populations of immunosuppressed patients. Oral imidazoles, especially fluconazole and itraconazole, may prove useful in preventing *Candida* colonization and deep *Candida* infections.

Fungal prophylaxis with fluconazole is increasing in ICU patients. There are three main reasons to use this regimen in the ICU: (1) many patients have risk factors for disseminated candidiasis and have persistent fevers; (2) cultures of sputum and urine are often positive, especially with Foley catheters and broad-spectrum antibiotics; and (3) there are no good diagnostic tests to prove or disprove invasive *Candida* infections. The problem with prophylaxis is the emergence of resistant *Candida* species, particularly *C. albicans* and *C. krusei*. Many patients on fluconazole have had cultures positive for these organisms. Resistance is inevitable if prophylaxis is allowed without strict guidelines for introduction.

Sinusitis

Five percent of nosocomial infections are caused by sinusitis.[121] The incidence in critically ill patients is ≥15% and is probably even higher in patients with nasogastric or nasotracheal tubes.[122] One study evaluated 162 patients with nasotracheal or oropharyngeal intubation extending more than 7 days. They found that only 25% of these patients had normal maxillary sinuses on computed tomography (CT) scans at 48 hours.[123] It is possible that mechanical ventilation or respiratory failure plays a role in the development of sinusitis in critically ill patients.

The risk factors for developing sinusitis are intubation, placement of nasogastric/nasotracheal tubes, and facial trauma. At this time, it is not known if soft feeding tubes or the Minnesota tubes are associated with sinusitis. Patients who are nasotracheally intubated develop sinusitis 95% of the time. They also develop it earlier and in both maxillary sinuses.

Pathogens/Pathogenesis

Impaired drainage of the maxillary sinus causes evolution of acute sinusitis. This event probably occurs secondary to local trauma and edema within the intubated nasal cavity and is promoted by limited head mobility, resulting in impaired drainage of the sinuses through the natural ostia.

Nosocomial sinusitis is usually polymicrobial. The most common organisms found are *Streptococcus, Pneumococcus, Staphylococcus,* or *Haemophilus influenzae.* Gram-negative enteric pathogens must also be considered in patients who are critically ill and intubated.

Diagnosis

Awake patients may complain of nasal congestion, purulent rhinorrhea, headache, and fever. Patients in the ICU who have an altered mental status may have only fever and leukocytosis, and some may have a foul-smelling nasal discharge. CT scans are the best diagnostic tool to ascertain if a patient has acute sinusitis. The scans give the most detail in the intubated patient. For those with positive scans (opacification, mucosal thickening, air-fluid level), aspiration should be performed. Infection is confirmed if a pathogen is identified along with neutrophils. For patients who cannot be moved, ultrasonography is becoming available for diagnosis and anatomic delineation. It has 100% specificity for identifying opacification of the maxillary sinus, which is consistent with acute sinusitis,[124] and may become a first-line diagnostic tool for this problem.

Treatment

Treatment of sinusitis starts with removal of all nasal tubes, topical decongestants, and maxillary sinus drainage and lavage. Decongestants and broad-spectrum antibiotics are the first line of defense. If the patient is not improving within 24 hours, a surgical drainage procedure may be justified. After an operative intervention, a specimen should be sent to the laboratory for Gram stain and culture. Antibiotics should then be tailored to the organisms' susceptibility profiles.

Flexible endoscopy has been used to visualize and débride diseased tissue in outpatients and in those with chronic sinusitis. Future studies may make this modality helpful in the ICU for diagnosis and treatment of sinusitis.

Prevention

Removal of all nasal tubes as soon as possible or oral intubation instead of nasal intubation may be helpful in preventing sinusitis. For patients who are immunocompromised or who require intubation for more than 7 days, the nasotracheal route is best avoided.[125]

Antibiotic-Associated Pseudomembranous Colitis

Critically ill patients are prone to antibiotic-associated diarrhea and pseudomembranous colitis because of the enormous doses of antibiotics to which they are exposed. The incidence of this infection is on the rise, especially in the ICU. This condition can be serious, but early recognition and intervention can avert mortality.

All antibiotics, except vancomycin, have the potential to cause these syndromes. Cephalosporins, clindamycin, and ampicillin have the highest association with pseudomembranous colitis. The incidence of antibiotic-associated diarrhea with these drugs ranges from 5% to 25%. There is a higher risk in older patients and those with prolonged use of antibiotics.

Pathogens/Pathogenesis

Clostridium difficile is the pathogen responsible for antibiotic-associated diarrhea and pseudomembranous colitis. This organism is cultured in up to 21% of all hospitalized patients.[126] *C. difficile* proliferates after the normal colonic bacterial flora has been suppressed by antibiotic therapy.[127] It then produces toxins, including toxin A (enterotoxin) and toxin B (cytotoxin), which damage the colonic epithelial cells and result in inflammation and impairment of normal fluid absorption by the colon.[128]

Diagnosis

Patients usually develop semiformed or liquid stools after receiving an antibiotic for 5–7 days, but these symptoms can arise after one dose or after discontinuing the antibiotic. If an ileus is present, the patient may not develop diarrhea. Fever, abdominal pain, and passage of bloody stool may be seen in moderate to severe cases. Toxic megacolon and perforation with generalized peritonitis are seen in severe cases and in association with pseudomembranous colitis.

Diagnosis is confirmed by fecal examination. Fecal leukocytes and red blood cells are usually present on Gram staining. *C. difficile* toxin assay is the best diagnostic test. False-positive tests have been described, but this problem can be overcome by restudying the stool. Sigmoidoscopy helps reveal the extent of disease. It can range from mild erythema to a granular, friable, hemorrhagic mucosa; or pseudomembrane colitis may be present.

Treatment

If the clinical picture permits, discontinuing the offending antibiotics is the first line of treatment. Fluid resuscitation and antibiotic therapy against *C. difficile* should then be instituted. For critically ill patients who require antibiotics, an alternative antibiotic regimen that is associated with a lower risk of antibiotic-associated colitis should be considered. Repeat stool specimens are obtained 2 weeks after a course of antibiotics to document eradication of the *C. difficile.* Twenty-five percent of patients have relapses, and these patients should be retreated. Operative management is reserved for those who present with or progress to fulminating colitis or toxic megacolon unresponsive to medical therapy and those with clinical signs of peritonitis suggesting perforation.

Prevention

Clostridium difficile can be transmitted in the ICU from staff to patient via hands, stethoscopes, or other inanimate objects. To prevent this from occurring, hand-washing, use of disposable gloves, isolation of patients with *C. difficile*, and daily cleaning of inanimate objects have been suggested.[129] Appropriate use of perioperative antibiotics, narrowing the spectrum as much as possible when treating an infection, and discontinuing antibiotics after an appropriate interval are of prime importance in preventing toxic sequelae.

Hospital-Acquired Ventriculitis and Meningitis

Ventricular catheters are used to diagnose and aid in the management of increased intracranial pressure (ICP). Venticulostomy catheters, subarachnoid catheters, or subarachnoid bolts are commonly used in patients who require ICP monitoring. Ventriculostomy has a greater risk of infection. The nosocomial infection rate for ventriculostomy is reported between 0% and 27%.[130] The overall risk of infection has been estimated at 1.5 infections per 100 monitoring days.[131]

Risk factors associated with the development of ventriculitis or meningitis after placement of a venticulostomy are a duration of ventricular catheterization of more than 5 days, irrigation of the system, ICP > 20 mmHg, intracerebral hemorrhage with intraventricular hemorrhage, and neurosurgical operations. Other possible risk factors are infections at other sites and a need for serial monitors.[132]

Pathogens/Pathogenesis

Staphylococcus is the most common organism to cause ventriculitis or meningitis with ventriculostomies. The etiology of the infection is thought to be contamination at the time of insertion, catheter contamination after insertion by poor aseptic technique, or multiple manipulations of the catheter.

Diagnosis

The diagnosis is suspected in patients who have the device and show signs of infection. Routine specimen collection for Gram stain, culture and sensitivity, cell count, glucose, and total protein should be done every 48 hours to monitor closely for developing signs of infection.[130] If the catheter is removed, the tip should be sent to the laboratory for Gram stain and cultures.

Treatment

Removal and culture of the catheter is mandatory when a patient has been diagnosed with ventriculitis or meningitis associated with a ventriculostomy. If continued monitoring is required, a second catheter should be placed at another location. Culture-directed antibiotics are used to treat the infection. Intrathecal antibiotics may also be necessary in patients with resistant organisms.

Prevention

Prevention has focused on maintaining a closed system, strict aseptic technique, and early removal. Studies are now being conducted on the efficacy of catheters impregnated with antibiotics. Hamilton et al. have shown that vancomycin-bonded, TDMAC-coated catheters can prevent infections without toxicity in rats.[133] This result has yet to be determined in patients. Other preventive measures include using fiberoptic devices rather than to fluid-filled tubing connected to a pressure transducer, which may reduce the frequency of manipulation, contamination, and infection. Prophylaxis with antibiotics has also proved to be of paramount importance for preventing the development of ventriculitis secondary to ventriculostomy, especially during the first 5 days of catheter placement.[130,134]

References

1. West JG, Trunkey DD, Lim RC: Systems of trauma care: a study of two counties. Arch Surg 1979;114:455–460.
2. Paneth N, Kiely JL, Wallenstein S, Marcus M, Pakter J, Susser M: Newborn intensive care and neonatal mortality in low-birth-weight infants: a population study. N Engl J Med 1982;307:149–155.
3. Baxt WG, Moody P: The impact of a physician as part of the aeromedical prehospital team in patients with blunt trauma. JAMA 1987;257:3246–3250.
4. Li TC, Phillips MC, Shaw L, Cook EF, Natanson C, Goldman L: On-site physician staffing in a community hospital intensive care unit: impact on test and procedure use and on patient outcome. JAMA 1984;252:2023–2027.
5. Knaus WA, Draper EA, Wagner DP, Zimmerman JE: An evaluation of outcome from intensive care in major medical centers. Ann Intern Med 1986;104:410–418.
6. Pollack MM, Getson PR, Ruttimann UE, et al: Efficiency of intensive care: a comparative analysis of eight pediatric intensive care units. JAMA 1987;258:1481–1486.
7. Ron A, Aronne LJ, Kalb PE, Santini D, Charlson ME: The therapeutic efficacy of critical care units: identifying subgroups of patients who benefit. Arch Intern Med 1989;149:338–341.
8. Fridkin SK, Welbel SF, Weinstein RA: Magnitude and prevention of nosocomial infections in the intensive care unit. Infect Dis Clin North Am 1997;11:479–496.
9. Fernandez-Crehuet R, Diaz-Molina C, de Irala J, Martinez-Concha D, Salcedo-Leal I, Mass-Calles J: Nosocomial infection in an intensive-care unit: identification of risk factors. Infect Control Hosp Epidemiol 1997;18:825–830.
10. Anonymous: Nosocomial infection rates for interhospital comparison: limitations and possible solutions: a report from the National Nosocomial Infections Surveillance (NNIS) system. Infect Control Hosp Epidemiol 1991;12:609–621.
11. Gross PA, Neu HC, Aswapokee P, Van Antwerpen C, Aswapokee N: Deaths from nosocomial infections: experience in a university hospital and a community hospital. Am J Med 1980;68:219–223.
12. Craven DE, Kunches LM, Kilinsky V, Lichtenberg DA, Make BJ, McCabe WR: Risk factors for pneumonia and fatality in patients

receiving continuous mechanical ventilation. Am Rev Respir Dis 1986;133:792-796.
13. Ruiz-Santana S, Garcia JA, Esteban A, et al: ICU pneumonias: a multi-institutional study. Crit Care Med 1987;15:930-932.
14. Graybill JR, Marshall LW, Charache P, Wallace CK, Melvin VB: Nosocomial pneumonia: a continuing major problem. Am Rev Respir Dis 1973;108:1130-1140.
15. Pezzarossi HE, Ponce DL, Calva JJ, Lazo de la Vega SA, Ruiz-Palacios GM: High incidence of subclavian dialysis catheter-related bacteremias. Infect Control 1986;7:596-599.
16. Stevens RM, Teres D, Skillman JJ, Feingold DS: Pneumonia in an intensive care unit: a 30-month experience. Arch Intern Med 1974;134:106-111.
17. Craven DE, Kunches LM, Lichtenberg DA, et al: Nosocomial infection and fatality in medical and surgical intensive care unit patients. Arch Intern Med 1988;148:1161-1168.
18. Craven DE, Steger KA, Barber TW: Preventing nosocomial pneumonia: state of the art and perspectives for the 1990s. Am J Med 1991;91:44S-53S.
19. Scheld WM, Mandell GL: Nosocomial pneumonia: pathogenesis and recent advances in diagnosis and therapy. Rev Infect Dis 1991;13(Suppl 9): S743-S751.
20. Hall JB, Schmidt GA, Wood LDH (eds): Principles of Critical Care Medicine, 2nd ed. New York, McGraw-Hill, 1998.
21. Abraham SN, Beachey EH, Simpson WA: Adherence of Streptococcus pyogenes, Escherichia coli, and Pseudomonas aeruginosa to fibronectin-coated and uncoated epithelial cells. Infect Immun 1983;41:1261-1268.
22. Woods DE, Bass JA, Johanson WGJ, Straus DC: Role of adherence in the pathogenesis of Pseudomonas aeruginosa lung infection in cystic fibrosis patients. Infect Immun 1980;30:694-699.
23. Tobin MJ, Grenvik A: Nosocomial lung infection and its diagnosis. Crit Care Med 1984;12:191-199.
24. Johanson WGJ, Pierce AK, Sanford JP, Thomas GD: Nosocomial respiratory infections with gram-negative bacilli: the significance of colonization of the respiratory tract. Ann Intern Med 1972;77:701-706.
25. Driks MR, Craven DE, Celli BR, et al: Nosocomial pneumonia in intubated patients given sucralfate as compared with antacids or histamine type 2 blockers: the role of gastric colonization. N Engl J Med 1987;317:1376-1382.
26. Palmer DL: Microbiology of pneumonia in the patient at risk. Am J Med 1984;76:53-60.
27. Fagon JY, Chastre J, Domart Y, et al: Nosocomial pneumonia in patients receiving continuous mechanical ventilation: prospective analysis of 52 episodes with use of a protected specimen brush and quantitative culture techniques. Am Rev Respir Dis 1989;139:877-884.
28. Fagon JY, Chastre J, Vuagnat A, Trouillet JL, Novara A, Gibert C: Nosocomial pneumonia and mortality among patients in intensive care units. JAMA 1996;275:866-869.
29. Tillotson JR, Finland M: Bacterial colonization and clinical superinfection of the respiratory tract complicating antibiotic treatment of pneumonia. J Infect Dis 1969;119:597-624.
30. Tillotson JR, Lerner AM: Characteristics of nonbacteremic Pseudomonas pneumonia. Ann Intern Med 1968;68:295-307.
31. Rello J, Torres A, Ricart M, et al: Ventilator-associated pneumonia by Staphylococcus aureus: comparison of methicillin-resistant and methicillin-sensitive episodes. Am J Respir Crit Care Med 1994;150:1545-1549.

32. Andrews CP, Coalson JJ, Smith JD, Johanson WGJ: Diagnosis of nosocomial bacterial pneumonia in acute, diffuse lung injury. Chest 1981;80:254-258.
33. Bell RC, Coalson JJ, Smith JD, Johanson WGJ: Multiple organ system failure and infection in adult respiratory distress syndrome. Ann Intern Med 1983;99:293-298.
34. Fagon JY, Chastre J, Hance AJ, et al: Detection of nosocomial lung infection in ventilated patients: use of a protected specimen brush and quantitative culture techniques in 147 patients. Am Rev Respir Dis 1988;138:110-116.
35. Johanson WGJ: Ventilator-associated pneumonia: light at the end of the tunnel [editorial, comment]? Chest 1990;97:1026-1027.
36. Meduri GU: Ventilator-associated pneumonia in patients with respiratory failure: a diagnostic approach. Chest 1990;97:1208-1219.
37. Bartlett JG, Alexander J, Mayhew J, Sullivan-Sigler N, Gorbach SL: Should fiberoptic bronchoscopy aspirates be cultured? Am Rev Respir Dis 1976;114:73-78.
38. Delclaux C, Roupie E, Blot F, Brochard L, Lemaire F, Brun-Buisson C: Lower respiratory tract colonization and infection during severe acute respiratory distress syndrome: incidence and diagnosis. Am J Respir Crit Care Med 1997;156:1092-1098.
39. Lode H, Schaberg T, Raffenberg M, Mauch H: Lower respiratory tract infections in the intensive care unit: consequences of antibiotic resistance for choice of antibiotic. Microb Drug Resist 1995;1:163-167.
40. Bone RC, Balk R, Slotman G, et al: Adult respiratory distress syndrome: sequence and importance of development of multiple organ failure; the Prostaglandin E_1 Study Group. Chest 1992;101:320-326.
41. Stanley E, Lieschke GJ, Grail D, et al: Granulocyte/macrophage colony-stimulating factor-deficient mice show no major perturbation of hematopoiesis but develop a characteristic pulmonary pathology. Proc Natl Acad Sci USA 1994;91:5592-5596.
42. Kollef MH: The role of selective digestive tract decontamination on mortality and respiratory tract infections: a meta-analysis. Chest 1994;105:1101-1108.
43. Brochard L, Mancebo J, Wysocki M, et al: Noninvasive ventilation for acute exacerbations of chronic obstructive pulmonary disease. N Engl J Med 1995;333:817-822.
44. Kelley RE, Vibulsresth S, Bell L, Duncan RC: Evaluation of kinetic therapy in the prevention of complications of prolonged bed rest secondary to stroke. Stroke 1987;18:638-642.
45. Gentilello L, Thompson DA, Tonnesen AS, et al: Effect of a rotating bed on the incidence of pulmonary complications in critically ill patients. Crit Care Med 1988;16:783-786.
46. Fink MP, Helsmoortel CM, Stein KL, Lee PC, Cohn SM: The efficacy of an oscillating bed in the prevention of lower respiratory tract infection in critically ill victims of blunt trauma: a prospective study. Chest 1990;97:132-137.
47. DeBoisblanc BP, Castro M, Everret B, Grender J, Walker CD, Summer WR: Effect of air-supported, continucus, postural oscillation on the risk of early ICU pneumonia in nontraumatic critical illness. Chest 1993;103:1543-1547.
48. Mahul P, Auboyer C, Jospe R, et al: Prevention of nosocomial pneumonia in intubated patients: respective role of mechanical subglottic secretions drainage and stress ulcer prophylaxis. Intensive Care Med 1992;18:20-25.
49. Valles J, Artigas A, Rello J, et al: Continuous aspiration of subglottic secretions in preventing ventilator-associated pneumonia. Ann Intern Med 1995;122:179-186.

50. Klick JM, du Moulin GC, Hedley-Whyte J, et al: Prevention of gram-negative bacillary pneumonia using polymyxin aerosol as prophylaxis. II. Effect on the incidence of pneumonia in seriously ill patients. J Clin Invest 1975;55:514–519.
51. Feeley TW, du Moulin GC, Hedley-Whyte J, Bushnell LS, Gilbert JP, Feingold DS: Aerosol polymyxin and pneumonia in seriously ill patients. N Engl J Med 1975;293:471–475.
52. Klastersky J, Hensgens C, Noterman J, Mouawad E, Meunier-Carpentier F: Endotracheal antibiotics for the prevention of tracheobronchial infections in tracheotomized unconscious patients: a comparative study of gentamicin and aminosidin-polymyxin B combination. Chest 1975;68:302–306.
53. Klastersky J, Cappel R, Noterman J, Snoeck J, Geuning C, Mouawad E: Endotracheal gentamicin for the prevention of bronchial infections in patients with tracheotomy. Int J Clin Pharmacol 1973;7:279–286.
54. Rouby JJ, Poete P, Martin dL, et al: Prevention of gram negative nosocomial bronchopneumonia by intratracheal colistin in critically ill patients: histologic and bacteriologic study. Intensive Care Med 1994;20:187–192.
55. Johanson WG: Pneumonia prevention: a step backwards [editorial, comment]. Intensive Care Med 1994;20:173.
56. Rumbak MJ, Cancio MR: Significant reduction in methicillin-resistant Staphylococcus aureus ventilator-associated pneumonia associated with the institution of a prevention protocol. Crit Care Med 1995;23:1200–1203.
57. Johanson WGJ, Seidenfeld JJ, de los Santos R, Coalson JJ, Gomez P: Prevention of nosocomial pneumonia using topical and parenteral antimicrobial agents. Am Rev Respir Dis 1988;137:265–272.
58. Flynn DM, Weinstein RA, Nathan C, Gaston MA, Kabins SA: Patient's endogenous flora as the source of "nosocomial" Enterobacter in cardiac surgery. J Infect Dis 1987;156:363–368.
59. Mandelli M, Mosconi P, Langer M, Cigada M: Prevention of pneumonia in an intensive care unit: a randomized multicenter clinical trial. Intensive Care Unit Group of Infection Control. Crit Care Med 1989;17:501–505.
60. Norwood S, Jenkins G: An evaluation of triple-lumen catheter infections using a guidewire exchange technique. J Trauma 1990;30:706–712.
61. Snyder RH, Archer FJ, Endy T, et al: Catheter infection: a comparison of two catheter maintenance techniques. Ann Surg 1988;208:651–653.
62. Bahnson RR: Urosepsis. Urol Clin North Am 1986;13:627–635.
63. Seiler WO, Stahelin HB: Practical management of catheter-associated UTIs. Geriatrics 1988;43:43–50.
64. Heyland DK, Cook DJ, Jaeschke R, Griffith L, Lee HN, Guyatt GH: Selective decontamination of the digestive tract. an overview. Chest 1994;105:1221–1229.
65. Hurley JC: Prophylaxis with enteral antibiotics in ventilated patients: selective decontamination or selective cross-infection? Antimicrob Agents Chemother 1995;39:941–947.
66. Vandenbroucke-Grauls CM, Vandenbroucke JP: Effect of selective decontamination of the digestive tract on respiratory tract infections and mortality in the intensive care unit. Lancet 1991;338:859–862.
67. Hoyt JW: Controversy regarding hospital-acquired pneumonia [editorial, comment]. Crit Care Med 1993;21:1267–1268.
68. Hammond JM, Potgieter PD, Saunders GL, Forder AA: Double-blind study of selective decontamination of the digestive tract in intensive care. Lancet 1992;340:5–9.
69. Jarvis WR: Nosocomial outbreaks: the Centers for Disease Control's Hospital Infections Program experience, 1980–1990: Epidemiology Branch, Hospital Infections Program. Am J Med 1991;91:101S–106S.
70. Smith RL, Meixler SM, Simberkoff MS: Excess mortality in critically ill patients with nosocomial bloodstream infections. Chest 1991;100:164–167.
71. Maki DG, Ringer M: Evaluation of dressing regimens for prevention of infection with peripheral intravenous catheters: gauze, a transparent polyurethane dressing, and an iodophor-transparent dressing. JAMA 1987;258:2396–2403.
72. Mermel LA, Maki DG: Epidemic bloodstream infections from hemodynamic pressure monitoring: signs of the times. Infect Control Hosp Epidemiol 1989;10:47–53.
73. Mermel LA, Maki DG: Infectious complications of Swan-Ganz pulmonary artery catheters: pathogenesis, epidemiology, prevention, and management. Am J Respir Crit Care Med 1994;149:1020–1036. Erratum. Am J Respir Crit Care Med 1994;150:290.
74. Maki DG: Infections Associated with Indwelling Medical Devices, 2nd ed. Washington, DC, American Society for Microbiology, 1994.
75. Maki DG, McCormack KN: Defatting catheter insertion sites in total parenteral nutrition is of no value as an infection control measure: controlled clinical trial. Am J Med 1987;83:833–840.
76. Snydman DR, Murray SA, Kornfeld SJ, Majka JA, Ellis CA: Total parenteral nutrition-related infections: prospective epidemiologic study using semiquantitative methods. Am J Med 1982;73:695–699.
77. Cercenado E, Ena J, Rodriguez-Creixems M, Romero I, Bouza E: A conservative procedure for the diagnosis of catheter-related infections. Arch Intern Med 1990;150:1417–1420.
78. Maki DG, Cobb L, Garman JK, Shapiro JM, Ringer M, Helgerson RB: An attachable silver-impregnated cuff for prevention of infection with central venous catheters: a prospective randomized multicenter trial. Am J Med 1988;85:307–314.
79. Snydman DR, Gorbea HF, Pober BR, Majka JA, Murray SA, Perry LK: Predictive value of surveillance skin cultures in total-parenteral-nutrition-related infection. Lancet 1982;2:1385–1388.
80. Flowers RH, Schwenzer KJ, Kopel RF, Fisch MJ, Tucker SI, Farr BM: Efficacy of an attachable subcutaneous cuff for the prevention of intravascular catheter-related infection: a randomized, controlled trial. JAMA 1989;261:878–883.
81. Armstrong CW, Mayhall CG, Miller KB, et al: Clinical predictors of infection of central venous catheters used for total parenteral nutrition. Infect Control Hosp Epidemiol 1990;11:71–78.
82. Bjornson HS, Colley R, Bower RH, Duty VP, Schwartz-Fulton JT, Fischer JE: Association between microorganism growth at the catheter insertion site and colonization of the catheter in patients receiving total parenteral nutrition. Surgery 1982;92:720–727.
83. Sitges-Serra A, Linares J, Garua J: Catheter sepsis: the clue is the hub. Surgery 1985;97:355–357.
84. Linares J, Sitges-Serra A, Garau J, Perez JL, Martin R: Pathogenesis of catheter sepsis: a prospective study with quantitative and semiquantitative cultures of catheter hub and segments. J Clin Microbiol 1985;21:357–360.
85. Henderson DK: Intravascular device-associated infection: current concepts and controversies. Infect Surg 1988;7:365.
86. Kovacevich DS, Faubion WC, Bender JM, Schaberg DR, Wesley JR: Association of parenteral nutrition catheter sepsis with urinary tract infections. JPEN J Parenter Enteral Nutr 1986;10:639–641.

87. Pettigrew RA, Lang SD, Haydock DA, Parry BR, Bremner DA, Hill GL: Catheter-related sepsis in patients on intravenous nutrition: a prospective study of quantitative catheter cultures and guidewire changes for suspected sepsis. Br J Surg 1985;72:52–55.
88. Maki DG, Rhame FS, Mackel DC, Bennett JV: Nationwide epidemic of septicemia caused by contaminated intravenous products. I. Epidemiologic and clinical features. Am J Med 1976;60:471–485.
89. Peters G, Locci R, Pulverer G: Adherence and growth of coagulase-negative staphylococci on surfaces of intravenous catheters. J Infect Dis 1982;146:479–482.
90. Maki DG, Weise CE, Sarafin HW: A semiquantitative culture method for identifying intravenous-catheter-related infection. N Engl J Med 1977;296:1305–1309.
91. Wormser GP, Onorato IM, Preminger TJ, Culver D, Martone WJ: Sensitivity and specificity of blood cultures obtained through intravascular catheters. Crit Care Med 1990;18:152–156.
92. Dugdale DC, Ramsey PG: Staphylococcus aureus bacteremia in patients with Hickman catheters. Am J Med 1990;89:137–141.
93. Burchard KW, Minor LB, Slotman GJ, Gann DS: Fungal sepsis in surgical patients. Arch Surg 1983;118:217–221.
94. Emori TG, Gaynes RP: An overview of nosocomial infections, including the role of the microbiology laboratory. Clin Microbiol Rev 1993;6:428–442.
95. Haley RW, Culver DH, White JW, Morgan WM, Emori TG: The nationwide nosocomial infection rate: a new need for vital statistics. Am J Epidemiol 1985;121:159–167.
96. Warren JW: Urethral catheters, condom catheters, and nosocomial urinary tract infections [editorial]. Infect Control Hosp Epidemiol 1996;17:212–214.
97. Green MS, Rubinstein E, Amit P: Estimating the effects of nosocomial infections on the length of hospitalization. J Infect Dis 1982;145:667–672.
98. Givens CD, Wenzel RP: Catheter-associated urinary tract infections in surgical patients: a controlled study on the excess morbidity and costs. J Urol 1980;124:646–648.
99. Carson CC: Nosocomial urinary tract infections. Surg Clin North Am 1988;68:1147–1155.
100. Seiler WO, Stahelin HB: Practical management of catheter-associated UTIs. Geriatrics 1988;43:43–50.
101. Shapiro M, Simchen E, Izraeli S, Sacks TG: A multivariate analysis of risk factos for acquiring bacteriuria in patients with indwelling urinary catheters for longer than 24 hours. Infect Control 1984;5:525–532.
102. Harding GK, Nicolle LE, Ronald AR, et al: How long should catheter-acquired urinary tract infection in women be treated? A randomized controlled study. Ann Intern Med 1991;114:713–719.
103. Ronald AR: Optimal duration of treatment for kidney infection [editorial]. Ann Intern Med 1987;106:467–468.
104. Stamm WE, McKevitt M, Counts GW: Acute renal infection in women: treatment with trimethoprim- sulfamethoxazole or ampicillin for two or six weeks; a randomized trial. Ann Intern Med 1987;106:341–345.
105. Wise GJ, Kozinn PJ, Goldberg P: Amphotericin B as a urologic irrigant in the management of noninvasive candiduria. J Urol 1982;128:82–84.
106. Rivett AG, Perry JA, Cohen J: Urinary candidiasis: a prospective study in hospital patients. Urol Res 1986;14:183–186.
107. Galgiani JN: Fluconazole, a new antifungal agent. Ann Intern Med 1990;113:177–179.
108. Johnson JR, Roberts PL, Olsen RJ, Moyer KA, Stamm WE: Prevention of catheter-associated urinary tract infection with a silver oxide-coated urinary catheter: clinical and microbiologic correlates. J Infect Dis 1990;162:1145–1150.
109. Stamm WE: Catheter-associated urinary tract infections: epidemiology, pathogenesis, and prevention. Am J Med 1991;91:65S–71S.
110. Safran DB, Dawson E: The effect of empiric and prophylactic treatment with fluconazole on yeast isolates in a surgical trauma intensive care unit. Arch Surg 1997;132:1184–1188.
111. Wey SB, Mori M, Pfaller MA, Woolson RF, Wenzel RP: Hospital-acquired candidemia: the attributable mortality and excess length of stay. Arch Intern Med 1988;148:2642–2645.
112. Wey SB, Mori M, Pfaller MA, Woolson RF, Wenzel RP: Risk factors for hospital-acquired candidemia: a matched case-control study. Arch Intern Med 1989;149:2349–2353.
113. Kountakis SE, Burke L, Rafie JJ, Bassichis B, Maillard AA, Stiernberg CM: Sinusitis in the intensive care unit patient. Otolaryngol Head Neck Surg 1997;117:362–366.
114. Solomkin JS, Flohr AB, Quie PG, Simmons RL: The role of Candida in intraperitoneal infections. Surgery 1980;88:524–530.
115. Talluri G, Mangone C, Freyle J, Shirazian D, Lehman H, Wise GJ: Polymerase chain reaction used to detect candidemia in patients with candiduria. Urology 1998;51:501–505.
116. Nassoura Z, Ivatury RR, Simon RJ, Jabbour N, Stahl WM: Candiduria as an early marker of disseminated infection in critically ill surgical patients: the role of fluconazole therapy. J Trauma 1993;35:290–295.
117. Pittet D, Monod M, Suter PM, Frenk E, Auckenthaler R: Candida colonization and subsequent infections in critically ill surgical patients. Ann Surg 1994;220:751–758.
118. Pfaller MA, Jones RN, Doern GV, Sader HS, Hollis RJ, Messer SA: International surveillance of bloodstream infections due to Candida species: frequency of occurrence and antifungal susceptibilities of isolates collected in 1997 in the United States, Canada, and South America for the SENTRY Program; the SENTRY participant group. J Clin Microbiol 1998;36:1886–1889.
119. Pfaller MA, Jones RN, Messer SA, Edmond MB, Wenzel RP: National surveillance of nosocomial blood stream infection due to Candida albicans: frequency of occurrence and antifungal susceptibility in the SCOPE Program. Diagn Microbiol Infect Dis 1998;31:327–332.
120. Martins MD, Rex JH: Resistance to antifungal agents in the critical care setting: problems and perspectives. New Horiz 1996;4:338–344.
121. Caplan ES, Hoyt NJ: Nosocomial sinusitis. JAMA 1982;247:639–641.
122. Holzapfel L, Chevret S, Madinier G, et al: Influence of long-term oro- or nasotracheal intubation on nosocomial maxillary sinusitis and pneumonia: results of a prospective, randomized, clinical trial. Crit Care Med 1993;21:1132–1138.
123. Rouby JJ, Laurent P, Gosnach M, et al: Risk factors and clinical relevance of nosocomial maxillary sinusitis in the critically ill. Am J Respir Crit Care Med 1994;150:776–783.
124. Lichtenstein D, Biderman P, Meziere G, Gepner A: The "sinusogram," a real-time ultrasound sign of maxillary sinusitis. Intensive Care Med 1998;24:1057–1061.
125. Seiden AM: Sinusitis in the critical care patient. New Horiz 1993;1:261–270.
126. Tedesco FJ: Pseudomembranous colitis: pathogenesis and therapy. Med Clin North Am 1982;66:655–664.

127. Manabe YC, Vinetz JM, Moore RD, Merz C, Charache P, Bartlett JG: *Clostridium difficile* colitis: an efficient clinical approach to diagnosis. Ann Intern Med 1995;123:835–840.
128. Impallomeni M, Galletly NP, Wort SJ, Starr JM, Rogers TR: Increased risk of diarrhoea caused by Clostridium difficile in elderly patients receiving cefotaxime. BMJ 1995;311:1345–1346.
129. Cleary RK: *Clostridium difficile*-associated diarrhea and colitis: clinical manifestations, diagnosis, and treatment. Dis Colon Rectum 1998;41:1435–1449.
130. Bader MK, Littlejohns L, Palmer S: Ventriculostomy and intracranial pressure monitoring: in search of a 0% infection rate. Heart Lung 1995;24:166–172.
131. Kanter RK, Weiner LB, Patti AM, Robson LK: Infectious complications and duration of intracranial pressure monitoring. Crit Care Med 1985;13:837–839.
132. Clark WC, Muhlbauer MS, Lowrey R, Hartman M, Ray MW, Watridge CB: Complications of intracranial pressure monitoring in trauma patients. Neurosurgery 1989;25:20–24.
133. Hamilton AJ, Orozco J, Narotam P, Bowersock T: Efficacy of vancomycin/tri-iododecyclemethyl ammonium chloride-coated ventriculostomy catheters in reducing infection. Neurosurgery 1997;40:1043–1049.
134. Hickman KM, Mayer BL, Muwaswes M: Intracranial pressure moinitoring: review of risk factors associated with infection. Heart Lung 1990;19:84–90.

33
Modulation of the Hypermetabolic Response After Trauma and Burns

Art Sanford and David N. Herndon

A hypermetabolic physiologic response characterizes the human response to major trauma. The complex process of maintaining homeostasis can be upset by a variety of perturbations. As the pathways and mechanisms begin to be understood, it is possible to think of modulating them under conditions of stress due to burn or blunt trauma to eliminate the deleterious components and restore the organism to a more normal state quickly. This possibility was recognized initially by Cuthbertson,[1] who identified the stress response after traumatic injuries that resulted in a period of negative nitrogen balance. Building on this foundation is the idea that manipulations can be done clinically to limit the deleterious effects of the systemic response to inflammatory mediators.

Physiology

In the event of a traumatic or burn injury, the body responds to the stress by releasing catabolic hormones that prepare the body to preserve its most basic functions. The perturbations of metabolism seen after burn injury appear to be mediated, at least in part, by a realignment of metabolic set points in the hypothalamus.[2] The signal that stimulates this "morbid cascade" is pain and direct cellular damage, with the resulting release of inflammatory cytokines, free oxygen radicals, and catecholamines. The chemicals released include complement components C3, C3a, terminal complement complex, thromboxanes A_2 and B_2, C-reactive protein, elastase, neopterin, histamine, prostaglandins, bradykinins, and serotonin.[3] Fluid loss and these mediators lead to a period of shock with resulting tissue hypoperfusion, creating further cellular damage. This repetitious system can become amplified out of control to the detriment of the injured.

Once this cascade has begun to develop, dysfunction occurs in systems well removed from the initial location of injury. With burns, body surface injuries of more than 30% produce increased capillary permeability throughout the body (including the lungs) and perturbations in cell membrane potentials that cause impaired sodium and water regulation, with resulting tissue edema.[4] Immune suppression has also been demonstrated that puts a patient with such trauma at increased risk of further insult from secondary infections that occur in hospital.[5]

The hypothalamic reset is manifested by increased plasma concentrations of catecholamines, glucagon, and cortisol. These substances function to create an environment of free substrates throughout the organism by promoting hyperglycemia, lipolysis, and proteolysis. As a point of demonstration, the hypermetabolic state can be reproduced in normal volunteers be combined infusion of epinephrine, glucagon, and cortisol.[6] Gluconeogenic substrate production is the goal of these physiologic responses. If the glucose supply is inadequate, excessive protein catabolism results, highlighting the need to provide as much carbohydrate as tolerated. However, hypermetabolic patients begin to have difficulty metabolizing glucose when infused supplements exceed 4 mg/kg/min.[7] Catecholamines are released from chromaffin granules in the sympathetic nerve terminals of the adrenal medulla in response to the stress of injury. Their biologic effects are mediated through interactions with specific receptors. These receptors are termed alpha (α) and beta (β), and each has a different affinity for catecholamines; moreover, their density is different in selected tissues. From a metabolic standpoint, catecholamine stimulation causes an increase in hepatic gluconeogenesis, hepatic glycogenolysis, and peripheral lipolysis.

Although patients with thermal injury usually have elevated blood glucose levels, their serum insulin levels are not depressed and, in fact, are elevated compared to controls without burn.[8] The hyperglycemia that results from a burn injury is due to elevation of serum glucagon and cortisol concentrations to a disproportionately greater degree than the serum insulin concentration.[9] Cortisol produces a similar result on substrate generation but also causes insulin resistance. The goal of this glucose production is to provide fuel for inflammatory cells and neural tissue.

Muscle proteolysis provides alanine to the liver for use in the tricarboxylic acid (TCA) cycle to produce energy, substrates to perform gluconeogenesis, and constituents of acute-phase proteins. Muscle proteolysis also provides glutamine to the gut and immune system for direct metabolism. Peripheral lipolysis results from the action of catecholamines, cortisol, and glucagon stimulating lipases that cause the adipocyte to release free fatty acids and glycerol,[10] which are used by the liver to produce energy by oxidation, are deposited in the liver after reesterification, or recirculated as very low density lipoproteins. Fatty liver develops in the severely injured patient because normal processing enzymes become overloaded, or there is downregulation of mechanisms to handle the abundance of fatty acids.[11]

The nitrogen losses after starvation are markedly different from the catabolism that follows injury or illness. During starvation fat utilization is maximized. Hypoglycemia resulting from inadequate intake causes the release of catecholamines and glucagon, signaling the liver to shift from glucose storage to glucose production. Substrates are generated for gluconeogenesis by peripheral lipolysis and proteolysis. Acetyl-coenzyme A (CoA) combines with oxaloacetate to produce energy via the TCA cycle; but when glucose is needed the oxaloacetate is diverted, making it no longer available for this pathway. The acetyl-CoA is unused and goes on to form the ketone bodies acetate, acetoacetate, and 3-hydroxybutyrate (Fig. 33.1). High concentrations of ketone bodies inhibit proteolysis and decrease glucose utilization. In contrast to the hypermetabolic response to trauma, plasma ketone bodies are lowered by their preferential use as an energy source by brain and cardiac muscle. Inadequate sources of oxygen further disturb the TCA cycle by depressing oxidative phosphorylation and causing the buildup of lactic acid, which impedes glycolysis. Metabolic stress that persists causes glucagon, catecholamine, and cortisol levels to remain high; it promotes acute-phase (protein-based) metabolism and prevents the shift to the more efficient lipid-based metabolism.[12]

With both trauma and burn injuries there is a direct correlation between the magnitude of the injury and the resulting hypermetabolic response. The severity of injury after blunt trauma is typically related to physiologic parameters (e.g., systolic blood pressure), the number of organ systems involved, and the death rate associated with specific injuries. In the case of burns it is easier to quantify, as the percentage of body surface area burned is measured objectively. That is what makes the study of burns a convenient model for studying the manipulations of this response. Ultimately, it is the initial resuscitation and degree of preventable cell damage that occurs that determines the degree of the hypermetabolic response.

The typical postinjury response is characterized by an "ebb" phase followed by a "flow" phase made up of catabolic and anabolic components. The "ebb" phase demonstrates decreased metabolic rate, hypothermia, and low cardiac output. Inadequate treatment at this stage exacerbates the injury. If fluid resuscitation is successful, cardiac output returns toward a normal level and overshoots previous normals to go on to a hypermetabolic state. This is the "flow" phase, where cardiac output and oxygen consumption are high and there is increased heat production and hyperglycemia. Early in the "flow" phase the hormonal milieu causes the net negative nitrogen balance that characterizes this catabolic phase. As the organism begins to return to homeostasis, the anabolic phase ensues in an attempt to restore the previously lost constitutional proteins. In

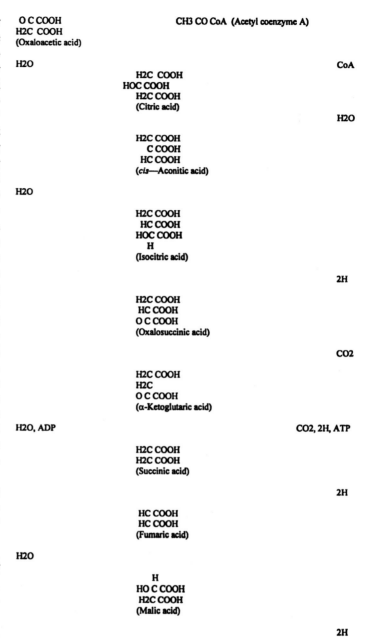

FIGURE 33.1. Tricarboxylic acid cycle.

the case of burn wounds, this increased resting energy expenditure persists even after all wounds have closed.

Many processes have been implicated in the development of this hypermetabolic response. In burned experimental models (rats, sheep, pigs) the process of bacterial translocation occurs.[13] Bacteria migrate from inside the lumen of the intestinal tract into the lymphatic channels that drain the intestine or the portal venous circulation. Traumatic injuries facilitate this process by causing atrophy of the mucosal lining secondary to the diversion of blood flow from this "nonvital" system during early shock. Early enteral feeding of burned animals has been shown to prevent mucosal atrophy and translocation of bacteria and to decrease the hypermetabolic response to injury.[14] Interestingly, this effect is not seen if enteral feedings are not initiated within 24 hours of the burn, emphasizing the importance of early enteral feeds.[15] The burn model for initiation of the hypermetabolic response also includes bacterial contamination of the wound. In an animal model, burn wounds contaminated by bacteria at the onset of injury become hypermetabolic sooner than do uncontaminated wounds.[16] The rate of increase of the metabolic rate was also found to be proportional to the degree of contamination.[17] Topical antimicrobial agents, which delay the onset of burn wound colonization, also appear to slow the rate of increase to a hypermetabolic condition. The triggers for this hypermetabolic response are less well defined but, in addition to the aforementioned, include infectious etiology (pulmonary or occult abscess) and sterile sepsis: "the systemic inflammatory response."

Modulation

The hormonal and metabolic response to a burn or traumatic injury results in hypermetabolism, progressive weight loss, increased susceptibility to infection, and poor wound healing. Modulation by environmental, nutritional, and pharmacologic means can eliminate some of the negative outcomes that would normally result.

Environmental Support

Control of room temperature alone is one of the easiest therapeutic maneuvers available to decrease some of the hypermetabolic demands of a burn patient. By raising the ambient temperature of the room from 25°C to 33°C, metabolic rates decreased significantly in a group of burned men from 2.0 times normal to 1.4 times normal.[18] Importantly, those who were not able to mount the higher metabolic rate at the lower temperature were more likely to die from their burn. The futile cycling that accompanies shivering adds energy wasting to an already hypermetabolic patient. Furthermore, the heat of water evaporative loss is 0.576 kcal/ml, with evaporative losses of 200 ml/m^2 body surface area burn (TBSA)/hr; if the energy to replace this loss does not come from the environment, it must come from the patient.[19] Although controlling the ambient temperature can attenuate the hypermetabolic state, the body is still trying to maintain a significantly higher core temperature than normal (38.5°C vs. 37°C) and requires additional nutritional support.

Nutritional Support

Nutritional support is another easy way to help modulate the hypermetabolic condition. Wound healing is impaired and mortality increased when inadequate nutrition results in a 20% weight loss. Tissue breakdown causes production of nitrogen at 30 g/day in an attempt to provide substrates for gluconeogenesis, but this loss can be limited by a dietary supply of carbohydrate.[18,20] Oral intake is seldom adequate to meet these needs, and early attempts to supplement with parenteral nutrition met with increased mortality rates,[21] shown to be secondary to a negative effect on the immune system.[22] Early postburn nutritional support may be given by the enteral route, limiting postburn hypermetabolism[23] and preserving mucosal gut integrity to limit bacterial translocation.[24,25] Protein metabolism in the hypermetabolic state has shown increased protein breakdown throughout but is significantly increased during the early posttrauma, or "flow," phase, when there is increased urea production, indicating that synthesis does not keep up with breakdown.[26] The switch to subsequent net protein anabolism from net protein catabolism seen later during recovery occurs in the setting of continued elevated protein turnover as synthetic mechanisms are restored.

Protein supplementation, including branched-chain amino acid-, arginine-, and glutamine-rich diets, have been attempted. Children with a more than 60% TBSA burn fed high-protein diets were found to have better indices of immunity,[27] higher protein levels, fewer days when bacteremia was seen, and improved survival.[28] Adults with more than 70% TBSA burns have also been studied at different protein intake rates, with administration of 1.4 g/kg/day producing balanced protein synthesis and catabolism; increased protein intake at 2.2 g/kg/day did not result in net synthesis, although the absolute rates of protein synthesis and catabolism were both stimulated to an equal degree. Branched-chain amino acid supplementation to nutritional support has also been attempted, but nitrogen balance measurements were not significantly altered when compared to intact protein.[29,30] Arginine supplementation, on the other hand, has been shown to be of benefit, with the optimal concentration at 2% of total protein.[31] In rat and guinea pig models of sepsis, it stimulated T cell immunity.[32,33] Wound healing and immune function were both stimulated in the elderly.[34] It appears that arginine exerts its effects via the hypothalamic-pituitary axis by causing stimulation of insulin, glucagon, prolactin, and growth hormone, as the response is absent in hypophysectomized rats. Glutamine is the most common amino acid in the body and may become an essential amino acid under stress conditions when it becomes a preferred fuel for rapidly dividing hypermetabolic cells.[35,36] Because of the high metabolic rate of the gut mucosa, a decrease in blood flow after selective shunting away from the bowel during shock would make supplementation with glutamine a logical practice, but there are no adequate data to support this practice. Supplementation of adenine nucleotides has also been proposed to enhance immune function in the stressed patient,[37] but human data are inadequate here as well.

Most dietary fats in enteral feeding formulas consist of linoleic acids, which lead to production of the immunodepressive prostaglandin E6 (PGE$_6$). Early data using tube feeding enriched with omega-3 fatty acids plus being linoleic-restricted, high-protein, and supplemented with arginine, cysteine, histidine, and vitamins was compared to two standard tube feedings. This protocol showed a trend toward reduced wound infections, shortened hospital stay, and preserved muscle mass; but larger patient participation is required to show statistical significance.[38]

Enteral feeding, when possible—given early with 20% protein and 50% carbohydrates compounded with low linoleic acid containing fats to meet measured metabolic needs—seems ideal. Polymeric protein diets function as well as more elemental diets, so long as they are tolerated. Inexpensive, readily available cow's milk has been used extensively to good effect.

Hormonal Modulation

After burn injury the sympathetic-adrenal axis assumes control of the metabolic rate from the thyroid gland with the previously described catecholamine surge that occurs in the hypermetabolic response, as evidenced by the fact that adrenalectomy limits the increase in metabolic rate after a burn but thyroidectomy does not.[39] The resulting low triiodothyronine (T_3) level following burn injury in the face of hypermetabolism results in a sick euthyroid syndrome, with the thyroid remaining responsive to thyroid-stimulating hormone (TSH).[40] Thyroid function or supplementation has not been shown to alter burn survival or response with hypermetabolism, but it has resulted in improved quality of scar formation in T_3-treated burn models.[41,42]

Growth Factors

Several growth factors have been identified, all with great diversity in terms of the site of origin and cross-reactivity. Platelet-derived growth factor (PDGF) is thought to be a regulator of other hormones but is itself chemotactic to fibroblasts and inflammatory cells. Clinical studies have shown topical PDGF to enhance healing of chronic ulcers and nonhealing wounds.[43] Collagen synthesis is also affected by PDGF, although the mechanism of action remains to be elucidated. Fibroblast growth factor (FGF) is a family of seven proteins that stimulate vascular endothelium and are mitogenic for fibroblasts and keratinocytes.[44] Transforming growth factors α and β (TGF) are released at extremes of pH, as would be found in wounds; in-vivo studies have demonstrated their usefulness for enhancement of wound healing and tensile strength.[45] Epidermal growth factor (EGF) and TGF are structurally similar,[46] and both have been shown to enhance in vivo reepithelialization.[47] EGF has also been shown to be effective in other areas of wound healing, including venous stasis and corneal ulcers.[48,49] Although studies on the topical application of these agents are promising, assessment of wound healing and application protocols are not uniform, so claims of benefit should be made with caution.

Growth Hormone

Despite reports of increased mortality in general intensive care unit (ICU) patients receiving growth hormone (GH),[50] beneficial metabolic effects have been demonstrated in burn patients for some time.[51-54] GH is a potent anabolic agent that induces net protein synthesis directly or indirectly with insulin-like growth factor-1 (IGF-1) as a mediator.[55-59] It has systemic effects, including increased appetite, decreased nitrogen loss, increased retention of nitrogen and potassium, weight gain, more rapid wound healing, increased oxygen utilization, and decreased respiratory quotient.[60,61]

Growth hormone (0.2 mg/kg/day) has been shown to increase protein turnover, with elevation of both protein synthesis and breakdown but with synthesis exceeding breakdown in a group of approximately 70% TBSA burned hypermetabolic adolescents, with a 50% net reduction in protein loss compared to controls.[62] Infusion of stable amino acid isotopes revealed that the treatment improved leg blood flow significantly, but there was no change in an already hyperdynamic cardiac output. Urinary nitrogen was also decreased in the treated group; and despite a 30-fold increase in GH levels and a 3-fold increase in IGF-1 levels, there was no change in insulin, resistance and inhibition of glucose uptake relative to the availability of insulin.[63] Rates of glucose use were similar between the experimental and control groups, but the hyperglycemia implies that glucose transport is impaired in the presence of GH. As counterregulation, plasma levels of insulin rise to attempt to maintain euglycemia. About one-third of patients treated with GH require therapeutic insulin for 2-3 days, whereafter borderline hyperglycemia persists but usually not at a level requiring insulin treatment. Investigation of the effects of GH on other stress hormones during the hyperdynamic, hypermetabolic period after a burn revealed that there were significantly elevated levels of catecholamines, glucagon, and insulin—above already elevated controls[64] (Table 33.1). Despite these mediators being elevated, protein anabolism resulted; and the metabolic rate/resting energy expenditure was not increased by these hormonal changes as

TABLE 33.1. Hormonal and Metabolic Parameters with Growth Hormone Treatment.

Parameter	Controls ($n = 8$)	Growth hormone ($n = 6$)
Growth hormone (normal < 8 mg/ml)	2.3 ± 0.3	30.4 ± 19.9*
Insulin-like growth factor-1 (normal 22–138 U/ml)	56 ± 15	168 ± 24*
Free fatty acids (normal 0.19–0.90 mEq/L)	0.59 ± 0.04	0.74 ± 0.01*
Glucose (normal 60–115 mg/dl)	129 ± 13	133 ± 16
Insulin (normal: 5–25 µU/ml)	25 ± 3	33 ± 3*
Total catecholamines (normal 120–450 pg/ml)	1117 ± 137	1817 ± 177*
Glucagon (normal 50–200 pg/ml)	158 ± 22	215 ± 18*
Cortisol (normal 7–27 mg/dl)	21.3 ± 1.6	28.4 ± 5.4

Data are presented as the mean ± SEM.
*Significantly different at $p < 0.05$.

TABLE 33.2. Donor Site Healing Times of Infants and Late Presenters.

Treatment	No.	Age (years)	TBSA burn (%)	Healing time (days)
GH at < 2 years	9	1.4 ± 0.2	56 ± 5	6.0 ± 4*
GH late	6	5.2 ± 1.2	57 ± 7	6.0 ± 0.7*
Control	26	8.4 ± 0.9	67 ± 3	8.5 ± 0.5

TBSA, total body surface area; GH, growth hormone.
Data are presented as the mean ± SEM.
*Significantly different at $p < 0.05$.

would be expected if the increased levels of stress hormones were clinically significant.

Skin is a target for GH, either by direct receptor-ligand interaction on the surface of epidermal and dermal cells or indirectly via circulating IGF-1.[65,66] GH has been demonstrated to cause increased collagen content and tensile strength of skin and granulation tissue in animal models.[67-69] Also, a significant increase in skin thickness was noted when 12 previously healthy men, aged 61–81 years, who had subnormal IGF-1 levels were given GH three times per week.[70] Use of GH at 0.2 mg/kg/day in massively burned children demonstrated significantly accelerated wound healing of the skin graft donor site, with the result that they could be returned to the operating room 2 days earlier than the controls[71] (Table 33.2). The clinical implication of this finding was the ability to close a 60% TBSA burn in 32 days with treatment, in contrast to 46 days without GH. The authors found no antibodies to the preparation of recombinant human GH administered in these studies. Not included in these prospective randomized studies were extremely young children and children with delayed presentation to burn centers. Infants less than 2 years of age were shown to have the same benefits as the older treated patients, without adverse effects. Patients presenting late in the course of hypermetabolism also were able to benefit from GH administration with significantly more rapid donor site healing times despite generalized appearances of poor nutrition and cachexia[72] (Table 33.3). Adults also show this 2-day decrease in time for donor site healing.[73]

Children, after 40% TBSA burns, exhibit profound growth retardation and do not exhibit "catch-up" growth spurts for as long as 3 years after the injury, despite the short-term administration of GH.[74] This is in contrast to other forms of pediatric trauma, where the victims overcome the metabolic stress of the injury and grow rapidly for a period of return to comparable peer-group growth patterns.[75] Preliminary data indicate that this trend may be reversed with long-term GH administration, but it awaits final analysis.[76]

Use of GH shows many benefits in the postburn individual, including significant cost savings. GH use in an American pediatric burn center with bed costs of US $1600 per day, although decreased hospitalization times due to faster wound healing and netted an 18% overall cost reduction.[77]

Insulin-Like Growth Factor-1

The mechanism of action of GH involves the mediator IGF-1, and attempts have been made to use it directly to avoid any possibly harmful effects of GH. In an animal model, administration of IGF-1 caused a decrease in oxygen consumption and a significant increase in body weight compared to the control group.[78] In humans, 3-day administration of IGF-1 demonstrated decreased protein oxidation and promotion of glucose uptake; the resting energy expenditure and nitrogen balance were not changed, providing evidence of the anabolic effects of IGF-1.[79] Importantly, the IGF response to GH is diminished relative to the severity of trauma or burn,[80,81] and in certain circumstances (e.g., sepsis) GH has been shown not to increase IGF-1 levels. The activity of IGF-1 is dependent not only on its tissue concentration but its interaction with specific binding proteins; repeated administration of IGF-1 has resulted in lower amounts of insulin-like growth factor binding protein-3 (IGFBP-3). Levels of IGFBP-3 are regulated by GH and IGF-1 feedback loops, and administration of IGF-1 causes downregulation of GH release and indirectly downregulates IGFBP-3.[12]

The use of recombinant human IGF-1 overcomes the previously discussed side effect of hypoglycemia by combining it with one of the naturally occurring binding proteins, IGFBP-3, in clinical application. This complex has been demonstrated to increase net protein synthesis across the isolated leg of severely burned adults.[82,83]

β-Adrenergic Receptor Blocking Agents

Catecholamine excess accompanies the hypermetabolic response to a burn injury. Tachycardia is persistent and can contribute to postburn mortality. Total catecholamine absence in 60% burned rats, resulting from adrenalectomy or chronic reserpine administration, decreased hypermetabolism but also resulted in increased mortality.[84]

Catecholamines stimulate peripheral lipolysis after a burn injury, and administration of β-blocking agents could promote protein breakdown by eliminating this source of energy substrate. A decrease in metabolic rate has been demonstrated with combined α- and β-blockade, and with β-blockade alone.[18] Reducing the pulse, blood pressure, minute ventilation, and free fatty acid production decreased the metabolic rate. An important finding from this study was that cold stress increased urinary catecholamine release and the metabolic rate in

TABLE 33.3. Donor Site Healing Times.

Treatment	Healing time (days)		
	First harvest	Second harvest	Third harvest
Placebo	9.0 ± 0.4	9.0 ± 0.7	8.0 ± 1.0
Growth hormone (0.2 mg/kg/day)	7.0 ± 0.5*	6.0 ± 0.4*	6.0 ± 1.0

Data are presented as the mean ± SEM.
*Significantly different at $p < 0.05$.

survivors; but those who were unable to meet the extra demands of cold stress died. Based on these findings, adrenergic blockade that precludes a cold stress response is best avoided.

Propanolol, given at 2 mg/kg/day per seven days reduced the heart rate by 20%, the left ventricular stroke work index by 22%, and the rate pressure product by 36%. Plasma glucose, free fatty acids, triglyceride, and insulin levels remained unchanged.[85] The propanolol level required to accomplish this blockade was 700 ± 500 mg/ml. Catecholamine levels were not affected by this treatment, but blood urea nitrogen levels were elevated in the treatment group owing to measured increases in the production of urea from unopposed α-adrenergic stimulation.

Septic burn patients (82 ± 11% TBSA) who received propanolol under monitored conditions also showed beneficial effects of β-adrenergic blockade. The pressure–work index and rate–pressure product were significantly decreased, as the cardiac index, oxygen delivery index, and oxygen consumption were improved without adversely affecting overall oxygen delivery or total body oxygen consumption. The dose necessary to drop the heart rate 25% was still able to permit appropriate responses to the cold stress.[86]

Metoprolol (B_1 selective) has been compared to nonselective blockade with propanolol at equivalent doses to reduce the heart rate by 18%. Using protein infusion studies, metoprolol had no effect on protein or lipid metabolism, whereas propanolol produced a decrease in lipolysis with no change in urea production.[87]

Selective $β_1$-blockade is a metabolically inactive, cardiovascularly safe means of limiting the postburn hyperdynamic response. Metoprolol would then be the choice for burn-induced hypertension.[88] Selective $β_2$-agonists have known protein anabolic effects.[89] Postsurgical rats and burned rats showed increased muscle mass and body weight after using clenbuterol, as well as evidence of increased hypermetabolism.

Anabolic Steroids

Agents that could counteract the muscle-wasting effects of the hypermetabolic state include anabolic steroids. Endogenous testosterone is diminished after induction of hypermetabolism, and supplemental testosterone is rapidly metabolized.[90] This finding demonstrates how the anabolic stimulus is greatly reduced under these conditions. Hepatotoxicity is a possible side effect of many of the synthetic replacements, limiting their usefulness.[91] Oxandrolone is an exception, being apparently free of hepatotoxicity but still with adequate pharmacokinetics to be worked out in the hypermetabolic population. Use of oxandrolone in debilitated patients has resulted in significant improvements in muscle mass and even altered mortality statistics.[92,93] The use of combining oxandrolone with a high calorie (35 cal/kg/day), high protein 2 g/kg/day) diet and an exercise program in an attempt to restore muscle mass has also been tested.[94] Addition of oxandrolone was shown to promote weight gain significantly, from 7.5 pounds to 14.5 pounds. Unfortunately, the investigators were unable to perform nitrogen balance studies to determine the etiology of the gain.

Conclusions

Many things can be done to modulate and attenuate the postinjury hypermetabolic state to aid in wound healing before deleterious results occur. A few of the regulatory pathways we have begun to manipulate are discussed here. With further understanding of the physiology that incites this condition, new focuses for control points surely will be elucidated.

References

1. Cuthbertson DP: The disturbance of metabolism produced by bony and non-bony injury, with modes of certain abnormal conditions of bone. Biochemistry 1930;24:144.
2. Wilmore DW, Long JM, Mason AD Jr, Pruitt BA Jr: Stress in surgical patients as a neurophysiologic reflex response. Surg Gynecol Obstet 1976;142:257.
3. Roumen RMH, Long JM, Schlag G, et al: Inflammatory mediators in relation to the development of multiple organ failure in patients after severe blunt trauma. Crit Care Med 1995;23:474–475.
4. Arturson G: Capillary permeability in burned and nonburned areas in dogs. Acta Chir Scand 1961;274(Suppl):55.
5. Heidman M, Bengtsson A: The immunologic response to thermal injury. World J Surg 1992;16:53–56.
6. Bessey PQ, Watters JM, Aoki TT, Wilmore DW: Combined hormonal infusion simulates the metabolic response to injury. Ann Surg 1984;200:264.
7. Wolfe RR, Durkot MJ, Allsop JR, Burke JK: Glucose metabolism in severely burned patients. Metabolism 1979;28:1031.
8. Shuck JM, Eton RP, Shuck LW, Wachtel TL, Schade BS: Dynamics of insulin and glucagon secretions in severely burned patients. J Trauma 1977;17:706.
9. Waymack JP, Rutan RL, Herndon DH: Burn management for general surgery. In: Ritchie WR, Steele G, Dean RH (eds) General Surgery. Philadelphia, Lippincot, 1995.
10. Steinberg D, Khoo JC: Hormone sensitive lipase in adipose tissue. Fed Am Soc Exp Biol Proc 1977;36:1986–1990.
11. Wolf RR, Klein S, Herndon DN, Jahoor F: Substrate cycling in thermogenesis and amplification of net substrate flux in human volunteers and burned patients. J Trauma 1990;30:86–89.
12. Wolf SE, Barrow RE, Herndon DN: Growth hormone and IGF-1 therapy in the hypercatabolic patient. Bailliercs Clin Endocrinol Metab 1996;10:447–451.
13. Tokyay R, Ziegler ST, Traber DL, et al: Postburn gastrointestinal vasoconstriction increases bacterial and endotoxin translocation. J Appl Physiol 1993;74:1521–1527.
14. Mochizuki H, Trocki O, Dominioni L, Alexander JW: Reduction of post-burn hypermetabolism by early enteral feeding. Curr Probl Surg 1985;42:121.
15. Mochizuki H, Trocki O, Dominioni L, Brackett KA, Joffe SN, Alexander JW: Mechanism of prevention of post-burn hypermetabolism and catabolism by early enteral feeding. Ann Surg 1984;200:297.
16. Aulick LH, McManus AT, Mason AD Jr, Pruitt BA Jr: Effects of infection on oxygen consumption and core temperature in experimental thermal injury. Ann Surg 1986;204:48.

17. Aulick LH, Wroczyski FA, Coil JA, Mason AD Jr: Metabolic and thermoregulatory responses to burn wound colonization. J Trauma 1989;29:478.
18. Willmore DW, Long JM, Mason AD, Skreen RW, Pruitt BA: Catecholamines: mediator of the hypermetabolic response to thermal injury. Ann Surg 1974;180:653–669.
19. Barr PO, Birke G, Liljedahl SO, et al: Oxygen consumption and water loss during treatment of burns with warm dry air. Lancet 1968;1:164–168.
20. Sonhoff HS, Pearson E, Artz CP: An estimation of nitrogen requirements for equilibrium in burn patients. Surg Gynecol Obstet 1961;112:159.
21. Herndon DN, Barrow RE, Stein M, et al: Increased mortality with intravenous supplemental feeding in severely burned patients. J Burn Care Rehabil 1989;10:309–313.
22. Moore FA, Feliciano DV, Andrassy RJ, et al: Early enteral feeding, compared with parenteral, reduces post operative septic complications: the results of a meta-analysis. Ann Surg 1992;216:172–183.
23. Mochizuki H, Trocki O, Dominioni L, et al: Mechanism of prevention of postburn hypermetabolism and catabolism by early enteral feeding. Ann Surg 1991;200:297–310.
24. Herndon DN, Ziegler ST: Bacterial translocation after thermal injury. Crit Care Med 1993;21:S50–S54.
25. Saito H, Trocki O, Alexander JW, Kopcha R, Heyd T, Jnfee SN: The effect of route of nutrient administration on the nutritional state, catabolic hormone secretion, and gut mucosal integrity after burn injury. J Parenter Enteral Nutr 1987;11:7.
26. Jahoor F, Desai M, Herndon DN, Wolfe RR: Dynamics of the protein metabolic response after a burn injury. Metabolism 1988;37:330–337.
27. Neely AW, Petra AB, Holloman GH, Rustitan FW, Turner MD, Hardy JD: Researches on the cause of burn hypermetabolism. Ann Surg 1974;179:291–294.
28. Alexander JW, MacMillan BG, Stinnett JD, et al: Beneficial effects of aggressive protein feeding in severely burned children. Ann Surg 1980;192:505–517.
29. Yu Y-M, Wagner DA, Walesreswski JC, Burke SF, Young VR: A kinetic study of leucine metabolism in severely burned patients: comparison between a conventional and branched chain amino acid-enriched nutritional therapy. Ann Surg 1988;207:421–429.
30. Trocki O, Moehizuri H, Dominioni L, Alexander JW: Intact protein versus free amino acids in the nutritional support of thermally injured animals. J Parenter Enteral Nutr 1986;10:139–145.
31. Alexander JW, Gottschlich MM: Nutritional immunomodulation in burn patients. Crit Care Med 1990;18:S149–S153.
32. Madden HP, Breslin RJ, Wasserkmg HL, Efron G, Barboh A: Stimulation of T cell immunity by arginine enhances survival in peritonitis. J Surg Res 1988;41:658–663.
33. Saito H, Trocki O, Wang SL, Gonce SS, Joffe SN, Alexander JW: Metabolic and immune effects of dietary arginine supplementation after burn. Arch Surg 1987;122:784–789.
34. Kirk SJ, Hurson M, Regan MC, Host DR, Wasserkrug HL, Barbul A: Arginine stimulates wound healing and immune function in elderly human beings. Surgery 1993;114:155–160.
35. Souba WW, Smith RJ, Wilmore DW: Glutamine metabolism by the intestinal tract. J Parenter Enteral Nutr 1985;9:608–615.
36. Lacey J, Wilmore D: Is glutamine a conditionally essential amino acid? Nutr Rev 1990;48:297–310.
37. Daly JM, Lieberman MD, Goldfine J, et al: Enteral nutrition with supplemental arginine, RNA, and omega-3 fatty acids in patients after operation: immunologic, metabolic, and clinical outcome. Surgery 1992;112:56–67.
38. Gottschlich MM, Jenkins M, Warden GD, et al: Differential effects of three enteral dietary regimens on selected outcome variables in burn patients. J Parenter Enteral Nutr 1990;14:225–236.
39. Herndon DN, Wilmore DW, Mason AD, Pruitt BA: Humoral mediators of nontemperature dependent hypermetabolism in 50% burned adult rats. Surg Forum 1977;28:37–39.
40. Aun F, Medeiros-Neto GA, Younes RN, Birogini D, Ramos de Oliveira M: The effect of major trauma on the pathways of thyroid hormone metabolism. J Trauma 1983;23:1048–1050.
41. Herndon DN, Wilmore DW, Mason AD, Curreri PW: Increased rates of wound healing in burned guinea pigs treated with triiodothyronine. Surg Forum 1979;30:95–97.
42. Mehregan AH, Zamick P: The effect of triiodothyronine in healing of deep chemical burns and marginal scars of skin grafts: a histologic study. J Cutan Pathol 1974;1:113–116.
43. Robson MC, Phillips LG, Thomason A, Robson LE, Pierce GF: Platelet derived growth factor BB for the treatment of chronic pressure ulcers. Lancet 1992;339:23–25.
44. Schweigerer L, Neufield G, Friedman J, et al: Capillary endothelial cells express basic fibroblast growth factor, a mitogen that promoted their own growth. Nature 1987;325:257–259.
45. Quaglino D, Nanney LB, Ditesheim JA, Davidson JM: Transforming growth factor beta stimulates wound healing and modulates extracellular matrix gene expression in pig skin: incisional wound model. J Invest Dermatol 1991;97:34–42.
46. Derynk R: Transforming growth factor. Cell 1988;54:593–595.
47. Martin PM, Wooley IH, McCluskey J: Growth factors and cutaneous wound repair. Prog Growth Factor Res 1992;4:25–44.
48. Falanga V, Eaglstein WH, Bucalo B, Katz MH, Hams B, Carson P: Topical use of human recombinant epidermal growth factor (h-EGF) in venous ulcers. J Dermatol Surg Oncol 1992;18:60–66.
49. Brown GL, Curtsinger L, Jurkiewicz A, et al: Stimulation of healing of chronic wounds by epidermal growth factors [see comments]. Plast Reconstr Surg 1991;88:189–194.
50. Public Communications from Pharmacia & Upjohn Pharmaceuticals and Rolf Gunnarsson, M.D. to all industry and medical community involved with the use or potential use of recombinant human growth hormone, October 31, 1997.
51. Soroff HS, Rozin RR, Mooty Jr, et al: Role of human growth hormone in the response of trauma: metabolic effects following burns. Ann Surg 1967;166:739–752.
52. Liljadahl SO, Gemzell CA, Plantin LO, et al: Effect of human growth hormone in patients with severs burns. Acta Chir Scand 1961;1221:1–4.
53. Wilmore DW, Moyland JA Jr, Bristow BF, Mason AD, Pruitt BA: Anabolic effects of growth hormone and high caloric feedings following thermal injury. Surg Gynecol Obstet 1974;138:875–884.
54. Soroff HS, Pearson E, Green NL, Artz CE: The effect of growth hormone on nitrogen balance at various levels of intake in burned patients. Surg Gynecol Obstet 1960;111:259–273.
55. Soroff HS, Rozin RR, Mooty J, et al: Role of human growth hormone in response to trauma: metabolic effects following burns. Ann Surg 1967;166:739–752.

56. Liljadhal SO, Gemzel CA, Plantin LO, Birke G: Effect of human growth hormone in patients with severe burns. Acta Chir Scand 1961;122:1–4.
57. McManson JM. Smith RJ, Wilmore DW: Growth hormone stimulates protein synthesis during hypocaloric parenteral nutrition. Ann Surg 1988;208:136–149.
58. Wolfe RR, Jahoor K, Hartl WH: Protein and amino acid metabolism after injury. Diabetes Metab Rev 1989;5:149–164.
59. Finkelstein JW, Roffward HP, Boyer RM, Kream J, Hellman L: Age related change in the twenty-four hour spontaneous secretion of growth hormone. J Clin Endocrinol Metab 1972;35:665–670.
60. Roe CF, Kinky J: The influence of human growth hormone on energy sources in convalescence. Surg Forum 1962;13:369–371.
61. MacGorman LR, Rizza R, Gerich JE: Physiological concentrations of growth hormone exert insulin like and insulin antagonistic effect on both hepatic and extra hepatic tissues in man. J Clin Endocrinol Metab 1981;53:556–559.
62. Gore DC, Honeycult D, Jahoor F, Wolfe R, Herndon DN: Effect of exogenous growth hormone on whole-body and isolated limb protein kinetics in burned patients. Arch Surg 1991;126:38–43.
63. Gore DC, Honeycutt D, Jahoor E, Rutan T, Wolfe R, Herndon DN: Effect of exogenous growth hormones on glucose utilization in burn patients. J Surg Res 1991;51:518–523.
64. Fleming RYD, Rutan RI, Jahoor F, Barrow RE, Wolfe RR, Herndon DN: Effect of recombinant human growth hormone on catabolic hormones and free fatty acids following thermal injury. J Trauma 1992;32:698–703.
65. Gabrilove JL, Schwartz A, Chung J: Effect of hormones on the skin in endocrinologic disorders. J Clin Endocrinol Metab 1962;22:688–692.
66. Tavakkol A, Elder JT, Griffiths CEM, et al: Expression of growth hormone receptor, insulin-like growth factor I (IGF-I) and IGF-I receptor mRNA and proteins in human skin. J Invest Dermatol 1992;99:343–349.
67. Jorgensen PH, Andreassen TT, Jorgensen KD: Growth hormone influences collagen deposition and mechanical strength of intact rat skin: a dose-response study. Acta Endocrinol (Copenh) 1989;120:767–772.
68. Jorgensen PH, Andreassen TT: A dose-response study of the effects of biosynthetic human growth hormone on formation and strength of granulation tissue. Endocrinology 1987;121:1637–1641.
69. Jorgensen PH, Andreassen TT: The influence of biosynthetic human growth hormone on biomechanical properties and collagen formation in granulation tissue. Horm Metab Res 1988;20:490–493.
70. Rudman A, Feller AG, Nagraj HS: Effect of human growth hormone in men over 60 years old. N Engl J Med 1990;323:1–6.
71. Herndon DN, Barrow RE, Kunkel KR, Broemeling L, Rutan RL: Effects of recombinant human growth hormone on donor-site healing in severely burned children. Ann Surg 1990;212:424–431.
72. Gilpin DA, Barrow RE, Rutan RL, Broemeling BSN, Herndon DN: Recombinant human growth hormone accelerates wound healing in children with large cutaneous burns. Ann Surg 1994;220(I):19–24.
73. Sherman SK, Demling RH, Lalonde C, et al: Growth hormone enhances reepithelialization of human split thickness skin graft donor sites. Surg Forum 1989;40:37–39.
74. Rutan RI, Herndon DN: Growth delay in postburn pediatric patients. Arch Surg 1990;125:392–395.
75. Prader A: Catch-up growth. Postgrad Med J 1978;54(Suppl):133–146.
76. Low JFA, Herndon DN, Barrow RE: Effect of growth hormone on growth delay in burned children: a 3-year follow-up study. Lancet 1999;354:1789.
77. Rutan R, Herndon DN: Justification for the use of growth hormone in a pediatric burn center. In: Proceedings of the American Burn Association, Orlando, FL, 1994.
78. Strock LL, Singh H, Abdullah A, et al: The effect of insulin-like growth factor I in postburn hypermetabolism. Surgery 1990;108:161–164.
79. Cioffi WG, Gore DC, Rue LW III, et al: Insulin-like growth factor-I lowers protein oxidation in thermally injured patients. Ann Surg 1994;220:310–316.
80. Kimbrough TD, Sheman S, Ziegler TR, et al: Insulin-growth factor-1 response is comparable following intravenous and subcutaneous administration of growth hormone. J Surg Res 1991;51:472–476.
81. Dahn MS, Lange MP, Jacobs LA: Insulin-like growth factor-I production is inhibited in human sepsis. Arch Surg 1988;123:1409–1414.
82. DebRoy MA, Zhang XJ, Wolfe SE, et al: Anabolic effects of administration of recombinant human insulin-like growth factor I/binding protein 3 on protein metabolism in adult burn patients. Surg Forum 1998;49:56–57.
83. DebRoy MA, Wolf SE, Zhang XJ, et al: Anabolic effects of insulin-like growth factor in combination with insulin-like growth factor binding protein-3 in severely burned adults. J Trauma (in press).
84. Herndon DN: Mediators of metabolism. J Trauma 1981;21:701–705.
85. Herndon DN, Barrow RE, Rutan TC, Minifee P, Jahoor F, Wolfe RR: Effect of propanolol administration on hemodynamic and metabolic responses of burned pediatric patients. Annals Surg 1998;208:484–492.
86. Honeycutt D, Barrow R, Herndon DN: Cold stress response in patients with severe burns after beta-blockade. J Burn Care Rehabil 1992;13:181–186.
87. Herndon DN, Nguyen TT, Wolfe RR, et al: Lipolysis in burned patients is stimulated by the beta 2-receptor for catecholamines. Arch Surg 1994;129:1301–1305.
88. Popp MB, Silverstein EB, Srivastaver LS, Laggie JMH, Knowles HC, MacMillan BG: A pathophysiologic study of the hypertension associated with burn injury in children. Ann Surg 1981;193:817–824.
89. Choo JJ, Horan MA, Little RA, et al: Anabolic effects of clenbuterol on skeletal muscle are mediated by beat-2 adrenoreceptor activation. Am J Physiol 1992;263(Endocrinol Metab 26):E50–E56.
90. Moore FD: Responses to starvation and stress. In: Metabolic Care of the Surgical Patient. Philadelphia, Saunders 1989;202–275.
91. Kanti A, Ranney RE, Zagarella BA, et al: Oxandrolone disposition and metabolism in man. Clin Pharmacol Ther 1973;14:862–866.
92. Mendenhall CL, Anderson S, Garcia-Pont P, et al: Short term and long term survival in patients treated with oxandrolone and prednisone. N Engl J Med 1984;311:1464–1470.
93. Mendenhall CL, Anderson S, Garcia-Pont P, et al: A study of oral nutritional support with oxandrolone in malnourished patients with alcholic hepatitis: results of the Department of Veterans Cooperative Study. Hepatology 1993;17:564–570.
94. Demliing RH, DeSanti L: Oxandrolone, an anabolic steroid significantly increases the rate of weight gain in the recovery phase after major burns. J Trauma 1997;43:47–51.

Part V
Specific Remote Organ Failures

34
Circulation

Jean-Louis Vincent

The circulation is perhaps not always thought of as an individual organ and, indeed, is not a compact, well defined structure as are many other organs, such as the heart, liver, kidney, and brain. Instead, it is composed of some 60,000 miles of vessels of various size, capacity, and function. Together these vessels form a unique organ that provides the body with the means of transporting oxygen, nutrients, and waste products around the body. The circulation thus functions to maintain an appropriate environment in all tissues for optimal cellular activity and survival; and efficient and effective circulatory function is essential for normal body function. In fact, the circulation could perhaps be considered the most important organ in the development of multiple organ failure, as its function is vital for the normal function of all other organs; if the circulation fails, everything fails. This chapter discusses the various causes of circulatory failure and the available therapeutic interventions used to treat it.

Etiology and Definition

Classification of Circulatory Failure

The circulation is normally tightly regulated, so blood flow through each organ is adapted according to its function and needs at any particular moment. Failure of the circulation results in failure of tissue perfusion and an inadequate supply of oxygen and nutrients to the tissues. Consequent cellular dysfunction proceeds to organ dysfunction, organ failure, and death if the circulatory insufficiency is not corrected. Circulatory failure can be regional (e.g., following arterial thrombosis, vasospasm, mesenteric infarction); but if it is generalized and clinically evident, circulatory failure is synonymous with shock. Initial features and physiologic alterations may differ according to the initiating event; but as shock becomes established, a common pattern is seen related to the consequences of inadequate tissue perfusion.

Various types of circulatory failure have been defined with differing hemodynamic features. They are generally characterized into four groups (Table 34.1).

1. *Hypovolemic*: the result of acute blood or fluid loss, usually with a decrease in circulating blood volume of at least 30%. Fluid losses can be exogenous (e.g., hemorrhage, burns, diarrhea, vomiting) or endogenous (e.g., anaphylaxis, inflammation).
2. *Cardiogenic*: the result of failure of the cardiac pump. Impaired pump function may result from myocardial infarction (the most common cause), advanced cardiomyopathy, or valvular dysfunction. Severe cardiac arrhythmias can also result in cardiogenic shock.
3. *Obstructive*: the result of an obstruction to normal blood flow (e.g., pulmonary embolism, cardiac tamponade, or dissecting aneurysm).
4. *Distributive*: the primary mechanism in sepsis, anaphylaxis, and pancreatitis. Unlike the other types of shock, it is typically associated with a normal or high cardiac output.

Although this list provides a useful means of classification, as in many areas of medicine, the story is not quite so simple; many types of shock are in reality a mixture of two or more of the four classic forms. For example, the patient with septic shock may combine distributive and hypovolemic features and may also have evidence of myocardial impairment. Similarly, following trauma a patient may have mixed hypovolemia and distributive shock. In addition, the category of shock into which any patient initially falls may alter with time and therapy.

Signs of Circulatory Failure

Regardless of the underlying mechanism, the cardinal sign is hypotension, considered to be a systolic blood pressure of less than 90 mmHg (mean arterial pressure less than 60 mmHg), or a fall in systolic blood pressure of 30 mmHg. Blood pressure determines tissue perfusion and is itself dependent on cardiac output and vascular resistance. Cardiac output is determined by heart rate and stroke volume, which is the balance between preload, afterload, and myocardial contractility. Vascular resistance is dependent on the size and length of the vessels and the viscosity of blood. In essence, arteriolar smooth muscle tone is the most important factor in the control of vascular resistance and is regulated by local and systemic humoral and neural

TABLE 34.1. Principal Causes and Characteristics of Circulatory Shock.

Primary defect and causes	AP	CVP/RAP	PAP	PAOP	CO	SvO$_2$
Hypovolemic defect						
Hemorrhage	↓	↓	↓	↓	↓	↓
Diarrhea, vomiting	↓	↓	↓	↓	↓	↓
Extensive burns	↓	↓	↓	↓	↓	↓
Inflammation	↓	↓	↓	↓	↓	↓
Cardiogenic defect						
Myocardial infarction	↓	↑	↑	↑	↓	↓
(right ventricular)	↓	↑	N	N	↓	↓
Valvular disease	↓	↑	↑	↑	↓	↓
Cardiomyopathy	↓	↑	↑	↑	↓	↓
Arrhythmias	↓	↑	↑	↑	↓	↓
Obstructive defect						
Pericardial tamponade	↓	↑	↑	↑	↓	↓
Massive pulmonary embolism	↓	↑	↑	N	↓	↓
Distributive defect						
Septic shock	↓	↓N↑	↑	↓N↑	↑	↑
Acute adrenal insufficiency	↓	↓N↑	↑	↓N↑	↑	↑
Drug overdose	↓	↓N↑	↑	↓N↑	↓N↑	↓N↑
Pancreatitis	↓	↓N↑	↑	↓N↑	↓N↑	↓N↑

AP, arterial blood pressure; CVP, central venous pressure; RAP, right arterial pressure; PAP, pulmonary artery pressure; PAOP, pulmonary artery occlusion pressure; CO, cardiac output; SvO$_2$, mixed venous oxygen saturation; ↑, ↓, N, increased, decreased, normal, respectively.

components. Microcirculatory factors related to endothelial dysfunction, such as enhanced leukocyte and platelet adhesion, can also influence tissue perfusion during shock.[1]

Hypotension per se is an inadequate indicator of shock; evidence of organ hypoperfusion must also be present. Such indications of inadequate perfusion include decreased skin turgor, altered mental status, and decreased urine output. Abnormal cellular metabolism with anaerobic glycolysis also results in the production of lactate, and blood lactate levels are elevated. The end result of circulatory failure is organ dysfunction and death; and the duration of shock, as assessed by the duration of hyperlactatemia, has been associated with the degree of organ failure and worsened mortality rates[2–4] (Fig. 34.1).

Oxygen Uptake/Supply Dependence

In the normal, stable situation, oxygen uptake (VO$_2$) equals oxygen demand and is independent of oxygen delivery (DO$_2$); it remains stable even when the DO$_2$ varies over a wide range of values. This independence is achieved by mechanisms in the microvasculature that enables oxygen extraction to be adjusted at the tissue level. However, a critical point is reached, below which the increase in oxygen extraction is insufficient to compensate for a further fall in DO$_2$, and the VO$_2$ starts to decrease, becoming DO$_2$-dependent. This situation is termed physiologic supply dependence and is a feature of all forms of circulatory failure. Below the critical DO$_2$, tissue oxygenation is compromised and lactate levels rise.[5,6] The exact value of the critical DO$_2$ is difficult to determine in humans; but Ronco et al.,[7] by taking sequential measurements of DO$_2$ and VO$_2$ as

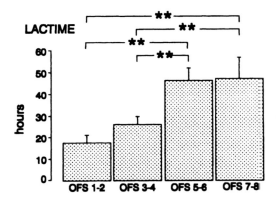

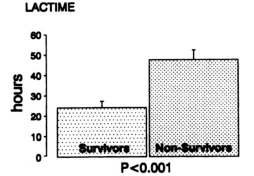

FIGURE 34.1. Association of organ failure score (OFS, top panel) and mortality (lower panel) with lactime (time during which blood lactate levels exceeded 2.0 mmol/l) in patients with circulatory failure due to sepsis. **$p < 0.01$. (Adapted from Bakker et al.,[4] with permission.)

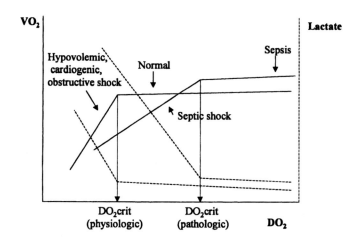

FIGURE 34.2. Relation of DO_2 with VO_2 and blood lactate levels during acute circulatory failure. VO_2 remains independent of DO_2 over a wide range of DO_2 values until a critical point is reached (DO_2 crit), at which point the VO_2 falls, becoming DO_2-dependent, and blood lactate levels rise. During sepsis the DO_2 crit occurs at a higher level (pathologic VO_2/DO_2 dependence).

DO_2 was reduced in patients in whom terminal life support was being discontinued, found a definable critical DO_2 of 3.8–4.5 ml/min/m². With septic shock tissue oxygen extraction is altered and less efficient, and the critical DO_2 level is higher, with the VO_2 remaining dependent on the DO_2 at higher levels than in physiologic supply dependence (Fig. 34.2), leading to the term pathologic supply dependence.[8,9] There has been some debate about the existence of pathologic supply dependence, with suggestions that the dependence seen is in fact artifactual. Proponents of this concept argue that use of the same parameters to calculate VO_2 and DO_2 cause mathematic coupling of data sufficient to account for the apparent pathologic supply dependence.[10] We do not believe that mathematic coupling of data is sufficient to account for the observed supply dependence for several reasons.[11] First, good correlation has been shown between direct and indirect measurements of VO_2 in various groups of patients.[12,13] Second, several studies have identified supply VO_2/DO_2 dependence in some patients but not in others using the same measurement technique.[14,15] Third, supply dependence can still be observed when assessing the VO_2/DO_2 relation using the relation between cardiac index and oxygen extraction, which avoids any possibility of mathematic coupling, as the parameters are determined independently.[16] The presence of supply dependence is an indicator of inadequate tissue oxygenation, and its presence should be taken as an indication that urgent treatment is necessary to promote tissue perfusion.

Therapy

As outcome is related to the length of a shock episode, it is logical to attempt to reduce the duration of circulatory shock. The basic rules of resuscitation must be applied and attention paid to the VIP (ventilation, infusion, pump) principles, as initially proposed by Weil and Shubin.[17]

Ventilation

Oxygen must be administered routinely to ensure that arterial oxygen pressures (PaO_2) are maintained as close as possible to normal and certainly above 60 mmHg. Endotracheal intubation and mechanical ventilation should be considered early and used without hesitation when mask oxygen is not adequate. Mechanical ventilation can have additional beneficial effects by reducing the oxygen demand of respiratory muscles.

Infusion

Fluid replacement plays a vital role in the treatment of acute circulatory failure, and fluids must be administered early and in sufficient volume. The type of fluid is probably less important than the quantity, and clinical studies have failed to demonstrate benefits of one type of fluid over another. In general, colloids are preferred for acute circulatory failure as small quantities provide the same effect as crystalloids, and the risk of edema is therefore reduced.[18] Ideally, fluids are administered until no further increase in cardiac index is observed. The presence of anemia is now considered less important than previously. The general consensus that red blood cell transfusions should be administered to maintain a hematocrit above 30–35% and a hemoglobin level higher than about 10 g/dl is now being questioned. A multicenter, randomized study in Canada[19] showed that a liberal transfusion strategy was associated with a higher mortality rate than a restricted transfusion strategy. In any case, hemoglobin levels above 10 g/dl have no further benefit in terms of oxygen delivery, and the increase in blood viscosity may in fact impair oxygen delivery. Stored red blood cells may lose their deformability and hence promote tissue ischemia.[20] Fresh blood cells are therefore preferable when possible.

Pump

Fluids may not be sufficient to restore perfusion pressure, and it may be necessary to use vasopressors in addition to fluids. There is no evidence that any drug is superior to another, but excessive vasoconstriction should be avoided, as it may further impair tissue perfusion. Dopamine is generally the preferred first-line agent for its combined α and β effects. At low to moderate doses (<10 μg/kg/min), β-adrenergic effects predominate, increasing cardiac contractility and maintaining cardiac output. At higher doses, α-adrenergic effects predominate, resulting in vasoconstriction and a greater rise in blood pressure. At very low doses (<2 μg/kg/min) dopamine also activates dopaminergic receptors, and theoretically one would expect this to increase blood flow to the splanchnic and renal regions more than to other areas. Low dose, "renal dose" dopamine has been and is used by many physicians for just this purpose. Although low dose dopamine can indeed increase renal and hepatosplanchnic blood flow in healthy volunteers and animal models,[21,22] the situation in the critically ill is less clear. There is no consistent evidence suggesting a beneficial effect of low dose dopamine as a renal or gastrointestinal protective agent. Although some still advocate its use,[23] there is insufficient evidence to support this viewpoint; and the routine use of low dose dopamine for renal protection is not recommended.[24–30]

Although dopamine is generally considered the vasopressor with the most desirable pharmacologic profile, it (as all drugs) has important potential side effects. They include the risk of tachyarrhythmias related to its β effects, a decrease in the release of prolactin with possible risk of immunosuppression,[31,32] and possible redistribution of blood flow within the gut layers resulting in decreased perfusion of the gut mucosa.[33] Some investigators have therefore advocated replacing dopamine with norepinephrine.[34,35]

Norepinephrine is an endogenous catecholamine with potent α-agonist effects, moderate β_1 activity, and minimal β_2 effects. It is therefore a stronger vasoconstrictor than dopamine, and vascular tone is rapidly restored with a resultant rise in blood pressure, although cardiac output is usually maintained especially at lower doses. Despite its potent vasoconstrictive action, deleterious effects on renal function are often not seen, and urine output may even be restored owing to increased renal perfusion pressure.[36,37] Although the role of these agents is still being reviewed and perhaps norepinephrine given early will prove to be beneficial in certain patients with circulatory failure (e.g., septic shock), with the available evidence we currently prefer to reserve norepinephrine for patients who fail to respond to maximum doses of dopamine (20–25 $\mu g/kg/min$).

With any vasopressor the risk of excessive vasoconstriction with a decreased cardiac output remains, and dobutamine is therefore often added to the protocol to increase cardiac output and oxygen delivery (DO_2).[38] Dobutamine is a synthetic catecholamine with predominant β activity but some α activity. It increases myocardial contractility with no increase in mean arterial pressure or heart rate. Dopexamine was developed as an alternative inotropic agent more than a decade ago, but, it is still considered an investigational agent and is commercially available in only a few European countries. It combines β_2-agonist effects with dopaminergic effects: it has minimal β_1 effects and no α-adrenergic activity. The combination of inotropic and vasodilating effects has led to the term "inodilator." It increases cardiac output, due in part to its effects of increasing the heart rate, which limits its use at high doses.[39] With its dopaminergic effects, a potential advantage of dopexamine over dobutamine might lie in its potential to increase hepatosplanchnic blood flow. However, studies have given conflicting results; and although in experimental studies dopexamine appears fairly consistently to improve splanchnic blood flow, effects on gastric intramucosal pH (pHi) are less conclusive, and results from clinical trials are scarce.[40]

Phosphodiesterase inhibitors, (e.g., milrinone, enoximone, amrinone) are also inodilators that act by inhibiting the degradation of cyclic adenosine 3',5'-monophosphate. Their vasodilating effects can, however, result in a fall in blood pressure; and with their long half-life this is a potential problem. Although conceptually phosphodiesterase inhibitors could be useful in combination with strong vasopressors such as norepinephrine,[41] clinically these drugs have little place in the management of acute circulatory failure.

In summary, then, adequate fluid and oxygen administration are vital first steps in the resuscitation of the patients with acute circulatory failure, whatever the cause. To restore perfusion pressure, adrenergic agents may be required. We recommend starting with dopamine and adding norepinephrine if high doses of dopamine fail to have the desired effect. Dobutamine should also be administered to increase cardiac output and oxygen delivery.

"Supranormal DO_2" Debate

The presence of VO_2/DO_2 dependence as discussed above indicates inadequate tissue perfusion, and attempts should be made to increase the DO_2 by manipulating any of its three components: PaO_2, hemoglobin level, or cardiac output. Once PaO_2 reaches physiologic values of 90–100 mmHg, with the oxygen saturation in arterial blood (SaO_2) around 97%, further increases do not significantly increase the DO_2. Increasing hemoglobin levels may not reliably increase DO_2 because cardiac output usually decreases in relation to the increased viscosity; moreover, there may be other risks associated with transfusion, as discussed above. Hence DO_2 is generally increased by increasing the cardiac output.

What is the optimal level of DO_2 for which we should aim? Several studies have supported using aggressive attempts to increase DO_2 to supranormal levels,[42–45] but this approach is a subject of debate and has been challenged by two randomized studies.[46,47] Gattinoni et al.[47] included all patients with an APACHE II score greater than 11, and Hayes et al.[46] included all high risk patients. Studies demonstrating a benefit from this approach used more homogeneous groups, for example, trauma patients,[43,44] or patients with sepsis or acute respiratory distress syndrome (ARDS).[45] In fact, the data from all these studies are compatible. While the overall mortality remained unchanged in the study by Gattinoni et al.,[47] this likely represents a balance between an improved mortality rate in some patients and a worsened outcome in others, as suggested by the data of Hayes et al.[46] It is indeed likely that stable patients do not require additional fluids and vasoactive agents and, indeed, may be harmed by this approach; unnecessary fluid administration carries the risk of worsening pulmonary edema, high doses of adrenergic agents potentially causing tachyarrhythmias, or alteration of blood flow distribution. Therapy in critically ill patients with cardiocirculatory failure therefore must be individually tailored and titrated according to response. We make the following recommendations (Fig. 34.3).

Stable Patients

No further fluids should be administered if the patient is stable and if there is any risk of pulmonary edema; in fact, diuretics

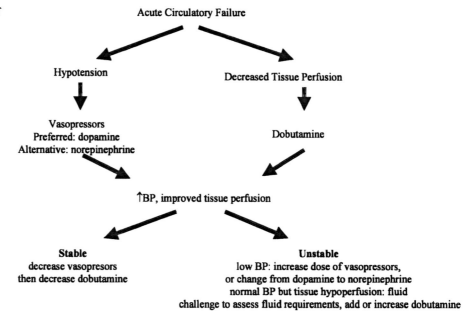

FIGURE 34.3. Basic schema for treatment of patients with acute circulatory failure.

may be administered to stabilized patients with ARDS. No additional vasoactive agents should be given; and in septic patients, who typically have a high cardiac output, no adrenergic agent is required.

Unstable Patients

Rapid correction of the circulatory deficit in unstable patients is required to minimize tissue damage and organ dysfunction. Therapy must be tailored according to the following parameters.

1. *Clinical evaluation*: Blood pressure monitoring alone is insufficient. It must be combined with other markers of tissue perfusion, including urine output, skin turgor, and mental status, although the latter may not be possible in patients prescribed sedative agents.

2. *Hemodynamic parameters*: If a pulmonary artery catheter is in place, mixed venous oxygen saturation (SvO_2) should be monitored and kept above 65%. A fall in SvO_2 indicates an imbalance between VO_2 and DO_2 and is a global indicator of poor oxygenation. It should, however, be considered in conjunction with other parameters, including the cardiac index. The relation between cardiac index and oxygen extraction may provide a useful means of assessing the more complicated patient.[16] Monitoring critically ill patients has been covered in detail in Chapter 25.

3. *Blood lactate*: A normal value is around 1 mEq/l, and values of 2 mEq/l or more can be considered to indicate inadequate tissue oxygenation; unless they are falling rapidly, it is suggested that treatment be altered to improve DO_2. When interpreting blood lactate levels, other possible causes, including decompensated diabetes, extensive malignant tumors, severe malnutrition, persistent shivering or fits, and inherent metabolic deficiencies, must be excluded, but they are rare in the intensive care patient.

Abnormal liver function can prolong the clearance of lactate, thereby slowing the fall in lactate levels with treatment; but it cannot by itself cause hyperlactatemia. During sepsis high lactate levels are probably the result of abnormal cellular metabolism in addition to tissue hypoxia, with decreased pyruvate dehydrogenase activity being suggested as one mechanism.[48] Elevated lactate levels have been associated with a poor prognosis due to various forms of circulatory failure.[2–4,49–51] The trend in lactate levels is of more importance than any individual raised level.[2]

4. *Gastric intramucosal pH (pHi) or PCO_2*: If gastric tonometry is available, the pHi provides useful additional prognostic information.[50] Increasingly, the PCO_2 gap, defined as the difference between gastric PCO_2 ($PgCO_2$) and arterial PCO_2 ($PaCO_2$), is being used as a valuable indicator of the adequacy of regional (gastric) perfusion.[52] Although clinical data are limited, a PCO_2 gap of >6–7 mmHg is currently considered to indicate gastric mucosal hypoperfusion.

If the patient is hypotensive despite fluids, vasopressor support should be given as discussed above. If arterial pressure is acceptable, however, but there is evidence of tissue underperfusion, the situation is less clear. Pouring in fluids is of no benefit if they are having no clear effect; hence the benefits should be assessed by a fluid challenge, which involves monitoring the response to a rapid infusion (500–1000 ml/hr) of small aliquots of fluid. If there is no improvement in oxygenation parameters, no further benefit can be gained with fluids. If some improvement is seen, further challenges should be administered so long as there is no excessive increase in filling pressures.

Dobutamine should also be considered. Again, liberal doses of dobutamine are of no benefit if there is no effect; and in general, doses of 5 μg/kg/min are generally sufficient, although occasionally doses of 10 and even 15 μg/kg/min may be warranted. Despite the downregulation of β-receptors during sepsis, the response is usually evident even in these patients. Adding dobutamine often decreases the need for vasopressor agents, so it may then be possible to reduce the dosage or stop them entirely.

Conclusions

Acute circulatory failure is a key factor in the development of multiple organ failure. Regardless of the initiating factor, its key features are hypotension associated with inadequate tissue perfusion. The basics of resuscitation (i.e., ventilation, infusion, pump) must be respected, with an adequate supply of oxygen, sufficient fluid administration, and appropriate adrenergic support when necessary. Aggressive attempts to improve DO_2 to supranormal levels are not warranted in all critically ill patients. Individualized treatment is preferred, with treatment titrated based on the hemodynamic status and indicators of tissue perfusion. There is some evidence that the mortality rates associated with shock, particularly septic shock, are finally improving.[53] To continue this trend, the physician must be attentive to the risks of acute circulatory failure and act early to restore tissue perfusion and limit the negative effects of prolonged tissue hypoxia. Early treatment shortens the duration of shock, reduces the related organ dysfunction, and hence improves outcome.

References

1. Vincent JL, Preiser JC, Friedman G, et al: Endothelial cell function in the critically ill. In: Reinhart K, Eyrich K, Sprung C (eds) Sepsis: Current Perspectives in Pathophysiology and Therapy. Heidelberg, Springer, 1994;174–180.
2. Vincent JL, Dufaye P, Berre J, et al: Serial lactate determinations during circulatory shock. Crit Care Med 1983;11:449–451.
3. Manikis P, Jankowski S, Zhang H, et al: Correlation of serial blood lactate levels to organ failure and mortality after trauma. Am J Emerg Med 1995;13:619–622.
4. Bakker J, Gris P, Coffernils M, et al: Serial blood lactate levels can predict the development of multiple organ failure following septic shock. Am J Surg 1996;171:221–226.
5. Cain SM, Adams RP: Appearance of excess lactate in anesthetized dogs during anemic and hypoxic hypoxia. Am J Physiol 1965;209:604–608.
6. Bakker J, Vincent JL: The oxygen supply dependency phenomenon is associated with increased blood lactate levels. J Crit Care 1991;6:152–159.
7. Ronco JJ, Fenwick JC, Tweeddale MG, et al: Identification of the critical oxygen delivery for anaerobic metabolism in critically ill septic and nonseptic humans. JAMA 1993;270:1724–1730.
8. Nelson DP, Samsel RW, Wood LD, et al: Pathological supply dependency of systemic and intestinal O_2 uptake during endotoxemia. J Appl Physiol 1988;64:2410–2419.
9. Zhang H, Vincent JL: Oxygen extraction is altered by endotoxin during tamponade-induced stagnant hypoxia in the dog. Circ Shock 1993;40:168–176.
10. Phang PT, Cunningham KF, Ronco JJ, et al: Mathematical coupling explains dependence of oxygen consumption on oxygen delivery in ARDS. Am J Respir Crit Care Med 1994;150:318–323.
11. Vincent JL, De Backer D: Oxygen uptake/oxygen supply dependency: fact or fiction? Acta Anaesthesiol Scand Suppl 1995;107:229–237.
12. Hankeln KB, Gronemeyer R, Held A, et al: Use of continuous noninvasive measurement of oxygen consumption in patients with adult respiratory distress syndrome following shock of various etiologies. Crit Care Med 1991;19:642–649.
13. De Backer D, Moraine JJ, Berre J, et al: Effects of dobutamine on oxygen consumption in septic patients: direct vs indirect determinations. Am Rev Respir Crit Care Med 1994;150:95–100.
14. Vincent JL, Roman A, De Backer D, et al: Oxygen uptake/supply dependency: effects of short-term dobutamine infusion. Am Rev Respir Dis 1990;142:2–8.
15. Kruse JA, Haupt MT, Puri VK, et al: Lactate levels as predictors of the relationship between oxygen delivery and consumption in ARDS. Chest 1990;98:959–962.
16. Silance PG, Simon C, Vincent JL: The relation between cardiac index and oxygen extraction in acutely ill patients. Chest 1994;105:1190–1197.
17. Weil MH, Shubin H: The "VIP" approach to the bedside management of shock. JAMA 1969;207:337–340.
18. Haupt MT, Rackow EC: Colloid osmotic pressure and fluid resuscitation with hetastarch, albumin and saline solutions. Crit Care Med 1982;10:159–163.
19. Hebert PC, Wells G, Blajchman MA, et al: A multicenter, randomized, controlled clinical trial of transfusion requirements in critical care. N Engl J Med 1999;340:409–417.
20. Marik PE, Sibbald WJ: Effect of stored-blood transfusion on oxygen delivery in patients with sepsis. JAMA 1993;269:3024–3029.
21. Bersten AD, Holt AW: Vasoactive drugs and the importance of renal perfusion pressure. New Horiz 1995;3:650–661.
22. Richer M, Robert S, Lebel M: Renal hemodynamics during norepinephrine and low-dose dopamine infusion in man. Crit Care Med 1996;24:1150–1156.
23. Carcoana OV, Hines RL: Is renal dose dopamine protective or therapeutic? Yes. Crit Care Clin 1996;12:677–685.
24. Duke GJ, Bersten AD: Dopamine and renal salvage in the critically ill patient. Anaesth Intensive Care 1992;20:277–287.
25. Thompson BT, Cockrill BA: Renal-dose dopamine: a siren song? Lancet 1994;344:7–8.
26. Maynard ND, Bihari DJ, Dalton RN, et al: Increasing splanchnic blood flow in the critically ill. Chest 1995;108:1648–1654.
27. Olson D, Pohlman A, Hall JB: Administration of low-dose dopamine to nonoliguric patients with sepsis syndrome does not raise gastric intramucosal pH nor improve creatinine clearance. Am J Respir Crit Care Med 1996;154:1664–1670.
28. Cottee DB, Saul WP: Is renal dose dopamine protective or therapeutic? No. Crit Care Clin 1996;12:687–695.
29. Chertow GM, Sayegh MH, Allgren RL, et al: Is the administration of dopamine associated with adverse or favorable outcomes in acute renal failure. Am J Med 1996;101:49–53.
30. Juste RN, Moran L, Hooper J, et al: Dopamine clearance in critically ill patients. Intensive Care Med 1998;24:1217–1220.
31. Devins SS, Miller A, Herndon BL, et al: Effects of dopamine on T-lymphocyte proliferative responses and serum prolactin concentrations in critically ill patients. Crit Care Med 1992;20:1644–1649.
32. Bailey AR, Burchett KR: Effect of low-dose dopamine on serum concentrations of prolactin in critically ill patients. Br J Anaesth 1997;78:97–99.

33. Giraud GD, MacCannell KL: Decreased nutrient blood flow during dopamine and epinephrine induced intestinal vasodilation. J Pharmacol Exp Ther 1984;230:214–220.
34. Martin C, Papazian L, Perrin G, et al: Norepinephrine or dopamine for the treatment of hyperdynamic septic shock? Chest 1993;103:1826–1831.
35. Marik PE, Mohedin J: The contrasting effects of dopamine and norepinephrine on systemic and splanchnic oxygen utilization in hyperdynamic sepsis. JAMA 1994;272:1354–1357.
36. Desjars P, Pinaud M, Bugnon D, et al: Norepinephrine therapy has no deleterious renal effects in human septic shock. Crit Care Med 1989;17:426–429.
37. Marin C, Eon B, Saux P, et al: Renal effects of norepinephrine used to treat septic shock patients. Crit Care Med 1990;18:282–285.
38. Vincent JL, Roman A, Kahn RJ: Dobutamine administration in septic shock: addition to a standard protocol. Crit Care Med 1990;18:689–693.
39. Vincent JL, Reuse C, Kahn RJ: Administration of dopexamine, a new adrenergic agent, in cardiorespiratory failure. Chest 1989;96:1233–1236.
40. Silva E, De Backer D, Creteur J, et al: Effects of vasoactive drugs on gastric intramucosal pH. Crit Care Med 1998;26:1749–1758.
41. De Boelpaepe C, Vincent JL, Contempre B, et al: Combination of norepinephrine and amrinone in the treatment of endotoxin shock. J Crit Care 1989;4:202–207.
42. Shoemaker WC, Appel PL, Kram HB, et al: Prospective trial of supranormal values of survivors as therapeutic goals in high-risk surgical patients. Chest 1988;94:1176–1186.
43. Fleming A, Bishop M, Shoemaker W, et al: Prospective trial of supranormal values as goals of resuscitation in severe trauma. Arch Surg 1992;127:1175–1179.
44. Bishop MH, Shoemaker WC, Appel PL, et al: Prospective, randomized trial of survivor values of cardiac index, oxygen delivery, and oxygen consumption as resuscitation endpoints in severe trauma. J Trauma 1995;38:780–787.
45. Yu M, Burchell S, Hasaniya NWMA, et al: Relationship of mortality to increasing oxygen delivery in patients >50 years of age: a prospective randomized trial. Crit Care Med 1998;26:1011–1019.
46. Hayes MA, Timmins AC, Yau EH, et al: Elevation of systemic oxygen delivery in the treatment of critically ill patients. N Engl J Med 1994;330:1717–1722.
47. Gattinoni L, Brazzi L, Pelosi P, et al: A trial of goal-oriented hemodynamic therapy in critically ill patients. N Engl J Med 1995;333:1025–1032.
48. Vary TC: Sepsis-induced alterations in pyruvate dehydrogenase complex activity in rat skeletal muscle: effects on plasma lactate. Shock 1996;6:89–94.
49. Bakker J, Coffernils M, Leon M, et al: Blood lactate levels are superior to oxygen derived variables in predicting outcome in human septic shock. Chest 1991;99:956–962.
50. Friedman G, Berlot G, Kahn RJ, et al: Combined measurements of blood lactate concentrations and gastric intramucosal pH in patients with severe sepsis. Crit Care Med 1995;23:1184–1193.
51. Marecaux G, Pinsky MR, Dupont E, et al: Blood lactate levels are better prognostic indicators than TNF and IL-6 levels in patients with septic shock. Intensive Care Med 1996;22:404–408.
52. Vincent JL, Creteur J: Gastric mucosal pH (pHi) is definitely obsolete: please tell us more about gastric mucosal PCO_2 ($PgCO_2$). Crit Care Med 1998;26:1479–1481.
53. Friedman G, Vincent JL: Has the mortality of septic shock changed with time? Crit Care Med 1998;26:2078–2086.

35
Effect of Inflammatory Conditions on the Heart

A.B.J. Groeneveld and L.G. Thijs

The heart plays a central role in multiple organ failure associated with inflammatory conditions during the course of sepsis or after cardiac surgery.[1] Although appearing dissimilar at first, the conditions may have in common the generalized inflammatory state and the circulatory (i.e., cardiac) response to it (Fig. 35.1). This chapter describes the epidemiology, pathogenesis, and therapeutic approach to myocardial dysfunction associated with sepsis and cardiopulmonary bypass surgery.

Sepsis

Epidemiology and Diagnosis

Septic shock is a life-threatening condition, particularly during the course of some other illness; it often affects elderly patients, who may have coronary artery disease.[1] The prevalence of myocardial dysfunction during the course of sepsis, which is usually characterized, particularly after fluid loading, by a hyperdynamic circulation with a supranormal cardiac output, is virtually unknown.[1-7] Myocardial dysfunction may occur early or late in the course of sepsis, but it is unclear whether it contributes to outcome independently from other failing organs, even though myocardial dysfunction may be less severe or ameliorate during the course of disease in survivors and may be more severe or deteriorate further in ultimate nonsurvivors of the syndrome.[3,5,6,8-14] In fact, the early outcome of septic shock is determined by the peripheral hemodynamic abnormalities, including systemic hypotension and vasodilation-associated defective global O_2 extraction, rather than by cardiac output; thus hyperdynamic circulation maintained by fluid loading and inotropic agents may hardly improve outcome if hypotension persists.[11,14,15] Cardiac dysfunction may therefore be a marker, rather than a primary mediator, of progression to multiple organ failure and death from septic shock. Nevertheless, cardiac dysfunction could contribute to an adverse outcome, as the peripheral abnormalities may make O_2 uptake more than normally dependent on O_2 delivery.[8,14] Otherwise, both the peripheral and cardiac abnormalities of septic shock may be relatively refractory to the vasoactive agents administered to treat the syndrome.[15,16]

The myocardial dysfunction of septic shock manifests clinically as a relatively flat cardiac function curve so, particularly in patients destined to die, ventricular stroke work is relatively low and filling pressure is high[5,8,13,17,18] (Table 35.1). Hence a subnormal response of stroke work to fluid loading may denote myocardial dysfunction, and this response may be further exacerbated during the course of disease in nonsurvivors and may improve in survivors.[5,13] Because of hypotension and a reduced afterload, stroke volume can still be normal to supranormal. Hence myocardial dysfunction may be relatively difficult to recognize early using conventional hemodynamic measurements unless stroke work, the product of arterial pressure and stroke volume, has been calculated and found to be subnormal for a given filling pressure.[5,8,11,13,18]

The most specific measure of myocardial contractility, the relation between maximal end-systolic pressure and volume (elastance), is also decreased with septic shock and more so in nonsurvivors than in survivors.[12] Volumetric measurements allows us to distinguish preload due to end-diastolic volume from that due to pressure, which may be confounded by compliance changes and thereby less representative of true cardiac preload. Volumetric measurement techniques include nuclear angiography, (transesophageal) echocardiography, or the rapid response thermodilution technique for right ventricular ejection fraction measurements.

Myocardial dysfunction may be characterized by, in addition to decreased elastance, ventricular dilatation, a low ejection fraction, and wall motion abnormalities that can even be segmental, particularly in areas affected by prior coronary artery disease.[2-4,7,9-12,17,19-24] Evaluation of end-diastolic volume allow us to evaluate the stroke work/end-diastolic volume relation (preload-recruitable stroke work), a function that is relatively specific for cardiac contractility; the slope of the relation has been shown to decline during septic shock.[2,17,20,21,23,25] Indeed, endotoxin infusion in healthy volunteers results in a decline in both elastance and preload-recruitable stroke work, even in the presence of an elevated cardiac output; and the absence of severe hypotension suggests that the myocardial dysfunction of sepsis can be an early phenomenon.[17,19,21,23,25]

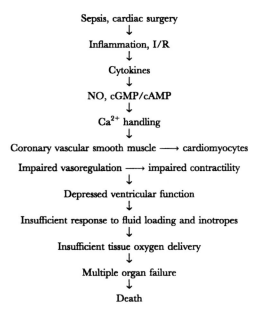

FIGURE 35.1. Common pathways of sepsis and cardiopulmonary bypass surgery in terms of inflammatory and circulatory pathways, myocardial dysfunction, and patient outcome. NO, nitric oxide; cAMP, cyclic adenosine or cGMP, guanosine monophosphate; I/R.

Of note, the ventricular ejection fraction is not load-independent, so even if the left ventricular ejection fraction is normal myocardial dysfunction may occur as a consequence of peripheral vasodilation and a reduced left ventricular afterload.[3,7,9,10] Investigators have documented a subnormal ejection fraction from the beginning of sepsis that improved concomitantly with reversal of hypotension in survivors, indicating reversal of myocardial dysfunction, during the first week of recovery; the low ejection fraction also improved somewhat, concurrently with unrelenting hypotension in nonsurvivors, showing progressive myocardial dysfunction.[3,4,7,9,11]

Hence serial measurements may be helpful for elucidating the severity and course of the myocardial dysfunction of sepsis.[3,4,7,9–11,17] There may be a circulating marker of the myocardial depression of sepsis, (i.e., troponin I), a contractile protein that is more cardiospecific than the creatine kinase MB fraction and is released upon cardiac injury.[26,27]

Many animal models of endotoxemia and sepsis are characterized by a fall in contractility, as determined (via conductance catheters, ultrasonic/piezoelectric crystals, and radionuclide methods) from a fall in the maximal or end-systolic pressure-to-volume/dimension ration (elastance) and in the stroke work-to-end-diastolic volume relation during fluid loading.[6,28–46] Again, these indices are more specific indicators of contractility and less dependent on loading conditions than indices such as the ejection fraction and the rate of pressure development, which have been used to assess the effect of endotoxin on heart function in the past.[6,32,33,36,39,42,47–51] The myocardial dysfunction may be present, irrespective of the phase of shock (i.e., during both hyperdynamic and hypodynamic phases), characterized by a subnormal and supranormal cardiac output, respectively, and during normotensive and hypotensive phases.[32] Indeed, low dose, continuously administered endotoxin or bacteria, fecal inoculation, or cecal ligation and puncture is more likely to induce subacute or chronic sepsis and shock (particularly if accompanied by fluid loading, with a rise in cardiac output, as is usually encountered in humans) than a large intravenous bolus of endotoxin or bacteria in nonresuscitated models; it rapidly results in fatal pulmonary hypertension and hypodynamic arterial hypotension.[28,32,50,52] Both models may be characterized, however, by early myocardial dysfunction, even though it is less severe in chronic models than in acute models; it appears transiently in surviving animals and progressively in the nonsurvivors.[28,29,32–34,50–53] Obviously, the species studied and the type and depth of the anesthesia may also affect the response to bacteria/endotoxin, so increases in myocardial function following endotoxin administration have been reported as well.[48,54–56] Nevertheless, heart muscle removed (even early) from endotoxemic/septic animals may show depressed function during alterations in preload, afterload, or Ca^{2+} perfusate concentration, so compensation mechanisms can mask myocardial depression in vivo.[5,6,31,48,55,57,58]

During the course of septic shock, diastolic dysfunction may concur with systolic dysfunction.[3,4,9,24,28,42,59,60] The cardiac dysfunction during the course of human septic shock may be accompanied, according to some, by a rise in myocardial compliance, leading to ventricular dilatation; this may be viewed as a means to maintain stroke volume in the presence of diminished contractility.[3,4,7,9,20,25,28,60] It also implies that ventricular dilatation is accompanied by a relatively low filling pressure, even though in other patients' dilatation has been reported to be associated with high filling pressures.[4,20,60] Indeed, ventricular filling pressures and volumes, for instance, may hardly correlate.[60] A fall in compliance, particularly at high ventricular end-diastolic volumes, may also be explained by fluid overloading and reduced distensibility at high volumes rather than by sepsis per se.[20,34,59] Conversely, an inability to dilate following impaired ventricular relaxation and decreased compliance, particularly in patients with coronary artery disease, may contribute to a diminished cardiac output reserve,

TABLE 35.1. Clinical Indicators of Global Myocardial Dysfunction In Vivo.

Conventional hemodynamic indices
  Low cardiac output (stroke volume) at high PAOP
  Low left ventricular stroke work–PAOP relation
  Subnormal response of left ventricular stroke work to volume loading for a given rise in filling pressure
  Supranormal decrease in cardiac output upon a rise in arterial blood pressure
  Higher CVP than PAOP in the presence of right ventricular overload

Volumetric indices
  Low ejection fraction and high end-diastolic volume/dimension
  Subnormal response of ventricular stroke work to volume loading for a given rise in end-diastolic volume
  Low end-systolic or maximal pressure–volume relation
  Abnormal diastolic pressure–volume relation (compliance)

PAOP, pulmonary artery occlusive pressure; CVP, central venous pressure.

rendering output more dependent on atrial systole. This sequence may be predominantly encountered in patients with a fatal outcome.[3,9,19,28,59] Similarly, some subacute or chronic animal models of endotoxemia or sepsis may be characterized by a rise (and in nonsurvivors a subsequent fall) in left ventricular compliance.[28,34]

The right ventricle often faces a moderate rise in afterload during septic shock, as moderate pulmonary hypertension is a common feature of the syndrome in animals and humans.[10,11,20,21,30,44,46,60-67] It is often associated with acute lung injury or the adult respiratory distress syndrome (ARDS), a common complication of sepsis and shock. Even in the absence of diminished right ventricular contractility, the rise in right ventricular afterload leads to end-systolic and end-diastolic dilatation, so the ejection fraction declines in an attempt to maintain stroke volume; these phenomena are relatively common during septic shock.[10,11,20,60-62,64,66] Systemic and thus coronary hypotension may impair coronary vasodilation and perfusion of the right ventricle, thereby creating a mismatch between O_2 supply and demand, eliciting right ventricular dysfunction and further dilatation.[61,62] This situation can be surmised clinically on the basis of conventional hemodynamics, by a central venous pressure (CVP) higher than the pulmonary artery occlusion pressure (PAOP), and a greater rise in the former with little or no increase in cardiac output during fluid loading.[20,60,62] A fall in the right ventricular ejection fraction concomitantly with right ventricular dilation and an increased subnormal stroke volume during fluid loading, as judged from measurements with help of the rapid response thermistor thermodilution technique, for instance, indicate right ventricular overloading and herald failure.[20,60] It may also prognosticate a poor outcome.[10,11,63]

Others, however, have decided that dysfunction of the right ventricle was equal to that of the left ventricle during experimental and human septic shock, and that it was relatively independent of increased afterload.[10,20,21] Recognition of right ventricular overloading and failure may have therapeutic consequences, as amelioration of hypotension and an increase in arterial (coronary perfusion) pressure may overcome the vicious cycle of overload, dilatation, and hypoperfusion of the right heart.[63] Multiple factors may play a role in the development of pulmonary hypertension and right heart overload, including endothelial changes with increased endothelin and reduced nitric oxide responses, increased platelet-activating factor (PAF) and thromboxane A_2, reduced prostacyclin release, hypercapnia, and metabolic (lactic) acidosis.[30,35,64,67-70]

Pathogenesis

Several factors may play a role in the development and course of septic myocardial dysfunction (Table 35.2).

Inflammatory Mediators and Negative Inotropic Factors

The myocardial dysfunction of sepsis may relate to multiple circulating factors, factors released from coronary endothelium and affecting underlying heart muscle, factors produced by cardiomyocytes themselves upon circulating stimuli, or combinations (Table 35.3). Indeed, coronary and endocardial endothelium normally regulates the contractility of underlying cardiac myocytes by producing nitric oxide (NO), via constitutive NO synthase (cNOS), or endothelin, a Ca^{2+}-dependent positive inotropic substance.

In the past, various authors have found circulating factors released during the course of several types of experimental and human septic shock, with negative inotropic properties on the heart; mostly these factors have been found in vitro, but the origin and nature of these "myocardial depressant factors" vary from study to study, and their existence has even been seriously doubted.[6,22,71,72] Some authors suggested a splanchnic or pancreatic origin. Some of the factors are dialyzable.[22,71] Serum obtained from septic patients has myocardial depressant actions in vitro, and the substances responsible may be tumor necrosis factor-α (TNFα) and interleukin-1 (IL-1).[73]

Indeed, animal experiments have suggested that endotoxin and cytokines released during sepsis and shock may be partly responsible for the myocardial diastolic and systolic dysfunction via upregulation of inducible NOS (iNOS) in the coronary arteries and cardiomyocytes, as shown in vitro. They may also be responsible for the formation of NO, which activates guanylate cyclase and causes production of cyclic guanosine monophosphate (cGMP), thereby enhancing relaxation and impairing contractility via an effect on sarcoplasmic membrane Ca^{2+} currents, myofilament Ca^{2+} sensitivity, or both.[43,50,58,72-80]

TABLE 35.2. Mechanisms Involved in Myocardial Depression of Sepsis and After Cardiopulmonary Bypass Surgery.

Microcirculatory and myocardial inflammation and edema
Altered coronary vascular reactivity and maldistribution of blood flow
Pulmonary hypertension and right ventricular overload
Postischemic dysfunction (stunning)
Negative inotropic factors
Metabolic abnormalities

TABLE 35.3. Humoral Factors with Positive and Negative Inotropic Properties on the Heart.

Positive inotropic properties
  Endothelin
  β-Adrenergic receptors
  cAMP
  Calcium

Negative inotropic properties
  Activated complement
  Cytokines: TNFα, IL-1β, IL-2, IL-6
  NO, cGMP
  α-ANP
  "Myocardial depressant factor"
  Arachidonic acid metabolites
  Neutrophil products, oxygen free radicals

TNF, tumor necrosis factor; IL, interleukin; NO, nitric oxide; cAMP, cGMP, cyclic adenosine or guanosine monophosphate; ANP, atrial natriuretic peptide.

In fact, circulating end-products of NO are elevated during septic shock, and a portion of these factors may come from the heart.[50] However, the effects of endotoxin on cardiac dysfunction and Ca^{2+} handling may be independent of cytokines, NO, and cGMP.[57] Blockade of NO synthesis by L-arginine analogues in conditions mimicking sepsis may enhance myocardial function in vitro and in vivo, even though the response (mostly observed in vivo) includes a rise in systemic (and pulmonary arterial) blood pressure and a detrimental fall in cardiac output.[43,57,77,80–82] Otherwise, physiologic basal concentrations of NO may be more positive inotropic than negative inotropic,[46,83,84] particularly during β-adrenergic stimulation, Hence L-arginine blockade may be detrimental for cardiac contractility.

Finally, the cytokines and lipids that may be involved in the iNOS upregulation in the heart and impaired cardiac contraction during sepsis include TNFα, IL-1, IL-2, IL-6, and PAF; and the cardiac effects of these substances can mimic those of endotoxin.[39,44,73,75,82,85–88] In fact, anti-TNFα and PAF receptor antagonists may partially prevent the decreased contractility seen with endotoxemia in animals.[39,44,85] The negative inotropic properties of TNFα and PAF may also be mediated in part by released prostaglandins.[86] Finally, activated complement products may activate neutrophils in the coronary circulation, liberate coronary vasoconstricting prostaglandins, and thereby compromise cardiac perfusion and function, although anaphylatoxins may also adversely affect cardiac contractility directly.[89,90] Even though liberated during experimental and human septic shock, the role of complement and prostaglandins in myocardial dysfunction remains incompletely defined.[23,30,35,86,91]

There is also some human evidence that the myocardial dysfunction of septic shock involves cytokine-activate NO in the heart. In fact, circulating end-products of NO are elevated during human septic shock, as in animals.[92] The serum may contain substances that inhibit contraction of rat cardiac myocytes in vitro, and they have been characterized as TNFα and IL-1.[73] Anti-TNFα or methylene blue administration to septic shock patients may inhibit guanylate cyclase, but the cAMP stimulator pentoxifylline, which attenuates neutrophil and macrophage activation, may not increase myocardial function.[23,93,94] Also, L-arginine analogues, used to competitively block iNOS-induced NO synthesis, may hardly ameliorate myocardial dysfunction during sepsis and allied conditions.[81,95] Administration of these drugs during human septic shock, as in experimental conditions, often induces a detrimental decrease in cardiac output associated with a rise in arterial blood pressure and afterload and perhaps inadvertent coronary vasoconstriction, so the left ventricular stroke work–filling pressure relation does not improve.[81,95]

The myocardial dysfunction of sepsis, in animals and humans, may be further characterized by a diminished response to β-adrenergic stimulation. Endotoxin, cytokines, and iNOS may contribute to diminished sensitivity to adrenergic agents via the β-receptor, the inhibitory G-proteins, adenylate cyclase, and cyclic adenosine monophosphate (cAMP) pathways.[6,15,16,18,33,40,76,77,96–99] In some endotoxin experiments, β-adrenergic receptors may be phosphorylated and internalized, thereby decreasing the active number of receptors at the cell surface.[53] Indeed, lymphocytes of patients with septic shock have a downregulated number of β-receptors as well as uncoupling (i.e., a postreceptor defect in signal transduction for cAMP production).[18,100] This may have been caused in part by prior treatment with β-adrenergic agents and may coincide with diminished dobutamine responsiveness of the heart.[16,18] The defects in the postreceptor pathway may be attributed to cGMP stimulation by cytokine-induced NO, induction of inhibitory G-proteins leading to a reduction of adenylate cyclase, reduced cAMP action, or induction of cAMP-cleaving phosphodiesterase.[97,99] In fact, increased concentrations of inhibitory G-proteins have been found in the hearts of patients dying from catecholamine-refractory septic shock.[16]

Circulating α-atrial natriuretic peptide (ANP) concentration may increase during experimental and human septic shock,[64,94,101] probably as a consequence of cardiac dysfunction, dilatation, and increased wall stress. Endothelin may also contribute to its release. Because α-ANP may negatively affect contractility through cGMP formation in the heart,[101] circulating α-ANP not only may serve as a marker but may also be a mediator of the myocardial depression of septic shock. Indeed, infusion of α-ANP antagonists may improve myocardial function in various animal sepsis models.[101] O_2 free radicals released by activated neutrophils have also been implicated in the myocardial dysfunction of sepsis.[31,32,45,102] Neutrophils may become entrapped in the coronary circulation during sepsis; and allied conditions and their activation and extravasation could contribute to coronary and cardiomyocyte alterations.[45]

Finally, the opioid system is activated during experimental endotoxin and human septic shock, which may also contribute to myocardial dysfunction, as infusion of the opioid receptor antagonist naloxone may increase mean arterial pressure at unchanged or even increased cardiac output and thereby stroke work; cardiac filling seems unchanged.[103,104]

Compensatory Factors

Positive inotropic factors may be released during septic shock, possibly including endothelium-derived endothelin.[67,70,92] Circulating endothelin and NO end-products are simultaneously elevated during experimental and human septic shock.[67,69,92] Endothelin release is stimulated by cytokines acting on the endothelium, which may counteract increased NO production.[70] This interaction also occurs in the heart. Hence both endothelin and NO production may increase in the septic heart. The myocardial dysfunction of septic shock therefore must be predominantly affected by negative, rather than positive, inotropic factors. Also, systemic release of endothelin could contribute to pulmonary vasoconstriction, thereby placing a load on the right ventricle.[67,69,70] Finally, sympathetic (baroreceptor) activation during sepsis and shock increases circulating catecholamines, which may have positive chronotropic and inotropic effects, in case some β-adrenergic responsiveness persists.[100,105] Endogenous sympathetic activation may mask septic myocardial dysfunction in vivo.[48,56]

Coronary Insufficiency

Arterial hypotension could lead to coronary hypoperfusion when coronary vasodilation is exhausted. On the other hand, the global workload for the left ventricle decreases during hypotension. Nevertheless, severe hypotension could endanger the O_2 supply to demand balance in the subendocardium of the left ventricle, particularly in the presence of coronary artery disease. In fact, some severely septic and hypotensive patients may have electrocardiographic (ECG) changes suggestive of ischemia.[106] In most cases, however, the myocardial dysfunction of sepsis seems independent of coronary blood flow, which tends to increase, rather than decrease, following inappropriate vasodilation.[31,47,52,54,107-110] In most animal models coronary blood flow and O_2 delivery, even if decreasing, are inappropriately high for the amount of external work performed, which decreases following hypotension; in hypodynamic models there is also decreased cardiac output. Hence myocardial dysfunction seems independent of coronary blood flow.[31,32,38,42,47,52,54,109-111] Nevertheless, the coronary blood flow reserve may diminish.[52,54,112] The global myocardial O_2 extraction is relatively low, and uptake is high for the amount of work performed, so contractile efficiency is low.[32,38,52,107-109,113,114] The latter may be due to cytokines and myofilament insensitivity, but the role of NO is controversial.[80,114,115] Nevertheless, there may be focal decreases in blood flow despite the absence of global hypoperfusion. There may be redistribution of heterogeneous coronary blood flow throughout the heart during endotoxin shock in dogs and pigs, reflecting maladaptation of regional coronary blood flow to regional differences in metabolic demand, with focal over- and underperfusion relative to demand.[38,109] This may also include a steal phenomenon of blood flow from hypoperfused areas to areas with maximal vasodilation. In fact, the endocardial/epicardial blood flow ratio may fall, albeit not in all studies, making the heart vulnerable to subendocardial ischemia.[38,47,109]

Indeed, there is evidence that the vasoregulatory function of endothelial coronary cells is altered in sepsis and allied conditions, whereas vascular smooth muscle function is generally well preserved.[50,116-118] This change may be caused by activated neutrophils, among others, and result in diminished vasoconstrictor and vasodilator responses.[118] Endothelium-dependent, adrenergic receptor- or acetylcholine-mediated vasorelaxation may be impaired.[118] The latter may imply diminished cNOS or increased endothelin, which may be the result of circulating activated complement or cytokines.[86,89,90] Other authors have noted that after endotoxin/septic challenge the coronary artery may have upregulated NOS, thereby producing excess amounts of vasorelaxing NO. The NO, in turn, may decrease vasoconstrictor tone and increase pressure dependence of the coronary blood flow.[50,113,116,117,119] Inhibition with L-arginine analogues may then ameliorate the increase in coronary blood flow during endotoxemia and attenuate impaired autoregulation, but they may also induce focal ischemia owing to local vasoconstriction.[57,113,117] The metabolic (auto) regulation of coronary vascular tone and blood flow during changes in blood O_2 content or myocardial workload and O_2 demand seems less than normal, but this theory is not supported by other studies, which have shown that the rise in coronary blood flow during endotoxemia or sepsis was appropriate for the rise in metabolic demand and O_2 uptake, and it changed in parallel with the changing workload.[36,52,54,110,112,119-121]

There is usually no indication of globally diminished aerobic energy production, an inhibited tricarboxylic acid cycle, and the resultant lactate production in the septic heart of animals or humans,[36,38,54,57,107-109,111,120] even though a fall in lactate extraction may not exclude focal hypoperfusion.[108,109] The global concentrations of substrates and energy-rich substances usually remain unchanged, although others have reported decreases in energy stores.[31,33,36,47,54,56,57,108,110,111] In fact, NO may inhibit mitochondrial respiration, which may contribute to impaired contractility and decreased energy levels.[80,114,115,122]

Ischemia/Reperfusion

Sepsis, endotoxemia, or cytokinemia may, like a prior episode of hypoperfusion (preconditioning), partially protect the heart from ischemia/reperfusion (I/R) injury and postischemic dysfunction (stunning).[49,123,124] Conversely, prior I/R or endotoxin increases the resistance of the heart to a subsequent endotoxin challenge.[125] Preconditioning is probably mediated by induction of heat shock proteins and protective enzymes such as antioxidants.[125,126] Adenosine release probably plays a central role in this preconditioning, and some authors have indeed shown that adenosine can mimic preconditioning and protect the heart from the harmful effect of endotoxin or I/R and the resultant TNFα expression.[124,127]

Intrinsic Changes in the Myocardial Structure

Myocardial edema, whether interstitial or intracellular, may be associated with capillary compression and cell damage, respectively; and changes in sarcolemnal and mitochondrial membrane structures have been noted after endotoxin shock in some studies. These changes have been attributed in part to activated neutrophils and O_2 radicals[6,34,36,45,47,58,74,111] The role of these alterations in the development of myocardial dysfunction and stiffness is unclear.[34,36,47,49,51] Membrane changes may include phosphorylation and altered Ca^{2+} handling and ATPase activity.[53,74,79,128]

Alterations in External Milieu

Metabolic (lactic) acidosis may have a negative inotropic effect on the heart,[68] but alkali therapy may not ameliorate dysfunction of the ischemic heart.[129] Elevated insulin and glucagon levels may have inotropic effects as well.[47,55] Finally, hypocalcemia and hypophosphatemia may impair, and correction may improve, the hemodynamic stability of septic shock patients.[130]

Potential Therapeutic Implications

The standard treatment of sepsis and shock is still aimed at maintaining a "compensated hyperdynamic circulation"[14] —characterized by a high cardiac output and absence of hypotension—until the infection has been eradicated and the circulatory abnormalities have abated. It is accomplished by infusion of fluids and administration of inotropic and vasopressor drugs.

Glucocorticoids, among their other actions, depress TNFα, endothelin, and iNOS expression and thus NO synthesis in the heart; they could thereby increase contractility, as shown in many in vitro experiments.[76,114] Nevertheless, their use for treatment of sepsis and shock has been abandoned, as multicenter studies did not show a benefit of such treatment.[131] Other substances that aim at reducing the inflammatory response are the immunomodulators such as anti-TNF, soluble TNF receptors, IL-1 receptor antagonist, PAF antagonists, prostaglandin synthesis inhibitors, and the phosphodiesterase inhibitor and cAMP stimulator pentoxifylline, which attenuates neutrophil and macrophage activation. Most of these substances have generally failed to decrease cardiac alterations, morbidity and mortality due to sepsis,[23,131,132] even if they were successful in experimental animal models of sepsis, ameliorating, among other problems, myocardial dysfunction.[39,44,87,127] Anti-TNFα administration to septic shock patients may increase myocardial function, however.[93] Relative unresponsiveness to β-adrenergic agents may be circumvented by treatment with cAMP-enhancing phosphodiesterase inhibitors; amrinone, for instance, has been shown to ameliorate the fall in end-systolic elastance in canine endotoxin shock.[42,88] Rapid infusion of insulin may, particularly when combined with hypertonic glucose and potassium, transiently increase myocardial contractile indices during experimental endotoxin administration and clinical septic shock.[47,55]

L-Arginine analogues, used to competitively block iNOS-induced NO synthesis,[43,81,82,95] may increase blood pressure during experimental and human septic shock. However, it may be accompanied by a detrimental fall in cardiac output, with myocardial dysfunction hardly ameliorated, possibly as a consequence of coronary vasoconstriction or right ventricular overload following pulmonary vasoconstriction.[43,81,95] The left ventricular stroke work—filling (pressure) relation may not improve.[81,82,95] However, methylene blue to inhibit guanylate cyclase may be used as an adjuvant treatment and may increase myocardial function.[94] Inhalation of NO may ameliorate right ventricular overload via selective pulmonary vasodilation.[133] Inhibitors or receptor blockers of endogenous vasoconstrictors such as endothelin are being evaluated experimentally.[67] Blockade of endothelin receptors and cyclooxygenase and lipoxygenase inhibitors may ameliorate pulmonary hypertension and right heart overload during bacteremia and endotoxemia, but the effects on left ventricular dysfunction are controversial.[30,35,67,70,91] The merits of these interventions in terms of decreasing morbidity and mortality remain largely unknown.[70,81,94]

A new approach involves renal replacement techniques, such as continuous arterio/venovenous hemofiltration/dialysis (CAVH, CAVHD, CVVH), whereby relatively large volumes of plasma water can be exchanged for saline via filters with pore sizes of 30–50 kDa.[37,41,134–140] Particularly large ultrafiltration volumes may help remove "toxic substances" from the circulation in septic patients needing such treatment for other reasons, including renal failure and fluid overload.[37,134,138] Indeed, use of high volume filtration or large pore sizes (100 kDa) may improve cardiac function during endotoxemia/bacteremia in animals. The plasma ultrafiltrate from endotoxemic pigs depresses myocardial function in normal pigs, but the effect on survival in these models remains controversial.[37,41,134,139] Hemofiltration in animals and humans has been shown to filter from plasma the activated complement products (anaphylatoxins), PAF, "myocardial depressant factor," and other small molecular mediators that may adversely affect the circulation. However, effective removal from plasma of large molecular TNFα, interleukins, prostaglandins, and adhesion molecules remains controversial.[22,135–138] The relative importance of clearance and membrane absorption is controversial as well.[137,138,140] Finally, the technique may remove circulating antiinflammatory substances, but the artificial kidney membrane itself may induce a local inflammatory response.[140] The techniques have not yet been proven to decrease morbidity and mortality during treatment of septic shock in patients, although anecdotal data suggest more rapid reversal from shock when applied early, even in the absence of overt acute renal failure.

A rise in right ventricular afterload and resultant dysfunction can be alleviated by selective pulmonary vasodilation, as afforded by vasodilating NO inhalation for the treatment of severe ARDS in mechanically ventilated patients.[65] There is even some experimental evidence that it may ameliorate left ventricular dysfunction as well.[46] Alternatively, various intravenous vasodilators have been evaluated, carrying the disadvantage of spillover into the systemic circulation and inadvertent vasodilation, as well as worsening of ventilation and perfusion matching in the lung with resultant hypoxemia.[61] Finally, a rise in the systemic blood pressure with vasoconstrictors, rather than administration of positive inotropic drugs, may ameliorate coronary hypoperfusion, thereby forcing the right ventricle to cope with an increased afterload.[62]

Antioxidants could be used to ameliorate oxidative damage of the heart. *N*-Acetylcysteine (NAC) and L-2-oxothiazolidine-4-carboxylic acid replete the endogenous antioxidant glutathione. They are safe drugs that may increase myocardial function in experimental septic shock, but their (cardiac) effects in human septic shock are still controversial.[102,141,142] Indeed, antioxidants such as NAC may also potentiate NO and sometimes aggravate, rather than ameliorate, myocardial dysfunction.[143]

Postcardiac Surgery

Epidemiology and Diagnosis

Although most patients exhibit an uneventful course after coronary artery bypass grafting (CABG) or valve replacement involving hypothermic cardioplegia and cardiopulmonary bypass (CPB), some patients have postoperative (segmental) myocardial dysfunction at the time of recovery and admittance to the intensive care unit (ICU).[4,8,144–152] It may be only partly related to underlying heart disease and might relate to the surgical procedure itself. For instance, the risk might increase with prolonged bypass and ischemia times.[148,149,153] Myocardial dysfunction may manifest as hypotension and a low cardiac output "syndrome" in the ICU. In fact, some patients, particularly when elderly, need inotropic or vasopressor support (or both) to maintain arterial blood pressure after surgery.[147,151] The need and intensity of such therapy is associated with multiple organ failure, a long stay in the ICU, and ultimate death.[148,153,154] Nevertheless, cardiac dysfunction after cardiac surgery involving cardioplegic arrest and CPB can be reversed in part within 48 hours after surgery in most patients. Primary myocardial dysfunction should be differentiated from a pericardial tamponade due to postoperative bleeding and a postoperative myocardial infarction, which may rarely complicate the postoperative course.[148,155,156] The postoperative course of creatine kinase-myocardial band (CK-MB) plasma levels does not accurately distinguish patients having myocardial infarction after surgery from the large group without myocardial injury; serial determinations of troponin I may be helpful in this respect, particularly (as is often the case), when the ECG is inconclusive.[26,27,155,156]

Techniques such as transesophageal echocardiography and the right ventricular ejection fraction catheter (or implanted ultrasonic crystals) enable more precise evaluation of heart function than conventional tests of hemodynamics.[144,145,157,158] In fact, volumetric assessments allow estimates of end-systolic and maximal elastances, preload-recruitable stroke work, and diastolic compliance, which show a decline directly after otherwise uneventful coronary artery surgery involving bypass, in children and adults.[145,157,159] The left and right ventricles may be involved. Right coronary artery disease and pulmonary hypertension, aggravated by surgery for malfunctioning valves or congenital malformations, may contribute to predominantly right ventricular dysfunction after surgery.[144,145,158]

Pathogenesis

Ischemia/Reperfusion

After surgery the heart resumes its function, the extracorporeal circuit is disconnected, and the patient is rewarmed. Hence CPB-involving cardiac surgery is associated with I/R, particularly of the heart. Cardiac dysfunction after cardiac surgery involving cardioplegic arrest and CPB has been attributed in part to transient postischemic dysfunction (i.e., myocardial stunning), affecting both ventricles.[150] During CPB and cardioplegic cardiac arrest, hypothermia can be applied to minimize the damaging effect of hypoperfusion. However, "cold" cardioplegia may not dramatically help prevent cardiac dysfunction after cardiac surgery.[158,160] Particularly "cold," rather than "warm," cardioplegia and CPB may impose oxidative stress on the heart, but it may not affect postoperative heart function.[160]

The direct effect of I/R and the liberated cascades may modulate cardiac functional recovery.[161] I/R, among its effects, increases O_2 radical formation, TNFα, and iNOS expression, which may contribute to post-I/R tissue injury and dysfunction.[127] Other mediators include activated complement, IL-2, IL-6, and IL-8, which may help recruit and activate neutrophils for removal of damaged tissue. Inflammation evoked by I/R may contribute, together with alterations in Ca^{2+} handling, to postischemic myocardial dysfunction (stunning) and ultimate residual dysfunction.[150] The processes of necrosis, apoptosis, and survival after ischemic lesions are also controlled by the inflammatory process evoked by I/R. Finally, coronary vascular reactivity is transiently altered after CPB-associated I/R,[162] which may be associated with O_2 radical-mediated endothelial injury and relate to defects in adrenergic signaling.

On the one hand, NO may ameliorate postischemic stunning by promoting coronary relaxation and inhibiting neutrophil aggregation. There is experimental evidence for reduced NO after I/R and a beneficial effect of NO donation during reperfusion after cardioplegic/ischemic arrest, associated with less neutrophil-endothelium interactions.[16,163,164] On the other hand, NO may also potentiate, via a reaction with reactive O_2 species, the formation of cytotoxic hydroxyl peroxynitrite, thereby inhibiting mitochondrial respiration and aggravating post-I/R dysfunction and injury.[122,123,164,165] Hypoxia/reoxygenation during CPB in pigs resulted in increased myocardial NO production, injury, and diminished contractility; the reaction was attenuated by NO inhibition or O_2 radical scavengers, indicating that NO contributed to harmful peroxynitrite and hydroxyl ion production and stunning during reoxygenation.[123,164] Although a brief episode of hypoperfusion may precondition the heart to better tolerate a second episode of hypoperfusion, ischemic preconditioning prior to cardiac surgery (slightly hypothermic) with bypass in human did not have such a protective effect and even injured the heart.[126] In contrast, mimicking the effect of preconditioning by adding adenosine to the cardioplegic solution may have a protective effect. The human allograft heart may exhibit increased iNOS expression, which may contribute to diminished contractile function after heart transplantation.[98]

Inflammatory Mediators

Cardiopulmonary bypass may incur a systemic inflammatory host response that involves the systemic release of activated complement, cytokines, and other substances and may be a function of time spent on the bypass.[146,147,161,165,167] Part of the circulating inflammatory response may originate from the heart itself, (i.e., from coronary and endocardial endothelium).[166] Release of mediators may lead to activated neutrophil–endothelial interaction, in remote organs and in the heart.[161,165,167] Circulating NO derivation products are somewhat elevated after cardiac surgery involving CPB, and increased vessel wall NO production may be associated in part with vasodilation.[168,169] Endothelin may also be released, but not to the levels encountered during sepsis.[69,166,169] Endothelin may contribute to postoperative pulmonary hypertension, particularly in children operated for congenital heart disease.[166,169,170] Some circulating inflammatory mediators may correlate with cardiac dysfunction after CPB surgery, suggesting that these mediators, including activated complement products and TNFα have an adverse effect on the coronary circulation and cardiomyocyte function, with impaired coronary reactivity and myocardial stunning after CPB surgery, respectively.[146,147,161,166] It is also believed that part of the inflammatory response is induced by translocating endotoxin and bacteria that bypass the liver as a consequence of bypass-associated gut hypoperfusion and increased epithelial permeability.[147,149,166,168,171]

There is some evidence that β-adrenergic receptors and cAMP-dependent secondary signaling systems are inhibited during and after cardiac surgery involving CPB, so the contractile response to β-adrenergic stimulation is subnormal, but this hypothesis is controversial.[172,173] Cardiac surgery involving cardioplegia and CPB may also evoke myocardial edema, but its role in postoperative heart dysfunction is unclear.[174] Increasing contractility by dobutamine may facilitate resolution of edema postoperatively.[174]

Therapeutic Implications

The mainstay of treatment for post-CPB cardiac dysfunction is to rule out reversible (ischemic) abnormalities amenable to treatment and to support the circulation with a judicious fluid regimen and continuous infusion of vasoactive and inotropic drugs. The latter may include phosphodiesterase inhibitors, which may bypass the β-adrenergic system and thereby increase contractility more than β-adrenergic agonists can in the case of β-receptor downregulation or uncoupling.[152]

It has been surmised that hemofiltration techniques in patients after cardiac bypass surgery could remove circulating inflammatory and negative inotropic substances in addition to ameliorating fluid overload and pulmonary and cardiac edema. They would thereby exert a positive effect on the heart and circulation, attenuating "low cardiac output" hypotension.[159,166,169,175,176] In some series decreased pulmonary hypertension, increased myocardial systolic and diastolic function, and decreased morbidity and mortality have been reported with this procedure, particularly in children after surgery for congenital heart disease complicated by pulmonary hypertension.[159,169,175,176] Hemofiltration techniques have also been started during surgery for, among other reasons, adjustment of fluid balance.[169] Nevertheless, the nature and extent of removed substances in the blood remains unclear but may include prostaglandins and endothelin.[166,169] There are few controlled clinical trials.[169]

Other substances that have been evaluated include corticosteroids, pentoxifylline, antiendotoxin, antioxidants, selective gut decontamination, heparin-coated tubing, and pumps. These agents have also been claimed to reduce, to varying degrees, the systemic inflammatory response, hemodynamic instability, and morbidity after CBP surgery.[166,167,177] These measures have generally failed to decrease the mortality rate.[166,167,177]

Treatment of pulmonary hypertension and right ventricular overload, particularly that occurring after surgery for congenital heart disease or valve replacement, can be accomplished by inhaling NO as a selective pulmonary vasodilator. The effect on morbidity, and mortality, however, remains unclear.[178] L-Arginine or endothelin receptor blockers are also being evaluated.[166,170]

Conclusions

During the course of sepsis and after cardiopulmonary bypass surgery, the systemic inflammatory host response may adversely affect cardiac function. Although based on multiple factors, cardiac depression may increase morbidity and mortality. Adjunctive measures to improve myocardial function, in addition to standard fluid loading and the use of inotropes to maintain tissue O_2 delivery, are being explored.

References

1. Groeneveld ABJ, Schneider AJ, Thijs LG: Cardiac alterations in septic shock: pathophysiology, diagnosis, prognostic and therapeutic implications. In: Vincent J-L (ed) Update in Intensive Care and Emergency Medicine, vol 14. Berlin, Springer, 1991; 126–136.
2. Calvin JE, Driedger AA, Sibbald WJ: An assessment of myocardial function in human sepsis utilizing ECG gated cardiac scintigraphy. Chest 1981;80:579–586.
3. Parker MM, Shelhamer JH, Bacharach SL: Profound but reversible myocardial depression in patients with septic shock. Ann Intern Med 1984;100:483–490.
4. Ellrodt AG, Riedinger MS, Kimchi A, et al: Left ventricular performance in septic shock: reversible segmental and global abnormalities. Am Heart J 1985;110:402–409.
5. Rackow EC, Kaufman BS, Falk JL, Astiz ME, Weil MH: Hemodynamic response to fluid repletion in patients with septic shock: evidence for early depression of cardiac performance. Circ Shock 1987;22:11–22.
6. Abel FL: Myocardial function in sepsis and endotoxin shock. Am J Physiol 1990;257:R1265–R1281.
7. Jardin F, Brun-Ney D, Auvert B, Beauchet A, Bourdarias P: Sepsis-related cardiogenic shock. Crit Care Med 1990;18:1055–1060.
8. Weisel RD, Vito D, Dennis RC, Valeri CR, Hechtman HB: Myocardial depression during sepsis. Am J Surg 1977;133:512–521.
9. Parker MM, Suffredini AF, Natanson C, Ognibene FP, Shelhamer JH, Parrillo JE: Responses of left ventricular function in survivors and nonsurvivors of septic shock. J Crit Care 1989;4:19–25.

10. Parker MM, McCarthy KE, Ognibene FP, Parrillo JE: Right ventricular dysfunction and dilatation, similar to left ventricular changes, characterize the cardiac depression of septic shock in humans. Chest 1990;97:126–131.
11. Vincent J-L, Gris P, Coffernils M, Leon M, Pinsky M, Reuse C, Kahn RJ: Myocardial depression characterizes the fatal course of septic shock. Surgery 1992;111:660–667.
12. Parker MM, Ognibene FP, Parrillo JE: Peak systolic pressure/end-systolic volume ratio, a load-independent measure of ventricular function, is reversibly decreased in human septic shock. Crit Care Med 1994;22:1955–1959.
13. Metrangolo L, Fiorillo M, Friedman G, et al: Early hemodynamic course of septic shock. Crit Care Med 1995;23:1971–1975.
14. Hayes MA, Timmins AC, Yau EHS, Palazzo M, Watson D, Hinds CJ: Oxygen transport patterns in patients with sepsis syndrome or septic shock: influence of treatment and relationship to outcome. Crit Care Med 1997;25:926–936.
15. Groeneveld ABJ, Bronsveld W, Thijs LG: Hemodynamic determinants of mortality in human septic shock. Surgery 1986;99:140–152.
16. Böhm M, Kirchmayer R, Gierschik P, Erdmann E: Increase of myocardial inhibitory G-proteins in catecholamine-refractory septic shock or in septic multiorgan failure. Am J Med 1995;98:183–186.
17. Ognibene FP, Parker MM, Natanson C, Shelhamer JH, Parrillo JE: Depressed left ventricular performance: response to volume infusion in patients with sepsis and septic shock. Chest 1988;93:903–910.
18. Silverman HJ, Penaranda R, Orens JB, Lee NH: Impaired β-adrenergic receptor stimulation of cyclic adenosine monophosphate in human septic shock: association with myocardial hyporesponsiveness to catecholamines. Crit Care Med 1993;21:31–39.
19. Raper RF, Sibbald WJ: The effect of coronary artery disease on cardiac function in nonhypotensive sepsis. Chest 1988;94:507–511.
20. Schneider AJ, Teule GJJ, Groeneveld ABJ, Nauta JJP, Heidendal GAK, Thijs LG: Biventricular performance during volume loading in patients with early septic shock, with emphasis on the right ventricle: a combined hemodynamic and radionuclide study. Am Heart J 1988;116:103–112.
21. Raper R, Sibbald WJ, Driedger AA, Gerow K: Relative myocardial depression in normotensive sepsis. J Crit Care 1989;4:9–18.
22. Reilly JM, Cunnion RE, Burch-Whitman C, Parker MM, Shelhamer JH, Parrillo JE: A circulating myocardial depressant substance is associated with cardiac dysfunction and peripheral hypoperfusion (lactic acidemia) in patients with septic shock. Chest 1989;95:1072–1080.
23. Martich GD, Parker MM, Cunnion RE, Suffredini AF: Effects of ibuprofen and pentoxifylline on the cardiovascular response of normal humans to endotoxin. J Appl Physiol 1992;73:925–931.
24. Poelaert J, Declerck C, Vogelaers D, Colardyn F, Visser CA: Left ventricular systolic and diastolic funciton in septic shock. Intensive Care Med 19997;23:553–560.
25. Suffredini AF, Fromm RE, Parker MM, et al: The cardiovascular response of normal humans to the administration of endotoxin. N Engl J Med 1989;321:280–287.
26. Kollef MH, Ladenson JH, Eisenberg PR: Clinically recognized cardiac dysfunction: an independent determinant of mortality among critically ill patients: is there a role for serial measurements of cardiac troponin I? Chest 1997;111:1340–1347.
27. Noble JS, Reid AM, Jordan LVM, Glen ACA, Davidson JAH: Troponin I and myocardial injury in the ICU. Br J Anaesth 1999;82:41–16.
28. Natanson C, Danner RL, Fink MP, et al: Cardiovascular performance with E. coli challenges in a canine model of human sepsis. Am J Physiol 1988;254:H558–H569.
29. Pasque MK, Van Trigt P, Pellom GL, Freedman BM, Wechsler AS: Assessment of the intrinsic contract status of the heart during sepsis by myocardial pressure-dimension analysis. Ann Surg 1988;208:110–117.
30. Schützer K-M, Haglund U, Falk A: Cardiopulmonary dysfunction in a feline septic shock model: possible role of leukotrienes. Circ Shock 1989;29:13–25.
31. Adams HR, Parker JL, Laughlin MH: Intrinsic myocardial dysfunction during endotoxemia: dependent or independent of myocardial ischemia? Circ Shock 1990;30:63–76.
32. Goldfarb RD, Lee KJ, Andrejuk T, Dziuban SW: End-systolic elastance as an evaluation of myocardial function in shock. Circ Shock 1990;30:15–26.
33. Raymond RM: When does the heart fail during shock? Circ Shock 1990;30:27–41.
34. Stahl TJ, Alden PB, Ring WS, Madoff RC, Cerra FB: Sepsis-induced diastolic dysfunction in chronic canine peritonitis. Am J Physiol 1990;258:H625–H633.
35. Fujioka K, Sugi K, Isago T, et al: Thromboxane synthase inhibition and cardiopulmonary function during endotoxemia in sheep. J Appl Physiol 1991;71:1376–1381.
36. Solomon MA, Correa R, Alexander HR, et al: Myocardial energy metabolism and morphology in a canine model of sepsis. Am J Physiol 1994;266:H757–H768.
37. Freeman BD, Yatsiv I, Natanson C, et al: Continuous arteriovenous hemofiltration does not improve survival in a canine model of septic shock. J Am Coll Surg 1995;180:286–292.
38. Herbertson MJ, Werner HA, Russell JA, Iversen K, Walley KR: Myocardial oxygen extraction ratio is decreased during endotoxemia in pigs. J Appl Physiol 1995;79:479–486.
39. Herbertson MJ, Werner HA, Goddard CM, et al: Anti-tumor necrosis factor-α prevents decreased ventricular contractility in endotoxemic pigs. Am J Respir Crit Care Med 1995;152:480–488.
40. Karzai W, Reilly JM, Hoffman WD, Cunnion RE, Danner RL, Natanson C: Hemodynamic effects of dopamine, norepinephrine, and fluids in a dog model of sepsis. Am J Physiol 1995;268:H692–H702.
41. Mink SN, Wang R, Yang J, Jacobs H, Light RB: Effect of continuous arteriovenous hemofiltration combined with systemic vasopressor therapy on depressed left ventricular contractility and tissue oxygen delivery in canine Escherichia coli sepsis. Anesthesiology 1995;83:178–190.
42. Werner HA, Herbertson MJ, Walley KR: Amrinone increases ventricular contractility and diastolic compliance in endotoxemia. Am J Respir Crit Care Med 1995;152:496–503.
43. Herbertson MJ, Werner HA, Walley KR: Nitric oxide synthase inhibition partially prevents decreased contractility during endotoxemia. Am J Physiol 1996;270:H1979–H1984.
44. Herbertson MJ, Werner HA, Walley KR: Platelet-activating factor antagonism improves ventricular contractility in endotoxemia. Crit Care Med 1997;25:221–226.
45. Granton JT, Goddard CM, Allard MF, Van Eeden S, Walley KR: Leukocytes and decreased left-ventricular contractility

during endotoxemia in rabbits. Am J Respir Crit Care Med 1997;155:1977–1983.
46. Ishihara S, Ward JA, Tasaki O, et al: Inhaled nitric oxide prevents left ventricular impairment during endotoxemia. J Appl Physiol 1998;85:2018–2024.
47. Bronsveld W, Van Lambalgen AA, Van Velzen D, Van den Bos GC, Koopman PAR, Thijs LG: Myocardial metabolic and morphometric changes during canine endotoxin shock before and after glucose-insulin-potassium. Cardiovasc Res 1985;19:455–464.
48. Kober PM, Thomas JX, Raymond RM: Increased myocardial contractility during endotoxin shock in dogs. Am J Physiol 1985;249:H715–H722.
49. Piper RD, Yan Li F, Lee Myers M, Sibbald WJ: Structure-function relationships in the septic rat heart. Am J Respir Crit Care Med 1997;156:1473–1482.
50. Forfia PR, Zhang X, Ochoa F, et al: Relationship between plasma NOx and cardiac and vascular dysfunction after LPS injection in anesthetized dogs. Am J Physiol 1998:274:H193–H201.
51. Zhou M, Wang P, Chaudry IH: Cardiac contractility and structure are not significantly compromised even during the later, hypodynamic stage of sepsis. Shock 1998;9:352–358.
52. Bloos FM, Morisaki HM, Neal AM, Martin CM, Ellis CG, Sibbald WJ: Sepsis depresses the metabolic oxygen reserve of the coronary circulation in mature sheep. Am J Respir Crit Care Med 1996;153:1577–1584.
53. Tang C, Yang J, Wu L-L, Dong L-W, Liu M-S: Phosphorylation of beta-adrenergic receptor leads to its redistribution in rat heart during sepsis. Am J Physiol 1998;274:R1078–1086.
54. Rumsey WL, Kilpatrick L, Wilson DF, Erecinska M: Myocardial metabolism and coronary flow: effects of endotoxemia. Am J Physiol 1988;255:H1295–H1304.
55. Law WR, McLane MP, Raymond RM: Insulin and β adrenergic effects during endotoxin shock: in vivo myocardial interactions. Cardiovasc Res 1990;24:72–80.
56. Pawlush DG, Musch TI, Bannar SM, Martin LF: Cardiac dysfunction in a rat model of chronic bacteremia. Circ Shock 1990;31:269–279.
57. Decking UKM, Flesche CCW, Godecke A, Schrader J: Endotoxin-induced contractile dysfunction in guinea pig hearts is not mediated by nitric oxide. Am J Physiol 1995;268:H2460–H2465.
58. Rigby SL, Hofmann PA, Zhong J, Adams HR, Rubin LJ: Endotoxemia-induced myocardial dysfunction is not associated with changes in myofilament Ca^{2+} responsiveness. Am J Physiol 1998;274:H580–H590.
59. Munt B, Jue J, Gin K, Fenwick J, Tweeddale M: Diastolic filling in human severe sepsis: an echocardiographic study. Crit Care Med 1998;26:1829–1833.
60. Dhainaut J-F, Pinsky MR, Nouria S, Slomka F, Brunet F: Right ventricular function in human sepsis: a thermodilution study. Chest 1997;112:1043–1049.
61. Schneider AJ, Teule GJJ, Kester ADM, et al: Effects of vasodilators prostaglandin E_1 and methylprednisolone on pulmonary hypertension and right ventricular performance during volume loading in porcine septic shock: a combined invasive and radionuclide study. Circ Shock 1987;22:141–154.
62. Schneider AJ, Groeneveld ABJ, Teule GJJ, Nauta J, Heidendal GAK, Thijs LG: Volume expansion, dobutamine, and noradrenaline for treatment of right ventricular dysfunction in porcine septic shock: a combined invasive and radionuclide study. Circ Shock 1987;23:93–106.
63. Schreuder WO, Schneider AJ, Groeneveld ABJ, Thijs LG: The effect of dopamine versus noradrenaline on hemodynamics in septic shock, with emphasis on right ventricular function. Chest 1989;95:1282–1288.
64. Redl G, Woodson L, Traber LD, et al: Mechanism of immuno-reactive atrial natriuretic factor release in an ovine model of endotoxemia. Circ Shock 1992;38:34–41.
65. Uchida T, Ichikawa K, Yokoyama K, Mitaka C, Toyooka H, Amaha K: Inhaled nitric oxide improved the outcome of severe right ventricular failure caused by lipopolysaccharide administration. Intensive Care Med 1996;22:1203–1206.
66. D'Orio V, Lambermont B, Detry O, et al: Pulmonary impedance and right ventricular-vascular coupling in endotoxin shock. Cardiovasc Res 1998;38:375–382.
67. Wanecek M, Rudehill A, Hemsén A, Lundberg JM, Weitzberg E: The endothelin receptor antagonist, bosentan, in combination with the cyclooxygenase inhibitor, diclofenac, counteracts pulmonary hypertension in porcine endotoxin shock. Crit Care Med 1998;25:848–857.
68. Teplinsky K, O'Toole M, Olman M, Walley KR, Wood LDH: Effect of lactic acidosis on canine hemodynamics and left ventricular function. Am J Physiol 1990;258:H1193–H1199.
69. Pittet J-F, Morel DR, Hemsén A, et al: Elevated plasma endothelin-1 concentrations are associated with the severity of illness in patients with sepsis. Ann Surg 1991;213:261–264.
70. Battistini B, Forget M-A, Leight D: Potential roles for endothelins in systemic inflammatory response syndrome with a particular relationship to cytokines. Shock 1996;5:167–183.
71. Bessayag C, Christeff N, Auclair M-C, et al: Early released lipid-soluble cardiodepressant factor and activated oestrogenic substances in human septic shock. Eur J Clin Invest 1984;14:288–294.
72. Hallström S, Koidl B, Müller U, Werdan K, Schlag G: A cardiodepressant factor isolated from blood blocks Ca^{2+} current in cardiomyocytes. Am J Physiol 1991;260:H869–H876.
73. Kumar A, Thota V, Deel L, Olson J, Uretz E, Parrillo JE: Tumor necrosis factor-α and interleukin 1β are responsible for in vitro myocardial depression induced by human septic shock serum. J Exp Med 1996;183:949–957.
74. Mohammed FI, Liu M-S: Impairment in the phosphorylation of canine cardiac sarcoplasmatic reticulum following endotoxin administration. J Mol Cell Cardiol 1990;22:587–598.
75. Kinugawa K-I, Takahashi T, Kohmoto O, et al: Nitric oxide-mediated effects of interleukin-6 on $[Ca^{++}]i$ and cell contraction in cultured chick ventricular myocytes. Circ Res 1994;75:285–295.
76. Balligand J-L, Cannon PJ: Nitric oxide synthases and cardiac muscle: autocrine and paracrine influences. Arterioscler Thromb Vasc Biol 1997;17:1846–1858.
77. Yasuda S, Lew WYW: Lipopolysaccharide depresses cardiac contractility and β-adrenergic contractile response by decreasing myofilament response to Ca^{2+} in cardiac myocytes. Circ Res 1997;81:1011–1020.
78. Zhong J, Hwang T-C, Admas HR, Rubin LJ: Reduced L-type calcium current in ventricular myocytes from endotoxemic guinea pigs. Am J Physiol 1997;273:H2312–H2324.
79. Powers FM: Cardiac myofilament protein function is altered during sepsis. J Mol Cell Cardiol 1998;30:967–978.
80. Suto N, Mikuniya A, Okuba T, Hanada H, Shinozaki N, Okumura K: Nitric oxide modulates cardiac contractility and

oxygen consumption without changing contractile efficiency. Am J Physiol 1998:275:H41–H49.
81. Kilbourn RG, Szabo C, Traber DL: Beneficial versus detrimental effects of nitric oxide synthase inhibitors in circulatory shock: lessons learned from experimental and clinical studies. Shock 1997;7:235–246.
82. Quezado ZMN, Karzai W, Danner RL, et al: Effects of L-NMMA and fluid loading on TNF-induced cardiovascular dysfunction in dogs. Am J Respir Crit Care Med 1998;157:1397–1405.
83. Preckel B, Kojda G, Schlack W, et al: Inotropic effects of glyceryl trinitrate and spontaneous NO donors in the dog heart. Circulation 1997;96:2675–2682.
84. Prendergast BD, Sagach VF, Shah AM: Basal release of nitric oxide augments in the Frank-Starling response in the isolated heart. Circulation 1997;96:1320–1329.
85. Massey CV, Kohout TA, Gaa ST, Lederer WJ, Rogers TB: Molecular and cellular actions of platelet-activating factor in rat heart cells. J Clin Invest 1991;88:2106–2116.
86. Pugsley MK, Salari H, Walker MJA: Actions of platelet-activating factor on isolated rat hearts. Circ Shock 1991;35:207–214.
87. Kapadia S, Torre-Amione G, Yokoyama T, Mann DL: Soluble TNF binding proteins modulate the negative inotropic properties of TNF-α in vitro. Am J Physiol 1995;268:H517–H525.
88. Kumar A, Kosuri R, Kandula P, Dimou C, Allen J, Parrillo JE: Effects of epineprhine and amrinone on contractility and cyclic adenosine monophosphate generation of tumor necrosis factor-α-exposed cardiac myocytes. Crit Care Med 1999;27:286–292.
89. Amsterdam EA, Rendig SV, Longhurst JC: Contractile actions of C5a on isolated porcine myocardium. Am J Physiol 1992;263:H74–H745.
90. Del Balzo U, Engler RL, Ito BR: Complement C5a-mediated myocardial ishcemia and neutrophil sequestration: two independent phenomena. Am J Physiol 1993;264;H336–H344.
91. Heard SO, Baum TD, Feldman HS, Latka C, Fink MP: Lipopolysaccharide-induced myocardial depression is not mediated by cyclooxygenase products. Crit Care Med 1991;19:723–727.
92. Groeneveld ABJ, Hartemink KJ, De Groot MCM, Visser J, Thijs LG: Circulating endothelin and nitrate/nitrite relate to haemodynamic and metabolic variables in human septic shock. Shock 1999;11:160–166.
93. Vincent J-L, Bakker J, Marcaux G, Schandene L, Kahn RJ, Dupont E: Administration of anti-TNF antibody improves left ventricular function in septic shock patients: results of a pilot study. Chest 1992;101:810–815.
94. Daemen-Gubbels CRGM, Groeneveld PHP, Groeneveld ABJ, Van Kamp GJ, Bronsveld W, Thijs LG: Methylene blue increases myocardial function in septic shock. Crit Care Med 1995;23:1363–1370.
95. Avontuur JAM, Tutein Nolthenius RP, Buijk SLCE, Kanhai KJK, Bruining HA: Effect of L-NAME, an inhibitor of nitric oxide synthesis, on cardiopulmonary function in human septic shock. Chest 1998;113:1640–1646.
96. Jones SB, Romano FD: Myocardial beta adrenergic receptor coupling to adenylate cyclase during developing septic shock. Circ Shock 1990;30:51–61.
97. Campbell KL, Forse RA: Endotoxin-exposed atria exhibit G protein-based deficits in inotropic regulation. Surgery 1993;114:471–479.
98. Paulus WJ, Kästner S, Pajudas P, Shah AM, Drexler H, Vanderheyden M: Left ventricular contractile effects of inducible nitric oxide synthase in the human allograft. Circulation 1997;96:3436–3442.
99. Joe EK, Schussheim AE, Longrois D, et al: Regulation of cardiac myocyte contractile function by inducible nitric oxide synthase (iNOS): mechanisms of contractile depression by nitric oxide. J Mol Cell Cardiol 1998;30:303–315.
100. Bernardin G, Strosberg AD, Bernard A, Mattei M, Marullo S: β-Adrenergic receptor-dependent and -independent stimulation of adenylate cyclase is impaired during severe sepsis in humans. Intensive Care Med 1998;24:1315–1322.
101. Hinder F, Booke M, Traber LD, Traber DL: The atrial natriuretic peptide receptor antagonist HS 142-1 improves cardiovascular filling and mean arterial pressure in a hyperdynamic ovine model of sepsis. Crit Care Med 1997;25:820–826.
102. Poon BY, Goddard CM, Leaf CD, Russell JA, Walley KR: L-2-Oxothiazolidine-4-carboxylic acid prevents endotoxin-induced cardiac dysfunction. Am J Respir Crit Care Med 1998;158:1109–1113.
103. Thijs LG, Balk E, Tuynman HARE, Koopman PAR, Bezemer PD, Mulder GH: Effects of naloxone on hemodynamics, oxygen transport, and metabolic variables in canine endotoxin shock. Circ Shock 1983;10:147–160.
104. Safani M, Blair J, Ross D, Waki R, Li C, Libby G: Prospective, controlled, randomized trial of naloxone infusion in early hyperdynamic septic shock. Crit Care Med 1989;17:1004–1009.
105. Jones SB, Romano FD: Dose- and time-dependent changes in plasma catecholamines in response to endotoxin in conscious rats. Circ Shock 1989;8:59–68.
106. Terradellas JB, Bellot JF, Saris AB, Gil CL, Torrallardona AT, Garriga JR: Acute and transient ST segment elevation during bacterial shock in seven patients without apparent heart disease. Chest 1982;81:444–448.
107. Cunnion RE, Schaer GL, Parker MM, Natanson C, Parrillo JE: The coronary circulation in human septic shock. Circulation 1986;73:637–644.
108. Dhainaut J-F, Huyghebaert M-F, Monsallier JF: Coronary hemodynamics and myocardial metabolism of lactate, free fatty acids, glucose and ketones in patients with septic shock. Ciruclation 1987;75:533–541.
109. Groeneveld ABJ, Van Lambalgen AA, Van den Bos GC, Bronsveld W, Thijs LG: Maldistribution of heterogeneous coronary blood flow during canine endotoxin shock. Cardiovasc Res 1991;25:80–88.
110. Van Lambalgen AA, Van Kraats AA, Mulder MF, Teerlink T, Van den Bos GC: High-energy phosphates in heart, liver, kidney, and skeletal muscle of endotoxemic rats. Am J Physiol 1994;266:H1581–H1587.
111. Hotchkiss RS, Song S-K, Neil JJ, et al: Sepsis does not impair tricarboxylic acid cycle in the heart. Am J Physiol 1991;260:C50–C57.
112. Fox GA, Bersten A, Lam C, et al: Hematocrit modifies the circulatory control of systemic and myocardial oxygen utilization in septic sheep. Crit Care Med 1994;22:470–479.
113. Avontuur JAM, Bruining HA, Ince C: Inhibition of nitric oxide synthesis causes myocardial ischemia in endotoxemic rats. Circ Res 1995;76:418–425.
114. Panas D, Khadour FH, Szabo C, Schulz R: Proinflammatory cytokines depress cardiac efficiency by a nitric oxide-dependent mechanism. Am J Physiol 1998;275:H1016–H1023.

115. Kelm M, Schäfer S, Dahmann R, et al: Nitric oxide induced contractile dysfunction is related to a reduction in myocardial energy generation. Cardiovasc Res 1997;36:185–194.
116. Shibano T, Vanhoutte PM: Induction of NO production by TNF-α and lipopolysaccharide in porcine coronary arteries without endothelium. Am J Physiol 1993;264:H403–H407.
117. Myers PR, Gupta M, Rogers S, Mattox ML, Adams HR, Parker JL: Chronic endotoxemia and endothelium-dependent vasodilation in coronary arteries. Shock 1996;6:267–273.
118. Wang SY, Cameron EM, Fink MP, Sellke W: Chronic septicemia alters α-adrenergic mechanisms in the coronary circulation. J Surg Res 1997;69:61–66.
119. Avontuur JAM, Bruining HA, Ince C: Nitric oxide and dysfunction of coronary autoregulation in endotoxemic rats. Cardiovasc Res 1997;35:368–376.
120. Bersten AD, Sibbald WJ, Hersch M, Cheung H, Turledge FS: Interaction of sepsis and sepsis plus sympathomimetics on myocardial oxygen availability. Am J Physiol 1992;262: H1164–H1173.
121. Raper RF, Sibbald WJ, Hobson J, Neal A, Cheung H: Changes in myocardial blood flow rates during hyperdynamic sepsis with induced changes in arterial perfusing pressures and metabolic need. Crit Care Med 1993;21:1192–1199.
122. Xie Y-W, Wolin MS: Role of nitric oxide and its interaction with superoxide in the suppression of cardiac muscle mitochondrial respiration: involvement in response to hypoxia/reoxygenation. Circulation 1997;94:2580–2586.
123. Matheis G, Sherman MP, Buckberg GD, Haybron DM, Young HH, Ignarro LJ: Role of L-arginine-nitric oxide pathway in myocardial reoxygenation injury. Am J Physiol 1992;262: H616–H620.
124. Ismail JA, McDonough KH: The role of coronary flow and adenosine in postischemic recovery of septic rat hearts. Am J Physiol 1998;275:H8–H14.
125. Meng X, Brown JM, Ao L, et al: Endotoxin induces cardiac HSP70 and resistance to endotoxemic myocardial depression in rats. Am J Physiol 1996;271:C1316–C1324.
126. Perrault LP, Menasché P, Bel A, et al: Ischemic preconditioning in cardiac surgery: a word of caution. J Thorac Cardiovasc Surg 1996;112:1378–1386.
127. Cain BS, Meldrum DR, Dinarello CA, Meng X, Banerjee A, Harken AH: Adenosine reduces cardiac TNF-α production and human myocardial injury following ischemia-reperfusion. J Surg Res 1988;76:117–123.
128. Grocott-Mason RM, Shah AM: Cardiac dysfunction is sepsis: new theories and clinical implications. Intensive Care Med 1988;24:286–295.
129. Mazer CD, Naser B, Kamel KS: Effect of alkali therapy with $NaHCO_3$ or THAM on cardiac contractility. Am J Physiol 1996;270:R955–R962.
130. Bollaert P-E, Levy B, Nace L, Laterre P-F, Larcan A: Hemodynamic and metabolic effects of rapid correction of hypophosphatemia in patients with septic shock. Chest 1995;107: 1698–1701.
131. Natanson C, Esposito CJ, Banks SM, Magnuson WG: The sirens' songs of confirmatory sepsis trials: selection bias and sampling error. Crit Care Med 1998;26:1927–1931.
132. Staudinger T, Presterl E, Graninger W, et al: Influence of pentoxifylline on cytokine levels and inflammatory parameters in septic shock. Intensie Care Med 1996;22:888–893.
133. Weitzberg E, Rudehill A, Modin A, Lundberg JM: Effect of combined nitric oxide inhalation and N^G-nitro-L-arginine infusion in porcine endotoxin shock. Crit Care Med 1995;23: 909–918.
134. Grootendorst AF, Van Bommel EFH, Van Leengoed LAMG, Van Zanten AR, Huipen HJC, Groeneveld ABJ: Infusion of ultrafiltrate from endotoxemic pigs depresses myocardial performance of normal pigs. J Crit Care 1993;8:161–169.
135. Bottoms G, Fessler J, Murphey E, et al: Efficacy of convective removal of plasma mediators of endotoxic shock by continuous veno-venous hemofiltration. Shock 1996;5:149–154.
136. Heering P, Morgera S, Schnitz FJ, et al: Cytokine removal and cardiovascular hemodynamics in septic patients with continuous venovenous hemofiltration. Intensive Care Med 1997;23: 288–296.
137. Hoffmann JN, Hartl WH, Deppisch R, Faist E, Jochum M, Inthron D: Effect of hemofiltration on hemodynamics and systemic concentrations of anaphylatoxins and cytokines in human sepsis. Intensive Care Med 1996;22:1360–1367.
138. Kellum JA, Johnson JP, Kramer D, Palevsky P, Brady JJ, Pinsky MR: Diffusive vs. convective therapy: effects of mediators of inflammation in patients with severe systemic inflammatory response syndrome. Crit Care Med 1988;26:1995–2000.
139. Lee PA, Weger GW, Pryor RW, Matson JR: Effects of filter pore size on efficacy of continuous arteriovenous hemofiltration therapy for staphylococcus aureus-induced septicemia in immature swine. Crit Care Med 1998;26:730–737.
140. Tetta C, Cavaillon J-M, Schulze M, et al: Removal of cytokines and activated complement components in an experimental model of continuous plasma filtration coupled with sorbent absorption. Nephrol Dial Transplant 1998;13:1458–1464.
141. Spies CD, Reinhart K, Witt I, et al: Influence of N-acetylcysteine on indirect indicators of tissue oxygenation in septic shock patients: results from a prospective, randomized, double-blind study. Crit Care Med 1994;22:1738–1746.
142. Zhang H, Spapen H, Nguyen DN, Benlabed M, Buurman WA, Vincent J-L: Protective effects of N-acetyl-cysteine in endotoxemia. Am J Physiol 1994;266:H1746–1754.
143. Peake SL, Moran JL, Leppard PI: N-Acetyl-L-cysteine depresses cardiac performance in patients with septic shock. Crit Care Med 1996;24:1302–1310.
144. Boldt J, Kling D, Bormann B, Scheld H, Hempelmann G: Influence of PEEP ventilation immediately after cardiopulmonary bypass on right ventricular function. Chest 1988;94: 566–571.
145. Gorscan J, Gaisor TA, Mandarino WA, Deneault LG, Hattler BG, Pinsky MR: Assessment of the immediate effects of cardiopulmonary bypass on left ventricular performance by on-line pressure-area relations. Circulation 1994;89:180–190.
146. Hennein HA, Ebba H, Rodriguez JL, et al: Relationship of proinflammatory cytokines to myocardial ischemia and dysfunction after uncomplicated coronary revascularization. J Thorac Cardiovasc Surg 1994;108:626–635.
147. Te Veldhuis H, Jansen PGM, Oudemans-van Straaten HM, Sturk A, Eijsman L, Wildevuur CRH: Myocardial performance in elderly patients after cardiopulmonary bypass is suppressed by tumor necrosis factor. J Thorac Cardiovasc Surg 1995;110: 1663–1669.
148. Turner JS, Morgan CJ, Thakrar B, Pepper JR: Difficulties in predicting outcome in cardiac surgery patients. Crit Care Med 1995;23:1843–1850.

149. Bennett-Guerrero E, Ayuso L, Hamilton-Davies C, et al: Relationship of preoperative antiendotoxin core antibodies and adverse outcomes following cardiac surgery. JAMA 1997;277:646–650.
150. Bolli R: Basic and clinical aspects of myocardial stunning. Prog Cardiovasc Dis 1998;40:477–517.
151. Butterworth JF, Legault C, Royster RL, Hammon JW: Factors that predict the use of positive inotropic drug support after cardiac valve surgery. Anesth Analg 1998;86:461–467.
152. Rathmell JP, Prielipp RC, Butterworth JF, et al: A multicenter, randomized, blind comparison of amrinone with milrinone after elective cardiac surgery. Anesth Analg 1998;86:683–690.
153. Thompson MJ, Elton RA, Sturgeon KR, et al: The Edinburgh cardiac surgery score survival prediction in the long-stay ICU cardiac surgical patients. Eur J Cardiothorac Surg 1995;9:419–425.
154. Ryan TA, Rady MY, Bashour A, Leventhal M, Lytle B, Starr NJ: Predictors of outcome in cardiac surgical patients with prolonged intensive care stay. Chest 1997;112:1035–1042.
155. Alyanakian M-A, Dehoux M, Chatel D, et al: Cardiac troponin I in diagnosis of perioperative myocardial infarction after cardiac surgery. J Cardiovasc Vasc Anesth 1998;12:288–294.
156. Gensini GF, Fusi C, Conti AA, et al: Cardiac troponin I and Q-wave perioperative myocardial infarction after coronary artery bypass surgery. Crit Care Med 1998;26:1986–1990.
157. McKenney PA, Apstein CS, Mendes LA, et al: Increased left ventricular diastolic chamber stiffness immediatley after coronary artery bypasss surgery. J Am Coll Cardiol 1994;24:1189–1194.
158. Christakis GT, Buth KJ, Weisel RD, et al: Randomized study of right ventricular function with intermittent warm or cold cardioplegia. Ann Thorac Surg 1996;61:128–134.
159. Davies MJ, Nguyen K, Gaynor JW, Elliott MJ: Modified ultrafiltration improves left ventricular systolic function in infants after cardiopulmonary bypass. J Thorac Cardiovasc Surg 1998;115:361–370.
160. Biagioli B, Borrelli E, Maccherini M, et al: Reduction of oxidative stress does not affect recovery of myocardial function: warm continuous versus cold intermittent blood cardioplegia. Heart 1997;77:465–473.
161. Menasché P: The inflammatory response to cardiopulmonary bypass and its impact on postoperative myocardial funciton. Curr Opion Cardiol 1995;10:597–604.
162. Wang SY, Friedman M, Johnson RG, Weintraub RM, Sellke FW: Adrenergic regulation of coronary microcirculation after extracorporeal circulation and crystalloid cardioplegia. Am J Physiol 1994;267:H2462–H2470.
163. Amrani M, Gray CC, Smolenski RT, Goodwin AT, Lodon A, Yacoub MH: The effect of L-arginine on myocardial recovery after cardioplegic arrest and ischemia under moderate and deep hypothermia. Circulation 1997;96(Suppl II):274–279.
164. Nonami Y: The role of nitric oxide in cardiac surgery. Surg Today Jpn J Surg 1997;27:583–592.
165. Igarashi J, Nishida M, Hoshida S, et al: Inducible nitric oxide synthase augments injury elicited by oxidative stress in rat cardiac myocytes. Am J Physiol 1998;274:C245–C255.
166. Wan S, LeClerc J-L, Vincent J-L: Inflammatory responses to cardiopulmonary bypass. Chest 1997;112:676–692.
167. Jansen NJG, Van Oeveren W, Van de Broek L, et al: Inhibition by dexamethasone of the reperfusion phenomena in cardiopulmonary bypass. J Thorac Cardiovasc Surg 1991;102:515–525.
168. Myles PS, Leong CK, Currey J: Endogenous nitric oxide and low systemic vascular resistance after cardiopulmonary bypass. J Cardiothorac Vasc Anesth 1997;11:571–574.
169. Bando K, Turrentine MW, Vijay P, et al: Effect of modified ultrafiltration in high-risk patients undergoing operations for congenital heart disease. Ann Thorac Surg 1998;66:821–828.
170. Reddy VM, Hendricks-Munoz KD, Rajasinghe HA, Petrossian E, Hanley FL, Fineman JR: Postcardiopulmonary bypass pulmonary hypertension in lambs in lambs with increased pulmonary blood flow: a role for endothelin 1. Circulation 1997;95:1054–1061.
171. Sinclair DG, Haslam PL, Quinlan GJ, Pepper JR, Evans TW: The effect of cardiopulmonary bypass on intestinal and pulmonary endothelial permeability. Chest 1995;108:718–724.
172. Dupuis J-Y, Li K, Calderone A, et al: β-Adrenergic signal transduction and contractility in the canine heart after cardiopulmonary bypass. Cardiovasc Res 1997;36:223–235.
173. Booth JV, Landolfo KP, Chesnut LC, et al: Acute depression of myocardial β-adrenergic receptor signaling during cardiopulmonary bypass: impairment of the adenylyl cyclase moiety. Anesthesiology 1998;89:602–611.
174. Allen SJ, Geissler HJ, Davis KL, et al: Augmenting cardiac contractility hastens myocardial edema resolution after cardiopulmonary bypass and cardioplegic arrest. Anesth Analg 1997;85:987–992.
175. Coraim FJ, Coraim HP, Ebermann R, Stellwag FM: Acute respiratory failure after cardiac surgery: clinical experience with the application of continuous arteriovenous hemofiltration. Crit Care Med 1986;14:714–718.
176. Rivera ES, Kimball TR, Bailey WW, Witt SA, Khoury PR, Daniels SR: Effect of veno-venous ultrafiltration on myocardial performance immediately after cardiac surgery in children: a prospective randomized study. J Am Coll Cardiol 1998;32:766–772.
177. Hoffmann H, Markewitz A, Kreuzer E, Reichert K, Jochum M, Faist E: Pentoxifylline decreases the incidence of multiple organ failure in patients after major cardiothoracic surgery. Shock 1998;9:235–240.
178. Snow DJ, Gray SJ, Ghosh S, et al: Inhaled nitric oxide in patients with normal and increased pulmonary vascular resistance after cardiac surgery. Br J Anaesth 1994;72:185–189.

36
Lung

R. Phillip Dellinger

Triggering of the systemic inflammatory response syndrome (SIRS) by conditions such as sepsis, multisystem trauma, shock (and massive transfusions), burns, and pancreatitis produces a pulmonary vascular flood of products of the activated humoral cascade system, where inflammatory cells, bacterial toxins, and toxin-produced cellular mediators clearly assume responsibility. Depending on its severity this diffuse injury is characterized as acute lung injury (ALI) or acute respiratory distress syndrome (ARDS). ALI is a syndrome of inflammation and increased permeability that leads to physiologic, radiologic, and clinical abnormalities. When ALI is severe, ARDS is the term used to describe the condition. The consensus definition of ALI includes (1) acute onset; (2) $PaO_2/FiO_2 \leq 300$; (3) bilateral infiltrates on frontal chest radiograph; and (4) pulmonary artery wedge pressure ≤ 18 mmHg, or in the absence of a pulmonary artery catheter no clinical evidence of left atrial hypertension.[1] The consensus definition of ARDS is ALI with $PaO_2/FiO_2 \leq 200$. Although ARDS can be primary (due to direct causes such as pneumonia and gas inhalation), it is more strongly linked to outside lung events, which appear to trigger the systemic inflammatory syndrome (SIRS). This type of ARDS is called secondary (or indirect) and is often associated with the multiple organ dysfunction syndrome (MODS).

Acute Respiratory Distress Syndrome

Etiology and Association with MODS

Garber et al. in 1996 reported a meta-analysis of 83 studies related to risk factors for ARDS.[2] The strongest evidence for cause and effect in this study was demonstrated by SIRS associated with sepsis. Of the other four links to cause and effect (aspiration, multisystem trauma, multiple transfusions, and disseminated intravascular coagulation) three of the four were likely SIRS-related as well.

Sepsis represents the most common cause of SIRS-induced ARDS. Sepsis-induced ARDS usually occurs in the context of MODS. Bell et al. demonstrated nonpulmonary organ failure in 85% of patients with ARDS and noted a significant relation between the development of organ dysfunction and infection.[3] Knaus et al. found that 76% of ARDS patients (with sepsis as the most frequent cause) exhibited nonpulmonary organ dysfunction.[4] Shock, metabolic acidosis, and altered mentation were the most common organ dysfunctions. Nonsurvivors had a significantly larger number of organ dysfunctions. Herbert et al. reported a series of 154 consecutive septic patients and demonstrated that ALI and ARDS were the most common forms of organ dysfunction (74 patients).[5] In this study pulmonary dysfunction correlated poorly with the likelihood of death. Estimation of the incidence of SIRS-induced ARDS is difficult because authors have used different clinical criteria for its definition. The ability to define incidence and outcome more precisely, however, has been significantly improved by consensus definitions of ALI and ARDS. The incidence of ARDS is likely to be 3/100,000 to 74/100,000 population.[6]

Pathophysiology

The SIRS-associated inflammatory response manifested in the lung involves a multitude of humoral mediator systems, inflammatory cells, and bacterial toxins.[6] Neutrophilic infiltrates predominate in histologic samples from the lungs of patients with ARDS. Bronchoalveolar lavage (BAL) demonstrates high neutrophil counts and high concentrations of neutrophil degranulation products. Neutrophil-associated oxidant activity increases. Oxidant injury is likely an important component of SIRS-related lung injury. This has been demonstrated in animal models following gut ischemia/reperfusion. Defective surfactant activity may result through oxidant attack on lipid or lipoprotein components, inhibition by plasma-derived proteins that gain access to the alveolar space, or direct type 2 pneumocyte injury.

The complex interaction between endothelial cells and neutrophils leads to endothelial cell damage with formation of pulmonary edema and production of vasomotor disturbances of the pulmonary circulation. Toxin-induced formation of tumor necrosis factor (TNF) and interleukin-8 (IL-8) by macrophages is important in this response. The primary function of IL-8 is neutrophil activation and chemotaxis. TNF promotes neutrophil adherence to the endothelium and pulmonary circulatory vasoconstriction. Lipid mediators such as platelet-activating factor, leukotrienes, and prostanoids are also important in augmenting inflammation and producing vascular reactivity.

There is much current interest in the role of coagulation cascade activation in the production of ARDS in patients with SIRS. Activation of the coagulation system by TNF, IL-1, and plasminogen activator inhibitor may be important in the development of ARDS. In the injured alveolar compartment, fibrin deposition is initiated by increased activity of the intrinsic coagulation pathway (tissue factor associated with factor VII) and the contact coagulation pathways is also activated. Local fibrinolysis is generally impaired.

The perpetuating inflammation at the gas-exchange level is responsible for lung pathophysiology, which is characterized by interstitial and alveolar edema, hyaline membrane formation, atelectasis, gas-exchange abnormalities, increased pulmonary vascular resistance, and microthrombi. Clinical changes include hypoxemia, increased deadspace, and markedly reduced lung compliance.

Various patterns of organ dysfunction may occur with SIRS-induced lung injury. In some patients early onset of interstitial and alveolar edema predominate, whereas in others serious gas-exchange disturbances characterized by ventilation-perfusion mismatch may be accompanied by only moderate edema formation, seen on radiologic examination.

Neutrophil recruitment to the lung is accomplished through vascular adhesion molecules, which are upregulated in SIRS. There is direct linkage between cytokines such as TNF and IL-1 and expression of vascular adhesion molecules such as intracellular adhesion molecule-1 (ICAM-1). Complement activation also has diverse effects on the expression of endothelial adhesion molecules. Endothelial changes in SIRS-induced ARDS contribute to regional increases in vascular resistance and hypoperfusion. Multiple inflammatory stimuli synergistically promote neutrophil-mediated tissue injury through priming and activation. Platelet-activating factor is important in this priming process. The lung has the ability to autoregulate, and the importance of antiinflammatory cytokines such as IL-10 in containment of the inflammatory response is now recognized.

Nonsepsis SIRS-Induced ARDS

The adverse effects of hypothermia, hypotension, shock, and multiple transfusions on coagulation are well documented. After major trauma, hemorrhagic shock, or surgical procedures characterized by major blood loss, the concentrations of TNF, IL-1, and IL-6 are increased. High concentrations found during the early postinjury period are associated with increased risk of ARDS development and mortality. In addition, in patients with accidental trauma severe injury produces rapid, large increases in circulating concentrations of cytokines that may contribute to the development of ARDS. An increase in the level of urinary leukotriene E_4 has been demonstrated in burn patients with severe injuries and SIRS who develop ARDS.

Most patients undergoing cardiopulmonary bypass (CPB) recover uneventfully. However, in a small percentage of these patients ARDS complicates the postoperative period; and when it occurs it may be profound. Mortality is high when MODS develops in these patients. The cause and pathophysiology of post-CPB complications are not clear. Sinclair and colleagues calculated the protein accumulation index (PAI) as a BAL marker of integrity of the alveolar capillary membrane following CPB.[7] Changes in the integrity of the gut barrier membrane was also documented in this study. An elevated PAI was found to correlate with both longer operative bypass time and the postoperative serum myeloperoxidase level. This study confirmed that significant microvascular injury complicates CPB even in the absence of significant clinical sequelae, as only 1 of the 20 patients developed ARDS.

Acute respiratory distress syndrome may be seen during pregnancy and is associated with maternal mortality similar to that of nonpregnant patients. The main risks for development of ARDS are hemorrhage, infection, and toxemia. When maternal deaths occur, they are typically in the setting of ARDS plus other organ dysfunctions (MODS).

Predictors of Development

There is an association between massive transfusion and ARDS. That transfused blood is foreign protein and that it is often passed through sophisticated machines and devices, such as during CPB and autotransfusion, may also be important. We should be reminded of the statement by Lister in 1863: "I have only lately been aware of the great influence exerted upon the blood by exposure for a very short time to a foreign solid, and I feel that many of my own experiments, and many performed by others, have been vitiated for want of this knowledge."

Acute respiratory distress syndrome is seen in a significant percentage of patients during the early post-bone marrow transplant (engraftment) period. It is a major cause of morbidity and mortality. This type of ARDS has been linked to a generalized capillary leak syndrome. Some have suggested that the endothelial damage may be related to graft-versus-host disease (GVHD), whereas others have demonstrated release of TNF and IL-2 unrelated to GVHD preceding development of this injury.

General Studies

Bone and colleagues studied the serial development of organ dysfunction in patients admitted to an intensive care unit (ICU).[8] They noted that lung dysfunction dominated the early clinical course. When respiratory function was supported, other organ dysfunctions developed. In 1982 Pepe and colleagues studied clinical predictors of ARDS.[9] They selected eight conditions that were thought to put the patient at risk for ARDS: (1) sepsis syndrome, (2) aspiration of gastric contents, (3) pulmonary contusion, (4) multiple emergency transfusions, (5) multiple major fractures, (6) near-drowning, (7) pancreatitis, and (8) prolonged hypotension. The greatest risk was associated with sepsis syndrome (38%), followed by documented aspiration of gastric contents (30%), and multiple emergency transfusions (24%). The risk approximately doubled with each increase from one to two to three risk factors. They found that risk factors were more predictive than the injury severity score (ISS) used in this study. Hudson and colleagues studied another cohort of patients who developed ARDS.[10] Again, sepsis syndrome was the greatest risk factor followed by multiple emergency transfusions and then multiple trauma. Secondary factors of risk included the Acute Physiology and Chronic Health Evaluation (APACHE II) score in patients with sepsis and increased APACHE II and ISS scores in trauma patients.

Scoring Systems for Prediction of ARDS

Roumen and colleagues studied the ability of seven scoring systems and sequential lactate concentrations to predict the development of ARDS.[11] Severity systems include the ISS, Trauma Score (TS), Trauma Score and Injury Severity Score (TRISS), Glasgow Coma Scale (GCS), Polytrauma Score (PTS), APACHE II, and Sepsis Severity Score (SSS). By stepwise regression analysis the authors demonstrated that ISS, SSS, and lactate level at day 3 were the most significant variables for predicting development of ARDS. All patients had multiple trauma. Slotman and Quinn evaluated multiple regression modeling for predicting pulmonary dysfunction in critically ill patients with severe sepsis.[12] Modeling equations used physiologic and clinical laboratory measurements, circulating levels of eicosanoids and cytokines obtained when severe sepsis criteria were first met, and organ dysfunction indicators measured at 24, 48, and 72 hours. A PaO_2/FiO_2 ratio of ≤ 150 and lung injury score of ≥ 7 were used as thresholds. Multivariate prediction of the onset of pulmonary dysfunction in patients without lung dysfunction at baseline was highly sensitive but lacked specificity. When multivariate prediction was used for continued lung dysfunction in patients with lung dysfunction at baseline, it was a poor predictor of PaO_2/FiO_2 changeover time, lacking both sensitivity and specificity. Although the sensitivity and specificity for predicting a lung injury score of ≥ 7 was poor at 7 hours, it increased at 48 hours and became highly sensitive and specific when predicting 72-hour changes.

Specific Serum Factors as Predictors

The ability of serum ferritin to predict ARDS seems rational, as proinflammatory cytokines increase ferritin synthesis as it relates to increased oxidative stress (patients at risk for ARDS might liberate iron from ferritin, thus accelerating toxic hydroxyl radical [·OH] formation). Using this hypothesis to guide their experimented design, Connelly et al. demonstrated a correlation between ferritin levels and being at risk for ARDS.[13] Donnelly and colleagues demonstrated that within minutes of a trauma event there is evidence of enhanced neutrophil degeneration as measured by elevated levels of immunoreactive neutrophil elastase in the peripheral blood.[14] This elevation correlates with the degree of subsequent lung injury. Douzinas studied transpulmonary gradients of cytokines and lactate and demonstrated an increase in these measurements across the pulmonary vascular bed in patients with multiple organ failure (MOF) that included ARDS, whereas there was a drop in levels in patients with MOF that included hepatic injury but not ARDS.[15] This supports the concept of lung production of cytokines and lactate in patients with ARDS and clearance in other non-ARDS states of multiple organ dysfunction. Roumen et al. demonstrated that the concentration of lipofuscin as a measurement of oxidative stress correlated positively with the development of ARDS.[16]

Predictors of Mortality

Table 36.1 summarizes 12 articles published between 1985 and 1998 that demonstrated predictors of mortality for patients with ARDS.[17-26]

Radiologic Assessment

Chest radiographic infiltrates develop almost immediately after the onset of gas-exchange abnormalities of ARDS. The early occurrence of bilateral, symmetric, patchy, dense peripheral infiltrates, predominantly acinar in appearance, is progressively replaced by a diffuse ground-glass appearance. Substantial asymmetry may be seen in the presence of preexisting lung disease (bullae, pulmonary emboli) or if the patient has had a decubitus. Barotrauma in SIRS-induced ARDS is most commonly observed in ARDS during the chronic support phase (weeks 1–4). In patients who demonstrate a path of resolution of ARDS following reversal of the initial insult, radiographic densities tend to reverse over 10–14 days. Some patients, however, develop progressive disease despite apparent control of the triggering process. Most ARDS survivors show near-normal pulmonary function and a near-normal radiographic appearance by 1 year after resolution of ARDS. A smaller proportion of survivors, 20–25%, have both residual fibrosis and persistent significant pulmonary function abnormalities (most notably a diffusion abnormality and restrictive defect).

The portable chest radiograph has limited reliability of radiographic information but is usually all that is available for critically ill patients with ARDS. Variations in technique from day to day can have a significant impact on observer interpretation of improvement or worsening of infiltrates. Attempts to standardize technique as much as possible are desirable. Diuresis tends to alleviate infiltrates, and volume overload worsens infiltrates independent of improvement or worsening of the underlying ARDS. Chest computed tomography (CT) may offer significant advantages in patients with ARDS. It affords improved evaluation of the pleural space (pneumothorax and pleural effusion) and identification of discrete parenchymal abnormalities. It also assists in proper chest tube positioning. It may, however, be a risk to the patient during transport to the radiology department.

Management of ARDS Due to Severe SIRS

General Management Principles

Fluid Balance

In the absence of a need for high left ventricular preload to maintain oxygen delivery it is desirable to maintain a low

TABLE 36.1. Predicting Mortality in Patients with ARDS.

Study	Year	No. of patients	Studied	Results
Montgomery[16]	1985	277 Consecutive patients with risk factors for ARDS, 47 developed ARDS	Mortality in ARDS versus non-ARDS ICU patients	68% Mortality in ARDS patients and 35% in controls; 16% of ARDS deaths due to irreversible respiratory failure; most late deaths due to severe sepsis.
Russell[17]	1990	40 ARDS patients	Oxygen delivery, oxygen consumption, left ventricular preload	Survivors of ARDS had greater oxygen delivery and oxygen consumption than nonsurvivors; greater oxygen delivery appeared related to higher stroke volume index due to greater LV end-diastolic volume.
Suchyta[18]	1992	215 ARDS patients	Cause of ARDS, organ dysfunction, demographics	Deaths of 40% of patients were directly related to respiratory failure. MODS, sepsis, and age increased the chance of mortality from ARDS.
Clark[19]	1995	117 ARDS patients, 6 healthy controls	Studied type III procollagen peptide	Increased levels of type III procollagen in BAL fluid was strongly associated with fatal outcome independent of other variables.
Donnelly[20]	1996	28 ARDS patients, 9 ventilated non-ARDS controls	TNF, IL-1β, IL-8, IL-10, IL-1 receptor antagonist	Low concentration of antiinflammatory cytokines (IL-10, IL-RA) and not high concentrations of proinflammatory cytokines are associated with higher mortality in ARDS.
Headley[21]	1997	34 ARDS patients with conventional treatment and 9 with glucocorticoid therapy for fibroproliferative ARDS	Clinical variables, etiology of ARDS, and inflammatory cytokines (TNF, IL-1, IL-2, IL-4, IL-6, IL-8) in plasma and BAL fluid	Plasma inflammatory cytokine levels but not clinical criteria or precipitating cause of ARDS correlated with patient outcome.
Milberg[22]	1995	918 ARDS patients	Fatality rates by etiology of ARDS and age	Significant decrease in fatality rates predominantly in patients younger than 60 years and those with severe sepsis as etiology. Overall fatality rates decreased to 36% in 1993.
Abel[23]	1998	ARDS patients 41: 1990–1993 78: 1993–1997	Mortality 1990–1993 (period 1) compared to 1993–1997 (period 2) with relation to age, pulmonary physiology, and severity score	Between periods 1 and 2 mortality decreased from 66% to 34%. Postulated to be multifactorial and attributable to general patient management strategies and use of new therapeutic strategies for ARDS. During period 2 the APACHE II score and PaO_2/FiO_2 predicted survival.
Zilberberg[24]	1998	107 Consecutive ALI patients	Studied chronic disease, age, severity of illness, lung injury score, etiology, preceding nonlung organ dysfunction	Predictors of death were age >65, organ transplantation, HIV infection, cirrhosis, active malignancy, and sepsis.
Hudson[10]	1995	695 Patients	Patients with risk factors who developed ARDS vs. those who did not develop ARDS	Overall mortality with ARDS was 62% in those who developed ARDS vs. 19% in those who did not develop ARDS; with trauma 56% vs. 13%; with sepsis 69% vs. 49%.

ICU, intensive care unit; TNF, tumor necrosis factor; IL, interleukin; LV, left ventricular; BAL, bronchoalveolar lavage; ILRA, interleukin receptor antibody; ALI, acute lung injury; HIV, human immunodeficiency virus.

normal capillary pressure in ARDS due to severe SIRS. Hypovolemia should be avoided. Keeping the patient "a little on the dry side" may be associated with a better prognosis.[26] Maintaining a low wedge pressure at the expense of compromising oxygen delivery and organ perfusion, however, is inappropriate. Adequate urine output is usually a good indicator of adequate left ventricular preload.

Increased Airflow Resistance

Airflow resistance may be elevated in patients with ARDS. If airways resistance is increased to a clinically significant degree (evidenced by a large difference between peak and plateau airway pressures not explained by endotracheal tube resistance) or if there is wheezing at the time of physical examination, aerosolized bronchodilator therapy should be considered.

Cardiovascular Support

Increased levels of circulating cytokines have been reported in severe SIRS, and the hemodynamic profile may be the same as that of severe sepsis (increased cardiac output with decreased systemic vascular resistance). The presence of this profile therefore does not necessarily imply sepsis. In ARDS patients who might require vasodilator therapy for other indications, it should be remembered that some vasodilators (nitroglycerin and nitroprusside) have been associated with significantly increased shunting in low ventilation–perfusion areas, leading to significant drops in PaO_2. Cardiac output may also become compromised with treatment of ARDS owing to a combination of high intrathoracic pressure compromising right ventricular filling and increased pulmonary vascular resistance producing right heart dysfunction.

Prevention and Diagnosis of Pneumonia

Ventilation-acquired pneumonia (VAP) is a leading cause of morbidity and mortality in patients with ARDS. The primary risk factors are the presence of the endotracheal tube and the weakened capability of the lungs (and of the patient in general) to deal with bacterial invasion. Although no prospective controlled trials have definitively established clinical outcome differences, there are data, especially in surgical ICU patients, to indicate the ability of selective gut decontamination to decrease the incidence of pneumonia.[27,28] The trade-offs are the possibility of developing resistant organisms and the cost of therapy. Likewise, continuous aspiration of subglottic secretions has also been shown to decrease the incidence of VAP by decreasing the chronic microaspirations around the cuff of the endotracheal tube.[29]

Diagnosing VAP is difficult because patients with ARDS have baseline bilateral infiltrates and frequently other vital sign abnormalities seen with pneumonia. The use of semiquantitative cultures has been advocated by investigators[30,31] but it is controversial especially when patients are already on antibiotics.[32,33] Cutoffs for supporting the diagnosis of pneumonia are typically $\geq 10^3$ colony counts after fiberoptic bronchoscopy (FOB) with a protected catheter brush and $\geq 10^4$ colony counts for FOB. The use of quantitative cultures from blind endotracheal tube aspirates may be a less expensive option than FOB.[32]

Other Therapies to Decrease Morbidity Associated with ARDS and Prolonged Mechanical Ventilation

Patients with ARDS should receive prophylaxis for deep vein thrombosis with some combination of low dose heparin and intermittent compression devices based on the risk for bleeding and additional risks for thromboembolic disease. Enteral nutrition should be instituted on day 1 unless absolute contraindications exist (mechanical obstruction, mesenteric ischemia). Promotility agents and postpyloric placement of the feeding tube may facilitate success. The use of total parenteral nutrition (TPN) should be considered for enteral feeding failures, although the ability of TPN to alter outcome is controversial.[34]

Mechanical Ventilation: Lung Protection Strategy

Minimal (Optimal) Positive End-Expiratory Pressure

The lower inflection point is the midpoint of the transition from the flat portion of the pressure–volume curve to the steeper, more compliant area. With ARDS this point typically represents an area where lung units (alveoli) are collapsing at end-expiration and reopening during the next inspiration. When this is allowed to occur, animal studies suggest that a shearing force is exerted on the endothelial and epithelial cells in collapsed lung that is adjacent to an open lung.[35] It is expected to produce further lung injury. During early ARDS the application of that level of positive end-expiratory pressure (PEEP) at or slightly above the lower inflection point to prevent collapse of acinar units seems reasonable to protect the lung from shear force injury. Each breath would begin on a steeper portion of the pressure–volume curve, leading to improved compliance. The lowest PEEP that gives the best compliance is typically regarded as the optimal PEEP.[36] This PEEP would be expected to maximize recruitment of collapsed alveoli and be assumed to maximize oxygenation from PEEP effect on lung recruitment. In hypoxemic ARDS patients, oxygenation can be increased by optimizing PEEP, increasing mean airway pressure, raising FiO_2, or increasing alveolar ventilation. The latter two items are the least efficient mechanisms. Higher PEEP levels, if resulting in improved oxygenation, may be doing so by increasing mean airway pressure only. Early in the ARDS disease process, sufficient total PEEP that prevents tidal closure of alveolar units (usually 8–15 cmH_2O) may therefore improve compliance and oxygenation as well as decrease injury from repeated opening and closing of unstable lung units.

The lower inflection point (LIP) can be located by constructing a static pressure–volume curve (requires patient paralysis), or it may be inferred by using pressure-controlled ventilation to ascertain the lowest PEEP value that gives the highest tidal volume with a fixed pressure application. This is true only if the inspiratory time is prolonged enough to ensure a no-flow state at end-inspiration and if the applied inspiratory pressure is low enough to avoid the upper deflection zone (see discussion to follow). More frequently, PEEP is titrated to the value between 8 and 15 cmH$_2$O that provides the best oxygenation. Another approach is to increase the PEEP based on FiO$_2$ requirements using PEEP levels of 8–18 cmH$_2$O as FiO$_2$ requirements increase between 0.4 and 1.0.

Limiting Alveolar Overinflation

Animal studies suggest that lung injury may be due to alveolar hyperinflation, even if barotrauma does not occur.[37] This injury is called "volutrauma." Understanding volutrauma necessitates understanding the forces determining alveolar inflation and their relation to inspiratory plateau pressure (IPP), the best readily available correlate of transalveolar pressure, the true determinant of alveolar distension. Inflation of alveolar units beyond total lung capacity has been shown to produce hemorrhagic edema in animal lungs. An IPP of 35 cmH$_2$O is thought to approximate total lung capacity in normally compliant lungs. CT scans of patients with ARDS show that the upper portions of nondependent lung are almost normal in appearance and would be expected to have near-normal compliance.[38] Therefore ARDS patients mechanically ventilated with IPP > 35 cmH$_2$O are at risk for volutrauma. Using >35 cmH$_2$O IPP as a cutoff for the risk of volutrauma assumes the presence of normal pleural space, a normal chest wall, and normal abdominal compliance. Therefore in the presence of an edematous chest wall, massive ascites, or large bilateral pleural effusions, a considerably higher IPP may be necessary to reach alveolar distension equal to total lung capacity.[39] Overinflation of lungs is associated with decreased compliance; and as overinflation is approached and exceeded, an upper deflection zone is created on the pressure–volume curve.

Ventilatory strategy can be developed to limit peak alveolar pressure. Measurement of the IPP requires delaying expiration at the end of inspiration (inspiratory hold), allowing pressure to equilibrate in the lung at end-inspiration. This measurement is possible on most modern mechanical ventilators. Lung protective strategy involves the selection of smaller tidal volumes, directly setting it on volume-cycled ventilators or lowering the delivered pressure on time-cycled ventilators. It must be remembered that although the risk of volutrauma (and barotrauma) is defined by the IPP level, it is the increase or decrease in tidal volume that changes this value. Decreasing tidal volume results in a decrease in alveolar ventilation, an increase in PaCO$_2$, and a decrease in pH, which explains the derivation of the name "permissive hypercapnia" as a route to lowering IPP.[40,41] So long as the decrease in pH is not severe ($\geq$ 7.25), hypercapnia does not usually cause clinical problems (exceptions include patients with increased intracranial pressure). The tidal volume can be incrementally decreased (by decreasing the applied pressure or the tidal volume directly) to as low as 6 ml/kg. Rises in PaCO$_2$ of 1 mmHg/hr are usually well tolerated so long as the pH remains at 7.25 or higher. In addition, the renal response to PaCO$_2$-induced decreases in pH is to retain bicarbonate and over time allow greater reductions in tidal volume at the same pH. The use of iatrogenic metabolic alkalosis to allow more aggressive lowering of the tidal volume in ARDS patients is controversial (although in general it is supported for permissive hypercapnia in those with severe status asthmaticus).

The strategy of limiting the IPP by decreasing the tidal volume directly with volume-controlled ventilators or indirectly with pressure-controlled ventilators results in a decrease in mean airway pressure. A decrease in mean airway pressure may be associated with a fall in PaO$_2$, which can usually be countered by holding the tidal volume constant and increasing either the inspiratory time or the rate. Either of these maneuvers increases the mean airway pressure without raising the IPP so long as auto-PEEP is not induced. The inspiration/expiration ratio may be increased to more than 1:1 (inverse ratio ventilation). Auto-PEEP is defined as the positive recoil pressure at end-expiration when there is insufficient time for the lung to return to its functional residual capacity. It is common in patients with chronic obstructive pulmonary disease or with one-lung ventilation.

Clinical Trials

Two clinical trials have been published in peer review journals that target lung protection strategy for potential benefit in ARDS. The first of these studies, by Stewart and colleagues, targeted prevention of overinflation of lung units by utilization of permissive hypercapnia.[42] This study evaluated ventilation strategy to prevent barotrauma in patients at high risk for ARDS. A total of 120 patients were randomized, 60 to each group. Tidal volumes were 7.2 ml/kg in the limited-ventilation group, and 10.8 ml/kg in the control group. Peak inspiratory pressures were 23.6 in the limited-ventilation group and 34.0 in the control group. The incidence of barotrauma, mortality, and highest multiple organ dysfunction scores were the same in the two groups. Paralytic agents were used more frequently in the limited-ventilation group, and dialysis for renal failure was instituted more often. The other two studies (presented in abstract form) also failed to show benefit of limiting inspiratory plateau pressure with use of permissive hypercapnia in ARDS.

The second study, by Amato and colleagues, looked at the effect of protective ventilation strategy on mortality in ARDS.[43] This study, however, targeted not only limitation of inspiratory plateau pressure but also institution of minimal PEEP targeted at the lower inflection point. A total of 53 patients were included in the study: 29 in the protective ventilation group and 17 controls. Mortality at 28 days was 38% in the lung protection group and 71% in the conventional ventilator group. Rates of weaning from mechanical ventilation favored the protective ventilation group by 66% versus 29%. Rates of barotrauma were 7% in the protective ventilation group and 42% in controls. The difference in survival to hospital discharge, however, was not significant, with 45% mortality in the protective ventilation group and 71% in the conventional

TABLE 36.2. Consensus Conference Recommendations for Goals of Ventilatory Management.

1. Ensure appropriate O_2 delivery and sufficient CO_2 removal.
2. Minimize oxygen toxicity: take aggressive steps to lower fraction of FiO_2 when $FiO_2 > 0.65$.
3. Target PEEP toward obliteration of lower inflection point. Use the lowest mean airway pressure that accomplishes oxygenation goals. Full PEEP effects may not be immediately realized.
4. Strategies that keep IPP ≤ 30–40 cmH_2O should be employed.
5. Prevent atelectasis: periodically employ higher volume, longer-duration breaths to forestall atelectasis.
6. Use sedation/hyperanalgesic drugs judiciously and avoid paralytic agents if possible. If paralytic agents are required, use should be as brief as possible and the depth of blockade periodically assessed.

PEEP, positive end-expiratory pressure; IPP, intermittent positive pressure.

ventilation group ($p = 0.37$). This small study, although encouraging for use of a combination of minimal PEEP and limitation of overinflation, needs validation with additional studies. It should also be noted that 71% mortality in the conventional ventilation group is high and is the reason for the difference between the two groups.

Preliminary data from the U.S. National Heart, Lung, and Blood Institute (NHLBI) ARDS Clinical Trial Group study on lung protection strategy in ARDS were recently presented at the annual meeting of the American Thoracic Society. The data revealed a significant reduction in mortality with the 6 ml/kg tidal volume arm of the study compared to the 12 ml/kg arm. Both groups had PEEP titrated upward relative to the severity of hypoxemia. The American-European Consensus Conference on ARDS (Part 2) current recommendations are listed in Table 36.2.[44]

Inverse Ratio (Reverse I:E) Ventilation

A typical inspiratory/expiratory (I:E) ratio selection for mechanical ventilator support is 1:2. The I:E ratio is determined by how much of each minute is required for inspiration; what is left is the expiratory time. Inspiratory time with volume-cycled ventilation is determined by peak inspiratory flow, rate, and tidal volume and with time-cycled ventilation (pressure control) by rate and the direct setting of the inspiratory time for breath delivery. Patients with ARDS require little expiratory time because of the decreased compliance and associated increase in elastic recoil of the lungs. An I:E ratio of 1:1 or higher is feasible in this patient group.[45–47] A potential advantage of such an I:E ratio would be to allow longer inspiratory times to facilitate better filling of noncompliant areas of the lung with prolonged time constants for filling. By increasing the inspiratory time the mean airway pressure, a primary determinant of oxygenation, is also increased. The use of inverse-ratio ventilation to increase mean airway pressure is an option to increase the mean airway with higher inflation pressures, which may be associated with less volutrauma and barotrauma. This mode of ventilation may be tried in patients who cannot be oxygenated with conventional mechanical ventilation and PEEP or in the presence of prohibitively high peak airway pressures. Inverse ratios of up to 3:1 have been utilized. Concerns with inverse-ratio ventilation include barotrauma due to excessive auto-PEEP, hemodynamic compromise due to excessive auto-PEEP or increases in mean airway pressure, and patient tolerance.

High-Frequency Jet Ventilation

High-frequency jet ventilation delivers small tidal volumes (1–5 ml/kg) at rates of 60–3600 cycles per minute. It would be predicted to offer ventilation advantages by ventilating between lower and upper inflection points of the pressure–volume curve in patients with severe ARDS. Thus far no ARDS trials in adults have shown clinical outcome benefit.

Extracorporeal Gas Exchange

Extracorporeal gas exchange theoretically separates oxygenation (extracorporeal membrane oxygenation, or ECMO) and extracorporeal carbon dioxide removal (ECO_2R), although overlap occurs as it relates to clinical usage.[48] During ECMO a high partial pressure of oxygen on one side establishes a concentration gradient for diffusion of oxygen through a semipermeable membrane. Adequate oxygen delivery depends on high blood flow through the circuit. Effective ECO_2R is accomplished when gas flows are high across the membrane relative to blood flow because of the high solubility of CO_2 in blood. Systemic anticoagulation during extracorporeal gas exchange is essential. Extracorporeal gas exchange is morbid, cumbersome, and costly; and it is not recommended for routine use in ARDS patients. Problems encountered include blood loss related to anticoagulation, thrombocytopenia, and a need for frequent patient monitoring. Although there is justifiable enthusiasm for using the technique in infants and children, the results are not as impressive as in adults. Advanced ARDS responds poorly. It seems appropriate to consider it salvage therapy (patients not responding to other therapy). New methods of intracorporeal gas exchange such as the intravenous oxygenation device (IVOX) have also been disappointing thus far.

Prone Positioning

The CT scans obtained in patients with severe ARDS reveal severe basilar atelectasis and consolidation. Ventilation is therefore primarily directed to the more compliant nondependent areas of the lung. Significant perfusion, however, still goes to the more dependent atelectatic lung areas. Ventilation–perfusion (V/Q) matching is therefore poor, with the presence of low V/Q and shunt areas. The primary benefit of prone positioning demonstrated in some patients appears to be a shift from the previous nondependent open areas of lung to a dependent area where perfusion would be better, thereby improving V/Q matching. One could also postulate that reversal of the dorsal atelectasis would occur owing to improved drainage in the nondependent position. Atelectasis and consolidation would be expected to shift to the now-dependent anterior regions; thus a rationale for rotating the patient back and forth between prone and supine positions has been offered.

The normal smaller size of dependent alveoli relative to nondependent alveoli at functional residual capacity predisposes the lower dependent lung regions to atelectasis in the presence of disease. This gradient may be less severe in the prone position than in the supine position because of differences in the pleural pressure gradient.

In addition, teleologically there may be a better distribution of blood flow relative to ventilation in the prone position. This is because dorsal blood flow may be better preserved than ventral blood flow in the nondependent position. Studies indicate that this is the most likely reason for the improvement in oxygenation, especially as consolidation of the new dependent area and aeration of the new nondependent area occur rapidly.

Prone positioning has been shown to improve oxygenation in some patients.[49-51] If prone positioning is to be used, the earlier the better. With the initial turning to the prone position, oxygenation may temporarily deteriorate prior to improving. Not all patients improve with prone positioning. Prone positioning is difficult for maintenance of lines, tubes, and monitors. Pressure points are problematic, and both shoulders and pelvis should be cushioned with pillows.

Inhaled Nitric Oxide

When inhaled as a gas at low levels, nitric oxide (NO) selectively dilates the pulmonary circulation and may offer physiologic benefit in patients with ARDS.[52-54] Significant systemic vasodilation does not occur because NO is inactivated by rapidly binding to hemoglobin. Furthermore, in patients with ARDS inhaled NO produces greater vasodilation in areas of well ventilated lung units and may "steal" blood flow away from poorly ventilated regions, creating better V/Q matching. This reduces intrapulmonary shunting and improves arterial oxygenation. In patients with ARDS, inhaled NO reduces pulmonary hypertension and improves arterial oxygenation without reducing systemic arterial pressure. Tachyphylaxis due to inhaled nitric oxide (iNO) has not been observed. Although additional chronic toxicology studies are needed, significant pulmonary toxicity has not been observed at inhaled low concentrations. Methemoglobin is not clinically elevated at these concentrations. NO_2 is formed when NO interacts with oxygen, and NO_2 levels in the inspiratory limb are typically monitored. Inhaled NO improves oxygenation in most patients with ARDS.[55] The rationale for iNO therapy is that an improvement in PaO_2 would be associated with decreased mechanical ventilation-related lung injury. In addition, the predominance of animal data and one human study suggests an antiinflammatory effect of inhaled NO that could offer potential benefit in humans.[56-58] Because inhaled NO decreases the increased pulmonary vascular resistance in ARDS, it also decreases pulmonary capillary pressure and could decrease capillary leak.[59]

The first double-blind, placebo-controlled clinical trial of inhaled NO in ARDS was completed in 1995.[55] This multicenter study enrolled 177 patients who met the American-European consensus definition of ARDS [PaO_2/FiO_2 200 mmHg (26 kPa)]. Patients were randomized to inhaled NO at concentrations of 1, 1.25, 5, 20, 40, or 80 ppm. Investigators agreed to guidelines for prioritizing mechanical ventilatory support. Attempts to discontinue the treatment gas were made when the FiO_2 was ≤0.4 and PEEP was ≤5 cmH_2O. In most patients the etiology of ARDS was pneumonia or aspiration. Mechanical ventilation was held constant over the first 4 hours of treatment to evaluate the acute physiologic effects of NO. Approximately 60% of patients receiving inhaled NO met the defined criteria for a response (PaO_2 increase of >20%). By 4 hours, 24% of placebo patients also met the criteria for response. The response rate varied considerably over time and was not associated with outcome measures. Overall mortality was 30% for placebo and pooled inhaled NO groups. Additional outcome parameters evaluated include the number of days alive after reaching oxygenation criteria for extubation, number of days alive and off mechanical ventilation, and the percent of patients alive and off mechanical ventilation at day 28. In terms of the percent of patients alive and off mechanical ventilation at day 28, there were no significant differences noted except for a difference (by post hoc analysis) between the placebo group and the 5 ppm group. There were no significant differences in rates of adverse events across the placebo and the inhaled NO groups.

An open, randomized, parallel group study was performed at 43 sites in Europe; it was stopped in 1997 before full enrollment was completed.[60] A total of 267 patients with acute lung injury (ALI) and unilateral or bilateral pulmonary infiltrates were recruited based on criteria of intubation and mechanical ventilation for 18-96 hours, PaO_2 < 165 mmHg (22 kPa), and PEEP ≥ 5 cmH_2O. Patients were randomized to treatment groups based on their response to 2, 10, and 40 ppm NO inhaled for 10 minutes. An increase of PaO_2 of ≥25% on any dose resulted in 180 responders being randomized to conventional treatment ($m = 87$) or inhaled NO treatment ($m = 93$). The concentration of NO used was the lowest clinically effective dose as determined by the physician. Most patients received 10 ppm NO. The primary endpoint of ALI reversal [PaO_2/FiO_2 > 210-225 mmHg (28-30 kPa)] in preliminary reports was 60% in both treatment groups. Additional endpoints of survival and percent of patients alive and off mechanical ventilation of 30 days were not significantly different between conventional and inhaled NO therapy.

A multicenter, double-blind study of inhaled NO was also completed in France in 1997.[61] A total of 203 patients were enrolled in 24 centers based on Murray score of 2.5-3.0 after therapeutic optimization for 24 hours. Patients received placebo (N_2) or inhaled NO 10 ppm. One shift of gas was allowed for objective deterioration. Patients were weaned from the treatment gas when the PaO_2/FiO_2 was >250 mmHg (33 kPa) on FiO_2 1.0 for at least 4 hours. Preliminary results showed that the primary endpoint of weaning from ventilatory support at 28 days was reached in 31% with inhaled NO and 34% with placebo. Inhaled therapy was discontinued in 62% receiving inhaled NO and 56% receiving placebo. Mortality was not significantly different between the treatment groups.

A case series of 10 consecutive patients with ARDS that developed after pulmonary resection treated with inhaled NO (10–20 ppm) demonstrated significant improvement in oxygenation and good outcome.[62] Although inhaled NO improves right ventricular function in ARDS, it does not typically produce an increase in cardiac output.[63] Although not recommended for routine use in ARDS, inhaled NO should be considered for salvage therapy in patients not responding to traditional ventilation therapy. Other inhaled vasodilators, prostaglandin E_1, and prostaglandin G_2 have also been demonstrated to improve PaO_2 in patients with ARDS.[64,65] No large clinical trials have been performed to judge the effect of these agents on clinical outcome.

Partial Liquid Ventilation

Partial liquid ventilation consists of using a perfluorocarbon as a vehicle to transfer oxygen to blood and eliminate carbon dioxide in patients with severe ARDS.[66] Perfluorocarbon has relatively high density and low surface tension, and it is an efficient carrier of oxygen and carbon dioxide. Partial liquid ventilation is employed by filling the lungs to functional reserve capacity with perfluorocarbon followed by conventional mechanical ventilation of ARDS. The high density and low surface tension of perfluorocarbon appear to enhance recruitment of atelectatic lung regions. This produces a better match between pulmonary blood flow, which is primarily dependent, and ventilation. At the same time blood may be displaced to the better aerated nondependent portion of the lung. Other potential benefits of partial liquid ventilation include mobilization of debris and a possible direct antiinflammatory effect. Complications include the possibility of mucous plug formation and pneumothorax. Clinical trials have thus far been disappointing

Status of Innovative Pharmacologic Therapy

No innovative pharmacologic therapies are currently considered standard therapy, despite much interest and many clinical trials. Although clinical trials using steroids during the early phase of ARDS failed to show any benefit, some investigators now advocate the use of steroids in the later stages of ARDS, the so-called fibroproliferative phase, to decrease progression to fibrosis. Toward the end of the first week of ARDS, nonsurvivors (compared to survivors) have histologic evidence of more intense inflammatory and fibrotic activity with maladaptive lung repair.[67] Furthermore, in patients with persistent ARDS compatible with an overly exuberant fibrotic response, persistently high cytokine levels can be demonstrated in blood and BAL fluid.[68] A single-center study, somewhat handicapped by small numbers (24 patients), significant crossover, and sophisticated statistical analysis, demonstrated rather profound results in favor of steroid treatment for patients with "unresolving ARDS."[69]

Although results from this trial are promising, larger clinical trials are needed to validate this therapy.

Although ARDS may have normal amounts of surfactant, it is often dysfunctional. The potential benefit of surfactant replacement includes reduced airway pressures, improved ventilation, and reduced instances of nosocomial pneumonia. Clinical trials in adults with ARDS thus far have failed to show a significant impact of exogenous surfactant on clinical outcome.[70,71] Clinical research continues in this area.

Acetylcysteine, an oxygen scavenger, has been studied in clinical trials of ARDS and has not been shown to have an impact on clinical outcome.[72] Nonsteroidal antiinflammatory drugs, such as ibuprofen and indomethacin, inhibit prostaglandin pathways. A clinical trial in ARDS did not show benefit in clinical outcome.[73] Finally, antiendotoxin and anticytokine therapy might be expected to ameliorate ARDS by decreasing the cytokine and secondary mediator response. Thus far, multiple clinical trials in severe sepsis have not indicated any improvement in clinical outcome related to ARDS.[74]

Clinical trials in ARDS patients have been judged unsuccessful or as failures based on endpoints of mortality or days alive and off assisted ventilation. Some argue that these endpoints are unrealistic and difficult to obtain with most therapies, even if they are beneficial.[75] This position is controversial.[76]

Conclusions

The lung remains the primary affected organ in SIRS. Although the direct contribution of pulmonary dysfunction to mortality is less clear, the inability to quickly transition the patient to liberation from mechanical ventilation has major implications for iatrogenic complications and morbidity during the ICU stay. Much has been learned about the inflammatory milieu that produces and sustains ALI and ARDS. Thus far interventions targeted toward ameliorating that response have been unsuccessful. New therapies and better understanding may yet lead to success in this area. Our understanding of the potential for ventilation-induced lung injury has led to consensus recommendations on ventilation management. Several therapies that are not recommended for routine therapy of ARDS should be considered for salvage therapy. Prophylaxis to avoid iatrogenic complications during the ICU stay is important, as is adequate nutritional support.

References

1. Bernard GR, Artigas A, Brigham KL, et al: The American-European consensus conference on ARDS: definitions, mechanisms, relevant outcomes, and clinical trial coordination. Am J Respir Crit Care Med 1994;149:818–824.
2. Garber BG, Herbert PC, Yelle JD, et al: Adult respiratory distress syndrome: a systemic overview of incidence and risk factors. Crit Care Med 1996;24:687–695.
3. Bell RC, Coalson JJ, Smith JD: Multiple-organ system failure and infection in the adult respiratory distress syndrome. Ann Intern Med 1983;99:293–298.

4. Knaus WA, Sun X, Hakim RB, Wagner DP: Evaluation of definitions for adult respiratory distress syndrome. Am J Respir Crit Care Med 1994;150:311–317.
5. Herbert PC, Drummond AJ, Singer J, et al: A simple multiple system organ failure scoring system predicts mortality of patients who have sepsis syndrome. Chest 1993;104:230–235.
6. Temmesfeld-Wollbrück B, Walmrath D, Grimminger F, Seeger J: Prevention and therapy of the adult respiratory distress syndrome. Lung 1995;173:139–164.
7. Sinclair DG, Haslam PL, Quinlan GJ, et al: The effect of cardiopulmonary bypass on intestinal and pulmonary endothelial permeability. Chest 1995;108:718–724.
8. Bone RC, Balk R, Slotman G, et al: Adult respiratory distress syndrome: sequence and importance of development of multiple organ failure. Chest 1992;101:320–326.
9. Pepe PE, Potkin RT, Reus DH, et al: Clinical predictors of the adult respiratory distress syndrome. Am J Surg 1982;144:124–129.
10. Hudson LD, Milberg JA, Anaardi D, Maunder RJ: Clinical risks for development of the acute respiratory distress syndrome. Am J Respir Crit Care Med 1995;151:293–301.
11. Roumen RMH, Redl H, Schlat G, et al: Scoring systems and blood lactate concentrations in relation to the development of adult respiratory distress syndrome and multiple organ failure in severely traumatized patients. J Trauma 1993;35:349–355.
12. Slotman GJ, Quinn JV: Multivariate regression modeling for the prediction of inflammation, systemic pressure, and end-organ function in severe sepsis. Shock 1997;8:225–231.
13. Connelly KG, Moss M, Parsons PE, et al: Serum ferritin as a predictor of the acute respiratory distress syndrome. Am J Respir Crit Care Med 1997;155:21–25.
14. Donnelly SC, MacGregor I, Zamani A, et al: Plasma elastase levels and the development of the adult respiratory distress syndrome. Am J Respir Crit Care Med 1995;151:1428–1433.
15. Douzinas EE, Tsidemidou PD, Piteridis NT, et al: The regulation and production of cytokines and lactate in sepsis related multiple organ failure. Am J Respir Crit Care Med 1997;55:53–59.
16. Roumen RMH, Hendriks T, De Man BM, Goris RJA: Serum lipofuscin as a prognostic indicator of adult respiratory distress syndrome and multiple organ failure. Br J Surg 1994;81:1300–1305.
17. Montgomery AB, Stager MA, Carrico CJ, Hudson LD: Causes of mortality in patients with the adult respiratory distress syndrome. Am Rev Respir Dis 1985;132:485–489.
18. Russell JA, Ronco JJ, Lockhat D, et al: Oxygen delivery and consumption and ventricular preload are greater in survivors than in nonsurvivors of the adult respiratory distress syndrome. Am Rev Respir Dis 1990;140:659–665.
19. Suchyta RM, Clemmer TP, Elliott CG, et al: The adult respiratory distress syndrome: a report of survival and modifying factors. Chest 1992;101:1074–1079.
20. Clark JG, Milbert JA, Steinberg KP, Hudson LD: Type III procollagen peptide in the adult respiratory distress syndrome: association of increased peptide levels in bronchoalveolar lavage fluid with increased risk for death. Ann Intern Med 1995;122:17–23.
21. Donnelly SC, Strieter RM, Reid PT, et al: The association between mortality rates and decreased concentrations of interleukin-10 and interleukin-1 receptor agonist in the lung fluids of patients with the adult respiratory syndrome. Ann Intern Med 1996;125:191–196.
22. Headley AS, Tolley E, Meduri GU: Infections and the inflammatory response in acute respiratory distress syndrome. Chest 1997;111:1306–1321.
23. Milberg JA, Davis DR, Steinberg KP, Hudson LD: Improved survival of patients with acute respiratory distress syndrome (ARDS): 1983–1993. JAMA 1995;273:306–309.
24. Abel SJC, Finney SJ, Brett SJ, et al: Reduced mortality in association with the acute respiratory distress syndrome (ARDS). Thorax 1998;53:292–294.
25. Zilberberg MD, Epstein SK: Acute lung injury in the medical ICU: comorbid conditions, age, etiology, and hospital outcome. Am J Respir Crit Care Med 1998;157:1159–1164.
26. Humphrey H, Hall J, Sznajder I, et al: Improved survival in ARDS patients associated with a reduction in pulmonary capillary wedge pressure. Chest 1990;97:1176–1180.
27. Cerra FB, Maddaus MA, Dunn DL, et al: Selective gut decontamination reduces nosocomial infections and length of stay but not mortality or organ failure in surgical intensive care unit patients. Arch Surg 1992;127:163–169.
28. Garcia MS, Cambronero JA, Diaz JL, et al: Effectiveness and cost of selective decontamination of the digestive tract in critically ill incubated patients. Am J Respir Crit Care Med 1998;158:908–916.
29. Vallés J, Artigas A, Rello J, et al: Continuous aspiration of subglottic secretions in preventing ventilator-associated pneumonia. Ann Intern Med 1995;122:179–186.
30. Chastre J, Fagon JY: Invasive diagnostic testing should be routinely used to manage ventilated patients with suspected pneumonia. Am J Respir Crit Care Med 1994;150:570–574.
31. Bonten MJM, Bergmans CJJ, Stobberingh EE, et al: Implementation of bronchoscopic techniques in the diagnosis of ventilator-associated pneumonia to reduce antibiotic use. Am J Respir Crit Care Med 1997;156:1820–1824.
32. Niederman MS, Torres A, Summer W: Invasive diagnostic testing is not needed routinely to manage suspect ventilator-associated pneumonia. Am J Respir Crit Care Med 1994;150:565–569.
33. Souweine B, Veber B, Bedos JP, et al: Diagnostic accuracy of protected specimen brush and bronchoalveolar lavage in nosocomial pneumonia: impact of previous antimicrobial treatments. Crit Care Med 1998;26:236–244.
34. Heyland DK, MacDonald S, Keefe L, Drover JW: Total parenteral nutrition in the critically ill patient: a meta-analysis. JAMA 1998;280:2013–2019.
35. Mead J, Takishima T, Leith D: Stress distribution in lungs: a model of pulmonary elasticity. J Appl Physiol 1970;28:596–608.
36. Marini JJ: Ventilation of the acute respiratory distress syndrome: looking for Mr. Goodmode [editorial]. Anesthesiology 1994;80:972–974.
37. Slutsky AS, Tremblay LN: Multiple system organ failure: is mechanical ventilation a contributing factor? Am J Respir Crit Care Med 1998;157:1721–1725.
38. Desai SR, Hansell DM: Lung imaging in the adult respiratory distress syndrome: current practice and new insights. Intensive Care Med 1997;23:7–15.
39. Marini JJ: Tidal volume, PEEP and barotrauma: an open shut case [editorial]? Chest 1996;109:302–304.

40. Tuxen DV: Permissive hypercapnic ventilation. Am J Respir Crit Care Med 1994;150:870–874.
41. Balk R: Permissive hypercapnia: an alternative ventilatory mode for the management of acute lung injury and acute airflow obstruction. Clin Pulm Med 1997;4:29–33.
42. Stewart TE, Meade MO, Cook DJ, et al: Evaluation of a ventilation strategy to prevent barotrauma in patients at high risk for acute respiratory distress syndrome. N Engl J Med 1998;338:255–361.
43. Amato MBP, Barbas CSV, Medeiros DM, et al: Effect of a protective-ventilation strategy on mortality in the acute respiratory distress syndrome. N Engl J Med 1998;338:347–354.
44. Artigas A, Bernard GR, Carlet J, et al: The American-European consensus conference on ARDS. Part 2. Ventilatory, pharmacologic, supportive therapy, study design strategies, and issues related to recovery and remodeling. Am J Respir Crit Care Med 1998;157:1332–1347.
45. Armstrong BW, MacIntyre NR: Pressure-controlled, inverse ratio ventilation that avoids air trapping in the adult respiratory distress syndrome. Crit Care Med 1995;23:279–285.
46. Rappaport SH, Shpiner R, Yoshihara G, Wright J, Chang P, Abraham E: Randomized, prospective trial of pressure-limited versus volume-controlled ventilation in severe respiratory failure. Crit Care Med 1994;22:22–32.
47. Tharratt RS, Allen RP, Albertson TE: Pressure controlled inverse ratio ventilation in severe adult respiratory failure. Chest 1988;94:755–762.
48. Barie PS: Organ-specific support in multiple organ failure: pulmonary support. World J Surg 1995;19:581–591.
49. Marini JJ: Down side up—a prone and partial liquid asset. Intensive Care Med 1995;21:963–965.
50. Pappert D, Rossaint R, Slama K, Gruning T, Falke KJ: Influence of positioning on ventilation-perfusion relationships in severe adult respiratory distress syndrome. Chest 1994;106:1511–1516.
51. Pelosi P, Tubiolo D, Mascheroni D, et al: Effects of the prone position on respiratory mechanics and gas exchange during acute lung injury. Am J Respir Crit Care Med 1998;157:387–393.
52. Dellinger RP: Inhaled nitric oxide in cardiopulmonary disease. In: Cernaianu AC (ed) Critical Issues in Surgery. New York, Plenum (in press).
53. Rossaint R, Falke, KF, Lopez F, et al: Inhaled nitric oxide for the adult respiratory distress syndrome. N Engl J Med 1993;328:399–405.
54. Puybasset L, Rouby JJ, Mourgeon E, et al: Inhaled nitric oxide in acute respiratory failure: dose-response curves. Intensive Care Med 1994;20:319–327.
55. Dellinger RP, Zimmerman JL, Taylor RW, et al: Effects of inhaled nitric oxide in patients with acute respiratory distress syndrome: results of a randomized phase II trial. Crit Care Med 1998;26:15–23.
56. Kavanagh B, Mouchawar A, Goldsmith J, Pearl R: Effects of inhaled NO and inhibition of endogenous NO synthesis in oxidant-induced acute lung injury. J Appl Physiol 1994;76:1324–1329.
57. Poss W, Timmons O, Farrukh I, et al: Inhaled nitric oxide prevents the increase in pulmonary vascular permeability caused by hydrogen peroxide. J Appl Physiol 1995;79:886–891.
58. Chollet-Martin S, Gatecel C, Kermarrec N, et al: Alveolar neutrophil functions and cytokine levels in patients with adult respiratory distress syndrome during nitric oxide inhalation. Am J Respir Crit Care Med 1996;153:985–990.
59. Benzing A, Brautigam P, Geiger K, et al: Inhaled nitric oxide reduces pulmonary transvascular albumin flux in patients with acute lung injury. Anesthesiology 1995;83:1153–1161.
60. Lundin S, Mang H, Smithies M, et al: Inhalation of nitric oxide in acute lung injury: preliminary results of a European multicenter study. Intensive Care Med 1997;23(Suppl 1):S2.
61. Groupe d'Etude sur le NO Inhale' au Course le l'ARDS (GENOA): Inhaled NO ARDS: presentation of double blind randomized multicentric study [abstract]. Am J Respir Crit Care Med 1996;153:A590.
62. Mathisen DJ, Kuo EY, Hahn C, et al: Inhaled nitric oxide for adult respiratory distress syndrome after pulmonary resection. Ann Thorac Surg 1998;65:1–9.
63. Rossaint R, Slama K, Steudel W, et al: Effects of inhaled nitric oxide on right ventricular function in severe acute respiratory distress syndrome. Intensive Care Med 1995;21:97–203.
64. Meyer J, Theilmeier G, Van Aken H, et al: Inhaled prostaglandin E_1 for treatment of acute lung injury in severe multiple organ failure. Anesth Analg 1998;86:753–758.
65. Pappert D, Busch T, Gerlach G, et al: Aerosolized prostacyclin versus inhaled nitric oxide in children with severe acute respiratory distress syndrome. Anesthesiology 1995;82:1507–1511.
66. Hirschl RB, Pranikoff T, Wise C, et al: Initial experience with partial liquid ventilation in adult patients with the acute respiratory distress syndrome. JAMA 1996;275:383–389.
67. Meduri GU: The role of the host defense response in the progression and outcome of ARDS: pathophysiological correlations and response to glucocorticoid treatment. Eur Respir J 1996;9:2650–2670.
68. Headley AS, Tolley E, Meduri GU: Infections and the inflammatory response in acute respiratory distress syndrome. Chest 1997;111:1306–1321.
69. Meduri GU, Headley AS, Golden E, et al: Effect of prolonged methylprednisolone therapy in unresolving acute respiratory distress syndrome. JAMA 1998;280:159–165.
70. Anzueto A, Baughman RP, Guntupalli KK, et al: Aerosolized surfactant in adults with sepsis-induced acute respiratory distress syndrome: Exosurf Acute Respiratory Distress Syndrome Sepsis Study Group. N Engl J Med 1996;334:1417–1421.
71. Arnold J: Surfactant replacement in acute lung injury—the saga continues. Crit Care Med 1999;27:31–32.
72. Jepsen S, Herlevsen P, Knudsen P, Bud MI, Klausen NO: Antioxidant treatment with N-acetylcysteine during adult respiratory distress syndrome: a prospective, randomized, placebo-controlled study. Crit Care Med 1992;20:918–923.
73. Bernard GR, Wheeler AP, Russell JA, et al: The effects of ibuprofen on the physiology and survival of patients with sepsis. N Engl J Med 1997;336:912–918.

74. Dellinger RP: Severe sepsis: any hope? In: Cernaianu AC (ed) Critical Issues in Surgery. New York, Plenum (in press).
75. Fuhrman BP, Abraham E, Dellinger RP: Futility of randomized, controlled ARDS trials: a new approach is needed. Crit Care Med 1999;27:431–433.
76. Bernard G: Research in sepsis and acute respiratory distress syndrome: are we changing course? Crit Care Med 1999;27:434–436.

37
Renal Function and Dysfunction in Multiple Organ Failure

Richard J. Mullins

This chapter is a review of renal function and dysfunction within the context of the inflammatory response to injury, ischemia, and infection. Available information with direct applicability to clinical circumstances is emphasized. A brief, selective summary of renal function is included to provide a framework of comparison when dysfunction is described. The role of therapies that modify the inflammatory response to benefit patients is examined from the perspective of effectiveness against systemic manifestations and renal toxicity.

Renal Dysfunction and Renal Failure: Historical Perspective

The onset of acute renal failure (ARF) in a critically ill intensive care unit (ICU) patient has remained a lethal complication for 50 years. Despite substantial investigative efforts to develop treatments that salvage the damaged nephron, once established ARF usually requires renal replacement therapy during the days to weeks required for recovery of renal function.[1] Hemodialysis has been perfected, and new renal replacement techniques have been developed; but they have not improved survival.[2,3] Patients burdened with ARF have a more than 50% probability of death.[4,5] An increasing proportion of patients in the ICU who develop ARF have multiple organ failure associated with sepsis.[6-8] In these patients the onset of ARF follows a systemic inflammatory response syndrome (SIRS), and a principal goal for physicians and surgeons must be effective treatment to prevent ARF during the early phases of SIRS. Many patients with ARF have a prodromal period of renal function deterioration related to ischemia; and adjuvant interventions that restore renal perfusion, when accomplished promptly, can preserve renal function.

The concept that renal dysfunction/failure is a secondary consequence of events remote from the kidney is well established. During World War II, when renal failure as a distinct phenomenon was noted among London's citizens with extremities crushed by falling debris, the concept that a remote organ injury could mediate renal toxicity was defined by careful clinical observation and postmortem study. Rhabdomyolysis was established as a cause of renal failure early during the war.[9]

By the end of World War II, the death rate for wounded soldiers who developed renal failure exceeded 80%.[10] Autopsy studies of patients with ARF, after being resuscitated from hemorrhage with blood transfusion, were noted to have a characteristic renal lesion, initially termed "lower nephron nephrosis" but subsequently widely designated "acute tubular necrosis".[11] The principal role of ischemia as the adverse event causing renal failure was recognized, prompting development of the concept that "prerenal" mechanisms lead to ischemia, renal dysfunction (oliguria), and when severe, renal failure (anuria). The therapeutic implications of recognizing that ischemia is a principal cause of ARF were clear to surgeons resuscitating patients in shock. Prompt, effective restoration of intravascular volume to restore renal perfusion was essential to avert ARF.

With the introduction of renal replacement therapy during the late 1940s, there was hope that death rates for patients who developed ARF would improve. The efficacy of dialysis for managing short-term problems such as potassium intoxication and uremia was established;[10] however, dialysis did not regularly enable patients with ARF to have a better than 50% chance of long-term survival. It was clear from careful study of wounded soldiers aggressively treated during the Korean War who developed ARF that infection was a condition frequently associated with death.[12] The association of infection and renal dysfunction was advanced by other investigators. Strauch et al., in the Clinical Shock Trauma Unit at the University of Maryland, noted in 1967 that patients in septic shock with renal dysfunction had a decreased glomerular filtration rate, which they attributed to a decrease in renal blood flow. Renal failure was directly linked to death in these patients.[13] At the same time, reports from Southeast Asia on treatment of military personnel who developed renal failure concluded that "infection was the direct cause in 72% of deaths."[14]

Renal Failure as a Component of Multiple Organ Failure Syndrome

Two clinical reports regarding ARF published during the early 1970s reported that the nature of renal failure in surgical practice was changing. Berne and Barbour noted that renal failure patients most commonly expired with sepsis, gastrointestinal (GI) bleeding, and pulmonary insufficiency.[15] Tilney et al. reported that patients who developed renal failure after successful surgery on a ruptured abdominal aortic aneurysm died not of their renal failure but of irreversible deterioration in the function of other organ systems.[16] In a 1975 editorial, Fischer and Polk pronounced that gram-negative sepsis had displaced hemorrhagic shock as the principal etiology of ARF.[17] Renal failure, although manageable with hemodialysis, was a highly lethal complication when it developed in patients after surgery. It was apparent that successful treatment of the site of infection, often an intraabdominal infection, was an essential therapeutic goal.

In 1975 Baue described the three essential characteristics of what he proposed were the weak links in the capability of ICUs to treat injured patients: failure of multiple organs in a progressive or sequential manner that culminates in an overwhelming, fatal insult.[18] As the pathophysiology for multiple system organ failure was investigated, the prevalence of uncontrolled infection and dominance of lung failure, or adult respiratory distress syndrome (ARDS), was identified.[19] Faist et al. reviewed a cohort of trauma patients, principally individuals with multiple injuries following motor vehicle collisions, and defined two patterns of organ failure. Early organ failure was rapidly progressive, associated with irreversible shock, and designated by the authors as the single-phase syndrome. The two-phase syndrome of multiple organ failure they described occurred in patients typically recovering from their initial insult when a second septic insult led to deterioration of organ function. In the series reported by Faist et al. 19% of patients developed organ failure; and of these, 27% had renal failure with a 61% mortality rate.[20] The authors corroborated an observation previously made by Eiseman et al. that a common theme in the clinical course of patients with organ failure was identifiable errors in management.[21] During the 1980s a hypothesis regarding the cause of multiple organ failure that came to be widely supported proposed that organ damage was the consequence of the excessive endogenous inflammatory response to an insult that was commonly, but not always, culture-proven infection.[22,23] A new challenge to providing optimal critical care to seriously ill or injured patients was to develop methods for modulating or blunting the adverse influence of a systemic response to infection without simultaneously depriving the patient of immunocompetence to resist pathogenic invasion.

Renal Dysfunction Leads to Renal Failure

Renal failure is a component of multiple organ failure syndrome in 20–40% of patients who develop the syndrome[24] (Table 37.1). In most series patients with renal failure are stratified based on the maximum elevation of their serum creatinine level: mild (1–2 mg/dl), moderate (2–4 mg/dl), or severe (>5 mg/dl) renal dysfunction and failure. Most patients have oliguria. In addition to the endogenous inflammatory insult, there can be multiple specific causes of renal failure in these critically ill patients, including toxicity caused by drugs or contrast agents, hypovolemic shock, or the abdominal compartment syndrome. Most patients with renal failure have oliguria that can progress to anuria. The serum creatinine level as an indication of impaired glomerular filtration is useful in circumstances where events occur over several days. However, serum creatinine is less useful as an immediate indicator of renal dysfunction because there is a delay in creatinine level rise in the presence of acute onset of impaired renal function.

Impaired renal function occurs over a range of severity, and patients who meet the criteria of the most severe loss of renal function are those in acute renal failure requiring renal replacement therapy for survival. Liano et al. reported a mean maximal elevation in serum creatinine of 5.2 ± 2.3 mg/dl among a cohort of patients treated in regional ICUs around Madrid, Spain who developed renal impairment.[25] More than 70% of these patients

TABLE 37.1. Prevalence of Renal Failure in At-Risk Patients.

Year	Author	Population characteristics	% Organ failure	% Renal failure (of organ failure group)	Comments
1980	Fry	Emergency surgical	7	—	Cause was uncontrolled infection
1983	Faist	Multiple trauma	19	27 (mortality 61)	As the number of failed organs increases, death rate increases
1991	Martin	Postoperative patients with shock or sepsis	54	64	
1991	Ruokonen	Septic shock	3 early, 8 late		
1996	Zimmerman	ICU patients	46, 14	42	No substantial change in mortality over 8 years of study
1996	Moore	High risk trauma	15	37 early, 9 late	One organ failure
1996	Cohen	Septic patients	63 one organ 44 two or more	26 of survivors with ARF	Early and late second hit

ARF, acute renal failure.

had renal function deterioration to a level requiring dialysis. In most cases the pathologic diagnosis for these patients was acute tubular necrosis (ATN), and the authors designated "sepsis" as the cause of ATN in 35% of patients, although they added the caveat that in some cases the cause was multifactorial. The duration of renal impairment among the patients who survived was 17 ± 17 days. The average duration of dialysis was 2 weeks, and the mortality rate was 71% for this group of patients. Recovery of renal function was the rule for those who survived. Among patients discharged alive from the hospital, 90% had return of renal function by 45 days. The range of renal impairment is consistent with the concept that the injury to tissue in patients with multiple organ dysfunction is proportional to the intensity of activation of inflammatory mediators.[24]

Clinical Diagnosis of SIRS and Renal Failure

Consensus Conference Definition of SIRS

In 1991 the American College of Chest Physicians and the Society of Critical Care Medicine co-sponsored a consensus conference chaired by Richard C. Bone. The conference intended to bring together experts in critical care for the purpose of defining the relation between SIRS, infection, and organ failure.[26] Variability in the terminology used by investigators was identified as an impediment to making informed comparisons among clinical studies, and members of the conference deliberated and produced a glossary. There was agreement that the problem for many patients with life-threatening infection was a combination of invasive destruction of an infected organ and the patient's own systemic inflammatory response, producing dysfunction in multiple organs remote from the site of infection. The SIRS hypothesis held that an induced inflammatory response that resulted in organ damage remote from the site of infection was as much a threat to the patient as the infection itself.

Members of the consensus conference agreed on definitions for the essential terminology of SIRS.[26] They thought that investigators speaking the same language are more efficient and reliable in their communication. *Infection* was defined as the circumstance of microbial invasion. In response to infection, the organism can mount a systemic response, *sepsis*, characterized by fever, tachycardia, tachypnea, and an elevated white blood cell count with a shift of immature neutrophils of more than 10%. The *systemic inflammatory response syndrome* has characteristics identical to those of sepsis but is a process in response to events other than infection.

A fundamental concept of this conference was that SIRS is a phenomenon involving the entire body, and that it is this endogenous inflammatory response that mediates organ failure. A critical distinction made at this conference was that infection-based *sepsis* or other proinflammatory insults (i.e., pancreatitis, burns, trauma, sterile peritonitis) are capable of inducing the SIRS response.

The consensus conference further elaborated on a range of severity in patients with *sepsis* (SIRS due to infection) and proposed terms to account for the range of severity. *Bacteremia* was defined as the circumstance of viable bacteria being cultured from blood. *Severe sepsis* was sepsis characterized by organ dysfunction attributable to hypoperfusion. Severely septic patients show evidence of inadequate oxygen delivery even with normal vital signs. This evidence includes acidosis, oliguria, and decreased mental status. *Septic shock* is a quantum increase in severity from severe sepsis in which hypotension persists despite adequate intravascular volume resuscitation. The consensus conference referred to clinical series where these distinctions applied to populations of hospitalized patients in ICUs and enabled the populations to be categorized—even on the first day of ICU admission—into subpopulations with graded risks for morbidity and mortality.

The consensus conference members advocated use of the term multiple organ dysfunction syndrome (MODS) to represent the circumstance of an acutely ill patient with SIRS whose organ dysfunction requires medical therapy to sustain homeostasis. MODS was further qualified to encompass a continuum ranging from mild disruptions of normal function to total organ failure. Conference members further emphasized that primary MODS is the direct result of the inciting insult (renal failure due to rhabdomyolysis), whereas secondary MODS differs; secondary MODS is the consequence of the inflammatory response of the host with infection, *sepsis*, *septic shock*, or another proinflammatory event capable of causing SIRS, such as trauma, pancreatitis, or burns. In either circumstance the patient's outcome often becomes more dependent on successful management of the MODS than of the primary event. On the other hand, timely, effective therapy of the primary event causing MODS is often the most effective intervention for ameliorating the host inflammatory response causing MODS.

Natural History of Patients with SIRS

The definitions developed at the consensus conference on SIRS were rigorously evaluated by Rangel-Frausto et al. in a prospective cohort analysis of patients in a tertiary care hospital[27] (Table 37.2). Diligent examination of medical records revealed 2527 patients who met the criteria of SIRS. Among those with SIRS, only 26% had culture-proven infection and thus could be classified as having sepsis. A fundamental concept to the conclusions of the consensus conference was that the endogenous inflammatory response is a continuum ranging from the relatively benign SIRS through stages with increasing risk of morbidity and mortality designated by the terms *sepsis*, *severe sepsis*, and *septic shock*. The authors confirmed the hypothesis that clinical progression occurred; patients first noted to meet the criteria of a lower risk category were later noted to meet criteria for a higher risk category. The SIRS population studied could be divided into 26% with *sepsis*, 18% with *severe sepsis*, and 4% with *septic shock*. This study also supported the hypothesis of graded risk by category. Hospital death rates ranged from 7% among those with SIRS to 16%, 20%, and 46% for the patients

TABLE 37.2. Prevalence of Renal Dysfunction and Failure Among 2527 Patients with Two or More Criteria of SIRS, Divided into the Four Stages of the MOF Syndrome.

Syndrome[a]	Acute renal failure (%)
SIRS	
Two criteria (100%)	9
Three criteria	13
Four criteria	19
Sepsis	
Culture-positive (26%)	19
Culture-negative (35%)	5
Severe sepsis	
Culture-positive (18%)	23
Culture-negative (21%)	16
Septic shock	
Culture-positive (4%)	51
Culture-negative (3%)	38

Modified from Rangel-Frausto et al.,[27] with permission.
[a]Numbers in parentheses represent the percent of the population defined as having SIRS.
*$p < 0.05$ compared to culture-negative population.

categorized, respectively, as having *sepsis*, *severe sepsis*, and *septic shock*. Furthermore, there was an additional substantial risk of death after hospital discharge for patients with SIRS. An important distinction made in this study was the high prevalence of patients who met criteria for having *sepsis*, *severe sepsis*, and *septic shock* but did not have cultures confirming infection. The prospective study of Rangel-Frausto et al. described a natural history to SIRS in their population of patients in a tertiary care hospital.[27]

Normal Renal Structure and Function

This section provides a brief overview of the structure and functional aspects of the kidney to develop a background to the discussion of renal dysfunction associated with multiple organ failure syndromes. The two kidneys in the normal adult contain more than 2 million nephrons. The nephron is the fundamental structural unit of renal function. Functionally, the nephron begins at the interface of the endothelium of the renal glomerular capillaries and the visceral epithelium of Bowman's capsule. These two luminal surfaces adhere to a glomerular basement membrane. A critical structural characteristic of the endothelium and epithelium in the renal glomerulus are the fenestrae, or slit-like openings, which cover more than 10% of the capillary surface area and are sites of high permeability. The fenestrae allow filtration of plasma, which is the cardinal function of the nephron. The glomeruli are visible in the outer cortical layer of the bivalved kidney as renal corpuscles. The filtrate in Bowman's capsule flows into a proximal convoluted tubule and then through the loop of Henle, which descends toward the renal hilum in the medullary, or inner, layer of the kidney before reversing completely to return to the cortex and the distal convoluted tubule. A segment of the distal convoluted tubule returns to the hilum of the glomerulus and forms the juxtaglomerular apparatus with the afferent and efferent vessels; this structure is important in nephron regulation. The distal convoluted tubule continues until it fuses with an embryologic extension of the ureteric bud and becomes confluent with the collecting ducts. The collecting ducts descend through the medullary portion of the kidney adjacent to the loop of Henle before the filtrate is delivered into the renal pelvis for excretion.

Glomerular filtration is the cardinal event of renal function. Blood flows through afferent arterioles into the glomerular capillary tufts. The selective filtration of water and small solutes into the Bowman's capsule is quantitatively determined by the hydrostatic pressure in the capillaries. Normally, albumin is not filtered owing to the electrostatic characteristics of the matrix constituting the basement membrane. Efferent arterioles end in a second capillary network surrounding the tubules, which enables retrieval of a high percentage of filtered water and sodium back to the plasma compartment. The adjacent proximity of the vascular endothelium and tubular epithelium in nephrons enables filtration and reabsorption to occur. The permeability characteristics of the capillary are not fixed. Mesangial cells in the interstices of the glomerular tuft adhere to the basement membrane. Receptors to many of the paracrine mediators produced by the endothelium and juxtaglomerular apparatus have been identified on the surfaces of these interstitial mesangial cells. Actin and myosin fibers within the mesangial cells contract, alter the shape of the cells of the glomerular filtration barrier, and reduce permeability characteristics of the barrier. This mechanism joins with adjustments in afferent and efferent arteriolar tone as the means for intrarenal regulation of the glomerular filtration rate (GFR).

As blood flows from the glomerulus into the efferent arteriole, the plasma protein concentration and consequently the colloid pressure increase. The increased oncotic pressure in blood flowing into efferent arterioles, which drain the glomerular capillary tufts, provides a driving force for reabsorption of selected filtrate back into the plasma compartment. However, aerobic metabolism is the essential first step in sustaining active sodium reabsorption from the tubular lumen. The oxygen consumption of the tubular cells is used to generate the large amounts of energy consumed by enzyme-supported active reabsorption of selected solutes. The substantial oxygen needs of these cells helps explain why renal blood flow is disproportionate to total cardiac output. Insufficient oxygen delivery stresses these tubular cells, and this shock can rapidly lead to impaired function.

Renal mass is 0.5% of the total body mass, whereas renal blood flow is more than 20% of the cardiac output. This disproportionate blood flow enables sufficient filtration of plasma to occur to achieve a plasma clearance that easily accomplishes purification of water in both the intracellular and extracellular compartments. In a 70- to 75-kg adult renal blood flow is 1000–1200 ml/min, corresponding to the approximately 700 ml/min of renal plasma flow. Twenty percent of the plasma is filtered, and thus a normal GFR lies between 120 and 140 ml/min (7200–8400 ml of filtrate per hour). The urine output of 50–100 ml/hr corresponds to water and solutes not reabsorbed from the filtrate. The selective reabsorption of more than 95% of water and sodium filtered by the glomerulus, along with other solutes, is the physiologic mechanism that enables purification of the extracellular fluid. The filtration and immediate reabsorption of filtered plasma is also the basis for renal control of the size and composition of the extracellular space, including the plasma compartment.

Glomerular filtration is a closely regulated process. The vascular tone of the afferent and efferent arterioles determines the hydrostatic pressure in the glomerular capillaries, which is the driving force for filtration. Adjustments in the resistance of afferent or efferent arterioles (or both) enable the glomerular capillary pressure to be maintained over a wide range of systemic pressures. This autoregulation of the GFR is accomplished through multiple mediators. If the systemic arterial pressure drops, afferent arterioles can vasodilate and glomerular filtration is sustained. The myogenic response of the afferent arteriole is a stretch-activated vasoconstriction of these vessels in reaction to increased intraluminal pressure. The myogenic response prevents the glomerular capillary pressure from becoming high when systemic pressure is elevated. Glomerular filtration pressure regulation is additionally influenced by adjusted changes in efferent arteriolar tone. Specifically, vasoconstriction of these vessels distal to the glomerulus causes a retrograde increase in the pressures driving glomerular filtration. Hormones and other mediators of both vasoconstriction and vasodilation of the afferent and efferent arterioles have been identified. The regulation of glomerular filtration is complex, and the vascular tone of the afferent and efferent arterioles is the summation of multiple antagonistic influences.

The reabsorption of filtered sodium from tubular fluid occurs via several mechanisms of active transport along the length of the nephron's tubules. Active transport is accomplished by oxygen consumption. Most sodium is transported with chloride in the proximal tubule. In the distal tubule, exchange of tubular sodium for potassium or a proton enables the kidney to modulate the extracellular potassium concentration and acid–base balance. The loop of Henle segment of the nephron in the medullary portion of the kidney enables function of a countercurrent mechanism and produces hyperosmolar interstitium. This hyperosmolarity acts as the driving force to produce concentrated urine—conserving the body's water—when the presence of adequate levels of arginine vasopressin facilitate water transport back to the plasma compartment from the filtrate in tubules.

The kidney is an endocrine organ by several criteria. Cells in the juxtaglomerular apparatus produce the hormone renin, which, following a series of steps, leads to production of the potent vasoconstrictor angiotensin II. Aldosterone is released from the adrenal gland in response to angiotensin II and directs the distal tubules to retrieve more sodium from the filtrate. The paracrine function of the tubuloglomerular feedback has an important regulatory function; as the amount of sodium delivered to the macula densa segment of the distal tubule increases, vasoconstrictors are locally released that increase afferent arteriolar tone and reduce glomerular filtration. Less filtration reduces sodium loss into the filtrate. This feedback loop is an important method for preventing a renal-caused critical reduction in extracellular volume.

Renal Pathophysiology in SIRS

Renal Ischemia

Renal ischemia, with all of its manifestations, can occur in patients with SIRS. Patients who develop *septic shock* are at highest risk for renal dysfunction. The decline in renal perfusion can be attributed to the systemic hypotension that develops in these patients. The low blood pressure characteristic of septic shock occurs for several reasons.[28]

A commonly reported observation in hypotensive patients with septic shock is hyperdynamic circulation. These patients have cardiac outputs severalfold greater than normal. The diffuse vasodilation of the systemic circulation is attributed to a release of cytokines and the secondary mediators of smooth muscle relaxation they generate. The hypotension of the hyperdynamic circulation in sepsis reduces perfusion pressure in the renal artery; and when compensatory adjustments in the afferent and efferent arterioles fail to sustain glomerular filtration pressure, the filtration rate declines.[29] Lower perfusion pressure also corresponds to the adverse circumstance of insufficient blood flow to the renal medullary segments, where the susceptible tubular cells become hypoxic and dysfunctional. The mechanism of renal dysfunction in the ischemic kidney varies depending on the severity of the hypoxic insult to the tubule cells. With profound renal ischemia, the tubule cells necrose and slough into and occlude the renal tubules, producing a blockade of tubule filtrate flow. In the less severe ischemic circumstances of reduced blood flow into the efferent arteriole due to vasoconstriction, there are more subtle structural and functional changes in the oxygen-deprived tubule cells. The consequence is not necrosis but failure of the active transport of sodium from tubular fluid. As large amounts of sodium are delivered to the macula densa located in the juxtaglomerular apparatus, there is marked paracrine-directed vasoconstriction of the afferent arteriole, which further shuts down glomerular filtration and exacerbates tubular cell hypoxia. Thus a hyperdynamic circulation may indicate inadequate renal perfusion pressures and account for renal dysfunction and failure.

The syndrome of acute tubular necrosis as a consequence of hypovolemic shock is a recognized complication.[30] With hypovolemic shock, the patient's compensatory mechanisms lead to profound vasoconstriction, in contrast to the vasodilation of septic shock. The profound vasoconstriction is mediated through circulating vasoconstrictors such as arginine vasopressin and epinephrine. Increased sympathetic nervous system tone leads to the release of norepinephrine and α-adrenergic-mediated vasoconstriction. Hypotensive SIRS patients are often hypovolemic, and their mean arterial pressures improve if given intravenous fluid and blood. Septic patients develop hypovolemia following substantial extravasation of plasma proteins and fluid into edema and fluid collections related to infection. These findings therapeutically imply it is essential to restore intravascular volume by fluid infusion to restore renal function.

The inflammatory cascade induced by infection includes the production of the cytokines tumor necrosis factor-α (TNFα) and interleukin-6 (IL-6). The association of elevated levels of these mediators and renal dysfunction has been demonstrated. Navasa et al. examined a group of patients with spontaneous bacterial peritonitis and cirrhosis of the liver.[31] They reported elevated levels of TNFα and IL-6 measured in the ascites fluid and plasma of patients with spontaneous bacterial peritonitis. The three independent factors in a prediction model that indicated risk for renal impairment were the existence of preexisting renal impairment, elevated IL-6 levels in ascites fluid, and hypotension. This and other studies support the pathophysiologic role of cytokines as initial mediators of the lethal organ failure syndrome in patients with severe sepsis and septic shock.[32,33]

Mixed Role of Nitric Oxide in SIRS-Related Renal Impairment

Nitric oxide (NO) is a potent mediator of several cellular functions, including vasodilation[34,35] (Table 37.3). NO is a small gas molecule generated from L-arginine and oxygen in an enzyme-directed reaction described as NO synthesis. Two categories of nitric oxide synthase have been identified. The constitutive form is found in endothelial cells (eNOS) and produces NO in nanomolar concentrations. This amount of NO is sufficient to accomplish modest arteriole vasodilation through cyclic guanosine monophosphate (cGMP), and constitutive eNOS is a mechanism for maintaining vasomotor tone in normal circumstances. The inducible form of nitric oxide synthase (iNOS) is made as part of an inflammatory response through stimulation of the macrophage nucleus when cytokines bind to the inflammatory cell surface. The amount of NO produced by the iNOS isoform is several magnitudes greater than the NO produced by eNOS. At these relatively large concentrations, NO acts as a vasodilator but also prevents platelet and leukocyte adhesion. NO in large concentrations can have a direct toxic effect on cells. NO is normally cleared rapidly by conversion to nitrate and nitrite compounds; and its brief duration means its effectiveness as a mediator depends on the function of the isoforms of NOS. These enzymes have been the focus of pharmacologic manipulation.

Considerable evidence has accumulated that NO is a mediator of events, both adverse and beneficial, in septic shock. Experimental studies of animal models of septic shock have depended on measurement of nitrate and nitrite concentrations. When drugs that blocked both eNOS and iNOS were given to sheep with a hyperdynamic circulation in response to endotoxemia, the hyperdynamic state was reversed without evidence of impaired oxygen metabolism with less oxygen delivery.[36] This and similar studies suggest that blockade of NO may have therapeutic benefit. Human studies of patients with SIRS, sepsis syndrome, and septic shock have supported the hypothesis that hemodynamic changes of lowered systemic vascular resistance and hypotension are associated with increased NO synthesis.[35,37] Currently, studies are being conducted to determine if blockade of iNOS improves the survival rate of patients with septic shock and a hyperdynamic circulation.

There is experimental and some clinical evidence that NO can have a direct role as a toxic mediator in SIRS that causes renal dysfunction. The nanomolar amounts of NO produced by constitutive eNOS help to sustain glomerular filtration pressure over a range of perfusion pressures. The effects of this constitutive NOS in normal human volunteers was examined by Bech et al. in a study of renal plasma flow, GFR, and urinary sodium excretion before and after administration of a specific competitive inhibitor of NOS.[38] Suppression of NO synthesis led to a reduction in renal plasma flow and a 10% decline in GFR. The urine flow rate and sodium excretion was suppressed by more than 30%. The authors concluded that NO is a tonic vasodilator of the renal vasculature in normal circumstances, and that the micromolar amounts of NO produced by inflammatory cells are pathologic.

There are two mechanisms by which NO impairs renal function. The hyperdynamic circulation with low systemic vascular resistance (SVR) and hypotension in septic patients with systemic activation of iNOS carries the consequence that perfusion pressure in the renal circulation is inadequate to sustain glomerular filtration. This mechanism has been supported by the clinical observation that modest doses of α-adrenergic vasoconstrictors in septic patients with low SVR improve the systolic pressure sufficiently to restore renal function.

There are also directly toxic changes in the nephron caused by NO that may explain the severe renal dysfunction and renal failure of septic shock patients. Groeneveld et al. reported that patients with *severe sepsis* have elevated serum nitrate levels that correlate with the magnitude of renal dysfunction.[39] Serum nitrate is a by-product of effervescent NO. The authors concluded that a transient insult occurs during the initial phase of septic shock which initiates events that subsequently become evident as renal dysfunction. They speculated that excessive NO levels in renal circulation and urine may be directly toxic to

TABLE 37.3. Vasomotor Control of Glomerular Filtration.

Anatomic site	Vasodilation	Vasoconstriction
Afferent arteriole	eNOS → ↑ NO iNOS → ↑ NO Less TGF	Adenosine Myogenic response More TGF Angiotensin II
Efferent arteriole	Adenosine PGE$_2$, prostacyclin NO	Angiotensin II Norepinephrine (sympathetic)

NO, nitric oxide; eNOS, iNOS, constitutive nitric oxide synthetase; TGF, tubuloglomerular feedback in which the more sodium delivered to the distal tubule, the more the macula densa mediates afferent arteriole vasoconstriction; PGE$_2$, prostaglandin E$_2$.

renal tubular cells. These observations imply that antagonist therapy directed against NO must be instituted early during the septic insult to be effective.

Spain et al. have examined the influence of NOS blockade on renal microcirculation in the rat using a model of videomicroscopy that measures the diameter of afferent arterioles.[40] In control rats, blockade of NOS caused a 26% reduction in renal afferent arteriole diameter. This vasoconstriction was attributed to the action of the drug on eNOS. The investigators produced a hyperdynamic sepsis model and noted that the afferent arteriole was vasoconstricted despite increased cardiac output, indicating paradoxical renal vasoconstriction during sepsis despite generalized vasodilation. The authors carried their investigation one step further by administering NOS blockade to septic rats and noted profound vasoconstriction in the afferent arteriole. The role of NO as a mediator that sustains renal perfusion in these septic rats led the authors to speculate that anti-NOS therapy may have adverse consequences on the renal function of humans.

Schwartz et al. studied renal function in rats treated with endotoxin and examined if selective blockade of either eNOS or iNOS was preferentially beneficial in sustaining renal function. These investigators confirmed that iNOS-generated NO impaired nephron function and glomerular filtration persisted when it was blocked, and eNOS could still affect afferent arteriole vasodilation.[41]

Vasomotor Nephropathy and Renal Failure

Several mechanisms have been identified for adjusting the vasomotor tone of the afferent and efferent arterioles: the sympathetic nervous system; circulating vasoactive agents such as epinephrine and arginine vasopressin; local paracrine factors released from endothelial, mesangial, and tubular cells that influence the vascular smooth muscle cells; and the inflammatory mediator released from macrophages and leukocytes. Clearly the renal vascular tone in the afferent and efferent arterioles are the consequence of a balance of mediators. The renal dysfunction and renal ischemia of SIRS and sepsis can be perceived as the consequence of disharmony of these balancing forces. Several specific vasomotor agents have been identified in experimental studies to be associated with renal dysfunction.

Endothelin-1

Endothelin-1 is a potent vasoconstrictor peptide released by the endothelial cell following stimulation by cytokines. First identified in 1988, at least four distinct molecular forms of endothelin have been identified as have several receptor sites. Endothelin-1 participates in a paracrine response where the endothelial cell synthesizes and releases the peptide that binds to adjacent vascular smooth muscle and causes a shift of Ca^{2+} into the cell and muscle cell contraction.[42] In addition to vasoconstriction, endothelin-1 may reduce the GFR by contracting mesangial cells in the glomerulus, which has a direct effect on the surface area available for filtration.[43] The plasma endothelin-1 level was elevated in humans with sepsis compared to that in healthy volunteers.[44] In animal experiments, the renal circulation was vasoconstricted when infused with endothelin-1, and the GFR dropped substantially. Pittet et al. reported a correlation of plasma endothelin-1 and creatinine concentrations ($r = 0.80$) in septic patients, which these authors interpreted as evidence that endothelin-1 mediates vasoconstriction of renal arterioles and may be a mechanism of renal dysfunction in septic patients.[44]

Endotoxin-induced declines in GFR were reversed by anti-endothelin-1 antibodies in experiments conducted in rats.[30] Mitaka et al. reported renal function preservation benefits of anti-endothelin therapy using a nonselective receptor antagonist.[45] Dogs exposed to lipopolysaccharide (LPS) developed renal ischemia. Depressed renal blood flow improved and creatinine clearance increased when the antagonist drug was administered prior to exposure to LPS, which blocked endothelin-1. These observations support the expectation by investigators interested in preserving renal function during SIRS that an effective therapy may be linked to anti-endothelin-1.[30] Various intracellular events are induced within cells by surface binding of endothelin-1, depending on which of the several receptors on the vascular smooth muscle cell surface the endothelin binds, and tailored therapy may be developed in which individual receptors are blocked.

Platelet-Activating Factor

Platelet-activating factor (PAF) is a lipid mediator produced by inflammatory cells and glomerular endothelial cells.[30] Patients with sepsis have increased levels of PAF in their plasma.[46] PAF is released from macrophages and leukocytes when these cells are exposed to toxins or the inflammatory mediators TNF and IL-1. PAF stimulates through binding to receptors on and within endothelial cells, with the result that the cells release vasoactive agents. Release of both the vasodilator NO and the vasoconstrictor thromboxane A_2 have been linked to PAF.[47]

An amplification mediator in septic shock, PAF enhances the release of secondary mediators, some of which lead to renal dysfunction. Antagonist therapy directed against PAF was developed by synthesis of molecules that bind to the PAF intracellular receptors. In animal models where toxin infusion leads to a sepsis-like syndrome and renal dysfunction, treatment with PAF receptor agonists preserved renal function.[48,49] A clinical trial of PAF receptor antagonist given to patients with sepsis failed to reduce mortality, although subset analyses suggested possible survival benefit.[50] Experimental evidence suggests that therapy against PAF may be more effective if it is directed against the actions of PAF within leukocytes and endothelial cells.[49,51]

Arachidonic Acid Metabolites

Arachidonic acid is the progenitor lipid to a family of eicosanoids with a range of effects in the inflammatory response. Phospholipase A_2 is a key enzyme that triggers release from the cell membrane of arachidonic acid. This lipid is altered by either the cyclooxygenase pathway to prostaglandins (PGs) (prostacyclin, thromboxane) or the lipoxygenase pathway to leukotrienes (LTC_4, LTD_4, LTE_4). Dormant circulating leukocytes are activated during SIRS and adhere to endothelium. During SIRS the endothelial cell expression for leukocyte adhesion molecules is upregulated, contributing to leukocyte recruitment to the kidney microcirculation.[42] Activated leukocytes adhere to endothelium and synthesize leukotrienes, which are potent vasoconstrictors. These mediators may account for the vasoconstriction that reduces the GFR.

In experimental studies monoclonal antibodies that block adhesion molecule sites show promise for protecting the nephron from dysfunction during endotoxemia.[51] Leukotrienes are also effective for reducing the GFR by acting on mesangial cells.[30,52] Septic shock and renal dysfunction have been attributed to disharmony of the complex relation of the eicosanoid mediators produced from arachidonic acid.[53] The clinical significance of the complex relation among eicosanoids was evident in an observation made by Fink et al. that cyclooxygenase inhibitors in dogs with peritonitis resulted in further deterioration of renal function and not the anticipated benefit.[54]

Thromboxane A_2 is a product of the cyclooxygenase pathway and a potent vasoconstrictor. Experimental evidence indicates that several cell types in the renal cortex produce thromboxane A_2 when exposed to endotoxin, and renal ischemia and GFR decline results.[52] Specific antagonists of this vasoconstrictor have protected animals exposed to endotoxin from renal ischemia. Successful therapy for cyclooxygenase-mediated renal dysfunction apparently depends on developing specific antagonists to vasoconstriction mediator receptors. Alternative therapy may include enhancement of the production of vasodilatory prostaglandins such as PGE_2 and prostacyclin.[30]

In humans with sepsis, trial administration of ibuprofen, a cyclooxygenase inhibitor, reduced fever, tachycardia, and lactic acid levels.[55] The excretion of prostacyclin and thromboxane metabolites was substantially suppressed in patients treated with ibuprofen, proving the drug had the intended effect. However, the drug did not effectively improve clinical outcome; specifically, renal failure did not improve. Hemodialysis was required to manage acute renal failure in 3% of ibuprofen-treated patients and 6% of placebo-treated patients ($p = 0.11$).

Thrombosis and Renal Failure

Microvascular thrombosis of glomerular capillaries is an unusual cause of ARF among septic patients who came to autopsy following their deaths with multiple organ failure syndrome. Thrombosis obstructs nutritive blood flow, which results in irreversible necrosis of renal tissue. In contrast, vasomotor nephropathy syndrome is the more common (and reversible) cause of ARF. Essentially, afferent arteriole constriction reduces glomerular filtration pressure, and adequate blood flow persists to deliver oxygen to the tubular cells of the nephron. Sublethal tubular cell structural changes—not the "tubular cell necrosis" noted in some victims of lethal renal failure—have been identified. Recovery of renal function can occur when vasodilation enables perfusion pressure to sustain glomerular filtration and tubular cells receive sufficient oxygen to sustain active sodium transport.

The pathophysiology of microvascular thrombosis in sepsis is linked to disseminated activation of the coagulation and fibrinolytic systems. The pathophysiology of patients with disseminated intravascular coagulation (DIC) is a balance between two opposing actions. Activation of the coagulation cascade favors intravascular thrombosis, whereas with DIC there is simultaneous activation of plasmin (which lyses clots). Overwhelming fibrinolysis leads to consumption of coagulation factors and a bleeding disorder. If there is more coagulation, clots can lead to generalized ischemic necrosis, as described for the Schwartzman reaction.[42] Schwartzman described the essential components of this pathologic condition as a "priming" exposure to a toxin followed by a second exposure that produces intravascular thrombosis and tissue necrosis. Although clinical examples of ARF attributed to Schwartzman reactions are not common, the lesions have relevance in some forms of renal dysfunction caused by sepsis. Linas et al. described a model of renal failure in which primed leukocytes, activated by exposure to endotoxin, had no effect when infused into normal kidneys, whereas the same cells caused renal failure when infused into kidney that had been subjected to mild ischemia (ischemia insufficient itself to cause renal impairment).[56]

Endothelial cell function is pivotal in the renal microcirculation thrombosis syndrome. Endothelial cells have at least three types of coagulation-mediated response to stimulation by the cytokines TNF and IL-1.[42] Tissue factor, synthesized and expressed on the endothelial cell surface, activates the extrinsic coagulation cascade and results in fibrin formation. Endothelial cells normally produce plasmin, which lyses new clots; and this plasmin is suppressed in response to cytokines. Cytokines also suppress production of activated protein C, which normally functions as a potent anticoagulant in the presence of thrombin-thrombomodulin. In patients with SIRS there may also be platelet activation that enhances the adhesion of these cells to endothelium and thus facilitates microvascular thrombosis. In summary, it is clear there are complex relations between multiple pro- and anticoagulation pathways in patients, which under normal circumstances favor an anticoagulant environment on the surface of endothelial cells but can be disrupted in favor of clot formation by multiple mediators produced in response to sepsis.

Treatment to Avert Renal Dysfunction and Failure

Prevention of SIRS

The magnitude of the endogenous inflammatory response to SIRS determines in proportion the extent to which organs become dysfunctional. For clinicians this relation between intensity of inflammation and organ injury implies that rapid, effective elimination of the cause of the inflammatory response reduces the duration and deterioration of MODS. Thus a vigilant physician treating a patient with impending serious infection must intervene early to eradicate, or at least reduce, the systemic load of toxins that initiate SIRS. For example, a grade IIIB fracture of an extremity indicates disruption of soft tissue, bone, and major arteries. There are often compelling reasons to attempt to preserve the extremity, and these reasons may also justify conservative débridement of injured tissue needed to cover the fracture and for vessel repairs. However, the surgeon's enthusiasm to embark on a sequence of treatments intended to achieve extremity salvage must be tempered by knowledge that a compromised extremity could develop rapidly progressive invasive infection with overwhelming toxemia. Evidence indicates that a "second hit" of infection in injured patients already primed by the first stimulus (being injured) results in amplification of the inflammatory response that causes severe SIRS or *septic shock*. Control of infection by both antibiotics and excision of sites of potential toxemia are interventions that can prevent MODS. Organ failure is a consequence of inflammatory events beginning hours before the clinician first notes organ dysfunction. Prevention is the most cost-effective therapy for MODS.

Neutralizing or Blocking Primary Inflammatory Mediators

Substantial research into the mechanisms of injury active in patients with SIRS and associated conditions has identified multiple sites where antagonist drugs can be effective. These interventions intend to reduce injury to organs caused by inflammatory cascades. Such treatments can be classified as blockade or amelioration of primary mediator cascades or as direct neutralization of inflammatory agents.

Blockade of Primary Mediators

The toxin-mediated initiation of inflammatory cytokines has been a prime target of therapy. Antibodies directed against endotoxin were developed using bioengineering methodology; and infusion of these agents to neutralize endotoxin—the trigger of the SIRS response—was attempted in high risk patients with sepsis. The initial success seen in selected populations has not been confirmed in large, randomized control trials.[57,58] Therapies intended to neutralize the secondary agents of injury have not been effective in clinical trials.

Hypotension in SIRS patients causes renal dysfunction and enables emergence of renal failure. Thus treatment of hypotension is of paramount importance for preserving renal function. The patient's response to therapy for shock has been used to categorize patients with SIRS. For patients in the severe sepsis category of SIRS, infusion of intravenous fluid is effective and can reverse hypotension.[27] Rangel-Frausto et al. reported that in a prospective cohort of ICU patients severe sepsis occurred in 39% of the SIRS population. Patients whose hypotension was not reversed by an adequate expansion of intravascular volume—a criterion that indicated *septic shock*—constituted 9% of the population studied.[27] Many patients in *septic shock* are oliguric. Therapy that increases the mean arterial pressure and intends to restore glomerular capillary hydrostatic pressure and blood flow can be monitored by restoration of urine flow. Inducing diuresis in an oliguric SIRS patient with powerful natriuretic drugs, which only alter tubular cell function, can be imprudent. The physician masks of a salutary diuresis which indicates a favorable response to therapy to restore renal perfusion.

Interventions

Three interventions are available to the physician treating a SIRS patient with shock. Each has different physiologic consequences, and a pulmonary artery catheter that enables measurement of cardiac performance may be required to indicate the most appropriate therapy in complex cases. The three therapeutic interventions are intravascular volume expansion to increase end-diastolic volume in the right and left ventricle, infusion of inotropic drugs, and infusion of vasoconstricting drugs to increase systemic vascular resistance.

Intravascular Volume Expansion

The intravascular compartment of a SIRS patient can be depleted for several reasons. Vomiting, diarrhea, peritonitis, and wound edema (formed as an inflammatory transudate) all deplete the plasma volume and plasma protein content. Hemorrhage is a commonly associated condition in patients with serious infection. Physiologic hypovolemia can develop not by depletion but by venous dilation induced by vasoactive mediators of SIRS, which expand the size of the vascular compartment. Thus what was an adequate volume must increase to fill the largely expanded venous reservoirs. Restoration of intravascular volume should be accomplished in the hypotensive SIRS patient by prompt, vigorous infusion of replacement fluids. Balanced electrolyte solutions are effective and recommended by many authors. Some clinicians prefer colloid solutions, which may have a superior capability to expand the blood volume, transiently but have never been demonstrated to provide superior survival commensurate with the added cost.[28,59] Substantial fluid volumes are often required to resuscitate patients with preexisting hypovolemia who develop *severe sepsis*. Ognibene predicted that 10–20 liters of crystalloid may be required during the first 24 hours of resuscitation of some patients with septic shock.[60]

Volume infusion can be guided by measuring filling pressures in the cardiac ventricles. The central venous pressure is measured relatively easily, and a reading less than 10 mmHg provides a useful indication that the patient requires greater expansion of the blood volume. For complex patients, many clinicians rely on the pulmonary artery wedge pressure, which several authors advocate should be increased to a level of 15–18 mmHg by repeated intravenous infusions of 500–1000 ml of balanced electrolyte solutions.[60,61] There is evidence that routine reliance on pulmonary artery catheters to provide information guiding resuscitation carries detrimental consequences.[62] The Pulmonary Artery Catheter Consensus Conference held in December 1996 recommended that selective use of pulmonary artery catheters was appropriate when patients with sepsis/septic shock failed to respond to initial trials of intravascular volume expansion and low doses of cardiovascular drugs.[63] Reversal of oliguria is an important indication that adequate filling pressure has been restored with adequate organ perfusion in hypotensive patients with severe sepsis.

Infusion of Inotropic Drugs

The therapeutic consequence of vascular volume expansion should be high-normal end-diastolic volumes in the right and left ventricle and increased cardiac output. Patients with *severe sepsis* typically develop a hyperdynamic circulation, and the cardiac index may increase severalfold. Detailed studies of the ventricular performance of patients with hyperdynamic sepsis have revealed impaired myocardial performance. Cardiac dysfunction during *severe sepsis* and *septic shock* contributes to refractory hypotension, which impairs renal function. Specifically, the ventricular walls are stiff, and the ejection fraction is reduced.[61] The right ventricle must cope with marked increases in pulmonary artery resistance that develop in septic patients. Hypocalcemia and hypophosphatemia are electrolyte abnormalities noted in patients with sepsis that contribute to impaired contractility but can be easily reversed.

Most patients with impaired cardiac contractility should receive an intravenous infusion of inotropic agents. Dopamine infused at doses of under 10 μg/kg/min can improve contractility by binding to unique dopaminergic receptors. β-Agonist drugs, specifically dobutamine or low doses of epinephrine, are also effective inotropic drugs for treatment of *severe sepsis* and *septic shock*. Duke et al. reported that dobutamine was superior to dopamine in improving creatinine clearance among critically ill patients.[64] Ognibene concluded that β-agonists and their resultant vasodilation should be avoided as the first drugs for inotropic support in hypotensive septic patients.[60]

Infusion of Vasoconstrictor Drugs

Hypotensive patients with *severe sepsis* and *septic shock* frequently have low systemic vascular resistance. Hypotension caused by vasodilation in patients with septic shock can be refractory to inotropic drug infusion and thus lethal.[65] Systemic vascular resistance—calculated from cardiac output and the difference in arterial and central venous pressures—is a parameter to follow during vasoconstrictor treatments intended to reverse arteriolar vasodilation.

α-Adrenergic Agonists. α-Adrenergic agonists are the principal drugs infused to reverse septic shock via vasoconstriction. Norepinephrine is a potent α-adrenergic agonist and a moderate $β_1$- and $β_2$-agonist; the clinical effectiveness of this drug, including reversal of renal dysfunction, has been reported.

Desjars et al. determined in patients with septic shock refractory to dopamine (15 μg/kg/min) that infusion of norepinephrine (0.5–1.0 μg/kg/min) improved mean arterial pressure and urine flow rates and contributed to 58% survival.[66] Meadows et al. infused norepinephrine alone at rates of 0.03–0.89 μg/kg/min into patients with refractory septic shock and observed improved mean arterial pressures (to 89 ± 10 mmHg) and reversal of oliguria.[67] Hesselvik and Brodin specifically reported merit from norepinephrine infusion (0.03–0.50 μg/kg/min) as a renal-sparing therapy, although they confirmed that vasoconstriction therapy can adversely aggravate the oxygen debt in septic patients with an associated worsening of lactic acidosis.[68] Martin et al. concluded, that norepinephrine (0.5–5.0 μg/kg/min) was superior to dopamine (2.5–25.0 μg/kg/min). Norepinephrine did not have an adverse effect on renal function in this trial. The authors concluded that norepinephrine was the preferred vasopressor for *septic shock*.[69] Redl-Wenzl et al. measured creatinine clearance in patients in refractory septic shock infused with norepinephrine (0.1–2.0 μg/kg/min). They noted that creatinine clearance increased after 24 hours of adjusted-dose infusion of norepinephrine given to sustain the mean arterial pressure.[70]

The summary results of these clinical studies indicate that norepinephrine infusion has merit. Norepinephrine infusion carries risk because it is a potent vasoconstrictor, and in high doses it causes sufficient vasoconstriction of the renal vascular bed to reduce or terminate the GFR. The hemodynamic pattern in septic patients is vasodilation of the peripheral circulation to all organs, including skin and skeletal muscle. The renal benefits of norepinephrine infusion relate to the differential vasoconstriction of the vasculature to less critical tissue. Clinical studies report a wide range of doses that benefit individuals; furthermore, different formulas of associated inotropic infusions have been reported. Thus proper use of norepinephrine to support renal function in many patients requires invasive, continuous hemodynamic monitoring.

"Renal Dose" Dopamine. Infusion of dopamine at doses of 1–3 μg/kg/min has been demonstrated to increase renal blood flow and induce a natriuresis and associated diuresis in normal humans.[71] The effect of dopamine is mediated through specific receptors D_1 and D_2. D_1 receptors are located on the renal vasculature and mediate vasodilation, including afferent arterioles, with the result that the drug can increase the GFR in circumstances of excessive vasoconstriction. This property has made low-dose dopamine a popular drug for preventing further deterioration of renal dysfunction and, in circumstances where ARF becomes established, converting oliguric renal failure to the more easily managed polyuric renal failure. Dopamine receptors on tubular cells provide a mechanism for dopamine-mediated natriuresis. In most carefully controlled trials of dopamine infusion into high risk patients, a statistically significant improvement over no dopamine infusion could not be demonstrated.[72] In a group of chronically ill patients with MODS and ARF, Chertow et al. were unable to demonstrate that infusion of low-dose dopamine had a statistically significant

beneficial influence on survival or need for dialysis. These authors concluded that as of 1996 there was insufficient evidence to support routine infusion of low-dose dopamine to improve renal function in patients with high risk circumstances.[73] Dopamine as a selective vasodilator of the renal circulation may have specific benefit in patients infused with norepinephrine to counter the systemic vasodilation characteristics of SIRS.[74]

In summary, the benefits of "renal dose" dopamine are inconsistently reported in the medical literature and, as with many interventions in patients with the complex physiology of SIRS, may not have the isolated effect demonstrated in normal, healthy volunteers. The use of dopamine in these patients should be limited to circumstances where continuous monitoring can determine the specific benefit or lack of effect of this drug.

Treatment of Patients with Renal Failure and SIRS

New methods of renal replacement therapy have been developed as alternatives to hemodialysis for support of patients with ARF.[2] Continuous hemofiltration carries the purported advantage that patients with hyperdynamic sepsis have less hypotension. Barzilay et al. reported that survival of patients with multiple organ dysfunction and renal failure was greater when continuous arteriovenous hemofiltration techniques were employed. The authors speculated that one advantage of this form of therapy might be removal of the mediators that cause organ dysfunction.[75]

McCarthy examined the survival of adult patients with new onset of renal failure (patients with preexisting chronic renal failure were excluded from these analyses) treated at hospitals associated with the Mayo Clinic.[76] Compared to those treated a decade earlier, patients treated during 1991–1992 had improved hospital survival (52%), although only 30% of the initial renal failure group were alive at 1 year. This improvement was not shared by patients who had sepsis and ARF, whose 80% mortality rate remained unchanged. The authors did report that among the survivors of acute renal failure more than 80% had recovery of renal function. In another small series of patients with sepsis and shock, the addition of continuous arteriovenous hemofiltration did clear TNF but not IL-6, both of which were substantially elevated in plasma; however, survival was only 23%.[77] Although the capacity to treat renal impairment in an ICU is substantial, optimal management currently depends on an early diagnosis of SIRS and preemptive interventions to neutralize SIRS-related mechanisms of renal injury.

The other organ systems that fail in patients with multiple organ dysfunction cumulatively contribute to their risk of death.[24] Respiratory failure is defined as a sustained need for mechanical ventilation. Cardiovascular failure is sustained hypotension, although the specific defects may be a decline in systemic vascular resistance and a decrease in cardiac contractility. Hepatic failure is most directly measured as jaundice, although not all patients with an elevated bilirubin level suffer critical dysfunction in hepatic synthesis function. Other organ systems compromised in MODS are neurologic and hematologic.

Patients who develop MODS have a risk of death proportional to the number of organs that fail. In the ICU cohort studied by Liano et al., the death rate for patients with isolated ARF was 30%. Adding one, two, or three or more organ failure burdens increased mortality rates to 53%, 80%, and >91%, respectively.[25] Greater mortality from multiple organ failure suggests that patients with overwhelming physiologic dysfunction are more difficult to sustain with organ replacement or support therapy, perhaps because of the complex dependence of these organs on the function of one another.

References

1. Spurney RF, Fulkerson WJ, Schwab SJ: Acute renal failure in critically ill patients: prognosis for recovery of kidney function after prolonged dialysis support. Crit Care Med 1991;19:8–11.
2. Mehta RL: Therapeutic alternatives to renal replacement for critically ill patients in acute renal failure. Semin Nephrol 1994;14:64–82.
3. Forni LG, Hilton PJ: Continuous hemofiltration in the treatment of acute renal failure. N Engl J Med 1997;336:1303–1309.
4. Levy EM, Viscoli CM, Horwitz RI: The effect of acute renal failure on mortality. JAMA 1996;275:1489–1494.
5. Brady HR, Singer GG: Acute renal failure. Lancet 1995;346:1534–1540.
6. Thadhani R, Pascual M, Bonventre JV: Acute renal failure. N Engl J Med 1996;334:1448–1460.
7. Bivet FG, Kleinknecht D, Loirat P, et al: Acute renal failure in intensive care units—causes, outcome, and prognostic factors of hospital mortality: a prospective, multicenter study. Crit Care Med 1996;24:192–198.
8. Cioffi WG, Ashikaga T, Gamelli RL: Probability of surviving postoperative acute renal failure: development of a prognostic index. Ann Surg 1984;200:205–211.
9. Bywaters EGL, Beall D: Crush injuries with impairment of renal function. BMJ 1941;1:427–432.
10. Smith LH, Post RS, Teschan PE, et al: Post-traumatic renal insufficiency in military casualties. Am J Med 1955;18:187–198.
11. Locke B: Lower nephron nephrosis (renal lesions of the crush syndrome, of burns, transfusions, and other conditions which affect the lower segment of the nephrons). Milit Surg 1946;99:371–396.
12. Balch HH, Meroney WH, Sako Y: Observations on the surgical care of patients with posttraumatic renal insufficiency. Surg Gynecol Obstet 1955;100:439–452.
13. Strauch M, McLaughlin JS, Mansberger A, et al: Effects of septic shock on renal function in humans. Ann Surg 1967;165:536–543.
14. Lordon RE, Burton JR: Post-traumatic renal failure in military personnel in Southeast Asia. Am J Med 1972;53:137–147.
15. Berne JV, Barbour BH: Acute renal failure in general surgical patients. Arch Surg 1971;102:594–597.
16. Tilney NL, Bailey GL, Morgan AP: Sequential system failure after rupture of abdominal aortic aneurysms: an unsolved problem in postoperative care. Ann Surg 1973;178:117–122.
17. Fischer RP, Polk HC Jr: Changing etiologic patterns of renal insufficiency in surgical patients. Surg Gynecol Obstet 1975;140:85–86.
18. Baue AE: Multiple, progressive, or sequential systems failure. Arch Surg 1975;110:779–781.

19. Fry DE, Pearlstein L, Fulton RL, et al: Multiple system organ failure: the role of uncontrolled infection. Arch Surg 1980;115:136–140.
20. Faist E, Baue AE, Dittmer H, et al: Multiple organ failure in polytrauma patients. J Trauma 1983;23:775–787.
21. Eiseman B, Beart R, Norton L: Multiple organ failure. Surg Gynecol Obstet 1977;144:323–326.
22. Goris RJ, Boekkorst TPA, Nuytinck JKS, et al: Multiple-organ failure: generalized autodestructive inflammation? Arch Surg 1985;120:1109–1115.
23. Bone RC, Fisher CJ, Clemmer TP, et al: Sepsis syndrome: a valid clinical entity. Crit Care Med 1989;17:389–393.
24. Breen D, Bihari D: Acute renal failure as a part of multiple organ failure: the slippery slope of critical illness. Kidney Int 1998;53 (Suppl 66):S25–S33.
25. Liano F, Junco E, Pascual J, et al: The spectrum of acute renal failure in the intensive care unit compared with that seen in other settings. Kidney Int 1998;53(Suppl 66):S16–S24.
26. American College of Chest Physicians/Society of Critical Care Medicine Consensus Conference: definitions for sepsis and organ failure and guidelines for the use of innovative therapies in sepsis. Crit Care Med 1992;20:864–875.
27. Rangel-Frausto M, Pitter D, Costigan M, et al: The natural history of the systemic inflammatory response syndrome (SIRS), a prospective study. JAMA 1995;273:117–123.
28. Wheeler AP, Bernard GR: Treating patients with severe sepsis. N Engl J Med 1999;340:207–214.
29. Lucas CE, Rector FE, Werner M, et al: Altered renal homeostasis with acute sepsis. Arch Surg 1973;106:444–449.
30. Thijs A, Thijs LG: Pathogenesis of renal failure in sepsis. Kidney Int 1998;53(Suppl 66):S34–S37.
31. Navasa M, Follo A, Filella X, et al: Tumor necrosis factor and interleukin-6 in spontaneous bacterial peritonitis in cirrhosis: relationship with the development of renal impairment and mortality. Hepatology 1998;27:1227–1232.
32. Girardin E, Grau GE, Dayer J, et al: Tumor necrosis factor and interleukin-1 in the serum of children with severe infectious purpura. N Engl J Med 1988;319:397–400.
33. Waage A, Halstensen A, Espevik T: Association between tumour necrosis factor in serum and fatal outcome in patients with meningococcal disease. Lancet 1987;1:355–357.
34. Thiemermann C: Nitric oxide and septic shock: a review. Gen Pharmacol 1997;29:159–166.
35. Ketteler M, Cetto C, Kirdorf M, et al: Nitric oxide in sepsis-syndrome: potential treatment of septic shock by nitric oxide synthase antagonists. Kidney Int 1998;53(Suppl 64):S27–S30.
36. Meyer J, Lentz CW, Stothert JC, et al: Effects of nitric oxide synthesis inhibition in hyperdynamic endotoxemia. Crit Care Med 1994;22:306–312.
37. Goode HF, Howdle PD, Walker BE, et al: Nitric oxide synthetase activity is increased in patients with sepsis syndrome. Clin Sci 1995;88:131–133.
38. Bech JN, Nielsen CB, Pedersen EB: Effects of systemic NO synthesis inhibition on RPF, GFR, and U_{Na}, and vasoactive hormones in healthy humans. Am J Physiol 1996;270:F845–F851.
39. Groeneveld PHP, Kwappenberg KMC, Langermans JAM, et al: Nitric oxide (NO) production correlates with renal insufficiency and multiple organ dysfunction syndrome in severe sepsis. Intensive Care Med 1996;22:1197–1202.
40. Spain DA, Wilson MA, Garrison RN: Nitric oxide synthase inhibition exacerbates sepsis-induced renal hypoperfusion. Surgery 1994;116:322–331.
41. Schwartz D, Mendonca M, Schwartz I, et al: Inhibition of constitutive nitric oxide synthase (NOS) by nitric oxide generated by inducible NOS after lipopolysaccharide administration provokes renal dysfunction in rats. J Clin Invest 1997;100:439–448.
42. Pober JS, Cotran RS: Cytokines and endothelial cell biology. Physiol Rev 1990;70:427–451.
43. Badr KF, Murray JJ, Dreyer MD, et al: Mesangial cell, glomerular and renal vascular responses to endothelin in the rat kidney: elucidation of signal transduction pathways. J Clin Invest 1989;83:336–342.
44. Pittet JF, Morel DR, Hemsen A, et al: Elevated plasma endothelin-1 concentrations are associated with the severity of illness in patients with sepsis. Ann Surg 1991;213:261–264.
45. Mitaka C, Hirata Y, Yokoyama K, et al: Improvement of renal dysfunction in dogs with endotoxemia by a nonselective endothelin receptor antagonist. Crit Care Med 1999;27:146–153.
46. Lopez Diez F, Nieto ML, Fernandez-Gallardo S, et al: Occupancy of platelet receptors for platelet-activating factor in patients with septicemia. J Clin Invest 1989;83:1733–1740.
47. Szabo C, Wu CC, Mitchell JA, et al: Platelet-activating factor contributes to the induction of nitric oxide synthase by bacterial lipopolysaccharide. Circ Res 1993;73:991–999.
48. Wang J, Bunn MJ: Platelet-activating factor mediates endotoxin-induced acute renal insufficiency in rats. Am J Phys 1987;253:F1283–F1289.
49. De Kimpe SJ, Thiemermann C, Vane JR: Role for intracellular platelet-activating factor in the circulatory failure in a model of gram-positive shock. Br J Pharmacol 1995;116:3191–3198.
50. Tenaillon A, Dhainaut JF, Letulozo Y, et al: Efficacy of PAF antagonist (BN52021) in reducing mortality of patients with severe gram-negative sepsis. Am Rev Respir Dis 1993;147:A196.
51. Steward AG, Dubbin PN, Harris T, et al: Platelet-activating factor may act as a second messenger in the release of eicosanoids and superoxide anions from leukocytes and endothelial cells. Proc Natl Acad Sci USA 1990;87:3215–3219.
52. Badr KR: Novel mediators of sepsis-associated renal failure. Semin Nephrol 1994;14:3–7.
53. Foex BA, Quinn JV, Little RA, et al: Differences in eicosanoid and cytokine production between injury/hemorrhage and bacteremic shock in the pig. Shock 1997;8:276–283.
54. Fink MP, MacVittie TJ, Casey LC: Effects of nonsteroidal anti-inflammatory drugs on renal function in septic dogs. J Surg Res 1984;36:516–525.
55. Bernard GR, Wheeler AP, Russell JA, et al: The effects of ibuprofen on the physiology and survival of patients with sepsis. N Engl J Med 1997;336:912–918.
56. Linas SL, Whittenburg D, Parsons PE, et al: Ischemia increases neutrophil retention and worsens acute renal failure: role of oxygen metabolites and ICAN 1. Kidney Int 1995;48:1584–1591.
57. Greenman RL, Schein RM, Martin MA, et al: A controlled clinical trial of E5 murine monoclonal IgM antibody to endotoxin in the treatment of gram-negative sepsis: the XOMA sepsis study group. JAMA 1991;266:1097–1102.
58. Bone RC, Balk RA, Fein AM, et al: A second large controlled clinical study of E5, a monoclonal antibody to endotoxin: results of a prospective, multicenter, randomized, controlled trial: the E5 sepsis study group. Crit Care Med 1995;23:989–991.

59. Rackow EC, Falk JL, Fein IA, et al: Fluid resuscitation in circulatory shock: a comparison of the cardiorespiratory effects of albumin, hetastarch, and saline solutions in patients with hypovolemic and septic shock. Crit Care Med 1983;11:839–850.
60. Ognibene FP: Hemodynamic support during sepsis. Clin Chest Med 1996;17:279–287.
61. Bunnell E, Parrillo JE: Cardiac dysfunction during septic shock. Clin Chest Med 1996;17:237–248.
62. Connors AF Jr, Speroff T, Dawson NV, et al: The effectiveness of right heart catheterization in the initial care of critically ill patients. JAMA 1996;276:889–897.
63. Pulmonary Artery Catheter Consensus Conference: consensus statement. Crit Care Med 1997;25:910–925.
64. Duke GJ, Briedis JH, Weaver RA: Renal support in critically ill patients: low-dose dopamine or low-dose dobutamine? Crit Care Med 1994;22:1919–1925.
65. Parker MM, Shelhamer JH, Natanson C, et al: Serial hemodynamic patterns in survivors and non-survivors of septic shock in humans: heart rate as an early predictor of prognosis. Crit Care Med 1987;15:923–929.
66. Desjars P, Pinaud M, Potel G, et al: A reappraisal of norepinephrine therapy in human septic shock. Crit Care Med 1987;15:134–137.
67. Meadows D, Edwards JD, Wilkins RG, et al: Reversal of intractable septic shock with norepinephrine therapy. Crit Care Med 1988;16:663–666.
68. Hesselvik JF, Brodin B: Low-dose norepinephrine in patients with septic shock and oliguria: effects on afterload, urine flow and oxygen transport. Crit Care Med 1989;17:179–180.
69. Martin C, Papzian L, Perrin G, et al: Norepinephrine or dopamine for the treatment of hyperdynamic septic shock? Chest 1993;103:1826–1831.
70. Redl-Wenzl EM, Armbruster C, Edelmann G, et al: The effects of norepinephrine on hemodynamics and renal function in severe septic shock states. Intensive Care Med 1993;19:151–154.
71. Lee MR: Dopamine and the kidney: ten years on. Clin Sci 1993;84:357–375.
72. Denton MD, Chertow GM, Brady HR: "Renal-dose" dopamine for the treatment of acute renal failure: scientific rationale, experimental studies and clinical trials. Kidney Int 1996;49:4–14.
73. Chertow GM, Sayegh MH, Allgren RL, et al: Is the administration of dopamine associated with adverse or favorable outcomes in acute renal failure? Am J Med 1996;101:49–53.
74. Richer M, Robert S, Lebel M: Renal hemodynamics during norepinephrine and low-dose dopamine infusions in man. Crit Care Med 1996;24:1150–1156.
75. Barzilay E, Kessler D, Berlot G, et al: Use of extracorporeal supportive techniques as additional treatment for septic-induced multiple organ failure patients. Crit Care Med 1989;17:634–637.
76. McCarthy JT: Prognosis of patients with acute renal failure in the intensive care unit: a tale of two eras. Mayo Clin Proc 1996;71:117–126.
77. Tonnesen E, Hansen MB, Hohndorf K, et al: Cytokines in plasma and ultrafiltrate during continuous arteriovenous haemofiltration. Anaesth Intensive Care 1993;21:752–758.

38
Metabolic Depletion and Failure: Muscle Cachexia During Injury and Sepsis

Timothy A. Pritts, David R. Fischer, and Per-Olof Hasselgren

Severe injury and sepsis are associated with metabolic changes in virtually all organs and tissues and include alterations in carbohydrate, lipid, and protein metabolism.[1,2] One of the most prominent metabolic consequences of critical illness is the catabolic response in skeletal muscle. Metabolic depletion and failure in skeletal muscle result in muscle atrophy, weakness, and fatigue, preventing ambulation and delaying recovery in these patients. When respiratory muscles are involved in the catabolic response,[3] difficulties arise when weaning the patient from the ventilator. In addition, muscle weakness increases the risk for aspiration and pneumonia.

Muscle cachexia after severe injury and during sepsis is mainly caused by increased protein breakdown, particularly degradation of myofibrillar proteins,[4,5] although reduced protein synthesis and inhibited amino acid uptake contribute as well.[6] This chapter focuses on intracellular and molecular mechanisms as well as mediators of injury- and sepsis-induced muscle cachexia. Prevention and treatment are also discussed.

Mediators

Proinflammatory Cytokines

Several lines of evidence support a role for proinflammatory cytokines in the catabolic response to injury and sepsis.[7] In particular, tumor necrosis factor (TNF) and interleukin-1 (IL-1) participate in the regulation of muscle protein breakdown.

Increased production of TNF and IL-1 was reported in a number of previous studies in injured and septic patients and experimental animals.[7] In other studies administration of recombinant TNF or IL-1 to rats resulted in stimulated total and myofibrillar protein breakdown in skeletal muscle,[8] and sepsis-induced muscle proteolysis was inhibited or blunted by treatment with anti-TNF antibody[9] or IL-1 receptor antagonist.[10] Taken together, these reports suggest that TNF and IL-1 regulate muscle protein degradation during sepsis and probably other catabolic conditions as well.

There is evidence that TNF and IL-1 stimulate muscle protein degradation by different mechanisms. Thus whereas the catabolic effects of TNF were abolished by adrenalectomy[11] or treatment with the glucocorticoid receptor antagonist RU38486,[8] these treatments did not influence the catabolic effects of IL-1.[8] The results are consistent with the concept that TNF exerts its catabolic effects in skeletal muscle mainly through glucocorticoids, whereas IL-1 stimulates muscle proteolysis through a glucocorticoid-independent mechanism. Because treatment of incubated muscles or cultured muscle cells with TNF or IL-1, even at high concentrations, did not stimulate protein degradation, it is not likely that the cytokines have a direct effect on muscle protein breakdown.[12–14] The factor(s) that mediate the catabolic effects of IL-1 are not known at present.

In addition to TNF and IL-1, IL-6 is produced and released at a high rate during sepsis and other critical illness.[15] The role of IL-6 in the regulation of muscle protein breakdown is controversial. Muscle atrophy in IL-6 transgenic mice[16] and improved muscle protein balance after treatment of tumor-bearing mice with anti-IL-6 antibody[17] support a role of IL-6 in the development of muscle cachexia. In contrast, in a study from our laboratory the catabolic effects of sepsis were almost identical in IL-6 knockout and wild-type mice, suggesting that IL-6 is not required for the development of muscle cachexia, at least not under those experimental conditions.[18] In the same study, treatment of normal mice with repeated doses of IL-6 and of cultured myotubes with high concentrations of IL-6 did not stimulate protein degradation, further supporting the concept that IL-6 does not regulate muscle protein breakdown. Results indicating that IL-6 does not regulate muscle proteolysis have been reported by others as well.[19,20]

Glucocorticoids

Plasma levels of cortisol are increased in patients with sepsis and severe injury,[21] and there is evidence that the increased levels of glucocorticoids are an important factor in the development of muscle cachexia in these conditions. Treatment of healthy humans with cortisol[22] or of normal rats with corticosterone or dexamethasone[23,24] resulted in increased muscle protein degradation. In other studies, treatment of rats with the glucocorticoid receptor antagonist RU38486 blocked the sepsis-induced increase in total and myofibrillar protein breakdown.[25] In more recent experiments we found that this effect of RU38486 reflected inhibited energy/ubiquitin-dependent muscle proteolysis.[24] Glucocorticoids regulate muscle protein breakdown in other catabolic conditions as well, including burn injury,[26] fasting,[27] and renal failure with metabolic acidosis.[28]

In vitro experiments suggest that glucocorticoids have a direct effect on skeletal muscle. Thus treatment of incubated intact muscles from rats or mice[29] or of cultured muscle cells[30] with dexamethasone resulted in increased protein degradation. In recent studies we found that the effect of dexamethasone on protein degradation in cultured L6 myotubes was mainly due to increased ubiquitin/proteasome-dependent proteolysis, although calcium-dependent proteolysis was also involved.[31]

Cytokines and Glucocorticoids

Proinflammatory cytokines and glucocorticoids interact with each other at several levels. Cytokines, particularly TNF and IL-1, stimulate the hypothalamic–pituitary–adrenal axis resulting in increased production of ACTH and adrenal production of glucocorticoids.[32] Conversely, glucocorticoids inhibit the production of several proinflammatory cytokines, providing a negative feedback mechanism by which dangerously high cytokine levels can be prevented.[33] The role of glucocorticoids in TNF-induced muscle cachexia was discussed above. In addition, there is evidence that glucocorticoids and TNF interact at the cellular level to induce muscle breakdown.[34] A simplified scheme of the interaction between TNF, IL-1, and glucocorticoids in the regulation of muscle protein breakdown during sepsis is provided in Fig. 38.1.

Other Cachectic Factors

Tisdale[35] provided evidence of a cachectic factor (proteolysis-inducing factor, or PIF) produced by certain tumors and excreted in the urine of patients with cancer. This factor is a sulfated glycoprotein with a molecular weight of approximately 24 kDa.[36] Unlike TNF and IL-1, it seems to have a direct effect on skeletal muscle because it is capable of stimulating protein breakdown in incubated muscle tissue. It should be noted that this proteolysis-inducing factor is not present in all cancers, and its potential role in injury- and sepsis-related muscle proteolysis is not known. Interestingly, the presence of PIF was reported in patients with sepsis almost 20 years ago by Clowes et al.[37] The PIF reported by Clowes et al.[37] was a much smaller molecule (approximately 4 kDa) than Tisdale's PIF and was believed to be a cleavage product of IL-1.

Although studies have provided insight into mediators of muscle protein breakdown in catabolic conditions, particularly TNF, IL-1, and glucocorticoids, little is known about the intracellular signaling pathways that regulate protein turnover in skeletal muscle. In a review article, Thompson and Palmer[38] discussed the potential role of protein kinase C, phospholipase D, and the transcription factors NF-κB and AP-1 in the regulation of muscle protein metabolism, but there is no information available at present regarding these mechanisms and muscle cachexia in regard to sepsis and injury.

Intracellular Mechanisms

Intracellular protein breakdown is regulated by a number of proteolytic mechanisms, including lysosomal, calcium-dependent, and ubiquitin/proteasome-dependent protein degradation. Some of the intracellular proteolytic pathways and enzymes regulating the various mechanisms are shown in Table 38.1. Studies from our and other laboratories suggest that the ubiquitin-proteasome mechanism is particularly important in cachectic muscle.[39–42] In addition, there is evidence that calcium-dependent, calpain-mediated proteolysis may play a role in the regulation of sepsis-induced muscle proteolysis.[43]

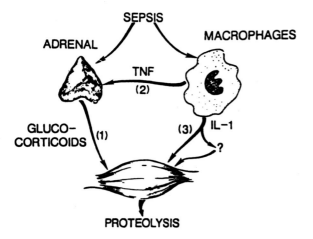

FIGURE 38.1. Proposed interaction between (1) glucocorticoids, (2) tumor necrosis factor (TNF), and (3) interleukin-1 (IL-1) in the regulation of sepsis-induced muscle proteolysis. The effect of TNF on muscle proteolysis is mainly mediated by glucocorticoids, whereas IL-1 regulates muscle proteolysis by glucocorticoid-independent pathway(s).

TABLE 38.1. Intracellular Proteolytic Pathways and Some of the Enzymes Regulating the Pathways.

Lysosomal pathway
  Cathepsins

Ca^{2+}-dependent pathway
  m-Calpain
  μ-Calpain
  p94

Energy/ubiquitin-dependent pathway
  E1, E2, E3
  26S proteasome

Ubiquitin/Proteasome-Dependent Muscle Proteolysis

The ubiquitin-proteasome proteolytic pathway has been reviewed elsewhere[44,45] and is discussed here only briefly. This proteolytic mechanism has two important features: (1) protein breakdown in this pathway is energy-dependent; and (2) proteins are conjugated to multiple molecules of ubiquitin before they are degraded (Fig. 38.2). Ubiquitination of a protein is regulated by multiple enzymes, including the ubiquitin-activating enzyme E1, the ubiquitin-conjugating enzyme E2, and the ubiquitin-protein ligase E3. In skeletal muscle the predominant E2 is the 14-kDa ubiquitin-conjugating enzyme $E2_{14k}$, and the predominant E3 is $E3\alpha$.[46] The ubiquitinated substrate protein is recognized by the 26S proteolytic complex; and after binding and unfolding, the substrate is funneled through the 20S proteasome, which is the catalytic core of the 26S proteasome. The 20S proteasome (Fig. 38.3) is a barrel-shaped particle composed of four stacked rings with each ring consisting of seven subunits.[47] The subunits of the outer rings are called α subunits and those of the inner rings β subunits. The proteolytic activity is confined to the inner surface of some of the β subunits.

Measurement of protein breakdown rates after inhibition of various proteolytic pathways can give information about which proteolytic pathway is responsible for increased muscle proteolysis in catabolic conditions. We incubated extensor digitorum longus muscles from septic rats in the presence of inhibitors of lysosomal or calcium-dependent protein degradation or in energy-depleting medium.[39] Results from those experiments suggested that sepsis-induced muscle proteolysis is mainly energy-dependent, not mediated by lysosomal enzymes, and is calcium-independent. Of particular interest was the finding that the increase in myofibrillar protein breakdown, measured as release of 3-methylhistidine, reflected energy-dependent proteolysis. This finding was significant because in other studies evidence was found that the myofibrillar proteins are particularly vulnerable to the effects of sepsis.[4] Because the gene expression of ubiquitin and the amount of ubiquitinated proteins were increased in septic muscles, the results were interpreted as indicating that muscle catabolism during sepsis at least in part reflects ubiquitin-dependent protein breakdown.[39]

Voisin et al.[43] found that in addition to ubiquitin-dependent proteolysis, activation of calcium-dependent and lysosomal systems may also be important for the regulation of muscle protein breakdown, particularly during the late and chronic phases of sepsis. Thus although energy/ubiquitin-dependent protein breakdown may be the most important mechanism of sepsis-induced muscle catabolism, other mechanisms may be involved as well. This was further supported by studies in which we found evidence that calcium-dependent, calpain-mediated release of myofilaments from Z-disks may be an early event in sepsis-related muscle catabolism (further discussed below).

Burn injury is associated with pronounced metabolic changes similar in magnitude to those seen during sepsis. In addition, infection and sepsis are common complications in burned patients, further aggravating the catabolic response. Using an experimental approach similar to that described above (i.e., incubating muscle in the presence of inhibitors of various proteolytic pathways), experiments in our laboratory have provided evidence that muscle protein breakdown following burn injury is mainly energy/ubiquitin-dependent, although a calcium-dependent mechanism contributes to the burn-induced muscle breakdown.[48] Thus the intracellular mechanisms and pathways involved in the catabolic response to sepsis and injury are similar, though not identical.

Ubiquitin-Proteasome Gene Expression in Cachectic Muscle

A severalfold increase in muscle ubiquitin mRNA levels has been noted in septic[39,43] and burned[48] rats. In addition to increased levels of ubiquitin mRNA, the expression of several other components of the ubiquitin-proteasome pathway is

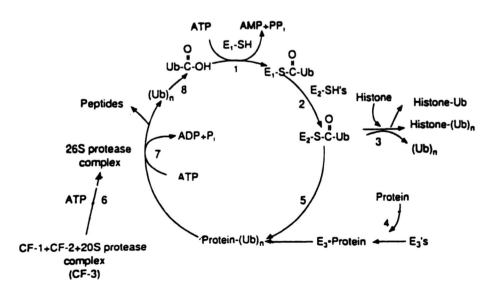

FIGURE 38.2. Ubiquitin-proteasome proteolytic pathway as described by Hershko and Ciechanover.[45] Substrate proteins are conjugated to multiple molecules of ubiquitin, after which they are recognized and degraded by the 26S protease complex (proteasome). See text for further details. (From Hershko and Ciechanover,[45] with permission.)

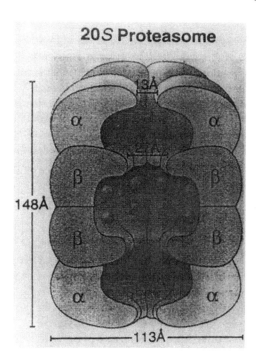

FIGURE 38.3. Cross section of the 20S proteasome. The 20S proteasome is composed of four stacked, seven-member rings. The rings form a central channel through which the substrate protein is funneled and degraded. The catalytic sites are located on the inner side of some of the β subunits, as indicated. (From Weissman et al.,[47] with permission.)

increased in septic muscle. For example, we found that mRNA levels for several 20S proteasome α and β subunits were increased in muscle from septic rats, and this response was associated with stimulated proteolytic activity of isolated 20S proteasomes.[49] In the same experiments, protein levels for the proteasome subunit RC 9 were unchanged in the catabolic muscles, indicating that the amount of proteasomes was not increased. Thus injury and sepsis may result in increased specific activity of the 20S proteasome.

Most proteins degraded by the proteasome in muscle during sepsis and after injury are ubiquitinated. The conjugation of ubiquitin to the target protein, regulated by the $E2_{14k}$ enzyme in skeletal muscle, has been proposed to be the rate-limiting step in ubiquitin-dependent protein breakdown.[46,50] We have found evidence that the gene expression of $E2_{14k}$ was increased in fast-twitch muscle of septic[51] and burned (unpublished observation) rats. A similar response was observed in a more chronic model of sepsis,[43] further supporting the role of the ubiquitin-proteasome pathway in muscle cachexia caused by sepsis and injury.

The observation that mRNA levels for several of the ubiquitin-proteasome pathway components are increased in catabolic muscle must be interpreted with caution for several reasons. First, it is not known from increased steady-state levels of mRNA if gene transcription is increased. Although we found that the stability of ubiquitin mRNA was not altered in muscle from septic and burned rats,[52,53] it was only indirect evidence that transcription of the ubiquitin gene was upregulated. Second, the relation between elevated mRNA levels and the proteins has not been established for most of the ubiquitin-proteasome pathway components. It is possible that some of the proteins are increased in parallel with increased mRNA levels, for example ubiquitin itself,[39] whereas other proteins are not increased despite increased mRNA (e.g., the 20S proteasome subunit RC 9).[49] Third, even if protein levels of the various components of the pathway are increased, it does not necessarily mean that their activities are stimulated. For example, it remains to be determined if the increased mRNA level of $E2_{14k}$ in septic muscle[51] is reflected by increased enzyme activity. An additional important question is whether the ubiquitin/proteasome-dependent mechanism is the cause or rate-limiting component of injury- and sepsis-induced muscle proteolysis.

One way to better define the role of the ubiquitin-proteasome pathway in sepsis- and burn-induced muscle proteolysis is to use metabolic inhibitors specific for the mechanism. The development of more or less specific inhibitors of the proteasome has made such studies possible.

Proteasome Blockers

Various proteasome inhibitors and their use in cell biology research have been reviewed.[54] Treatment of septic muscles in vitro with LLnL, a peptide aldehyde that reversibly blocks the proteasome chymotryptic and peptidylglutamine peptidase activities, reversed most of the increase in total protein breakdown noted in muscles from septic rats.[41] Because LLnL is not a completely specific proteasome blocker, but inhibits some cathepsins and calpains as well,[54] additional experiments were performed in which septic muscles were treated with lactacystin, a more specific proteasome blocker than LLnL.[55] This treatment inhibited the sepsis-induced increase in both total and myofibrillar muscle protein breakdown. A similar inhibition of protein degradation in septic muscle by proteasome blockers has been reported by others as well.[56]

In related studies we found that proteasome inhibitors blocked the increase in total and myofibrillar protein breakdown in skeletal muscle after burn injury.[57] In that study, we also examined the effect of the lactacystin β-lactone derivative, which is the active form of the inhibitor.[58] LLnL, lactacystin, and β-lactone all blocked the burn-induced increase in muscle protein breakdown.

Muscle Cachexia in Injured and Septic Patients

Most previous studies implicating the ubiquitin-proteasome pathway in injury- and sepsis-induced muscle proteolysis (and other catabolic conditions as well) have been conducted in experimental animals (mainly rats). Studies suggest that similar mechanisms are involved in the regulation of protein degradation in human muscle as well. Thus in a study of patients with head injury, the gene expression of several components of the ubiquitin-proteasome pathway was increased in muscle tissue concomitant with evidence of negative nitrogen balance and muscle catabolism.[59]

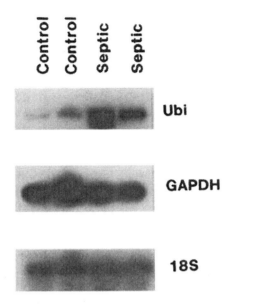

FIGURE 38.4. Ubiquitin (Ubi) mRNA levels (determined by Northern blotting) in muscle tissue from two control and two septic patients. Similar results were observed in nine additional controls and five additional septic patients. (From Tiao et al.,[40] with permission.)

Results in a study from our laboratory suggest that ubiquitin/proteasome-dependent proteolysis is accountable for muscle cachexia in septic patients as well.[40] In that study, mRNA levels for ubiquitin and the 20S proteasome subunit HC3 were increased severalfold in muscles from patients with sepsis (Figs. 38.4, 38.5) concomitant with elevated tissue levels of tyrosine and 3-methylhistidine. In other studies, we found upregulated gene expression of the ubiquitin-proteasome pathway in muscle from patients with cancer,[60] another condition characterized by significant muscle breakdown.

Although there is evidence of a similar role of the ubiquitin-proteasome pathway in catabolic muscle from humans and rats, it must be noted that there is not an absolute correlation between findings in experimental animals and patients. For example, whereas the role of glucocorticoids in the regulation of protein degradation and expression of the ubiquitin-proteasome pathway is well established in muscles from rats,[61,62] mRNA levels for ubiquitin, $E2_{14k}$, and several proteasome subunits were not increased in patients with Cushing syndrome.[63] In another report, the expression of ubiquitin and the proteasome subunit C2 was not increased in muscle from patients with chronic renal failure[64] despite a number of previous reports of upregulated expression of ubiquitin and 20S proteasome subunits in muscle from rats with chronic renal failure.[65]

N-End Rule Pathway and Muscle Protein Breakdown

Although much research has been performed to define the expression and activity of the ubiquitin-proteasome pathway in cachectic muscle during sepsis and other catabolic conditions, surprisingly little is known about the substrates for the proteolytic pathway. In previous studies Varshavsky et al.[66,67] found evidence that there is a relation between the half-life of a protein and the identity of its N-terminal residue, the "N-end rule." Proteins with basic N-terminal residues (Arg, Lys, His), bulky hydrophobic N-terminal residues (Phe, Leu, Trp, Tyr, Ile), or acidic N-termini that have undergone arginyl/tRNA-dependent N-terminal arginylation are recognized by the ubiquitin-protein ligase E3α, which is the predominant E3 enzyme in skeletal muscle. The ubiquitin-conjugating enzyme associated with E3α is $E2_{14k}$. Reports of increased expression of $E2_{14k}$ in muscles from septic rats[43,51] and burned rats (unpublished observations in our laboratory) support the concept that the N-end rule pathway (substrates with destabilizing N-terminal residue, $E2_{14k}$, E3α) at least in part accounts for sepsis-induced ubiquitin/proteasome-dependent protein breakdown in skeletal muscle; but more experiments are needed to further define the role of the N-end rule pathway in catabolic muscle. The cloning of mouse and human genes encoding E3α[68] will hopefully provide tools in the near future to perform studies aimed at determining the role of the N-end rule pathway in muscle cachexia associated with sepsis, severe injury, and other catabolic conditions.

Studies by Solomon et al.[69,70] suggest that the N-end rule pathway does indeed participate in the degradation of muscle proteins. In those experiments, various inhibitors of the E3α enzyme were used, and results were interpreted as indicating that 50–60% of soluble muscle proteins undergo E3α-dependent proteolysis. Although the E3α-dependent protein degradation was increased in atrophic muscle, one remaining "problem" is the fact that only a minor portion (approximately 10–15%) of actin and myosin underwent E3α-dependent breakdown.[69] This indicates that modification of the myofibrillar proteins may be needed before they become suitable substrates for the N-end rule pathway. It is possible that a rate-limiting step in the degradation of the long-lived muscle proteins is a slow exo- or endoproteolytic cleavage that exposes a destabilizing N-terminal residue. Such a modification in vivo could even be a regulated mechanism that triggers the acceleration of muscle proteolysis in fasting or other

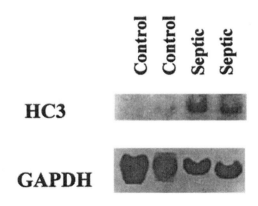

FIGURE 38.5. mRNA levels for the 20S proteasome subunit HC3 in muscle tissue from two control and two septic patients. Similar results were observed in nine additional controls and five additional septic patients. (From Tiao et al.,[40] with permission.)

catabolic states. Based on results in recent experiments (see below), we propose that calcium-dependent, calpain-mediated release of myofilaments from the Z-disks is just such a rate-limiting step in sepsis-induced muscle protein degradation.

Sepsis-Induced Disintegration of Z-disks and Calcium-Dependent Release of Myofilaments in Skeletal Muscle

We found electron microscopic evidence that sepsis resulted in morphologic changes in skeletal muscle consisting of partial to complete disintegration of a large portion of Z-disks.[71] As a result, many sarcomeres lost their normal alignment with each other and were out of register. In the same muscles, the fraction of "easily releasable myofilaments" was increased, indicating that the anchorage of actin and myosin to the Z-disks had been disrupted. The expression of m- and μ-calpain and the muscle-specific calpain p94 was increased three- to fourfold and the increase in myofilament release was blocked by treating the septic rats with the calcium antagonist dantrolene.

Because in subsequent experiments we found evidence that dantrolene inhibits the sepsis-induced increase in cytoplasmic calcium levels and total and myofibrillar protein breakdown (unpublished observations), the results are consistent with the concept that sepsis results in calcium-dependent, calpain-mediated Z-disk disintegration and release of myofilaments. It may be speculated that the detachment of actin and myosin from the Z-disks exposes destabilizing N-terminal residues, making the released myofilaments suitable substrates for the N-end rule pathway. If this mechanism is involved in sepsis-induced muscle cachexia, the role of the ubiquitin-proteasome pathway may have to be reevaluated. Thus it is possible that the upregulated expression and activity of this proteolytic mechanism is the result, rather than the cause, of muscle breakdown during sepsis, and that the ubiquitin pathway serves the purpose of ridding the cell of "abnormal" proteins (i.e., myofilaments released into the cytoplasm and having destabilizing N-terminal residues). If this is the case, trying to block sepsis-induced muscle proteolysis with proteasome inhibitors, as proposed by ourselves and others,[41,56] may actually be harmful, allowing accumulation of abnormal proteins. Inhibition of a more "proximal," calcium-dependent release of myofilaments from the Z-disks may prove more fruitful in the prevention and treatment of muscle cachexia associated with severe injury, sepsis, and perhaps other catabolic conditions as well.

Prevention and Treatment

The best prevention and treatment of sepsis- and injury-related muscle cachexia, of course, are to prevent and treat the underlying cause of the catabolic response in skeletal muscle. For example, drainage of abscesses and débridement of necrotic tissue are the mainstays for treating patients with sepsis caused by intraabdominal abscesses and devitalized tissue. Other therapeutic avenues that have been explored to reduce the catabolic response to sepsis and injury in clinical trials and experimental animals include treatment with anabolic hormones, cytokine antibodies, and various nutritional formulas.

Hormones

Among the anabolic hormones, insulin, growth hormone (GH), and insulin-like growth factor-I (IGF-I) are the most widely studied hormones in catabolic patients and experimental animals. The protein-sparing effects of insulin have been well characterized for years. The mechanism of the insulin action varies in different cells and tissues. For example, in liver the most important effect of insulin is inhibition of lysosomal protein breakdown,[72] whereas in skeletal muscle insulin exerts its anabolic effect by stimulating protein synthesis and inhibiting proteolysis.[73] Insulin has not gained widespread acceptance for treating septic or injured patients, one reason being the complicating hypoglycemia associated with this treatment. Another reason is that insulin has not been successful in reversing the catabolic response to sepsis and severe injury, most likely reflecting the development of insulin resistance in patients with some of these conditions.[74]

In previous studies we treated incubated muscles from nonseptic and septic rats with increasing concentrations of insulin and measured protein synthesis and breakdown rates as well as amino acid uptake.[75] Insulin stimulated protein synthesis and cellular uptake of α-aminoisobutyric acid, transported mainly by system A, in a dose-dependent manner with no difference in the hormone effect between nonseptic and septic muscle. In contrast, the inhibitory effect of the hormone on protein breakdown was less pronounced in septic than in nonseptic muscle, and the dose-response curves were consistent with a reduced responsiveness to insulin. This result, in combination with an unaltered effect of insulin on protein synthesis and amino acid uptake in septic muscle, is consistent with postreceptor insulin resistance of protein breakdown in skeletal muscle during sepsis. The mechanism of insulin resistance with regard to the regulation of muscle protein breakdown in septic muscle is not known but is an important area for future research.

Interestingly, other studies suggest that insulin resistance is not universal to all catabolic conditions. For example, burn injury did not alter the response to insulin in skeletal muscle with regard to the regulation of protein synthesis or breakdown.[76]

Previous studies provided evidence that treatment of burned or injured patients with GH improved whole-body nitrogen balance and protein synthesis, and although muscle protein turnover rates were not specifically measured in those studies, it was assumed that the anabolic effect of GH reflected an improved protein balance in skeletal muscle.[77] Further support for that interpretation was the improved muscle strength noted in GH-treated patients after major operations.[78] Additional benefits of GH in burned patients include improved wound healing, decreased wound infection rates, and decreased length of hospital stay. The side effects of GH administration include hyperglycemia, fluid retention, and insulin resistance. Of note is a report from two European phase III prospective, randomized, double-blind trials examining GH as a supplement in the treatment of burned and critically ill patients. It indicated that GH administration was associated with increased mortality.[79] In contrast, a report from a major pediatric burn center in the United States concluded that the use of GH in severely burned children is safe and effective.[80]

Because the anabolic effects of GH are mainly mediated by IGF-I, the effect of this hormone has attracted special interest. In experiments in our laboratory, treatment of incubated muscles from burned rats restored the burn-induced reduction of protein synthesis and blocked the increase in protein degradation.[81] In another study, we found that treatment of burned rats with IGF-I in vivo improved the catabolic condition in skeletal muscle.[82] Although the anabolic effects of IGF-I in certain cell types, particularly in the hepatocyte, may be secondary to cell swelling, the protein-sparing effects of the hormone in skeletal muscle are probably caused by other mechanism(s).[83]

Interestingly, the effects of IGF-I on protein turnover in septic muscle are different from those seen after burn injury. Thus when muscles from septic rats were treated with increasing concentrations of IGF-I in vitro, protein synthesis was stimulated but protein degradation was not reduced[84] (Figs. 38.6, 38.7). The results suggest that muscle protein breakdown becomes resistant to IGF-I during sepsis and that this resistance is at the postreceptor level, similar to the situation for insulin.[75] A study in our laboratory suggested that IGF-I resistance in septic muscle is not an in vitro phenomenon only but occurs in vivo as well. When septic rats were infused with IGF-I in vivo, the sepsis-induced reduction in protein synthesis was blunted (though not completely reversed), whereas the increase in protein breakdown was not affected by the hormone (unpublished observations). The results discussed here suggest that treatment with IGF-I (and perhaps insulin as well) may be efficacious in treating or preventing muscle cachexia in some (e.g., burn injury) but not all (e.g., sepsis) catabolic conditions. The difference in regulation of protein degradation by IGF-I in muscles from septic and burned rats is an interesting observation in itself because it suggests that intracellular signaling pathways accounting for stimulated proteolysis may vary among catabolic conditions.

Related to treatment with anabolic hormones is treatment designed to block the effects of catabolic hormones. In previous studies we found that treatment of rats with the glucocorticoid receptor antagonist RU38486 blocked the sepsis-induced increase in muscle proteolysis[25] and that this effect of the receptor antagonist mainly reflected inhibited energy/ubiquitin-dependent protein breakdown.[24] Similar results were observed after treatment of burned rats with RU38486.[85] It should be noted that in those studies RU38486 was used to elucidate the role of glucocorticoids in sepsis-induced muscle breakdown, and the implications of the results with regard to the potential use of the drug to reduce the catabolic response in septic or injured patients are not known at present.

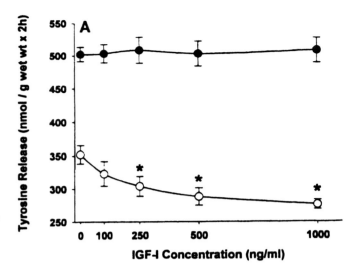

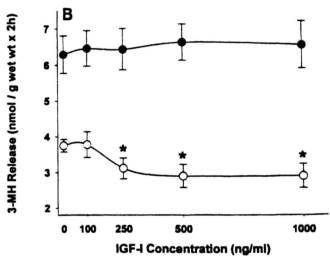

FIGURE 38.6. Effect of various concentrations of insulin-like growth factor-I (IGF-I) on total (A) and myofibrillar (B) protein breakdown in muscles from sham-operated rats (open circles) and septic rats (filled circles): $n > 7$ for each data point. $^*p < 0.05$ versus no IGF-I. (From Hobler et al.,[84] with permission.)

Anticytokine Treatment

Because of the important role of proinflammatory cytokines in the development of sepsis and the systemic inflammatory response syndrome (SIRS), a number of studies have been reported in which various treatments to block the effects of some of these cytokines were tested. Although clinical studies using this approach in septic patients have been disappointing so far,[86,87] blocking the effects of proinflammatory cytokines has been successful in reducing or inhibiting sepsis-induced muscle cachexia.

In studies in our laboratory, treatment of rats with anti-TNF antibody prevented a sepsis-induced increase in muscle protein breakdown, supporting the role of TNF as an essential mediator of muscle proteolysis.[9] In other experiments we found that treatment of septic rats with IL-1 receptor antagonist abolished

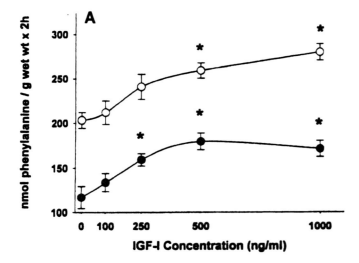

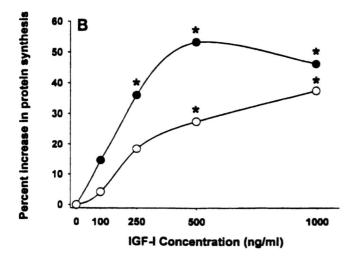

FIGURE 38.7. Effect of various concentrations of IGF-I on protein synthesis in muscles from sham-operated rats (open circles) and septic rats (filled circles). Results are given as nanomoles of phenylalanine per gram wet weight over 2 hours (A) or percent increase in protein synthesis (B); $n = 7$ or 8 for each data point. $^*p < 0.05$ versus no IGF-I. (From Hobler et al.,[84] with permission.)

the increase in muscle protein degradation.[10] Reports from other laboratories provided evidence that pentoxifylline, a substance that inhibits TNF release during sepsis and endotoxemia, improved the catabolic situation in skeletal muscle.[88]

It should be noted that even if treatment with cytokine antibodies or receptor antagonists can effectively block sepsis-induced muscle proteolysis, the interpretation of those results with regard to potential clinical applicability must be done with caution. The cytokine cascade is a complex response to sepsis and injury and probably has both positive and negative effects. Manipulation of this response therefore must be done extremely carefully, and previous failures of clinical trials suggest that anticytokine treatment does not play an important role in the prevention of muscle cachexia in these patients. The most important role of this treatment will probably continue to be as a tool to define mediators and mechanisms of the catabolic response in skeletal muscle.

Nutritional Support

A large number of previous studies have addressed the role of nutritional support in injured and septic patients. Three major areas have been the subject of research: (1) the composition of the nutritional support; (2) the timing (i.e., early versus delayed nutrition); and (3) the route of administration (i.e., enteral versus parenteral nutrition). Most authors seem to agree that early administration of nutrition is better than late treatment, and that enteral is better than parenteral nutrition, although some controversy exists. Most previous reports on the role of nutrition in injured and septic patients examined morbidity (e.g., infectious complications, anastomotic leaks), length of hospital stay, and mortality, surprisingly little information is available with regard to the specific influence on muscle protein balance in these patients.

In early studies parenteral nutrition enriched with high concentrations of branched-chain amino acids (leucine, isoleucine, valine) was used in an attempt to reduce the catabolic response in skeletal muscle and to improve the whole-body protein balance.[89] Those studies were in part based on in vitro observations that the branched-chain amino acids reduced protein breakdown and stimulated protein synthesis in incubated rat skeletal muscles.[90] Although some beneficial effects were noted, most studies did not show a significant improvement of nitrogen balance after administration of branched-chain amino acid-enriched solutions to patients with sepsis and other critical illness.[89] One reason for the lack of effect of this treatment may be that the anabolic effects of the branched-chain amino acids seen in normal muscle were not present in septic muscle, suggesting that catabolic muscles are resistant to the effects of these amino acids.[91]

Glutamine is probably the most extensively studied (and perhaps the most controversial) individual component of enteral and parenteral nutrition. The use of glutamine to improve muscle cachexia is based on in vitro experiments in rat skeletal muscle. In those studies treatment of incubated or perfused rat muscles with glutamine increased protein synthesis and inhibited protein breakdown.[92,93] In other studies, muscle glutamine levels were reduced in catabolic muscles,[94] further supporting the concept that administration of this amino acid to patients with injury or sepsis would improve muscle protein balance. Although some studies have reported improved nitrogen balance and stimulated muscle protein synthesis after administration of glutamine-enriched solutions, most of those studies were performed in patients with only mild trauma (e.g., elective cholecystectomy).[95] There is evidence that with more severe muscle catabolism, as seen during sepsis, glutamine may not be efficacious.[96] In addition, the role of glutamine in the regulation of muscle protein turnover was challenged by experiments in which manipulation of intracellular glutamine levels over a wide range of concentrations was not accompanied by changes in protein synthesis or breakdown rates.[97]

The role of enteral feeding in the metabolic care of critically ill patients has attracted great attention in recent years. One potential mechanism by which enteral feeding may be superior to parenteral feeding is the inhibited release of proinflammatory cytokines.[98] So-called immunonutrition (i.e., provision of specific nutrients that can influence immune function, in particular arginine, glutamine, omega-3 fatty acids, and RNA) has been intensively investigated in recent years.[99-101] Results from several of those studies suggest that enteral administration of these substances to patients with critical illness may improve the metabolic situation, reduce infectious complications, and shorten the length of stay in the ICU. The effect of immunonutrition on muscle protein metabolism in these patients is not known at present.

It should be noted that although many authorities are in agreement that enteral feeding is superior to parenteral feeding, an extensive review of the literature offered a different view of the subject.[102] The author of that review concluded that with the exception of decreased cost and potentially reduced septic morbidity in patients with acute abdominal trauma the available literature does not support the concept that enteral feeding is better than parenteral nutrition in humans.

Acknowledgments. Supported in part by NIH grant DK 37908 and by grants from the Shriners of North America, Tampa, FL. T.A.P. was supported by NIH training grant 1T32GM008478 and D.R.F. by a Research Fellowship from the Shriners of North America.

References

1. Hasselgren PO: Mediators, hormones, and control of metabolism: regulation of protein, carbohydrate, and lipid metabolism in critical illness. In: Fischer JE (ed) Nutrition and Metabolism in the Surgical Patient, 2nd ed. Boston: Little, Brown, 1996; 57–104.
2. Hill AG, Hill GL: Metabolic response to severe injury. Br J Surg 1998;85:884–890.
3. Reid WD, MacGowan NA: Respiratory muscle injury in animal models and humans. Mol Cell Biochem 1998;179:63–80.
4. Hasselgren PO, James JH, Benson DW, et al: Total and myofibrillar protein breakdown in different types of rat skeletal muscle: effects of sepsis and regulation by insulin. Metabolism 1989;38:634–640.
5. Long CL, Birkhahn RH, Geiger JW, et al: Urinary excretion of 3-methylhistidine: an assessment of muscle protein catabolism in adult normal subjects and during malnutrition, sepsis, and skeletal trauma. Metabolism 1981;30:765–776.
6. Vary TC, Kimball SR: Sepsis-induced changes in protein synthesis: differential effects on fast- and slow-twitch muscles. Am J Physiol 1992;262:C1513–C1519.
7. Chang HR, Bistrian B: The role of cytokines in the catabolic consequences of infection and injury. JPEN J Parenter Enteral Nutr 1998;22:156–166.
8. Zamir O, Hasselgren PO, Higashiguchi T, et al: Tumor necrosis factor and interleukin-1 induce muscle proteolysis through different mechanisms. Mediat Inflamm 1992;1:247–250.
9. Zamir O, Hasselgren PO, Kunkel SL, et al: Evidence that tumor necrosis factor participates in the regulation of muscle proteolysis during sepsis. Arch Surg 1992;127:170–174.
10. Zamir O, O'Brien W, Thompson R, et al: Reduced muscle protein breakdown in septic rats following treatment with interleukin-1 receptor antagonist. Int J Biochem 1994;26:943–950.
11. Mealy K, van Lanschot JJB, Robinson BG, et al: Are the catabolic effects of tumor necrosis factor mediated by glucocorticoids? Arch Surg 1990;125:42–48.
12. Moldawer LL, Svaninger G, Gelin J, et al: Interleukin-1 and tumor necrosis factor do not regulate protein balance in skeletal muscle. Am J Physiol 1987;253:C766–C773.
13. Goldberg AL, Kettelhut IC, Furano K, et al: Activation of protein breakdown and prostaglandin E_2 production in rat skeletal muscle in fever is signaled by a macrophage product distinct from interleukin-1 or other known monokines. J Clin Invest 1988;81:1378–1383.
14. Hasselgren PO, James JH, Benson DW, et al: Is there a circulating proteolysis-inducing factor during sepsis? Arch Surg 1990;125:510–514.
15. Damas P, Ledoux D, Nys M, et al: Cytokine serum level during severe sepsis in human: IL-6 as a marker of severity. Ann Surg 1992;215:356–362.
16. Tsujinaka T, Ebisui C, Fujita J, et al: Muscles undergo atrophy in association with increase of lysosomal cathepsin activity in interleukin-6 transgenic mouse. Biochem Biophys Res Commun 1995;207:168–174.
17. Strassman G, Fong M, Kenney JS, et al: Evidence for the involvement of interleukin-6 in experimental cancer cachexia. J Clin Invest 1992;89:1681–1684.
18. Williams A, Wang JJ, Wang L, et al: Sepsis in mice stimulates muscle proteolysis in the absence of IL-6. Am J Physiol 1998;275:R1983–R1991.
19. Garzia-Martinez C, Lopez-Soriano FJ, Argiles JM: Interleukin-6 does not activate protein breakdown in rat skeletal muscle. Cancer Lett 1994;76:1–4.
20. Espat NJ, Auffenberg T, Rosenberg JJ, et al: Ciliary neurotrophic factor is catabolic and shares with IL-6 the capacity to induce an acute phase response. Am J Physiol 1996;271:R185–R190.
21. Vaughan GM, Becker RA, Allen JP, et al: Cortisol and corticotrophin in burned patients. J Trauma 1982;22:263–273.
22. Darmann D, Matthews DE, Bier DM: Physiological hypercortisolemia increases proteolysis, glutamine and alanine production. Am J Physiol 1988;255:E366–E373.
23. Kayali AG, Young VR, Goodman MN: Sensitivity of myofibrillar proteins to glucocorticoid-induced muscle proteolysis. Am J Physiol 1987;252:E621–E626.
24. Tiao G, Fagan J, Roegner V, et al: Energy-ubiquitin-dependent muscle proteolysis during sepsis in rats is regulated by glucocorticoids. J Clin Invest 1996;97:339–348.
25. Hall-Angeras M, Angeras U, Zamir O, et al: Effect of the glucocorticoid receptor antagonist RU38486 on muscle protein breakdown in sepsis. Surgery 1991;109:468–473.
26. Fang CH, James JH, Ogle CK, et al: Influence of burn injury on protein metabolism in different types of skeletal muscle and the role of glucocorticoids. J Am Coll Surg 1995;180:33–42.
27. Wing SS, Goldberg AL: Glucocorticoids activate the ATP-ubiquitin-dependent proteolytic system in skeletal muscle during fasting. Am J Physiol 1993;264:E668–E676.

28. Savary I, Debras E, Dardavet D, et al: Effect of glucocorticoid excess on skeletal muscle and heart protein synthesis in adult and old rats. Br J Nutr 1998;79:297–304.
29. Odedra BR, Bates PC, Millward DJ: Time course of the effect of catabolic doses of corticosterone on protein turnover in rat skeletal muscle and liver. Biochem J 1983;214:617–627.
30. Hong DH, Forsberg NE: Effects of dexamethasone on protein degradation and protease gene expression in rat L8 myotube cultures. Mol Cell Endocrinol 1995;108:199–209.
31. Wang L, Luo GJ, Wang JJ, et al: Dexamethasone stimulates proteasome- and calcium-dependent proteolysis in cultured L6 myotubes. Shock 1998;10:298–306.
32. Del Ray A, Besedovsky HO: Metabolic and neuroendocrine effects of pro-inflammatory cytokines. Eur J Clin Invest 1992;22:10–15.
33. Kern JA, Lamb RJ, Reed JC, et al: Dexamethasone inhibition of interleukin-1 beta production by human monocytes. J Clin Invest 1988;81:237–244.
34. Hall-Angeras M, Angeras U, Zamir O, et al: Interaction between corticosterone and tumor necrosis factor stimulated protein breakdown in rat skeletal muscle, similar to sepsis. Surgery 1990;108:460–466.
35. Tisdale MJ: New cachexic factors. Curr Opin Clin Nutr Metab Care 1998;1:253–256.
36. Todorov PT, Deacon M, Tisdale MJ: Structural analysis of a tumor-produced sulfated glycoprotein capable of initiating muscle protein degradation. J Biol Chem 1997;272:12279–12288.
37. Clowes GHA, George BC, Villee CA, et al: Muscle proteolysis induced by a circulating peptide in patients with trauma and sepsis. N Engl J Med 1983;308:545–552.
38. Thompson MG, Palmer RM: Signaling pathways regulating protein turnover in skeletal muscle. Cell Signal 1998;10:1–11.
39. Tiao G, Fagan JM, Samuels N, et al: Sepsis stimulates non-lysosomal energy-dependent proteolysis and increases ubiquitin mRNA levels in rat skeletal muscle. J Clin Invest 1994;94:2255–2264.
40. Tiao G, Hobler SC, Wang JJ, et al: Sepsis is associated with increased mRNAs of the ubiquitin-proteasome proteolytic pathway in human skeletal muscle. J Clin Invest 1997;99:163–168.
41. Hobler SC, Tiao G, Fischer JE, et al: The sepsis-induced increase in muscle proteolysis is blocked by specific proteasome inhibitors. Am J Physiol 1998;274:R30–R37.
42. Attaix D, Taillandier D: The critical role of the ubiquitin-proteasome pathway in muscle wasting in comparison to lysosomal and calcium-dependent systems. Adv Mol Cell Biol 1998;27:235–266.
43. Voisin L, Breuille O, Combaret L, et al: Muscle wasting in a rat model of long lasting sepsis results from the activation of lysosomal, calcium-activated, and ubiquitin-proteasome proteolytic pathways. J Clin Invest 1996;97:1610–1617.
44. Hasselgren PO, Fischer JE: The ubiquitin-proteasome pathway: review of a novel intracellular mechanism of muscle protein breakdown during sepsis and other catabolic conditions. Ann Surg 1997;225:307–316.
45. Hershko A, Ciechanover A: The ubiquitin system for protein degradation. Annu Rev Biochem 1992;61:761–807.
46. Wing SS, Banville D: 14-kDa ubiquitin-conjugating enzyme: structure of the rat gene and regulation upon fasting and by insulin. Am J Physiol 1994;267:E39–E48.
47. Weissman JS, Sigler PB, Horwich AL: From the cradle to the grave: ring complexes in the life of a protein. Science 1995;268:523–524.
48. Fang CH, Tiao G, James JH, et al: Burn injury stimulates multiple proteolytic pathways in skeletal muscle, including the ubiquitin-energy-dependent pathway. J Am Coll Surg 1995;180:161–170.
49. Hobler SC, Williams AB, Fischer D, et al: The activity and expression of the 20S proteasome are increased in skeletal muscle during sepsis. Am J Physiol 1999;277:R434–R440.
50. Wing SS, Bedard N: Insulin-like growth factor I stimulates degradation of an mRNA transcript encoding the 14 kDa ubiquitin conjugating enzyme. Biochem J 1996;319:455–461.
51. Hobler SC, Wang JJ, Williams AB, et al: Sepsis is associated with increased ubiquitin conjugating enzyme E2-14kDa mRNA in skeletal muscle. Am J Physiol 1999;276:R468–R473.
52. Tiao G, Lieberman MA, Fischer JE, et al: Intracellular regulation of protein degradation during sepsis is different in fast- and slow-twitch muscle. Am J Physiol 1997;272:R849–R856.
53. Fang CH, Li BG, Tiao G, et al: The molecular regulation of protein breakdown following burn injury is different in fast- and slow-twitch skeletal muscle. Int J Mol Med 1998;1:163–169.
54. Lee DH, Goldberg AL: Proteasome inhibitors: valuable new tools for cell biologists. Trends Cell Biol 1998;8:397–403.
55. Fenteany G, Standaert RF, Lane WS, et al: Inhibition of proteasome activities and subunit-specific amino-terminal threonine modification by lactacystin. Science 1995;268:726–731.
56. Tawa NE, Odessey R, Goldberg AL: Inhibitors of the proteasome reduce the accelerated proteolysis in atrophying rat skeletal muscles. J Clin Invest 1997;100:197–203.
57. Fang CH, Wang JJ, Hobler S, et al: Proteasome blockers inhibit protein breakdown in skeletal muscle after burn injury in rats. Clin Sci 1998;95:225–233.
58. Dick LR, Cruikshank AA, Grenier L, et al: Mechanistic studies on the inactivation of the proteasome by lactacystin: a central role for clasto-lactacystin beta-lactone. J Biol Chem 1996;271:7273–7276.
59. Mansoor O, Beaufrere B, Boirie Y, et al: Increased mRNA levels for components of the lysosomal, calcium-activated, and ATP-ubiquitin-dependent proteolytic pathways in skeletal muscle from head trauma patients. Proc Natl Acad Sci USA 1996;93:2714–2718.
60. Williams AB, Sun X, Fischer JE, et al: The expression of genes in the ubiquitin-proteasome proteolytic pathway is increased in skeletal muscle from patients with cancer. Surgery (in press).
61. Tiao G, Fagan J, Roegner V, et al: Energy-ubiquitin-dependent muscle proteolysis during sepsis in rats is regulated by glucocorticoids. J Clin Invest 1996;97:339–348.
62. Auclair D, Garrel DR, Zerouala AC, et al: Activation of the ubiquitin pathway in rat skeletal muscle by catabolic doses of glucocorticoids. Am J Physiol 1997;272:C1007–C1016.
63. Ralliere C, Tauveron I, Taillandier D, et al: Glucocorticoids do not regulate the expression of proteolytic genes in skeletal muscle from Cushing's syndrome patients. J Clin Endocrinol Metab 1997;82:3161–3164.
64. Roberts RG, Redfern CPF, Goodship THJ: Changes in the expression of proteolytic enzymes following correction of acidosis in humans with renal failure [abstract 1]. Presented at the Fourth International Symposium on Amino Acid/Protein Metabolism in Health and Disease, Padova, Italy, April 1996.

65. Price SR, England BK, Bailey JK, et al: Acidosis and glucocorticoids concomitantly increase ubiquitin and proteasome subunit mRNAs in rat muscle. Am J Physiol 1994;267:C955–C960.
66. Madura K, Dohmen RJ, Varshavsky A: N-recognin/Ubc2 interactions in the N-end rule pathway. J Biol Chem 1993;268:12046–12054.
67. Varshavsky A: The N-end rule pathway of protein degradation. Genes Cells 1997;2:13–28.
68. Kwon YT, Reiss Y, Fried VA, et al: The mouse and human genes encoding the recognition component of the N-end rule pathway. Proc Natl Acad Sci USA 1998;95:7898–7903.
69. Solomon V, Lecker SH, Goldberg AL: The N-end rule pathway catalyzes a major fraction of the protein degradation in skeletal muscle. J Biol Chem 1998;273:25216–25222.
70. Solomon V, Barracos V, Sarraf P, et al: Rates of ubiquitin conjugation increase when muscles atrophy, largely through activation of the N-end rule pathway. Proc Natl Acad Sci USA 1998;95:12602–12607.
71. Williams A, de Courten-Myers GM, Fischer JE, et al: Sepsis stimulates release of myofilaments in skeletal muscle by a calcium-dependent mechanism. FASEB J 1999;13:1435–1443.
72. Kimball SR, Vary TC, Jefferson LS: Regulation of protein synthesis by insulin. Annu Rev Physiol 1994;56:321–348.
73. Hasselgren PO, Fischer JE: Regulation by insulin of muscle protein metabolism during sepsis and other catabolic conditions. Nutrition 1992;8:434–439.
74. Thorell A, Nygren J, Hirschman MF, et al: Surgery-induced insulin resistance in human patients: relation to glucose transport and utilization. Am J Physiol 1999;276:E754–E761.
75. Hasselgren PO, Warner BW, James JH, et al: Effect of insulin on amino acid uptake and protein turnover in skeletal muscle from septic rats: evidence for insulin resistance of protein breakdown. Arch Surg 1987;122:228–233.
76. Hinton PS, Littlejohn SP, Allison FP, et al: Insulin and glucose to reduce the catabolic response to injury in burned patients. Lancet 1971;17:767–769.
77. Wilmore DW, Moylan JA, Briston B, et al: Anabolic effects of human growth hormone and high caloric feedings following thermal injury. Surg Gynecol Obstet 1974;138:855–884.
78. Jiang SM, He GZ, Zhang SY, et al: Low-dose growth hormone and hypocaloric nutrition attenuate the protein-catabolic response after major operation. Ann Surg 1989;210:513–524.
79. Public communication from Pharmacia & Upjohn Pharmaceuticals and Rolf Gunnarsson, M.D., to all industry and medical community involved with the use or potential use of recombinant human growth hormone, October 1997.
80. Ramirez RJ, Wolf SE, Barrow AE, et al: Growth hormone treatment in pediatric burns: a safe therapeutic approach. Ann Surg 1998;228:439–448.
81. Fang CH, Li BG, Wang JJ, et al: Insulin-like growth factor I (IGF-I) stimulates protein synthesis and inhibits protein breakdown in muscle from burned rats. JPEN J Parenter Enteral Nutr 1997;21:245–251.
82. Fang CH, Li BG, Wang JJ, et al: Treatment of rats with insulin-like growth factor I inhibit the catabolic response in skeletal muscle following burn injury. Am J Physiol 1998;275:R1091–R1098.
83. Fang CH, Li BG, James JH, et al: The anabolic effects of IGF-I in skeletal muscle are not caused by increased cell volume. JPEN J Parenter Enteral Nutr 1998;22:115–119.
84. Hobler SC, Williams A, Fischer JE, et al: Insulin-like growth factor I (IGF-I) stimulates protein synthesis but does not inhibit protein breakdown in muscle from septic rats. Am J Physiol 1998;274:R571–R576.
85. Fang CH, James JH, Ogle C, et al: Influence of burn injury on protein metabolism in different types of skeletal muscle and the role of glucocorticoids. J Am Coll Surg 1995;180:33–42.
86. Fisher CJ, Dhainhaut JFA, Opal SM, et al: Recombinant human interleukin-1 receptor antagonist in the treatment of patients with sepsis syndrome: results from a randomized, double-blind, placebo-controlled trial. JAMA 1994;271:1836–1843.
87. Zeni F, Freeman B, Natanson C: Anti-inflammatory therapies to treat sepsis and septic shock: a reassessment. Crit Care Med 1997;25:1095–1100.
88. Breuille D, Farge MC, Rose R, et al: Pentoxifylline decreases the body weight loss and muscle protein wasting during chronic sepsis. Am J Physiol 1994;268:E636–E641.
89. Sax HC, Talamini MA, Fischer JE: Clinical use of branched-chain amino acids in liver disease, sepsis, trauma, and burns. Arch Surg 1986;121:358–366.
90. Buse MG, Reid SS: Leucine: a possible regulator of protein turnover in muscle. J Clin Invest 1975;56:1250–1261.
91. Hasselgren PO, James JH, Warner BW, et al: Protein synthesis and degradation in skeletal muscle from septic rats: response to leucine and alpha-ketoisocaproic acid. Arch Surg 1988;123:640–644.
92. MacLennan PA, Brown RA, Rennie MJ: A positive relationship between protein synthetic rate and intracellular glutamine concentration in perfused rat skeletal muscle. FEBS Lett 1987;215:187–191.
93. MacLennan PA, Smith K, Weryk B, et al: Inhibition of protein breakdown by glutamine in perfused rat skeletal muscle. FEBS Lett 1988;237:133–136.
94. Roth E, Funovics J, Muhlbacher F, et al: Metabolic disorders in severe abdominal sepsis: glutamine deficiency in skeletal muscle. Clin Nutr 1982;1:25–41.
95. Hammarqvist F, Wernerman J, Ali R, et al: Addition of glutamine to total parenteral nutrition after elective abdominal surgery spares free glutamine in muscle, counteracts the fall in muscle protein synthesis, and improves nitrogen balance. Ann Surg 1989;209:455–461.
96. Karner J, Roth E, Ollenschlager G, et al: Glutamine-containing dipeptides as infusion substrates in the septic state. Surgery 1989;106:893–900.
97. Fang CH, James JH, Fischer JE, et al: Is muscle protein turnover regulated by intracellular glutamine during sepsis? JPEN J Parenter Enteral Nutr 1995;19:279–285.
98. Kiyama T, Witte MB, Thornton FJ, et al: The route of nutrition support affects the early phase of wound healing. JPEN J Parenter Enteral Nutr 1998;22:276–279.
99. Evoy D, Lieberman MD, Fahey TJ, et al: Immunonutrition: the role of arginine. Nutrition 1998;14:611–617.
100. Wilmore DW, Shabert JK: Role of glutamine in immunologic responses. Nutrition 1998;14:618–626.
101. Alexander JW: Immunonutrition: the role of omega-3 fatty acids. Nutrition 1998;14:627–633.
102. Lipman TO: Grains or veins: is enteral nutrition really better than parenteral nutrition? A look at the evidence. JPEN J Parenter Enteral Nutr 1998;22:167–182.

39
Immunomodulation of Cell-Mediated Responses: Is It Feasible?

Eugen Faist and M.W. Wichmann

We know that the endogenous provisions of the organism to survive after major trauma are not sufficient and require exogenous support. Immunomodulatory strategies should prevent the conversion from systemic inflammatory response syndrome (SIRS) to bacterial sepsis and septic shock. Several strategies have been evaluated, including the blockade of mediators, particularly if their levels or effects become excessive and threaten the individual. Clinical trials with anti-tumor necrosis factor (TNF) antibodies, soluble TNF receptors, interleukin-1 (IL-1) receptor antagonists, and anti-lipopolysaccharide (LPS) monoclonal antibodies have been carried out, but no significant treatment benefit was observed.

Severe trauma is a vital threat to each patient; the threat lies not only in the trauma itself but the complications seen during the subsequent clinical course due to ensuing immunologic dysregulation. We have previously reported that 50% of all patients with an Injury Severity Score (ISS) ≥ 30 who survived the immediate posttraumatic phase suffered from a complicated clinical course due to inflammatory or infectious episodes.[1] Furthermore, a significantly increased incidence of SIRS and multiple organ failure as well as an increased postoperative mortality rate (35%) have been observed in patients with a postoperative Acute Physiology and Chronic Health Evaluation (APACHE II) score ≥ 19.[2,3]

Inflammatory and infectious complications may ultimately result in sepsis and multiple organ failure, which are known to be associated with a mortality rate of up to 80%.[4] Reasons for these severe posttraumatic complications are believed to be extended tissue necrosis, hemorrhagic shock, and bacterial translocation from the gut. Moreover, significant alterations of the posttraumatic mediator release, including cytokines, have been observed. A number of laboratory and clinical studies have demonstrated the close relation between trauma, shock, SIRS, and sepsis. These studies show that trauma and hemorrhagic shock may induce SIRS, which results in severe depression of immunologic functions and gives way to the development of multiple organ failure, severe sepsis, or septic shock.[5–11]

Macrophages and lymphocytes contribute to the severity of the systemic inflammatory response through increased release of a number of cytokines.[12,13] The overwhelming inflammatory response results from an uncontrolled immune reaction with overactivation of nonspecific reaction and paralysis of specific reactions, thereby inducing an autodestructive process.[14] This systemic process may finally result in dysfunction of organs that were not affected primarily by the trauma mechanism itself.[15] Multisystem organ failure (MOF) usually occurs in a cascade that affects the lungs prior to the liver, gut, and kidneys.[16] Circulatory failure usually is a late symptom of this disease process.

Immunologic Alterations Following Severe Trauma

The immunologic response to severe trauma and hemorrhagic shock, which starts within minutes, is characterized by the immediate activation of monocytes. This activation leads to the increased synthesis and release of inflammatory mediators.[17–19] Under physiologic conditions there is a delicate balance between pro- and antiinflammatory cytokines (Table 39.1) that is easily disrupted under adverse conditions. In correlation with the severity of trauma and the duration of the hypotension, not only a localized inflammatory response for the initiation of tissue repair may be observed but also systemic induction of a generalized inflammatory process.[16] This first phase of the inflammatory response is mediated by the coagulation and complement activation cascade.[20] Activated macrophages then contribute to the severity of the inflammatory response. The overwhelming immune response to trauma may induce SIRS and MOF, which is observed in up to 30% of all trauma patients and is known to result in up to 80% mortality.[21,22] Because of the systemic inflammation, not only organs affected by the trauma itself fail but remote organ failure may be observed as well.[16] MOF therefore may be considered the major complication of severe trauma and hemorrhagic shock.[23]

Significant depression of cell-mediated and humoral immune functions have been described following soft tissue trauma, bone fracture, and hemorrhagic shock.[10–12,24–28] Furthermore, an increased risk of septic complications has been observed following hemorrhagic shock.[29] The observed changes of

TABLE 39.1. Proinflammatory and Antiinflammatory Mediators.

Proinflammatory mediators
  TNFα
  IL-1
  IL-6
  IL-8

Antiinflammatory mediators
  IL-4
  IL-10
  IL-11
  IL-13
  TGFβ

specific and nonspecific immune functions following severe trauma are shown in Table 39.2.

A number of hormones and mediators have been described that may influence host immunity following trauma-hemorrhage. Melatonin and prolactin were observed to exert protective effects, whereas male sex steroids have been shown to be detrimental to posttraumatic immune functions (Table 39.3).[30–36]

Cytokine Levels After Trauma

Trauma and shock with subsequent ischemia/reperfusion and burn trauma activate immunocompetent cells and induce the release of proinflammatory mediators.[17,18] Nonetheless, the exact trauma-induced alterations of cytokine plasma levels and their physiologic implications are not completely understood. Moreover, contradictory findings regarding the detectable levels of pro- and antiinflammatory cytokines following adverse conditions have been reported. These observations support the notion that not only the circulating levels of

TABLE 39.2. Immune Dysfunctions Observed Following Hemorrhagic Shock and Soft Tissue Trauma.

Specific immune functions
  Lymphopenia
  CD4/CD8 ratio < 1
  T and B cell proliferation ↓
  B cell differentiation ↓
  Natural killer (NK) cell activity ↓
  Lymphokine production ↓ (IL-2, IL-3, IFNγ)
  IL-2 receptor expression ↓
  IL-4 and IL-10 production ↑
  HLA-DR expression ↓
  DTH skin test ↓

Nonspecific immune functions
  Monocytosis
  IL-6 (and TNFα?) plasma levels ↑
  Acute-phase protein synthesis ↑
  MØ IL-1 production ↓
  MØ PGE$_2$ production/plasma level ↑
  Granulocyte function ↓ (chemotaxis, phagocytosis)
  Neopterin plasma level ↑

TABLE 39.3. Hormones with Immunomodulatory Potential.

Hormone	Immunologic effects
Melatonin	Stimulation of posttraumatic cell-mediated immunity; improved survival of polymicrobial sepsis
Prolactin	Stimulation of posttraumatic cell-mediated immunity; improved survival of polymicrobial sepsis
Testosterone	Decreased posttraumatic immune function
Serotonin	Dose-dependent improvement of granulocyte function

immunologic mediators are of special interest; local concentrations of these mediators at the site of inflammation should be measured as well, although they are difficult if not impossible to obtain.

It is well documented that the initial overactivation of monocytes/macrophages results in initial immunologic paralysis, which is only partially compensated after 3–5 days owing to the influx of new and immature monocytes/macrophages.[37] Overactivation of immunocompetent cells results in the increased release of proinflammatory mediators, for which measurements were attempted in a number of studies.

Immediately following severe trauma decreased synthesis and release of cytokines [i.e., IL-2, IL-3, interferon-γ (IFNγ)] have been observed. Furthermore, IL-2 receptors and HLA-DR are downregulated on the surface of monocytes. A positive correlation between the decreased expression of HLA-DR and the incidence of septic complications in trauma patients has been reported.[38]

Plasma IL-6 and TNF levels were measured following trauma and elective surgery. Significantly increased IL-6 levels were followed by a significant increase of C-reactive protein (CRP), but there were no significant changes in the TNF levels.[39] Moreover, there was no correlation between the measured cytokine levels and the development of complications.[39] Additional studies confirmed the association between increased IL-6 and CRP levels.[40,41] Another study evaluated the importance of elevated IL-6 and TNFα levels in trauma patients and showed a positive correlation between increased levels of these cytokines and poor prognosis in patients with multiple system organ failure.[42] A rapid, significant increase of plasma IL-6 and IL-8 levels within 12 hours of resuscitation was observed in trauma patients.[22] These levels remained significantly increased for more than 5 days in patients with a trauma score (ISS) higher than 25.[22] Schinkel et al.[18] showed immediate activation of chemotactic cytokines (IL-8, ENA-78) and soluble adhesion molecules (sE-selectin, sP-selectin) following severe trauma within minutes after trauma, but they did not correlate with the incidence of infection or patient outcome.[18]

Immunomodulatory Approach

The immunomodulatory intervention following severe trauma or hemorrhagic shock aims to ameliorate the early hyperinflammatory phase (SIRS) with the massive release of mediators to avoid the development of sepsis. At the same time a possibly developing phase of compensation (CARS) must be detected and treated with immunoenhancing measures. Immunomodulation therefore must prevent lymphocytes and macrophages as well as granulocytes and endothelial cells from overactivation. Because of the multitude of therapeutic goals it is obvious that not a single drug or intervention can be useful in the immunomodulatory approach. The intervention must address several issues.

1. Excessive stimulation of macrophages through circulating endotoxins or exotoxins must be avoided.
2. Short-term limitation of the inflammatory response of immunocompetent cells must be achieved (<72 hours).
3. Posttraumatic immunoparalysis must be overcome via reactivation of cell-mediated immunity.[43]

A number of laboratory and clinical studies have been carried out to evaluate the immunomodulatory potential of various drugs and hormones following trauma and hemorrhagic shock.

Immunomodulation in Laboratory Animal Studies

Positive immunologic effects were observed following the experimental use of interferon,[44,45] ATP-MgCl$_2$,[46–48] n-3 unsaturated fatty acids,[49] ibuprofen,[50] chloroquine,[51–53] TNF antibodies,[54] diltiazem,[55] chemically modified/nonanticoagulant heparin,[56,57] pentoxifylline,[58] platelet-activating factor (PAF) antagonists,[59] prolactin,[35] and melatonin.[33,34] A number of these agents were less effective in clinical trials, particularly IFNγ,[60] TNF antibodies,[61] and PAF antagonists.[62] It appears that the disappointing results so far are due in part to difficulties with the study design and data evaluation. Pentoxifylline, however, was shown to exert beneficial immunologic effects even in clinical studies.[63,64] The other mentioned therapeutic interventions are still under clinical evaluation or have not yet been tested.

Influence of Sex Steroids

Data from animal research suggest the importance of male and female sex steroids for cell-mediated immune functions. These studies focused on the immunologic relevance of male and female sex steroids following soft tissue trauma and hemorrhagic shock as well as during severe sepsis following cecal ligation and puncture (CLP). Our laboratory studies were initiated because of the better outcome of female patients regarding the incidence of and mortality due to septic complications following trauma and hemorrhagic shock observed in a small number of clinical and epidemiologic studies.[65–67]

Zellweger et al. reported significantly better immune functions and better survival rates in female mice than in males following induction of polymicrobial sepsis (CLP).[68,69] Subsequent studies comparing male mice with proestrus and diestrus female mice following hemorrhagic shock showed significantly increased levels of IL-1 and IL-3 release from lymphocytes and splenocyte proliferative capacity in female mice.[70] Male mice, on the other hand, suffered from significantly decreased release of IL-1, IL-2, IL-3, and IL-6 from macrophages and lymphocytes. Subsequently, male mice were subjected to castration to elucidate the contribution of testosterone to the immune dysfunction observed in males following hemorrhagic shock. These studies showed significant depression of splenocyte proliferation and IL-2 and IL-3 release in sham-castrated mice following hemorrhagic shock and soft tissue trauma.[30] Castrated males with no detectable circulating testosterone, in contrast, showed conservation of cell-mediated immunity. Similar observations were made with IL-1 and IL-6 release from splenic and peritoneal macrophages.[32]

These observations indicate the important role of testosterone in the observed immune dysfunction in male mice following trauma-hemorrhage. To study whether castration itself prior to trauma-hemorrhage contributed to the observed immune protection, a testosterone receptor antagonist, flutamide, was administered following trauma-hemorrhage. At 72 hours after soft tissue trauma and hemorrhagic shock, similar protection of the cell-mediated immunity was observed in flutamide-treated mice.[31] Peritoneal and splenic macrophage IL-1 release as well as lymphocyte IL-2 and IL-3 release were preserved in a dose-dependent fashion following trauma-hemorrhage. This observation indicates the important influence of testosterone and testosterone receptors on immunocompetent cells in mediating immune dysfunction in male mice following soft tissue trauma and hemorrhagic shock. Subsequent studies revealed the potential of the testosterone receptor antagonist flutamide to protect male mice from the lethal effects of CLP following hemorrhagic shock.[71]

A clinical investigation by Wichmann et al.,[72] studying almost 4000 surgical intensive care unit (ICU) patients, was unable to demonstrate gender differences regarding mortality due to severe sepsis in humans, although a significantly lower incidence of sepsis was observed in female patients. Schröder et al.,[73] on the other hand, observed in far smaller patient population significantly lower mortality in female patients with severe sepsis. Whether the observed influence of sex steroids translates into an immunologic advantage for mostly postmenopausal female surgical ICU patients remains to be determined.

Despite the contradictory clinical findings, we suggest that sex steroids play an important role in modulating immune functions following severe trauma and hemorrhagic shock. Furthermore, these findings led us to conclude that sex steroids, receptor antagonists, or both could be used as adjuncts for the treatment of immune dysfunction observed after severe trauma.

Influence of the Brain-Immune Axis

The central nervous system (CNS) and the endocrine system modulate immune functions via release of neurotransmitters, neuropeptides, and endocrine hormones.[74] Mediators released by immunocompetent cells, on the other hand, also have a significant influence on CNS and endocrine functions.[74]

A number of studies reported modulation of immune functions by the CNS, and it has been shown that isolated severe head injury is associated with suppressed cellular immunity. The observed suppression of IL-2 receptor expression and decreased lymphocyte blastogenesis may be partly responsible for increased rates of infection in these patients.[75]

Opioids play a major role in the so-called brain-immune axis, and opioid-induced modulation of the immune system is known to be a complex phenomenon that involves opioid receptors, central and sympathetic neural pathways, and catecholamine receptors.[76] The precise neural pathways and the physiologic relevance of endogenous opioid immune modulation are not well understood.[76] In terms of opioid receptors being involved in the modulation of immunity through mediators released by the CNS, we were able to show that administration of the opioid receptor antagonist naloxone after hemorrhagic shock did not have a beneficial effect on cell-mediated immune functions.[77] In contrast to these findings, other investigators observed functional naloxone-sensitive opioid receptors on lymphocytes that may mediate morphine-induced immunologic dysfunction.[78] In addition to these findings it has been observed that the opioid methionine-enkephalin has significant effects on cell-mediated and humoral immune functions.[79] It was shown that low doses of this opioid have immune-enhancing effects, and high doses suppress immune functions.[79]

In regard to hormones of the hypothalamic-pituitary-adrenal (HPA) axis being part of the immune response to trauma and hemorrhagic shock, Zellweger et al. studied the effects of prolactin on cell-mediated immunity following trauma-hemorrhage. They reported significant beneficial effects on splenocyte proliferation and splenocyte IL-2 and IL-3 release in mice treated with 100 μg prolactin subcutaneously following severe hemorrhagic shock.[35] Significantly improved macrophage IL-1 and IL-6 release following hemorrhagic shock and better survival after severe sepsis (CLP) were observed in additional studies.[36] Finally, administration of metoclopramide, which is known to increase circulating prolactin levels, was shown to exert comparable beneficial effects on cell-mediated immunity (macrophage and lymphocyte cytokine release and proliferation) following hemorrhagic shock.[80] Wichmann et al. studied the effects of melatonin administration on cell-mediated immunity following trauma-hemorrhage. Melatonin, the major hormone released by the pineal gland, has been reported to protect mice subjected to severe hemorrhage and soft tissue trauma from significant depression of immune functions.[33] Furthermore, there was better survival of animals with short-term treatment following hemorrhage prior to the induction of severe sepsis.[34] It is of interest that long-term treatment continued after the induction of sepsis resulted in significantly increased mortality.[34]

These findings allow us to propose that the CNS has significant influence on cell-mediated and humoral immune functions under normal conditions as well as following trauma and hemorrhagic shock. Several immunoregulatory cytokines, including IL-1, IL-2, IL-6, INFγ, and TNF, are produced not only in the immune system but in the neuroendocrine system as well.

Immunomodulation in Clinical Studies

Among the various antiinflammatory therapeutic approaches, several new immunomodulatory strategies have been promoted recently. The use of various growth factors to accelerate wound healing has been suggested; in particular, the sepsis prophylactic property of granulocyte colony-stimulating factor (G-CSF) is of great interest. Suppression of lipopolysaccharide (LPS)-inducible TNFα and IL-1β release by about 50% within 20 hours after treatment was observed, as was a substantial increase of sTNF-R, p75, and IL-1 receptor antagonist. From these findings, it has been concluded that G-CSF treatment switches peripheral leukocyte behavior toward antiinflammatory activity. Another promising approach for attenuating an excessive systemic inflammatory response is the use of xanthine derivatives such as pentoxifylline, which selectively inhibits the formation of TNFα, probably by causing accumulation of intracellular cyclic adenine monophosphate (cAMP).

In one of our most recent investigations, we observed that the addition of human recombinant IL-13 (hrIL-13), a T cell lymphokine, to cell cultures of macrophages from patients after multiple trauma, burns, or major surgical procedures resulted in effective downregulation of the synthesis of proinflammatory mediators such as TNFα, IL-1β, IL-6, and IL-8 as well as nitric oxide.[81] In addition to its antiinflammatory functional properties, hrIL-13 supports a cell-mediated immune response in terms of upregulation of major histocompatibility complex class II antigen-presenting capacity and IFNγ synthesis from large granular lymphocytes.[82] Comparison of the influence of hrIL-13 administration with the effects of hrIL-10 administration to macrophage cultures revealed massive suppression of inflammatory cytokine release by IL-10, whereas the downregulatory effect of IL-13 was moderate. Earlier reports about the biologic properties of IL-10 indicated that this cytokine (unlike IL-13) also acts as a major suppressor factor for T cell performance (proliferation, IL-2 synthesis), has macrophage antigen-presenting capacity, and prompts IFN synthesis and B cell function, resulting in an overall immunosuppressive capacity.[83,84] Our observations and the previously reported findings have raised doubts about the utility of IL-10 as a biologic response modifier for states of posttraumatic SIRS and sepsis, as suggested by others.[85] Taking into account the coexistence of the two immunomechanistic entities—hyperinflammation and depression of cell-mediated immune responses—we believe that IL-13 rather than IL-10 has the characteristics required for an integrated, concerted response in terms of target-seeking counterregulation.

Because adequate macrophage activation and forward-regulatory function depend on sufficient delivery of IFN to these cells, it appeared reasonable to substitute this lymphokine during trauma-induced states of IFN deficiency. IFNγ has been used in two large clinical studies. The first study did not show any differences regarding infection rate or mortality following traumatic immunodepression.[86] The second study, however, demonstrated comparable infection rates following severe trauma but a decreased infection-related mortality rate in the treatment group.[87] These findings agree with those from a number of experimental studies showing that IFN administration in patients with surgical infections is associated with improved outcome; it decreases translocation following transfusion and thermal injury, and it reduces susceptibility to sepsis following hemorrhagic shock. However, under certain conditions IFN mediates the lethality of endotoxin and TNFα via its overwhelming inductive capacity for TNFα release in LPS-activated macrophages.[88]

We have demonstrated that IFN can induce production of its own promoting cytokine IL-12 within a positive feedback mechanism. Studies by Mannick and Rodrick demonstrated that exogenous IL-12 can restore T-helper-1 (Th1) cell cytokine production and resistance to infection under traumatic stress. We agree with these authors that therapeutic administration of IL-12 may be a powerful weapon for counterregulation of trauma-induced immunodeficiency.[9]

Most recently, another compound, CNI-1493, a tetravalent guanylhydrazone, has been suggested to be a "macrophage pacifying agent." Acting through suppression of translation efficiency, it effectively inhibits macrophage nitric oxide and cytokine production (TNF) and therefore should attenuate the sequelae of sepsis, septic shock, and acute inflammation in animal models. One of the latest "early blockade" strategies attempts to prevent sepsis by administration of IL-11. IL-11, a cytokine produced by fibroblasts in the bone marrow, maintains gut epithelial membrane integrity and attenuates endotoxin-induced proinflammatory cytokine production.

Following severe trauma or hemorrhagic shock, prostaglandin E$_2$ (PGE$_2$) mediates the disruption of the T cell–macrophage interaction and thereby induces disruption of cell-mediated immunity. Mediators of posttraumatic immune dysfunction such as PGE$_2$ have an effect on the phosphokinase A/phosphokinase C pathway via cAMP. An immunomodulatory intervention against PGE$_2$-mediated immune dysfunction could block cAMP or enhance the protective cyclic guanosine monophosphate (cGMP). These effects could be mediated through the cyclo-oxygenase blocker indomethacin or the cGMP-stimulating agent thymopentin.

In patients with open heart surgery in vitro lymphocyte proliferation and the delayed-type hypersensitivity (DTH) skin response were significantly improved by perioperative subcutaneous application of 50 mg thymopentin-5 (TP-5) compared to that in placebo-treated patients.[89] Indomethacin administration in patients following gastrectomy or aortic surgery resulted in improved postoperative monocytosis and conservation of IL-2 receptor expression on T lymphocytes.[90]

Combined application of thymopentin and indomethacin in patients with open heart surgery resulted in conservation of cell-mediated immunity (IL-1 and IL-2 production, IL-2-receptor expression, lymphocyte proliferation, IFNγ production) and the in vivo skin reaction to recall antigens.[91] Furthermore, a reduced macrophage-mediated acute-phase reaction was achieved, which could be demonstrated by decreased plasma IL-6 levels and neopterin levels.[92]

Hematopoietic growth factors are so-called colony-stimulating factors (CSF) and erythropoietin. CSFs are hematopoietic growth factors that regulate granulocyte and monocyte growth. Four CSFs have been described: G-CSF, macrophage CSF (M-CSF), granulocyte/macrophage CSF (GM-CSF), and IL-3 (multi-CSF). CSFs may exert their effects through stimulating growth and initiating maturation. Furthermore, it has been reported that CSFs may prevent apoptosis of hematologic precursor cells.[93] Through the use of G-CSF peripheral leukocytes were observed to have antiinflammatory properties.[94] CSFs are in clinical use for the prophylaxis of septic complications in neutropenic patients and in patients with agranulocytosis.[95] Cioffi et al.[96] were able to improve leukocyte function and the leukocyte count in burn patients using GM-CSF. The potential interaction of the hematopoietic growth factors with immunocompetent cells are illustrated in Fig. 39.1.

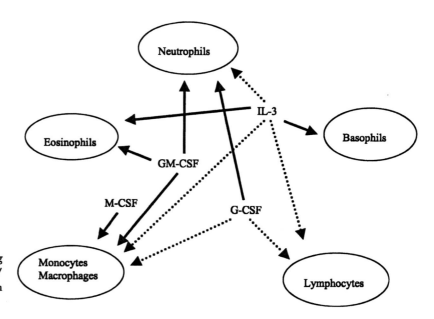

FIGURE 39.1. Interaction of granulocyte colony-stimulating factor (G-CSF), macrophage CSF (M-CSF), granulocyte/macrophage CSF (GM-CSF), and IL-3 (multi-CSF) with immunocompetent cells.

The immunomodulatory properties of the xanthine derivate pentoxifylline and its therapeutic potential in patients suffering from SIRS and MOF resulted in major interest in this hemorheologic drug.[97] Decreased endotoxin-induced TNFα production was observed in human macrophages following pentoxifylline administration.[98,99] Improved hemodynamic parameters and oxygen extraction were demonstrated in septic pentoxifylline-treated patients.[100] Furthermore, in a randomized, double-blind, placebo-controlled study of patients with severe sepsis, Staubach et al. observed a significantly improved MODS score and PaO_2/FiO_2 ratios, but there was no reduction of sepsis mortality.[64] In patients at risk after cardiac surgery there was a significant reduction of the incidence of MOF following pentoxifylline administration.[63]

The therapeutic approach at another level of the pathomechanisms of organ failure following severe trauma and shock is the administration of antithrombin III (AT III). Exogenous administration of the thrombin inhibitor AT III was shown to improve lung function and to prevent the development of kidney and liver failure.[101]

Future immunomodulatory therapy for posttraumatic/hemorrhage-induced immune dysfunction will consist of a combination of drugs (e.g., pentoxifylline, PAF antagonists, AT III, TP-5), hormones (e.g., melatonin, prolactin, sex steroids), growth factors (e.g., G-CSF), and cytokines (e.g., IFNγ). This "cocktail" must be applied at the right time during the developing immune dysfunction following trauma-hemorrhage (SIRS or CARS?), and all cellular components of the immune system (e.g., lymphocytes, macrophages, granulocytes, endothelial cells) must be protected.

References

1. Faist E, Schinkel C, Zimmer S, Kremer JP, Donnersmarck GH, Schildberg FW: Inadequate interleukin-2 synthesis and interleukin-2 messenger expression following thermal and mechanical trauma in human is caused by defective transmembrane signalling. J Trauma 1993;36:1–9.
2. Kreuzer E, Kääb S, Piltz G, Werdan K: Early prediction of septic complications after cardiac surgery by APACHE II score. Eur J Cardiothorac Surg 1992;6:524–527.
3. Pilz G, Kreuzer E, Kääb S, Appel R, Werdan K: Early sepsis treatment with immunoglobulins after cardiac surgery in score-identified high risk patients. Chest 1994;105:76–82.
4. Baker CC, Oppenheimer L, Lewis FR, Trunkey DD: The epidemiology of trauma death. Am J Surg 1980;140:144–150.
5. Chaudry IH, Ayala A: Immunological Aspects of Hemorrhage. Austin, TX, Medical Intelligence Unit, R.G. Landes Company, 1992.
6. Alexander JW: Mechanism of immunologic suppression in burn injury. J Trauma 1990;30:S70–S75.
7. Faist E, Kupper TS, Baker CC, Chaudry IH, Dwyer J, Baue AE: Depression of cellular immunity after major injury: its association with post traumatic complications and its restoration with immunomodulatory agents. Arch Surg 1986;121:1000–1005.
8. Faist E, Mewes A, Strasser T, et al: Alteration of monocyte function following major injury. Arch Surg 1988;123:287–292.
9. O'Sullivan ST, Lederer JA, Horgan AF, Chin DHL, Mannick JA, Rodrick ML: Major injury leads to predominance of the T helper-2 lymphocyte phenotype and diminished interleukin-12 production associated with decreased resistance to infection. Ann Surg 1995;222:482–492.
10. Wichmann MW, Zellweger R, Williams C, Ayala A, DeMaso CM, Chaudry IH: Immune function is more compromised following closed bone fracture and hemorrhagic shock than hemorrhage alone. Arch Surg 1996;131:995–1000.
11. Wichmann MW, Remmers D, Ayala A, Chaudry IH: Der Beitrag von Weichteiltrauma und/oder Knochenfraktur zur Immundepression nach haemorrhagischem Schock im Tierexperiment [The contribution of soft-tissue trauma and/or bone fracture to depressed immunity following hemorrhagic shock in an experimental setting]. Unfallchirurg 1998;101:37–41.
12. Glauser MP, Zanetti G, Baumgartner JD, Cohen J: Septic shock: pathogenesis. Lancet 1991;338:732–736.
13. Bone RC: The pathogenesis of sepsis. Ann Intern Med 1991;115:457–469.
14. Baue AE: Multiple Organ Failure. Patient Care and Prevention. St. Louis, Mosby, 1990.
15. Baue AE: The horror autotoxicus and multiple-organ failure. Arch Surg 1992;127:1451–1462.
16. Rose S, Marzi I: Pathophysiologie des Polytraumas [Pathophysiology of polytrauma]. Zentralbl Chir 1996;121:896–913.
17. Harris BH, Gelfand JA: The immune response to trauma. Semin Pediatr Surg 1995;4:77–82.
18. Schinkel C, Faist E, Zimmer S, et al: Kinetics of circulating adhesion molecules and chemokines after mechanical trauma and burns. Eur J Surg 1996;162:763–768.
19. Guirao X, Lowry SF: Biologic control of injury and inflammation: much more than too little or too late. World J Surg 1996;20:437–446.
20. Lampl L, Helm M, Specht A, Bock KH, Hartel W, Seifried E: Gerinnungsparameter als prognostische Faktoren beim Polytrauma: Konnen klinische Kenngrossen fruhzeitig eine diagnostische Hilfestellung geben? [Blood coagulation parameters as prognostic factors in multiple trauma: can clinical values be an early diagnostic aid?] Zentralbl Chir 1994;119:683–689.
21. Goris RJ, TeBoekhorst T, Nuytinck J, Gimbrere JS: Multiple-organ failure: generalized auto destructive inflammation. Arch Surg 1985;120:1109–1115.
22. Hoch RC, Rodriguez R, Manning T, et al: Effects of accidental trauma on cytokine and endotoxin production. Crit Care Med 1993;21:839–845.
23. Baue AE: MOF/MODS, SIRS: an update. Shock 1996;6:S1–S5.
24. McRitchie DI, Girotti MJ, Rotstein OD, Teodorczyk-Injeyan JA: Impaired antibody production in blunt trauma. Arch Surg 1990;125:91–96.
25. Faist E, Ertel W, Mewes A, Alkan S, Walz A, Strasser T: Trauma-induced alterations of the lymphokine cascade. In: Faist E, Ninnemann J, Green D (eds) Immune Consequences of Trauma, Shock, and Sepsis: Mechanisms and Therapeutic Approaches. Berlin, Springer, 1989;79–94.
26. Stephan RN, Mitsuyoski S, Conrad PJ, Dean RE, Geha AS, Chaudry IH: Depressed antigen presentation function and membrane interleukin-1 activity of peritoneal macrophages after laparotomy. Surgery 1987;102:147–154.
27. Stephan RN, Kupper TS, Geha AS, Baue AS, Chaudry IH: Hemorrhage without tissue trauma produces immunosuppres-

sion and enhances susceptibility to sepsis. Arch Surg 1987; 122:62–68.
28. Chaudry IH, Ayala A, Ertel W, Stephan RN: Editorial review: hemorrhage and resuscitation: immunological aspects. Am J Physiol 1990;259:R663–R678.
29. Ayala A, Perrin MM, Wagner MA, Chaudry IH: Enhanced susceptibility to sepsis following simple hemorrhage: depression of Fc and C3b receptor mediated phagocytosis. Arch Surg 1990;125:70–75.
30. Wichmann MW, Zellweger R, DeMaso CM, Ayala A, Chaudry IH: Mechanisms of immunosuppression in males following trauma-hemorrhage: critical role of testosterone. Arch Surg 1996;131:1186–1192.
31. Wichmann MW, Angele MK, Ayala A, Cioffi WG, Chaudry IH: Flutamide: a novel agent for restoring the depressed cell-mediated immunity following soft-tissue trauma and hemorrhagic shock. Shock 1997;8:242–248.
32. Wichmann MW, Ayala A, Chaudry IH: Male Sex-steroids are responsible for depressing macrophage immune function after trauma-hemorrhage. Am J Physiol 1997;273:C1335–C1340.
33. Wichmann MW, Zellweger R, DeMaso CM, Ayala A, Chaudry IH: Melatonin administration attenuates depressed immune functions after trauma-hemorrhage. J Surg Res 1996;63:256–262.
34. Wichmann MW, Haisken JM, Ayala A, Chaudry IH: Melatonin administration following hemorrhagic shock decreases mortality from subsequent septic challenge. J Surg Res 1996;65: 109–114.
35. Zellweger R, Wichmann MW, Ayala A, DeMaso CM, Chaudry IH: Prolactin: a novel and safe immunomodulating hormone for the treatment of immunodepression following severe hemorrhage. J Surg Res 1996;63:53–58.
36. Zellweger R, Zhu XH, Wichmann MW, Ayala A, DeMaso CM, Chaudry IH: Prolactin administration following hemorrhagic shock improves macrophage cytokine release capacity and decreases mortality from subsequent sepsis. J Immunol 1996; 157:5748–5754.
37. Faist E, Storck M, Hueltner L, et al: Functional analysis of monocyte activity through synthesis patterns of proinflammatory cytokines and neopterin in patients in surgical intensive care. Surgery 1992;112:562–572.
38. Casals-Stenzel J: Triazolodiazepines are potent antagonists of platelet activating factor (PAF) in vitro and in vivo. Arch Pharm (Weinheim) 1987;335:351–355.
39. Pullicino EA, Carli F, Poole S, Rafferty B, Malik STA, Elia M: The relationship between the circulating concentrations of interleukin 6 (IL-6), tumor necrosis factor (TNF) and the acute phase response to elective surgery and accidental injury. Lymphokine Res 1990;9:231–238.
40. Yoshizaki K: Clinical significance of cytokines-interleukin 6 in disease. Rinsho Byori 1990;38:375–379.
41. Wortel CH, van Deventer SJ, Aarden LA, et al: Interleukin-6 mediates host defense responses induced by abdominal surgery. Surgery 1993;114:564–570.
42. Svoboda P, Kantorova I, Ochmann J: Dynamics of interleukin 1, 2, and 6 and tumor necrosis factor alpha in multiple trauma patients. J Trauma 1994;36:336–340.
43. Faist E, Wichmann M, Kim C: Immunosuppression and immunomodulation in surgical patients. Curr Opin Crit Care 1997;3:293–298.
44. Ayala A, Wang P, Chaudry IH: Insights into the mechanism by which interferon-gamma improves macrophage function following hemorrhage and resuscitation. J Surg Res 1993; 54:322–327.
45. Ertel W, Morrison MH, Ayala A, Dean RE, Chaudry IH: Interferon-gamma attenuates hemorrhage-induced suppression of macrophage and splenocyte functions and decreases susceptibility to sepsis. Surgery 1992;111:177–187.
46. Chaudry IH, Ohkawa M, Clemens MG: Improved mitochondrial function following ischemia and reflow by ATP-MgCl$_2$. Am J Physiol 1984;246:R799–R804.
47. Chaudry IH: Use of ATP following shock and ischemia. Ann NY Acad Sci 1990;603:130–141.
48. Wang P, Ba ZF, Morrison MH, Ayala A, Dean RE, Chaudry IH: Mechanism of the beneficial effects of ATP-MgCl$_2$ following trauma-hemorrhage and resuscitation: downregulation of inflammatory cytokine (TNF, IL-6) release. J Surg Res 1992;52: 364–371.
49. Ertel W, Morrison MH, Ayala A, Chaudry IH: Modulation of macrophage membrane phospholipids by n-3 polyunsaturated fatty acids increases interleukin-1 release and prevents suppression of cellular immunity following hemorrhagic shock. Arch Surg 1993;128:15–21.
50. Ertel W, Morrison MH, Meldrum DR, Ayala A, Chaudry IH: Ibuprofen restores cellular immunity and decreases susceptibility to sepsis following hemorrhage. J Surg Res 1992;53:55–61.
51. Ertel W, Morrison MH, Ayala A, Chaudry IH: Chloroquine attenuates hemorrhagic shock-induced immunosuppression and decreases susceptibility to sepsis. Arch Surg 1992;127:70–76.
52. Ertel W, Morrison MH, Ayala A, Chaudry IH: Chloroquine attenuates hemorrhagic shock induced suppression of Kupffer cell antigen presentation and MHC class II antigen expression through blockade of tumor necrosis factor and prostaglandin release. Blood 1991;78:1781–1788.
53. Zhu X, Ertel W, Ayala A, Morrison MH, Perrin MM, Chaudry IH: Chloroquine inhibits macrophage tumor necrosis factor-α mRNA transcription. Immunology 1993;80:122–126.
54. Ertel W, Morrison MH, Ayala A, Perrin MM, Chaudry IH: Anti-TNF monoclonal antibodies prevent haemorrhage induced suppression of Kupffer cell antigen presentation and MHC class II antigen expression. Immunology 1991;74:290–297.
55. Meldrum DR, Ayala A, Chaudry IH: Mechanism of diltiazem's immunomodulatory effects after hemorrhage and resuscitation. Am J Physiol 1993;265:C412–C421.
56. Wang P, Ba ZF, Chaudry IH: Chemically modified heparin improves hepatocellular function, cardiac output, and microcirculation after trauma-hemorrhage and resuscitation. Surgery 1994;116:169–176.
57. Zellweger R, Ayala A, Zhu X, Holme KR, DeMaso CM, Chaudry IH: A novel nonanticoagulant heparin improves splenocyte and peritoneal macrophage immune function after trauma-hemorrhage and resuscitation. J Surg Res 1995;59: 211–218.
58. Wang P, Ba ZF, Zhou M, Chaudry IH: Pentoxifylline restores cardiac output and tissue perfusion following trauma-hemorrhage and decreases susceptibility to sepsis. Surgery 1993;114:352–359.
59. Zellweger R, Ayala A, Schmand JF, Morrison MH, Chaudry IH: PAF-antagonist administration after hemorrhage-resuscitation prevents splenocyte immunodepression. J Surg Res 1995; 59:366–370.
60. Mock CN, Dries DJ, Jurkovich GJ, Maier RV: Assessment of two clinical trials: interferon-gamma therapy in severe injury. Shock 1996;5:235–240.

61. Deitch EA: Animal models of sepsis and shock: a review and lessons learned. Shock 1998;9:1-11.
62. Mathiak G, Szewczyk D, Abdullah F, Ovadia P, Rabinovici R: Platelet-activating factor (PAF) in experimental and clinical sepsis. Shock 1997;7:391-404.
63. Hoffmann H, Markewitz A, Kreuzer E, Reichert K, Jochum M, Faist E: Pentoxifylline decreases the incidence of multiple organ failure in patients after major cardiothoracic surgery. Shock 1998;9:235-240.
64. Staubach KH, Schröder J, Stüber F, Gehrke K, Traumann E, Zabel P: Effect of pentoxifylline in severe sepsis: results of a randomized, double-blind, placebo-controlled study. Arch Surg 1998;133:94-100.
65. McGowan JE, Barnes MW, Finland N: Bacteremia at Boston City Hospital: occurrence and mortality during 12 selected years (1935-1972) with special reference to hospital-acquired cases. J Infect Dis 1975;132:316-335.
66. Centers for Disease Control: Mortality patterns—United States 1989. MMWR 1992;41:121-125.
67. Bone RC: Toward an epidemiology and natural history of SIRS (systemic inflammatory response syndrome). JAMA 1992; 268:3452-3455.
68. Zellweger R, Wichmann MW, Ayala A, Stein S, DeMaso CM, Chaudry IH: Females in proestrus state maintain splenic immune functions and tolerate sepsis better than males. Crit Care Med 1997;25:106-110.
69. Wichterman KA, Baue AE, Chaudry IH: Sepsis and septic shock: a review of laboratory models and a proposal. J Surg Res 1980;29:189-201.
70. Wichmann MW, Zellweger R, DeMaso CM, Ayala A, Chaudry IH: Enhanced immune responses in females as opposed to decreased responses in males following hemorrhagic shock and resuscitation. Cytokine 1996;8:853-863.
71. Angele MK, Wichmann MW, Ayala A, Cioffi WG, Chaudry IH: Testosterone receptor blockade after hemorrhage in males: restoration of the depressed immune functions and improved survival following subsequent sepsis. Arch Surg 1997;132: 1207-1214.
72. Wichmann MW, Inthorn D, Schildberg FW: Incidence and mortality of severe sepsis in surgical intensive care: influence of gender on disease process and out-come [abstract]. Shock, 1998;10:3.
73. Schröder J, Kahlke V, Staubach KH, Zabel P, Stüber F: Gender differences in human sepsis. Arch Surg 1998;133:1200-1205.
74. Qiu Y, Peng Y, Wang J: Immunoregulatory role of neurotransmitters. Adv Neuroimmunol 1996;6:223-231.
75. Quattrocchi KB, Frank EH, Miller CH, Dull ST, Howard RR, Wagner FC Jr: Severe head injury: effect upon cellular immune function. Neurol Res 1991;13:13-20.
76. Brinkman WJ, Hall DM, Suo JL, Weber RJ: Centrally-mediated opioid-induced immunosuppression: elucidation of sympathetic nervous system involvement. Adv Exp Med Biol 1998;437:43-49.
77. Wichmann MW, Faist E, Chaudry IH: Naloxon verschlechtert die zellvermittelte Immunfunktion nach haemorrhagischem Schock [abstract]. Langenbecks Arch Chir 1997;585-588.
78. Carr DJ, Carpenter GW, Garza HH Jr, Baker ML, Gebhardt BM: Cellular mechanisms involved in morphine-mediated suppression of CTL activity. Adv Exp Med Biol 1995;373:131-139.
79. Jankovic BD, Radulovic J: Enkephalins, brain and immunity: modulation of immune responses by methionine-enkephalin injected into the cerebral cavity. Int J Neurosci 1992; 67:241-270.
80. Zellweger R, Wichmann MW, Ayala A, Chaudry IH: Metoclopramide: a novel and safe imunomodulating agent for restoring the depressed macrophage immune function following hemorrhage. J Trauma 1998;44:70-77.
81. Kim C, Schinkel C, Fuchs D, et al: Interleukin-13 effectively down-regulates the monocyte inflammatory potential during traumatic stress. Arch Surg 1995;130:1330-1336.
82. DeWaal Malefyt R, Figdor CG, Huijbens R, et al: Effects of IL-13 on phenotype, cytokine production, and cytotoxic function of human monocytes. J Immunol 1993;151:6370-6381.
83. DeWaal Malefyt R, Yssel H, Roncaralo MG, Spits H, de Vries J: Interleukin-10. Curr Opin Immunol 1992;4:314-320.
84. Ayala A, Lehman DL, Herdon CD, Chaudry IH: Mechanism of enhanced susceptibility to sepsis following hemorrhage: interleukin (IL)-10 suppression of T-cell response is mediated by eicosanoid induced IL-4 release. Arch Surg 1994;129: 1172-1178.
85. Napolitano LM, Campbell C: Nitric oxide inhibition normalizes splenocyte interleukin-10 synthesis in murine thermal injury. Arch Surg 1994;129:1276-1282.
86. Polk HC Jr, Cheadle WG, Livingston DH, et al: A randomized prospective clinical trial to determine the efficacy of interferon-gamma in severely injured patients. Am J Surg 1992:163: 191-196.
87. Babcock GF, Rodeberg DA, White-Owen C: Changes in neutrophil function following major trauma or thermal injury [abstract]. J Intensive Care Med 1994;20:172.
88. Silva AT, Cohen J: Role of Interferon-gamma in experimental gram-negative sepsis. J Infect Dis 1992;166:331-335.
89. Faist E, Ertel W, Salmen B, et al: The immune-enhancing effect of perioperative thymopentin administration in elderly patients undergoing major surgery. Arch Surg 1988;123:1449-1453.
90. Faist E, Ertel W, Cohnert T, Huber P, Inthorn D, Heberer G: Immunoprotective effects of cyclooxygenase inhibition in patients with major surgical trauma. J Trauma 1990;30:8-18.
91. Faist E, Markewitz A, Fuchs D, Lang S, Zarius S, Schildberg FW: Immunomodulatory therapy with thymopentin and indomethacin: successful restoration of interleukin-2 synthesis in patients with major surgery. Ann Surg 1991;214:264-274.
92. Markewitz A, Faist E, Weinhold C, et al: Alterations of cell-mediated immune response following cardiac surgery. Eur J Cardiothorac Surg 1993;7:193-199.
93. Van Furth R: Cell biology of mononuclear phagocytes. In: Van Furth R (ed) Hemopoietic Growth Factors and Mononuclear Phagocytes. Basel, R. Karger, 1993;1-9.
94. Hartung T, Döcke WD, Gantner F, et al: Effect of granulocyte colony-stimulating factor treatment on ex-vivo blood cytokines response in human volunteers. Blood 1995;85:2482-2489.
95. Bonilla MA, Gillio AP, Ruggiero M, et al: Effects of recombinant human granulocyte colony-stimulating factor on neutropenia in patients with congenital agranulocytosis. N Engl J Med 1989;320:1574-1580.
96. Cioffi WG Jr, Burleson DG, Jordan BS, et al: Effects of granulocyte-macrophage colony-stimulating factor in burn patients. Arch Surg 1991;126:74-79.
97. Mandell G: ARDS, neutrophils, and pentoxifylline. Am Rev Respir Dis 1988;136:1103-1105.
98. Strieter RM, Remick DG, Ward PA, et al: Cellular and molecular regulation of tumor necrosis factor-alpha production

by pentoxifylline. Biochem Biophys Resun Commun 1998; 155:1230–1236.
99. Endres S, Fulle HJ, Sinha B, et al: Cyclic nucleotides differentially regulate the synthesis of tumour necrosis factor-alpha and interleukin-1 beta by human mononuclear cells. Immunology 1991;72:56–60.
100. Bacher A, Mayer N, Klimscha W, Oismüller C, Steltzer H, Hammerle A: Effects of pentoxifylline on hemodynamics and oxygenation in septic and nonseptic patients. Crit Care Med 1997;25:795–800.
101. Inthorn D, Hoffmann JN, Hartl WH, Mühlbayer D, Jochum M: Antithrombin III supplementation in severe sepsis: beneficial effects on organ dysfunction. Shock 1997;8:328–334.

40
Central Nervous System Failure: Neurotrauma Trials

Jamie S. Ullman and Anthony H. Sin

Traumatic brain injury accounts for approximately 52,000 deaths each year in the United States. The incidence of severe head injury (SHI) is about 10–50 per 100,000 population.[1] Although SHI accounts for only about 10% of all head injuries, it is still one of the most common entities seen in neurosurgical practice. Historically, SHI has been a black box of uncertain outcome, generating medical frustration.

During the 1970s closed SHI mortalities in hospital were reported to be about 45–50%.[2,3] However, even during this time period patients treated with intensive care management, including intracranial pressure (ICP) monitoring, showed a mortality of 30–36%.[4–6] By the 1990s SHI mortality rates were less than 30%.[7,8] There has been an evolution in SHI treatment paralleling innovations in radiologic diagnosis, intensive care treatment, and neuromonitoring.[9] Through new technologies there has been improved understanding of the pathophysiologic mechanisms influencing outcome. The ultimate goal of SHI management is to reduce mortality and improve functional outcome. This chapter highlights significant trials that have influenced current closed SHI management.

Pathophysiology

Severe head injury occurs as a result of an impact to or disruption of the intracranial contents. The injury can be blunt, involve rotational and acceleration/deceleration forces, or be penetrating. The primary injury may result in bleeding around or within the brain substance, shearing of neuronal axons, or vascular injury producing varying degrees of damage.

The formidable enemy to SHI recovery is the secondary injury process. From the moment of impact onward, regional or global changes in blood flow can occur,[10] resulting in neuronal damage extending beyond the area of primary structural damage. Autopsy studies have revealed microscopic evidence of ischemia.[11,12]

Ischemia leads to a cascade of molecular events resulting in cellular breakdown. Calcium influx is one of the primary culprits. Calcium channels become opened. Release of excitatory amino acid (EAA) neurotransmitters (glutamate, aspartate), which activate receptor-mediated calcium channels including the N-methylaspartate (NMDA) and α-amino-3-hydroxy-5-methyl-4 isoxazole propionic acid (AMPA) receptors, activate this influx. Calcium enters the cell, resulting in reduced mitochondrial phosphorylation and adenosine triphosphate (ATP) production. Anaerobic glycolysis ensues. There is an increase in membrane permeability owing to phospholipase, proteinase, and myelinase activation. Free fatty acid release leads to activation of the cyclooxygenase and lipoxygenase arachidonic acid pathways resulting in the release of prostaglandins and leukotrienes, leading to edema formation. Thromboxane production leads to vasoconstriction and platelet aggregation, further compromising blood flow and oxygen delivery. An inflammatory response from substances such as tumor necrosis factor can result in further diffuse neuronal damage.[13,14] The ongoing ischemic process is the target of most of our present-day therapies.

Despite injury severity, the brain can maintain its ability to autoregulate.[15,16] Autoregulation is the process by which cerebral blood flow (CBF) remains constant in the face of environmental changes. CBF is maintained according to Poiseuille's law:

$$Q = \frac{CPP \pi r^4}{8 l \eta}$$

where CPP is the transmural pressure gradient, or cerebral perfusion pressure [mean arterial pressure minus intracranial pressure (MAP − ICP)]; r is the radius; l is the vessel length; and η is the blood viscosity.

Ischemia results in reflex vasodilation of the pial arterioles to maintain CBF. Normal CBF is approximately 50 ml/100 g/min. When CBF falls below approximately 20 ml/100 g/min, neuronal paralysis occurs but ion pump function is preserved. This cessation of activity is reversible so long as blood flow can be restored prior to falling below approximately 10 ml/100 g/min, at which point membrane breakdown occurs, leading to cell death. Increasing the CPP can improve CBF.[17]

The CBF in head-injured patients can be compromised within the early hours after impact.[10,18] There is a correlation between low CBF and outcome.[19–22] Hemodynamic compro-

40. Central Nervous System Failure: Neurotrauma Trials

TABLE 40.1. Glasgow Coma Score.

Points	Eye opening	Verbal response	Motor response
6	—	—	Follows commands
5	—	Oriented	Localizes to pain
4	Spontaneous	Confused	Withdraws to pain
3	To voice	Inappropriate	Flexor (decorticate)
2	To pain	Incomprehensible	Extensor (decerebrate)
1	None	None	

From Teasdale and Jennett,[24] with permission.
Total maximum = 15 points; total minimum = 3. Head injury severity: mild, 13–15; moderate, 9–12; severe 3–8.

mise due to shock and interventions such as hyperventilation may further compromise blood flow.[19]

Clinically, other factors have been shown to correlate with outcome after SHI. A poor postresuscitation Glasgow Coma Score (GCS)[23] (Table 40.1), hypotension and hypoxia,[25,26] abnormal pupillary responses,[23] and increasing age[27] have been shown to correlate negatively with outcome. Computed tomography (CT) characteristics of compressed basal cisterns, midline shift, and the presence of subarachnoid blood are negative predictors for survival[28] (Fig. 40.1).

Neurotrauma Trials

Cerebral Perfusion Pressure Management

Cerebral perfusion pressure (CPP) is the transmural pressure gradient across the cerebral blood vessel wall. CPP is an important component of CBF. The normal CPP is approximately 50 mmHg, below which CBF becomes passively dependent on CPP (Fig. 40.2).[16] Above 50 mmHg the CBF remains constant, defining autoregulation.[16,29]

As the regional CBF can differ after severe head injury, there may be areas within the brain that are operating below the autoregulatory threshold.[15] These areas are in danger of irreversible ischemic damage.[30] Although autoregulation is regionally impaired, it is often restored when CBF is augmented. CPP becomes a critical factor in this restorative process.[16] This property was recognized during the 1970s, inferring that blood pressure augmentation can improve CBF.[29,31] Heilbrun et al.[31] suggested that measuring CPP in addition to ICP can be beneficial for meeting cerebral hemodynamic requirements.

In 1984 Rosner et al.[32] observed in normal animals that plateau waves (prolonged ICP elevation), classically described by Lundberg as "A" waves,[33] were precipitated by a slow decline in SBP, causing reactive vasodilation and a consequent ICP elevation due to increased cerebral blood volume. Resolution of these waves was initiated by a spontaneous rise in systemic blood pressure, a normal autoregulatory response. The authors concluded that plateau waves are the "expected and logical consequence of an unstable CPP acting upon a generally intact cerebrovascular bed in the face of elevated ICP and decreased compliance."[33]

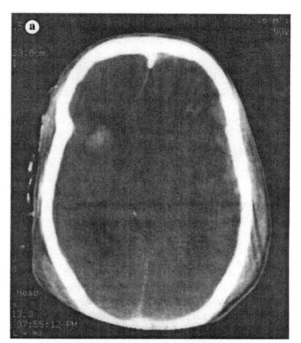

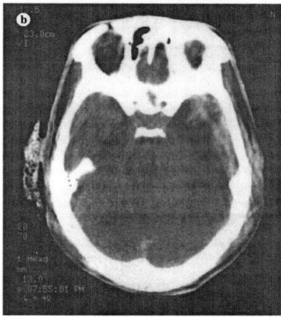

FIGURE 40.1. Computed tomography scan of a 26-year-old man involved in a motor vehicle accident. (a) Left subdural hematoma, left hemispheric swelling, left and right frontal contusions are present. There is a significant midline shift. (b) Left temporal contusions and subdural hematoma are present on an inferior cut. There is an absence of perimesencephalic cisterns. The above findings are among the poor prognostic signs reported by Eisenberg et al.[28] The patient was treated with hypothermia for refractory intracranial pressure (ICP) control but eventually expired.

These observations prompted the "vasodilatory" and "vasoconstriction cascade" models.[16] Hemodynamic mechanisms can lead to reduced perfusion and CBF, which increases ischemia

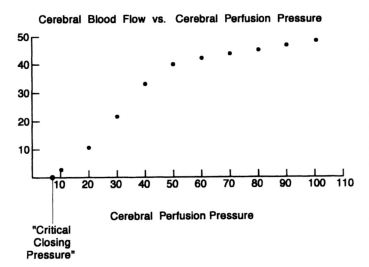

FIGURE 40.2. In normal subjects the cerebral blood flow (CBF) remains relatively constant over a wide range of cerebral perfusion pressure (CPP) over 50 mmHg. Below this level pial arterioles become maximally dilated, resulting in CBF dependence CPP. The critical closing pressure is the CPP level at which the blood flow through the cerebral vessel is zero. This curve shifts to the right with severe head injury. (From Andrews BT, ed., Neurosurgical Intensive Care, New York: McGraw-Hill, 1993:57–112, with permission of The McGraw-Hill Companies.)

and consequently brain edema, resulting in increased tissue pressure. Vasodilation in response to CBF reduction can lead to increased cerebral blood volume and ICP (Fig. 40.3). Increasing perfusion and blood flow via various mechanisms (Fig. 40.4) can potentially reverse these processes.[16] Arterial hypertension has been shown to normalize tissue oxygenation in ischemic areas in SHI.[34] Head injury and chronic hypertension can increase the minimal perfusion requirements through increased cerebrovascular resistance.[8,16,35] Clinical reviews have demonstrated poor outcomes related to reduced CPP (<60), with the more significant culprit being a reduction in systolic blood pressure.[35] In 1985 Schrader et al.[37] demonstrated improved intracranial volume tolerance to epidural balloon inflation in hypertension-induced animals.

Although ICP reduction is an important factor in maintaining CPP, it may not always be feasible to maintain strict control below 25 mmHg. CPP-directed management emphasizes CPP maintenance above 70 mmHg regardless of absolute ICP value. If adequate perfusion can be maintained, perhaps the functional outcome can be improved.

In 1995 Rosner et al.[8] published results of 158 patients with a GCS of 3–7 treated with CPP maintenance as the primary goal. This report was an expansion of an earlier one.[38] CPP was kept under optimal control with ventricular drainage and mannitol, usually prompted by an ICP rise, reducing the CPP below 70 mmHg. Volume expansion and vasopressors augmented blood pressure. Barbiturates, hypothermia, craniectomy, and lobar resection were not used for ICP control.

The overall mortality for this group was 29%, with 59% achieving a favorable outcome as defined by the Glasgow Outcome Score (GOS) (Table 40.2). The average CPP was 83 mmHg. Forty percent of the patients required vasopressors; these patients had a lower average GCS (4.7 vs. 6.4; no vasopressors) and a higher initial ICP (28.7% vs. 17.5%). The mortality among this subgroup was also higher (47% vs. 18%).

When comparing outcome stratified by GCS to historical controls from the Traumatic Coma Data Bank (TCDB),[23] CPP patients showed significant improvements. Interestingly, GCS 3 patients had 52% mortality with 35% favorable recovery compared to 78% versus 7% for the TCDB subgroup.

Management of CPP as a general, intensive medical treatment paradigm has produced encouraging results with improvements over previously published outcome data. The exact level of CPP maintenance is not well defined, but CPP > 70 mmHg

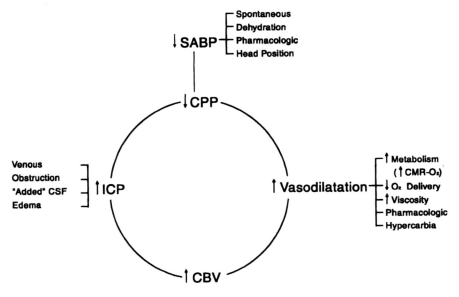

FIGURE 40.3. "Complex vasodilatory cascade" demonstrates the various environmental factors that could precipitate ultimate intracranial hypertension. Reflex pial arteriolar vasodilation from reduced blood flow can result in increased cerebral blood volume (CBV) and, consequently, ICP. Elevating the head of the bed may result in a decrement in systemic blood pressure (SABP) at the level of the internal carotid artery. CMR-O_2, cerebral metabolic rate of oxygen consumption. (From Andrews BT, ed., Neurosurgical Intensive Care, New York: McGraw-Hill, 1993:57–112, with permission of The McGraw-Hill Companies.)

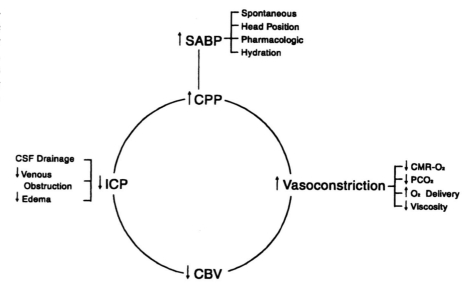

FIGURE 40.4. "Complex vasoconstriction cascade" represents the interventions that increase CPP, enabling restoration of autoregulatory vasoconstriction resulting in reduced CBV and, consequently, decreasing ICP. (From Andrews BT, ed., Neurosurgical Intensive Care. New York: McGraw-Hill, 1993:57–112, with permission of The McGraw-Hill Companies.)

appears to be the threshold noted in several studies [40–41] and is the current *Guidelines for the Management of Severe Head Injury* recommendation.[43] Vasopressors (i.e., norepi-nephrine) for CPP maintenance have been shown to increase CPP effectively without changes in ICP or oxygen extraction.[44,45]

Hypothermia

Profound hypothermia has been utilized for cerebral protection during cardiac bypass surgery.[46] Circulatory arrest with hypothermia has also been used during repair of difficult cerebral aneurysms.[47] Without bypass, profound hypothermia (<28°C) results in impaired cardiac contractility, decreased cardiac output, and ventricular fibrillation. Increased serum viscosity and coagulopathy also can occur.

Hypothermia has been shown to decrease the number of necrotic or damaged neurons and axons after experimental head injury.[48–51] The concept of hypothermic cerebral protection after severe head injury began during the 1950s.[52,53] Hypothermia has now been subjected to randomized/controlled trials addressing the question of whether it can improve functional outcome when induced during the early postinjury period.

After severe head injury there is often an early decrease in cerebral blood flow,[10,18] with rises in the cerebral metabolic rate of oxygen ($CMRO_2$), glucose consumption, and lactate production.[54,55] Hypothermia lowers cerebral metabolism, perhaps resulting in better coupling with blood flow and thereby reducing ischemic damage. Other postulated mechanisms for neuronal protection are the reduction of EAA release, especially, glutamate, and inflammatory response suppression, noted by decreased cerebrospinal fluid (CSF) interleukin-1β.[7,56]

Clifton et al.[57–59] reported that moderate hypothermia (32°–34°C) is well tolerated and relatively safe. When instituted within 6 hours of injury and maintained for 48 hours, there was a trend toward improved favorable outcome compared to that of normothermic controls.

Marion et al.[7] randomized 82 patients, GCS 3–7, to normothermia and hypothermia (32°–33°C) groups. Hypothermia was initiated within 6 hours of injury and maintained for 24 hours. Overall length of stay and mortality were approximately the same (21%) for the two groups. A significant benefit for hypothermia was found in patients with GCS 5–7. Favorable outcome (GOS 4 and 5) at 6 months was 75% versus 35%. Although favorable outcome was 73% versus 39% at 12 months, the difference was calculated to be not significant when adjusting for severity of CT findings, which are known to influence outcome independently. The overall conclusion was that hypothermia improved outcome at 3 and 6 months after severe closed head injury in patients above GCS 4. The authors reported no major complications during hypothermia. Mild hypokalemia and clinically insignificant partial thromboplastin times were noted.

Hypothermia has been used to reduce an ICP > 20 refractory to hyperventilation, fluid restriction, and high-dose barbiturates. Shiozaki et al.[60] divided 33 patients into two groups: those with hypothermia to 33.5°C and normothermic controls. Hypothermia was continued for 2 days or until ineffective. If the ICP increased during rewarming, hypothermia was reinstituted until the ICP remained below 20 mmHg for at least 24 hours. Hypothermia was successful in reducing the ICP (mean 10.4 mmHg) and increasing the CPP (mean 14 mmHg). CBF and $CMRO_2$ were also decreased. The mortality rates for the hypothermia group versus the controls were 50% and 82%, respectively. Among the hypothermia patients, 38% achieved a

TABLE 40.2. Glasgow Outcome Score.

Score	Outcome
5	Good recovery with minor deficits
4	Moderate disability with independence
3	Severe disability with dependence
2	Persistent vegetative state
1	Death

From Jennett and Bond,[39] with permission.
Outcome: favorable 4 and 5; unfavorable 1–3.

favorable outcome compared to 6% of controls. Complication rates were not statistically significant between the groups. A later study demonstrated the ineffectiveness of hypothermia for improving outcomes in patients with ICP > 40 mmHg and patients with GCS 3 or 4.[61]

Hypothermia to 33°C is associated with a decrease in cardiac index, hypokalemia, elevated serum lipase, pancreatitis, and thrombocytopenia and can mask infection. Coagulation profiles tend to be unchanged.[55,59] Peripheral vasodilation after rewarming has resulted in significant hypotension.[60] Rewarming should be performed slowly at a rate of 1°C per hour.[7] There is evidence that patients with initially lower brain temperatures have worse outcomes[9] and may suffer adverse consequences from induced hypothermia. Hypothermia should not be undertaken without invasive hemodynamic and cerebral metabolic monitoring.

Hyperventilation

Hyperventilation is extremely effective for achieving rapid ICP reduction in the acute herniation syndrome. By reducing the PCO_2, the increase in pH results in cerebral vasoconstriction, which decreases cerebral blood volume and consequently the ICP. Prolonged hyperventilation may become ineffective owing to its diminished effect on cerebrospinal fluid (CSF) pH and arteriolar diameter after 24 hours.[62] Rapid cessation of hyperventilation may cause increased pCO_2 with consequent vasodilation and a rebound ICP rise.[63]

With severe head injury, CBF is regionally and globally reduced in many patients. Despite this fact, cerebral vasoresponsivity and autoregulation are largely intact.[15,21] Profound hyperventilation may result in vasoconstriction and restriction of blood flow to critically ischemic areas. In addition, hyperventilation can worsen ischemic effects due to posttraumatic vasospasm.[63]

Traditionally, SHI patients have routinely been hyperventilated to PCO_2 25 mmHg prophylactically to prevent intracranial hypertension. Hyperventilation has also been the first-line therapy for treatment of new-onset intracranial hypertension. Muizelaar et al.[62] reported a prospective, randomized trial regarding prolonged, prophylactic routine use of hyperventilation in 113 SHI patients. Forty-one patients were treated with normocapnia (35 mmHg), 26 with hyperventilation (25 mmHg), and 36 with hyperventilation with the buffer tromethamine (THAM). They found that patients with GCS 4 or 5 treated with hyperventilation alone had significantly worse outcomes at 3- and 6-month follow-ups than controls or those treated by hyperventilation with THAM.

It has been thought that profound hyperventilation can help reduce an elevated ICP resulting from significant cerebral hyperemia,[64] especially in children. Such therapy, however, still runs the risk of creating severe ischemia, even in such patients. Schneider et al.[65] demonstrated brain tissue PO_2 reduction with hyperventilation.

The current recommendation is to maintain normocapnia at 35 mmHg.[43] The first-line therapy for reducing ICP include CSF drainage, muscle relaxants and sedation, and optimization of blood rheology with mannitol. Mild hyperventilation is undertaken after these steps prove ineffective. Monitoring jugular venous saturations can help determine if such therapy is resulting in global ischemia.[66,67] Jugular saturation of less than 50% is an indicator of high cerebral oxygen extraction as a result of global ischemia;[68] however, regional ischemic effects cannot be accounted for with this method. These regional measurements methods are expensive and not widely available.

In summary, routine prophylactic hyperventilation is counterproductive in certain SHI patients. Hyperventilation should be administered cautiously when needed. Cerebral metabolic monitoring is useful.

Pharmacologic Methods

Agents Aimed at the Ischemic Cascade

As previously described, calcium entry into the neuron precipitates of cascade eventually leading to cell death. Studies with experimental head injury and focal ischemia models have reported reduced ischemic damage when agents that ultimately block calcium entry are used. In this regard, clinical studies using calcium channel lockers, NMDA receptors, and inhibitors of glutamate release have been initiated.

Calcium Channel Blockers

Prophylactic, 21-day administration of the calcium channel blocker nimodipine for aneurysmal subarachnoid hemorrhage (SAH) has become routine. According to Allen et al.,[39] nimodipine reduced the occurrence of severe neurologic deficits and possibly the severity of arterial spasm. In a small double-blind study, nicardipine was shown to decrease transcranial Doppler flow velocities in head injury patients with presumed vasospasm. No effect on outcome was demonstrated.[70]

Ischemic damage after head injury could be potentially reduced by calcium channel blockade. The European Study Group on Nimodipine in Severe Head Injury failed to show effectiveness of nimodipine on outcome. However, a trend toward improvement was noted in patients with SAH.[71]

Eisenberg et al.[28] reported that CT evidence of SAH was an independent, negative outcome predictor in SHI patients postulated to be a result of ischemic damage due to vasospasm. Delayed ischemic deficits due to traumatic SAH and vasospasm have been documented.[72] Harders et al.[73] further studied the effect of nimodipine on traumatic SAH in a multicenter placebo-controlled study of 123 patients. Although the mortality rates were not significant different, there was a decrease in unfavorable outcomes in the survivors.

In our institution, nimodipine is administered to all trauma patients with cisternal SAH. Transcranial Doppler measurements are routinely undertaken to assess for increased cerebral artery vessel velocities indicating vasospasm. Nimodipine is sometimes associated with hypotension requiring dose reduction or discontinuation.

EAA Release and Receptor Inhibitors

A plethora of experimental brain injury and ischemia models have been used to test the efficacy of EAA inhibitors and receptor blockers. The results have been promising, with evidence of a significant reduction in ischemic damage and mortality and improved outcome.[56,74,75]

A number of compounds have been developed. They can be classified as NMDA receptor antagonists (competitive or noncompetitive) and modulators, AMPA receptor modulators, and EAA release inhibitors.[75,76] Several of these compounds are currently undergoing randomized clinical trails, although lack of statistically significant improvements in outcome has forced some of these trials to be discontinued. Their effectiveness under controlled laboratory environment has not been extrapolated to the clinical setting.[77]

With human head injury there is considerable heterogeneity regarding brain impact and ischemia. Environmental and extracerebral factors are multiple and variable, affecting individual patients differently. To account for all of these factors is a formidable task. The best that can be done is to standardize the in-hospital management. It is becoming increasingly clear that the above-mentioned drugs, when given alone, are insufficient to counteract these variables. Trials using these compounds in association with other "neuroprotective" measures (i.e., hypothermia) may be warranted.

Steroids

Steroids have long been used in neurosurgery as effective agents for reducing the vasogenic edema associated with brain and spinal cord tumors.[78] High-dose methylprednisolone has been shown to have some favorable effect on outcome for acute spinal cord injury.[79,80] Lipid peroxidation reduction and free-radical scavenging are the postulated mechanisms. Efficacy has not been proven in head injury.

During the 1960s and 1970s encouraging reports showed that high-dose dexamethasone reduced mortality, shortened length of recovery, and improved outcome in SHI patients.[81-83] The number of patients in these studies were small, however, and data reanalysis revealed no statistical significance.[84]

Gudeman et al.[85] found no influence of high-dose methylprednisolone on ICP and brain compliance in 20 patients. Others have confirmed this finding.[84,86] One might conclude from these results that steroids have little effect on reducing cerebral edema.

Randomized, prospective, double-blind trials have been performed with increased patient numbers.[49,86,87] All showed no effect of steroids, at any dosage, on outcome after head injury. In addition, there was no significant difference in medical complications among the groups. Saul et al.[88] found that steroids had a negative effect in patients who did not respond to SHI treatment. Steroids seem to have little place in the management of head injury in terms of ICP, edema, and outcome. Because of the potential complications, the risk/benefit ratio for these drugs may be considered high in certain cases; such therapy, at present, is outmoded.

Marshall et al.[89] reported the results of a randomized trial using the 21-aminosteroid triliazad, which has antioxidant effects. This agent had been promising in experimental studies. The multicenter study included a cohort of 1120 patients with GCS 4–12. Although safe, there was no significant difference in outcome between the treatment and placebo groups. There appeared to be, however, an imbalance in the predictive variables in the population studied. There was a suggestion of improved survival in male patients with SAH, a finding that warrants further investigation.

Barbiturates

Barbiturates have become important for cerebral protection during neuroanesthetic induction and neurovascular procedures requiring temporary vascular occlusion. Given prior to the onset of ischemia, barbiturates can reduce the area of resulting damage.[90] Routine prophylactic use for SHI has not been supported, however.[91]

Barbiturates rapidly reduce intracranial hypertension.[90] Because of this property these agents have been used frequently in the intensive care unit (ICU) setting to reduce high ICP refractory to other medical or surgical means. The likely reasons for ICP reduction are several. Barbiturates reduce neuronal activity, cerebral metabolism, and brain temperature. Vasoconstriction in autoregulated regions of the brain may shunt blood flow to more damaged areas. Barbiturates, especially thiopental, may act as free radical scavengers.[92] It appears that barbiturates are more effective when autoregulation is intact.[93,94] Lactate production and EAA release also seem to be tempered by these agents.[95]

High-dose barbiturate therapy, or "barbiturate coma," has seemingly improved outcome in various studies.[96-98] Eisenberg et al.[99] studied high-dose pentobarbital in 73 patients with ICP elevation refractory to "conventional" treatment methods. The overall result indicated a twofold benefit in successful control of intracranial hypertension. When cardiovascular complications were present (prerandomization hypotension, acute or chronic hypertension), no significant effect was noted. In the absence of these complications, barbiturates were four times as effective as conventional methods for controlling ICP. Furthermore, of the 12 patients whose ICP responded to barbiturates 8% died, in contrast to 83% of 22 nonresponders. This study, though small in patient number, suggests that patients with intracranial hypertension without cardiac complications have a higher likelihood of responding to high-dose barbiturates.

For many, barbiturate coma is a last-resort method for ICP control and should not be undertaken lightly. These agents are well known to induce cardiac depression and hypotension and to reduce systemic vascular resistance and gut motility.[100] Patients undergoing such treatment require intensive hemodynamic monitoring with intravascular volume maintenance and possible vasopressor support to maintain adequate cerebral perfusion pressure. Endpoints of therapy include ICP reduction and electrocerebral burst suppression. Pentobarbital,[101] with its intermediate half-life, is currently the preferred agent for ICU use.

Hypertonic Saline

Interest in resuscitating trauma victims with hypertonic saline (HS) has mounted. Evidence points to a positive effect on achieving increased, sustained blood pressure with small doses of fluids containing HS and HS with dextran.[102–106]

There is evidence to support an increase in ICP when infusing hypotonic fluids.[107] Ideally, isotonic or hypertonic fluids would have no significant or beneficial effect on ICP. When administering HS, the intravascular osmotic gradient is increased, drawing more fluid into the intravascular space, which may explain the beneficial effects on blood pressure using small volumes. HS with dextran has not been shown to improve cardiodynamic parameters.[108] Like mannitol,[109] HS has been shown to reduce cerebral water content in uninjured brain.[110] Rheologically, mannitol[111] produces a decrease in cerebral blood volume through vasoconstriction of pial arterioles and a consequent decrease in ICP.[112] A similar analysis of HS is warranted.

The effect of HS in experimental injury has been promising.[113–117] One study reported that 7.5% saline was as effective as 20% mannitol in reducing ICP.[113] Relatively few human studies have been performed. The studies currently available have small patient numbers and lack sufficient analysis of the associated variables for SHI outcome. Despite these shortcomings, some inferences can be drawn.

Vassar et al.[102] reported a randomized trial of 7.5% HS with dextran versus lactated Ringer's solution given to 166 trauma patients undergoing prehospital transport. Smaller volumes of HS were required for adequate resuscitation. Although overall outcomes were not significant between the groups, the subset of SHI patients given HS with dextran showed improved survival until discharge. The dose was 250 ml of 7.5% HS with additional lactated Ringer's solution as needed. In a similar cohort there appeared to be no significant survival benefit from added dextran versus HS alone.[103]

Shackford et al.[118] studied the routine use of 1.6% HS versus hypotonic solutions in moderately and severely head-injured patients. The HS was used to restore systolic blood pressure to >90 mmHg or to maintain urine output at >0.5 ml/kg/hr, with normal saline as the maintenance solution. The hypotonic patients received lactated Ringer's solution for the above criteria and 0.45 N saline for maintenance. In the HS group, a sodium level of 157 mEq/L and serum osmolality of 357 mosm/L was tolerated without consequence. The mean ICP and CPP were not significantly different for the two groups. However, the mean maximal ICP was higher in the HS group during the first day with a significant negative change in ICP in contrast to a positive change seen in this parameter for the lactated Ringer's solution group, suggesting a positive effect of HS on cerebral compliance. The problem with this study lies in the small patient numbers, inclusion of those with moderate head injuries, and a relative disparity between mean GCS score (4.7 for the HS group and 6.7 for the lactated Ringer's solution group).

Several clinical studies have demonstrated that HS is effective for reducing refractory ICP in some brain-injured patients.[119–122] Radiographic improvement in brain shift has been reported.[119] Schatzmann et al. showed similar effects with a 100-ml bolus of 10% HS in patients.[121]

Hypertonic saline administration is associated with hyperchloremic metabolic acidosis, hypokalemia, and decreased systemic vascular resistance and peripheral dilation.[108,114] In clinical studies these effects were nondetrimental. Vassar et al.[102] found no evidence of increased intracranial bleeding in patients given HS with dextran. Central pontine myelolysis, which usually occurs with rapid correction of hyponatremia, has not been reported.

Endpoints of HS management may be best measured through serum osmolality and sodium levels. Bingham[123] found increased fatalities among head-injured patients treated with dehydration when the sodium concentration and osmolality exceeded 155 mEq/L and 340 mosm/kg, respectively. In euvolemic patients given hyperosmolar therapy the tolerated levels may be higher. It is likely safest to aim for a sodium level of 145–155 mEq/L and an osmolality of 325 mosm/kg, based on the few clinical studies available.

In summary, HS appears to be an effective general resuscitative fluid for acute trauma, requiring smaller volumes than conventional fluids. There is benefit in decreasing the ICP in such patients with associated severe head injuries. The effect on overall outcome has yet to be determined.

SHI with Associated Systemic Injuries

Often SHI is associated with other systemic injuries, complicating the management and contributing negatively to the outcome.[124] Long-bone orthopedic injuries are the most frequent injury concurrent with head injury. A large retrospective study of 386 head injury patients with or without extracranial injuries not suffering from shock found no significant difference in mortality between two groups.[125]

Jaicks et al.[126] showed an increased incidence of hypotension, hypoxemia, and poor neurologic outcome from early fracture fixations in SHI patients. In addition, there was an increased incidence of acute respiratory distress syndrome (ARDS) when early fixation was done in patients with major thoracic injury along with other systemic injuries.[127] In contrast, some studies have recommended operating less than 24 hours after the injury to facilitate mobility and prevent pulmonary complications, including ARDS.[128–131]

We undertook a retrospective review of 62 recently treated SHI, GCS ≤ 8 patients to determine the characteristics of those with multitrauma (group A) and those with isolated head injury (group B), including morbidity and mortality. The immediate outcome was rated using the GOS. Our study included patients who had suffered hypotension or hypoxia after injury. Patient characteristics and outcome are summarized in Table 40.3 and Fig. 40.5.

The averaged admitting GCS and age in the two groups were similar despite discrepancies in sample sizes. The leading associated injury in group A was a combination of tibia/fibula

TABLE 40.3. Patient Characteristics of Two Study Groups: Multiple Trauma with SHI and SHI Alone.

Characteristic	Group A (multiple trauma with SHI)	Group B (SHI alone)
No. of patients	14	48
Average age (years)	43	40
Admission GCS	5.71	5.73
Admission GCS among survivors	6.2	6.0
Leading mechanism of injury	Pedestrian struck	Fall
Leading long-bone fracture	Tibia/fibula	None
Leading infectious complication	Pneumonia	Pneumonia
Discharge GOS among survivors	3.8	3.7
Leading cause of mortality	Brain death	Brain death
Incidence of ARDS	21%	0%
Overall mortality*	64%	27%

SHI, severe head trauma; GCS, Glasgow coma score; GOS, Glasgow outcome score; ARDS, acute respiratory distress syndrome.
*$p = 0.036$.

fractures, followed closely by femoral and pelvic fractures. Most of the group A patients (64%) were pedestrians struck by an automobile, whereas a fall was the leading mechanism of injury in group B.

Infectious complications were more prevalent in group A (43%) than group B (27%), led by pulmonary infections (A 14%, B 23%). A significant difference in overall immediate mortality of groups A and B was noted: 64% versus 27%, respectively ($p = 0.036$). Most suffered brain death (A 67%, B 77%). Three patients (21%) in group A died from ARDS; no one in group B developed ARDS. The overall incidence of death due to a non-central nervous system (CNS) cause was 33% and 23%, respectively. Among the survivors, approximately 60% (A and B) were referred for inpatient rehabilitation. The isolated head injury patients also had better outcomes measured by GOS at the time of discharge (A 2 vs. B 2.9; $p = 0.054$). Although there is a large disparity in patient number among the groups, the multitrauma patients with SHI had 2.4 times higher mortality than those with isolated head injury. Brain death was the main cause of death in both groups.

Current Management Strategies: Putting It All Together

In an effort to reduce variability when managing SHI, evidence-based guidelines have been published and disseminated among neurosurgeons.[43,132] These guidelines provide a framework for treating SHI, ensuring maximal protection against secondary injury; and they cover various treatment aspects from resuscitation to nutritional support.

Dissemination of *Guidelines* has resulted in increased awareness and understanding among neurosurgeons. In a 1997 survey of board-certified neurosurgeons, 83% performed ICP monitoring in contrast to 28% in a similar survey performed in 1991. Prophylactic hyperventilation had declined in usage from 83% to 36% in 1997. Also in 1997 about 97% believed that CPP should be maintained at >70 mmHg.[133]

In our institution, SHI has been treated according to a protocol initiated in July 1996. This protocol utilizes *Guidelines* recommendations with emphasis on CPP maintenance. We have found success in treating difficult patients such as the one in Fig. 40.6. The protocol is outlined in Table 40.4. After 2 years the SHI mortality rate has been approximately 27%. Whether this represents an improvement over mortality for patients treated prior to this protocol, when management was variable, is part of an ongoing analysis.

Conclusions

Current treatment of severe head injury is aimed at arresting the ongoing cellular damage that occurs after the primary impact. This battle starts during the prehospitalization period. Avoidance of hypotension and hypoxia is the first step. Neurotrauma trials have greatly enhanced our understanding of SHI mechanisms. It is evident from the declining mortality rates that we are beginning to open that black box. The greater our understanding and commitment for aggressive treatment, the easier it will be to meet the challenges of restoring such patients to society.

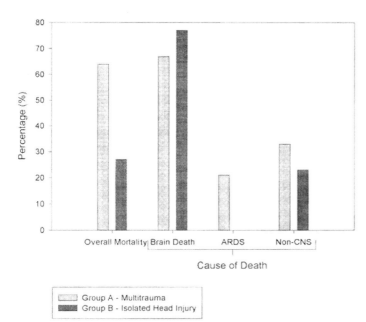

FIGURE 40.5. Mortality and causes of death in a retrospective comparison of severe head injury patients with and without concurrent systemic injuries.

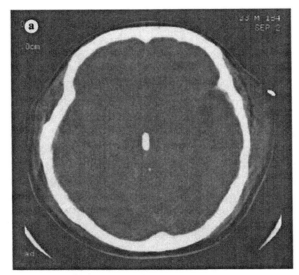

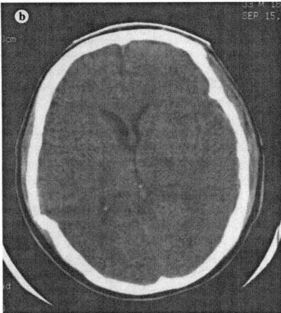

FIGURE 40.6. Computed tomography scans of a 33-year-old man with severe head injury after a fall, having developed a subdural hematoma necessitating craniotomy. (a) Postoperative day 2. Midline hyperdense object is an intraventricular catheter. Both ventricles are compressed, and cortical sulci are absent, representing diffuse cerebral swelling. The patient experienced intracranial hypertension treated with a CPP-directed protocol. (b) Twelve days later. Alleviation of brain swelling is seen with reexpansion of the ventricle and reappearance of the cortical sulci. This patient awoke from coma with good function and was discharged to a rehabilitation center.

TABLE 40.4. Protocol for Managing Severe Head Injury.

EMERGENCY ROOM
1. Advanced Trauma Life Support protocol
    a. ABCs: airway, breathing, circulation
    b. Intubation using cerebral protection and short-acting muscle relaxants and sedatives
2. GCS assessment: initial and after resuscitation
3. Prompt head CT and preliminary cervical spine clearance
4. Normotension, normovolemia, normocapnea
    a. Ideal MAP > 90 mmHg
    b. Iso/hypertonic fluids
5. Avoid prolonged hypoxia (SaO_2 < 90%)/hypotension (SBP < 90 mmHg)
6. In cases of suspected intracranial hypertension (pupil abnormality, focal deficit)
    a. Avoid interference with systemic hypertension (Cushing's response)
    b. Mannitol 1 g/kg
        i. Avoid intravascular fluid depletion by replacement
        ii. Monitor strict intake/output (I/O) by urinary catheter
    c. Mild hyperventilation (PCO_2 30–35 mmHg)

SURGICAL/ANESTHETIC MANAGEMENT
1. Prompt surgical evacuation of mass lesions
2. Normotension, normovolemia, normal/mild hypocapnia
    a. Iso/hypertonic fluids or colloids
    b. Vasopressors available
3. Early hypothermia currently discretionary—not routine

CRITICAL CARE MANAGEMENT
General
1. Intracranial pressure (ICP) monitor: ventriculostomy preferred
2. Cerebral perfusion pressure (CPP) ≥ 70 mmHg, maintained at least 96 hours after injury when ICP is normal
3. Normovolemia—iso/hypertonic fluids or colloids; strict I/O monitoring
    a. Central venous pressure (CVP) at > 8–10 mmHg
    b. Pulmonary artery occlusion pressure (PAOP) 12–15 mmHg
4. Avoid hypoxia and maintain hematocrit at 28–33%

Management of intracranial hypertension (ICP > 20–25 or CPP < 70 mmHg)
    ICP limit may change depending on ability to maintain CPP
    CPP limit may increase depending on ICP response
1. If persistent, pulmonary artery catheter is placed for fluid management
2. Retrograde jugular bulb catheter
    a. $SJVO_2$ < 50%: rule out hypoxia, hypocarbia, anemia, hypotension
    b. $SJVO_2$ > 85%: rule out hyperemia (Doppler), hypercarbia, optimize CPP
3. Head of bed flat to ensure accurate CPP
4. Management withdrawn slowly when ICP < 20 mmHg for 48 hours
5. Sequence for management
    a. Optimize sedation
    b. Ensure adequate CPP using volume or vasopressors (phenylephrine, Levophed)
    c. Ventricular drainage
    d. Mannitol 0.25–1.00 g/kg, replacing volume loss: may be repeated 12.5–25.0 g every 6 hours for ICP or CPP limit set by neurosurgeon
    e. Muscle relaxants
    f. Mild hyperventilation to PCO_2 30–35 mmHg
    g. Prompt CT scan to assess for new mass lesion: consider possible lobar resection/craniectomy if warranted by clinical condition
    h. High-dose barbiturates
    i. Consider hypothermia
    j. PCO_2 < 30 mmHg, only in presence of jugular bulb catheter to evaluate for ischemia, oxygen extraction

MISCELLANEOUS
1. Daily weight
2. Nutrition commencing within 72 hours; may be withheld if there is persistant intracranial hypertension, hypothermia, or barbiturate coma
3. Blood glucose 80–200 mg/dl (hypo/hyperglycemia can potentiate neuronal damage)
4. Nimodipine 60 mg every 4 hours by gastric tube if traumatic subarachnoid hemorrhage present
5. Transcranial Doppler measurements to assess for vasospasm, hyperemia

References

1. Torner JC, Choi S, Barnes TY: Epidemiology of head injuries. In: Marion DW (ed) Traumatic Brain Injury. New York, Thieme, 1999:9–25.
2. Turazzi S, Bricolo A, Pasut ML: Review of 1000 consecutive cases of severe head injury treated before the advent of CT scanning. Acta Neurochir (Wien) 1984;72:167–195.
3. Jennett B, Teasdale G, Galbraith S, et al: Severe head injuries in three countries. J Neurol Neurosurg Psychiatry 1977;41:291–298.
4. Becker DP, Miller DJ, Ward JD, et al: The outcome from severe head injury with early diagnosis and intensive management. J Neurosurg 1977;47:491–502.
5. Bowers SA, Marshall L: Outcome in 200 consecutive cases of severe head injury treated in San Diego County: a prospective analysis. Neurosurgery 1980;6:237–242.
6. Miller JD, Butterworth J, Guideman SK, et al: Further experience in the management of severe head injury. J Neurosurg 1981;54:289–299.
7. Marion DW, Penrod LE, Kelsey SF, et al: Treatment of traumatic brain injury with moderate hypothermia. N Engl J Med 1997; 336:540–546.
8. Rosner MJ, Rosner S, Johnson AH: Cerebral perfusion pressure: management protocol and clinical results. J Neurosurg 1995;83:949–962.
9. Zauner A, Doppenberg E, Soukup J, et al: Extended neuromonitoring: new therapeutic opportunities? Neurol Res 1998;20 (Suppl 1):S85–S90.
10. Marion DW, Darby J, Yonas H: Acute regional cerebral blood flow changes caused by severe head injuries. J Neurosurg 1991;74:407–414.
11. Graham DI, Adams JH: Ischaemic brain damage in fatal head injuries. Lancet 1971;1:265–266.
12. Graham DI, Adams J, Doyle D: Ischaemic brain damage in fatal non-missile head injuries. J Neurol Sci 1978;39:213–234.
13. Grady MS, Shapira Y: Pathophysiology of head injury: primary central nervous system effects. In: Lam AM (ed) Anesthetic Management of Acute Head Injury. New York, McGraw-Hill, 1995;11–24.
14. McIntosh TK, Juhler M, Raghupathi R: Secondary brain injury: neurochemical and cellular mediators. In: DW M (ed) Traumatic Brain Injury. New York, Thieme, 1999;39–54.
15. Marion DW, Bouma G: The use of stable xenon-enhanced computed tomographic studies of cerebral blood flow to define changes in cerebral carbon dioxide vasoresponsivity by a severe head injury. Neurosurgery 1991;29:869–873.
16. Rosner MJ: Pathophysiology and management of increased intracranial pressure. In: Andrews BT (ed) Neurosurgical Intensive Care. New York, McGraw-Hill, 1993;57–112.
17. Ullman JS, Bederson JB: Hypertensive, hypervolemic, hemodilutional therapy for aneurysmal subarachnoid hemorrhage: is it efficacious? Yes. Crit Care Clin 1996;12:697–707.
18. Bouma GJ, Muizelaar JP, Stringer WA, et al: Ultra-early evaluation of regional cerebral blood flow in severely head injury patients using xenon-enhanced computerized tomography. J Neurosurg 1992;77:360–368.
19. Bouma GJ, Muizelaar JP, Choi SC, et al: Cerebral circulation and metabolism after severe traumatic brain injury: the elusive role of ischemia. J Neurosurg 1991;75:685–693.
20. Bouma GJ, Muizelaar JP: Cerebral blood flow, cerebral blood volume, and cerebrovascular reactivity after severe head injury. J Neurotrauma 1992;9(Suppl 1):S333–S348.
21. Obrist WD, Gennarelli TA, Segawa H, et al: Relationship of cerebral blood flow to neurological status and outcome in head-injured patients. J Neurosurg 1979;51:292–300.
22. Uzzell BP, Obrist WD, Dolinskas CA, et al: Relationship of acute CBF and ICP findings to neuropsychological outcome in severe head injury. J Neurosurg 65;65:630–635.
23. Marshall LF, Eisenberg HM, Jane JA, et al: The outcome of severe closed head injury. J Neurosurg 1991;75:S28–S36.
24. Teasdale G, Jennett B: Assessment of coma and impaired consciousness. Lancet 1974;2:81–83.
25. Pitts LH: Brain trauma and ischemia. In: Weinsten PR FA (ed) Protection of the Brain from Ischemia. Baltimore, Williams & Wilkins, 1990;171–181.
26. Marmarou A, Anerson RL, Ward JD: Impact of ICP instability and hypotension in outcome in patients with severe head trauma. J Neurosurg 1991;75:S59–S66.
27. Vollmer DG, Torner JC, Eisenberg HM, et al: Age and outcome following coma: why do older patients fare worse? J Neurosurg 1991;75:S37–S49.
28. Eisenberg HM, Gary HE, Aldrich EF, et al: Initial CT findings in 753 patients with severe head injury: a report from the NIH Traumatic Coma Data Bank. J Neurosurg 1990;73:688–698.
29. Gobiet W, Grote W, Boke WJ: The relation between intracranial pressure, mean arterial pressure, and cerebral blood flow in patients with severe head injury. Acta Neurochir (Wien) 1975;32:13–24.
30. Overgaard J, Tweed W: Cerebral circulation after head injury. Part 4. Functional anatomy and boundary-zone flow deprivation in the first week of traumatic coma. J Neurosurg 1983;59:439–446.
31. Heilbrun MP, Jorgensen PB, Boysen G: Relationships between cerebral perfusion pressure and regional cerebral flow in patients with severe neurological disorder. Stroke 1972;3:181–195.
32. Rosner MJ, Becker DP: Origin and evolution of plateau waves: experimental observations and a theoretical model. J Neurosurg 1984;60:312–324.
33. Lundberg N: Continuous recording and control of ventricular fluid pressure in neurosurgical practice. Acta Psychiatr Scand 1960;36(Suppl 149):1–193.
34. Stocchetti N, Chieregato A, De Marchi, et al: High cerebral perfusion pressure improves low values of local brain tissue O_2 tension ($PtiO_2$) in focal lesions. Acta Neurochir Suppl (Wien) 1998;71:162–165.
35. Gray WJ, Rosner MJ: Pressure-volume index as a function of cerebral perfusion pressure. Part 2. The effects of low cerebral perfusion pressure and autoregulation. J Neurosurg 1987;67:377–380.
36. Marmarou A, Saad A, Rigsbee M: Contribution of raised ICP and hypotension to CPP reduction in severe brain injury: correlation to outcome. J Neurotrauma 1995;12:378.
37. Schrader H, Lofgren J, Zwetnow NN: Influence of blood pressure on tolerance to an intracranial expanding mass. Acta Neurol Scand 1985;71:114–126.
38. Rosner MJ, Daughton S: Cerebral perfusion pressure management in head injury. J Trauma 1990;30:933–941.
39. Jennett B, Bond M: Assessment of outcome after severe brain damage: a practical scale. Lancet 1975;1:480–484.

40. Chan KH, Miller JD, Dearden NM, et al: The effect of changes in cerebral perfusion pressure upon middle cerebral artery blood flow velocity and jugular bulb venous oxygen saturation after severe brain injury. J Neurosurg 1992;77:55–61.
41. Chan KH, Dearden NM, Miller JD, et al: Multimodality monitoring as a guide to treatment of intracranial hypertension after severe head injury. Neurosurgery 1993;32:547–552.
42. Rosner MJ, Coley I: Cerebral perfusion pressure: a hemodynamic mechanism of mannitol and the post mannitol hemogram. Neurosurgery 1987;21:147–156.
43. Bullock R, Chestnut RM, Clifton G, et al: Guidelines for the Management of Severe Head Injury. Brain Trauma Foundation and The American Association of Neurological Surgeons, 1995.
44. Biestro A, Barrios E, Baraibar J, et al: Use of vasopressors to raise cerebral perfusion pressure in head injured patients. Acta Neurochir Suppl (Wien) 1998;71:5–9.
45. Myburgh JA, Upton RN, Grant C, et al: A comparison of the effects of norepinephrine, epinephrine, and dopamine on cerebral blood flow and oxygen utilisation. Acta Neurochir Suppl (Wien) 1998;71:19–21.
46. Tharion J, Johnson DC, Celermajer JM: Profound hypothermia with circulatory arrest: nine year's clinical experience. J Thorac Cardiovasc Sirg 1982;84:66–72.
47. Solomon RA, Smith CR, Raps EC, et al: Deep hypothermic circulatory arrest for the management of complex anterior and posterior circulation aneurysms. Neurosurgery 1991;29:732–738.
48. Connolly E, Solomon R: Hypothermic cardiac standstill for cerebral aneurysm surgery. Neurosurg Clin North Am 1998;9:681–695.
49. Dietrich WD, Alonso O, Busto R, et al: Post-traumatic brain hypothermia reduces histopathological damage following concussive brain injury in the rat. Acta Neuropathol (Berl) 1994;87:250–258.
50. Koizumi H, Povlishock J: Posttraumatic hypothermia in the treatment of axonal damage in animal model of traumatic axonal injury. J Neurosurg 1998;89:303–309.
51. Laptook AR, Corbett RJT, Sterett R, et al: Modest hypothermia provides partial neuroprotection when used for immediate resuscitation after brain ischemia. Pediatr Res 1997;42:17–23.
52. Rosmonoff HL, Shulman K, Raynor R, et al: Experimental brain injury and delayed hypothermia. Surg Gynecol Obstet 1960;110:27–32.
53. Drake CG, Jory TA: Hypothermia in the treatment of critical head injury. Can Med Assoc J 1962;84:887–891.
54. Marion DW, Obrist WD, Carlier PM, et al: The use of moderate therapeutic hypothermia for patients with severe head injuries: a preliminary report. J Neurosurg 1993;79:354–362.
55. Metz C, Holzscuh M, Bein T, et al: Moderate hypothermia in patients with severe head injury: cerebral and extracerebral effects. J Neurosurg 1996;85:533–541.
56. Myseros JS, Bullock R: The rationale for glutamate antagonists in the treatment of traumatic brain injury. Ann NY Acad Sci 1995;765:262–271.
57. Clifton G: Hypothermia and hyperbaric oxygen as treatment modalities for severe head injury. New Horiz 1995;3:474–478.
58. Clifton GL, Allen S, Barrodale P, et al: A phase II study of moderate hypothermia in severe brain injury. J Neurotrauma 1993;10:263–271.
59. Clifton G, Allen S, Berry J, et al: Systemic hypothermia in treatment of brain injury. J Neurotrauma 1992;9:S487–S495.
60. Shiozaki T, Sugimoto H, Taneda M, et al: Effect of mild hypothermia in uncontrollable intracranial hypertension after severe head injury. J Neurosurg 1993;79:363–368.
61. Shiozaki T, Sugimoto H, Taneda M, et al: Selection of severely head injured patients for mild hypothermia therapy. J Neurosurg 1998;89:206–211.
62. Muizelaar JP, Marmarou A, Ward JD, et al: Adverse effects of prolonged hyperventilation in patients with severe head injury: a randomized clinical trial. J Neurosurg 1991;75:731–739.
63. Marion DW, Firlik A, McLaughlin MR: Hyperventilation therapy for severe head injury. New Horiz 1995;3:439–447.
64. Bruce DA, Gennarelli TA, Langfitt TW: Resuscitation from coma due to head injury. Crit Care Med 1978;6:254–269.
65. Schneider GH, Sarrafzadeh AS, Keining K, et al: Influence of hyperventilation on brain tissue: PO_2, PCO_2, and pH on patients with intracranial hypertension. Acta Neurochir Suppl (Wien) 1998;71:62–65.
66. Ausina A, Baguena M, Nadal M, et al: Cerebral hemodynamic changes during sustained hypocapnia in severe head injury: can hyperventilation cause cerebral ischemia? Acta Neurochir Suppl (Wien) 1998;71:1–4.
67. Sheinberg M, Kanter MJ, Robertson CS, et al: Continuous monitoring of jugular venous oxygen saturation in head-injured patients. J Neurosurg 1992;76:212–217.
68. Gopinath SP, Robertson CS, Contant CF, et al: Jugular venous desaturation and outcome after head injury. J Neurol Neurosurg Psychiatry 1994;57:717–723.
69. Allen GS, Ahn HS, Preziosi TJ, et al: Cerebral arterial spasm — a controlled trial of nimodipine in patients with subarachnoid hemorrhage. N Engl J Med 1983;308:619–624.
70. Compton JS, Lee T, Jones NR, et al: A double blind placebo controlled trial of the calcium entry blocking drug, nicardipine, in the treatment of vasospasm following severe head injury. Br J Neurosurg 1990;4:9–16.
71. European Study Group on Nimodipine in Severe Head injury: A multicenter trial of the efficacy of nimodipine on outcome after severe head injury. J Neurosurg 1994;80:797–804.
72. Ullman JS, Morgan BC, Eisenberg HM: Traumatic subarachnoid hemorrhage. In: Bederson J (ed) Subarachnoid Hemorrhage: Pathophysiology and Management. Park Ridge, IL, American Association of Neurological Surgeons, 1997;225–237.
73. Harders A, Kakareika A, Braakman R, et al: Traumatic subarachnoid hemorrhage and its treatment with nimodipine. J Neurosurg 1996;85:82–89.
74. Kroppenstedt SN, Schneider GH, Tomale UW, et al: Protective effects of aptinagel HCl (Cerestat) following controlled cortical impact injury in rat. J Neurotrauma 1998;15:191–197.
75. Smith DH, Casey K, McIntosh TK: Pharmacological therapy for traumatic brain injury: experimental approaches. New Horiz 1995;3:562–572.
76. Marshall LF, Marshall SB: Pharmacologic therapy: promising clinical investigations. New Horiz 1995;3:573–580.

77. Doppenberg EMR, Shoi SC, Bullock R: Clinical trials in traumatic brain injury: what can we learn from previous studies. Ann NY Acad Sci 1997;825:305–322.
78. French L: The use of steroids in the treatment of cerebral edema. Bull NY Acad Med 1966;42:301–311.
79. Bracken MB, Shepard MJ, Collins WF, et al: A randomized, controlled trial of methylprednisolone or naloxone in the treatment of acute spinal-cor injury. N Engl J Med 1990;322:1405–1411.
80. Bracken MB, Shepard MJ, Holford TR, et al: Methylprednisolone or tirilazad mesylate administration after acute spinal cord injury: 1-year follow up. J Neurosurg 1998;89:699–706.
81. James HE, Madauss WC, Tibbs PA, et al: The effect of high dose dexamethasone in children with severe close head injury. Acta Neurochir (Wien) 1979;45:225–236.
82. Kelly D: Steroids in head injury. New Horiz 1995;3:453–455.
83. Sparacio RR, Lin TH, Cook AW: Methylprednisolone sodium succinate in acute cerebral trauma. Surg Gynecol Obstet 1965;121:513–516.
84. Cooper PR, Moody S, Clark WK, et al: Dexamethasone and severe head injury: a prospective double-blind study. J Neurosurg 1979;51:307–316.
85. Gudeman SK, Miller JD, Becker DP: Failure of high-dose steroid therapy to influence intracranial pressure in patients. J Neurosurg 1979;51:301–306.
86. Dearden NM, Gibson JS, McDowall DG, et al: Effect of high-dose dexamethasone on outcome from severe head injury. J Neurosurg 1986;64:81–88.
87. Braakman R, Schouten HJA, Blaauw-van Dishoeck M, et al: Megadose steroids in severe head injury: results of a prospective double-blind clinical trial. J Neurosurg 1983;58:326–330.
88. Saul TG, Ducker TB, Salcman M, et al: Steroids in severe head injury: a randomized clinical trial. J Neurosurg 1981;54:596–600.
89. Marshall LF, Maas AIR, Marshall SB, et al: A multicenter trial on the efficacy of using triliazad mesylate in cases of head injury. J Neurosurg 1998;89:519–525.
90. Shapiro HM: Barbiturates in brain ischemia. Br J Anaesth 1985;57:82–95.
91. Ward JD, Becker DP, Miller JD, et al: Failure of prophylactic barbiturate coma in the treatment of severe head injury. J Neurosurg 1985;62:383–388.
92. Smith DS, Rehncrona S, Siesjo BK: Barbiturates as protective agents in brain ischemia and as free radical scavengers in vitro. Acta Physiol Scand Suppl 1980;492:129–134.
93. Messeter K, Nordstrom CH, Sundbarg G, et al: Cerebral hemodynamcis in patients with acute severe head trauma. J Neurosurg 1986;64:231–237.
94. Miller JD: Barbiturates and raised intracranial pressure. Ann Neurol 1979;6:189–193.
95. Goodman JC, Valadka AB, Gopinath SP, et al: Lactate and excitatory amino acids measured by microdialysis are decreased by pentobarbital coma in head-injured patients. J Neurotrauma 1996;13:549–556.
96. Marshall LF, Smith RW, Shapiro HM: The outcome with aggressive treatment in severe head injuries. Part II. Acute and chronic barbiturate administration in the management of head injury. J Neurosurg 1979;50:26–30.
97. Nordby HK, Nesbakken R: The effect of high dose barbiturate decompression after severe head injury: a controlled clinical trial. Acta Neurochir (Wien) 1984;72:157–166.
98. Rockoff MA, Marshall LF, Shapiro HM: High-dose barbiturate therapy in humans: a clinical review of 60 patients. Ann Neurol 1978;6:194–199.
99. Eisenberg HM, Fankowski RF, Contant CF, et al: High-dose barbiturate control of elevated intracranial pressure in patients with severe head injury. J Neurosurg 1988;69:15–23.
100. Traeger SM, Henning RJ, Dobkin W, et al: Hemodynamic effects of pentobarbital therapy for intracranial hypertension. Crit Care Med 1983;11:697–701.
101. Bayliff CD, Schwarta ML, Hardy BG: Pharmacokinetics of high-dose pentobarbital in severe head trauma. Clin Pharmacol Ther 1985;38:457–461.
102. Vassar MJ, Perry CA, Gannaway WL, et al: 7.5% Sodium chloride/dextran for resuscitation of trauma patients undergoing helicopter transport. Arch Surg 1991;126:1065–1072.
103. Vassar MJ, Perry CA, Holcroft JW: Prehospital resuscitation of hypotensive trauma patients with 7.5% NaCl versus 7.5% NaCl with added dextran: a controlled trial. J Trauma 1993;34:622–633.
104. Velasco IT, Pontieri V, Silva RE, et al: Hyperosmotic NaCl and severe hemorrhagic shock. Am J Physiol 1980;239:H664–H673.
105. Mattox K, Maningas PA, Moore EE, et al: Prehospital hypertonic saline/dextran infusion for posttraumatic hypotension. Ann Surg 1991;213:482–490.
106. Monafo WW, Halverson JD, Schechtman K: The role of concentrated sodium solutions in the resuscitation of patients with severe burns. Surgery 1984;95:129–135.
107. Prough DS, DeWill DS, Zornow MH: Fluid management and resuscitation in neurological trauma. In: Abrams KJ, Grahame CM (eds) Trauma Anesthesia and Critical Care of Neurological Injury. Armonk, NY, Futura, 1997;189–226.
108. Ogino R, Susuki K, Kohno M, et al: Effects of hypertonic saline and dextran 70 on cardiac contractility after hemorrhagic shock. J Trauma 1998;44:59–69.
109. Nath F, Galbraith S: The effect of mannitol in cerebral white matter water content. J Neurosurg 1986;65:41–43.
110. Wisner DH, Schuster L, Quinn C: Hypertonic saline resuscitation of head injury: effects on cerebral water content. J Trauma 1990;30:75–78.
111. Burke AM, Quest DO, Chien S, et al: The effects of mannitol on blood viscosity. J Neurosurg 1981;55:550–553.
112. Muizelaar JP, Wei EP, Kontos HA, et al: Mannitol causes compensatory vasoconstriction and vasodilation in response to blood viscosity changes. J Neurosurg 1983;59:822–828.
113. Freshman SP, Battistella FD, Matteucci M, et al: Hypertonic saline (7.5%) versus mannitol: a comparison for treatment of acute head injuries. J Trauma 1993;35:344–348.
114. Battistella FD, Wisner DH: Combined hemorrhagic shock and head injury: effects of hypertonic saline (7.5%) resuscitation. J Trauma 1991;31:182–188.
115. Prough DS, Whitley JM, Tayor CL, et al: Regional cerebral blood flow following resuscitation from hemorrhagic shock with hypertonic saline. Anesthesiology 1991;75:319–327.
116. Prough DS, Johnson JC, Poole GV, et al: Effects on intracranial pressure resuscitation from hemorrhagic shock with hypertonic saline versus lactated Ringer's solution. Crit Care Med 1985;13:407–411.

117. Gunnar W, Jonasson O, Merlotti G, et al: Head injury and hemorrhagic shock: studies of the blood brain barrier and intracranial pressure after resuscitation with normal saline solution, 3% saline solution and dextran-40. Surgery 1988;103:398–407.
118. Shackford SR, Bourguignon PR, Wald SL, et al: Hypertonic saline resuscitation of patients with head injury: a prospective, randomized clinical trial. J Trauma 1998;44:50–58.
119. Qureshi AI, Suarez JI, Bahardwaj A, et al: Use of hypertonic saline (3%) saline acetate infusion in the treatment of cerebral edema: effect on intracranial pressure and lateral displacement of the brain. Crit Care Med 1998;26:440–446.
120. Simma B, Burger R, Falk M, et al: A prospective, randomized, controlled study of fluid management in children with severe head injury: lactated Ringer's solution versus hypertonic saline. Crit Care Med 1998;26:1265–1270.
121. Schatzmann C, Heisseler HE, Konig K, et al: Treatment of elevated intracranial pressure by infusion of 10% saline in severely head injured patients. Acta Neurochir Suppl (Wien) 1998;71:31–33.
122. Worthley LIG, Cooper DJ, Jones N: Treatment of resistant intracranial hypertension with hypertonic saline. J Neurosurg 1988;68:478–481.
123. Bingham WF: The limits of cerebral dehydration in the treatment of head injury. Surg Neurol 1986;25:340–345.
124. Alvarez M, Nava JM, Rue M, et al: Mortality prediction in head trauma patients: performance of Glasgow Coma Score and general severity systems. Crit Care Med 1998;26:142–148.
125. Baltas I, Gerogiannis N, Sakellariou P, et al: Outcome in severely head injured patients with and without multiple trauma. J Neurosurg Sci 1998;42:85–88.
126. Jaicks RR, Cohn SM, Moller BA: Early fracture fixation may be deleterious after head injury. J Trauma 1997;42:1–6.
127. Pape HC, Auf'm'Kolk M, Paffrath T, et al: Primary intramedullary femur fixation in multiple trauma patients with associated lung contusion: a cause of posttraumatic ARDS? J Trauma 1993;34:540–548.
128. Bone L, McNamara K, Shine B, et al: Mortality in multiple trauma patients with fractures. J Trauma 1994;37:262–265.
129. Goris R, Gimbrere J, Van Neikerk J, et al: Early osteosynthesis and prophylactic mechanical ventilation in the multitrauma patient. J Trauma 1982;22:895–903.
130. Hoffman P, Goris R: Timing of osteosynthesis of major fractures in patients with severe head injury. J Trauma 1991;31:261–263.
131. Johnson KD, Cadambi A, Seibert GB: Incidence of adult respiratory distress syndrome in patients with multiple musculoskeletal injuries: effect of early operative stabilization of fractures. J Trauma 1985;25:375–384.
132. Maas AIR, Dearden M, Teasdale GM, et al: EBIC-guidelines for management of severe head injury in adults. Acta Neurochir (Wein) 1997;139:286–294.
133. Marion DW: Management of traumatic brain injury: past, present, and future. Clin Neurosurg 1999;45:184–191.

41
Stress Gastritis: Is It a Disappearing Disease?

Rodney M. Durham and Kelly Dreste

Stress gastritis is defined as acute superficial erosions of the gastric mucosa that occur secondary to physiologic stress. Because these erosions are superficial, complications of stress gastritis are primarily related to bleeding.[1] Other terms include hemorrhagic gastritis, erosive gastritis, stress ulceration, gastric erosions, and stress bleeding. During the 1960s and 1970s bleeding due to stress gastritis resulting in the death of a critically ill patient was not uncommon.[2] Research during this period was directed toward defining the pathophysiology of stress gastritis and its prevention. Recommendations that all critically ill patients receive prophylactic acid-reducing therapy were based on these trials.[3] However, many of the early studies used heme-positive gastric aspirates to diagnose stress gastritis even though this finding is rarely clinically significant. During the 1980s most patients admitted to an intensive care unit (ICU) received stress prophylaxis, and research was directed toward defining the efficacy of prophylactic agents and complications of those agents.[4]

During the late 1980s and early 1990s it became apparent that stress erosions were found on endoscopy in most critically ill patients, but most patients remained asymptomatic and the erosions resolved spontaneously when the stress was removed.[5] Currently an impression exists that clinically significant bleeding has decreased during the last decade,[6] attributed to improvements in care of critically ill patients. This impression has led to a change in focus, so current research is directed toward defining the incidence of clinically important bleeding in various critical illnesses to identify patients who will benefit most from stress prophylaxis.

Pathophysiology

The lesions associated with stress gastritis are located primarily in the fundic mucosa of the stomach. The process may involve the antral mucosa and less frequently the duodenal mucosa, but isolated involvement of these areas has not been seen without fundic involvement.[7] In 42 trauma patients, endoscopic examination performed within 72 hours of injury showed multiple gastric erosions predominantly in the fundus in all patients.[2] Initial lesions were small punctate erosions 1–2 mm in diameter with a central area of pallor surrounded by an area of hemorrhage. Over a 48-hour period the lesions can enlarge up to 25 mm; and some spread to involve the entire stomach.[8]

Injury to the gastric mucosa occurs when acid and pepsin overcome gastric mucosal defenses owing either to excessive acid secretion or a breakdown in the gastric mucosal barrier. Hydrogen ions in the gastric lumen are a prerequisite for stress-related mucosal injury, but impairment of the gastric mucosal barrier is the etiology of stress gastritis in most patients.[9,10] The barrier allows the stomach to maintain a large pH gradient between the gastric lumen and the epithelial cell surface. The gastric mucosal barrier is not a single anatomic structure but a number of physiologic mechanisms, including (1) secretion of mucus and bicarbonate, forming a protective layer between the epithelial surface and luminal acid; (2) cell membranes that allow passage of lipid-soluble molecules but not water-soluble hydrogen ions; (3) rapid regeneration of the epithelial cell surface by progenitor cells located in the basal lamina; (4) endogenous prostaglandins, which increase mucosal blood flow, stimulate epithelial cell regeneration, increase mucus and bicarbonate secretion, and suppress gastric acid secretion; and (5) gastric mucosal blood flow.

Disruption of any of these mechanisms may result in damage to the gastric mucosa, but the initial event leading to stress erosions is thought to be decreased gastric mucosal blood flow. Menguy demonstrated a decrease in gastric mucosal adenosine triphosphate (ATP) after hemorrhagic shock.[11] Decreases in cellular ATP are most prominent in the gastric fundus, the most common location for stress erosions. This energy deficit decreases secretion of mucus, bicarbonate, and acid by the cell. Paradoxically, cells that are actively secreting acid are more resistant to luminal acid than resting cells,[12] due in part to the alkaline tide. As hydrogen ion is secreted into the gastric lumen, bicarbonate is produced and secreted into the mucosal capillaries. As long as mucosal blood flow is adequate, this bicarbonate can neutralize any acid that diffuses back through the cellular membrane. Systemic acidosis seen during shock may further compromise the ability of the gastric mucosa to deal with back-diffusion of acid from the lumen.

Patients who develop stress-related mucosal ulceration have commonly been in shock, resulting in alterations of gastric mucosa blood flow.[13] Gut perfusion is sacrificed with shock to enhance flow to the brain and heart. Most of the increased systemic vascular resistance to maintain blood pressure to vital core organs during hypovolemia occurs in the splanchnic bed with a decrease in intestinal blood flow, which is particularly severe and selective for the gastric mucosa.[14] It impairs the ability of the microcirculation to dispose of hydrogen ions, resulting in intramural acidosis, cell death, and mucosal ulcerations. If these ulcerations extend beyond the basal laminae, the ability of the mucosa to regenerate is compromised.[12] Aggressive, early fluid resuscitation is necessary to optimize oxygen delivery, restore splanchnic perfusion, and prevent persistent hypoperfusion of the gastric mucosa. Adequate perfusion of all organs, including the splanchnic bed and the gastric submucosa, requires maintaining appropriate cardiac preload and monitoring cardiac index, O_2 delivery, and O_2 consumption.[15] Monitoring the intramucosal gastric pH by gastric tonometry may prevent subacute splanchnic hypoperfusion secondary to inadequate volume resuscitation.[16]

Despite the importance of mucosal blood flow, gastric erosions do not occur after ischemia in the absence of luminal acid.[17] Several investigators have suggested that acidification of the gastric mucosa plays a key role in the development of stress ulceration. In cases of acidosis or other alterations in intramucosal pH, back-diffusion of luminal hydrogen ions may be a cause of the stress ulcer. The mucosa can be protected by supplying systemic bicarbonate to the mucosal capillaries or neutralizing luminal acid. Kivilaakso et al. showed that maintaining the intraluminal pH > 7 prevents intracellular acidosis and decreases stress erosions.[18]

Although luminal acid plays an important role in stress gastritis, gastric acid secretion is normal or decreased in most patients.[19] However, acid hypersecretion occurs in some patients with burns (Curling ulcers) or intracranial disease (Cushing ulcers). In burn patients these ulcers tend to be single, chronic, and penetrate deeper into the mucosa than stress ulcers. These chronic lesions can perforate and are pathologically different from typical stress ulcerations.[20] Cushing's ulcers in neurosurgical patients tend to be deep, often full-thickness erosions of the esophagus, stomach, or duodenum. Hypersecretion of gastrin and pepsin are common in neurosurgical patients but unusual in stress ulcer patients. In a rat model, stress activates α-adrenergic stimulation to the stomach through the hypothalamus. This controls intragastric blood flow and serotonin release. Specific peptides (bombesin, calcitonin, corticotropin-releasing factor, neurotensin, opioid) may act in the central nervous system (CNS) to induce or prevent the formation of ulceration or to alter gastric secretory and motor function. Several autonomic neurotransmitters, such as dopamine, epinephrine, and norepinephrine, promote mucosal resistance. These animal models may explain in part the different clinical manifestations of stress ulcer disease in neurosurgical patients, but the relevance of these models to stress ulceration in humans is uncertain.[21]

Diagnosis

The diagnosis of stress ulcers depends on the identification of upper gastrointestinal bleeding in critically ill patients. Guaiac testing of nasogastric aspirates is neither sensitive nor specific for the diagnosis of stress gastritis and is not clinically useful. Most studies now classify bleeding as overt or clinically important.[22] Overt bleeding is defined as hematemesis, melena, hematochezia, or aspiration of gross blood from the nasogastric tube. Aspiration of coffee-ground material is suggestive of bleeding but may not require further study without a decrease in hematocrit and if the patient is stable. Clinically important bleeding is defined as overt bleeding (1) with a decrease in blood pressure of 20 mmHg within 24 hours of bleeding; (2) and orthostasis with a change of heart rate of 20 beats/min; or (3) requiring transfusion.

The gold standard for the diagnosis of stress gastritis is endoscopy. All patients with clinically significant bleeding should undergo endoscopy to identify the source and exclude other sources of bleeding, such as ulcers and varices. Endoscopy allows treatment in these patients. Because it is invasive and expensive, it is usually reserved for patients with active bleeding.

Natural History

Depending on the patient's disease and severity of illness, stress erosions can be demonstrated by endoscopy in 70–100% of critically ill patients within 24 hours of the initial insult.[5] The clinical relevance of these findings is questionable, as most patients remain asymptomatic. When bleeding is defined as positive by guaiac testing of gastric aspirates, microscopic blood loss from a variety of sources, including erosions caused by the nasogastric tube, occurs in most ICU patients.[13,23]

Observations suggest that clinically significant bleeding due to stress gastritis has been decreasing over the last two decades.[6,24–26] Routine use of prophylaxis in all ICU patients has contributed to decreased bleeding, but better understanding of the pathogenesis of stress ulcers has led to the belief that routine prophylaxis may not be necessary in all patients. Comparisons of antacids and H_2-antagonists with placebo allows an estimation of gastritis in patients. Prior to 1978, clinically significant bleeding in patients not receiving prophylaxis ranged from 5.3% to 33.0%.[27] Clinical trials since then have reported widely varying incidences of clinically significant bleeding in patients not receiving prophylactic therapy. Ben-Menachem et al. found an average frequency of clinically significant bleeding of 6% in reports published between 1984 and 1994,[28] but the reported incidences ranged between 0.1% and 39.0%. Improvements in critical care appear to be partially responsible for the decreased incidence of clinically significant bleeding (Table 41.1). However, it is difficult to reach definitive conclusions based on these trials because studies have used different definitions of bleeding, have included patients with wide ranges in severity and etiology of critical illness, and did not accurately diagnose the source of bleeding in all patients.

TABLE 41.1. Factors for Improved Outcomes for Stress Gastritis.

Earlier resuscitation by ambulance and faster transportation to the hospital
Critical care specialists
Tissue oxygenation maintained
Correction of acid–base and fluid disorders
Prophylaxis with H_2-antagonists, antacids, or sucralfate

Adapted from Navab and Steingrub,[24] with permission.

To better define patient populations at risk for clinically significant bleeding, a number of risk factors have been identified. Statistically significant risk factors identified by Cook et al. in 1994 included the need for mechanical ventilation for more than 48 hours and coagulopathy.[29] (Table 41.2). However, about one-half of the patients in this study had had cardiovascular surgery, and it is not clear whether these results can be extrapolated to other patients. Other studies have reported that the risk of bleeding is increased in patients with three or more clinical risk factors, including shock, sepsis, multiple trauma, major organ dysfunction, burns over more than 35% of the body surface, and head injury.[27]

Clinically, stress gastritis is usually seen as one component of the larger syndrome of multiple organ failure (MOF). Improvements in resuscitation of critically ill patients and stress prophylaxis have been postulated to decrease the incidence of MOF and clinically significant stress bleeding.[9,30] In 756 trauma patients admitted to our ICU over a 2.5-year period clinically significant bleeding occurred in seven patients, all of whom had evidence of other organ failures. All patients received stress prophylaxis with H_2-blockers prior to the bleeding. In four patients, bleeding was from sources other than stress gastritis. One patient died from sepsis and organ failure before the source of bleeding could be documented, and two patients (0.2%) had endoscopically proven stress gastritis. Bleeding resolved in both of these patients with increased acid-reducing therapy.

Despite a decreased incidence of bleeding, mortality remains high among critically ill patients who bleed owing to stress gastritis, estimated to be 35–77%.[9,31] However, death is not related to bleeding but to the underlying disease process and MOF. In a meta-analysis of 1993 critically ill patients there were 821 patients who received no prophylaxis, and Lacroix et al. found only five deaths directly attributable to gastrointestinal hemorrhage.[32]

Reviews and Meta-Analyses of Clinical Trials of Prophylactic Therapy

Efficacy

A number of reviews and meta-analyses have attempted to resolve controversial issues. Although these studies suffer from the inherent limitations of meta-analysis, their findings provide a useful overview of stress gastritis.[33] Schuman et al. reviewed 16 prospective trials in 1987 and compared the incidence of microscopic (guaiac-positive nasogastric aspirate) and overt bleeding (hematemesis requiring transfusion, bright red blood per nasogastric tube, and melena) in patients receiving prophylaxis with antacids, cimetidine, or a placebo.[34] When any bleeding was the criterion for failure, it occurred in 3.4% of antacid patients 7.2% of cimetidine patients, and 17.5% of placebo patients. With overt bleeding, failure occurred in 3.3% with antacids, 2.7% with cimetidine, and 15% with placebo.

Because microscopic bleeding is of minimal clinical significance, later analyses examined only clinically important bleeding. Lacroix et al.[32] in 1989 reviewed many of the same trials reviewed by Shuman et al.[34] For overt bleeding, there was no difference between patients receiving antacids and those receiving cimetidine. Both treatments were superior to placebo. Hemorrhagic shock and death occurred in only 0.4% and 0.25%, respectively, of the 1993 patients studied.

In 1991 Tryba reported two meta-analyses of randomized and nonrandomized trials.[35,36] In the first meta-analysis overt bleeding or clinically important bleeding was used as the endpoint.[36] Fourteen trials compared H_2-blockers versus controls. Bleeding occurred in 5.3% in the H_2-blocker group compared with 16.1% in the control group. Bleeding occurred in 5.6% of an antacid group and 14.9% of the controls. Six trials compared sucralfate to H_2-blockers. A lower rate of bleeding was found with sucralfate. Ten trials compared antacids to sucralfate and found no significant differences in bleeding.

In a second meta-analysis in 1991, Tryba compared sucralfate to H_2-blockers (9 trials) and to antacids (10 trials) using significant bleeding as the endpoint.[35] A significantly lower rate of bleeding occurred with sucralfate than with H_2-blockers [odds ratio (OR) 0.532, confidence interval (CI) 0.303–0.933], and there was a trend toward less bleeding with sucralfate than with antacids (OR 0.868; CI 0.452–1.667).

Cook et al. in a meta-analysis in 1991 reviewed the incidence of overt bleeding with a 20 mmHg decrease in blood pressure within 24 hours of bleeding, a 10 mmHg decrease plus a 20 beat/min increase in heart rate on standing, or a decrease in hemoglobin of 2 g/dl with transfusion of 2 units of blood.[37] Only randomized, controlled trials were included. H_2-blockers

TABLE 41.2. Risk Factors for Clinically Important Gastrointestinal Bleeding.

Risk factor	Simple regression		Multiple regression	
	Odds ratio	p	Odds ratio	p
Respiratory failure	25.5	<0.001	15.6	<0.001
Coagulopathy	9.5	<0.001	4.3	<0.001
Hypotension	5.0	0.03	3.7	0.08
Sepsis	7.3	<0.001	2.0	0.17
Hepatic failure	6.5	<0.001	1.6	0.27
Renal failure	4.6	<0.001	1.6	0.28
Enteral feeding	3.8	<0.001	1.0	0.99
Glucocorticoid administration	3.7	<0.001	1.5	0.26
Organ transplantation	3.6	0.006	1.5	0.42
Anticoagulant therapy	3.3	0.004	1.1	0.88

Adapted from Cook et al.,[29] with permission.

alone were found to be effective in preventing clinically important bleeding when compared to controls (OR 0.35; CI 0.15–0.76). No difference in bleeding was found with antacids versus placebo, H_2-blockers versus antacids, antacids versus sucralfate, or H_2-blockers versus sucralfate.

To try to resolve the conflicting meta-analysis results, Cook et al. did a second meta-analysis in 1996.[22] Only randomized trials were included, and overt bleeding and clinically important bleeding were used as different endpoints. H_2-blockers decreased the incidence of both overt bleeding (OR 0.58; CI 0.42–0.79) and clinically important bleeding (OR 0.44; CI 0.22–0.88) compared with placebo. There was a trend toward a lower incidence of overt bleeding when antacids were compared to no therapy. With H_2-blockers and antacids there was a trend toward decreased clinically important bleeding compared to sucralfate. Cook's last meta-analysis is shown in Table 41.3. This study is one of the most comprehensive to date, but a major deficiency was that many of the clinical trials that were included did not use the same definition of clinically important bleeding that was used in the meta-analysis.

One of the largest randomized, blinded, placebo-controlled trials to date by Cook and the Canadian Critical Care Trials Group compared sucralfate to ranitidine for preventing stress bleeding in 1200 critically ill patients who required mechanical ventilation.[38] Most patients (61.9% in the ranitidine group and 58.8% in the sucralfate group) in the study were medical patients. Patients received sucralfate 1 g every 6 hours with an intravenous placebo given every 8 hours or ranitidine 50 mg every 8 hours with a nasogastric placebo every 6 hours. Clinically important bleeding occurred in 1.7% (10/596 patients) in the ranitidine group and 3.8% (23/604 patients) in the sucralfate group. This difference was statistically significant [relative risk (RR) 0.44; CI 0.21–0.92; $p < 0.02$]. The decision to perform endoscopy was made by the individual physician. Of the 33 patients who had clinically important bleeding, 17 underwent endoscopy; 14 of the 17 had documented bleeding from gastric, esophageal, or duodenal erosions. The source of bleeding was unclear in 8 patients in the ranitidine group and in 11 patients in the sucralfate group.

Nosocomial Pneumonia and Mortality

Cook et al.'s 1996 report analyzed 57 trials for bleeding.[22] Twenty-seven of these trials also evaluated nosocomial pneumonia as an outcome, although five did not report bleeding rates. With sucralfate there was a trend toward a lower incidence of pneumonia compared to that seen with antacids or H_2-blockers (Table 41.3) H_2-antagonists were associated with an increased incidence of pneumonia compared with placebo. Also sucralfate was associated with decreased mortality compared to antacids and H_2-blockers. However, this analysis suffered from variability in the criteria for the diagnosis of nosocomial pneumonia.

Mortality and nosocomial pneumonia were also studied by Cook and the Canadian Trails group.[38] Criteria for pneumonia in this study were a new radiographic infiltrate persisting at least 48 hours plus two or more of the following: temperature >38.5°C or <35°C, leukocyte count >10,000/mm³ or <3000/mm³, purulent sputum, or isolation of pathogenic bacteria from an endotracheal aspirate. Nosocomial pneumonia occurred in 19.1% with ranitidine and in 16.2% with sucralfate. The difference was not statistically significant. There was no difference in mortality (ranitidine 23.5%, sucralfate 22.8%) or in duration of ICU stay. Cook et al. concluded that ranitidine was associated with significantly less clinically important gastrointestinal bleeding than sucralfate, with no differences in pneumonia, duration of stay in the ICU, or mortality.

TABLE 41.3. Randomized Trials of Stress Ulcer Prophylaxis.

Comparison in trials	No. of trials	Common odds ratio (95% confidence interval)
Antacids vs. placebo/control		
Overt bleeding	7	0.66 (0.37–1.17)
Clinically important GI bleeding	3	0.35 (0.09–1.41)
Mortality rate	4	1.42 (0.82–2.47)
H_2-receptor antagonist vs. placebo/control		
Overt bleeding	20	0.58 (0.42–0.79)
Clinically important GI bleeding	10	0.44 (0.22–0.88)
Pneumonia	8	1.25 (0.78–2.00)
Mortality rate	15	1.15 (0.86–1.53)
H_2-receptor antagonist vs. antacids		
Overt bleeding	16	0.56 (0.37–0.84)
Clinically important GI bleeding	10	0.86 (0.46–1.59)
Pneumonia	3	1.01 (0.65–1.57)
Mortality rate	14	0.89 (0.66–1.21)
Sucralfate vs. placebo/control		
Overt bleeding	3	0.58 (0.34–0.99)
Clinically important GI bleeding	1	1.26 (0.12–12.87)
Pneumonia	2	2.11 (0.82–5.44)
Mortality rate	4	1.06 (0.67–1.67)
Sucralfate vs. H_2-receptor antagonist		
Overt bleeding	10	0.97 (0.62–1.51)
Clinically important GI bleeding	5	1.49 (0.42–5.27)
Pneumonia	6	0.80 (0.56–1.15)
Mortality rate	11	0.73 (0.54–0.97)
Sucralfate vs. H_2-receptor antagonists		
Overt bleeding	12	0.89 (0.63–1.27)
Clinically important GI bleeding	4	1.28 (0.27–6.11)
Pneumonia	11	0.78 (0.60–1.01)
Mortality rate	11	0.83 (0.62–1.09)

From Cook et al.,[22] with permission.
GI, gastrointestinal; H_2, histamine-2.
Statistically heterogeneous.

Prophylaxis

Enteral Nutrition

Early enteral nutrition may assist in preservation of gastric mucosal integrity by neutralizing acid and stimulating gastric mucosal blood flow.[39] Enteral feedings may also provide mucosal protection by stimulating endogenous prostaglandins and increasing the intragastric volume, which presumably decreases mucosal shear forces of gastric contractions.[40]

A decrease in upper gastrointestinal bleeding was reported when patients received enteral alimentation. Pingleton and Hadzima studied 43 mechanically ventilated patients. Twenty received antacids; 11 had microscopic bleeding, and 3 had bleeding requiring transfusion. Nine patients received cimetidine; seven had microscopic bleeding. Fourteen patients who received enteral alimentation had no evidence of bleeding.[39] The unknown type of enteral nutrition in patients who received antacids or cimetidine limits this study.

No large prospective studies examining the role of enteral feedings for the prevention of stress gastritis have been reported. The ability of feedings to maintain preset pH goals has not been demonstrated.[41] The effect of duodenal versus gastric feedings has not been fully explored. Presently most patients at high risk for stress gastritis receive other modes of prophylaxis in addition to enteral feedings.

Antacids

Hastings and colleagues in 1978 documented decreased gastrointestinal bleeding in critically ill patients treated with antacids to maintain the gastric pH higher than 3.5.[3] Intragastrically, pH 5 neutralizes 99.9% of acid produced.[42] (Table 41.4) Antacid-induced increases in gastric pH inhibit the proteolytic action of pepsin. The optimum pH for pepsin activity is 1.5–2.5, and progressive inhibition occurs as gastric pH increases. Above pH 4, the proteolytic activity of pepsin is minimal. Antacids, in decreasing order of their ability to neutralize a given amount of acid, are calcium carbonate, sodium bicarbonate, magnesium salts, and aluminum salts.

All antacids can potentially change the extent of absorption of other drugs by changing the transit time or through binding or chelation of the drug. A good rule is to wait 1 hour before administering the next medication. Increases in urinary pH may decrease the excretion of basic drugs (amphetamines, quinidine) and increase excretion of acidic drugs.[43]

Antacids are usually given as 30–60 ml through a nasogastric tube every 2–6 hours. Antacids in the fasting state reduce acidity for about 30 minutes. If administered after a meal, the effects last for about 3 hours. The longer duration of action after meals is due to a slower gastric emptying time. The effective neutralization quantity of antacids necessary to heal inflammation and ulceration of the gastroduodenal mucosa in most clinical settings is 180–400 mEq.[43] Problems associated with antacid administration vary based on the agent administered; they may include constipation, diarrhea, and electrolyte disorders (hypokalemia, hypermagnesemia, hypophosphatemia). Large volumes of antacids may increase the risk of aspiration, and nursing time is increased by the need to frequently monitor gastric pH.

H_2-Receptor Antagonists (H_2-Blockers): Cimetidine, Famotidine, Nizatidine, Ranitidine

The H_2-blockers competitively inhibit the action of histamine on the H_2-receptor of parietal cells, reducing gastric acid secretion.[43] Blockade of H_2-receptors inhibits activation of adenylcyclase, which decreases cyclic adenosine monophosphate (cAMP). In the parietal cell, cAMP is essential for the hydrogen/potassium/ATPase pump and acid secretion. Ranitidine is 3–10 times more potent on a molar basis than cimetidine in inhibiting stimulated gastric acid secretion. The potency of H_2-blockers varies 20- to 50-fold, with cimetidine being the least potent and famotidine the most.

A number of studies have demonstrated that antacids are superior to H_2-antagonists for controlling gastric pH, but pH control as an endpoint is not an accurate indicator of efficacy for prevention of bleeding. Poleski and Spanier compared antacids with cimetidine for preventing bleeding from stress erosions in 37 high risk patients.[44] Cimetidine was given in doses of 300 mg every 6 hours initially. If pH was not maintained above pH 4, the dose and interval were gradually increased up to a maximum of 400 mg every 4 hours. Mylanta II was initially given at a dose of 30 ml every hour and then increased to a maximum of 90 ml every hour until pH 4. Nasogastric aspirates were checked for the presence of occult or frank blood. All patients underwent endoscopy 72 hours after enrollment. No clinically significant bleeding occurred in either group. Endoscopy scores were similar in both groups. In the antacid group, pH was ≥4 in 97.9% of measurements compared with 79.5% in the cimetidine group. They concluded that Mylanta II controlled pH better than cimetidine, but they were equally effective in the prophylaxis of stress erosions. Thus even when cimetidine does not maintain pH > 4, it is effective in preventing bleeding. It has been suggested that pH monitoring is not necessary when standard doses of H_2-blockers are used. Monitoring may be needed when doses of these agents are adjusted for patients in renal failure.[27]

Drug interactions between H_2-blockers and magnesium and aluminum containing antacids are important. If given orally with antacids, H_2-blocker bioavailability is improved by 30–50% if antacid doses are separated by at least 2 hours.[45] The duration of inhibition of gastric acid appearance ranges from 4 to 13 hours for all the H_2-blockers. All of the H_2-blockers must be adjusted in the presence of renal impairment. Drug

TABLE 41.4. Significance of Intragastric pH Values.

pH	Activity
>3.5	Decreased incidence of bleeding
>4.5	Pepsin inactivated
5.0	99.9% Acid neutralization
<7.0	Clotting abnormalities
>9.0	Pepsin destroyed

Adapted from Peura,[42] with permission.

interactions are most common with cimetidine. Hepatic microsomal enzyme inhibition reduces metabolism of some drugs including coumadin anticoagulants, phenytoin, propanolol, some benodiazepines, lidocaine, metronidazole, triamterene, some tricyclic antidepressants, and theophylline, thus decreasing elimination and increasing blood concentrations. Famotidine and nizatidine can both be administered with food or antacids, with a decrease in bioavailability but no clinically significant effects or drug interactions. Ranitidine can also be administered with food or antacids without a change in bioavailability.[43]

Proton-Pump Inhibitors: Lansoprazole and Omeprazole

Lansoprazole and omeprazole are substituted benzamidazole antisecretory agents. They bind to hydrogen/potassium adenosine triphosphatase (H^+/K^+ exchanging ATPase) in gastric parietal cells. Inactivation of this enzyme system (also known as the proton, hydrogen, or acid pump) blocks the final step in secretion of hydrochloric acid. Thus gastric antisecretory agents such as lansoprazole are called proton-pump inhibitors.[43]

Lansoprazole and omeprazole are weak bases and are absorbed at an alkaline pH in the small intestine.[45] The degree of inhibition of gastric acid secretion is related to the dose and duration of therapy. Both lansoprazole and omeprazole are more potent inhibitors of acid secretion than the H_2-receptor antagonists. After 15 or 30 mg of lansoprazole orally, gastric acid inhibition occurs within 2–3 hours and 1–2 hours, respectively. After multiple daily doses, increased gastric pH occurs within 1 hour with 30 mg of lansoprazole and within 1–2 hours after 15 mg with oral omeprazole, gastric acid secretion inhibition occurs within 1 hour, peaks within 2 hours, and persists for up to 72 hours. Gastric acid secretion inhibition increases with continuous therapy and reaches a plateau after about 4 days. A 40 mg dose of omeprazole inhibits 58–80% of basal gastric acid secretion. After omeprazole is stopped, gastric acid secretion returns to baseline over a 3- to 5-day period. A 30 mg dose of lansoprazole inhibits 88% of acid secretion after 7 days of therapy. After lansoprazole is stopped, gastric acid secretion returns to baseline over a 2- to 4-day period.[43] No clinically significant drug interactions have been reported for lansoprazole or omeprazole. Dose adjustments are not necessary for patients with renal impairment, but hepatic dysfunction may warrant a lower dosage of both drugs.

Pantoprazole (Protium, Knoll) is a third proton-pump inhibitor that is currently available only in the United Kingdom.[46] Giving 40 mg of pantoprazole daily increases the 24-hour intragastric pH more than omeprazole (20 mg daily) and slightly less than lansoprazole (30 mg daily). These differences do not necessarily imply greater clinical efficacy. In the United Kingdom the pricing of pantoprazole is equal to that of lansoprazole. Both drugs cost slightly less than omeprazole.

Few data are available about proton-pump inhibitors being given for prevention of stress gastritis.[27,40] Proton-pump inhibitors prevent aspirin-induced mucosal damage in both animals and humans. They may offer little advantage over other prophylactic agents because bacterial colonization of the stomach has been demonstrated with their use even in normal volunteers. Although no definitive studies are available, these agents may be more useful in the management of patients with clinically significant bleeding.[47]

Sucralfate

Sucralfate is a basic, aluminum complex of sucrose sulfate that is structurally related to heparin but lacks anticoagulant activity. Sucralfate does not appreciably affect gastric acid output or concentration. Following oral administration, sucralfate rapidly reacts with HCl in the stomach to form a highly condensed, viscous, adhesive, paste-like substance with a minor capacity to buffer acid. The drug persists in this form in the proximal duodenum. Sucralfate adheres to the gastroduodenal mucosa and seems to locally protect an ulcer because it has a higher affinity for the ulcer site than for normal gastrointestinal mucosa. Binding to the ulcer crater is sucralfate's main therapeutic action.[43]

Secondary mechanisms may also contribute to protect the gastric mucosa. With gastric acid, an aluminum moiety is released that binds positively charged molecules such as peptides, proteins, glycoproteins, drugs, and metals. Physical, mechanical, absorbent, ion-exchange, and buffering properties of sucralfate may also contribute to its protective action. Finally, sucralfate may stimulate formation of prostaglandins by the gastric mucosa and exert a cytoprotecive effect similar to misoprostol.[45]

Standard doses of sucralfate are 1 g four times daily through a nasogastric tube. The medication must be delivered directly into the stomach. Administration of sucralfate with cimetidine, digoxin, ketoconazole, phenytoin, ranitidine, tetracycline, or theophylline results in a reduction in the bioavailability of those drugs. The clinical significance of these findings has not been determined in humans, but it has been recommended that sucralfate be given 2-hours before or after any of those drugs. Ciprofloxacin and norfloxacin have a 50% or more decrease in serum concentration with sucralfate use. The 2-hour dosing interval should be strictly adhered to with these fluoroquinolones.[43] Finally, sucralfate polymerization occurs best at pH < 4, so antacids or H_2-blockers probably should not be given with sucralfate.[48]

Misoprostol

Misoprostol is a synthetic analogue of prostaglandin E_1 (alprostadil) and is approved for use to prevent nonsteroidal antiinflammatory drug (NSAID)- and aspirin-induced gastric ulcers.[49] Misoprostol inhibits gastric acid secretion and protects the mucosa from the irritant or pharmacologic effects of these agents. Endogenous prostaglandins decrease acid secretion from parietal cells and increase mucus and bicarbonate secretion, thereby preventing disruption of the gastric mucosal barrier.

Inhibition or reduction of back-diffusion of hydrogen ions, regulation of mucosal blood flow, prevention of microvascular stasis, stabilization of lysosomal membranes with resultant reduction in enzyme release, and preservation of the mucosal capacity to regenerate cells are also functions of prostaglandins.

Misoprostol has a direct antisecretory effect that may represent its primary mode of action.[50] Gastric acid inhibition by misoprostol is proportional to dose. A 200-µg dose decreases 75–85% of meal-stimulated gastric acid secretions within 60–90 minutes and persists for about 3 hours. Misoprostol is contraindicated in pregnant women and relatively contraindicated in all women of childbearing age. It has been reported to produce uterine contractions and to stimulate uterine bleeding with total or partial expulsion of the products of conception in pregnant women. No drug interactions are noted, with the exception of magnesium-containing antacids increasing the occurrence of diarrhea.[43]

In a prospective, randomized, multicenter trial, misoprostol was compared to antacids for the prevention of stress bleeding in critically ill patients.[51] Misoprostal was given in an antisecretory dose of 20 µg every 4 hours. Gastric pH > 4 was maintained consistently in both groups, and no clinically significant bleeding occurred in either the antacid or the misoprostol group. Endoscopy did not reveal any difference in the number or severity of mucosal lesions in either group. Because of expense and failure to demonstrate improved efficacy, prostaglandins are not widely used for prophylaxis.

Treatment of Patients with Active Bleeding

Mortality among patients with active bleeding remains high but is most commonly related to the patient's underlying disease and not to hemorrhage. Schuster et al. reported clinically significant bleeding in 10 of 179 patients who were admitted to a medical intensive care unit and managed without stress prophylaxis.[31] Nine of these ten patients died, but death was related to hemorrhage in only one-third of them. Initial management of these patients is directed toward correcting the underlying physiologic stress if possible. Rapid resuscitation aids in restoring gastric mucosal blood flow. Acid–base imbalances and coagulopathies are corrected. Gastric lavage is instituted to remove clots from the stomach and to assess the rate of bleeding. Endoscopy should be performed early and may be therapeutic if other sources of bleeding such as peptic ulcers or bleeding esophageal varices are identified. For patients with confirmed stress gastritis, raising the gastric pH to > 7 may help improve local clotting mechanisms, and it may denature pepsin.[10,27] It can usually be accomplished with some combination of antacids, H_2-blockers, and proton-pump inhibitors. Most patients stop bleeding with medical management alone. Angiography or endoscopic control of bleeding sites is rarely of value because of the diffuse nature of the disease process. Surgical treatment has become increasingly rare and most reports describing operations are from the late 1970s and early 1980s. At that time, total gastrectomy was the procedure of choice for diffuse mucosal bleeding but was associated with a prohibitive mortality rate.[10,52,53]

Pharmacoeconomic Issues

For accurate estimation of the cost of prophylaxis for stress gastritis it is necessary to make a number of assumptions about clinical outcomes and cost of prophylaxis. Ben-Menachem and colleagues calculated the marginal cost-effectiveness of prophylaxis compared to no prophylaxis using sucralfate and cimetidine.[54] Marginal cost-effectiveness is defined as the additional cost of prophylaxis minus any cost savings due to prophylaxis divided by the number of bleeding episodes prevented. The results are reported as the cost per bleeding episodes averted. Baseline estimates assumed that the patient population studied had a 6% risk of developing stress-related hemorrhage (range 0.1–33.0%) and that prophylatic therapy reduced this risk by 50% (range 10–90%). In addition, the base case assumed that prophylactic therapy did not alter the incidence of nosocomial pneumonia, expressed as a 0% incidence of pneumonia compared to no prophylactic therapy (range 0–10%) Cost estimates included the cost of the medications, the cost of treating episodes of stress-related hemorrhage, and the cost of treating nosocomial pneumonia. Using these assumptions, the cost of sucralfate was $1144 per bleeding episode averted. The cost per bleeding episode averted was highly dependant on the risk of hemorrhage and the efficacy of sucralfate prophylaxis. The range of cost per bleeding episode averted was prohibitive at $103,725 for low-risk patients (0.1% incidence of bleeding) to cost savings for high-risk patients. The cost per bleeding episode averted also increased significantly as the risk of nosocomial pneumonia increased. The effect of pneumonia was greater for populations at low risk of hemorrhage. Assuming equal efficacy, the cost per bleeding episode averted by cimetidine was 6.5-fold higher than the cost per bleeding episode averted by sucralfate.

Richter et al.,[55] Maier et al.,[23] and the American Society of Health-System Pharmacists[27] (ASHAP) arrived at a similar conclusion, with the lowest cost with sucralfate. Assuming comparable efficacy, Maier et al. found that H_2-antagonists or antacids cause a three- to four-fold increase in costs compared with sucralfate. Richter et al. also found greater cost saving with sucralfate, with total costs savings of about $200,000 per 100 patients treated.

Cost analyses are difficult models to construct.[27] Costs are institution-specific, and each of the components considered is not consistent in these three studies. Applying such analyses to your institution may be more valuable. The cost of medication is a small part of prophylaxis. Nursing and pharmacy time, equipment (i.e., tubing, syringes, needles, ventilators), and the cost for an actual hemorrhage or nosocomial pneumonia must be calculated. The ASHAP has provided a template to aid institutions in their own analysis of the cost-effectiveness of stress gastritis prophylaxis.[27] The simplest and most straightforward reporting method for medication costs is the average wholesale price (AWP), as other factors vary depending on contracts with

TABLE 41.5. H_2-Receptor Blocker's Cost Comparison for Normal Renal Function.

Drug	Cost[a] for 24 hours
Cimetidine	
300 mg IV qid	$34.68
300 mg PO qid	$32.92
Famotidine	
20 mg IV bid	$ 7.96
20 mg PO bid	$ 3.40
Nazatidine	
150 mg PO bid	$ 3.40
Randitidine	
50 mg IV tid	$11.97
150 mg PO bid	$ 3.00

[a]Average of wholesale prices.

drug wholesalers and the hospitalization charges at the particular institution (Table 41.5 and 41.6).

Conclusions

With an apparent decrease in the incidence of stress bleeding in critically ill patients over the last two decades, the use of prophylaxis in all patients admitted to the ICU is no longer justified. Clinically significant bleeding is rare, occurring on average in about 6% of patients, often as one component of the larger syndrome of MOF. Even when bleeding does occur, it can usually be controlled with medical management after endoscopic confirmation of the source of bleeding. Giving prophylactic agents to all patients increases the cost of ICU care and may expose patients to an increased risk of complications, such as nosocomial pneumonia. Based on identified risk factors, stress gastritis prophylaxis is of primary benefit in patients with coagulopathy and in patients who require mechanical ventilation for more than 48 hours. It may also be of benefit in patients with multiple risk factors, head injuries, multiple trauma, burns, organ transplants, a history of gastrointestinal ulcers or bleeding, or who have had prolonged resuscitation after septic or hemorrhagic shock. Studies in these specific patient populations are necessary to define the risks of bleeding without prophylaxis.

In general, antacids are no longer used as prophylatic agents, as they are work-intensive and may increase gastroesophageal reflux. Although the risk of clinically important bleeding may be slightly greater with sucralfate, the related mortality and incidence of nosocomial pneumonia are similar to those seen with ranitidine. The decision of which prophylactic agent to use is based on institutional experience. If sucralfate is as effective as ranitidine, sucralfate is most cost effective. If ranitidine is assumed to be better and is associated with a similar incidence of nosocomial pneumonia, it may be most cost-effective.

With improvements in the care of critically ill patients there appears to have been a decrease in clinically important bleeding due to stress gastritis. However, additional well controlled clinical studies are necessary to further define cost-effective prophylaxis and to determine current rates of clinically significant bleeding in specific patient populations not receiving prophylaxis.

Addendum

The bacteria, Helicobacter pylori (H. pylori), is generally accepted as the cause for chronic inflammation of gastric mucosa, chronic gastric and duodenal ulcers, and probably gastric cancer. Little is known about H. pylori's role, if any, in stress ulceration. Now, Halm et al.[56] have completed a prospective study of patients with upper G.I. bleeding after cardiac operations. Stress ulcer prophylaxis was with I.V. vanitidine 150 mg total per day. They found that the presence of H. pylori was not associated with upper G.I. bleeding, and prophylactic eradication of H. pylori was not justified. The biggest risk factor for bleeding was prolonged mechanical ventilation.

References

1. Peura DA: Stress-related mucosal damage: an overview. Am J Med 1987;83:3–7.
2. Lucas C, Sugawa C, Riddle J, et al: Natural history and surgical dilemma of stress gastric bleeding. Arch Surg 1971;102:266–273.
3. Hastings P, Skillman J, Bushnell L, Silen W: Antacid titration in the prevention of acute gastrointestinal bleeding. N Engl J Med 1978;298:1041–1045.
4. Driks M, Craven D, Celli B, et al: Nosocomial pneumonia in intubated patients given sucralfate as compared with antacids or histamine type 2 blockers. N Engl J Med 1987;317:1376–1382.
5. Reusser P, Gyr K, Scheidegger D, et al: Prospective endoscopic study of stress erosions and ulcers in critically ill neurosurgical patients: current incidence and effect of acid-reducing prophylaxis. Crit Care Med 1990;18:270–274.
6. Pitimana-aree S, Forrest D, Brown G, et al: Implementation of a clinical practice guideline for stress ulcer prophylaxis increases appropriateness and decreases cost of care. Intensive Care Med 1998;24:217–223.
7. Silen W: The clinical problem of stress ulcers. Clin Invest Med 1987;10:270–274.
8. Weinstein W: Gastritis and inflammatory disorders of the stomach. In: Lamsback W (ed) Gastroenterologic Endoscopy. Philadelphia, Saunders, 1987;454–474.
9. Durham RM, Shapiro MJ: Stress gastritis revisited. Surg Clin North Am 1991;71:791–810.
10. O'Keefe G, Maier R: Current management of patients with stress ulcers. Adv Surg 1997;30:155–177.
11. Menguy R: Role of gastric mucosal energy metabolism in the etiology of stress ulceration. World J Surg 1981;5:175–180.

TABLE 41.6. Proton Pump Inhibitor and Sucralfate Cost Comparison.

Drug	Dose	Cost[a] for one dose
Lansoprazole	30 mg q day	$3.59
Omeprazole	20 mg q day	$3.87
Sucralfate	1 g qid	$0.77

[a]Average of wholesale prices.

12. Shorrock C, Rees W: Overview of gastroduodenal mucosal protection. Am J Med 1988;84:25–34.
13. Miller TA, Tornwall MS, Moody FG: Stress erosive gastritis. Curr Probl Surg 1991;28:453–509.
14. Haglund U: Gut ischemia. Gut 1994;35(Suppl 1):73–76.
15. Patel C, Durham R: ICU management. In: Longo W, Peterson G, Jacobs D (eds) Intestinal Ischemic Disorders: Pathophysiology and Management. St. Louis, Quality Medical Publishing, 1999;51–74.
16. Schenarts P, Prough D: Monitoring organ response during resuscitation in the systemic inflammatory response syndrome. Curr Opin Crit Care 1996;2:267–272.
17. Peterson WL: The role of acid in upper gastrointestinal haemorrhage due to ulcer and stress-related mucosal damage. Aliment Pharmacol Ther 1995;9(Suppl 1):43–46.
18. Kivilaakso E, Fromm D, Silen W: Relationship between ulceration and intramural pH of gastric mucosa during hemorrhagic shock. Surgery 1978;84:70–78.
19. Silen W: The clinical problem of stress ulcers. Clin Invest Med 1987;10:270–274.
20. Sevitt S: Duodenal and gastric ulceration after burning. Br J Surg 1967;54:32.
21. Bresailer R: The clinical significance and pathophysiology of stress-related gastric mucosal hemorrhage. J Clin Gastroenterol 1991;13(Suppl 2):35–43.
22. Cook DJ, Reeve BK, Guyatt GH, et al: Stress ulcer prophylaxis in critically ill patients: resolving discordant meta-analyses. JAMA 1996;275:308–314.
23. Maier RV, Mitchell D, Gentilello L: Optimal therapy for stress gastritis. Ann Surg 1994;220:353–360.
24. Navab F, Steingrub J: Stress ulcer: is routine prophylaxis necessary? Am J Gastroenterol 1995;90:708–712.
25. Schepp W: Stress ulcer prophylaxis: still a valid option in the 1990s? Digestion 1993;54:189–199.
26. Shiu-Kum L, Hui W: Is stress ulcer bleeding still and obnoxious killer in present day ICU? J Gastroenterol Hepatol 1992;7:553–555.
27. ASHP: ASHP therapeutic guidelines on stress ulcer prophylaxis. Am J Health Syst Pharm 1999;56:347–379.
28. Ben-Menachem T, Fogel R, Patel RV, et al: Prophylaxis for stress-related gastric hemorrhage in the medical intensive care unit: a randomized, controlled, single-blind study. Ann Intern Med 1994;121:568–575.
29. Cook DJ, Fuller HD, Guyatt GH, et al: Risk factors for gastrointestinal bleeding in critically ill patients. Canadian Critical Care Trials group. N Engl J Med 1994;330:377–381.
30. O'Keefe G, Maier RV: Current management of patients with stress ulceration. Adv Surg 1996;30:155–177.
31. Schuster D, Rowley H, Feinstein S: Prospective evaluation of the risk of upper gastrointestinal bleeding after admission to a medical intensive care unit. Am J Med 1984;76:623–630.
32. Lacroix J, Infante-Rivard C, Jenicek M: Prophylaxis of upper gastrointestinal bleeding in intensive care units: a meta-analysis. Crit Care Med 1989;17:862–869.
33. Fleiss J: The statistical basis of meta-analysis. Stat Methods Med Res 1993;2:121–145.
34. Schuman R, Schuster D, Zuckerman G: Prophylactic therapy for stress ulcer bleeding: a reappraisal. Ann Intern Med 1987;106:562–567.
35. Tryba M: Sucralfate versus antacids or H_2-antagonists for stress ulcer prophylaxis: a meta-analysis on efficacy and pneumonia rate. Crit Care Med 1991;19:942–949.
36. Tryba M: Prophylaxis of stress ulcer bleeding: a meta-analysis. J Clin Gastroenterol 1991;13(Suppl 2):44–55.
37. Cook DJ, Witt LG, Cook RJ, Guyatt GH: Stress ulcer prophylaxis in the critically ill: a meta-analysis. Am J Med 1991;91:519–527.
38. Cook D, Guyatt G, Marshall J, et al: A comparison of sucralfate and ranitidine for the prevention of upper gastrointestinal bleeding in patients requiring mechanical ventilation. Canadian Critical Care Trials group. N Engl J Med 1998;338:791–797.
39. Pingleton S, Hadzima S: Enteral alimentation and gastrointestinal bleeding in mechanically ventilated patients. Crit Care Med 1983;11:13–16.
40. Durham R, Shapiro M: Management of stress gastritis. J Intensive Care Med 1991;6:257–267.
41. Spilker C, Hinthorn D, Pingleton S: Intermittent enteral feeding in mechanically ventilated patients: the effect on gastric pH and gastric cultures. Chest 1996;110:243–248.
42. Peura D: Recognizing, setting therapeutic goals and selecting therapy for the prevention and treatment of stress-related mucosal damage. Pharmacotherapy 1987;7:95S–103S.
43. McEvoy G, Litvak K, Welsh O: Miscellaneous GI Drugs. Bethesda, American Society of Health-System Pharmacists, 1997;2263–2315.
44. Poleski M, Spanier A: Cimetidine versus antacids in the prevention of stress erosions in critically ill patients. Am J Gastroentrol 1986;81:107–111.
45. Sudhir D, Sood R: Clinical pharmacology of drugs used in GI disorders of critically ill patients. In: Chernow BA (ed) The Parmacologic Approach to the Critically Ill Patient, 3rd ed. Baltimore, Williams & Wilkins, 1994;614–620.
46. Anonymous: Pantoprazole—a third porton pump inhibitor. Drug Therapeutics Bull 1997;35(12):93–94.
47. Brunner G, Chang J: Intravenous therapy with high doses of ranitidine and omeprazole in critically ill patients with bleeding peptic ulcerations on the upper intestinal tract: an open randomized trial. Digestion 1990;45:217–225.
48. Sazabo S, Hollander D: Pathways of gastrointestinal protection and repair: mechanisms of action of sucralfate. Am J Med 1989;86:23–31.
49. Miller T: Protective effects of prostaglandins against gastric mucosal damage. Am J Physiol 1983;245:G601–G623.
50. Herting R, Nissen C: Overview of misoprostol. Dig Dis Sci 1986;31:47S–54S.
51. Zinner MJ, Rypins EB, Martin LR, et al: Misoprostol versus antacid titration for preventing stress ulcers in postoperative surgical ICU patients. Ann Surg 1989;210:590–595.
52. Primrose J, Gledhill T, Quirke P, Johnston D: Blind total gastrectomy for massive bleeding from the stomach. Br J Surg 1986;73:920–922.
53. Hubert JP Jr, Kiernan PD, Welch JS, et al: The surgical management of bleeding stress ulcers. Ann Surg 1980;191:672–679.
54. Ben-Menachem TA, McCarthy BR, Fogel RO: Prophylaxis for stress-related gastrointestinal hemorrhage: a cost effectiveness analysis. Crit Care Med 1996;24:238–245.
55. Richter J, Huse D, Thompsone D: Sucralfate suspension versus acid neutralization as stress-ulcer prophylaxis during mechanial ventilation: economic implications for critical-care medicine. Am J Gastroterol 1989;84:1168.
56. Halm U, Halm F, Thein D, et al: Helicobacter pylori infection: a risk factor for upper gastrointestinal bleeding after cardiac surgery? Crit Care Med 2000;28:110–113.

42
Gut and the Immune System: Enteral Nutrition and Immunonutrients

Stig Bengmark

Nutritional support is an important part of caring for critically ill patients. Total parenteral nutrition (TPN), established many years ago, was life-saving for many patients. It is recognized today that TPN produces many problems, although in certain patients it is necessary. In addition, the gastrointestinal (GI) tract, which was thought for years to remain quiescent in sick patients, undergoes many changes during illness. Disuse atrophy, permeability changes, bacterial translocation, and other changes may contribute to the illness. For this reason and others, enteral nutrition has become the best way to support the gut, prevent deleterious changes, and provide nutrients. Enteral nutrition, provided in the proximal small intestine by nasogastric-jejunal or transcutaneous-jejunal tubes is well tolerated in many sick patients during and after operations. It is currently recognized that the small intestine continues to function even when there may be ileus of the stomach and colon. Modulation of the inflammatory response, or the acute-phase response, by nutritional support may decrease the possibility of developing systemic inflammatory response syndrome (SIRS), multiple organ dysfunction syndrome (MODS), and multiple organ failure (MOF).

The importance of nutrients, saliva, and GI secretions for normal colonic function is emphasized herein. The importance of various key ingredients in a feeding formula are reviewed in this chapter, including antioxidants, nitric oxide producers, colonic food, and others. The immune-enhancing diets and ingredients and results of their use are reviewed in detail. It is important that nutritional support be continuous before operation and during the perioperative and postoperative periods. A tube has been developed and is described that passes easily and quickly from the stomach into the proximal jejunum. The importance of colonic flora (bacteria) for proper nutritional function is reviewed in detail in Chapter 44.

Acute-Phase Response

The acute-phase response (APR) after trauma or surgery is instant. Cytokines are released within seconds, changes in coagulation occur within minutes, and alterations in plasma levels of acute-phase proteins are observed in less than an hour. Many cytokines and other mediators reach their peaks within 2–4 hours after trauma/operation. If the aim is to modulate the early APR, attempts must be made, if possible, before induction of the stress/trauma, or as early as possible. For acutely ill patients, attempts to modulate the APR should begin as soon as the patient arrives in the emergency room (and for elective surgical patients immediately before, during, and immediately after the operation).

Trauma and surgery have two major, frequent complications—sepsis and thrombosis—and one major sequela—adhesion formation. There are good reasons to suggest that all three result from a prolonged and exaggerated APR and so are theoretically controllable by modulation of the APR and its related immune functions. Until recently it had not been realized that as much as 80% of the body's total immune function lies in the GI tract (Fig. 42.1),[1] which is where most of the body's immunoglobulin A (IgA) is produced. Also important is the fact that growth factors, such as epidermal growth factor (EGF), are to a large extent produced in the GI tract. Saliva is the main source of EGF. In recent years it has become clear that not only immune cells in the gut-associated lymphoid tissues (GALT) but also mucosal cells and flora are intimately involved in the APR and in the production of cytokines, coagulation and growth factors, antioxidants, immune-stimulating nutrients, and other modulators and mediators. Attempts to modulate APR and the immune response should be directed not only toward control of the classic immune cells but also the GI mucosa and its related glands, from the salivary glands to the pancreas, and toward commensal flora (see Chapter 44).

Most GI immune functions are in the two ends of the GI tract: the oral cavity (salivary glands) and the large intestine. Thus controlling the APR and regulating immune functions should include stimulation of GI secretion; promotion of rich salivation and normal gastric, pancreatic, and intestinal secretions; and facilitation of optimal colonic function, including commensal flora. To meet the optimal needs, enteral nutrition (EN) should contain food ingredients supplied especially for the colon. It has not always been recognized that the body has two separate digestive systems: (1) the system based on normal GI

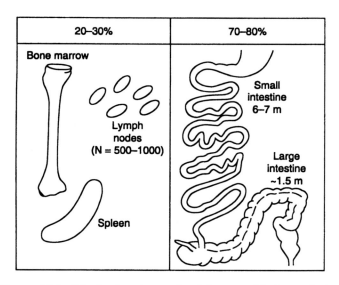

FIGURE 42.1. Distribution (percent) of immunoglobulin-producing immunocytes. All classes are included, but the respiratory and upper alimentary tracts are not taken into account. (From Brandzaeg et al.,[1] with permission.)

enzymes provided by GI secretions; and (2) a less well studied system that breaks down fibers and complex proteins enzymatically via commensal flora in the colon. It is essential to provide substrate for these commensal flora enzymes. At least 10% of calories, which roughly corresponds at 20% of the food volume, should consist of nutrients (plant fibers) destined for the large intestine (i.e., "colonic foods").

For management of perioperative and trauma patients, it is important to study and understand the immune response and cytokine actions so we can maintain the proper caloric and nitrogen balance. Immune functions are essential not only for controlling the APR but also for optimal utilization of exogenous nutrients. Cytokines such as interleukin-1 (IL-1), tumor necrosis factor-α (TNFα), and particularly IL-6 play central roles in initiation of the APR and in the loss of skeletal muscle protein.[2]

Attempts to control the APR and associated immune reactions by EN containing various nutritional ingredients have had conflicting results. Clinical studies have not always been successful, but data from numerous animal experiments support the use of EN to modulate the APR. Many of the human studies have lacked basic knowledge and an understanding of the complex physiology and immunology of the GI tract, EN is often undertaken without clear goals about which functions to influence. At least five cornerstones of such treatment must be considered if the goal is to control the APR and immune functions through EN.

1. EN should be instituted, if possible, before APR occurs and at least during the first minutes and hours after trauma/onset of disease or surgical operation. Most of the reported studies define early EN as within 48 hours and sometimes with elective surgery within 6 hours. However, because short postoperative enteral starvation follows 12–20 hours of preoperative and perioperative intestinal starvation, treatment instituted after 16–24 hours or later can, at best, be expected to influence only the further course or restitution of the disease.

2. As the dominant part of the immune system is in the large intestine, where the flora, mucosal cells, and GALT cells are immunologically active and produce APR-modulating cytokines, EN should contain substrate (fiber) for fermentation by commensal flora and local production of the needed immunoregulatory nutrients [e.g., short-chain fatty acids (SCFAs), polyamines, amino acids, antioxidants, vitamins]. Most studies so far have not included fiber in the EN formulas. The type of fiber is equally important, because flora can produce the various nutrients, antioxidants, coagulation, and growth factors needed only if the substrate is right (see Chapter 44).

3. Saturated fat is avoided, as it is known to be immunodepressive. Fat in the diet has been shown to influence the outcome significantly (see below).

4. The use of flora-reducing antibiotics should be avoided or at least limited, and if necessary the flora resupplied when it is lost (see Chapter 44).

5. Production of free radicals consumes large amounts of antioxidants (see below).

Sepsis Control: Unresolved Issue

Nosocomial infection remains the largest threat to success during treatment of postoperative and trauma patients. Each year about 2 million Americans (6%) suffer from nosocomial infections, and about half the infections occur in people over age 65,[3] who most likely have suboptimal immune function. Other frequent victims are neutropenic patients, transplantation patients, those receiving myelosuppressive chemotherapy, those with malignancies, and those suffering from decompensated liver cirrhosis, diabetes mellitus, or malnutrition. In the United States as many as one-third of patients suffer infection after liver or pancreas resection, one-fifth after gastric or colonic resection, and every tenth patient after coronary bypass surgery. The conditions in Europe and other countries with a similar, so-called Western life style are identical or worse; they may be better in countries with different life styles, as in Asia (as observed in Japanese patients).

One study, based on 1327 hospitalized patients, reported that 40–55% of the patients were either malnourished or at risk of malnutrition, and up to 12% were severely malnourished.[4] A similar study reported that 43% of 129 patients admitted to an intensive care unit (ICU) were malnourished.[5] The figures are not much different in Europe, and a study in England reported that 40% of patients admitted to hospital to have a body mass index (BMI) of < 20, and another 34% are overweight (BMI > 25)[6]; both groups had reduced immune function.

Venous thrombosis remains an unresolved problem. Clinical manifestations of venous thrombosis may still occur in more than 10% of patients after surgery, especially if nourished by parenteral nutrition (PN). We are able to suppress the major clinical manifestations of the disease with modern anticoagulation therapy, although if phlebography is performed subclinical signs of thrombosis, are still detected in most cases (40–70%).[7] Major thrombotic events such as pulmonary emboli, right atrial thrombosis, and superior vena cava thrombosis are found in about 35% of children receiving long-term total PN (TPN).[8] Parenteral nutrition is associated with enhanced activation of coagulation, Van der Poll et al. said that "one common complication (bacterial infection) may facilitate the occurrence of another common complication (venous thrombosis) by synergistic stimulation of the coagulation system."[9]

Visceral and synovial adhesions are seen with the APR, manifesting as activation of coagulation and production and deposition of fibrinogen at mesothelial and synovial surfaces. Peritoneal adhesions occur in more than 90% of patients who undergo abdominal surgery. This hidden and often neglected complication/sequela of surgery is important, as it makes reoperations more difficult and sometimes impossible. It is responsible for more than 60% of intestinal obstructions and at least half of female infertility. About 400,000 adhesiolysis operations are yearly performed in the United States alone, consuming more than a million hospital days and $2 billion (US). Antiadhesion prophylaxis, if available, could be used in up to two million general surgery patients and another two million gynecology patients. Prevention of adhesions has large economic implications.[10]

Gut and Liver: Central to APR

The APR is part of our alarm system and is seen with microbial invasion, allergic reactions, surgical operations, trauma, burns, tissue ischemia, tissue infarction, strenuous exercise, and childbirth. The gut is a central organ in APR, but most of the reactions are modulated by the liver, which: (1) Modulates the APR through synthesis of acute-phase proteins (APPs); (2) Regulates activation (production) and inactivation of other mediators, such as prostaglandins and leukotrienes; and (3) Eliminates toxins. Both the gut and the liver are involved in the early events leading to development of MOF. During the early phase of APR gut-derived bacteria, toxins, and various signal substances (bacteriokines, cytokines) influence gut mucosal function. Moreover, the GALT system, free macrophages, T cells, B cells, natural killer (NK) cells, fixed macrophages in the liver (Kupffer cells) and spleen, and hepatocytes participate in neuroendocrine activation. Cytokines not only are involved in initiation and resolution of inflammation, but with various growth factors and nitric oxide they regulate splanchnic blood flow (from mucosal to hepatic), bile production, and various regeneration processes. All these functions, can be greatly influenced by nutrients, antioxidants, probiotic bacteria, and fiber.

Modern laboratory technologies, such as the polymerase chain reaction (PCR) has made it possible to establish the presence of specific infectious agents, which has led to a suggestion that eventually all diseases are infectious.[11] Even if not infectious, most diseases today do involve inflammation. Excessive production of APPs and cytokines has been linked to acute and chronic inflammatory conditions, not only those of septic origin but also allergies such as bronchial asthma and autoimmune conditions such as rheumatoid arthritis. Increased APR also occurs with chronic conditions, such as arteriosclerosis, neurodegenerative diseases such as multiple sclerosis, and Alzheimer's disease. Prolonged elevations of circulating cytokines such as IL-6 are observed after trauma, burns, surgical operations, various septic conditions, acute respiratory distress syndrome (ARDS), and MOF.

Interleukin-6 is a potent inducer of APP synthesis. It also increases adhesion of polymorphonuclear neutrophils (PMNs) to endothelium through stimulation of the intracellular adhesion molecule-1 (ICAM-1),[12] and it delays PMN apoptosis through generation of platelet-activating factor (PAF).[13]

High Morbidity with Metabolic Syndrome X

An "environmental disease," metabolic syndrome X has been identified and studied. This syndrome, which affects up to 20% of the population in Western countries, is related to abuse of life style, long prevalent in Western countries, and it is now spreading to developing countries. It is associated with reduced physical inactivity, high intake of energy and fat, alcohol consumption, smoking, and stress. The metabolic syndrome consists of a cluster of related diseases, such as abdominal obesity, hypertension, arteriosclerosis, coronary heart disease, and diabetes (85% of the diabetes in Western countries is so-called non-insulin-dependent). Venous thrombosis, rheumatoid arthritis, mental depression, and neurodegenerative diseases are frequent in these individuals. In a survey of 2458 nondiabetic US citizens no fewer than 12% had hyperinsulinemia, 13% impaired glucose tolerance, 28% hypertension, and 40% obesity.[14] Persons with this metabolic syndrome have a high risk of developing arteriosclerotic disease, diabetes, cancer, and other Western diseases.[15,16] They also have an unacceptably high risk of morbidity and mortality after surgery, trauma, burns, pancreatitis, and similar conditions. It is in this group of patients that ARDS, MODS, MOF, and SIRS most often develop.

Central to the metabolic syndrome is insulin resistance, glucose intolerance, dyslipidemia, and a prothrombotic state (impaired fibrinolysis). It has been suggested that hyperlipidemia, rather than hyperinsulinemia, may play the central role.[17] Sensitization to the hypothalamo-pituitary-adrenal axis (HPA) seems to be an initiating event in the syndrome, accompanied by inhibition of sex steroid and growth hormone secretions.[17] These individuals show an early increase in sympathetic and decreased parasympathetic tone, a constellation conducive to arrhythmias and sudden death.[18] Trophic hormones, including angiotension II and norepinephrine, two of the most potent trophic hormones, are usually increased. Most of the victims of the syndrome exhibit high serum cholesterol levels, especially high levels of low density lipoprotein (LDL) cholesterol and hypertriglyceridemia. These patients have increases in serum sialic acid, α_1 acid glycoprotein, C-reactive peptide, other APPs, and cytokines such as IL-6; all are indicators of an exaggerated and protracted APR, a condition eventually better named the chronic-phase response, which is similar or identical to the metabolic syndrome. Microalbuminuria is commonly observed in these patients.

Reduced Antioxidant Defense

Human immune functions deteriorate with aging, paralleled by an age-related decrease in endogenous antioxidants. In particular, catalases decrease in brain and kidney, glutathione transferase and peroxidase in the GI mucosa and kidney, and sodium dismutase in most if not all tissues.[19] Whether these changes result from an unfavorable life style related to the metabolic syndrome is not clear. It is well documented, though, that the negative effects of reduced endogenous antioxidant capacity can to a large extent be compensated for by restrictions in calorie intake and changing to a diet low in fat and cholesterol and high in polyunsaturated fat (emphasizing fresh fruits and vegetables). Few if any studies have looked at antioxidant status before surgery or trauma and its influence on outcome. To my knowledge no study has yet looked at surgical patients and the effects of supplying important fruit/vegetable-derived antioxidants such as flavonoids (polyphenols), some of which are known to have as much as 10-fold stronger antioxidant potential than conventional vitamins (e.g., vitamins C and E). Coumestrol, daidzein, genistein, and resverstrol are among the more than 4000 substances with unique antioxidant and phytoestrogen effects and in the future will be tried in various clinical conditions. A study performed in patients at risk of developing MOF demonstrated that on the day after admission not only cytokines (e.g., IL-6 and TNFα) and APPs (e.g., C-reactive protein) are significantly elevated, but plasma levels of vitamin C were significantly decreased (MOF 3.8 ± 1 vs. no MOF 11.2 ± 1.8).[20] Other biochemical markers of antioxidant activity, such as vitamin E, copper, and zinc, showed no difference between the groups.

Patients with skin anergy have high postoperative morbidity and mortality rates. Attention has been given to the reactivity of the patient's peripheral blood mononuclear cells when exposed to phytohemagglutinin (PHA), a well known T cell mitogen. Faist et al. found in 5 emergency patients and 14 patients with elective major surgery that the PHA response after 5–7 days was depressed in 11 of the 19 patients; 8 of the 11 later developed infectious complications.[21] Similar observations have been made in burn patients.[22] Patients with metabolic syndrome are no doubt overrepresented in the group with a depressed PHA response.

Saturated Fat and Immunodepression

Western food is far from ideal for optimal immune function (Table 42.1). Dietary fat influences immune functions; fish oil (omega-3) is known to reduce inflammatory reactions, and saturated fat promotes them. A study in mice found higher IgM

TABLE 42.1. Problems with "Western" Food.

Too much saturated fat
Too little polyunsaturated fat
Too much sodium (salt)
Too little fermentable fiber
Too much refined sugar
Too low antioxidant content: cooking, canning, and freezing destroy vitamins and antioxidants
Too high content of mutagens: frying and cooking produces mutagens
Too high content of animal-derived hormones and growth factors, which delays apoptosis and enhances tumor development
Too small content of probiotic microorganisms

and IgG antibody levels, shortened life-span, and worsened proteinuria in mice fed a high fat diet (200 g fat/kg food) compared to those fed a low fat diet (50 g fat/kg food).[22] In vitro lipopolysaccharide (LPS) stimulation of peritoneal macrophages from the two groups showed a significantly higher release of IL-6 (134 vs. 59, $p = 0.02$), TNFα (311 vs. 95, $p = 0.001$), and prostaglandin E_2 (PGE_2) (906 vs. 449, $p = 0.01$) in the group fed a high fat diet. However, a diet too rich in fish oil can depress immune functions. Studies in mice with standardized thermal injuries showed significantly increased mortality on challenge with *Pseudomonas aeruginosa* when 40% of total calories was supplied as fish oil.[23] Infusion of 20% intralipid in humans significantly potentiates endotoxin-induced coagulation activation.[24] Obesity is itself a risk factor during surgery and trauma, and the incidence of surgical infections increases steeply with the degree of obesity (Fig. 42.2).[25] A relation between fat consumption and disease is well documented for arteriosclerosis, coronary heart disease, and cancer. Patients on a fatty diet have

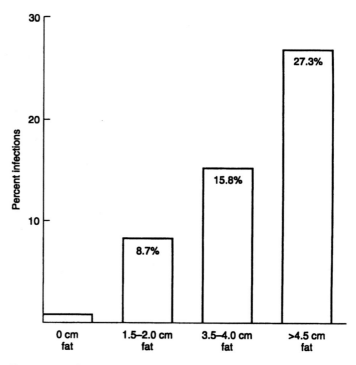

FIGURE 42.2. Wound infections after laparotomy correlated with the thickness of subcutaneous fat. (After Nyström et al.,[25] with permission.)

more aggressive tumor cell types,[26] earlier metastases,[26] and higher incidences of cancer and treatment failure. For each percent of saturated fat in the diet the risk of dying of breast cancer increases by 10%,[27] and the risk for treatment failure is 8%.[28] It is important to remember that polyunsaturated fats should be carefully supplemented, as an oversupply obviously has the same negative effects on immune function[29] as excess proteins and calories.[30,31]

Colonic Food

Colonic mucosa is mainly dependent on nutrients from the intestinal lumen for maintenance of its integrity and function. The short life cycle of GI mucosal cells (about 72 hours) indicates that only a few hours of reduced availability of luminal nutrients seriously affects mucosal regeneration and function. This, makes the lower part of the GI tract especially vulnerable to starvation. A period of 8–16 hours without food (as is routine before surgery), especially if combined with extensive intestinal cleansing and antibiotic therapy, is enough to reduce intestinal barrier function considerably and to promote septic complications. A continuous supply of foods for the colon is an important condition for optimal outcome. Moreover, it is essential for optimal GI immune function that the food supplied to the sick contains a reasonable proportion (>10 g) of ingredients destined for the colon (i.e., food that cannot be metabolized by GI secretion enzymes but reaches the colon intact, where it is metabolized by bacterial enzymes). Such foods include fruit and plant-derived fibers.

Another important source is the cellular debris from apoptotic mucosal cells and GI secretions, especially pancreatic secretions, the ingredients of which are reutilized after microbial fermentation. During this process important nutrients (e.g., various SCFAs, amino acids, polyamins, vitamins, antioxidants, and coagulation and growth factors) are locally produced and absorbed by the mucosal cells. The colon seems to be to the body what the afterburner is to an airplane: it is important for metabolic endurance and performance and essential for protein-sparing. Although an oral or enteral supply of individual free amino acids is important, it cannot fully replace what is locally produced and made available in the colon after disintegration of fermentable fibers. It is important that the nutrient fibers supplied are fresh, as many key nutrients such as glutamine and key antioxidants such as glutathione, as well as conventional vitamins, do not tolerate heating, drying, canning, or other methods used for preservation and storage. All these nutrients and antioxidants arrive normally in the body with fresh fruits and vegetables. A supply of fresh feeding formulas produced locally in the ward from fresh fruits and vegetables is an attractive supplement to commercial feeding formulas.

Sources of Key Nutrients

When medical use of fibers caught our interest 30 years ago it was mainly due to their bulk-increasing and motility-promoting

TABLE 42.2. Main sources of Three Amino Acids with Strong Effects on Immune System.

Amino acid	Content
Arginine (mg/100 g)	
Gelatin	6000
Pumpkin seeds	4030
Soya protein	3760
Peanuts	3600
Sesame seeds	3330
Soya beans	2730
Almonds	2500
Sunflower seeds	2400
Brazil nuts	2390
Peas, lentils	2050
Shrimp	2000
Baker's yeast	2000
Parmesan cheese	1560
Meat, fish	1500
Hamburgers	950
Cereals	~500
French fries	140
Ketchup	125
Vegetables	~100
Pulses	~100
Fruits	~50
Glutamic acid (mg/g)	
Parmesan cheese	9570
Gelatin	9150
Low-fat cheese	6490
Soya beans	6440
Peanuts	6350
Almonds	5930
Sunflower seeds	5580
Sesame seeds	4940
Lentils	3900
High-fat cheese	3770
Peas	3490
Oat	3000
Beans	2840
Cereals	~2500
Hamburgers	2060
Meat, fish	2000
Baker's yeast	1950
Ketchup	600
French fries	460
Vegetables	~100
Pulses	~100
Fruits	~50
Histidine (mg/100 g)	
Soya protein	2500
Parmesan cheese	1630
Tuna fish	1220
Sardines	950
Pheasant	940
Cheese 17%	940
Soya beans	930
Eel	880
Dry yeast	770
Beef	770
Peanuts	750
Pumpkin seeds	680
Sesame seeds	680
Lentils	650

TABLE 42.2 (Continued)

Amino acid	Content
Histidine (mg/100 g)	
Wheat germs	610
Hamburgers	590
Gelatin	580
French fries	60
Ketchup	25

As the author has not been successful finding data for glutamine, the contents of glutamic acid are instead presented. Histidine is known to be a strong antioxidant and to reduce inflammation and symptoms of autoimmune disease.[32]

effects, which were thought to prevent disease. Today, it is clear that the main function of dietary fibers is to supply the lower GI tract with substrate for its production of nutrients and antioxidants, for production of growth, for coagulation, and for other important functions. Most fibers in commercial EN solutions are chosen for their bulking abilities with little attention to their ability as substrates to produce special key nutrients. Table 42.2 lists foods with high contents of some key amino acids. It is clear that most of these rich foods are no longer consumed in significant quantities in Western countries. The Western food industry wishing to prolong the shelf life of products, has made strong efforts to decrease the amount of polyunsaturated fatty acids, especially those of the n-3 family.[33] Most Westerners have a relative deficiency in omega-3 fatty acids. Table 42.3 illustrates how difficult it is (sometimes impossible) to eat the

TABLE 42.3. Omega-3 Fatty Acids (Fish Oil) That Must Be Consumed Daily to Meet the Recommended Intake of 3 g.

Oils
 Fish oil 5 g
 Flaxseed oil 10 g
 Soybean oil 500 g
 Olive oil 500 g
Fish
 Salmon 30 g
 Canadian salmon 40 g
 Mackerel 60 g
 Herring 100 g
 Seafood or whitefish 1000 g
Nuts
 Walnuts 50 g
 Almonds 1000 g
Fruits and vegetables
 Cucumber 6500 g
 Apple 8000 g
Fast foods
 Hamburgers 3000 g
 French fries 15,000 g
 Ketchup 15,000 g

Hamburgers and french fries are chosen as examples of Western foods frequently consumed.

TABLE 42.4. Content and Antioxidant Potential of Some Natural Antioxidants. (Flavonoids, Phenylpronoids, and Carotenoids) Compared to Vitamins E and C.

Antioxidant	Sources	TEAC (mM)
Vitamins		
C	Fruits, vegetables	1.0 ± 0.02
E	Grains, nuts, vegetable oils	1.0 ± 0.03
Flavonols		
Quercitin	Onion, apple skin, black grapes, berries, broccoli, tea	4.7 ± 0.10
Epigallocatechin	Teas	3.8 ± 0.06
Epicatechin	Black grapes/red wine	2.4 ± 0.02
Flavonoids		
Anthocyanidins	Grapes, raspberries, strawberries, aubergine skin	4.4 ± 0.12
Oenine	Black grapes/red wine	1.8 ± 0.02
Hydrocinnamates		
p-Coumaric acid	White grapes, tomatoes, spinach, asparagus, cabbage	2.2 ± 0.06
Ferulic acid	Grains (oat), tomatoes, spinach, asparagus, cabbage	1.9 ± 0.02
Carotenoids		
Lycopene	Tomatoes	2.9 ± 0.15
β-Carotene	Carrots, sweet potato, tomatoes, paprika	1.9 ± 0.10
Xanthophylls		
β-Crytoxanthine	Mango, papaya, peaches, paprika, oranges	2.0 ± 0.02

After Rice-Evans and Miller,[34] with permission.
TEAC, Trolex equivalent antioxidant activity.

recommended daily supply of fish oil 3 g/day solely from food consumed in the Western world, especially with "fast food" or foods provided in cafeterias and hospitals. Fish oil supplements are needed in healthy individuals and even more so in the sick. Table 42.4 summarizes some important sources of these strong antioxidants.[34]

Narrow Therapeutic Window

Attempts to modulate the APR should be instituted if not before at least immediately on arrival at the emergency or postoperative room. In healthy humans the body temperature, serum norepinephrine and cortisol levels, and lactulose excretion (indicator of increased intestinal mucosa permeability) are significantly increased 1 hour after intravenous injection of endotoxin.[35] The platelet count and cytokines such as TNF and IL-6 increase almost immediately, with the highest peak at 2 hours.[36] The production of most APPs, including coagulation

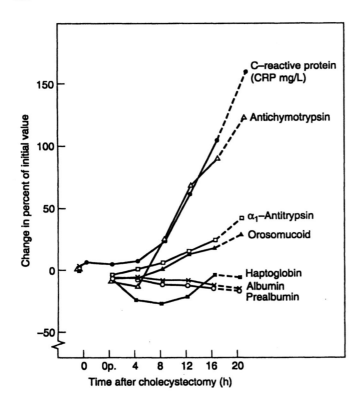

FIGURE 42.3. Fast quantitative changes in acute-phase reactants during the first 20 hours after cholecystectomy. (From Aronsen et al.,[37] with permission.)

factors, increases dramatically within minutes, some of them with up to 1000-fold. Fig. 42.3 shows the classic changes in APPs observed after a standardized elective cholecystectomy,[37] where some key APPs are significantly elevated 4–8 hours after the operation. In liver transplant patients[38] increases in cytokines such as TNF and IL-6 occurred during the late phase of the operation. If the elevation was six-fold or more, it suggested subsequent development of septic complications. After endoscopic retrograde cholangiopancreatography (ERCP) patients are prone to develop pancreatitis.[39] Significant elevations in IL-6 were observed 1 hour after the intervention in 9 of 61 patients who subsequently developed clinical post-ERP pancreatitis.[39] With experimental pancreatitis significant elevations in serum IL-6, IL-8, and amylase were observed at the earliest time of 30 minutes.[40,41] Reduced bowel motility and leakage of plasma proteins to the peritoneum were observed after 3 hours.[42] A decrease in anaerobic bacteria (especially lactobacilli) occurred after 6 hours in the ileum and colon.[43] In around 90% of animals these changes paralleled translocation of bacteria to both mesenteric lymph nodes (MLNs) and the inflamed pancreas.[44] A significant overgrowth of *Escherichia coli* occurred in the distal ileum and colon 12 hours after induction of pancreatitis.[43]

Norman[41] suggested that with acute pancreatitis there is a therapeutic window of not much more than 24 hours from the onset of the disease. Most likely such a narrow window exists with other conditions where the APR is involved. The observations discussed above and others support the assumption that immediate, aggressive efforts should be made to modulate the APR—if not possible before and during, at least immediately after the trauma/operation. Attempts to begin aggressive EN should be made immediately, when the patient arrives in the emergency or recovery room, and if possible before and during the operation.

Perioperative Enteral Starvation

Preoperative enteral starvation was introduced to avoid vomiting and aspiration during anesthesia, but such preoperative abstinence has largely lost its importance in preventing vomiting. Many studies have shown negative metabolic and psychological consequences of this old practice. Some studies indicate that it remains as "an amulet," or relic, in today's perioperative management. The time needed to obtain an empty stomach is often overestimated. Normally 50% of a liquid meal has left the stomach after 22 ± 3 minutes.[45]

It has been claimed that some groups of patients (e.g., the obese) more often have residues in the stomach, but one study found no differences in residual gastric content between lean and obese patients.[46] Early attempts to introduce a preoperative breakfast showed that the volume and median pH of gastric content, and the number of patients with pH > 3 did not differ when a light breakfast (buttered toast, tea/coffee, and milk) was given 3 hours before induction of anesthesia compared to patients who were fasted from midnight.[47] A survey of four British hospitals showed that elective patients are still fasted at least from midnight, and starvation periods of up to 12 hours are not rare.[48] In pediatric practice long starvation periods are reported (mean 10 hours).[49] This old practice does not offer optimal conditions, for barrier and immune functions. The reason for continuing this seemingly negligent attitude may be that many believe that PN can safely replace EN and a simple intravenous infusion of glucose is regarded as satisfactory. Children, the elderly, outpatients, and patients having major operations, especially those with reduced immune function, suffer the most. Many attempts to overcome the metabolic and psychological harm of preoperative enteral starvation, especially in children, and "new" regimens for preoperative enteral feeding have been tried, such as an enteral supply of glucose, eating porridge,[50] and "ultrashort" (≤ 2 hours) preoperative starvation.[51] Children were less irritable and obviously easier to deal with, and no other negative consequences were observed when the preoperative starvation period was reduced to 2 hours.[51] Despite these reports and recommendations from national professional organizations, this unsatisfactory routine remains unchanged. The time is ripe for strong efforts worldwide to "discontinue this imposition of avoidable psychological harm to patients who need surgical treatment under general anesthesia."[52]

Uninterrupted Enteral Nutrition

There are good reasons to believe that optimal control of the APR and immune functions is obtained if the enteral supply of nutrients is not discontinued. The concept of uninterrupted EN was developed for management of patients with thermal injuries, who within a short time often require repeat operations and who suffer metabolically from frequent interruptions in their enteral nutrition. Uninterrupted jejunal tube-feeding was tried in 47 patients, during the 1990s and no unwanted effects (including an increase in gastric residue) occurred at the end of the operation.[53] The authors concluded that "cessation of enteral feeding of even extensively burned patients during operation is not required."

A subsequent controlled study compared 40 patients uninterruptedly tube-fed during 161 surgical procedures with 40 patients who were managed traditionally with return to parenteral feeding during 129 operations.[54] The uninterruptedly enterally fed patients demonstrated, significant improvements despite slightly more extensive burns ($27.0 \pm 2.4\%$ vs. $22.0 \pm 2.9\%$; $p < 0.03$); they had a lower caloric deficit (cumulative caloric balance: $+2673 \pm 2147$ vs. -7899 ± 3123; $p < 0.006$), required less albumin supplementation to maintain a minimum serum level of 2.5 g/dl (732 ± 124 vs. 1528 ± 376 ml; $p < 0.04$), and demonstrated a lower incidence of wound infections (2/40 vs. 9/40 patients; $p < 0.02$). It seems reasonable to assume that if uninterrupted EN is beneficial in burn patients it should be expected to be beneficial in other critical conditions as well, including more extensive surgical interventions. Early reports from such attempts during extensive oropharyngeal, pancreatic, and hepatic operations are encouraging (G. Mangiante et al., personal communication).

Efficient Feeding Tubes

To make uninterrupted EN a widespread policy, efficient tubes are of utmost importance; such tubes should have a high rate of "spontaneous" postpyloric placement (without assistance by endoscopy or radiography) and with the tip reaching the region of the ligament of Treitz within a few minutes or hours. The rate of unintentional dislodgement (regurgitation or accidental removal) should then be reduced compared to that seen with conventional tubes. Spontaneous postpyloric placement with conventional tubes is only about 33% after 24 hours and about 66% after 72 hours. In addition, more than half of the conventional tubes are dislodged within 1 week.[55]

The lack of efficient tubes led me to develop a tube much different from all those on the market. Instead of a balloon or a heavy weight, this tube has in its tip a coil (Fig. 42.4) that is made to absorb the motility of the wall of the stomach and duodenum maximally for transport to the region of the ligament of Treitz.[56] The ability to absorb motility can be further maximized by providing the coil with thin, flexible fins at the outside and inside or by making the surface frosty or hairy.[57]

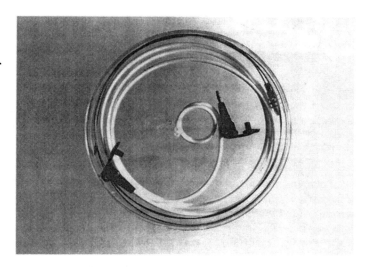

FIGURE 42.4. Autopositioning (self-propelling, self-anchoring) enteral feeding tube built to absorb the motility of the gastric wall during transportation and the coil for improved anchoring at the level of the ligament of Treitz.

After the coil is placed in the stomach with the aid of a guidewire, motility is stimulated by a small meal (e.g., a sandwich, pizza, spaghetti, orange). The tip of the tube (the coil) together with the eaten food is then transported to its final and optimal position more or less immediately. The tube is made not only to be self-propelling and for autopositioning, it is also self-anchoring.

Experience has shown that the rate of dislodgement is much less with this tube than with conventional tubes. Its position can be verified by pH measurements indicating that the tube has passed the pylorus and is ready for use. There is no reason nutrients should not be given immediately through the tube when it is positioned in the stomach; but it has become common practice to wait until the tip is properly placed in the duodenum or upper jejunum. (The tube is available in Europe from the Royal Numico/Nutricia/Pfrimmer group under the name of the Bengmark Flo-Care Tube.)

When introduced in a patient with normal motility, the tip of the tube is most often, without pharmacologic stimulation, positioned in its optimal position within a few minutes and always within 4 hours.[58] Although the tube was intended as a tool to be used only in patients with intact motility (e.g., introduced before and used in connection with elective surgery), it has been used increasingly in patients with reduced motility; and it is introduced with or without pharmacologically stimulated motility. Mangiante et al. reported successful intubation in ICU patients including 10 of 10 patients with pancreatitis and 6 of 6 patients with abdominal sepsis.[59] Motility was obviously reduced in these patients, but the tube reached optimal position within an average of 5.2 hours and always within 24 hours.

Importance of Saliva and GI Secretions

When the oral cavity and stomach are bypassed by jejunal feeding, it is important not to neglect stimulation of the immunologically important secretory activities of the salivary glands, stomach, and pancreas. Salivation is of the greatest importance, as saliva "possesses a multiplicity of defense systems antibacterial warfare that the Pentagon can envy."[60] It is rich in important immunologic factors such as IgA, lactoferrin, lactic dehydrogenase, lysozyme, mucins, and surfactants, it is also the main source of important growth factors such as EGF (Table 42.5).[61,62] The normally high nitrate content is of special interest, as this molecule acts as a donor molecule for gastric production of nitric oxide, essential for stimulation of GI motility and mucosal and splanchnic circulation, as well as for gastric bacteriostasis.[62]

The composition of saliva is close to that of human milk, and saliva is an important substitute through infancy to old age. Sialoadenectomy results in intestinal ulcerations and delayed healing of wounds of the skin, mouth, and stomach. Absence of salivation decreases liver regeneration. Salivary mucus/mucin is the main protective layer not only in the oral cavity but also in the upper GI tract. An 80% reduction of mucus/mucin in the lower esophagus is seen after sialoadenectomy. Normally more than 2 liters of saliva are produced per day, and children produce 0.5 liter saliva per day by age 5 years.[63] Saliva production is minimal during rest (in adults approximately 25 ml/hr) but increases about 20-fold on stimulation by chewing. It seems reasonable to assume that salivation in patients on jejunal tube feeding should be routinely stimulated by such simple measures as chewing gum. Salivation can also be significantly increased by chewing nitrate-rich vegetables (see below) or pharmacologically by repeat pilocarpine injections (5 mg × 3).[64] Unfortunately, standard ICU practice often inhibits salivation by use of drugs, with mouth dryness a side effect (Table 42.6).[61] The use of such drugs should be kept at an absolute minimum. One can assume that when salivation is inhibited other GI secretions are reduced as well.

Maintenance of low gastric pH constitutes an important protective mechanism against invading microorganisms. Inhibition of gastric secretion transforms the stomach into a microbial reservoir, especially for gram-negative bacilli, from the pharynx and respiratory tract. Also, the lower GI tract may be colonized. Inhibition of acidity is accompanied by inhibition of mucus secretion, which in turn decreases mechanical and immunologic protection of the gastric mucosa. Aggressive enteral feeding eliminates the need for routine use of H_2-blockers or proton inhibitors for protection against stress ulcerations.[65] If further enhancement of mucosa protection is desired, standard pectin can be administered orally/gastrically; this fiber has the unique ability to adhere to acidic surfaces and thereby form a protective layer. In animals it was proven to be as protective as modern gastroprotective drugs.[66] Also a stimulant of small intestinal mucosal growth, pectin is an excellent colonic food[67] and a strong antioxidant.[68]

TABLE 42.5. Salivary Constituents.

Proteins
  Albumin
  Amylase
  β-Glucuronidase
  Carbohydrases
  Cystatins
  Epidermal growth factor
  Esterases
  Fibronectin
  Gustin
  Histatins
  Immunoglobulin A
  Immunoglobulin G
  Immunoglobulin M
  Kallikrein
  Lactoferrin
  Lipase
  Lactic dehydrogenase
  Lysozyme
  Mucins
  Nerve growth factor
  Parotid aggregins
  Peptidases
  Phosphatases
  Proline-rich proteins
  Ribonucleases
  Salivary peroxidases
  Secretory component
  Secretory IgA
  Serum proteins (trace)
  Tyrosine-rich proteins
  Vitamin-binding proteins
Small organic molecules
  Creatinine
  Glucose
  Lipids
  Nitrogen
  Sialic acid
  Urea
  Uric acid
  Nitrate
Electrolytes
  Ammonia
  Bicarbonate
  Calcium
  Chloride
  Fluoride
  Iodide
  Magnesium
  Nonspecific buffers
  Phosphates
  Potassium
  Sodium
  Sulfates
  Thiocyanate

Nitric Oxide: Key to GI Motility and Blood Flow

Inhibition of both the inducible and constitutive forms of nitric oxide (NO) in animal endotoxin models has

TABLE 42.6. Drugs That Inhibit Saliva Secretion of Other Gastrointestinal Secretions.

Analgesics
 Meperedine HCl (Demerol)
 Alprazolam (Xanax)
 Diazepam (Valium)
 Triazolam (Halcion)

Anorexic (amphetamine) agent
 Methamphetamine HCl (Desoxyn)

Anorexic (nonamphetamine) agent
 Phendimetrazine tartrate (Adipex, Obezine, Trimtabs)

Antiacne preparation
 Isotretinoin (Accutane)

Antiarthritic agent
 Piroxicam (Feldene)

Anticholinergic/antispasmodic agents (GI)
 Atropine sulfate
 Clidinium bromide (Quarzan)
 Dicyclomine (Bentyl)
 Glycopyrrolate (Robinul)
 Hyoscyamine sulfate (Anaspaz)
 Propantheline bromide (Pro-Banthine)
 Combination drugs (Donnatal)

Anticholinergic/antispasmodic agents (urinary)
 Oxybutynin chloride (Ditropan)
 Combination drugs (Cytospaz, Urised)

Antidepressant agent
 Tricyclics (Elavil, Pamelor, Tofranil)

Antidiarrheal agent
 Diphenoxylate HCl and atropine (Lomotil)

Antihistamines
 Diphenhydramine HCl (Benadryl)
 Brompheniramine maleate (Dimetane, Veltane)
 Combination drugs (Triaminic, Historal, Dimetapp)

Antihypertensives
 Clonidine HCl (Catapres)
 Prozosin HCl (Minipress)

Antihypertensives/diuretics
 Clonidine HCl and chlorthalidone (Combipres)
 Naldolol and bendroflumethiazide (Corzide)
 Propranolol HCl and hydrochlorothiazide (Inderide)

Antiparkinsonian agents
 Biperiden HCl and biperiden lactate (Akineton)
 Benztropine mesylate (Cogentin)

Antipsychotic agents
 Lithium carbonate (Lithobid)
 Thioridazine (Mellaril)
 Trifluoperazine (Stelazine)

Diuretics
 Chlorothiazide (Diuril)
 Hydrochlorothiazide (Esidrix, HydroDiuril)
 Triamterene and hydrochlorothiazide (Dyazide)

Psychotherapeutic agents
 Alprazolam (Xanax)
 Diazepam (Valium)
 Triazolam (Halcion)

After Sreebny et al.,[61] with permission.

increased mortality. Moncada et al. suggested that NO, if released by only constitutive enzymes, protects the GI tract, at least during septic shock.[69] Maintenance of good mucosal and splanchnic blood flow is regarded as crucial to outcome. Intravenous infusion of methylene blue has been described as a safe option for eliminating the negative effects of NO and stimulating the positive effects of increased visceral circulation. Also, other NO donor molecules (e.g., nitroprusside counteract the reduction in splanchnic blood flow in burn patients and prevent microbial translocation.[70] Short-term intravenous infusion of methylene blue in patients with severe septic shock requiring adrenergic agents improves cardiac output, increases arterial pressure, and reduces the blood lactate concentration.[71]

In dogs with induced endotoxemia jejunal tube feeding using a standard commercially available EN formula increased hepatic artery, portal vein, and superior mesenteric artery blood flow and significant improved the mucosal and hepatic microcirculation, intestinal mucosal pH, and hepatic tissue oxygen pressure and energy charge (Fig. 42.5).[72] An enteral formula containing donor molecules for production of NO in both the upper and lower GI tracts should result in more pronounced, long-lasting effects. Nitrate/nitrite seems to be the important donor molecule for the upper GI tract, especially the stomach; but it might also complement arginine and play an important role in the lower GI tract especially the large bowel. Here NO is produced from arginine, a process in which commensal bacteria seem to play a key role. For optimal function these molecules should be supplied also in a "wrapped" form as colonic foods, important for local delivery to and function of the colon.

An important enterosalivary circulation of nitrate has been discovered.[62] Nitrate secreted by salivary glands, ingested nitrate, or both are reduced to nitrite by facultative anaerobic bacteria localized at the surface of the posterior third of the tongue. This reduction is not seen in germ-free animals and is significantly less when antibiotics are supplied. Nitrite swallowed into an acidified stomach (e.g., if the acidity has not been impaired by H_2-blockers or proton inhibitors) immediately leads to excess production of NO in the lumen of the stomach, the amount of which is said to be much larger than can be generated through intrinsic NO synthase.[73] At pH 2.0 about 600 nM of NO is produced, which is said to be several orders of magnitude greater than is required to stimulate mucosal blood flow or mucus formation, to influence motility, and for bacteriostasis. This production is important to prevent colonization of the stomach with pathogenic flora. Acidified nitrite is effective against not only *Candida albicans* and *Escherichia coli* but also *Shigella, Salmonella, Helicobacter pylori*, amebic dysentery, and chronic intestinal parasitism. One study demonstrated that adding 1 mM of nitrite in vitro to acidic solution (pH 2) completely killed *Helicobacter pylori* within 30 minutes, a phenomenon not seen when acid alone is administered ($p < 0.001$).[74]

In the future NO produced by acidified nitrite may be used not only to control microbial overgrowth but also to maintain

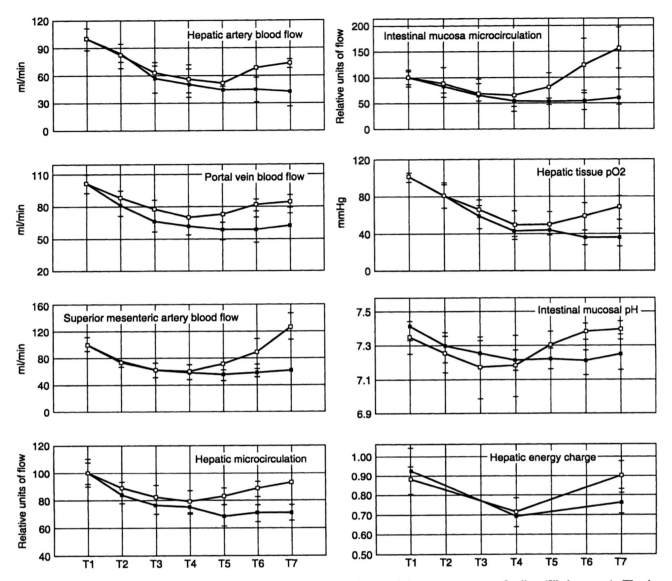

FIGURE 42.5. Alterations in splanchnic hemodynamics during the early phase after *Escherichia coli* lipopolysaccharide (LPS) induced by infusion of a commercial mixed nutrient meal (open squares) compared to infusion of the same amount of saline (filled squares). The interval between each time point is 30 minutes. (From Kazamias et al.,[72] with permission.)

and improve mucosal and splanchnic blood flow, stimulate gastrointestinal motility, and support the fast introduction of feeding tubes. An alternative option could be to let the patients chew fruits and vegetables rich in nitrate (Table 42.7) or let them slowly "wash the mouth" and swallow fresh juices especially made from nitrate-rich vegetables and fruits. Support for such a suggestion comes from a study in which animals with induced pancreatitis were treated with a 10% rhubarb decoction (rhubarb is rich in nitrate).[76] Significant reductions in translocation to mesenteric lymph nodes and pancreatic tissue (treated 25% vs. controls 100%), mortality (1/8 vs. 5/8 animals), and serum endotoxin levels (rhubarb-treated 5.41 ± 3.6 pg/L vs. controls 61.36 ± 28.3 pg/L; $p < 0.001$) were reported in the rhubarb-treated group. The authors concluded that: "remarkable inhibition of gut motility was observed in the control group, but gut motility was significantly improved by administration of rhubarb." Preliminary attempts to use rhubarb decoction to promote motility when introducing feeding tubes have been extraordinary successful.[77]

Special Immunomodulatory Nutrients

Goris et al. suggested in 1985 that MOF seen after trauma or surgery is due to a generalized inflammatory reaction, with activation of leukocytes and release of oxygen free radicals and other mediators, including cytokines, from the cells.[78] Numer-

TABLE 42.7. Vegetables Rich in Nitrate.

Vegetable	Nitrate content (mg/kg)
Fennel	3200
Head lettuce	2900
Celery	2700
Mangold	2600
Dill	2400
Spinach	1900
Beetroot	1700
Nettle	1600
Radish	1300
Chinese cabbage	1300
Savoy cabbage	1100
Leek	720
Rhubarb	700
Chives	670
White cabbage	620
Squash	580
Broccoli	490
Lettuce head	470
Horseradish	390

After Lönberg et al.,[75] with permission.

ous mediators have since been demonstrated to be deeply involved in the inflammatory reaction, and many attempts have been made to inhibit the catastrophic process. Most such attempts have supplied inhibitory molecules directed against a specific key mediator. These attempts have been largely unsuccessful.[79-81]

Such failure could be explained by the observation that most mediators function in large consortia "as instruments in a large immunomodulation orchestra." If so, monotherapies of individual inhibition of one or two, even if important, modulators could not be expected to help. Polytherapies, which are nonspecific as routine EN, have not always resulted in significant improvements.

An issue of Nutrition,[82] with participation of the world's leading experts, discussed in detail the potential key EN ingredients in the immunomodulation of perioperative and trauma patients. The need for antioxidants during the APR is extensive and the needs are usually not met in sick patients. Most studies so far limited their focus to changes in conventional antioxidants, such as vitamin C and E. To my knowledge no study in critically ill patients has considered the antioxidants provided by key fibers such as pectin, probiotic bacteria (see Chapter 44), or polyphenol antioxidants such as flavonoids. Nor has any study tried to satisfy the need for local production and delivery to the colon of key nutrients such as arginine, glutamine, polyamines, and polyunsaturated fatty acids. A supply of colonic food rich in antioxidants and in precursors of the various key nutrients is of special benefit to the sick. The EN solutions used in most clinical studies have not contained any fiber. Few attempts have been made so far to design nutrition solutions in terms of their richness in precursors important to the release/production in the colon of various antioxidants, nutrients, and growth factors, as discussed above (see Chapter 44).

Antioxidant/Glutamine Consumption During APR

Serum levels of key antioxidants such as glutathione and vitamin C are sensitive indicators of disease. Plasma vitamin C in healthy individuals averages 62 µmol/L (range 55-72 µmol/L); it decreases in patients with gastritis to about 47 µmol/L, in those with diabetes to 45 µmol/L, and in ICU patients to as low as 11.0 µmol/L (range 8-22 µmol/L).[83] It is even lower in those developing MOF. Another study found that not only key cytokines such as TNF and IL-6 were significantly elevated but also plasma concentrations of the antioxidants with an ability to trap peroxyl radicals in aqueous solutions, such as vitamin C were reduced to extremely low levels in patients who subsequently develop MOF (MOF group 3.8 ± 1.0 µmol/L vs. no-MOF group 12.0 ± 3.2 µmol/L).[20] No differences were observed in the antioxidants that trap free radicals in lipid phases, such as vitamin E (MOF group 15.1 ± 2.0 µmol/L vs. no-MOF group 11.2 ± 1.8 µmol/L).[83]

Hypoglutaminemia is a frequent observation in sick patients and may be more devastating than hypoglycemia.[84] Outcome seems often to depend on supplementation with glutamine. This amino acid is the most abundant free amino acid in the body and constitutes some 60% of the free intracellular amino acids in skeletal muscle. Muscle glutamine serves as an important source of nitrogen (ammonia) to the splanchnic area and immune system.[85] It is known that glutamine is an important donor of molecules used to synthesize purines and pyrimidines, which are essential for many functions and in many organ systems, including maintenance of muscles, preservation of GI tract integrity, the acid-base balance, and the immune system, commercial standard solutions usually do not contain glutamine. Muscles synthesize and store glutamine, but what is normally available, (about 100 g) is no more than what is needed solely by the immune cells over 24 hours. About 300 g of lymphocytes (total number 10^{12}) and 300 g of macrophages (fixed macrophages such as microglia and Kupffer cells included) each consume 50 g of glutamine per day. In the absence of an enteral supply, GI epithelial cells need a minimum of 50 g of glutamine, which makes the estimated daily requirement no less than 150 g/day in these patients.[84] It should be added that the synthesis of APPs, some of which (like C-reactive protein) increase up to 1000 times during the APR, is dependent on protein substrate for their production. Newsholme calculated that for production of six or seven such APPs at least 90 g protein/day, is needed.[84] It is not surprising that a protein loss of as much as 200 g/day is observed in patients such as those with severe burns.

A study in multiple-trauma patients found bacteremia episodes in 2 of 29 (7%) glutamine-supplemented patients compared to 13 of 31 (42%) control patients.[86] Only 1 of 29 patients in the glutamine-supplemented group developed clinical sepsis compared to 8 of 31 in the control group. This and other studies support the value of an exogenous supply of specific amino acids such as glutamine. Indiscriminant attempts to decrease protein degradation without maintaining normal plasma levels of glutamine not only might be of little value but could be "detrimental to the immune system and hence to the patient's recovery," as pointed out by Newsholme.[84]

Documented Benefits of Enteral Nutrition

That EN has definite advantages over PN in preventing critical illness is being increasingly accepted. There is a consensus that EN, if supplied early to perioperative/trauma patients, is more effective than PN. Although maintenance of body weight by nutrition therapy is no longer an important goal, it has thus far been believed that nutrition for these patients should meet, but not exceed, the energy requirements. This was often not the case in the past. EN solutions should contain adequate nitrogen to achieve an optimal balance but also contain sufficient nutrients, vitamins, and trace elements. A controlled study compared isocaloric and isonitrogenous EN and PN in patients with upper GI malignancies and found no signs of improved barrier function or clinical benefits from the use of the enteral route.[87] The enteral formula used Osmolite (Ross/Abbott), which contains, protein 45 g/L and fat 30% (the PN formula contained 55%) but no fiber. No statement about the time of introduction of EN was provided, although the dose administered is said to have begun with 30 ml/hr and slowly increased to 100 ml/hr depending on tolerance. The results of this study are in sharp contrast to the significant reduction in morbidity and mortality with EN in multiple-trauma patients.[88-90] It is tempting to speculate that the potential in immunostimulatory measures are greater in a group of patients who until a few hours before were healthy, well fed, and often young (e.g., trauma and burn patients), but significantly less when tried in the group of often old, and immunodepressed patients such as those suffering from cancer. Some indirect support for such a view can be obtained from a subsequent study by the same group comparing EN and PN performed in patients with acute pancreatitis[91] presenting within 48 hours after onset of disease. The design of this study was similar, and the nutrition formulas used were identical. Global improvement in SIRS, sepsis, organ failure, and ICU stay was observed in the EN group, paralleled by a more pronounced reduction in APACHE II scores ($p < 0.0001$), C-reactive protein (mean EN 84 vs. PN 141; $p < 0.0005$) and serum IgM anticore endotoxin antibodies (EN increase with 28.5%, PN decrease with 1.1%; $p < 0.05$). Furthermore, the total antioxidant increased capacity significantly in the EN group but decreased in the PN group (EN +27.7%, PN −32.6%; $p < 0.05$).

It is a demanding challenge to achieve successful modulation of APR and immune functions in elective surgical patients, especially in those suffering from neoplastic disease. Successful EN in patients suffering from hepatocellular carcinoma subjected to major liver resection was reported from Japan.[93] Both EN and PN groups received relatively equal amounts of protein and carbohydrate, but only the EN group had supplemental fat, although in small amounts (4.6 kcal/kg/day = approximately 15% of the total calories). No differences in nutritional parameters were observed between the two groups, such as the serum levels of retinol-binding protein, transferrin, prealbumin and 3-methylhistidine; but significant improvements were observed in the EN group in terms of changes from preoperative values of their immunologic parameters: NK activity (EN 10669, PN 4931; $p < 0.05$), lymphocyte numbers (EN 11468, PN 6626; $p < 0.05$), and PHA response (EN 10330, PN 7831; and $p < 0.05$). Most importantly the frequency of postoperative complications, mainly pneumonias and wound infections, was significantly reduced (EN 8%, PN 31%). They reported that institution of EN was delayed to the second postoperative day, and no fiber was included in the diet.

Immunoenhancement of EN Formulas Controversy

When tried separately, each of the nutrients (arginine, nucleic acids, omega-3 polyunsaturated FFAs, other nutrients, antioxidants) supports gut barrier function, improves immune functions, improves nitrogen balance, and improves wound healing. Attempts to improve the clinical outcome by supplying some of these combined nutrients resulted in an immunoenhancing formula. Several such commercial formulas are now on the market. They are all several times more expensive than conventional EN formulas, thereby requiring solid indications for their routine use. Barton, in two excellent, comprehensive, critical reviews, summarized the state of the art with immune-enhancing formulas.[93,94] These reviews and a commentary[95] to Burton's last review, summarizes well the experience with these formulas, which is controversial.

At least three more studies have now been reported. An Italian, well designed and controlled, seemingly isocaloric and isonitrogenous study compared enteral feeding using a standard EN solution (Novartis), an immune-enhancing enteral diet (Impact, Novartis), and standard PN in patients operated for upper GI cancer.[96] None of the diets contained fiber. There is no mention of antibiotic policy. Therapy started 6 hours after operation with a low rate (10 ml/hr) and was slowly increased over the next 3 days. A significant, but not impressive, difference in the rate of postoperative infections, mainly abdominal abscesses, was observed (Impact 15%, standard EN 23%, PN 28%). A similar German study in patients operated for upper GI cancer and with seemingly isocaloric and isonitrogenous groups compares one EN group receiving standard enteral nutrition (Novartis) and another EN group receiving the immunoenhancing diet (Impact, Novartis)[97] described in the previous study.[96] In this study the diet contained no fiber, and there was no reference to antibiotic policy. Enteral feeding was initiated late (i.e., not until 12–24 hours after surgery), and 20 ml/hr was administered in the beginning, increasing to 80 ml/hr on the fifth postoperative day. No statistically significant differences in postoperative complications were observed between the two groups, although fewer complications were observed during the late postoperative phase (i.e., after the fifth day) in the "immuno-enhanced" group.

Despite the fact that some compelling data have been presented in the literature, there is much to support the view of the reviewers[93–95] and others that, at least at present, *routine use of these formulas cannot be recommended*. Strong efforts should be made to design and undertake "objection-free," well controlled clinical studies. It is a must that such studies are designed to contain balanced isocaloric, isonitrogenous groups and similar amounts of fat. They can be expected to be more helpful if administered during the early phase of APR (i.e., immediately on conclusion of an operation) or, even better, in the form of uninterrupted nutrition. Furthermore, colonic food should be provided.

Preoperative nutritional support in the past has had little or no effect on outcome after surgery and has been regarded as not cost-efficient. It was therefore of special interest when a well controlled study looked at outcome after major GI cancer operations after a 7-day preoperative "immune-enhancing" diet (Impact, Novartis).[98] This attempt also failed. No differences in mean lymphocyte mitogenesis, mean peripheral blood mononuclear cell production of cytokines, or clinical outcome were observed.

Is Calorie Restriction Important?

Both overfeeding and underfeeding are detrimental to immune function and to resistance to disease. A large supply of glucose and fat is known to increase the oxidative processes in the body and the consumption of antioxidants. Overfeeding appears to be a much greater problem than underfeeding for regular daily life and more so for treatment of critically ill patients. The low density in Western food and in standard clinical nutrition formulas of natural antioxidants, phytochemicals, key nutrients, and fiber often leads to overconsumption of "empty calories" to obtain a reasonable supply of the various key factors needed. Caloric restriction is increasingly suggested as the main tool to produce resistance to the "chronic phase response"/metabolic syndrome X/environmental disease and might also be important in the APR. Table 42.8 summarizes the direct major metabolic, cellular, and hormonal effects of calorie restriction.[99]

Overfeeding macronutrients to the critically ill often leads to serious, sometimes fatal metabolic consequences.[100] A randomized, well designed study of 300 patients undergoing major general surgery compared TPN with 1000–1500 kcal/day only as glucose for up to 15 postoperative days.[101] The mortality and complication rates were no larger in any of the groups than are normally seen in other, similar studies. The nitrogen loss during the first week in the glucose group was reduced to about half

TABLE 42.8. Changes Known to Occur with Calorie Restriction.

General changes
  Body temperature—decreased
  Inflammatory response—decreased
Metabolic changes
  Blood glucose—unchanged or decreased
  Insulin secretion—decreased
  Hepatic gluconeogenesis activity—increased
Hormonal changes
  Serum corticosterone—increased
  Plasma ACTH—decreased
  Hepatic IGF-1—decreased
Cellular changes
  Cell proliferation—decreased
  Apoptosis—increased
  Leukopenia

After Frame et al.,[99] with permission.

that seen in the TPN group. The patients, who resumed normal eating within about 1 week, seemed to do well. However, TPN seemed to be life-saving for about 20% of the patients, who could not go back to normal eating after 2 weeks. Again, the general impression of the authors was that "overfeeding seemed to be a larger problem than underfeeding." A similar study from Memorial Sloan-Kettering Cancer Center arrived at similar conclusions. There 195 patients were randomized after resection for upper GI malignancies to two groups: one was given enteral supplementation with an immunoenhancing diet (Impact, Novartis), and the other was given traditional intravenous crystalloid infusions (CON).[102] The EN feeding is said to have started EN within 24 hours. No fiber was supplemented, and no statement is made on antibiotic policy. The caloric intake was low in both groups, 61% and 22% of the defined goals (25 kcal/kg/day) (e.g., in an 70-kg person: about 1000 kcal in the EN group and about 400 kcal in the CON group). No differences between the groups were observed in the number of minor (Impact 26/97, CON 16/98), major (Impact 27/97, CON 25/98), or infectious (20/97, CON 23/97) wound complications; nor was there a difference in mortality (Impact 2/97, CON 3/98) or length of stay in hospital (median 11 days for each group). In a study by the same group and published the same year, a significant decrease in fat oxidation and protein catabolism and an improved net nitrogen balance was observed in the "immune-enhanced" group.[103] Furthermore, statistically significant different hormone levels were observed in the "immune-enhanced" group on the fifth postoperative day, as both the insulin/glucagon quotient and the growth hormone level were increased. Another study adds to the confusion. This study was designed specifically to study respiratory functions and postoperative mobility in patients supplied early EN compared to those given PN.[104] Reduced vital capacity (day 6: EN 1.8 ± 1.0 L; PN 2.4 ± 0.6 L; $p < 0.05$), forced expiratory volume at 1 second (day 4: EN 1.1 ± 0.7, PN 1.5 ± 0.4; $p = 0.07$), and a statistically significant reduction in postoperative mobility and rate of recovery were reported for the EN group.

Recommendations for Nutritional Support of Trauma, Operated, and Sick Patients

1. Continuous enteral nutrition is begun as soon as possible. A special nasoenteric tube helps.
2. Enteral nutritional substrates should contain fiber, pectins, probiotic bacteria, polyphenol antioxidants, and glutamine, among others.
3. Saturated fat is to be avoided.
4. Flora-reducing antibiotics should be avoided or limited if possible.
5. Consider replacing colonic flora (see Chapter 44).
6. Add fresh fruits and vegetables (antioxidants) and fish oil supplements.
7. Saliva production should be stimulated, not depressed. Nitrate-containing foods (e.g., rhubarb) and gum chewing help.
8. The so-called immune-enhancing diets remain somewhat controversial. They have been helpful in certain circumstances. More and better controlled studies are needed. Many of the specific ingredients in the immune-enhancing diets seem helpful.

Conclusions

The stress response is responsible for many consequences of critical illness, including fluid overload, hypercatabolism, hypermetabolism, and glucose intolerance. More than 50 years ago Cuthbertson and Tilstone[105] described the stress response as a two-phase process, where the first (ebb) phase lasts only 24 hours and at the most 48 hours. Attempts to modulate such changes should be concentrated before and during this phase. There are reasons to suggest that a narrow therapeutic window exists, limited to the first minutes and hours after trauma, as there is a direct correlation between the time treatment is instituted and the results. Enteral nutrition solutions are constructed mainly to satisfy the need of effective nourishment so as to meet demand for calories and nitrogen and must less to modulate immune functions. It is often not realized that the most potent parts of the GI intestinal immune system are in the two ends of the GI tract: the oral cavity and the large intestine, two areas more or less neglected with routine EN regimens. Enteral nutrition formulas, or so-called immune-enhancing nutrition, are still designed mainly to meet nutritional needs and the needs of the small intestine. They rarely contain food for the colon, its mucosa and flora. A special fiber is not chosen for its ability to deliver key nutrients to the large intestine. The need of commensal flora to facilitate disintegration of fiber and production of key nutrients is rarely recognized. It is also rarely recognized that many antioxidants and some key nutrients can be supplied effectively only by fresh food, especially fruits and vegetables, as they do not tolerate freezing, drying, heating, or storage. This knowledge requires measures to be taken to provide some of the nutrients as "home-made" (i.e., produced on the ward or the ICU unit and administered as fresh and unprocessed as possible. The sickest patients should not continue to get the worst food. Overnutrition, especially of glucose and fat, should be avoided; and there must be special emphasis on supplying natural antioxidants.

It is regrettable that there are no simple methods to effect changes in mediators such is IL-6. Fast, "easy to operate" methods for direct measurements in ICU units will probably soon be made available. Hopefully such a development can help the clinician not only to follow but also successfully modulate the APR and immune reactions during the early minutes and hours after trauma, operations, or acute illness.

References

1. Brandtzaeg P, Halstensen TS, Kett K, et al: Immunobiology and immunopathology of human gut mucosa: humoral immunity and intraepithelial lymphocytes. Gastroenterology 1989;97:1562–1584.
2. Moldawer LL, Copeland EM: Proinflammatory cytokines, nutritional support, and the cachexia syndrome: interactions and therapeutic options. Cancer 1997;79:1828–1839.
3. Schwartz MN: Hospital-acquired infections; diseases with increasingly limited therapies. Proc Natl Acad Sci USA 1994;91:2420–2427.
4. Gallagher-Allred SR, Voss AC, Finn SC, McCamish MA: Malnutrition and clinical outcomes: the case for medical nutrition therapy. J Am Diet Assoc 1996;96:361–366, 369.
5. Giner M, Laviano A, Meguid MM, Gleason JR: In 1995 a correlation between malnutrition and poor outcome in critically ill patients still exists. Nutrition 1996;12:23–29.
6. McWhirter JP, Pennington CR: Incidence and recognition of malnutrition in hospital. BMJ 1994;308:945–948.
7. Brismar B, Hardsfeldt C, Malmborg AS: Bacteriology and phlebography in catherization for parenteral nutrition. Acta Chir Scand 1980;146:115–119.
8. Dollery CM, Sullivan ID, Bauraind O, et al: Thrombosis and embolism in long-term central venous access for parenteral nutrition. Lancet 1994;344:1043–1045.
9. Van der Poll T, Levi M, Braxton CC, et al: Parenteral nutrition facilitates activation of coagulation but not fibrinolysis during human endotoxemia. J Infect Dis 1998;177:793–795.
10. Bengmark S: Bioadhesive polymers that reduce adhesion formation. In: diZerega G (ed) Peritoneal Surgery. Springer, New York, 1999.
11. Lorber B: Are all disease infectious? Ann Intern Med 1996;125:844–851.
12. Barnett CC, Moore EE, Moore FA, et al: Intracellular adhesion molecule-1 promotes neutrophil-mediated cytotoxicity. Surgery 1995;118:171–175.
13. Biffl WL, Moore EE, Moore FA, et al: Interleukin-6 delays neutrophil apoptosis via mechanism involving platelet-activating factor. J Trauma 1996;40:575–578.
14. Meigs JB, D'Agostino RB Sr, Wilson PE, et al: Risk variable clustering in the insulin resistance syndrome: the Framingham offspring study. Diabetes 1997;46:1594–1600.
15. Manson JAE, Willett WC, Stampfer MJ, et al: Body weight and mortality among women. N Engl J Med 1995;333:677–685.

16. Grundy SM: Hypertriglyceridemia, atherogenic dyslipidemia, and the metabolic syndrome. Am J Cardiol 1998;26:18B–25B.
17. Zimmet PZ, McCarty DJ, DeCourten MP: The global epidemiology of non-insulin-dependent diabetes mellitus and the metabolic syndrome. J Diabetes Complications 1997;11:60–68.
18. Björnstorp P: Stress and cardiovascular disease. Acta Physiol Scand Suppl 1997;640:144–148.
19. Yu BP: Aging and oxidative stress: modulation by dietary restriction. Free Radic Biol Med 1996;21:651–668.
20. Borelli M, Roux-Lombard P, Grau GE, et al: Plasma concentrations of cytokines, their soluble receptors, and antioxidant vitamins can predict the development of multiple organ failure in patients at risk. Crit Care Med 1996;24:392–397.
21. Faist E, Kupper TS, Baker CC, et al: Depression of cellular immunity after major surgery: its association with posttraumatic complications and its reversal with immunomodulation. Arch Surg 1986;121:1000–1005.
22. Lin B-F, Huang C-C, Chiang B-L, Jeng S-J: Dietary fat influences Ia antigen expression, cytokines and prostaglandin E_2 production in immune cells in autoimmune-prone NZBxNZW F1 mice. Br J Nutr 1996;75:711–722.
23. Peck MD, Alexander JW, Ogla CK, Babcock GF: The effect of dietary fatty acids in response to Pseudomonas infection in burned mice. J Trauma 1990;30:445–452.
24. Van der Poll, Coyle SM, Levi M, et al: Fat emulsion infusion potentiates coagulation activation during human endotoxemia. Thromb Haemost 1996;75:83–86.
25. Nyström PO, Jonstam A, Höjer H, Ling L: Incisional infection after colorectal surgery in obese patients. Acta Chir Scand 1987;153:225–227.
26. Hislop TG, Band PR, Deschamps M, et al: Diet and histologic types of benign breast disease defined by subsequent risk of breast cancer. Am J Epidemiol 1990;131:263–270.
27. Jain M, Miller AB, To T: Premorbid diet and the prognosis of women with breast cancer. J Natl Cancer Inst 1994;86:1390–1397.
28. Holm LE, Nordevang E, Hjalmar ML, et al: Treatment failure and dietary habits in women with breast cancer. J Natl Cancer Inst 1993;85:32–36.
29. Shepard RJ, Shek PN: Immunological hazards from nutritional imbalance in athletes. Exerc Immunol Rev 1998;4:22–48.
30. Peck MD, Alexander JW, Gonce SJ, Miskell PW: Low protein diets improve survival from peritonitis in guinea pigs. Ann Surg 1989;209:448–454.
31. Klein CJ, Stanek GS, Wiles CE: Overfeeding macronutrients to critically ill adults: metabolic consequences. J Am Diet Assoc 1998;98:795–806.
32. Peterson JW, Boldogh I, Popov VL, et al: Anti-inflammatory and antisecretory potential of histidine in salmonella-challenged mouse small intestine. Lab Invest 1998;78:523–534.
33. Bengmark S: Ecoimmunonutrition: a challenge for the third millenium. Nutrition 1998;14:563–572.
34. Rice-Evans CA, Miller NJ: Antioxidant activities of flavonoids as bioactive components of food. Biochem Soc Transact 1996;24:790–795.
35. O'Dwyer ST, Michie HR, Ziegler TR, et al: A single dose of endotoxin increases intestinal permeability in healthy humans. Arch Surg 1988;123:1459–1464.
36. Santos AA, Rodrick ML, Jacobs DO, et al: Does the route of feeding modify the inflammatory response? Ann Surg 1994;220:155–163.
37. Aronsen KF, Ekelund G, Kindmark CO, Laurell CB: Sequential changes of plasma proteins after surgical trauma. Scand J Lab Invest 1972;29(Suppl 124):127–136.
38. Sautner T, Függer R, Götzinger P, et al: Tumour necrosis factor-α and interleukin-6: early indicators of bacterial infection after human orthotropic liver transplantation. Eur J Surg 1995;161:97–101.
39. Messmann H, Vogt W, Holstege A, et al: Post-ERP pancreatitis as a model for cytokine induced acute phase response in acute pancreatitis. Gut 1997;40:80–85.
40. Takács T, Farkas G, Czako L, et al: Time-course changes in serum cytokine levels in two experimental acute pancreatitis models in rats. Res Exp Med 1996;196:153–161.
41. Norman J: The role of cytokines in the pathogenesis of acute pancreatitis. Am J Surg 1998;175:76–83.
42. Leveau P, Wang X, Soltesz V, et al: Alterations in intestinal permeability and microflora in experimental acute pancreatitis. Int J Pancreatol 1996;20:119–125.
43. Andersson R, Wang X, Ihse I: The influence of abdominal sepsis on acute pancreatitis in rats: a study on mortality, permeability, arterial blood pressure and intestinal blood flow. Pancreas 1995;11:365–373.
44. De Souza LJ, Sampietre SN, Figueiredo S, et al: Bacterial translocation during acute pancreatitis in rats (in Portuguese, with English summary). Rev Hosp Clin Fac Med Sao Paolo 1996;51:116–120.
45. Bateman DN, Whittingham TA: Measurement of gastric emptying by real-time ultrasound. Gut 1982;23:524–527.
46. Harter RL, Kelly WB, Kramer MG, et al: A comparison of the volume and pH of gastric contents of obese and lean surgical patients. Anesth Analg 1998;86:147–152.
47. Miller M, Wishart HY, Nimmo WS: Gastric contents at induction of anesthesia: is a 4-hour fast necessary. Br J Anesth 1983;55:1185–1188.
48. Groves H: Preoperative patient fasting regimes. Br J Theatre Nurs 1994;4:14–16.
49. Maclean AR, Renwick C: Audit of pre-operative starvation. Anesthesia 1993;48:164–166.
50. Kushikata T, Matsuki A, Murakawa T, Sato K: Possibility of rice porridge for preoperative feeding in children. Matsui 1996;45:943–947.
51. Schreiber MS, Triebwasser A, Keon TP: Ingestion of liquids compared with preoperative fasting in pediatric outpatients. Anesthesiology 1990;72:593–597.
52. Hung P: Pre-operative fasting. Nurs Times 1992;25:57–60.
53. Buescher TM, Cioffi WG, Becker WK, et al: Perioperative enteral feedings [abstract]. Proc Am Burn Assoc 1992;22:162.
54. Jenkins ME, Gottschlich MM, Warden GD: Enteral feeding during operative procedures in thermal injuries. J Burn Care Rehabil 1994;15:199–205.
55. Bengmark S: Progress in perioperative enteral tube feeding. Clini Nutr 1998;17:145–152.
56. Bengmark S: Swedish patent 8700582; PTC patent 0278937; US patent 4.887.996.
57. Bengmark S: Swedish patent 507786 PTC application SE 98/00145.
58. Jeppsson B, Tranberg K, Bengmark S: Technical developments: a new self-propelling nasoenteric feeding tube. Clin Nutr 1992;11:373–375.
59. Mangiante G, Colucci G, Marinello P, et al: Bengmark's selfpropelling naso-jejunal tube: a new useful device for intensive

enteral nutrition [abstract]. Intensive Care Med 1998; 24:330.
60. Mandel ID: The function of saliva. J Dent Res 1987;66:623–627.
61. Sreebny LM, Bancozy J, Baum BJ, et al: Saliva: its role in health and disease. Int Dent J 1992;42:291–304.
62. Duncan C, Dougall H, Johnston P, et al: Chemical generation of nitric oxide in the mouth from the enterosalivary circulation of dietary nitrates. Nat Med 1995;1:546–551.
63. Watanabe S, Ohnishi M, Imai K, et al: Estimation of the total saliva volume produced per day in five-year-old children. Arch Oral Biol 1995;40:781–782.
64. Fox PC, van der Ven PF, Baum BJ, Mandel ID: Pilocarpine for the treatment of xerostomia associated with salivary gland dysfunction. Oral Surg 1986;61:243–248.
65. McDonald WS, Sharp CW, Deitch EA: Immediate enteral feeding in burn patients is safe and effective. Ann Surg 1991;214:177–183.
66. Bengmark S: Immunonutrition: the role of biosurfactants, fiber and probiotic bacteria. Nutrition 1998;14:585–594.
67. Vince AC, McNeil NI, Wager JD, Wrong OM: The effect of lactulose, pectin, arabinogalactan and cellulose on the production of organic acids and metabolism of ammonia by intestinal bacteria in a faecal incubation system. Br J Nutr 1990;63:17–26.
68. Kohen R, Shadmi V, Kakunda A, Rubinstein A: Prevention of oxidative damage in the rat jejunal mucosa by pectin. Br J Nutr 1993;69:789–800.
69. Wright CE, Rees DD, Moncada S: Protective and pathological roles of nitric oxide in endotoxin shock. Cardiovasc Res 1992;26:48–57.
70. Herndon DN, Ziegler ST: Bacterial translocation after thermal injury. Crit Care Med 1993;21:S50–S54.
71. Preiser JC, Lejeune P, Roman A, et al: Methylene blue administration in septic shock: a clinical trial. Crit Care Med 1995;23:259–264.
72. Kazamias P, Kotzampassi K, Koufogiannis D, Eleftheriadis E: Influence of enteral nutrition-induced splanchnic hyperemia on the septic origin of splanchnic ischemia. World J Surg 1998;22:6–11.
73. McKnight GM, Smith LM, Drummond RS: Chemical synthesis of nitric oxide in the stomach from dietary nitrate in humans. Gut 1997;40:211–214.
74. Dykhuizen RS, Fraser A, McKenzie H, et al: Helicobacter pylori is killed by nitrite under acidic conditions. Gut 1998;42:334–337.
75. Lönberg E, Everitt G, Mattson P: Nitrat i grönsaker [Nitrate in vegetables]. Var Foda 1985;37:316–322.
76. Chen X, Ran R: Rhubarb decoction prevents intestinal bacterial translocation during necrotic pancreatitis. J West China Univ Med Sci 1996;27:418–421.
77. Mangiante G, Marini P, Fratucello GB, et al: Perioperative nutrition: experiences in abdominal and oropharyngeal surgery [abstract] (in Italian). Riv Ital Nutr Parent Ent (RINPE) 1998;16:236.
78. Goris RJA, Boekhorst PA, Nuytink JKS, et al: Multiple organ failure: generalized autodestructive inflammation? Arch Surg 1985;120:1109–1115.
79. Abraham E, Anzueto A, Gutierrez G, et al: Double-blind randomized controlled trial of monoclonal antibody to human tumour necrosis factor in the treatment of septic shock. Lancet 1998;351:929–933.
80. Van Dissel JT, van Langevelde P, Westendorp RG, et al: Antiinflammatory cytokine profile and mortality in febrile patients. Lancet 1998;351:950–953.
81. Vincent JL: Search for effective immunomodulating strategies against sepsis. Lancet 1998;351:352.
82. Bengmark S (ed): Immunonutrition. Nutrition 1998;14:563–647.
83. Schorah CJ, Downing C, Piripitsi A: Total vitamin C, ascorbic acid, and dehydroascorbic acid concentrations in plasma in critically ill patients. Am J Clin Nutr 1996;63:760–765.
84. Newsholme EA: Hypercatabolism: metabolic causes and consequences. In: Lumley JSP, Craven JL (eds) Surgery, vol 8 [updated textbook] Abingdon, Oxon, UK, Medicine Publishing Company, 1998;190–192.
85. Deutz NEP, Reijven PLM, Athanasas G, Soeters PB: Postoperative changes in hepatic, intestinal, splenic and muscle fluxes of amino acids and ammonia in pigs. Clin Sci 1992;83:607–614.
86. Houdijk APJ, Rijnsburger ER, Jansen J: Randomised trial of glutamine-enriched enteral nutrition on infectious morbidity in patients with multiple trauma. Lancet 1998;352:772–776.
87. Reynolds JV, Kanwar S, Welsh FKS, et al: Does the route of feeding modify gut barrier function and clinical outcome in patients after major upper gastrointestinal surgery. JPEN 1997;21:196–201.
88. Moore FA, Moore EE, Jones TN, et al: TEN vs TPN following major abdominal trauma—reduced septic morbidity. J Trauma 1989;29:916–923.
89. Kudsk KA, Croece MA, Fabian TC, et al: Enteral versus parenteral feeding. Ann Surg 1992;215:503–513.
90. Moore FA, Feliciano DV, Andrassy RJ, et al: Early enteral feeding, compared with parenteral, reduces postoperative septic complications. Ann Surg 1992;216:172–183.
91. Windsor SCJ, Kanwar S, Li AGK, et al: Compared with parenteral nutrition, enteral feeding attenuates the acute phase response and improves disease severity in acute pancreatitis. Gut 1998;42:431–435.
92. Shirabe K, Matsumata T, Shimada M, et al: A comparison of parenteral hyperalimentation and early enteral feeding regarding systemic immunity after major hepatic resection: the result of a randomized prospective study. Hepatogastroenterology 1997;44:205–209.
93. Barton RG: Nutritional support in critical illness. Nutr Clin Pract 1994;9:127–139.
94. Barton RG: Immune-enhancing enteral formulas: are they beneficial in critically ill patients. Nutr Clin Pract 1997;12:51–62.
95. Dickerson RN: Immune-enhancing enteral formulas in critically ill patients. Nutr Clin Pract 1997;12:49–50.
96. Gianotti L, Braga M, Vignali A, et al: Effect of route of delivery and formulation of postoperative nutritional support in patients undergoing major operations for malignant neoplasms. Arch Surg 1997;132:1222–1230.
97. Senkal M, Mumme A, Eickhoff U, et al: Early postoperative enteral immunonutrition: clinical outcome and cost-comparison analysis in clinical patients. Crit Care Med 1997;25:1489–1496.

98. McCarter MD, Gentilini OD, Gomez ME, Daly JM: Preoperative oral supplement with immunonutrients in cancer patients. JPEN 1998;22:206–211.
99. Frame LT, Hart RW, Leakey JEA: Caloric restriction as a mechanism mediating resistance to environmental disease. Env Health Perspect 1998;(Suppl 14):313–324.
100. Klein CUJ, Stanek GS, Wiles CE: Overfeeding macronutrients to critically ill adults: metabolic complications. J Am Diet Assoc 1998;98:795–806.
101. Sandström R, Drott C, Hyltander A, et al: The effect of postoperative intravenous feeding (TPN) on outcome following major surgery evaluated in a randomized study. Ann Surg 1993;217:185–195.
102. Heslin MJ, Latkany L, Leung D, et al: A prospective randomized trial of early enteral feeding after resection of upper gastrointestinal malignancy. Ann Surg 1997;226:567–580.
103. Hochwald SN, Harrison LE, Heslin MJ, et al: Early postoperative enteral feeding improves whole body protein kinetics in upper gastrointestinal cancer patients. Am J Surg 1997;174:325–330.
104. Watters JM, Kirkpatrick SM, Norris SB, et al: Immediate postoperative enteral feeding results in impaired respiratory mechanisms and decreased mobility. Ann Surg 1997;226:369–380.
105. Cuthbertson DP, Tilstone WJ: Metabolism during post-operative period. Adv Clin Chem 1969;12:1–55.

43
Disseminated Intravascular Coagulation

J. Heinrich Joist

The hemostatic system designed to minimize bleeding in response to vascular injury comprises a complex system of integrated and intricately regulated reactions between endothelial cells, subendothelial cell vessel wall components, platelets, red blood cells (RBCs), white blood cells (WBCs), and a large number of plasma zymogens and cofactors. It provides a rapid formation of an appropriately sized, stable platelet–fibrin thrombus at the site of vessel injury. However, with a large number of pathologic conditions (Fig. 43.1) the hemostatic system may be activated excessively locally (e.g., aortic aneurysm or giant hemangioma) or systemically (e.g., septic shock, amniotic fluid embolism), overwhelming normal hemostatic regulatory mechanisms. Excessive hemostatic system activation may also be facilitated by inherited (e.g., protein C deficiency) or acquired (e.g., lupus anticoagulants) disorders of these control mechanisms. This imbalance between procoagulant and anticoagulant factors or mechanisms may lead to accelerated consumption and depletion of labile hemostatic blood components such as platelets, fibrinogen, and coagulation cofactors VIII and V, a condition commonly called disseminated intravascular coagulation (DIC), consumption coagulopathy (CC), CC with increased fibrinolysis (CCIF), or defibrination syndrome.[1-5] The clinical consequences of excessive hemostatic system activation may be abnormal bleeding, often from multiple sites and microvascular (and rarely macrovascular) thrombosis.

Thus DIC is not a disease in itself but a manifestation and sometimes serious, possibly life-threatening complication of various diseases or disorders. DIC is a dynamic process that may develop rapidly or slowly, resolve promptly once the triggering condition is resolved or eliminated, or persist and become more severe heralding poor patient outcome.

The term DIC is confusing and misleading for several reasons. First, it is commonly used for decompensated, excessive hemostatic system activation in association with conditions in which the activation and fibrin formation is localized (e.g., aortic aneurysm) and not widespread throughout the circulation. Second, DIC is frequently used as a clinical term for abnormal bleeding from multiple sites, which may occur with severe thrombocytopenia due to acute leukemia, aplastic anemia, or thrombotic thrombocytopenic purpura in the absence of accelerated intravascular coagulation (AIC), as reflected by increased levels in blood of molecular markers of enhanced thrombin formation [e.g., prothrombin fragment 1.2 (F1.2)] or thrombin activity [e.g., fibrinopeptide A (FPA), soluble fibrin (FnS), fibrin degradation product D-dimer, or thrombin/antithrombin III complexes (TAT)] (Fig. 43.2). Third, DIC is sometimes used as a term for AIC, the demonstration of which depends on specialized tests for these molecular markers of thrombin formation/activity (Fig. 43.2), which are not available in most clinical laboratories. Fourth, DIC is frequently referred to as a "clinical diagnosis"; that is, it is based on signs and symptoms of complications of excessive intravascular coagulation, such as abnormal bleeding from multiple sites as discussed above or microvascular thrombosis (e.g., multiple organ systems dysfunction, hypotension, shock, acidosis, and hypoxemia). None of these clinical manifestations of DIC is of course specific for or diagnostic of DIC, and their presence can only raise the suspicion of DIC. Because there is at present no internationally agreed on definition of DIC and to make the term clinically useful it is defined here more narrowly as excessive, decompensated AIC resulting in depletion of consumable coagulation factors to an extent that (1) the prothrombin time (PT), a global, robust coagulation screening test readily available in clinical laboratories on a 24-hour, rapid turnaround (stat) basis, is prolonged; (2) there is a decrease in blood of one or more consumable hemostatic factors such as platelets and fibrinogen; and (3) there is evidence of increased fibrin formation/degradation. Although this definition, which is similar to the one adopted by the Japanese Research Committee on DIC,[6] has some limitations (e.g., milder forms of excessive AIC may be missed, as discussed further below), it can be used readily in all medical practice settings and should provide a useful basis for decision making in regard to currently available options for patient management as well as monitoring therapy and prognosis. DIC may be further subdivided into acute, subacute (resolving), and chronic (low-grade) disease based on clinical and laboratory abnormalities.[3-5]

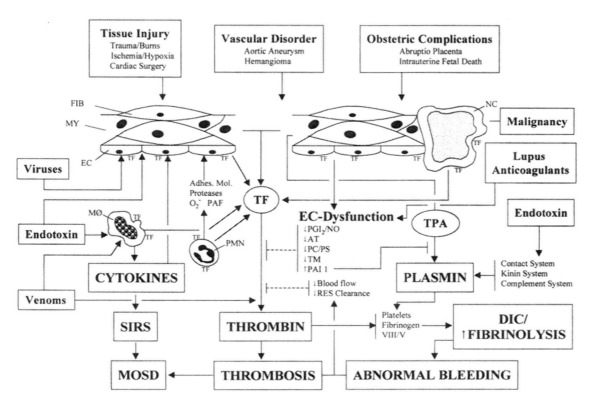

FIGURE 43.1. Mechanisms and factors involved in disseminated intravascular coagulation. Various triggering conditions and the critical roles of tissue factor, endothelial cell dysfunction, excess generation of thrombin and plasmin and cytokine-mediated amplification in the pathogenesis of DIC and the causation of abnormal bleeding, microvascular thrombosis, and multiple organ dysfunction are shown. Adhes. Mol., inducible adhesion molecules; AT, antithrombin III; DIC, disseminated intravascular coagulation; EC, endothelial cells; FIB, fibroblasts; MØ, monocytes; MOSD, multiple organ systems dysfunction; MY, myocytes; NC, neoplastic cells; NO, nitric oxide; O_2^-, oxygen radicals; PAF, platelet-activating factor; PAI1, plasminogen activator inhibitor 1; PC, protein C; PGI_2, prostaglandin I_2; PMN, polymorphonuclear leukocytes; PS, protein S; RES, reticuloendothelial system; SIRS, systemic inflammatory response syndrome; TF, tissue factor.

Pathophysiology

The pathogenesis of DIC is highly complex and variable depending on the precipitating or facilitating conditions involved (Fig. 43.1). Some of these conditions are briefly discussed here. More comprehensive reviews of causes of DIC are found elsewhere.[3-5] Elucidation of the mechanisms involved in DIC with different conditions has been greatly aided by the development of sensitive assays for specific intermediate or end products of coagulation and fibrinolytic system reactions (Fig. 43.2). With almost all conditions, including tissue injury due to trauma, burns, or cardiac surgery, obstetric complications, malignant disease, sepsis due to bacterial and viral infections, and cardiac surgery, excessive intravascular coagulation is triggered by exposure of circulating blood to tissue factor (TF) expressed on subendothelial cells, such as fibroblasts and myocytes, or damaged/activated endothelial cells (ECs) or associated with subendothelial connective tissue structures.[7,8] Whether and to what extent TF-containing, cell membrane-derived, phospholipoprotein particles (tissue thromboplastin) liberated from activated/damaged cells or tissues into the bloodstream plays a role in DIC with sepsis or massive trauma is uncertain.[9] TF functions as a powerful cofactor of factor VIIa in the initiation of the biologically predominant extrinsic pathway of coagulation capable of explosive generation of thrombin.[7,8] In contrast, activation of the intrinsic pathway of coagulation through activation of the contact system (high-molecular-weight kininogen, prekallikrein, factor XII) does not seem to play a major role in triggering DIC in conditions such as sepsis and septic shock,[10] but it may contribute to DIC in conditions such as cardiac surgery with cardiopulmonary bypass.[11]

Expression or exposure of TF and assembly of the TF-VIIa complex induced by inflammatory mediators (cytokines) may not only precipitate DIC[12] and amplify the cytokine-induced inflammatory response, it may also initiate excessive thrombin formation.[13] In experiments in primates, suppression of the TF-VIIa pathway by infusion of active site-inhibited VIIa or tissue factor pathway inhibitor (TFPI) protected against *Escherichia coli*-induced multiple organ systems failure (MOSD) and death, whereas suppression of DIC with active site-inhibited Xa did not.[13] Cytokines such as interleukin-1 (IL-1), IL-6, IL-8, tumor necrosis factor-α (TNF), and platelet-activating factor (PAF) play a powerful role in sepsis-associated fever, hypotension, and MOSD as well as in initiating and sustaining DIC during

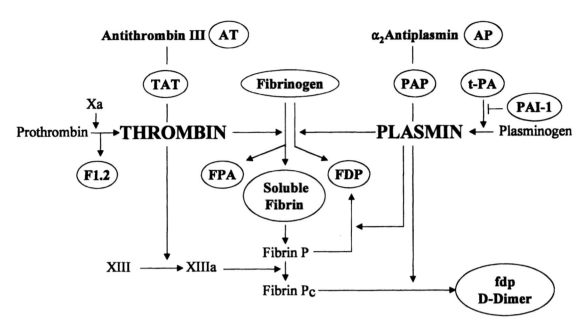

FIGURE 43.2. Molecular markers of increased generation and activity of thrombin and plasmin, the key enzymes involved in the pathogenesis of disseminated intravascular coagulation (DIC), and their inhibition. Molecules that can be quantitatively determined with routine or specialized tests are shown in ovals. F1.2, prothrombin fragment 1.2; FDP, fibrin/fibrinogen degradation products; FPA, fibrinopeptide A; PAI 1, plasminogen activator inhibitor 1; TAT, thrombin–antithrombin III complexes; t-PA, tissue plasminogen activator; Xa, activated coagulation factor X; XIII, coagulation factor XIII.

sepsis,[12–16] trauma, and perhaps other conditions.[9,12,13] Cytokines may not only activate ECs to express TF and release von Willebrand factor, they may also perturb and downregulate normal EC-associated hemostatic control mechanisms, such as production of prostacyclin (prostaglandin I_2, PGI_2) and nitric oxide (NO) (powerful inhibitors of platelet function), thrombomodulin function (a major scavenger of thrombin), the glycosaminoglycan–AT III system for neutralization of coagulation-active serine proteases (activated clotting factors), and the thrombin/thrombomodulin-dependent protein C/protein S system, which inactivates coagulation cofactors VIIIa and Va.[8,14,15] In addition, cytokines may induce EC expression of E-selectin and other leukocyte adhesion molecules[17] that may expose ECs to injurious substances produced by polymorphonuclear leukocytes (PMNs), such as proteases (e.g., cathepsin G, elastase), PAF, and oxygen radicals (O_2^-). They may also impair microcirculatory blood flow and thus clearance of activated coagulation factors.

Endothelial cell perturbation induced by mechanical, thermal, or hypoxic injury, endotoxin, viruses, or cytokines is also associated with complex alterations of the fibrinolytic system designed to prevent excessive accumulation of fibrin and thus thrombotic vessel occlusion.[1,3–5,18,19] In septic patients with DIC, the initial excess activation of fibrinolysis may be followed by inhibition.[15,19] Excess generation of plasmin may result from excess release of tissue plasminogen activator (t-PA) and urokinase-type plasminogen activator (u-PA) from ECs and other subendothelial cells due to either direct injury by the underlying condition (primary fibrinolysis) or DIC/microcirculatory thrombosis-mediated ischemia/hypoxia (secondary fibrinolysis). Excess plasmin may also be generated through increased activation of plasminogen via the coagulation contact system, the kinin system, and the complement system (endogenous or intrinsic fibrinolysis) induced by endotoxin and possibly other factors and mechanisms. Increased plasmin generation, particularly when associated with impaired fibrinolysis regulation (e.g., inadequate liberation from ECs and platelets or depletion of tissue plasminogen activator inhibitor (PAI1) or plasma $α_2$-antiplasmin (or both)) may lead to accelerated lysis of fibrin and fibrinogen,[18] degradation of factors VIII and V and platelet surface receptors (platelet dysfunction), and interference by fibrin and fibrinogen degradation products with normal fibrin polymerization.[1,3–5] Additional fibrinolytic activity may be generated in DIC as a result of liberation of proteases such as elastase from PMNs.[20] Laboratory evidence of excessive fibrinolysis, (e.g., shortened euglobulin clot lysis time or dilute whole blood clot lysis time, markedly increased plasmin–antiplasmin complexes) appears to be an important predictor of abnormal bleeding in DIC.[21] However, markedly increased D-dimer may be incorrectly interpreted as indicating excessive fibrinolysis (e.g., in septic patients) when in fact excessive PAI 1-mediated inhibition of fibrinolysis has already set in.[15,19]

The DIC process may be induced by mechanisms other than exposure of blood to excess TF[3–5] (Fig. 43.1). Examples are abruptio placentae with rapid intravasation of activated clotting factors from the retroplacental hematoma, snake and spider bites with exposure of blood to venomous substances which can directly activate factor X or prothrombin or convert fibrinogen to fibrin, and acute intravascular hemolysis with exposure of blood to large amounts of RBC-derived membrane particles rich in clotting active, polar phospholipids. DIC may also develop in patients with hypercoagulable states or thrombophilia, either inherited (e.g., homozygous protein C deficiency), in association with infections (purpura fulminans), or acquired (e.g., lupus anticoagulants/antiphospholipid antibody syndrome) and sometimes without apparent precipitating factors or conditions.[3-5]

Clinical Manifestations

The clinical manifestations of DIC are variable and generally nonspecific.[3-5] DIC is most often suspected in overtly ill, hospitalized patients with abnormal bleeding, particularly from multiple sites, such as skin (ecchymoses, petechiae), venipuncture or catheter insertion sites, mucous membranes (epistaxis, gingival bleeding, hematemesis, melena, hemoptysis), or with surgical or invasive procedures. Acral cyanosis, frequently symmetric ("blue finger syndrome," "blue toe syndrome") and sometimes affecting the nose or breasts, reflecting dermal microvascular thrombosis, may progress to infarction and gangrene requiring amputation. DIC should also be suspected in patients with progressive MOSD, particularly renal failure and neurologic or mental dysfunction.[3-5] Large-vessel, venous thromboembolic complications are rare. In some patients with DIC, as defined here, abnormal clinical signs and symptoms are absent. To what extent some or all of the above clinical manifestations can develop in patients without laboratory evidence of DIC (i.e., compensated AIC) is unclear and is difficult to determine; it requires careful, systematic patient evaluation for clinical signs and symptoms and laboratory evidence of MOSD, correlation with molecular markers of AIC, and tissue diagnosis of microvascular thrombosis.

Diagnosis

Acute DIC

None of the clinical manifestations of DIC (i.e., abnormal bleeding and microvascular thrombosis-associated tissue damage and organ dysfunction) are specific, tissue pathologic diagnosis is often not feasible and negative findings may be inconclusive (sampling error). The diagnosis of DIC thus depends on the documentation of characteristic laboratory abnormalities indicative of excessive, decompensated intravascular coagulation or consumption coagulopathy. Because DIC is suspected most commonly in acutely ill patients it must be confirmed or excluded expeditiously using readily available, routine tests. Because no single, specific test for DIC is currently available, a combination of tests (Table 43.1) is commonly used to demonstrate (1) coagulopathy (i.e., an abnormally prolonged, adequately sensitive, global coagulation test such as the PT) reflecting depletion of consumable coagulation factors; (2) depletion of one or more consumable hemostatic blood components (e.g., decreased platelets or fibrinogen); and (3) accelerated intravascular fibrin formation and fibrinolysis (e.g., increased degradation products of crosslinked fibrin (D-dimer)). The PT is preferred because it was shown to be more sensitive than the activated partial thromboplastin time (APTT) or thrombin time (TT) to detect coagulopathy in patients with the "clinical diagnosis" of DIC in several large studies.[3-5] A major limitation of the PT is its known variability, depending on the PT reagent/clot timer combination used, largely due to different sensitivity to decreases in factor VII and perhaps other common phase coagulation factors. Although standardization of the PT has been improved with expression of results in the International Normalized Ratio (INR) for monitoring patients on oral anticoagulant therapy, it is possible that this is not the case in patients with DIC, as has been shown for patients with liver disease.[22] Platelets are almost always

TABLE 43.1. Laboratory Tests Used for Diagnosis, Staging, and Differential Diagnosis of DIC.

Condition	Basic tests				Additional tests			
	↑PT	↓Plat	↓Fib	↑D-dimer	↑FnS	↓AT	↓FV	↓FVII
DIC								
Acute	+	+/−	−/+	+	+	+	+	−
Subacute (resolving)	+	+	−/+	+	+	+/−	+/−	−
Chronic	+	+/−	−/+	+	−/+	−/+	−/+	−
Vitamin K deficiency	+	−	−	−	−	−	−	+
Liver disease (severe)	+	+/−	−/+	−/+	−/+	+	+	+
Thrombocytopenia of sepsis	−	+	−	−	−	−	−	−
Massive RBC-Tx/hemodilution	+	+	+/−	−	−	+	+	+
TTP	−	+	−	−	−	−	−	−
HUS	+/−	+	−/+	−/+	−/+	−/+	−/+	−
Snake/spider bites	+	+/−	+	+/−	+	+/−	−/+	−

AT, antithrombin III; D-dimer, fibrin degradation products containing crosslinked D-dimer domains; FV, factor V; FVII, factor VII; Fib, fibrinogen; HUS, hemolytic uremic syndrome; Plat, platelets; PT, prothrombin time; Tx, transfusion; TTP, thrombotic thrombocytopenic purpura.

decreased mildly to moderately with acute and subacute DIC and less frequently with chronic DIC. Fibrinogen is frequently normal or increased with DIC, particularly in patients with trauma and sepsis, as it is an acute-phase reactant.[3-5] D-Dimer can be determined by commercial, simple semiquantitative latex agglutination slide tests, enzyme-linked immunosorbent assays (ELISAs), or fully automated Ligand Immunoassay (LIA) tests, which employ antibodies that specifically recognize neoantigens exposed on D-dimer-containing degradation products of thrombin/XIIIa-crosslinked fibrin.[23-26] D-Dimer testing is preferred over fibrin/fibrinogen degradation product (FDP) testing because it is, like the PT and fibrinogen assay, performed on citrated platelet-poor plasma (single blood specimen requirement, avoids false-positive tests with serum FDP due to incomplete clotting of blood specimen), and reflects the action of both thrombin (fibrinogen-fibrin conversion and factor XIIIa-mediated crosslinking of fibrin) and plasmin (Fig. 43.2). In contrast, increased FDP may result from increased lysis of fibrinogen (primary and secondary fibrinolysis) or fibrin (secondary fibrinolysis). In some patients with fulminant snake or spider bite-induced DIC due to direct venom-induced conversion of fibrinogen to fibrin (e.g., *Aghistrodon rhodostoma*) and massive fibrinolysis the D-dimer test may give misleading "false-normal" results, as fibrin is not crosslinked. In several studies D-dimer tests have been reported to have sensitivity and specificity for DIC, although there was considerable inhomogeneity in patient populations and criteria for diagnosis of DIC.[23-26] An elevated level of D-dimer, however, is not specific for DIC even when broader definitions of DIC are used, but may be observed in various clinical conditions, including deep vein thrombosis and pulmonary embolism, and after trauma, surgery, or myocardial infarction.[27,28] More recently developed ELISAs and LIA assays seem to have improved sensitivity and specificity for DIC but are not readily available in most laboratories. Based on published data, particularly the Japanese experience,[6] for confirmation of DIC it seems reasonable to require, in addition to a prolonged PT, that platelets or fibrinogen (or both) be decreased, and that these abnormalities not be explained by other causes (Table 43.1). These criteria may have to be modified in patients with thrombocytopenia due to other known causes such as leukemia and sepsis (often normal or increased fibrinogen). Although the schema depicted in Table 43.1 should be helpful in general for confirming or excluding DIC, staging and assessing the severity of DIC, and differentiating DIC from other conditions associated with abnormal bleeding and/or thrombosis that mimic DIC, uncertainties are likely to be encountered in individual patients. In such patients, additional tests (available in some large medical centers) may be useful (Table 43.1). In particular, measurement of soluble fibrin by ELISA using antibodies against neoepitopes generated by cleavage of fibrinopeptide A or B from fibrinogen by thrombin has been reported to be useful not only for confirming DIC suspected on clinical grounds[29,30] but also for predicting the development of DIC at an earlier stage than was possible with measurement of D-dimer.[29,31] Whether this holds true for more recently developed latex agglutination tests for soluble fibrin that can be performed more readily in routine clinical laboratories remains to be determined. There is also emerging evidence that tests for other molecular markers of hemostatic system activation can play a role; such tests, including measurements of thrombin/AT III complexes (TAT), plasmin/antiplasmin complexes (PAP), t-PA, F1.2, thrombomodulin, and PAI 1 (Fig. 43.2), may be useful in the diagnosis, staging, and prognosis prediction of DIC.[29-33] If it can be shown, for instance during sepsis, that the development of DIC as a marker for SIRS and MOSD and thus poor patient outcome can be reliably predicted with the use of one or more of these tests several days ahead of time, it may offer a means of selecting patients likely to benefit from early, targeted intervention. The diagnosis of DIC is a particular challenge in patients with advanced liver disease, which may produce similar laboratory abnormalities.[34] However, DIC appears to be rare even with severe liver disease except when it is complicated by acute blood loss or sepsis.[34] DIC may also be difficult to diagnose in sick, very low birth weight neonates with respiratory distress syndrome or septicemia; its importance may be difficult to assess even with the aid of tests for markers of AIC and fibrinolysis.[35,36]

Subacute DIC

Subacute DIC or DIC in resolution (e.g., following acute head trauma) is difficult to differentiate from acute DIC by basic laboratory tests (Table 43.1), but it may be suspected in patients who present with a prolonged PT, decreased platelets or fibrinogen (or both), and elevated D-dimer but normal FnS increased FnS is cleared within 6 hours of the cessation of thrombin generation, whereas the increased PT, decreased platelets/fibrinogen, and elevated D-dimer may persist several days after cessation of AIC. Additional adequately controlled and powered studies are required to assess the usefulness of FnS for distinguishing subacute from acute DIC and thus identifying patients who would not likely benefit from heparin therapy.

Chronic DIC

Hemostatic laboratory abnormalities consistent with or suggestive of (two or three criteria) mild to moderate DIC as described above may be observed in patients who do not appear to be acutely ill but are being evaluated for a recent history of recurrent, mild abnormal bleeding, such as easy bruising, frequent nose bleeds, or bleeding from gums. Conditions known to be associated with chronic DIC are metastatic malignancies (particularly of the lung, breast, and gastrointestinal tract), aortic aneurysm, promyelocytic leukemia, and dead fetus syndrome.

Differential Diagnosis

Conditions associated with clinical and hemostatic laboratory abnormalities similar to those seen in DIC are listed in Table 43.1. Most of these conditions can be readily distinguished from DIC by basic laboratory tests. Additional tests not generally available as rapid turnaround tests (e.g., assays for

FnS, antithrombin III, and factors VII and V) are useful in some patients (e.g., after cardiac surgery with infection and prolonged, parenteral alimentation, thrombocytopenia, increased PT and D-dimer) (DIC versus vitamin K deficiency? (Table 43.1)). Acute, fulminant, and advanced chronic liver disease may be associated with DIC-like hemostatic abnormalities: prolonged PT due to impaired coagulation factor synthesis, thrombocytopenia due to hypersplenism, increased D-dimer due to AIC, and impaired clearance of t-PA. Under certain circumstances (e.g., acute variceal gastrointestinal bleeding, trauma, infection, placement of peritoneovenous shunt), DIC may develop and be difficult to confirm or rule out even with the use of the additional tests listed in Table 43.1.[33]

Therapy

General Measures

In the absence of evidence from adequately powered, prospective clinical outcome studies, largely because of heterogeneity (different underlying conditions and clinical manifestations) and variable severity of DIC, treatment remains empiric.[3-5,37,38] Because DIC is an intermediary mechanism of disease and not a disease itself, treatment should be focused on (1) rapid identification and optimal management of the underlying disease or conditions (e.g., prompt administration of broad-spectrum antibiotics, abscess drainage, removal of a colonized intravascular catheter in bacterial sepsis, effective chemotherapy in acute promyelocytic leukemia, evacuation of the uterus with dead fetus syndrome); (2) aggressive fluid administration to restore/maintain adequate blood pressure and thus microcirculatory blood flow; and (3) restoration/maintenance of adequate tissue oxygenation by appropriate transfusion of red blood cells (to maintain hemoglobin at ≥10 g/dl)[39] and administration of oxygen. Persistence of DIC despite institution of the above measures indicates poor outcome.[3-5]

Replacement of Hemostatic Blood Components

Replacing hemostatic blood components, including platelets, fresh frozen plasma, and cryoprecipitate, is empiric. Because of the remaining, albeit small, risk of transmitting human immunodeficiency virus (HIV), hepatitis viruses, parvo B 19 virus, and other potentially pathogenic infectious agents, it should generally be considered only in patients with or at increased risk of serious bleeding with trauma, emergency surgery, or invasive procedures.

Platelet Concentrates

Platelet concentrates should be given as a single-donor pheresis product or six to eight random donor units to maintain the platelet count at >50,000–80,000/μl depending on the type/extent of surgery or invasive procedure or the extent and localization of trauma. The platelet count should be determined 30–60 minutes after transfusion of each batch of platelets and repeated every 4–6 hours to monitor platelet recovery and survival/consumption and to guide further transfusions until the platelet count has stabilized.

Fresh Frozen Plasma

Fresh frozen plasma (FFP), preferably obtained from repeatedly screened blood donors (donor-retested FFP, FFP-DR) or solvent/detergent-treated FFP (FFP-SD), contains all coagulation factors and natural coagulation inhibitors. FFP and FFP-DR should be infused at a rate of 10–12 ml/kg, FFP-SD at a dose of 12–15 ml/kg (20% less coagulation factor content than FFP) to maintain the PT-INR at <1.5 (prothrombin complex activity >30%), monitored at 4- to 6-hour intervals until stable. Prothrombin complex concentrates are not recommended, as all currently available preparations contain variable amounts of activated coagulation factors and thus are considered prothrombotic.

Cryoprecipitate

Cryoprecipitate (Cryo), which contains high concentrations of fibrinogen (~150 mg/bag), factor VIII (~150 units/bag), and von Willebrand factor (~200 units/bag) should be given in doses of 1 bag/5 kg in patients with severe DIC and a fibrinogen level <100 mg/dl. Close monitoring (every 6–12 hours depending on the severity of the DIC) of the complete blood count, PT, and fibrinogen level is required for guiding repeated blood component administration and assessing the course of DIC.

Antithrombin III

Concentrates of antithrombin III (AT) have been available for a number of years as products derived from human plasma as well as from recombinant DNA technology using in vitro animal cell cultures and transgenic animals. AT is an important regulatory protein of blood coagulation.[40] Inherited, heterozygous, partial deficiency (AT 50% of normal) is associated with a 20- to 40-fold increased risk of venous thromboembolism. Homozygous deficiency is apparently incompatible with extrauterine life. AT has also antiinflammatory properties.[41]

Antithrombin is decreased in DIC owing to irreversible complex formation with thrombin, factor Xa, and other clotting-active serine tissue proteases and clearance of the complexes,[40] as well as degradation by PMN-derived elastase.[20] A low AT level may be a predictor of MOSD[12] and increased mortality due to DIC.[8,12,14,42-44] Thus the rationale for AT supplementation in DIC is strong.[45] In addition to a number of case reports and retrospective studies, the findings of four prospective, controlled studies indicate that AT supplementation to achieve normal or supranormal levels decreases the severity and shortens the time to resolution of DIC in obstetric patients ($n = 77$),[46] adult patients with shock due to various causes ($n = 51$[47] and $n = 32$[48]), and septic shock ($n = 35$).[49] In the latter study[49] a 44% reduction in mortality was noted for AT-treated patients, but the difference was not statistically significant; and in the other studies overall survival was unaffected by AT supplementation. In a more recent multicenter study [50] of 120 patients with sepsis or postsurgical complications (or both), a survival advantage was found for AT-treated patients with septic shock, MOSD, and low AT levels. However, the number of patients with DIC was not stated. In none of these studies were major adverse events, including abnormal bleeding, attributable to AT. Given the large variability in the development and course of DIC in patients with sepsis and trauma, much larger and thus adequately powered and stratified prospective studies are likely required to determine the efficacy of AT supplementation for reducing mortality and long-term morbidity (e.g., chronic renal failure, patients with DIC associated with sepsis,[45] trauma, and other conditions). Some important questions need to be addressed in these studies: (1) Should AT be given early in patients at risk for DIC before DIC has developed? (2) Should AT be given to achieve normal or supranormal AT levels? (3) Should AT be given in combination with heparin or low-molecular-weight heparin? Until answers to such questions are available, costly treatment with AT cannot be generally recommended for patients with DIC.

Protein C

Protein C (PC), like AT an important natural anticoagulant (neutralization of activated factors VIII and V), is reduced in DIC and may contribute to morbidity and mortality during sepsis.[15,37] Human plasma-derived PC concentrate has been shown to be effective in preventing DIC and death in various animal models of gram-negative sepsis and in reversing DIC in humans with inherited PC deficiency.[37] Clinical trials are in progress.

Tissue Factor Pathway Inhibitor

Tissue factor pathway inhibitor (TFPI) is a natural anticoagulant that when combined with factor Xa effectively neutralizes the TF/factor VIIa complex; it thus shuts down the biologically predominant extrinsic coagulation pathway, which plays a major role in DIC. Supplementation with recombinant TFPI to achieve supranormal plasma levels is effective in preventing DIC and death in various animal models of sepsis.[37] Clinical trials are in progress.

Anticoagulant Drugs

Heparin

Anticoagulation with a rapidly acting agent such as heparin appears to be a rational approach to DIC and has been widely used. However, its safety and efficacy in reducing mortality and morbidity in DIC associated with sepsis, trauma, or other conditions have not been established in controlled clinical trials. There is particular concern about its safety (e.g., potential aggravation or precipitation of bleeding).[3-5,37] Conditions with DIC in which heparin has been used with apparent success as a bridge until more specific therapy of the condition becomes effective are acute promyelocytic leukemia, dead fetus syndrome, aortic aneurysm, purpura fulminans, carcinoma subject to cure or major palliation, and acral gangrene.[3-5,37,38]

Heparin therapy is initiated cautiously as a continuous intravenous infusion using doses 10–15 U/kg/hr, without bolus, followed by escalating doses until DIC laboratory abnormalities improve (e.g., thrombocytopenia, PT, fibrinogen monitored every 4-6 hours). Monitoring heparin therapy in patients with DIC is difficult, as the APTT may be prolonged at baseline. Moreover, the APTT therapeutic range in DIC is unknown and may vary among individual patients.

Low-Molecular-Weight Heparin

Low-molecular-weight heparin (LMWH) preparations have been shown to have potentially superior efficacy over heparin in preventing recurrent thromboembolic complications in patients with venous thromboembolism and acute coronary syndromes at similar or less risk of major abnormal bleeding.[51] Furthermore, it can be given subcutaneously once or twice a day and does not require laboratory monitoring, except in markedly obese patients, infants, and patients with renal failure. In a multicenter, double-blind, randomized study in patients with malignancies and DIC, LMWH was found to have greater efficacy than heparin in causing cessation of abnormal bleeding and an improved MOSD score.[52] LMWH is considerably more expensive than heparin, and additional studies are required.

Fibrinolytic Inhibitors

Increased fibrinolysis is a common feature of DIC and may contribute to abnormal bleeding;[19,21] if severe, it can predict poor patient outcome.[19] However, increased fibrinolysis is an important, normal defense mechanism against excessive fibrin accumulation/thrombosis. There are case reports of severe thromboembolic complications with the use of antifibrinolytic agents such as ε-aminocaproic acid and tranexamic acid.[3-5,37,38] There are no routine tests to distinguish appropriate and inappropriate or excessive fibrinolysis. There are, at present, no published data from controlled clinical trials concerning the safety and efficacy of these agents in patients with DIC for any conditions except cardiac surgery. Thus these agents are generally considered contraindicated for DIC except perhaps in patients with life-threatening bleeding not controlled with aggressive blood component therapy.[3-5,37,38]

Other Protease Inhibitors

Several broad-spectrum synthetic protease inhibitors active against thrombin, plasmin, and kallikrein, such as gabexate mesylate[53] and nafamostat mesylate,[54] have been used in Japan with promising results for treatment of DIC. Aprotinin appears to be relatively safe and effective for reducing blood and blood component transfusion during cardiac surgery, which is associated with DIC,[55,56] but there is at present no evidence from controlled studies as to its safety and efficacy for DIC with other conditions.

References

1. Müller-Berghaus G: Pathophysiologic and biochemical events in disseminated intravascular coagulation: dysregulation of procoagulant and anticoagulant pathways. Semin Thromb Hemost 1989; 15:58.
2. Müller-Berghaus G, Blombäck M, ten Cate JW: Attempts to define disseminated intravascular coagulation. In: Müller-Berghaus G, Madlener K, Blombäck M, ten Cate JW (eds) DIC: Pathogenesis, Diagnosis and Therapy of Disseminated Intravascular Fibrin Formation. Excerpta Medica International Congress Series. Amsterdam, Elsevier, 1993;3–8.
3. Marder VS, Feinstein DI, Francis CW, Colman RW: Consumptive thrombohemorrhagic disorders. In: Colman RW, Hirsh J, Marder VS, Salzman EW (eds) Hemostasis and Thrombosis. Basic Principles and Clinical Practice, 3rd ed. Philadelphia, Lippincott, 1994;1023–1063.
4. Seligsohn U: Disseminated intravascular coagulation. In: Beutler E, Lichtman MA, Coller BS, Kipps TV (eds) Williams Hematology, 5th ed. New York, McGraw-Hill, 1995;1497–1516.
5. Grosset AMB, Rodgers GM: Acquired coagulation disorders. In: Lee GR, Foerster J, Lukens J, Paraskevas F, Greer JP, Rogers GM (eds) Wintrobe's Clinical Hematology, 10th ed. Baltimore, Williams & Wilkins, 1999;1733–1780.
6. Kobayashi N, Maegawa K, Takada M, et al: Criteria for diagnosis of DIC based on the analysis of clinical and laboratory findings in 345 DIC patients collected by the Research Committee on DIC in Japan. Bibl Haematol 1987;49:265–275.
7. Wada H, Wakita Y, Shiku H: Tissue factor expression in endothelial cells in health and disease. Blood Coag Fibrinol 1995;6:S26–S31.
8. Mesters RM, Mannucci PM, Coppola R, et al: Factor VIIa and antithrombin III activity during severe sepsis and septic shock in neutropenic patients. Blood 1996;88:881–886.
9. Gando S, Nanzaki S, Sasaki S, Kemmotsu O: Significant correlations between tissue factor and thrombin markers in trauma and septic patients with disseminated intravascular coagulation. Thromb Haemost 1998;79:1111–1115.
10. Pixley RA, De La Cadena R, Page JD, et al: The contact system contributes to hypotension but not disseminated intravascular coagulation in lethal bacteremia. J Clin Invest 1993;91:61–68.
11. Despotis GJ, Joist JH, Goodnough LT: Monitoring of hemostasis in cardiac surgery patients: impact of point of care testing on blood loss and transfusion outcomes. Clin Chem 1997;43:1684–1696.
12. Gando S, Kameue T, Nanzaki S, Nakanishi Y: Disseminated intravascular coagulation is a frequent complication of systemic inflammatory response syndrome. Thromb Haemost 1996;75:224–228.
13. Taylor FB: Tissue factor and thrombin in post-traumatic systemic inflammatory response syndrome. Crit Care Med 1997;25:1774–1775.
14. Fourrier F, Chopin C, Goudemand J, et al: Septic shock, multiple organ failure and disseminated intravascular coagulation: compared patterns of antithrombin III, protein C, and protein S deficiencies. Chest 1992;101:816–823.
15. Levi M, van der Poll T, ten Cate H, et al: The cytokine mediated imbalance between coagulant and anticoagulant mechanisms in sepsis and endotoxemia. Eur J Clin Invest 1997;27:3–9.
16. Mayeux PR: Pathobiology of lipopolysaccharide. J Toxicol Environ Health 1997;51:415–435.
17. Okajima K, Uchiba M, Murakami K, et al: Plasma levels of E selectin in patients with disseminated intravascular coagulation. Am J Hematol 1997;54:219–224.
18. Takahashi H, Tatewaki W, Wada K, et al: Fibrinolysis and fibrinogenolysis in disseminated intravascular coagulation. Thromb Haemost 1990;63:340–344.
19. Verveot MG, Thijs LG, Hack CE: Derangements of coagulation and fibrinolysis in critically ill patients with sepsis and septic shock. Semin Thromb Hemost 1998;24:33–44.
20. Seitz R, Wolf M, Egbring R, et al: The disturbance of hemostasis in septic shock: role of neutrophil elastase and thrombin, effects of antithrombin and plasma substitution. Eur J Haematol 1989;43:22–28.
21. Stump DC, Taylor FB, Nesheim ME, et al: Pathologic fibrinolysis as a cause of clinical bleeding. Semin Thromb Hemost 1990;16:260–273.
22. Kovacs MJ, Wong A, MacKinnon K, et al: Assessment of the validity of the INR system for patients with liver impairment. Thromb Haemost 1994;71:727–730.
23. Whitaker AN, Rowe EA, Masci PP, Gaffney PJ: Identification of D-dimer E complex in disseminated intravascular coagulation. Thromb Res 1980;18:453–459.
24. Carr JM, McKinney M, McDonagh J: Diagnosis of disseminated intravascular coagulation: role of D-dimer. Am J Clin Pathol 1989;91:280–287.
25. Bredbacka S, Blombäck M, Wiman B, Pelzer H: Laboratory methods for detecting disseminated intravascular coagulation (DIC): new aspects. Acta Anesthesiol Scand 1993;37:125–30.
26. Charles L, Edwards T, Macik B: Evaluation of sensitivity and specificity of six D-Dimer latex assays. Arch Pathol Lab Med 1994;118:1102–1105.
27. Elias A, Haptel I, Huc B, et al: D-Dimer test and diagnosis of deep vein thrombosis: a comparative study of 7 assays. Thromb Haemost 1996;76:518–522.
28. Ginsberg JS, Wells PS, Kearon C, et al: Sensitivity and specificity of a rapid whole-blood assay for D-Dimer in the diagnosis of pulmonary embolism. Ann Intern Med 1998; 129:1006–1011.
29. Okajima K, Uchiba M, Murakami K, et al: Detection of plasma soluble fibrin using a new ELISA method in patients with disseminated intravascular coagulation. Am J Hematol 1996;51:186–191.
30. Wada H, Wakita Y, Nakase T, et al: Increased plasma-soluble fibrin monomer levels in patients with disseminated intravascular coagulation. Am J Hematol 1996;51:255–260.
31. Wada H, Sakurawaga N, Shiku H: Hemostatic molecular markers before onset of disseminated intravascular coagulation in leukemic patients. Semin Thromb Hemost 1998;24:253–297.
32. Wada H, Minamikawa, Wakita Y, et al: Increased vascular endothelial cell markers in patients with disseminated intravascular coagulation. Am J Hematol 1993;44:85–88.
33. Amano K, Tateyama M, Inaba H, et al: Fluctuations in plasma levels of thrombomodulin in patients with DIC. Thromb Haemost 1992;68:404–406.
34. Joist JH: Hemostatic abnormalities in liver disease. In: Colman RW, Hirsh J, Marder VJ, Salzman EW (eds) Hemostasis and Thrombosis. Basic Principles and Clinical Practice, 3rd ed. Philadelphia, Lippincott, 1993;906–920.
35. Aronis S, Platokouki H, Photopoulos S, et al: Indications of coagulation and/or fibrinolytic system activation in healthy and sick very-low-birth-weight neonates. Biol Neonate 1998;74:337–344.

36. Shirahata A, Shirakawa Y, Murakami C: Diagnosis of DIC in very low birth weight infants. Semin Thromb Hemost 1998;24:467–471.
37. De Jonge E, Levi M, Stoutenbeck CP, van Deventer SJH: Current drug treatment strategies for disseminated intravascular coagulation. Drugs 1998;55:767–777.
38. Colvin BT: Management of disseminated intravascular coagulation. Br J Haematol 1998;101(Suppl 1):15–17.
39. Goodnough LT, Brecher ME, Kanter MH, AuBuchon JP: Transfusion medicine; first of two parts: blood transfusion. N Engl J Med 1999;340:438–443.
40. Büller HR, ten Cate JW: Acquired antithrombin III-deficiency: laboratory diagnosis, incidence, clinical implications and treatment with antithrombin III concentrate. Am J Med 1989;87:445–455.
41. Okajma K, Uchiba M: The antiinflammatory properties of antithrombin III: new therapeutic implications. Semin Thromb Hemost 1998;24:27–32.
42. Lämmle B, Tran TH, Duckert F: Plasma prekallikrein, factor XII, antithrombin III, Cl-inhibitor and α_2 macroglobulin in critically ill patients with suspected disseminated intravascular coagulation (DIC). Am J Clin Pathol 1984;82:396–404.
43. Hellgren M, Egberg N, Eklund J: Blood coagulation and fibrinolytic factors and their inhibitors in critically ill patients. Intensive Care Med 1984;10:23–28.
44. Wilson RF, Mammen EF, Tyburski JG, et al: Antithrombin levels related to infection and outcome. J Trauma 1996;40:384–387.
45. Mammen EF: Antithrombin in DIC and sepsis. Biomed Progr 1997;10:57–61.
46. Maki M, Terao T, Ikenoue T, et al: Clinical evaluation of antithrombin III concentrate (BI 6.013) for disseminated intravascular coagulation in obstetrics: well-controlled multicenter trial. Gynecol Obstet Invest 1987;23:230–240.
47. Blauhut B, Kramer H, Vinazzer H, et al: Substitution of antithrombin III in shock and DIC: a randomized study. Thromb Res 1985;39:81–89.
48. Albert J, Blomquist H, Gastlund B, et al: Effect of antithrombin concentrate on haemostatic variables in critically ill patients. Acta Anaesthesiol Scand 1992;36:745–752.
49. Fourrier F, Chopin C, Huart JJ, et al: Double-blind, placebo-controlled trial of antithrombin III concentrates in septic shock with disseminated intravascular coagulation. Chest 1993;104:882–888.
50. Baudo F, Caimi TM, de Cataldo F, et al: Antithrombin III (ATIII) replacement therapy in patients with sepsis and/or postsurgical complications: a controlled, double-blind, randomized multicenter study. Intensive Care Med 1998;24:336–342.
51. Weitz JI: Low-molecular weight heparins. N Engl J Med 1997;337:688–698.
52. Sakuragawa N, Hasegawa H, Maki M, et al: Clinical evaluation of low-molecular weight heparin (FR-860) on disseminated intravascular coagulation (DIC): a multicentre cooperative double-blind trial in comparison with heparin. Thromb Res 1993;72:475–500.
53. Okamura T, Niho Y, Itoga T, et al: Treatment of disseminated intravascular coagulation and its prodromal stage with gabexate mesilate (FOY): a multi-center trial. Acta Haematol 1993;90:120–124.
54. Shibata A, Takahashi H, Aoki N, et al: Nafamostat mesilate as a therapy for disseminated intravascular coagulation (DIC): a well-controlled multicenter comparative study. Thromb Haemost 1989;62:371.
55. Bennett-Guerrero E, Sorohan VG, Gurevich MC, et al: Cost-benefit and efficacy of aprotinin compared with epsilon-aminocaproic acid in patients having repeated cardiac operation: a randomized, blinded clinical trial. Anesthesiology 1997;87:1373–1380.
56. Eberle B, Mayer E, Hafner G, et al: High-dose epsilon-aminocaproic acid versus aprotinin: antifibrinolytic efficacy in first-time coronary operations. Ann Thorac Surg 1998;65:667–673.

44
Refunctionalization of the Gut

Stig Bengmark

> As lactic fermentation serves so well to arrest putrification in general, why should it not be used for the same purpose within the digestive tube?
> —E. Metchnikoff,[1] Nobel Prize Laureate.

Ecoflora replacement therapy was suggested as early as the turn of the twentieth century by Metchnikoff. The concept of refunctionalization of the gut is to restore normal function after starvation, illness, stress, antibiotic-produced changes in colonic flora, and other alterations. This is done by providing an enteral diet and a program that enhances saliva and gastrointestinal (GI) secretion and production, including membrane lipids and mucus. Fiber is necessary, including pectin, oat gum, fructo-oligosaccharides, algal fibers, and glucomannan. Most important is provision of probiotic bacteria, such as *Lactobacillus plantarum*, to restore normal flora in the colon and reduce harmful bacteria. This action has also been called echo-immunonutrition. Probiotic bacteria are those organisms that help the gut function normally.

Microbe Organ

The "microbe organ" (the total bacterial population) in the human body has a weight similar to that of the liver (Table 44.1)[2] but contains far more cells than the liver. The human body is calculated to harbor 10 times more prokaryotic (bacterial) cells than eukaryotic cells,[3] and the human colon contains at least 10^{12} living bacterial cells. About 400–500 bacterial species have been identified, but no more than 30–40 species constitute 99% of the microbial cells in any one human. The bacterial cells have functions that are important for a high quality of life and optimal immune functions. In addition to manufacturing key nutrients and antioxidants, particularly for the colonic cells and the liver but also the rest of the body, the cells constituting the normal preventive (commensal) flora are also actively involved in production of cytokine-like molecules (bacteriokines) and coagulation and growth factors. Among the important nutrients released in the colon by commensal flora are various short-chain fatty acids (SCFAs), polyunsaturated fatty acids, amino acids, polyamines, peptides, vitamins, and various antioxidants such as flavonoids and carotenoids. It is generally accepted that for human food to contain enough precursors/donor substances at least 10% of the consumed calories (approximately 20% of the food volume) should be destined for the colon (e.g., foods that cannot be broken down by gastric, pancreatic, and small-intestinal enzymes but reaches the large intestine intact). These foods are mainly various plant fibers that are metabolized and various active nutrients and antioxidants released at the level of the large intestine.

There are several reasons impaired normal flora (dysbiosis) is frequently seen; insufficient colonization by commensal flora, loss of flora due to life style, disease and treatment with various synthetic drugs/pharmaceuticals, and antibiotics are among the most frequent. The idea of recolonization is not new. It was suggested almost 100 years ago by Metchnikoff,[1] but it is only in more recent years that it has been suggested as specific treatment in patients suffering from dysbiosis due to diarrhea of various etiology, human immunodeficiency virus/acquired immunodeficiency syndrome (HIV/AIDS), *Clostridium difficile* infections, pseudomembranous enterocolitis, ulcerative colitis, and multiple organ failure (MOF). Although general acceptance of bacteriotherapy by the medical community has run into significant difficulty, over the years there has been a small group of scientists and clinicians who have stubbornly promoted its use.[4]

There were many reasons for a hesitant attitude from the medical profession, but the most important was, without doubt, the lack of proper taxonomic instruments for properly identifying bacteria with specific activities. This problem was serious, as there are great genetic differences between different strains of lactic acid bacteria (LAB), and it has been claimed that the genetic difference between one LAB and another is sometimes greater than between a fish and a human. Without good taxonomic tools it is difficult to reproduce results. Furthermore, many studies undertaken in the past seem also to lack stringency regarding data interpretation and have inconsistencies with conclusions.[5] Another reason for limited enthusiasm for this form of therapy was that most efforts were based on the use of milk and yogurt bacteria, which are known to have only weak probiotic effects. Better results can be obtained by specific

TABLE 44.1. Microbe Organ: Relative Weights.

Site	Weight
Eyes	1
Nose	10
Mouth	20
Lungs	20
Vagina	20
Skin	200
Intestines	1000

After Gustafsson,[2] with permission.

fiber-fermenting LAB, common in fruit and vegetable ferments, in silage used for preservation of animal fodder, and in the human colon. The practice of preserving vegetables and fruits as ferments have, with the exception of Eastern Europe, disappeared during the twentieth century. It is tragic that during these years there has been no commercial interest in promoting studies using other LAB than those that make milk sour and tasteful. To improve the efficiency of bacteriotherapy in selective critically ill patients many physicians have tried to transfer whole feces from healthy individuals to those critically ill and in desperate need of gut reconditioning. During the last four to five decades several physicians reported successful treatment with bacteriotherapy, including such leading surgeons as Eiseman et al.,[6] and Wilmore.[7] The most important reason for the renewed interest in bacteriotherapy is the successful outcomes when tried. Also important are the increased insights into the microbiology and immunology of the gut and increasing awareness of the key role of flora for optimal gut immune function (see Chapter 41).

Reduced Daily Consumption of LAB

Physicians and nutritionists are convinced that the dietary habits over the past 100–200 years by Western society make an important etiologic contribution to dominant health problems in the Western world.[8] These problems are virtually unknown among the few surviving hunter-gatherer populations, whose way of life and eating habits most closely resemble those of preagricultural humans.[9,10] Not only did the diet of our paleolithic ancestors contain significantly less protein, saturated fatty acids, and sodium salts, it contained twice as much mineral content, four times as much plant fiber, ten times as much antioxidants, and sometimes up to fifty times as much omega-3 fatty acids. The largest difference, however, was the intake of LAB, which can be calculated to have been billions of times larger than what is available with today's food in most Western societies.

The main repository for food during the 6 to 12 million years that humans have existed on earth was the soil, where practically all food was kept. This is how we learned to produce fermented drinks such as wines and beers and fermented fishes, meats, vegetables, and fruits. Most of the food eaten (especially in northern parts of the globe with its seasonal variation in availability of fresh food) was kept in the soil; hence it fermented and became rich in LAB. With construction of the microscope a few hundred years ago, bacteria were identified. A dramatic decrease in LAB consumption thus began owing to sterilization/pasteurization. Another rich source of LAB, especially for children, was prechewed food, as parents, grandparents, and other people frequently helped the babies and infants by chewing the food for them and spitting it into their mouths.

Flora Reflects Life Style

Microbial flora of Westerners has altered during the last few hundred years. Persons living in rural areas in Africa,[11] and most likely also in Asia and South America, who consume large amount of lactobacilli and fiber with their daily diet have a flora rich in fiber-fermenting bacteria (e.g., *Lactobacillus plantarum* and *Lactobacillus rhamnosus*) and other LAB such as *Lactobacillus acidophilus*. These bacteria have often disappeared from the commensal flora of North Americans and Europeans. For example, *L. plantarum* exists in only about 25% of omnivorous North Americans, in contrast to two-thirds of the mainly vegetarian North American Seventh Day Adventists.[12] A study of healthy Swedish volunteers found *L. plantarum*, *L. rhamnosus*, and *L. paracasei* to be the most common lactobaculli on the rectal and oral mucosa, occurring in 52%, 26%, and 17% of individuals, respectively.[13] Other LAB, such as *L. reuteri*, *L. fermentum*, *L. acidophilus*, *L. oris*, and *L. vaginalis*, were found only occasionally.

There are also "acute" changes in flora, related to the food consumed. Thus formula-fed babies have a different flora than breast-fed babies.[14] Changing to an uncooked vegetarian diet, known as living food, and then returning to a conventional mixed Western diet induces major changes in the fecal microflora.[15,16] Western children, as a consequence of the "extreme" hygiene in child care, develop their commensal flora much later than and differently from children in the Third World. Western children sometimes have difficulty establishing a proper commensal flora. Proper flora is essential for programming the immune system and developing tolerance. This could be the reason for the increase in prevalence and severity of atopic diseases in industrialized countries with a market economy.[17] Swedish children have been shown to colonize their gut later than Pakistani children and with a significantly different flora.[18] Similarly, extensive colonization with enterobacteria have been found in Estonian but not Finnish neonates[19,20] and in Estonian but not Swedish infants.[21] Another factor contributing to the deranged microflora in Western countries is the frequent use of antibiotics.[22,23] Astronauts/cosmonauts on return to earth have not only lost their entire LAB flora but have acquired a high titer of pathogens in oral cavity and the colon (Table 44.2).[24] This derangement of flora is associated with poor quality food (dried, no fresh ingredients, sterilized) and stress, both factors with a profound influence on flora. Many people on earth like astronauts have difficulty maintaining a high quality commensal flora; hence they might need a daily "booster dose".

TABLE 44.2. Changes in Flora in Cosmonauts After Flights of Various Durations.

Condition	L. acidophilus	L. casei	L. plantarum	L. streptococcus
Saliva				
During preparation	1.8	1.2	0.3	4.2
After flights	0.9	0.9	0	3.0
After short flights	0.7	0.3	0	2.7
After long flights	1.3	1.7	0	3.5
During rehabilitation	0	1.5	0	6.8
Stool				
During preparation	4.0	3.5	2.6	4.9
After flights	1.7	0	0.5	4.8
After short flights	1.0	0	0.8	4.6
After long flights	2.9	0	0	5.1
During rehabilitation	0	4.0	1.7	8.5

After Lencner et al.,[24] with permission.
Results are the mean number (log/ml).

Influence on Immune Resistance

The gastrointestinal microflora is involved in numerous important functions in the body (Table 44.3), functions that are especially important for maintaining a very ill person. Supplementation of the normal flora with small amounts of LAB can significantly influence local and systemic immunity. Numerous animal studies and a few human studies support the observation of boosted immunity by oral or parenteral supplementation with live or dead LAB. The explanation for this dramatic effect is that the inoculum of LAB to a large extent targets host cells at levels that are not highly colonized, such as the jejunum. Peyer's patches (PPs) of the gut-associated lymphoid tissue (GALT) could be such special targets.[25] The epithelium of PPs contains specialized cells called M cells, known to be permeable to luminal components and to facilitate antigen sampling through contact and interaction with both luminal contents and immune cells. Increased antimicrobial activity of PP lymphocytes was observed after oral LAB.[26]

It is well documented that oral or parenteral administration of LAB strengthens resistance to infections, atopic diseases, and tumor development. Table 44.4 summarizes some of the immunomodulatory effects of LAB. Cells affected by LAB seem to be blood leukocytes, B and T lymphocytes, free and fixed

TABLE 44.3. Functions of Gastrointestinal Microflora.

Produces nutrients (e.g., SCFAs, PUFAs, polyamines, amino acids)
Produces vitamins and antioxidants
Produces coagulation and growth factors
Eliminates toxic substances
Eliminates mutagens
Increases mucosal apoptosis
Controls PPMs
Stimulates the immune system
Produces cytokine-like molecules/bacteriokines
Participates in regulation of mucus secretion, mucus utilization, nutrient absorption, GI motility, splanchnic blood flow

SCFAs, short-chain fatty acids; PUFAs, polyunsaturated fatty acids; GI, gastrointestinal; PPMs, Peyers Patches Meeks.

TABLE 44.4. Immunomodulatory Effects of Lactic Acid Bacteria.

Stimulate local cytokine production
Influence production of other mediators, such as prostaglandins and leukotrienes
Stimulate T, B, and natural killer cells
Increase mitogenic response
Increase macrophage activity
Increase antibody response to sheep red blood cells
Control infections
Have anticarcinogenic effects
Affect lactose utilization
Contribute to control of serum cholesterol

macrophages, other accessory cells of the immune system, intestinal mucosal cells, and bacterial cells in the lumen or adhering to the mucosal cells. Several bacterial moieties act as biologic response modifiers, including peptidoglucans, lipoteichoic acids, and endotoxin lipopolysaccharides.[27]

Maintaining T Cell (Th1/Th2) Balance

Conventional T cells, whose regulatory activity is mediated by cytokines, are essential to optimal functioning of the immune system. Cytokine production is not only harmful and associated with disease, it is also essential to health. A balance between T-helper-1 (Th1) lymphocytes, primarily associated with cellular immunity, and Th2 lymphocytes, mainly associated with humoral immunity, is essential to health and well-being. The balance between Th1 and Th2 activities can be nutritionally modulated, and LAB may play a role in this process. For example, T cell function is clearly suppressed in tumor-bearing mice, but the suppression can be abolished by administration of *Lactobacillus casei* and perhaps other LAB.

That LAB have special ability to stimulate defense mechanisms originates from observations during the 1920s that fermented mistletoe delays the development of cancer. Lactobacilli are gram-positive bacteria with a cell wall composed mostly of peptidoglucan, the main degradation product of which is muramyl peptides, known to be found in systemic tissues.[28] and known to have an important influence on such functions as sleep patterns, body temperature, and appetite[29] most likely through modulation of the acute-phase response (APR). Muramyl peptides are also known to be strong adjuvants that enhance immunologic reactivity.[30]

Mucosa: Not Only a Physical Barrier

The immune system is pluridimensional. It consists of the bone marrow/lymph nodes/splenic system and the mucosa-associated lymphoid system (MALT) with its two parts—GALT and the bronchus-associated lymphoid system (BALT)—which have somewhat different functions. There are two other components: the natural or innate immune system and the adaptive immune system. The natural immune system mediates nonspecific acute inflammatory responses; it involves the interaction of a relatively limited number of "foreign" molecules (LPS, peptidoglucan, lipoarabinomannan, bacterial polysaccharides) with a large number of effector cells. The adaptive immune system mediates antigen-specific immunity and has the ability to generate an almost unlimited variety of recognition molecules in the form of immunoglobulins and T cell receptors. This system recognizes potential pathogens and other antigens with great specificity. It has been found that intestinal epithelial cells secrete a spectrum of chemoattractant and proinflammatory cytokines after bacterial invasion.[31] Increased expression of genes encoding interleukin-8 (IL-8), tumor necrosis factor-α, (TNFα), monocyte chemotactic protein 1, and granulocyte/macrophage colony-stimulating factor (GM-CSF) have been observed.[31] The epithelial mucosal cells constitute a mechanical barrier to invasive bacteria and signal the presence of invasive pathogens to the mucosal cells and inflammatory cells.[31] Pathogenic and commensal bacteria participate with their cytokine-like molecules.[32,33] Hasselgren's group demonstrated that IL-6 is produced by murine enterocytes in response to endotoxin[34] and by human enterocytes in response to IL-1β.[35] Nuclear factor κB (NF-κB) is involved,[36] a factor known to activate several genes important for the inflammatory response, including the IL-6 gene in B cells, T cells, and monocytes.[37,38]

Too little is known about participation of LAB in these fundamental processes. Tannock said: "Investigation of the effect of *Lactobacillus* strains on the expression of cytokines by enterocytes should be an area of high priority for probiotic research."[39] Information on the influence of various LAB on the cytokine network is scarce. The only information we have is about yogurt bacteria, which are relatively weak immunomodulators. The activity of 2′-5′ synthetase, an expression of interferon-γ (IFN-γ) in blood mononuclear cells of healthy subjects, was found to be significantly increased (approximately 250%) 24 hours after a LAB-containing meal.[40] Increases in cytokine activity were observed when human mononuclear cells were incubated with yogurt bacteria (Yog)—*Lactobacillus bulgaricus* (BUL) and *Streptococcus thermophilus* (Ther)—combined or individually.

1. INFγ: Yog 570%, Bul 775%, Ther 2100%,
2. TNFα: Yog 970%, Bul 1020%, Ther 3180%
3. IL-1β: Yog 1920%, Bul 2120%, Ther 1540%

In each case there was strong, instant immunoactivation by LAB.[40] Another study demonstrated that heat-killed *Lactobacillus acidophilus* (LA 1), when exposed to mouse macrophages, increased the production of IL1-α (approximately 300%) and TNFα (approximately 1000%), which is considerably more than with other *L. acidophilus* strains and bifidobacteria but less than with *Escherichia coli*.[41]

Importance of LAB Colonization

The dairy industry has mainly expressed interest in promoting the health-improving potential of LAB. Their interest focused on such LAB that have the greatest potential for use in LAB-containing milks, yogurts, kefirs, and so on. One criterion for selection has obviously been palatability, which is why lactobacilli such as *L. acidophilus*, *L. casei*, and *L. delbruecki* and bifidobacteria such as *Bifidobacter adolescentis*, *B. bifidum*, *B. longum*, and *B. infantis* so far dominate. Little interest has been shown in the greater capacity of LAB to ferment plant fibers.

Only LAB with the ability to colonize the gut can be expected to have clinical effects. Colonization can be expected only by LAB with the ability to adhere to mucosal surfaces or to mucus. Such ability has been documented for a few LAB strains, but yogurt bacteria and most other LAB used in combination with milk do not adhere. Most *L. acidophilus*, *L. bulgaricus*, and *Bifidobacteria* strains do not have the ability to adhere to intestinal mucosa, at least not in vitro, where adhesion most often has been studied. On the other hand *L. rhamnosus* (GG) persists in feces 7 days after the last administration in at least one-third of individuals and *L. plantarum* (299) in two-thirds of individuals as long as 28 days. Whereas adherence of LAB is most often by protease-sensitive mechanisms or by lipid (lactosylceramid) receptors, *L. plantarum* has been shown to adhere via carbohydrate (mannose) adhesions (i.e., the same receptors used by gram-negative bacteria, such as *E. coli*, *Enterobacter*, *Klebsiella*, *Salmonella*, *Shigella*, *Pseudomonas*, and *Vibrio cholerae*.[42] This special feature makes it especially interesting to try to use *L. plantarum* and taxonomically related LAB as an alternative to antibiotics, making use of its potential to block receptor sites for gram-negative bacteria.

Lactobacillus plantarum and Related LAB

Lactobacillus plantarum and taxonomically related LAB are the major microbes in naturally fermented foods (vegetables, cereals, fish, meat, sourdough, green olives, natural wines, beers); they are also important ingredients in the food consumed in developing countries[11] and in the food of our paleolithic ancestors. They are dominant in fermented food products administered to farm animals (silage). It is thus not surprising that these bacteria are dominant LAB in the human GI tract when consumed.[13] Table 44.5 summarizes some of the unique features of *L. plantarum*.

Food products obtained through fermentation with *L. plantarum* better preserve key nutrients, such as omega-3 fatty acids, vitamins, and antioxidants as well as other sensitive nutrients, such as glutamine and glutathione, than foods obtained by modern preservation methods (e.g., freezing, drying, heating).[43] Another interesting characteristic of *L. plantarum* is its ability to utilize and eliminate nitrates. This factor should be a decisive criterion in the selection of LAB for bioconservation of vegetables.[44] All *L. plantarum* reduce the content of $NaNO_3$ in fermented cabbage and carrot juice, and some can eliminate it totally during a 7-day long fermentation process.[44] *L. plantarum* has the unique ability to facilitate production of nitric oxide (NO). Support for such an assumption is obtained by the fact that *L. plantarum* can metabolize only two amino acids, one of which is arginine, a well known donor molecule for NO production.[45] When added to tempeh, an Indonesian dish based on cooked, dehulled beans, prevents its

TABLE 44.5. Special Features of *Lactobacillus plantarum*.

Metabolizes tyrosine and arginine
Tolerates very low pH
Most common bacterium in natural ferments: vegetables, cereals, fish and meat, sourdough, green olives, natural wines and beers
Most common microbe in paleolithic diet
Most common microbe in rural African and Asian foods
Preserves n-3 and n-6 fatty acids better than other method of food preservation
Preserves vitamins and antioxidants better than other method of food preservation
Eliminates nitrate from the food
Eliminates PPMs from stored foods
Metabolizes semiresistant fibers such as oligofructans
Induces IFNα and IL-12 production
Suppresses IgE production

spoilage,[46] a unique ability used for preservation of other food products. The mechanisms are not known but can be expected to be via a direct antioxidant effect of the bacterium, bacteria-produced molecules such as plantaricins, NO production, or the low pH of *L. plantarum* ferments.

Oligofructans such as inulin and phleins are receiving increased attention as a nutritional fiber of importance. This fiber is difficult to ferment, and only a few LAB are able to do so. In a study of 712 LAB, only 16 were able to cleave and ferment the phlein type and 8 the inulin type.[47] Apart from *L. plantarum*, only three other LAB species—*L. paracasei* subsp. *paracasei*, *L. brevis*, and *Pediococcus pentosaceus*—were able to ferment these resistant fibers.

Allergic diseases are thought to be due to inappropriate generation of the Th2 response. In animal experiments using casein as the allergen, *L. plantarum* induced significant INFγ and IL-12 responses and suppressed anticasein immunoglobulin E (IgE).[48] Similar results were obtained with *L. casei* but not with *L. johnsonii* (LA-1) in a model using ovalbumin as the allergen.[49]

Availability of Fiber: Importance for Function

Our current knowledge of immunostimulatory amino acids such as arginine, glutamine, histidine, taurine, various sulfur and related amino acids, polyamines, omega fatty acids, vitamins, and other antioxidants has been summarized elsewhere.[50] For optimal effect not all amino acids should be delivered in a free form; a large proportion are delivered in a "wrapped" form and reach the colon untouched. Fibers are excellent as substrate for delivery of various compounds to the lower part of the GI tract, as most of them cannot be disintegrated by enzymes in the small intestine. It is never enough to supply only LAB; a daily supply of fibers is necessary, a fact often neglected in everyday medicine. One cannot expect compounds to be produced at the colonic level other than what is contained in the fiber supplied. The fiber must be chosen with knowledge and care. Key ingredients such as omega-3 fatty acids, glutamine, glutathione, and many other compounds do not tolerate processing or storage. Thus dried fiber does not contain large amounts of these compounds. They come only in fresh products. Whenever possible commercial formulas should be supplemented with fresh fruit and vegetable juices produced at the wards or ICU units. This practice has been promising whenever tried.

Not just one source of fiber but several should be used. Oat fiber is metabolized mainly in the proximal colon, whereas wheat fiber is fermented mainly in the distal part of the colon (i.e., where most cancers are localized). Oat has sepsis-reducing effects, and wheat has mainly been effective in cancer prevention. Table 41.2 shows various sources rich in three important amino acids: arginine, glutamic acid (little information exists on glutamine), and histidine. In general, seeds, nuts, beans, and peas are rich sources of them as are most other amino acids. Soya is a reliable source and is a good source of colonic food.

Oat Gum

Oats contain a series of interesting compounds, which is the reason why much of world production goes to the pharmaceutical and cosmetic industries. The amino acid pattern of oat is comparable to that of human muscle, so oat products can deliver most of the amino acids needed to build muscles. Oat is rich in water-soluble fibers, β-glucans, which are known to be antiseptic. Oats are rich also in natural antioxidants, particularly ferulic acid, caffeic acid, hydrocinnamic acid, and tocopherols. It was used extensively before synthetic antioxidants were available to preserve foods: milk, milk powder, butter, ice cream, fish, bacon, sausages, and other food products sensitive to fat oxidation. Another ingredient richly available in oats is inositol hexaphosphate (phytic acid), a strong antioxidant, particularly known to enhance natural killer (NK) cell activity and to suppress tumor growth.[51] In addition, oats are particularly rich in polyunsaturated fats/polar lipids such as phosphatidylcholine, which have been shown to have strong protective effects of mucosal surfaces.[52]

Pectin

Pectin is an interesting fiber, used extensively by the pharmaceutical and food industry. It forms gels and is commonly used as a carrier of pharmacologically active substances and in baby foods. Pectin is a strong antioxidant against the three most dominating mechanism of oxidation damage: peroxyl, superoxide, and hydroxyl radicals.[53] These effects might explain why pectin stimulates the GALT system and prevents disruption of intestinal microflora.[54,55]

We (Bengmark and Larsson, unpublished observations) observed that when the pH of the pectin solution in water is reduced to pH 1.0 (i.e., the pH of the stomach if not inhibited), a two-phase separation occurs, with formation of one gel phase and one watery phase. It is likely that when this separation occurs in the stomach, the gel phase adheres to the mucosal layer and increases the protective capacity of the mucus. Banana, especially when green and unripe, is rich in pectins and phospholipids and is known to protect against peptic ulcer.[56,57]

This knowledge led us to study the protective effect of pectin and phospholipids in animal models.[58,59] As shown in Fig. 44.1, strong protective effects can be obtained, especially when the concentrations are higher than normally found in fruits.[59] The protective and healing effects of pectin were similar to those of established drugs such as H_2-blockers, proton inhibitors, and surface-protection agents. Pectin appears ideal for perioperative use as it is effective, inexpensive, and eliminates the need for inhibiting stomach acidity, to prevent colonization of the stomach with pathogens. Pectin protects the whole GI tract and is fermented in the colon as an important colonic food. The only disadvantage with pectin is that it cannot be administered by feeding tubes, as it clogs the tube. It should be supplied orally with drinking water.

Oligofructans

Oligofructans are nondigestible oligomers of fructose and other saccharides; their contents are particularly rich in plants such as artichokes, onions, asparagus, and chicory. They display great gelling and thickening properties. Inulin, one such fructooligosaccharide is used in food items such as bread, baked goods, and dairy and cheese products. The daily intake in Western populations varies between 2 and 12 g/day. Like oats, it may have lipid-lowering ability. Several oligosaccharides are available today, and industry is interested in using them in clinical nutrition products. Only a few strains of LAB are able to metabolize the various oligofructans. Hence these LAB strains must be made available.[60] When oligofructans are administered, the number of fecal bifidobacteria increases. This could be a favorable situation, especially in very sick patients, as bifidobacteria produce (in the gut) and deliver various important vitamins such as thiamine, folic acid, nicotinic acid, pyridoxine, and vitamin B_{12}.[61]

Algal Fibers

Most algal fibers are resistant to hydrolysis by human endogenous digestive enzymes; however, they are fermented by colonic flora to variable degrees. The soluble fibers are lamarans (a sort of β-glucan associated with mannitol residues), fucans (sulfated polymers associated with xylose, galactose, and glucuronic acid), and alginates (mannuronic and glucuronic acid polymers); the insoluble polymers are mainly cellulose. It is questionable if fucans are fermentable, but fermentation of alginates produces a high yield of acetate (80%) and lamirans of butyrate (16%).[62] The physiologic effects of various algal fibers have just begun to be investigated.[63–65] Within a few years these fibers may be used in clinical enteral nutrition.

Glycomannans

Glycomannan, a glucose/mannose polymer derived from a plant, *Amorphophallus konjak*, is also called devil tongue, elephant yam, and umbrella arum. It has hydroscopic abilities. On contact with water it swells and forms a viscous gel, which delays gastric emptying and intestinal transit time. It is effective in delaying absorption of digestible energy.[66] It is presently used in Japan to treat diabetes,[67] hypertension, and hypercholesterolemia,[68,69] and it may soon be tried in clinical enteral nutrition. Konjak mannan has been shown to alter the flora and reduce tumorigenesis in experimental animals.[70]

Support from Animal Experiments

Table 44.6 summarizes the clinical effects of LAB. Following is a discussion of studies associated with trauma/infection and inflammation.

Experimental Colitis

Colitis was induced in rats by instilling a 4% acetic acid solution for 15 seconds in an exteriorized colonic segment. Colitis was produced with a threefold increase in myeloperoxidase activity

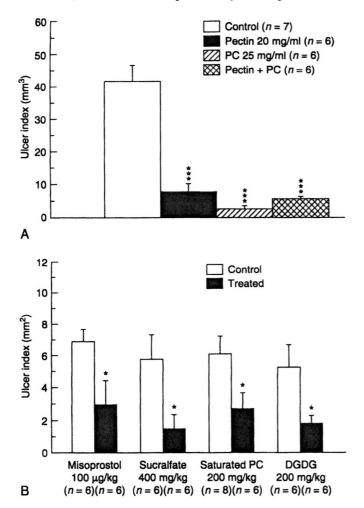

FIGURE 44.1. Peptic ulcer preventive effect in rats by an exogenous supply of pectin and phosphatidylcholine (PC) alone (A) or in combination (B) compared to pharmaceutical drugs on the market, such as misoprostol and sucralfate. DGDG, digalactodiacylglycerol. (After Dunjic et al.,[58,59] with permisson.)

TABLE 44.6. Clinical Effects of Dietary Lactic Acid Bacteria.

Reduce lactose intolerance
Reduce serum cholesterol
Eliminate luminal mutagens
Increase mucosal apoptosis and prevent cancer
Cure infant and "tourist" diarrheas
Prevent gastrointestinal infections

of the colonic tissue (index of neutrophil infiltration) and a sixfold increase in plasma exudation into the lumen (a sign of increased mucosal permeability). Intracolonic administration of species-specific *Lactobacillus reuteri* R2LC immediately after the acetic acid instillation, either as a pure bacterial suspension or a fermented oat soup, prevented the development of colitis.[71] The same treatment but delayed for 24 hours resulted in a significant but less pronounced healing effect. Intraperitoneal injection of methotrexate (MTX) (20 mg/kg body weight) was also used to induce enterocolitis. The animals were pretreated by a diet of *L. reuteri* R2LC or *L. plantarum* DSM 9843 and oat base with or without fermentation. Lactobacilli and oat base decreased the intestinal myeloperoxidase level, reestablished intestinal microecology, and reduced bacterial translocation to extraintestinal sites.[72] They also reduced plasma endotoxin levels. The effects were greater with fermentation. *L. plantarum* was more effective in reducing pathogens than *L. reuteri*. In another study using the same model, 4-day pretreatment with a 1% solution of pectin significantly reduced MTX-induced intestinal injury and improved bowel integrity.[73]

Experimental Intraabdominal Infection

Peritonitis was induced in rats by cecal ligation and puncture after 5 days of pretreatment with oral fermented or unfermented oat base or saline. On days 5 and 6 the animals were treated with intraperitoneal injections of either gentamicin or saline every 6 hours. No animal in the sham-operated group but 32 of 36 in the untreated control group demonstrated bacterial growth in blood, compared to 11 of 24, 8 of 20, and 12 of 24, respectively, in the *Lactobacillus*, gentamicin, and combined gentamicin/*Lactobacillus* groups.[74] The difference was statistically significant between the controls and the various treatment groups but not between the different treatment groups.

Chemical Hepatitis

Acute liver injury was induced by intraperitoneal injection of D-galactosamine (1.1 g/kg body weight) following 8 days pretreatment with rectal instillation of one of five lactobacilli, with and without a 2% arginine solution: *L. rhamnosus* DSM 6594 (strain 271), *L. plantarum* DSM 9843 (strain 299v), *L. fermentum* DSM 8740:3 (strain 245), and *L. reuteri* (strain 108). All lactobacilli, with or without added arginine, significantly reduced the extent of liver injury and reduced bacterial translocation. The most pronounced effect was with *L. plantarum* and arginine, which significantly reduced liver enzymes, hepatocellular necrosis, inflammatory cell infiltration, bacterial translocation, and the number of Enterobacteriaceae in the cecum and colon.[75] An oral supply of lactulose in the same model was highly effective in preventing liver injury and bacterial translocation.[76] Similar preventive effects can be obtained by intraperitoneal injections of endotoxin over 3 days before induction of liver injury;[77] oral *L. reuteri* for 3 days showed no beneficial effects. Endotoxin pretreatment rendered macrophages unresponsive to subsequent stimulation, which might explain the beneficial effects of endotoxin in D-galactosamine injury.[78]

Experimental Pancreatitis

Rats were pretreated with *L. plantarum* 299 (0.5×10^9 to 1.0×10^9 ml) for 4 days before induction of acute pancreatitis (isolation and ligation of the biliopancreatic duct). It was continued for 4 days after induction. Pathogenic bacteria could be cultivated from mesenteric lymph nodes in 14 of 20 animals and from pancreatic tissue in 10 of 20 untreated control animals. The dominating flora consisted of *Escherichia coli*, *Enterococcus faecalis*, *Pseudomonas*, and *Proteus*. When the animals received *L. plantarum* 299, only 4 of 20 animals demonstrated bacterial growth in mesenteric lymph nodes and 3 of 20 in pancreatic tissue.[79]

Human Experience: A Beginning

The demand for well controlled human studies is great. Although several human studies are underway, few have been completed, and the studies so far reported have dealt mainly with diarrhea or inflammatory bowel syndrome.[80,81] We gave *Lactobacillus* to five consecutive patients suffering from MOF after GI surgery (Table 44.7). The mean APACHE II score fell from 18 before treatment to 12 and 9 after 5 and 10 days of treatment, respectively. All patients were able to leave the ICU unit (see case studies below).

Patient 1

A 74-year-old man with Parkinson's disease (Fig. 44.2A) was admitted to a local hospital with upper GI bleeding. No source of the bleeding could be found during emergency laparotomy. Five days later he developed partial necrosis of the abdominal wall, wound dehiscence, and peritonitis. An emergency gastric resection was performed with a feeding jejunostomy. He was referred to the university hospital with pulmonary and renal insufficiency and sepsis. *Lactobacillus* and oat were administered

TABLE 44.7. Influence of APACHE II Scores After Enteral Supply of *Lactobacillus* and Oat Fiber.

Patient no.	APACHE II score		
	Before	After 5 days	After 10 days
1	16	5	4
2	20	12	8
3	21	17	13
4	20	18	16
5	15	9	3
Mean	18	12	9

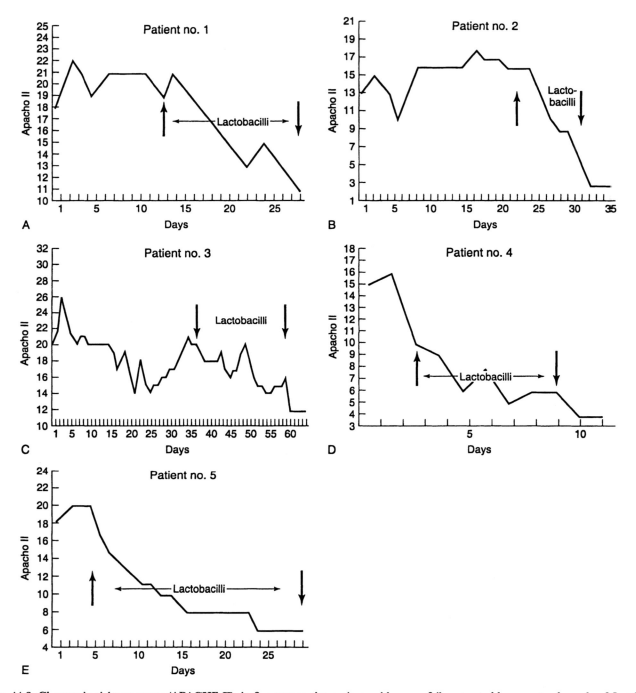

FIGURE 44.2. Changes in sickness scores (APACHE II) in five consecutive patients with organ failure treated by an enteral supply of *Lactobacillus* and oat fiber. Arrows indicate the period of treatment.

via the jejunal feeding tube. The patient was weaned from the ventilator after 10 days and left the ICU.

Patient 2

A 65-year-old man (Fig. 44.2B), developed pulmonary insufficiency and sepsis after a perforated duodenal ulcer and diffuse peritonitis. No abdominal abscess was found despite repeat computed tomography (CT) scans and two exploratory laparotomies. His general condition deteriorated, with increasing leukocytosis and plasma creatinine. At day 22 *Lactobacillus* and oat were given enterally, and the patient started to recover slowly. He left the ICU after 2 weeks of treatment.

Patient 3

A 52-year-old man (Fig. 44.2C) at a local hospital underwent emergency partial gastrectomy. He was referred to the university hospital because of a leaking duodenal stump. He was reoperated, with drainage of retroduodenal stump, a gastrostomy, and percutaneous transhepatic cholangiography. His condition deteriorated quickly, with a high fever, leukocytosis, and pulmonary, renal, and hepatic insufficiency. Treatment with *Lactobacillus* and oat was instituted after 45 days. He recovered slowly during the following 20 days. His organ functions improved, and he was weaned from the ventilator and left the ICU.

Patient 4

A 43-year-old man (Fig. 44.2D) at a local hospital underwent sigmoid resection because of perforated diverticulitis. After operation he developed anastomotic dehiscence and fecal peritonitis. A Hartmann procedure was performed, but the patient developed fever and ventilatory insufficiency and was referred to the university hospital. About 1 week after institution of *Lactobacillus* and oat the patient was able to leave the ICU.

Patient 5

A 63-year-old women with diabetes (Fig. 44.2E) underwent colectomy and ileostomy because of gangrene of the colon. She developed abdominal abscesses, wound dehiscence, and small-bowel fistulas, with subsequent circulatory, ventilatory, and renal insufficiencies. *Lactobacillus* and oat were administered, and after 24 days she was able to leave the ICU.

Comments

None of these patients had positive blood cultures before or during the treatment. Despite their being on antibiotic treatment, they developed clinical signs of sepsis. All had received total parenteral nutrition before the start of enteral nutrition with *Lactobacillus* and oat. TPN was often continued in parallel with the enteral nutrition. A dramatic improvement in their general condition and APACHE II scores occurred from the day the *Lactobacillus* and oat were instituted.

Impact of Antibiotics

The normal GI microflora is a remarkably stable ecosystem, although disease, hospitalization, drug treatment, and irradiation are associated with changes. The normal composition of the GI flora is shown in Fig. 44.3 and Table 44.8.[82] The most common cause of a disturbed gut flora is the use of antibiotics. Oral and parenteral antibiotics cause disturbances. Of the orally administered drugs those that are poorly absorbed have the most negative effects. Of the parenteral drugs, those secreted in saliva, bile, and intestinal secretions have the most negative effects on the flora. During operation there is usually no salivation or GI secretion, which is why one or two doses of antibiotics can be given safely. Suppression of the normal flora creates a microbiologic vacuum, which is readily filled by resistant microorganisms normally excluded from this site.[83]

Valuable information about antibiotics and their effects on flora has been obtained from the work of van Saene et al.

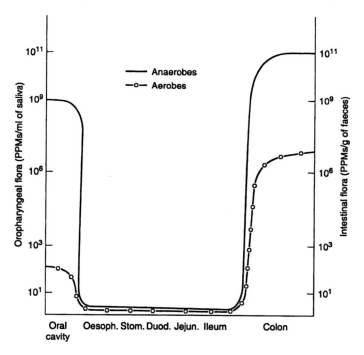

FIGURE 44.3. Distribution of flora in the human GI tract. (After van Saene et al.,[82] with permission.)

(Table 44.9).[82] Gismondo recently updated our information on the impact of antibiotics on intestinal microflora.[84] Ampicillin is incompletely absorbed and is associated with a high incidence of diarrhea. Piperacillin is excreted in bile and overgrowth of enterobacteria and *Bacteroides fragilis* resistant to

TABLE 44.8. Normal Values for Digestive Tract Flora.

Flora	Conc./ml[a]	Incidence (%)
Oropharyngeal cavity		
Anaerobes	10^7	100
Aerobes		
Streptococcus viridans	10^{5-7}	100
Staphylococcus aureus		
Streptococcus pneumoniae	10^3	10–40
Haemophilus influenzae		
Enterobacteriaceae	$\leq 10^3$	<10
Pseudomonadaceae	$\leq 10^3$	<1
Candida albicans	10^3	10–40
Gastrointestinal Canal		
Anaerobes	10^{11}	100
Aerobes		
Streptococcus faecalis	10^{5-7}	100
Staphylococcus aureus	10^3	10–40
Enterobacteriaceae		
Escherichia coli	10^{5-7}	100
Klebsiella spp.		
Proteus spp.	$\leq 10^3$	<20
Enterobacter spp.		
Pseudomonadaceae	$\leq 10^3$	<1
Candida albicans	10^3	10–40

[a] For the oropharyngeal cavity the concentration is per milliliter of saliva; for the gastrointestinal canal it is per gram of feces. (After van Saene et al.,[82] with permission.)

TABLE 44.9. Influence of Antimicrobial Agents on Colonization Resistance in the Human GI Tract.

Indifferent influence: cefaclor, cefradin, cefotaxime, ceftazidime, tobramycin, cotrimoxazole, doxycycline, amphotericin B, nystatin, polymyxins, metronidazoles, nalidixic acid, mecillinam, trimethoprim, cinoxacin
Decreases the count: penicillins, cephalosporins, aminoglycosides, erythromycin, tetracyclines, vancomycin, chloramphenicol, thioamphenicol, clindamycin, lincomycin

After van Saene et al.,[82] with permission.

piperacillin has been observed. No overgrowth was observed when it was combined with tazobactam. Fecal excretion of imipenem and meropenem is low, and only minor changes have been observed in the gut flora of patients receiving these antibiotics. Significant changes in both aerobic and anaerobic flora have been observed after administration of nitroimidazoles (metronidazole, ornidazole, timidazole), which were previously regarded as safe for the flora.

Because of the increasing awareness of the problems with antibiotic usage, it is suggested that probiotics be used to replace antibiotics in certain situations. One indication is perioperative infection prophylaxis. Such an attempt was recently made by L. Gianotti (personal communication). In a small pilot study two patients were pretreated enterally for 3 days with *L. Plantarum* 299 and oat fiber before colorectal surgery for cancer. Two other patients were treated conventionally with antibiotics and lavage. During operation biopsy specimens were obtained from the resected tissue for bacterial culture. No *Enterobacteriaceae* were found on the mucosa in the *L. plantarum*- and oat fiber-treated patients versus an average of 500 colonies/cm^2 in the controls.

Uncommon Causes of Bacteremia

Lactobacillus is rarely a human pathogen, although it has been reported in connection with pathologic conditions such as endocarditis.[85] However, the risk is small. Up to 1997 only 45 patients had been reported in the English-language literature. Most if not all patients with cancer or diabetes had depressed immune functions. They were often on immunosuppressive or antibiotic therapy or were receiving TPN. *Lactobacillus* bacteremia has also been reported recently in a small series of liver transplant recipients[86] and in patients with AIDS.[87] Although 31 of the 45 patients reported in the world literature died, only one death was attributed to *Lactobacillus* bacteremia. The view of Husni et al. is that when "*Lactobacillus* bacteremia occurs, it serves as a marker of a serious underlying illness and poor long-term prognosis for hospitalized patients."[85]

Conclusions

We have developed a nutritional formula based upon *Lactobacillus plantarum* and oat that, along with other nutrients, can best provide refunctionalization of the gut and restoration of normal GI function from saliva in the mouth through the small intestine to the colon. A group of us at Lund University, after a detailed analysis of the health-promoting potential of various probiotic bacteria in combination with various prebiotic fibers, developed an enteral nutritional formula obtained by fermentation of oatmeal with *L. plantarum* strains 299 and 299V. Nineteen human-specific *Lactobacillus* strains were studied in a group of healthy individuals. Mucosal biopsies from the jejunum and rectum, after administration of the formula, identified *L. plantarum* strains (as above) as the best. These strains also have a large capacity to ferment oat and have no difficulty surviving the acidity of the stomach and the bioacidity of the small intestine. Results of experimental and clinical observations suggest that this formula can stimulate gut immunity and help decrease the possibility of sepsis. Such an approach may be particularly helpful in such diseases as acute gastroenteritis, food allergy, atopic dermatitis, Crohn's disease, and rheumatoid arthritis, after pelvic radiotherapy, with intestinal inflammation, and after chemical exposure. The initial clinical evidence suggests that the use of probiotics, in combination with prebiotics (e.g., bacterial therapy and fiber), may be the future cornerstone for the prevention of gut inflammation and some infectious diseases. In addition, it could be a great stimulus in sick, injured, or operated patients to decrease the possibility of development of SIRS, MODS, and MOF.

Addendum

After submission of this review a randomized trial in human liver transplantation comparing perioperative enteral supply with live or heat-killed *Lactobacillus plantarum* and inulin fiber with selective bowel decontamination (SBD) was reported.[88] Each of the three groups consisted in 15 patients. In the group treated with SBD sepsis occurred in 40% (6/15 patients). When inulin fiber and heat-killed *Lactobacillus plantarum* was supplied the infection rate fell to 27% (4/15 patients), and in the group supplied inulin fiber and live *Lactobacillus plantarum* the infection rate was only 13% (2/15 patients). These findings support the conclusions made in this review.

References

1. Metchnikoff E: Prolongation of Life. New York, Putnam, 1908.
2. Gustafsson B: The Future of Germfree Research: New York Liss, 1985.
3. Tancrède C: Role of human microflora in health and disease. Eur J Clin Microbiol Infect Dis 1992;11:1012–1015.
4. Coconnier MH, Klaenhammar TR, Kernèis S, et al: Protein-mediated adhesion of *Lactobacillus acidophilus* BG2FO4 on human enterocyte and mucus-secreting cell lines in culture. Appl Environ Microbiol 1992;58:2034–2039.
5. Sanders ME: Lactic acid bacteria as promotors of human health. In: Goldberg I (ed) Functional Foods. New York, Chapman & Hall, 1994.
6. Eiseman B, Silen W, Bascom BS, Dauvar AJ: Fecal enema as an adjunct in the treatment of pseudomembranous enterocolitis. Surgery 1958;44:854–859.
7. Wilmore D: The surgeon and intestinal bacteria—reconsideration of our relationship. After Baue AE: The role of the gut in the

development of multiple organ dysfunction in cardiothoracic patients. Am Thorac Surg 1993;55:822–829.
8. Eaton SB, Konnor M: Paleolithic nutrition: a consideration of its nature and correct implications. N Engl J Med 1985;312:283–289.
9. Trowell H: Hypertension, obesity, diabetes mellitus and coronary heart disease. In: Trowell H, Burkitt D (eds) Western Diseases: Their Emergence and Prevention. Cambridge, Harvard University Press, 1981.
10. Lindeberg S: Apparent absence of cerebrocardiovascular disease in Melanesians. PhD thesis, Lund University, Lund, Sweden,1994.
11. Olasupo NA, Olukoya DK, Odunfa SA: Studies on bacteriocinogenic Lactobacillus isolated from selected Nigerian fermented foods. J Basic Microbiol 1995;35:319–324.
12. Finegold SM, Sutter VL, Mathisen GE: Normal indogenous intestinal flora. In: Hentges DJ (ed) Human Intestinal Microflora in Health and Disease. San Diego, Academic, 1983.
13. Ahrné S, Nobaek S, Jeppsson B, et al: The normal Lactobacillus flora of healthy human rectal and oral mucosa. J Appl Microbiol 1998;85:88–94.
14. Balmer SE, Scott PGH, Wharton BA: Diet and faecal flora in the newborn: casein and whey proteins. Arch Dis Child 1989;64:1678–1684.
15. Benno Y, Mitsuoka T: Effect of diet and aging on human fecal flora: comparison of Japanese and American diets. Am J Clin Nutr 1974;27:456–469.
16. Peltonen R, Ling WH, Hänninen O, Eerola E: An uncooked vegan diet shifts the profile of human fecal microflora: computerized analysis of direct stool sample gas–liquid chromatography profiles of bacterial cellular fatty acids. Appl Environ Microbiol 1992; 58:3660–3666.
17. Björksten B: Risk factors in early childhood for the development of atopic diseases. Allergy 1994;49:400–407.
18. Adlerberth I, Carlsson B, de Man P, et al: Intestinal colonization with Enterobacteriaceae in Pakistani and Swedish hospital-delivered infants. Acta Pediatr Scand 1991;80:602–610.
19. Mikelsaar M: Evaluation of the gastrointestinal microbial ecosystem in health and disease. Tartu Dissertationes Medicinae Universitatis Tartuensis, 1992.
20. Sepp E, Salminen S, Mikelsaar M: Effect of administration of Lactobacillus casei strain GG on the gastrointestinal microvbionta of newborns. Microb Ecol Health Dis 1993;6:309–314.
21. Sepp E, Julge K, Vasar M, et al: Intestinal microflora of Estonian and Swedish infants. Acta Pediatr 1997;86:956–961.
22. Hall MA, Cole CB, Smith SL, et al: Factors influencing the presence of faecal lactobacilli in early infancy. Arch Dis Child 1990;65:185–188.
23. Bennet R, Eriksson M, Tafari N, Nord CE: Intestinal bacteria of newborn Ethiopian infants in relation to antibiotic treatment and colonization by potentially pathogenic gram-negative bacteria. Scand J Infect Dis 1991;23:63–69.
24. Lencner AA, Lencner CP, Mikelsaar ME, et al: Die quantitative Zusammensetzung der Lactoflora des Verdauungstrakts vor und nach kosmischen Flugen unterschiedlicher Dauer. Nahrung 1984;28:607–613.
25. Schiffrin EJ, Brassart D, Servin AL, et al: Immune modulation of blood leukocytes in humans by lactic acid bacteria: criteria for strain selection. Am J Clin Nutr 1997;66:515S–520S.
26. De Simone C, Vesely R, Negri R, et al: Enhancement of immune response of murine Peyer's patches by a diet supplemented with yoghurt. Immunopharmacol Immunotoxicol 1987;98:87–100.
27. Standiford TJ, Arenberg DA, Danforth JM, et al: Lipoteichoic acid induces secretion of interleukin-8 from human blood monocyte: a cellular and molecular analysis. Infect Immun 1994;62:119–125.
28. Hoijer MA, Melief MJ, van Helden-Meeuwsen CG, et al: Detection of muramuric acid in carbohydrate fraction of human spleen. Infect Immun 1995;63:1652–1657.
29. Biberstine KJ, Rosenthal RS: Peptidoglucan fragment decrease food intake and body weight gain in rats. Infect Immun 1994;62:3276–3281.
30. Ellouz F, Adam A, Ciorbaru R, Lederer E: Minimal structural requirements for adjuvant activity of bacterial peptidoglucan derivates. Biochem Biophys Res Commun 1974;59:1317–1325.
31. Eckmann L, Kagnoff MF, Fierer J: Intestinal epithelial cells as watchdogs for the natural immune system. Trends Microbiol 1995;3:118–120.
32. Henderson B, Wilson M, Wren B: Are bacterial exotoxins cytokine network regulators? Trends Microbiol 1997;5:454–458.
33. Henderson B, Poole S, Wilson M: Microbial/host interactions in health and disease: who controls the cytokine network? Immunopharmacology 1996;35:1–21.
34. Meyer TA, Noguchi Y, Ogle CK, et al: Endotoxin stimulates interleukin-6 production in intestinal epithelial cells. Arch Surg 1994;129:1290–1295.
35. Parikh AA, Salzman AL, Fischer JE, Hasserlgren PO: Interleukin-1β and interferon-γ regulate interleukin-6 production in human intestinal cells. Shock 1997;8:249–255.
36. Parikh AA, Salzman AL, Kane CD, et al: IL-6 production in human intestinal epithelial cells following stimulation with IL-1β is associated with activation of the transcription factor NF-κB. J Surg Res 1997;69:139–144.
37. Liebermann TA, Baltimore D: Activation of interleukin-6 gene expression through the NF-κB transcription factor. Mol Cell Biol 1990;10:2327–2334.
38. Shimizu H, Mitomo K, Watanabe T, et al: Involvement of a NF-κB-like transcription factor in the activation of the interleukin-6 gene by inflammatory lymphokines. Mol Cell Biol 1990;10:561–568.
39. Tannock GW: Probiotic properties of lactic-acid bacteria: plenty of scope for fundamental R & D. Tibtech 1997;15:270–271.
40. Solis-Pereyra B, Aattouri N, Lemonnier D: Role of food in the stimulation of cytokine production. Am J Clin Nutr 1997;66:521S–525S.
41. Rangavajhyala N, Shahani KM, Sridevi G, et al: Nonlipopolysaccharide component(s) of Lactobacillus acidophilus stimulate(s) the production of interleukin-1 and tumor necrosis factor-α by murine macrophages. Nutr Cancer 1997;28:130–134.
42. Adlerberth I, Ahrné S, Johansson ML, et al: A mannose-specific adherence mechanism in Lactobacillus plantarum conferring binding to the human colonic cell line HT-29. Appl Environ Microbiol 1996;62:2244–2251.
43. Bengmark S: Ecoimmunonutrition: a challenge for the third millenium. Nutrition 1998;14:563–572.
44. Hybenová E, Drdák M, Guoth R, Gracák J: Utilisation of nitrates: a decisive criterion in the selection of lactobacilli for bioconservation of vegetables. Z Levensm Unters Forsch 1995;200:213–216.
45. Jonson S, Clausen E, Raa J: Amino acid degradation by a Lactobacillus plantarum strain from fish. Sys Appl Microbiol 1983;4:148–154.
46. Ashenafi M, Busse M: Growth of Bacillus cereus in fermenting tempeh made from various beans and its inhibition of Lactobacillus plantarum. J Appl Bacteriol 1991;70:329–333.

47. Muller M, Lier D: Fermentation of fructans by epiphytic lactic acid bacteria. J Appl Bacteriol 1994;76:406–411.
48. Murosaki S, Yamamoto Y, Ito K, et al: Heat-killed *Lactobacillus plantarum* L-137 suppresses naturally fed antigen-specific IgE production by stimulation of IL-12 production in mice. J Allerg Clin Immunol 1998;102:57–64.
49. Shida K, Makino K, Takamizawa K, et al: *Lactobacillus casei* inhibits antigen-induced IgE secretion through regulation of cytokine production in murine splenocyte cultures. Int Arch Allerg Immunol 1998;115:278–287.
50. Bengmark S (ed): Immunonutrition. Nutrition 1998;14:563–647.
51. Baten A, Ullah A, Tomazic VJ, Shamsuddin AM: Inositol-phosphate-induced enhancement of natural killer cell activity correlates with tumor suppression. Carcinogenesis 1989;10:1595–1598.
52. Bengmark S, Larsson K, Molin G: Gut mucosa reconditioning with species-specific lactobacilli, surfactants, pseudomucus and fibers: an invited review. Biotechnol Ther 1994–1995;5:171–194.
53. Kohen R, Shadmi V, Kakunda A, Rubinstein A: Prevention of oxidative damage in the rat jejunal mucosa by pectin. Br J Nutr 1993;69:789–800.
54. Zaporozhets TS, Besednova NN, Liamkin GP, et al: I. Antibacterial and therapeutic effectiveness of pectin from sea water grass zostera. Antibiot Khimioter 1991;36:24–26.
55. Zaporozhets TS, Besednova NN, Liamkin GP, et al: II. Immunomodulating properties of pectin from seawater grass zostera. Antibiot Khimioter 1991;36:31–34.
56. Best R, Lewis DA, Nasser N: The anti-ulcerogenic activity of the unripe banana (Musa species). Br J Pharmacol 1984;82:107–116.
57. Hills BA, Kirwood CA: Surfactant approach to the gastric mucosal barrier: protection of rats by banana even when acidified. Gastroenterology 1989;97:294–303.
58. Dunjic BS, Svensson I, Axelsson J, et al: Is resistance to phospholipase important to gastric mucosal protective capacity pf exogenous phosphatidylcholine? Eur J Gastroenterol Hepatol 1994;6:593–598.
59. Dunjic BS, Svensson I, Axelsson J, et al: Green banana protection of gastric mucosa against experimentally induced injuries in rats: a multicomponent mechanism? Scand Gastroenterol 1993;28:894–898.
60. Gibson GR, Beatty ER, Wang X, Cummings JH: Selective stimulation of bifidobacteria in the human colon by oligofructose and inulin. Gastroenterology 1995;108:975–982.
61. Deguchi Y, Morishita T, Mutai M: Comparative studies on synthesis of water-soluble vitamins among human species of bifidobacteria. Agrikc Biol Chem 1985;49:13–19.
62. Michel C, Lahaye M, Bonnet CH, et al: In Vitro fermentation of human faecal bacteria of total and purified dietary fibers from brown seaweeds. Br J Nutr 1996;75:263–280.
63. Anderson DMW, Brydon WG, Eastwood MA, Sedgwick DM: Dietary effects of sodium alginate in humans. Food Addit Contam 1991;8:225–236.
64. Anderson DMW, Brydon WG, Eastwood MA, Sedgwick DM: Dietary effects of propylene glycol alginate in humans. Food Addit Contam 1991;8:237–248.
65. Torsdottir I, Alpsten M, Holm G, et al: A small dose of soluble alginate-fiber affects postprandial glycemia and gastric emplyting in humans with diabetes. J Nutr 1991;121:795–799.
66. Biancardi G, Palmiero L, Ghirardi PE: Glucomannan in the treatment of overweight patients with osteoarthritis. Curr Ther Res Clin Exp 1989;46:908–912.
67. Doi K, Matssura M, Kowara A, Baba S: Treatment of diabetes with glucomannan. Lancet 1979;1:987–988.
68. Ebihara K, Masuhara R, Kiryama S: Effect of konjac mannan, a water-soluble dietary fiber, on plasma glucose and insulin responses in young men undergoing glucose tolerance test. Nutr Rep Int 1988;23:577–583.
69. Reffo GC, Ghirardi PE, Forattini C: Glucomannan is hypertensive outpatients: pilot clinical trial. Curr Ther Res Clin Exp 1988;44:22–27.
70. Mazutani T, Shimizu Y: Effect of konjak mannan on intestinal microflora and tumorigenesis. Gastroenterol Int 1998;11 (Suppl 1):52–55.
71. Fabia R, Ar'Rajab A, Johansson ML, et al: The effect of exogenous administration of *Lactobacillus reuteri* R2LC and oat fiber on acetic acid-induced colitis in the rat. Scand J Gastroenterol 1993;28:155–162.
72. Mao Y, Nobaek S, Kasravi B, et al: The effects of lactobacillus strains and oat fiber on methotrexate-induced enterocolitis in rats. Gastroenterology 1996;111:334–344.
73. Mao Y, Kasravi B, Nobaek S, et al: Pectin-supplemented enteral diet reduces severity of methotrexate induced enterocolitis in rats. Scand J Gastroenterol 1996;31:558–567.
74. Nobaek S, Klarin B, Jeppsson B, et al: Enteral administration of *Lactobacillus* R2LC and oat base changes blood clearance and organ distribution of *E. coli* cells in rats with experimental intraabdominal infection. In manuscript.
75. Adawi D, Kasravi FB, Molin G, Jeppsson B: Effect of *Lactobacillus* supplementation with and without arginine on liver damage and bacterial translocation in an acute liver injury model in the rat. Hepatology 1997;25:642–647.
76. Kasravi FB, Adawi D, Molin G, et al: Effect of oral supplementation of *lactobacilli* on bacterial translocation in acute liver injury induced by D-galactosamine. J Hepatol 1997;26:417–424.
77. Kasravi FB, Adawi D, Hagerstrand I, et al: The effect of pretreatment with endotoxin and lactobacillus on bacterial translocation in acute liver injury. Eur J Surg 1996;162:537–544.
78. Kasravi FB, Gebreselassie D, Adawi D, et al: The effect of endotoxin and *Lactobacillus* pretreatment on peritoneal macrophage behavior in acute liver injury in the rat. J Surg Res 1996; 62:63–68.
79. Mangiante G, Canepari P, Colucci G, et al: *Lactobacillus plantarum* reduces sepsis in exp pancreatitis. In manuscript.
80. Elmer GW, Surawics CM, McFarland LV: Biotherapeutic agents. a neglected modality for the treatment and prevention of selected intestinal and vaginal infections. JAMA 1996;275:870–876.
81. Kennedy RJ, Kirk SJ, Gardiner KR: Promotion of favourable gut flora in inflammatory bowel disease: a review article. In manuscript.
82. Van Saene HKF, Stoutenbeek CP, Miranda DR, Zandstra DF: A novel approach to infection control in the intensive care unit. Acta Anaesthesiol Belg 1983;3:193–208.
83. Cherbut C, Ferre JP, Corpet DE: Alterations of intestinal microflora by antibiotics: effects on fecal excretion, transit time and colonic motility in rats. Dig Dis Sci 1991;36:1729–1734.
84. Gismondo MR: Antibiotic impact on intestinal microflora. Gastroenterol Int 1998;11(Suppl 1):29–30.
85. Husni RN, Gordon SM, Washington JA, Longworth DL: Lactobacillus bacteremia and endocarditis: review of 45 cases. Clin Infect Dis 1997;25:1048–1055.
86. Patel R, Cockerill FR, Porayko MK, et al: Lactobacillemia in liver transplant patients. Clin Infect Dis 1994;18:207–212.
87. Horwitch CA, Furseth HA, Larson AM, et al: Lactobacillemia in three patients with AIDS. Clin Infect Dis 1995;21:1460–1462.
88. Rayes N, Hansen S, Müller AR, Bechstein WD, Bengmark S, Neuhaus P: SBD versus fibre containing enteral nutrition plus *lacrobacillus* or placebo to prevent bacterial infections after liver transplantation. European Transplant Society, 1999 meeting, Oslo, Norway, Abstract.

45
Liver: Multiple Organ Dysfunction and Failure

Arthur E. Baue

Hepatic failure and coma in patients with intrinsic liver disease, whether from cirrhosis, hepatitis, toxins, or congenital abnormalities have been studied extensively and are increasingly being treated in appropriate individuals by hepatic transplantation and other support mechanisms. What is known about liver failure as isolated or single organ failure and the hepatic support with an artificial liver are reviewed in depth in Chapter 46. Hepatic abnormalities occurring in otherwise normal individuals with previously normal livers who have had an injury or an operation require further study. I review here the place of liver dysfunction or failure as a part of multiple organ failure (MOF) and particularly as part of the domino effect leading to MOF.

Functional Changes in the Liver After Injury

Beecher originally measured a progressive low-grade rise in plasma bilirubin in battle casualties during World War II. He thought it was largely due to delayed resuscitation and the absorption of extravasated and hemolyzed blood.[1] In 1946 Bywaters described microscopic hepatocellular damage after injury.[2] Scott et al. reported on hepatic function in battle casualties in Korea, documenting that bilirubin levels frequently increased after injury and returned to normal or remained high in those who had complications.[3] Bromsulphalein retention was usually elevated and plasma prothrombin activity was depressed with abnormalities of cephalin flocculation and other changes. Thus a transient deficiency in hepatic function seemed to occur after injury. Nunes et al. found that moderate to severe jaundice developed in patients after shock and trauma 2–10 days after injury.[4] It suggested obstructive jaundice with conjugated hyperbilirubinemia and elevated alkaline phosphatase but no extrahepatic obstruction. In patients who survived, the jaundice usually resolved with no apparent residual liver injury. This situation resembled intrahepatic cholestasis. There was centrilobular congestion and necrosis. It was thought that it could be due to hepatic hypoxia. Champion et al. correlated peaks in bilirubin levels with transfusions, operations, hepatic dysfunction, sepsis, and septicemia.[5] Hepatic dysfunction was implicated in a large proportion of patients with posttraumatic jaundice that occurred as part of a spectrum of MOF. Biopsy specimens in patients at laparotomy or autopsy who had shock showed hepatocellular damage correlating with the jaundice peak. Rapid and progressively rising bilirubin levels implied a poor prognosis. Gottlieb et al. documented a marked reduction in hepatic blood flow after injury[6] that correlated with liver dysfunction.

Functional Changes in the Liver with Sepsis

Some years ago Neale et al. noted that abnormal liver function in seriously ill patients could be the result of extrahepatic infection.[7] Norton et al. found that more than one-third of patients with postoperative or postinjury hepatic failure had associated bacterial infection and that it carried a high mortality.[8] Royle and Kettlewell found that chronically ill patients with sepsis had abnormal hepatic function with lower concentrations of albumin and cholesterol and increased concentrations of alkaline phosphatase and serum glutamic oxalic transaminase (SGOT).[9] Striking abnormalities of the liver were found in patients who died of sepsis: midzonal and peripheral necrosis, acute inflammation, and cholestasis. Thus hepatocellular necrosis seems to be a characteristic of sepsis.

The mechanism for liver injury with sepsis is not completely understood. Part of the mechanism may be decreased blood flow in a patient with a hyperdynamic circulation in whom insufficient circulation is provided to the liver. Thus hepatocellular ischemia may be a factor. Second, cytokine- or mediator-induced damage to the liver could be a factor, as could oxidant injury. There are problems related to the reticuloendothelial system and the liver with immune complexes, complement activation, leukocyte clustering, leukoemboli, and a variety of other substances that may be circulating with the sepsis, such as permeability factors, elastase, coagulation factors, histamine, fibrinolysin, acid hydrolases from lysosomes, superoxides, fragment D, and others. In an extensive series of studies on hepatic blood flow and splanchnic oxygen consumption in injured and septic patients, Dahn et al. found that despite an increase in oxygen delivery to the splanchnic bed during sepsis there was regional hypermetabolism, increased metabolic demand, and an excessive discrepancy between splanchnic blood flow and the higher oxygen demand.[10-14] This situation may precipitate regional or central lobular ischemia within the liver.

The effect of liver disease on other organ systems has been studied extensively. It is now recognized that acute hepatic dysfunction due to many causes (particularly shock, injury, and sepsis) may adversely affect other organs.[10] Thus the liver may not only be damaged by the insult but may help perpetuate it. Some of it may be due to the production of cytokines, such as tumor necrosis factor by Kupffer cells of the liver.[15] Liver failure, whether acute or chronic, affects the central nervous system (hepatic coma), circulation (secondary hyperaldosteronism and other factors), kidney (hepatorenal syndrome),[16] metabolism, lungs,[17] and muscle, leading to loss of muscle mass. Thus, liver dysfunction may contribute to lung dysfunction and renal dysfunction and certainly affects metabolism in general. The lung and kidney can also adversely affect the liver.[18,19]

The relation of the liver and lungs in critically ill patients was confirmed in a study by Matuschak et al. in patients with severe liver disease.[17] The acute respiratory distress syndrome (ARDS) occurred in about 80% of patients. When ARDS and liver failure occurred together, the mortality approached 100%. The relation of these two may be due to the effects of sepsis, leukocyte activation, elastase, oxygen metabolites, and other factors on both organs.[18,19]

The arterial ketone body ratio (AKBR) is the ratio of acetoacetate to β-hydroxybutyrate in arterial blood. It is believed by many to be an excellent parameter for evaluating hepatic function and particularly the hepatic mitochondrial redox state. Hirasawa et al. found that the average AKBR among patients who survived was 0.62, and among nonsurvivors it was 0.37. There were no survivors among patients whose AKBR was <0.5. They used artificial liver support in patients with hepatic failure if the AKBR was <0.7.[20,21]

Therapy

Support of liver function after injury and sepsis is primarily prevention of hepatic damage. It requires rapid and adequate resuscitation with maintenance of adequate oxygen transport.[6] The evacuation or eradication of a septic focus, débridement of necrotic tissue to decrease the continuation of an inflammatory response, and early enteral nutritional support are extremely important for providing substrate for the liver through the gastrointestinal tract. In some circumstances selective decontamination of the digestive tract helps. Although there are approaches for applying mediator therapy, there is nothing specific now that helps the liver. Enteral nutrition has been associated with maintenance of normal metabolic energy expenditure and reduced stress hormone production (see Chapters 42, 44).

Conclusions

One can draw the following conclusions regarding liver alterations after injury whether the alterations are related to injury or to the complications of sepsis.[22,23] Markers of liver injury, particularly the bilirubin level, may not be evident initially. The same is true for other liver function tests and blood flows. With pulmonary failure the evidence is obvious, with hypoxia and labored ventilation. With the liver, however, the picture evolves only slowly. Although the injury may have occurred simultaneously in the lung, liver, and kidney, it is expressed late in the liver.

1. Early mild bilirubin elevations are associated with transfusions, hematomas, or anesthesia; they are transient and meaningless.
2. Increased bilirubin levels (>4 ml/dl, peaking at 8-12 days) indicate hepatic dysfunction from prior hypoxemic injury to hepatocytes and cellular injury with intrahepatic cholestasis.
3. Bilirubin levels that rise higher and remain high longer indicate sepsis and are associated with a greater incidence of MOF and increased mortality.

With jaundice there is cholestasis, biliary sludge, increased fat production, decreased liver redox potential, and increased ureagenesis with decreased hepatic amino acid clearance and reduced protein synthesis. There may be problems of endotoxin, cytokine, and other mediator clearance.

Posttraumatic hepatic insufficiency indeed contributes to morbidity and mortality in septic, injured, and postoperative patients. In the original description of MOF, I described hepatic dysfunction with peritonitis, inflammation, and decreased blood flow.[23] We have described many hepatic abnormalities produced by shock and trauma. Hepatic failure in patients with liver disease has been recognized for a long time. Now, however, we are aware of hepatic failure in patients with previously normal livers. The need to meet nutritional and energy requirements has been recognized. Jaundice after injury is common and has been recognized for years, but the recent identification of an early peak resulting from transfusions and hematomas, a second somewhat later peak related to hepatic dysfunction due to previous ischemia and hypoxemia of the liver, and a third peak caused by sepsis serve as a reminder of more serious underlying problems. The effects of shock and sepsis on the liver have been increasingly appreciated in altered hepatic metabolic activity and immune deficiency, as well as in other problems of synthetic activity of the liver. The best approach is prevention by rapid, adequate resuscitation, maintenance of high splanchnic blood flow, support of the lungs and kidneys, early adequate enteral nutrition to meet the metabolic needs of the patient and the liver, and prevention of sepsis or treating it early and adequately before MOF begins.

References

1. Beecher HK: The physiologic effect of wounds. In: Surgery in World War II. Washington, DC, Office of the Surgeon General, 1952.
2. Bywaters EG: Anatomical changes in the liver after trauma. Clin Surg 1946;6:19–39.
3. Scott R Jr, Howard JM, Olney JM Jr: Hepatic function of the battle casualty: the systemic response to injury. Int Abstr Surg 1956;102:209–222.
4. Nunes G, Blaisdell FW, Margaretten W: Mechanism of hepatic dysfunction following shock and trauma. Arch Surg 1970;100:546–556.
5. Champion HR, Jones RT, Trump BF, et al: A clinicopathologic study of hepatic dysfunction following shock. Surg Gynecol Obstet 1976;142:657–663.
6. Gottlieb ME, Sarfeh J, Stratton H, et al: Hepatic perfusion and splanchnic oxygen consumption in patients postinjury. J Trauma 1983;23:836–843.
7. Neale G, Coughey DE, Mollin DL, Booth CC: Effects of intrahepatic and extrahepatic infection on liver function. BMJ 1966;1:382–387.
8. Norton L, Moore G, Eiseman B: Liver failure in the postoperative patient: the role of sepsis and immunologic deficiency. Surgery 1975;78:6–13.
9. Royle GT, Kettlewell MGW: Liver function tests in surgical infection and malnutrition. Ann Surg 1980;192:192–194.
10. Dahn MS: Hepatic dysfunction in the critically ill and injured. Intensive Care World 1994;11(1):9–14.
11. Dahn MS, Mitchell RA, Lange P, Smith S, Jacobs LA: Hepatic metabolic response to injury and sepsis. Surgery 1994;117:520–530.
12. Dahn MS, Wilson RF, Lange P, Stone A, Jacobs LA: Hepatic parenchymal oxygen tension following injury and sepsis. Arch Surg 1990;125:441–443.
13. Dahn MS, Lange P, Lobdell K, Hans B, Jacobs LA, Mitchell RA: Splanchnic and total body oxygen consumption differences in septic and injured patients. Surgery 1986;101:69–80.
14. Dahn MS, Lange P, Wilson RF, Jacobs LA, Mitchell RA: Hepatic blood flow and splanchnic oxygen consumption measurements in clinical sepsis. Surgery 1990;107:295–301.
15. Bankey PE: Hepatic regulation of systemic inflammation following acute injury. Curr Opin Crit Care 1996;2:280–286.
16. Epstein M: The hepatorenal syndrome: newer perspectives. N Engl J Med 1992;327:1810–1811.
17. Matuschak GM, Rinaldo JE, Pincky MR, Gaalar JS, Van Thiel DH: Effect of endstage liver failure on the incidence and resolution of the adult respiratory distress syndrome. J Crit Care 1987;2:162–173.
18. Matuschak GM, Rinaldo JE: Organ interactions in the adult respiratory distress syndrome during sepsis. Chest 1988;94:400–406.
19. Callery MP, Kamdi T, Mangino MJ, Flye W: Organ interactions in sepsis: host defense and the hepatic-pulmonary macrophage axis. Arch Surg 1991;126:28–32.
20. Ohtake Y, Hirasawa H, Sugai T, et al: A study on arterial ketone body ratio (AKBR) and arterial ketone body concentration (KBC) in fulminant hepatitis. J Jpn Assoc Acute Med 1993;4:299–308.
21. Hirasawa H, Odaka M, Kobayashi H, et al: Serum osmolality gap and arterial ketone body ratio as indicators of the efficacy of plasma exchange in hepatic failure. Ther Plasmapheresis 1987;6:436–440.
22. Baue AE: Multiple organ failure: patient care and prevention. In: The Liver: Post-traumatic Hepatic Failure. St. Louis, Mosby-Year Book, 1990.
23. Baue AE: Multiple, progressive or sequential systems failure. Arch Surg 1975;110:779–781.

46
Liver: Hepatic Support and the Bioartificial Liver

Walid S. Arnaout and Achilles A. Demetriou

Severe liver failure continues to be one of the most challenging admitting diagnoses to an intensive care unit (ICU). Most patients present with an acute complication of a preexisting chronic liver disease such as gastrointestinal (GI) bleeding, hepatic encephalopathy, spontaneous bacterial peritonitis, or renal failure. In a smaller group, liver failure develops acutely without preexisting liver disease. These patients usually present with massive liver necrosis, profound coagulopathy, and encephalopathy often leading to deep coma and death. It is these patients who represent one of the most difficult therapeutic challenges in the ICU. This chapter outlines diagnostic and management issues in patients with acute liver failure.

Definitions

The definition of acute hepatic failure depends on the temporal relation between initial onset of illness and manifestation of jaundice, encephalopathy, and coagulopathy. The classic definition of Trey and Davidson for fulminant hepatic failure (FHF) is based on encephalopathy developing within 8 weeks from the onset of illness.[1] Bernau et al. defined FHF as acute hepatic failure complicated by encephalopathy occuring less than 2 weeks after the onset of jaundice; and the term subfulminant hepatic failure (SFHF) was introduced to describe acute hepatic failure complicated by encephalopathy developing between 2–12 weeks after the onset of jaundice.[2] Despite the various definitions and classifications of acute hepatic failure (Table 46.1), what all these definitions have in common is a lack of preexisting liver disease.

Etiology

The etiology of FHF falls in one of four major groups: viral, drug-induced, toxin-induced and miscellaneous. In the United States the most common etiology of FHF is acetominophen, particularly hepatitis B, which constituted approximately 20% of all cases in a recent multicenter combined series, followed by cryptogenic (15%) and idiosyncratic drug reactions (12%); viral hepatitis was less common.[3] Acetominophen is also the most common drug causing severe acute liver failure in Great Britain.[4]

Viral Hepatitis

Hepatitis A Virus

The incidence of fulminant and subfulminant hepatic failure in hepatitis A virus (HAV) infection is low, occuring in fewer than 0.01% of all causes.[2] Young patients with HAV infection rarely develop hepatic failure. The survival rate with medical therapy is relatively high, ranging from 40% to 60%.[5,6] Relapse of HAV occurs in 10% of patients, usually within 2–3 months after initial clinical improvement.[7] Relapse is recognized by an increase in serum transaminase and bilirubin levels with reappearance of the virus in the stool. If encephalopathy occurs during this period, the outcome is poor.[8]

Hepatitis B Virus

Fulminant and subfulminant hepatitis B virus (HBV) infections account for fewer than 1% of HBV infections, but it is the most common cause of virus-induced FHF.[9–11] As is the case for HAV infection, HBV infection results more commonly in FHF than SFHF.[2] Hepatitis B surface antigen (HBsAg) and HBV DNA are absent in some cases of HBV FHF.[12] These findings indicate that in FHF patients an enhanced immune response prevents further HBV replication and results in more rapid clearance of HBsAg. The survival rate in patients positive for HBsAg on presentation (17%) is much lower than that of patients who are HBsAg-negative (47%).[2] Clearance of HBsAg and HBV DNA results in better survival rates and a decreased incidence of recurrence after emergency liver transplantation.[13–16] In chronic carriers, reactivation of HBV is recognized by the reappearance of immunoglobulin M (IgM) anti-HBc antibody and HBV DNA.

Hepatitis D

Hepatitis D virus (HDV), a delta agent, is a defective virus that replicates only in the presence of HBsAg, which is used as the envelope protein. HDV RNA is detected only in 10% of patients

TABLE 46.1. Definitions of Liver Failure.

Parameter	Acute hepatic failure	Fulminant hepatic failure	Subfulminant hepatic failure	Hyperacute liver failure	Acute liver failure
Encephalopathy	No	Yes	Yes	Yes	Yes
Time from onset of jaundice to encephalopathy	None	<8 Weeks or <2 Weeks	2–12 Weeks	0–7 Days	8–28 Days
Cerebral edema	No	Frequent	Rare	Frequent	Frequent
Ascites	None	Rare	Frequent	Rare	Rare
Prognosis	Good	Poor to fair	Poor	Fair	Poor

with fulminant hepatitis D.[17] HDV can occur as either a co-infection with HBV or a superinfection in patients with chronic HBV.[18] HDV co-infection in an HBV patient increases the risk of FHF but decreases its associated mortality (52% vs. 73%).[19,20] In patients with fulminant HDV, co-infection occurs more often (53–77%) than superinfection (23–47%).[21] FHF due to HDV superinfection has a higher mortality rate (72% vs. 52%) and more often predisposes to chronic liver disease (54% vs. 31%) than FHF due to HDV co-infection.[22]

Hepatitis Non-A Non-B Non-C

Previously, FHF of indeterminate etiology was attributed to non-A non-B viral hepatitis. The extent of the contribution of HVC infection to the indeterminate group is unclear. In contrast to hepatitis A and B virus infections, SFHF is more common than FHF in hepatitis C patients. The ability to diagnose HCV infection has markedly improved with the detection of anti-HVC antibodies by enzyme-linked immunosorbent assay (ELISA II), recombinant immunoblot assay (RIBA) II, and HCV RNA by polymerase chain reaction (PCR).[23–25] Despite the availability of advanced serologic testing, there are still many cases of FHF and SFHF with indeterminate etiology.[2,26–28] These patients are placed in an NANBNC category, implying a viral etiology. A more accurate designation for this category is "indeterminate" because the etiology is unknown and it may or may not be due to undiagnosed viral hepatitis.

Drug-Induced Hepatotoxicity

Drug toxicity accounts for 15% of all cases of FHF and SFHF and usually runs a subfulminant course.[29] Drug ingestion results in liver injury in fewer than 1% of patients, with 20% of those patients developing FHF or SFHF. The risk of either FHF or SFHF increases with an increase in total drug dose, simultaneous ingestion of other drugs that induce or inhibit hepatic enzymes, and continuation of drug administration after the onset of liver disease.[2] Acetaminophen toxicity is the most common cause of drug-induced liver failure. Acetaminophen-induced FHF is usually associated with a better prognosis than FHF caused by nonacetaminophen drugs such as isoniazid, psychotropic drugs, antihistamines, and nonsteroidal antiinflammatory drugs.[30–35] Halothane-induced FHF occurs within 2 weeks of general anesthesia and is associated with high mortality.[36,37]

Toxins

Mushroom poisoning and industrial hydrocarbons are involved in most toxin cases. With mushroom poisoning the active agents are heat-stable and are not destroyed by cooking. Liver damage due to mushroom toxicity is delayed and is usually preceded by a few days of vomiting and diarrhea. Mushroom toxicity is associated with high mortality, up to 22% in one series.[38] Emergency liver transplantation can be successful.[29] Industrial hydrocarbons, such as carbon tetrachloride and trichloroethylene, are rare causes of FHF.[39] In Third World countries ingestion of aflatoxin and herbal medicines has been implicated as causes of FHF.

Miscellaneous Causes

Wilson's Disease

Wilson's disease may present as FHF or SFHF with intravascular hemolysis and renal failure.[40,41] A family history of liver and neurologic disease, Kayser–Fleischer rings, and low serum ceruloplasmin levels help establish the diagnosis. Mortality is high, and so early liver transplantation is indicated.[42,43]

Acute Fatty Liver of Pregnancy

Acute fatty liver of pregnancy is a rare cause of FHF, with a high mortality rate for both mother and infant. Delivery of the fetus results in regression of the microvesicular steatosis and abnormal liver tests. The risk of FHF is increased with misdiagnosis and continuation of the pregnancy. Liver transplantation has been performed successfully.[44]

In addition to the above-listed causes of FHF and SFHF, several other causes and disease processes known to cause liver failure in both adults and children are listed in Table 46.2.

Diagnosis and Treatment

Complications of Liver Failure

Liver failure is usually associated with multiple life-threatening complications and multisystem organ failure. Failure to recognize and aggressively treat these complications results in poor outcome. Patients at our institution are managed in a dedicated critical care unit, the Liver Support Unit (LSU), where all members of a multidisciplinary team have expertise in the treatment of severe forms of acute liver failure. Upon admission

TABLE 46.2. Common Causes of Fulminant and Subfulminant Hepatic Failure.

Infections
  Viruses
    Hepatitis A, B, C, D, E
    Hepatitis non-A-E (indeterminate)
    Herpes simplex, cytomegalovirus, Epstein-Barr virus, adenovirus
  Bacteria: Q fever
  Parasites: ameba

Drugs (acetominophen, nonacetominophen)

Toxins
  Mushrooms: *Amanita phalloides, A. verna, A. virosa; Lepiota* species
  Bacillus cereus
  Hydrocarbons: carbon tetrachloride, trichloroethylene, 2-nitropropane, chloroform
  Copper
  Aflatoxin
  Yellow phosphorus

Miscellaneous conditions
  Wilson's disease
  Acute fatty liver of pregnancy
  Reye syndrome
  Hypoxic liver cell necrosis
  Hypo- or hyperthermia
  Budd-Chiari syndrome
  Venoocclusive disease of the liver
  Autoimmune hepatitis
  Massive malignant infiltration of the liver
  Partial hepatectomy
  Liver transplantation
  Postjejunoileal bypass
  Galactosemia
  Hereditary fructose intolerance
  Tyrosinemia
  Erythropoietic protoporphyria
  Irradiation
  α_1-antitrypsin deficiency
  Niemann-Pick II (C)
  Neonatal hemochromatosis
  Cardiac tamponade
  Right ventricular failure
  Circulatory shock
  Tuberculosis

to the LSU, invasive monitoring including pulmonary artery catheter and arterial line placement, continuous pulse oximetry, and urinary catheter and nasogastric tube placement are instituted. Intracranial pressure (ICP) monitoring is initiated in patients suspected to have cerebral edema; endotracheal intubation is performed in patients who are comatose and require airway protection and mechanical ventilation. Neurologic assessment, including mental status and cognition evaluation, is performed frequently. Patients are placed in a quiet room, and sensory stimulation is kept at a minimum to avoid abrupt ICP elevations.

Fluid, Electrolyte, and Nutrition Management

Fluid management in FHF requires maintenance of euvolemia to avoid fluid overload, pulmonary edema, and dehydration. Extreme fluid shifts should be avoided; the presence of cerebral edema and intracranial hypertension require careful fluid administration to avoid expansion of the intravascular space and exacerbation of cerebral edema. Rapid bolus fluid administration should be avoided in favor of anticipatory adjustments in fluid delivery. Electrolyte and acid-base imbalances frequently occur in FHF. Most commonly seen are hyponatremia, hyperkalemia, hypocalcemia, hypophosphatemia, and hypomagnesemia. Calcium, phosphorus, and magnesium are supplemented as needed. Hyperkalemia could be multifactorial; usually it is secondary to liver necrosis, massive transfusion, acid-base imbalance, and renal failure. Acidosis results from increased lactic acid production and decreased hepatic handling of lactate by the failing liver. Compensatory respiratory alkalosis is present early; but if encephalopathy progresses, respiratory acidosis may result. GI losses of acid by a nasogastric tube or bicarbonate loss through diarrhea may further complicate the situation. Sodium or potassium bicarbonate infusions are used for severe acidosis. Acetate provides twice the bicarbonate load and is metabolized outside the liver. Thus continuous infusion of acetate salts can be utilized if sodium and potassium restrictions are severe.

The role of nutritional intervention in FHF is not clear. Hypoglycemia, if present, should be corrected rapidly by 50% dextrose infusion followed by a continuous intravenous infusion at 4 mg/kg/min. A 10% dextrose solution is usually an adequate vehicle, but higher concentrations of glucose should be considered with continued hypoglycemia or fluid restriction (or both). Caloric supplementation has not been extensively studied for FHF. Caloric requirements should be determined by indirect calorimetry, although patients rarely require more than 3000 kcal/day. Amino acids should be withheld initially to prevent excessive nitrogen load. Later, limited nitrogen supplementation (70-80 g protein/day) may be provided. FHF patients clinically demonstrate a high degree of catabolism leading to hypoalbuminemia, lymphopenia, and anergy.[45] Paradoxically, skeletal muscle catabolism releases amino acids and contributes to an increased plasma ammonia load. In this setting, supplemental nitrogen may offset the catabolic effect, which needs to be balanced with the risk of exacerbating hepatic encephalopathy. The type of proteins and amino acids delivered may be important. Aromatic amino acids are known neurotransmitter precursors; and it has been suggested that their products interfere with the activity of true neurotransmitters. The plasma branched-chain/aromatic amino acids ratio decreases steeply during encephalopathy.[46] Parenteral solutions of branched-chain amino acids have been utilized to favorably alter that ratio;[47] administration of branched-chain amino acid solutions has not been found to be beneficial when compared to use of conventional amino acid solutions.[48]

Hepatic Encephalopathy

The presence of hepatic encephalopathy and cerebral edema significantly influences the management and outcome of FHF patients. Autopsy studies demonstrate cerebral edema in 80% of patients who die from FHF.[49,50] Diagnosis of hepatic encephalopathy requires the recognition, and correction of other disorders affecting cerebral function, including electrolyte imbalance, azotemia, and hypoxia. Sedatives and paralytic agents should be avoided because of their effect on the central nervous system (CNS). If sedation or paralysis is required, use of short-acting agents is recommended, as the combination of poor hepatic function and shunting of blood away from the liver may greatly lengthen the drug elimination curve, complicating the interpretation of patient assessment.

The classic therapeutic objectives in hepatic encephalopathy have been to minimize ammonia formation, augment ammonia elimination, and correct factors that may result in deterioration of mental status and elevated intracranial pressure (ICP). Several studies demonstrated that increasing serum ammonia levels can induce hepatic encephalopathy.[51,52] Ammonia levels, however, do not correlate with the severity of encephalopathy, nor are they predictive of the development of encephalopathy. Additionally, ammonia is neuroexcitatory, and CNS depression is commonly seen with hepatic encephalopathy. Antibiotics and lactulose can be administered early in the course of the disease, though their efficacy in FHF-associated hepatic encephalopathy is not as established as in chronic liver disease.[48] Neomycin is a minimally absorbed antibiotic commonly used for gut decontamination. Lactulose is a synthetic disaccharide cathartic that can be delivered by the oral, nasogastric, or high enema route. The dosage is titrated to achieve two to four loose bowel movements per day. Lactulose is neither absorbed nor metabolized in the upper GI tract. Upon reaching the colon, bacterial degradation acidifies the luminal contents. This acidification inhibits coliform bacterial growth, thereby reducing ammonia production. Additionally, low intraluminal gut pH results in the conversion of ammonia to ammonium ions, which do not easily enter the bloodstream. The cathartic action of lactulose clears ammonium ions from the bowel. Aggressive lactulose therapy may induce volume depletion and result in severe electrolyte imbalance.

Neuroinhibitory processes may also contribute to the development of hepatic encephalopathy. The levels of the inhibitory neurotransmitter γ-aminobutyric acid (GABA) and its postsynaptic GABA receptor increased in a rabbit model of liver failure, but results were inconclusive in clinical studies.[53-55] Autopsies have demonstrated the presence of diazepam and desmethyldiazepam in brain tissue, indicating the existence of natural benzodiazepines.[56] Limited trials using fulmazenil, a pure benzodiazepine antagonist, suggest that hepatic encephalopathy can be transiently reversed.[57,58] This may allow one to test the neurologic integrity of comatose patients. However, lack of consistent response and the risk of seizure induction as a consequence of flumazenil administration, preclude the routine use of this medication and limit its usefulness.

Cerebral edema and intracranial hypertension develop rapidly in FHF and represent the leading cause of death in these patients. The cornerstone of management of cerebral edema is prevention, early recognition, and prompt treatment. Cerebral edema occurs in advanced stages of hepatic encephalopathy related to FHF and can be determined by clinical, radiologic or invasive methods. Clinical findings include decerebrate posturing, myoclonus, spastic rigidity, seizure activity, systolic hypertension, bradycardia, hyperventilation, and mydriasis with diminished pupillary response. Initially, the findings of cerebral edema are paroxysmal but later become persistent. Papilledema is usually a late finding. Noninvasive diagnostic modalities, including computed tomographic (CT) scanning, electroencephalographic (EEG) monitoring, and transcranial Doppler flow measurements, have not proved helpful for early detection or management of cerebral edema. CT scans of the brain are not sensitive for detecting early cerebral edema; 25–30% of patients with high ICP have no radiographic changes.[59-61] The CT scan, however, is useful for ruling out intracranial bleeding.

Currently, ICP monitoring is the best means for monitoring intracranial hypertension and is recommended for patients with grade III or IV encephalopathy to guide treatment. ICP can be measured using epidural, subdural, or intraventricular catheters. In a large comparative study, data from 262 patients with FHF were analyzed for incidence of bleeding or other complications. Although slightly less sensitive to ICP changes, epidural catheters had the lowest complication rate (3.8%) and lowest rate of fatal hemorrhage (1%).[62,63] Placement of an ICP monitor requires aggressive treatment of concomitant coagulopathy. Fresh frozen plasma (FFP) infusions are used to bring the prothrombin time to <20 seconds, and platelet transfusions are indicated if the patient is thrombocytopenic (<50,000/mm^3). Once ICP monitoring is established, FFP bolus administration is repeated as needed to keep the prothrombin time at $\leq$ 20 seconds.

The goal of invasive monitoring is to maintain the ICP at levels below 15 mmHg while maintaining a cerebral perfusion pressure (CPP) above 50 mmHg. CPP is calculated using the formula CPP = MAP − ICP, where MAP is the calculated mean arterial pressure. ICP monitoring allows aggressive management of cerebral edema; the same is true for measurement of CPP, which is a better predictor of outcome than ICP. The effect of either high ICP or low CPP on outcome following liver transplantation has not been studied in a randomized controlled fashion. However, it appears that elevated ICP secondary to severe cerebral edema is associated with an increased risk of developing irreversible brain damage and a grave outcome following liver transplantation.[64,65]

Management of elevated ICP involves use of hyperventilation, minimizing external stimulation, head elevation, maintenance of hemodynamic stability, and mannitol infusion. Dexamethasone administration has not been shown to have a beneficial effect.[66] Patients are usually sedated with a short-acting agent such as fentanyl in small boluses prior to any procedure, nascotracheal suction, venipuncture, or line placement. Mechanical hyperventilation lowers the ICP by lowering carbon dioxide pressure to 25–30 mmHg, which maximizes cerebral vascular constriction and reduces blood flow. This vascular effect progressively diminishes after 6 hours of therapy, though the clinical response is apparent for days. Mannitol infusions have an up to 80% response rate in patients without renal failure.[66] Serum osmolality should be measured frequently and maintained at 300–320 mosm. Mannitol should be withheld if osmolality is 320 mosm or higher, if renal failure occurs, or if oliguria and rising serum osmolality develop simultaneously. Repeated administration of mannitol may reverse the osmotic gradient. Thus mannitol should be discontinued if the ICP does not respond after the first few boluses.

Patients who fail to respond to conventional therapy could be placed in a barbiturate coma. Thiopental infusion has been shown to decrease cerebral metabolic activity, lower CNS oxygen demand, and protect the brain from ischemic injury secondary to decreased cerebral blood flow. In a retrospective, nonrandomized study thiopental infusion lowered the ICP and reduced mortality due to FHF.[67] In general, however, we find the effect of thiopental infusion on ICP transient and unpredictable.

Renal Impairment

Renal failure occurs in up to 50% of patients with FHF and has many etiologies.[68] Acute tubular necrosis is one of the most common causes of renal failure in patients with FHF, especially if the patient has not been resuscitated adequately, has experienced prolonged hypotension, or has ingested hepatotoxins that are also nephrotoxic (e.g., acetaminophen). Other causes of renal failure include hepatorenal syndrome and interstitial nephritis. Hepatorenal syndrome is the unexplained development of renal failure in both acute and chronic liver disease characterized by the development of azotemia, oliguria, low urinary sodium excretion (<10 mEq/day) and an increased urine/serum osmolality ratio in the absence of active urinary sediment.

Adequate urine volumes can be maintained with judicious use of loop diuretics and renal dose dopamine infusion. Depleted intravascular volume should be managed with administration of blood products, volume expanders, or both. Because plasma albumin is invariably low, salt-poor albumin solutions may be preferred over a carbohydrate-based volume expander. If oliguria is present, and especially if mannitol is administered to treat ICP, hemodialysis/hemofiltration may be needed to maintain optimal fluid volume.

Pulmonary Complications

Pulmonary complications, particularly pulmonary edema, aspiration pneumonia, and the development of adult respiratory distress syndrome (ARDS), occur frequently with FHF.[69] Pulmonary edema is seen in up to 40% of FHF patients. Supplemental oxygen and use of mechanical ventilation are always needed. Sedative and paralytic agents may be required to ensure tolerance of ventilation, but these measures should be used sparingly as they hinder neurologic evaluation. Aspiration pneumonia should be treated aggressively, as it could be a contraindication to transplantation.

Infectious Complications

Infection poses a serious threat to FHF patients: It places them at risk for sepsis and is a contraindication to liver transplantation. Immunologic defects include impaired opsonization, impaired chemotaxis, neutrophil and Kupffer cell function impairment, and complement deficiency.[70,71] Bacterial infection is reported to be prevalent in more than 80% of cases, usually with a respiratory or urinary source. Bacteria are seen in 25% of the patients, with *Staphylococcus* sp., *Streptococcus* sp., and gram-negative rods the most common pathogens.[72] Iatrogenic sources must be considered, as most patients have percutaneous lines and indwelling catheters. In one series fungal infections were found in a significant number of patients, with *Candida albicans* cultured from 33% of the patients studied.[73] These patients were predominantly in renal failure and had been treated with antibiotics for more than 5 days.

Despite the high prevalence of infection, prophylactic antibiotic administration is not advocated if there is no suspicion of active infection. The threshold for starting antibiotics should be low, however, as the usual clinical presentation with fever and leukocytosis is absent in 30% of FHF patients.[72] Specimens for surveillance cultures, looking for bacteria and fungi, must be obtained at frequent intervals from blood (peripheral and central lines), urine, sputum, and open wounds. Ascitic fluid is cultured if ascites is present. Additionally, chest radiographs are obtained to identify a developing infiltrate. High-dose, broad-spectrum antibiotics are started at the first sign of infection, narrowing the coverage as soon as an organism is identified. Special consideration is given to initiating amphotericin B or other antifungal therapy if there is a positive fungal culture or fever persists beyond 5 days especially in renal failure patients. The duration of antimicrobial therapy should be adjusted to the patient's situation. Follow-up cultures are recommended if a specific organism is isolated.

Coagulation and Hemorrhage

Bleeding is a frequent complication of FHF due to impaired hepatic synthesis of clotting factors, impaired platelet synthesis, and platelet dysfunction. GI bleeding is the most common clinical manifestation of coagulopathy and can be massive and life-threatening. Intracranial bleeding with neurologic sequelae is another devastating complication of coagulopathy in FHF.

Plasma activity of all clotting factors synthesized by the liver (II, V, VII, IX, X) is depressed with FHF. Factors II, VII, IX, and X are vitamin K-dependent; and factor V is synthesized independently of vitamin K availability. Factor 11, with a half-life of 2 hours, is the first to be depleted in the presence of hepatocellular dysfunction and is the first to be repleted with hepatocellular recovery. Increased consumption of clotting factors also may occur as a result of the development of disseminated intravascular coagulation (DIC). Thrombocytopenia and abnormalities of platelet function are frequently encountered with FHF. Acute splenomegaly, consumptive coagulopathy, and bone marrow suppression all contribute to the development of thrombocytopenia. Conversely, clearance of old platelets from the blood by the reticuloendothelial system is hindered, thereby creating an older, less effective platelet pool. In one study a mean platelet count of 50,000/mm^3 was associated with a high incidence of occurrence of GI hemorrhage.[73]

Presently, we transfuse platelets for thrombocytopenia (platelet count < 50,000/mm^3) or in cases of active bleeding.

The most common consequence of coagulopathy is GI bleeding. Though most episodes can be controlled, GI bleeding is associated with high morbidity and mortality. Bleeding in the lower GI tract is associated with a significant increase in plasma ammonia level and may exacerbate hepatic encephalopathy. H$_2$-receptor antagonists effectively control high acidity and reduce the incidence of GI hemorrhage. Cimetidine has been implicated as producing a high incidence of neurotoxicity, making ranitidine a preferred H$_2$-receptor antagonist in this setting. Proton-pump antagonists such as omeprazole have not been carefully studied in this setting.

In conclusion, medical management of FHF requires a multidisciplinary approach because of the complexity of the underlying disease. Hemodynamic and respiratory support plus prevention and treatment of cerebral edema are the major goals of medical therapy. Patients with rapidly deteriorating liver function require urgent orthotopic liver transplantation, as it remains the only effective therapeutic modality currently available.

Liver Transplantation

With the introduction of orthotopic liver transplantation (OLT) as the treatment of choice for irreversible severe acute liver failure, overall patients survival has improved from less than 20% to more than 60%.[74-78] As experience with OLT for FHF increased, it became obvious that appropriate patient selection was essential for a successful outcome. Patients with FHF should be considered for OLT prior to the development of irreversible brain injury or multisystem organ failure and sepsis. Patient selection for OLT must be based on a clear understanding of the natural history of the disease, the underlying etiology, and the likelihood of spontaneous recovery without transplantation.

Indications for OLT

Several prognostic criteria and indicators have been proposed in an attempt to predict OLT outcome in FHF patients. A number of variables have been found to be strongly related to prognosis, including: (1) etiology of the liver disease, such as acute hepatitis A or B infection or acetaminophen toxicity; (2) duration between onset of disease and encephalopathy; (3) degree of encephalopathy; (4) age of the patient; and (5) presence of cerebral edema. O'Grady and his associates at King's College in London have compiled the best criteria to predict a poor outcome following OLT (Table 46.3). These criteria have been validated in a prospective fashion in several series and have since been considered the standard for predicting outcome.[79]

In addition to biochemical and synthetic activities, investigators have considered assessment of the residual functional reserve of the liver as an indicator of prognosis. The acetoacetate/β-hydroxybutyrate ratio in an arterial blood sample (arterial ketone body ratio, or AKBR) is thought to reflect hepatic energy charge.[80] Galactose clearance is another func-

TABLE 46.3. King's College Hospital Early Indicators of Prognosis for Liver Transplantation for Fulminant Hepatic Failure.

Acetaminophen
  pH < 7.30 (irrespective of grade of encephalopathy) or
  Prothrombin time > 100 seconds (INR > 6.5)
  Serum creatinine > 3.4 g/dl
  Grade III or IV hepatic encephalopathy

Nonacetaminophen
  Prothrombin time > 100 seconds (INR > 6.5) (irrespective of grade of encephalopathy) or
  Any three of the following variables (irrespective of grade of encephalopathy)
    Age < 10 or > 40 years
    Etiology: non-A non-B hepatitis, halothane hepatitis, drug toxicity
    Duration of jaundice to encephalopathy > 7 days
    Prothrombin time > 50 seconds (INR > 3.5)
    Serum bilirubin > 17.6 g/dl

Data are from O'Grady et al.[79]

tional test that reflects both residual liver mass and hepatic blood flow.[81] It was considered a standard test of liver functional reserve in the past, and newer tests are often compared to it.

In summary, several schemes and prognostic criteria have been suggested and have been used in the clinical setting. Despite this wide variety of indicators, the King's College criteria remain the most widely used for predicting outcome in FHF patients. These criteria have been validated in several large series, and in most cases the prognosis could be predicted within a few hours of admission to a medical facility.

Patient Evaluation

As comprehensive ICU care is instituted, transplant surgeons and hepatologists assess a patient's overall condition, attempt to determine the underlying etiology of the disease, predict the chances of spontaneous recovery, and complete an emergency evaluation for liver transplantation. At our center the King's College criteria are used as a guideline to predict outcome without liver transplantation. In addition, we follow the general trend and degree of encephalopathy and changes in ICP and the degree of coagulopathy, metabolic acidosis, and renal failure. Once the initial assessment is made, an emergency evaluation for liver transplantation is completed often within 12-24 hours. Patients with FHF usually are not known to have underlying liver disease, and the evaluation workup must reveal the cause of the liver failure. The laboratory and diagnostic workup of patients with FHF is summarized in Table 46.4.

Bioartificial Liver Support System

As mentioned earlier, the morbidity and mortality of FHF remain exceptionally high, and liver transplantation is still the only effective therapeutic modality for most of the severe cases; however, the waiting period for transplantation remains long owing to the severe organ donor shortage. Therefore investigators have examined the use of "artificial liver support" systems to provide full metabolic, hemodynamic, physiologic support until

TABLE 46.4. Liver Transplant Evaluation for Fulminant and Subfulminant Hepatic Failure.

Laboratory workup
  CBC and differential
  Chemistry panel
  Coagulation profile
  24-Hour creatinine clearance
  Urinalysis
  Arterial blood gases
  Antinuclear antibodies, antimitochondrial antibody, ceruloplasmin, urinary copper, α_1-antitrypsin
  Tumor markers
  Rapid plasmin reagin test
  Thyroid function tests
  Alcohol and drug toxicology screen
Viral serologies
  Hepatitis A (IgM, IgG)
  Hepatitis B (HbsAg, HBcAb, HBV DNA)
  Hepatitis C
  Cytomegalovirus
  Epstein-Barr virus
  Human immunodeficiency virus
Cultures: bacterial, fungal, viral
  Blood
  Sputum
  Urine
  Ascites
12-Lead electrocardiography
Chest radiography
Pulmonary function tests
Abdominal ultrasonography with Doppler
Head CT scan

either the native liver regenerates or a liver becomes available for transplantation. During the past 30 years most therapeutic attempts focused primarily on the use of plasma detoxification, but they were either unsuccessful or not shown to have a significant impact on survival.[82-85]

With the severe shortage of human livers, several investigators have developed and tested a variety of xenogeneic-based liver support systems using whole-organ perfusion or isolated hepatocytes. We have developed a hybrid bioartificial liver (BAL) support system utilizing isolated porcine hepatocytes and charcoal in an extracorporeal perfusion circuit and have demonstrated its ability to provide detoxifying and synthetic functions in a series of in vitro and in vivo animal experiments. We subsequently initiated a clinical trial of the BAL support system for treating of patients with severe acute liver failure.

BAL Design

Hepatocytes

Methods of porcine hepatocyte isolation, purification, attachment to a collagen-coated matrix, cryopreservation, and storage have been previously described.[86,87] Five billion to seven billion viable (70–90%) fresh or cryopreserved hepatocytes were used for each patient treatment.

System Characteristics

The system has been standardized and modified and is currently manufactured by Circe Biomedical, Lexington, MA (HepatAssist "2000"). A detailed description of the system has been previously reported. The main components are (1) a plasmapheresis unit and a plasma reservoir; (2) activated cellulose-coated charcoal column; (3) oxygenator; (4) blood warmer; and (5) hollow-fiber module containing isolated microcarrier-attached porcine hepatocytes.[88] The module consists of an intracapillary chamber composed of several porous (0.2 μm) hollow fibers through which plasma flows and an extracapillary chamber surrounding the hollow fibers where the isolated hepatocytes are suspended. Plasma circulates through the fibers at 400 ml/min with free exchange of macromolecules across the surface of the fibers driven by a transmembrane pressure gradient. Following return from the BAL, plasma and blood cells are reconstituted and returned to the patient via a double-lumen venous dialysis catheter.

Patient Groups

All patients were admitted to the LSU. Three groups were studied: Group I ($n = 24$) patients had no previous history of liver disease, fulfilled all diagnostic criteria of FHF, and were candidates for OLT at the time of admission. Group II ($n = 3$) patients had undergone OLT and developed primary nonfunction (PNF) of the transplanted liver during the immediate postoperative period with rapid deterioration. Group III patients presented with acute exacerbation of known underlying chronic liver disease and were not candidates for OLT at the time of enrollment in the study ($n = 10$).

Patient Demographics

Patients were enrolled in the study when they developed stage III or IV encephalopathy while receiving optimal standard medical therapy. Table 46.5 and 46.6 summarize the demographic data and etiology of liver failure in all 37 patients.

TABLE 46.5. Patient Demographic Characteristics.

Group	Mean age (years)	Sex (M/F)	No. of ELS treatments	"Bridge time" (hours)
I	34.7 ± 13.0	11/13	2.3 ± 1.2	40.6 ± 28.0
II	48.3 ± 19.0	1/2	1.7 ± 1.1	83.0 ± 54.0
III	52.1 ± 11.0	7/3	1.8 ± 1.1	89.0 ± 31.0

ELS, extra-corporeal liver support.

TABLE 46.6. Disease Etiology.

Group	Virus	Indeterminate	Acetaminophen	Alcoholism	Ischemia	Autoimmune	Primary biliary cirrhosis
I	3	10	8	—	2	1	—
II	1	1	—	—	—	1	—
III	3	1	—	4	—	1	1

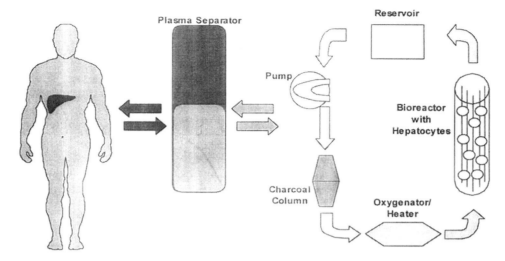

FIGURE 46.1. Bioartificial liver (BAL) circuit connected to plasma separator and patient. Blood is removed from the patient and is separated into plasma and blood cells in a plasma separator. Plasma is perfused through a charcoal column to reduce its toxicity before it perfuses a bioreactor hollow-fiber module containing five billion matrix-anchored viable porcine hepatocytes. A temperature regulator and oxygenator are included in the system to provide a physiologic environment for the cells. A volume reservoir allows high re-circulation flow through the circuit containing the porcine hepatocytes, thus enhancing the efficiency of the system.

Each BAL treatment lasted 6 hours. Plasma was separated and collected in a reservoir and recirculated through the BAL system at 400 ml/min. Finally, plasma was reconstituted with red blood cells and returned to the patient at the same rate at which it was removed (90–100 ml/min). Fig. 46.1 shows the BAL system with its main components.

Results

All patients who were OLT candidates were "bridged" successfully to OLT ($n = 18$). One patient with FHF and acute pancreatitis, initially a candidate for transplantation, underwent five treatments with the BAL and demonstrated remarkable neurologic recovery; however, he developed necrotizing pancreatitis and expired 21 days later with sepsis and multiorgan failure. Five additional patients with FHF secondary to acetaminophen toxicity treated with the BAL recovered fully without the need for liver transplantation. All 18 patients in group I and all 3 patients in group II were "bridged" to transplantation, experienced full neurologic and functional recovery, and were discharged from the hospital. Patients in group III experienced transient clinical improvement after BAL treatment. Two patients were able to recover enough native liver function to survive; they later became candidates for OLT and subsequently underwent successful OLT. The remaining eight patients died within 1–21 days (mean 7.1 days) following their last BAL treatment owing to variceal bleeding, sepsis, and multiorgan failure.

Neurologic Effects of the BAL

Patients in group I experienced remarkable neurologic improvement following BAL treatment(s) with reversal of the decerebrate posturing state, anisocoria, and sluggish pupillary reflex; moreover, the patients become more responsive to external stimuli. Brain stem function improved as shown by a higher Comprehensive Level of Consciousness Score (CLOCS). There was a significant reduction in ICP with a concomitant increase in cerebral perfusion pressure (CPP) (Table 46.7). It is important to note that when analyzing these data patients with ICP levels > 25 mmHg experienced the most dramatic reductions in ICP. Among patients with PNF, the impact of BAL treatments on the neurologic status was difficult to assess because they were in the postanesthetic period under the influence of paralyzing drugs; however, they did experience transient neurologic improvement after BAL treatments, manifested primarily by increased responsiveness.

TABLE 46.7. Effect of BAL on Neurologic Parameters.

Parameter	Pre-BAL	Post-BAL	p
Group I			
ICP (mmHg)	17.0 ± 1.5	10.9 ± 1.0	< 0.0002
CPP (mmHg)	70 ± 2	75 ± 2	< 0.04
GCS	6.8 ± 0.4	7.4 ± 0.4	< 0.01
CLOCS	24.7 ± 1.2	32.0 ± 1.1	< 0.000001
Group II			
GCS	5.0 ± 1.1	7.0 ± 1.4	< 0.2
CLOCS	29.7 ± 7.4	31.7 ± 7.9	< 0.5
Group III			
ICP (mmHg)	12.3 ± 0.9	14.0 ± 1.5	< 0.4
CPP (mmHg)	85 ± 1	98 ± 8	< 0.3
GCS	8.2 ± 0.7	8.4 ± 0.7	< 0.4
CLOCS	29.7 ± 2.3	34.0 ± 1.7	< 0.001

BAL, bioartificial liver; ICP, intracranial pressure; CPP, cerebral perfusion pressure; GCS, glasgow coma score; CLOCS, comprehensive level of consciousness score.

Metabolic Effects of the BAL

Metabolic effects of the BAL treatment on liver function, renal function, hematologic, and coagulation parameters are shown in Tables 46.8 and 46.9. Changes in serum transaminases, prothrombin time, and creatinine were noted. Plasma amino acid levels were measured at the beginning and end of each BAL treatment. There was a significant ($p < 0.01$) increase in the branched-chain/aromatic amino acids ratio (BCAA/AAA) from 0.75 ± 0.07 to 0.98 ± 0.07, which is one of the many possible reasons for the observed improvement in the degree of encephalopathy. This increase was primarily due to a reduction in AAA levels.

Toxic Liver Syndrome

Despite a multidisciplinary, aggressive approach, few patients with FHF develop a "toxic liver syndrome" characterized by severe intracranial hypertension, profound lactic acidosis, hemodynamic instability, and multisystem organ failure. This has led to the suggestion that removal of the necrotic liver may result in improved hemodynamic status and a decrease in ICP. In such extreme cases, a two-stage procedure has been applied: total hepatectomy with end-to-side portocaval shunt followed by liver transplantation when an allograft becomes available. The largest experience with this procedure was reported by Ringe et al.[89] Thirty-two adults with "toxic liver syndrome" underwent total hepatectomy and portocaval shunt. Thirteen patients did not show any signs of improvement after hepatectomy and died rapidly owing to multisystem organ failure, but 19 became more stable and underwent the full procedure. Patients were anhepatic for 987 ± 433 minutes (range 395–2489 minutes). Only seven patients remained alive at follow-up of 3–46 months.

We have used this approach to treat an 18-year-old female patient with uncontrollable cerebral edema secondary to FHF; she underwent total hepatectomy and portocaval shunt followed by OLT 14 hours later.[90] During the anhepatic period she was treated with the BAL. With artificial liver support, there was reversal of severe neurologic dysfunction, normalization of ICP, and a decrease in the serum ammonia level. The patient had a complete recovery with no neurologic deficit. A second patient with FHF has been treated with the same approach at our unit with a successful long-term outcome. It appears that in highly selected patients with severe "toxic metabolic state" and uncontrollable intracranial hypertension, total hepatectomy and portocaval shunt, preferably with some form of artificial liver support, followed by OLT may be considered a desperate measure to salvage these patients.

Conclusions

Liver failure remains a serious, liver-threatening condition for which there is still no fully effective therapy. In a small percentage of patients the native may regenerate, and patients recover with intense supportive management. Most patients do

TABLE 46.8. Effect of BAL on Liver Function Tests.

Test	Pre-BAL	Post-BAL	p
Group I			
AST (U/L)	1255 ± 261	879 ± 148	< 0.002
ALT (U/L)	1075 ± 184	674 ± 120	< 0.000005
Alkaline phosphatase (U/L)	116 ± 7	90 ± 5	< 0.0000001
Bilirubin (mg/dl)			
Total	17.9 ± 1.5	14.6 ± 1.2	< 0.000001
Direct	8.5 ± 1.0	6.4 ± 0.6	< 0.000001
Indirect	9.3 ± 0.8	7.9 ± 0.7	< 0.0000007
Group II			
AST (U/L)	5661 ± 2613	2821 ± 1291	< 0.1
ALT (U/L)	2139 ± 704	1633 ± 544	< 0.05
Alkaline phosphatase (U/L)	108 ± 15	83 ± 9	< 0.03
Bilirubin (mg/dl)			
Total	19.1 ± 2.2	14.7 ± 1.7	< 0.009
Direct	3.8 ± 1.3	3.1 ± 0.8	< 0.2
Indirect	15.3 ± 2.3	11.6 ± 1.3	< 0.05
Group III			
AST (U/L)	692 ± 374	723 ± 409	< 0.5
ALT (U/L)	349 ± 126	281 ± 114	< 0.06
Alkaline phosphatase (U/L)	117 ± 10	119 ± 22	< 0.9
Bilirubin (mg/dl)			
Total	26.0 ± 2.7	21.6 ± 2.2	< 0.000003
Direct	12.8 ± 1.5	10.3 ± 1.2	< 0.000006
Indirect	13.2 ± 1.8	11.3 ± 1.5	< 0.002

BAL, bioartificial liver; AST, aspartate aminotransferase; ALT, alanine aminotransferase.

TABLE 46.9. Effect of BAL on Metabolic and Renal Function Parameters.

Test	Pre-BAL	Post-BAL	p
Group I			
Glucose (mg/dl)	126 ± 5	175 ± 7	< 0.0000006
Ammonia (µmol/L)	160 ± 8	134 ± 6	< 0.0002
Lactate (mmol/L)	4.4 ± 0.7	4.2 ± 0.6	< 0.2
Albumin (g/dl)	3.12 ± 0.08	2.6 ± 0.10	< 0.0000006
BUN (mg/dl)	18.9 ± 2.5	17.0 ± 2.0	< 0.0000008
Creatinine (mg/dl)	1.5 ± 0.2	1.1 ± 0.1	< 0.000001
Group II			
Glucose (mg/dl)	117 ± 26	144 ± 24	< 0.06
Ammonia (µmol/L)	81 ± 9	91 ± 13	< 0.03
Lactate (mmol/L)	13.1 ± 2.9	13.2 ± 2.2	< 0.9
Albumin (g/dl)	3.7 ± 0.3	2.7 ± 0.1	< 0.01
BUN (mg/dl)	12.0 ± 2.4	11.5 ± 2.7	< 0.4
Creatinine (mg/dl)	1.6 ± 0.3	1.6 ± 0.3	< 1.0
Group III			
Glucose (mg/dl)	141 ± 9	171 ± 11	< 0.001
Ammonia (µmol/L)	173 ± 31	131 ± 15	< 0.08
Lactate (mmol/L)	5.7 ± 1.1	5.6 ± 0.9	< 0.9
Albumin (g/dl)	3.0 ± 0.1	2.6 ± 0.1	< 0.00003
BUN (mg/dl)	12.8 ± 1.5	35.5 ± 3.2	< 0.0004
Creatinine (mg/dl)	2.8 ± 0.3	2.2 ± 0.2	< 0.00002

BAL, bioartificial liver; BUN, blood urea nitrogen.

not recover, and liver transplantation is the only therapeutic alternative. Unfortunately, patients can die or develop irreversible brain damage while waiting for an organ. Thus in addition to comprehensive and dedicated ICU care, there is a need for a liver support system that can "bridge" these patients until a liver becomes available for transplantation or the native liver regenerates. The complexity of the liver is such that we are unable to provide full replacement of all liver functions for any significant length of time with any of the existing systems. The critical question then becomes: What are the critical liver functions that need to be supported to improve patient survival?

Intracranial hypertension and cerebral edema are the two most common causes of death among patients with FHF. Therefore for a liver support system to be effective, it has to arrest or reverse the rapid development of intracranial hypertension, which eventually leads to brain stem herniation, irreversible brain damage, and death. Our data suggest that treatment with the BAL along with aggressive, diligent medical management can result in a significant reduction in ICP. Based on the preliminary data presented here, the BAL appears to serve as a "bridge" to OLT. It is significant that treatment with the BAL alone (without OLT) was sufficient to support five patients until their native liver regenerated and ultimately recovered.

The remarkable survival obtained in our FHF patients is due to a combination of clinical teamwork with highly specialized skills and possibly the introduction of this innovative liver support technology. The role of the latter remains to be defined in a controlled randomized trial setting, which is currently in progress. For this or other liver support systems to play a meaningful role in the management of patients with exacerbation of underlying liver disease processes, such patients must be treated early while they have a residual liver mass that can potentially recover following the acute precipitating event.

References

1. Trey C, Davidson C: The management of fulminant hepatic failure. Prog Liver Dis 1970;3:282–298.
2. Bernuau J, Rueff B, Benhamou JP: Fulminant and subfulminant liver failure: definitions and causes. Semin Liver Dis 1986;6:97–106.
3. Schiodt FV, Atillasoy E, Shakil AO, et al: Etiology and outcome for 295 patients with acute liver failure in the United States. Liver Transplant Surg 1999;5:29–34.
4. O'Grady JG, Schalm SW, Williams R: Acute liver failure: redefining the syndrome. Lancet 1993;342:273–275.
5. Gimson AES, White YS, Eddleston ALWF, et al: Clinical and prognostic differences in fulminant hepatitis type A, B and non-A, non-B. Gut 1983;24:1194–1198.
6. Joshi YK, Gandhi BM, Tandon BN: Spectrum of hepatitis A virus infection in India [abstract]. Hepatology 1983;3:1060.
7. Sjogren MH, Tanno H, Fay O, et al: Hepatitis A virus in stool during clinical relapse. Ann Intern Med 1987;106:221–226.
8. Ritt DJ, Whelan G, Werner DJ, et al: Acute hepatic necrosis with stupor or coma: an analysis of 31 patients. Medicine 1969;48:151–172.
9. Redeker AG: Viral hepatitis. Am J Med Sci 1975;270:9–16.
10. Lettau LA, McCarthy JG, Smith MH, et al: Outbreak of severe hepatitis due to delta and hepatitis B virus in parenteral drug abusers and their contacts. N Engl J Med 1987;317:1256–1262.
11. Novick DM, Farci P, Croxson TS, et al: Hepatitis D virus and HIV antibodies in parenteral drug abusers who are hepatitis B surface antigen positive. J Infect Dis 1988;158:795–803.
12. Gimson AES, Tedder RS, White YS, et al: Serological markers in fulminant hepatitis B. Gut 1983;24:615–622.
13. Jones EA, Schafer DF. Fulminary hepatic failure. In: Zakim D, Boyer TD (eds) Hepatology: A textbook of liver disease. Philadelphia: Saunders, 1990:460–492.
14. Woolf IL, El Sheikh N, Cullens H, Lee WM, Eddleston AL, Williams R, et al: Enhanced HBsAb production in pathogenesis of fulminant viral hepatitis type B. Br Med J 1976;2(6037):669–671
15. Samuel D, Bismuth A, Mathieu D, Arulnaden JL, Reynes M, Benhamou JP, et al: Passive immunoprophylaxis after liver transplantation in HBsAg-positive patients. Lancet 1991;337(8745):813–815.
16. Todo S, Demetris AJ, Van Thiel D, Teperman L, Fung JJ, Starzl TE: Orthotopic liver transplantation for patients with hepatitis B virus-related liver disease [see comments]. Hepatology 1991;13(4):619–626.
17. Mas A, Buti M, Esteban R, Sanchez-Tapias JM, Costa J, Jardi R, et al: Hepatitis B virus and hepatitis D virus replication in HBsAg-positive fulminant hepatitis. Hepatology 1990;11(6):1062–1065.
18. Rizzetto M. The delta agent. Hepatology 1983;3(5):729–737.
19. Saracco G, Macagno S, Rosina F, Rizzetto M: Serologic markers with fulminant hepatitis in persons positive for hepatitis B surface antigen. A worldwide epidemiologic and clinical survey. Ann Intern Med 1988;108(3):380–383.
20. Govindarajan S, Chin KP, Redeker AG, Peters RL: Fulminant B viral hepatitis: role of delta agent. Gastroenterology 1984;86(6):1417–1420.
21. Smedile A, Farci P, Verme G, Caredda F, Cargnel A, Caporaso N, et al: Influence of delta infection on severity of hepatitis B. Lancet 1982;2(8305):945–947.
22. Purcell RH, Rizzetto M, Gerin JL: Hepatitis delta virus infection of the liver. Semin Liver Dis 1984;4(4):340–346.
23. Kotwal GJ, Baroudy BM, Kuramoto IK, McDonald FF, Schiff GM, Holland PV, et al: Detection of acute hepatitis C virus infection by ELISA using a synthetic peptide comprising a structural epitope. Proc Natl Acad Sci USA 1992;89(10):4486–4489.
24. Polito AJ, DiNello RK, Quan S, Andrews W, Rose J, Lee F, et al: New generation RIBA hepatitis C strip immunoblot assays. Ann Biol Clin (Paris) 1992;50(5):329–336.
25. Bukh J, Purcell RH, Miller RH: Importance of primer selection for the detection of hepatitis C virus RNA with the polymerase chain reaction assay. Proc Natl Acad Sci USA 1992;89(1):187–191.
26. Rakela J, Lange SM, Ludwig J, et al: Fulminant hepatitis: Mayo Clinic experience with 34 cases. Mayo Clinic Proc 1985;60:289–292.
27. Castells A, Salmeron JM, Navasa M, et al: Liver transplantation for acute liver failure: analysis of applicability. Gastroenterology 1993;105:532–538.
28. Gazzard BG, Portmann B, Murray-Lyon IM, et al: Causes of death in fulminant hepatic failure and relationship to quantitative histologic assessments of parenchymal damage. Q J Med 1975;44:615–626.

29. Bernuau J, Benhamou J-P: Fulminant and subfulminant hepatic failure. In: McIntyre N, Benhamou J-P, Bircher J, Rizzetto M, Rodes J (eds) Oxford Textbook of Clinical Hepatology. Oxford, Oxford Medical Publications 1991;921–942.
30. Dickinson DS, Bailey WC, Huschowitz BI, et al: Risk factors for isoniazid (INH)-induced liver dysfunction. J Clin Gastroenterol 1981;3:271–279.
31. Centers for Disease Control: Severe INH-associated hepatitis—New York, 1991-1993. MMWR 1993;42:545–547.
32. Danan G, Bernuau J, Moullot X, et al: Amitriptylline-induced fulminant hepatitis. Digestion 1984;30:179–184.
33. Rabinovitz G, Van Thiel DH: Hepatotoxicity of non-steroidal anti-inflammatory drugs. Am J Gastroenterol 1983;1696–1704.
34. Danan G, Trunet P, Bernuau J, et al: Pirprofen-induced fulminant hepatitis. Gastroenterology 1985;89:210–213.
35. Zimmerman HJ: Update of hepatotoxicity due to classes of drugs in common clinical use: non-steroidal drugs, anti-inflammatory drugs, antibiotics, antihypertensives, and cardiac and psychotropic agents. Semin Liver Dis 1990;10:322–338.
36. Carney FMT, Van Dyke RA: Halothane hepatitis: a critical review. Anesth Analg 1972;51:135–160.
37. Lewis JH, Zimmerman HJ, Ishak KG, et al: Enflurane hepatotoxicity: a clinicopathological study of 24 cases. Ann Intern Med 1983;98:984–992.
38. Floersheim GL: Treatment of human amatoxin mushroom poisoning: myths and advances in therapy. Med Toxicol 1987;2:1–9.
39. Ruprah M, Mant TGK, Flanagan RJ: Acute carbon tetrachloride poisoning in 19 patients: implications for diagnosis and treatment. Lancet 1985;1:1027–1029.
40. Rector WG Jr, Ushida T, Kanel GC, et al: Fulminant hepatitis and renal failure complicating Wilson's disease. Liver 1984;4:341–347.
41. McCullough AJ, Fleming CR, Thistle JL, et al: Diagnosis of Wilsons's disease presenting as fulminant hepatic failure. Gastroenterology 1983;84:161–167.
42. Peleman RP, Galavar JS, Van Thiel DH, et al: Orthotopic liver transplant for acute and subacute hepatic failure in adults. Hepatology 1987;7:484–489.
43. Stremmel W, Meyerose K-W, Niederau C, et al: Wilson disease: clinical prevention, treatment and survival. Ann Intern Med 1991;115:720–726.
44. Amon E, Allen SR, Petrie RH, et al: Acute fatty liver of pregnancy associated with preeclampsia: management of hepatic failure with postpartum liver transplantation. Am J Perinatol 1991;8:278–279.
45. O'Keefe SJ, El-Zayadi AR, Carraher TE, et al: Malnutrition and immunoincompetence in patients with liver disease. Lancet 1980;2:615–617.
46. Ansley JD, Isaacs JW, Rikkers LF, et al: Quantitative tests of nitrogen metabolism in cirrhosis: relation to other manifestations of liver disease. Gastroenterology 1978;75:570–579.
47. Ferenci P: Critical evaluation of the role of branched-chain amino acids in liver disease. In: Thomas JC, Jones EA (eds) Recent Advances in Hepatology. Edinburgh, Churchill Livingstone, 1986;137–154.
48. Marsano L, McClain C: How to manage both acute and chronic hepatic encephalopathy. J Crit Illness 1993;8:579–600.
49. Ware AJ, D'Agostina A, Combs B: Cerebral edema: a major complication of massive hepatic necrosis. Gastroenterology 1971;61:877–884.
50. Sik DBA, Hanid MA, Trewby PN, et al: Treatment of fulminant hepatic failure by polyacrylonitrile membrane hemodialysis. Lancet 1977;2:1–3.
51. Conn HO, Lieberthal MM: The Hepatic Coma Syndromes and Lactulose. Baltimore, Williams & Wilkins, 1979.
52. Gabuzda GL Jr, Philips GB, Davidson CS: Reversible toxic manifestation in patients with cirrhosis on the liver given cation-exchange resins. N Engl J Med 1952;248:124–130.
53. Minuk GY, Winder A, Burgess EJ, et al: Serum gamma-aminobutyric acid (GABA) levels in patients with hepatic encephalopathy. Hepatogastroenterology 1985;32:171–174.
54. Maddison JE, Dodd PR, Morrison M, et al: Plasma GABA, GABA-like activity and the brain: GABA-benzodiazepine receptor complex in rats with chronic hepatic encephalopathy. Hepatology 1987;7:621–628.
55. Levy LJ, Leek J, Losowsky MS: Evidence for gamma-aminobutyric acid binding in the plasma of humans with liver disease and hepatic encephalopathy. Clin. Science 1987;73:531–534.
56. Basile AS, Hughes KD, Harrison PM, et al: Elevated brain concentration of 1,4-benzodiazepines in fulminant hepatic failure. N Engl J Med 1991;325:473–478.
57. Grimm G, Ferenci P, Katzenschager R, et al: Improvement of hepatic encephalopathy treated with flumazenil. Lancet 1988;2:1392–1394.
58. Bansky G, Meier PJ, Riederer E, et al: Effects of the benzodiazepine receptor antagonist flumazenil in hepatic encephalopathy in humans. Gastroenterology 1989;97:744–750.
59. Munoz SJ, Robinson M, Northrup B, et al: Elevated intracranial pressure and computed tomography of the brain in fulminant hepatic failure. Hepatology 1991;13:209–212.
60. Lidofsky SD, Bass NM, Preger MC, et al: Intracranial pressure monitoring and liver transplantation for fulminant hepatic failure. Hepatology 1992;16:1–7.
61. Wijdicks EFM, Plevak DJ, Rakela J, et al: Clinical and radiologic features of brain edema in fulminant hepatic failure. Mayo Clin Proc 1995;70:119–124.
62. Sidi A, Mahla ME: Non-invasive monitoring of cerebral perfusion by transcranial Doppler during fulminant hepatic failure and liver transplantation. Anesth Analg 1995;80:194–200.
63. Blei AT, Olafsson S, Webster S, et al: Complications of intracranial pressure monitoring in fulminant hepatic failure. Lancet 1993;341:157–158.
64. Inagaki M, Shaw BW Jr, Schafer DF, et al: Advantages of intracranial pressure monitoring in patients with fulminant hepatic failure. Gastroenterology 1992;102:A826.
65. Jenkins JG, Glasgow JF, Black GW, et al: Reye's syndrome: assessment of intracranial pressure monitoring. BMJ 1987;294:337–338.
66. Canalese J, Gimson A, Davis C, et al: Controlled trial of dexamethasone and mannitol for the cerebral edema of fulminant hepatic failure. Gut 1982;23:625–629.
67. Forbes A, Alexander GJM, O'Grady JG, et al: Thiopental infusion in the treatment of intracranial hypertension complicating fulminant hepatic failure. Hepatology 1989;10:306–310.
68. Ring-Larsen H, Palazzo U: Renal failure in fulminant hepatic failure and in terminal cirrhosis: a comparison between incidence, types and prognosis. Gut 1981;22:585–591.
69. Trewby PN, Warren R, Contini S, et al: Incidence and pathophysiology of pulmonary edema in fulminate hepatic failure. Gastroenterolgoy 1978;74:859–865.

70. Bailey RJ, Woolf IL, Cullens H, et al: Metabolic inhibition of polymorphonuclear leukocytes in fulminate hepatic failure. Lancet 1976;1:1162–1163.
71. Imawari M, Hughes RD, Love CD, et al: Fibronectin and Kupffer cell function in fulminant hepatic failure. Dig Dis Sci 1985;30:1028–1033.
72. Rolando N, Harvey F, Brahm J, et al: Prospective study of bacterial infection in acute liver failure: an analysis of fifty patients. Hepatology 1990;11:49–53.
73. Rolando N, Harvey F, Brahm J, et al: Fungal infection: a common, unrecognized complication of acute liver failure. J Hepatol 1991;12:1–9.
74. O'Grady JG, Langley PG, Isola LM, et al: Coagulopathy in fulminant hepatic failure. Semin Liver Dis 1986;6:159–163.
75. Schafer DF, Shaw BW: Fulminant hepatic failure and orthotopic liver transplantation. Semin Liver Dis 1989;9:189–194.
76. Emond JC, Aran PP, Whitington PF, et al: Liver transplantation in the management of fulminant hepatic failure. Gastroenterology 1989;96:1583–1588.
77. Bismuth H, Samuel D, Gugenheim J, et al: Emergency liver transplantation for fulminant hepatitis. Ann Intern Med 1987;107:337–341.
78. Ascher NL, Lake JR, Emond JC, et al: Liver transplantation for fulminant hepatic failure. Arch Surg 1993;128:677–682.
79. O'Grady JG, Alexander GJM, Hayallar KM, et al: Early indicators of prognosis in fulminant hepatic failure. Gastroenterology 1989;97:439–445.
80. Saibara T, Onishi S, Sone J, et al: Arterial ketone body ratio as a possible indicator for liver transplantation in fulminant hepatic failure. Transplantation 1991;51:782–786.
81. Ranek L, Andreasen PB, Tygstrup N: Galactose elimination capacity as a prognostic index in patients with fulminant hepatic failure. Gut 1976;17:959–964.
82. Fox IJ, Langnas AN, Ozaki CF, et al: Successful application of extracorporeal liver perfusion for the treatment of fulminant hepatic failure; a technology whose time has come. Am J Gastroenterol 1993;88:1876–1881.
83. Gimson AES, Braude S, Mellon PJ, et al: Earlier charcoal hemoperfusion in fulminant hepatic failure. Lancet 1982;2:681–683.
84. Redeker AG, Yamahiro HS: Controlled trial of exchange transfusion therapy in fulminant hepatitis. Lancet 1973;1:3–6.
85. Cooper GN, Karlson KE, Clowes GHA, et al: Total body washout and exchange: a valuable tool in acute hepatic coma and Reye's syndrome. Am J Surg 1977;133:522–530.
86. Demetriou AA (Ed) Support of the Acutely Failing Liver. Medical intelligence Unit. Austin TX, RG Landes, 1994.
87. Morsiani E, Rozga J, Scott HC, et al: Automated liver cell processing facilitates large-scale isolation and purification of porcine hepatocytes. ASAIO J 1995;41:155–161R.
88. Watanabe FD, Claudy JP, Hewitt WR, et al: Clinical experience with a bioartificial liver (BAL) in the treatment of severe liver failure: a phase I clinical trial. Ann Surg 1997;225:484–494.
89. Ringe B, Pichlmayr R, Lubbe N, et al: Total hepatectomy as a temporary approach to acute hepatic or primary graft failure. Transplant Proc 1988;20:552–557.
90. Rozga J, Podesta L, LePage E, et al: Control of cerebral edema by total hepatectomy and extracorporeal liver support in fulminant hepatic failure. Lancet 1993;342:898–899.

Part VI
Therapeutic Horizons

47
Laboratory Markers to Support Early Diagnosis of Infection and Inflammation

Franz J. Wiedermann, Wolfgang Schobersberger, Bernhard Widner, Dietmar Fries, Barbara Wirleitner, Georg Hoffmann, and Dietmar Fuchs

Severe infection and sepsis with consecutive multiple organ dysfunction or failure (MODS) are major causes of morbidity and mortality in modern intensive care units (ICUs).[1] The four criteria for systemic inflammatory response syndrome (SIRS)—body temperature, leukocyte count, heart rate, respiration rate—may have an infectious or noninfectious etiology and are neither specific nor sensitive for sepsis.[2] Bacteriologic evidence of infection, although considered the gold standard, may have some drawbacks. Blood cultures are highly specific for detection of a septicemia but have an overall sensitivity of only 25–42%.[3] Negative blood cultures do not exclude sepsis, and multiple samples may be required over extended periods before positive cultures emerge.

In recent years a variety of laboratory and immunologic parameters have been proposed as possible markers for diagnosis and monitoring of infection and sepsis. C-reactive protein (CRP) is an acute-phase protein produced by the liver. Plasma concentrations are normally below 10 mg/L but increase severalfold after trauma, inflammation, and other stimuli that involve tissue damage.[4] Bacterial infection is also a potent stimulus, leading to rapid elevation of CRP as early as 4 hours after an inflammatory stimulus, attaining maximum levels within 24–72 hours.[5] Interleukin-6 (IL-6) is thought to be the main mediator stimulating CRP production, but other cytokines such as IL-1β and tumor necrosis factor (TNF) are also involved.[6] Two studies in critically ill patients showed that daily measurements of CRP were useful for detecting sepsis; CRP was more sensitive than body temperature and the white blood cell count and may be used to indicate successful treatment.[7,8]

Proinflammatory cytokines are undoubtedly involved in the pathophysiology of sepsis. For example, TNFα concentrations have been found to be significantly elevated in patients dying of acute meningococcal sepsis and malaria.[9,10] Plasma concentrations of IL-1β, the other suggested key initiator of the inflammatory response, have been shown to be increased in patients with septic shock[11] or not.[12] Calandra et al. reported that IL-6 was detected in 64% of patients at the onset of septic shock, but these levels diminished within 24 hours.[11]

Although high IL-6 levels at the onset of the disease were related to length of survival, they were not a useful indicator of outcome in patients with septic shock.[13] In a study of 251 nonselected patients admitted to the ICU plasma TNF concentrations were increased in 17%, plasma IL-1β in 6%, IL-6 in 77%, and IL-8 in 21% at presentation. There was no relation between bacteremia or the presence of SIRS and plasma cytokine concentrations.[14]

The laboratory diagnostic relevance of cytokine measurements is often hampered by the reliability of concentrations measured in body fluids. The biologic half-life of bioactive molecules such as cytokines may be short; and once the compounds are released into the circulation they may bind rapidly to cell-surface receptors or their soluble forms.[15] This may explain why cytokine measurements are often not satisfactory for clinical diagnostic use, even when they are considered to be the main players within the pathogenesis of, for example, sepsis. In addition, the stability of cytokines in serum of plasma specimens does not always agree with the requirements for laboratory diagnostic tests, as they often degrade rapidly. Serum soluble receptors of cytokines such as soluble IL-2 receptor or soluble TNF receptors (sTNFRs) turned out to be much better immune system parameters for diagnostic purposes,[16] although their biologic function is not yet fully understood. As for sTNFRs, soluble receptors on the one hand may have an antiinflammatory role by binding circulating cytokines, thereby counteracting their modulatory effects; alternatively, by this action they may also extend the half-life of cytokines in the circulation.

In addition to cytokines and cytokine receptors, a few other parameters have proved to be of predictive value in patients developing sepsis. Among them, procalcitonin and neopterin seem to represent powerful alternatives or additional means for immunologic monitoring in patients at risk for developing sepsis. Especially the combination of these two parameters seems to allow better decision making during the early phase and the later course of sepsis. Their analytic behavior circumvents the above-mentioned diagnostic limitations of short-lived compounds and allows routine application. These parameters allow insight into important aspects in the pathophysiology of sepsis. In this chapter measurement of procalcitonin and neopterin for early diagnosis and inflammation is being reviewed.

Procalcitonin

Procalcitonin (PCT), with a molecular mass of 13 kDa, is a polypeptide consisting of 116 amino acids. It is the precursor protein of the hormone calcitonin, which consists of 32 amino acids. Active calcitonin is produced from PCT by means of specific proteolytic enzymes in the C-cells of the thyroid gland. The synthesis of PCT and calcitonin starts with the transcription of a 141-amino-acid-containing peptide, so-called pre-PCT. This protein contains a signal sequence (amino acids 1–25), the N-terminal region PCT (N-ProCT), the sequence of calcitonin, and the C-terminal region of PCT called katacalcin. The signal sequence mediates uptake of the protein in the endoplasmic reticulum (ER), where the signal peptide is degraded and the remaining protein is PCT including the amino acid sequence of calcitonin in positions 60–91. Calcitonin is split off from PCT by further proteolysis.[3]

In healthy humans PCT levels are <0.1 ng/ml.[17] During severe infections (bacterial, parasitic, fungal) with systemic manifestations, the PCT level may rise to >100 ng/ml. After endotoxin injection, PCT begins to increase at 3–4 hours in the blood of healthy volunteers and then rises rapidly to reach a plateau at 6 hours, remaining elevated at least 24 hours (Fig. 47.1). The half-life is 25–30 hours. In the same patients, TNFα and IL-6 peak at 90 minutes and 3 hours and reach baseline concentrations at 6 and 8 hours, respectively. The fact that TNFα and IL-6 peaked before the appearance of PCT in plasma suggests that these cytokines play a role in inducing PCT formation and its release.[18] Calcitonin and PCT are both elevated in sera of patients with thyroid carcinoma in accordance with the transformation of PCT to calcitonin in thyroid C-cells.[19] The type of cells producing PCT during severe infection is not known yet. Thyroid is not the sole tissue involved in the secretion, as an infection-associated rise of PCT was shown in a thyroidectomized patient with septicemia.[17] The liver and neuroendocrine cells in the lung are possible sites of extrathyroidal PCT production in septic patients.[20]

It has been demonstrated that PCT mRNA is expressed by human mononuclear cells (MNCs) and modulated by lipopolysaccharide (LPS) and sepsis-related cytokines. Therefore MNCs may also be one of the sources for elevated plasma PCT levels in septic patients.[21] However, in a whole-blood model, LPS stimulation on blood samples from healthy volunteers showed no production of PCT, in contrast to large amounts of TNFα, IL-1β, IL-6 and IL-8.[22] Despite the markedly increased levels of PCT in severe systemic inflammation and sepsis, the mature calcitonin hormone remained normal or increased only slightly. One possible explanation relates to the intracellular processing of PCT to calcitonin. Hypothetically, either the massively increased biosynthesis of the prohormone overwhelms the cellular posttranslational capacity, or the processing enzymes are dysfunctional, deficient, absent, or inhibited by endotoxin and cytokines.[23]

The physiologic role of PCT in the human organism is not yet known. It is conceivable that the PCT that binds to the calcitonin receptor and appears to be active in osteoclast bioassays may exert biologic activity.[24,25] In a minimal-mortality hamster model of sepsis it was shown that the injection of PCT in humans (which in healthy animals was incapable of inducing death) causes augmentation of mortality in humans. More importantly, a significant reduction in mortality can be achieved in the hamster model of sepsis by administering a neutralizing antibody known to be reactive with endogenous PCT.[26]

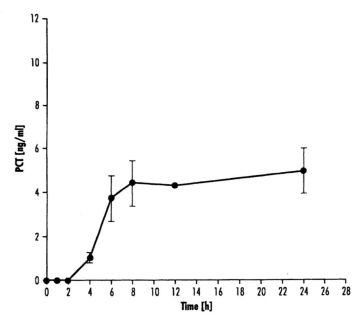

FIGURE 47.1. Serial procalcitonin concentrations in plasma of normal subjects injected with endotoxin (4 ng/kg body weight) at time zero. Note that procalcitonin was not detectable between 0 and 2 hours, but it became detectable in all subjects at 4 hours. Results are expressed as the mean ± SEM. There was only one reading at 12 hours, so there is no SEM. (From Dandona et al., Procalcitonin increase after endotoxin injection in normal subjects. J Clin Endocrinol Metab 1983;56:802–887; © The Endocrin Society.)

Measurement

Procalcitonin in blood specimens is usually determined using immunoassays (e.g., LUMItest PCT; Brahms Diagnostica, Berlin, Germany).[26] Serum or plasma specimens can be stored at −20°C until measured. The analytic sensitivity of this assays is 0.1 ng/ml, and the normal range of healthy controls without infection is 0.1–1.0 ng/ml. The sandwich assay involves two antibodies. The first antibody, which is of fixed to the test tubes, binds to the katacalcin sequence. The second antibody identifies the calcitonin sequence of PCT and is labeled with luminescence. When the reaction takes place the tracer is completely removed from the test tube, and the chemiluminescence measured is directly proportional to the PCT content.[27]

Clinical Applications

Differential Diagnosis of Viral and Bacterial Infections

During severe generalized bacterial infections with systemic manifestations, PCT levels may rise over 100 ng/ml. In contrast, an inflammatory response to viremia leads to only a small elevation in PCT levels.

Assicot et al. showed that children (newborns to age 12 years) with severe bacterial infections had high serum concentrations of PCT at diagnosis (range 6–53 ng/ml); and the levels decreased rapidly during antibiotic therapy. In contrast, patients with peripheral bacterial colonization or local infections without sepsis and patients with viral infections had concentrations within the normal range or slightly above normal (0.1–1.5 ng/ml).[17] Similar results were reported by Gendrel et al., who determined serum PCT in newborns at the time of admission to the pediatric or obstetric unit.[28] Their results are shown in Fig. 47.2. In children with meningitis the initial CRP, cerebrospinal fluid (CSF) proteins, and white blood cell (WBC) count in CSF were not sufficiently discriminative to distinguish between bacterial and viral meningitis. PCT was discriminative in all cases: The mean PCT in bacterial meningitis was 61 ng/ml (rang 4.8–335 ng/ml) and 0.33 ng/ml in viral meningitis (range 0–1.7 ng/ml).[29]

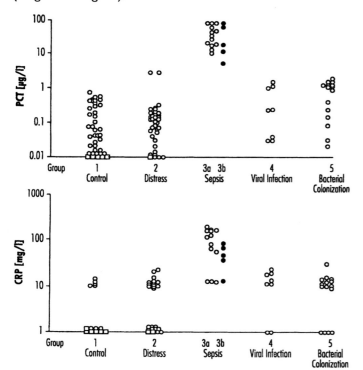

FIGURE 47.2. Comparison of C-reactive protein (CRP) and procalcitonin in 177 neonates. The low specificity of CRP in systemic bacterial infections compared to that of procalcitonin is seen in the distribution of CRP and procalcitonin values. There are five groups of patients: (1) controls ($n = 86$); (2) neonates with symptoms of distress without clinical signs of an infection ($n = 50$); (3) patients with clinical symptoms of sepsis and a positive blood culture (3a) or cerebrospinal fluid (3b) ($n = 13$); (4) patients with viral infections ($n = 8$, negative blood culture and positive isolation of the virus); (5) patients with bacterial colonization ($n = 15$, positive mucocutaneous cultures and negative blood and urine cultures). In the control group the procalcitonin levels were less than 0.71 ng/ml. Open square, 10 patients; open circles, 1 patient. (From Gendrel et al., Procalcitonin as a marker for the early diagnosis of neonatal infection. J Pediatr 1996;128:570–573.)

There are some limitations to the use of PCT for detecting neonatal infections because PCT peaks between 24 and 36 hours after birth (>2 ng/ml). During this time markedly increased concentrations and clear increases in comparison to the first hours of life can be observed in the absence of relevant bacterial infection.[30] In premature and term infants specific events (e.g., respiratory distress syndrome, hemodynamic failure) determined the PCT concentration during the first 10 days of life, independent of any bacterial infections.[31]

Procalcitonin seems to be a specific marker of bacterial sepsis in human immunodeficiency virus (HIV)-infected patients, as the baseline plasma level of PCT was low (0.50 ± 0.37 ng/ml), even during the latest stages of HIV disease. In HIV-infected patients with parasitic, viral, fungal, or mycobacterial infections and bacterial pneumonia or other localized bacterial infections, PCT levels were less than 2.1 ng/ml.[32]

Fungal Infections, Malaria, and Tropical Diseases

There are conflicting results regarding the diagnostic role of PCT in fungal infections. High serum PCT levels were reported during disseminated candidiasis in a patient after liver transplantation and in two patients with microbiologically documented *Candida* infection among 15 patients with septic shock.[33,34] After heart transplantation PCT was significantly elevated during bacterial, fungal, or protozoal infection.[35] In two immunodeficient patients there was a failure of PCT to indicate severe fungal infection (*Aspergillus fumigatus* and *Candida albicans*, respectively); and in two cases of disseminated aspergillosis after bone marrow transplantation there was only a moderate increase of PCT.[36,37] The above-mentioned study in HIV-infected patients also showed only a moderate increase of PCT in the presence of fungal infections. Why PCT synthesis is less impressive in fungal infections than in bacterial infections remains to be clarified. The low PCT values are probably associated with the immunodeficient or aplastic status of the patients.

Increased PCT plasma concentrations have been reported in patients with severe malaria. During the course of therapy the levels declined within a few days. In patients with suspected malaria the high specificity and negative predictive value suggest that PCT can serve as rapid exclusion test for acute malaria.[38]

Smith et al. described markedly elevated PCT plasma concentrations (up to >1000 ng/ml) in patients with melioidosis, a tropical disease caused by the gram-negative bacillus *Pseudomonas pseudomallei*. The plasma concentrations of PCT correlated well with the severity of the disease and with mortality.[39]

Sepsis and Multiorgan Dysfunction Syndrome

When PCT is compared with other routinely measured parameters for inflammation/infection, such as the WBC count, platelet count, or CRP levels, PCT seems to be more sensitive and specific for monitoring septic patients.[40,41] Al-Nawas et al. showed that 215 patients fulfilling SIRS criteria had a mean PCT level of 0.6 ng/ml; 53 patients with SIRS and microbiologically documented infection (but negative blood cultures) showed a mean level of 6.6 ng/ml; 49 patients with SIRS and a positive blood culture had a mean level of 8.5 ng/ml; and 20 patients with septic shock showed a mean level of 34.7 ng/ml. At a cutoff point of 0.5 ng/ml for infection, the sensitivity was 60%, specificity 79%, positive predictive value 61%, and negative predictive value 78%.[42] Elevated PCT levels dropped significantly within 48 hours in the case of successful surgical treatment of the septic focus. Persistence of elevated or increasing PCT levels were related to failure to eliminate the septic focus and were associated with high mortality (Fig 47.3).[43] In patients with peritonitis the kinetics of PCT levels had excellent prognostic value, with a sensitivity of 84% and a specificity of 91%, whereas single PCT levels do not allow prediction of the prognosis.[41] Another study showed that the value of procalcitonin was significantly elevated in nonsurvivors compared with survivors on the day sepsis was diagnosed. PCT increased continuously in nonsurvivors and decreased in survivors during severe inflammation.[44]

Pancreatitis

A clinical study showed that an increase in plasma PCT was closely related to biliary pancreatitis; the highest plasma PCT levels were found in patients with cholangitis. All patients with toxic pancreatitis (e.g., alcohol abuse) or idiopathic pancreatitis had normal PCT levels despite excessive increases in acute-phase proteins such as CRP and IL-6.[45]

The finding that elevated PCT levels are associated with a biliary origin of acute pancreatitis could not be confirmed by Rau et al. They assumed that the reported difference between biliary and toxic origin of pancreatitis was due to a lack of continuous serum PCT monitoring and proper morphologic stratification into infected/septic and noninfected patients. Their results showed that median concentrations of PCT were significantly higher in acute pancreatitis patients with infected necrosis than in those with sterile necrosis. In patients with edematous pancreatitis the overall median concentrations of PCT were low. After surgical treatment of infected necrosis, the median PCT values continued to be higher in patients with persisting pancreatic sepsis than in those having an uneventful postoperative course.[46]

Transplantation

The PCT values for patients with acute graft rejection after renal transplantation did not differ significantly from those of healthy transplant recipients. In contrast, PCT was clearly elevated during invasive bacterial infection or partial graft necrosis. Postoperatively, PCT rose to peak levels on the first and second days and mostly declined to normal within 1 week after renal transplantation.[47] After liver transplantation an increase in plasma PCT (up to 40 ng/ml) was observed without any clinical or laboratory signs of systemic infection. A continuous twofold daily reduction of this value down to 0.5 ng/ml was associated with a complication-free clinical course.[48] In patients after heart transplantation PCT levels were significantly elevated compared to those in allograft recipients without complications during bacterial, fungal, or protozoal infection. PCT was not elevated during acute rejection and was not affected by immunosuppressive drugs.[35]

Autoimmune Disorders and Neoplastic Disorders

In patients with systemic lupus erythematosus (SLE) and with systemic antineutrophil cytoplasm antibody (ANCA)-associated vasculitis but without systemic infection, serum PCT

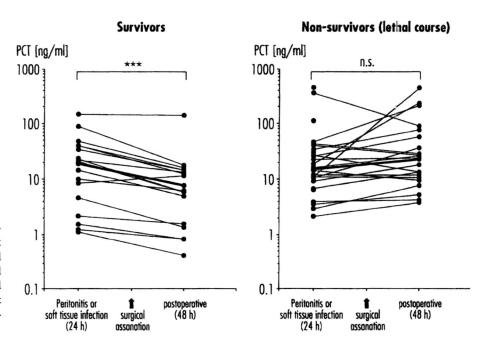

FIGURE 47.3. Procalcitonin serum concentrations in patients with peritonitis or deep soft tissues infections who survived ($n = 17$) and those with a lethal course ($n = 25$). A surgical operation was performed on day 1 in all patients. Wilcoxon-test: ***$p > 0.001$; n.s., not significant. (From Gramm et al.,[43] with permission of S. Karger AG, Basel.)

levels were within the normal range (i.e., <0.5 ng/ml), whereas the values for neopterin, IL-6, and CRP were elevated in patients with active underlying disease. Systemic bacterial infections were associated with PCT levels that were markedly elevated.[49] Another study confirmed normal PCT levels (<0.5 ng/ml) in patients with active rheumatoid arthritis and SLE but recommended that PCT levels of <1 ng/ml be the cutoff for invasive infections in patients with ANCA-positive vasculitis.[50]

In cases of active Wegener's granulomatosis (WG) most of the patients during active WG and all during inactive WG had PCT levels in the normal range. In 3 of 26 patients who had highly active WG but definitely no infection, serum PCT concentrations were markedly elevated (0.8–3.3 ng/ml).[51]

Some malignant tumors synthesize PCT or similar peptides as a paraneoplastic phenomenon: medullary C-cell carcinoma of the thyroid and small-cell carcinoma of the lung. These malignant cells may synthesize both calcitonin and PCT, and increased concentrations are present in the plasma.[52]

PCT Plasma Levels after Surgery and Trauma

After minor and aseptic operations (e.g., total hip replacement, peripheral vascular surgery, or herniotomy) and minor abdominal surgery (e.g., cholecystectomy) increased PCT concentrations were detected in 32% of the patients, but they were rarely (< 8%) above 1 ng/ml. After cardiac and thoracic surgery, PCT elevations above 2 ng/ml occurred in only 8% of the patients and remained below 0.5 ng/ml in 41% of the patients. Interestingly, after abdominal surgery with anastomosis of the intestine 95% of patients had increased PCT; the concentrations were above 2 ng/ml in 25% of the patients in this group. High PCT concentrations were also observed occasionally after major abdominal operations (e.g., Whipple) and abdominothoracic surgery affecting the mediastinum or retroperitoneum (e.g., esophagectomy, abdominal or thoracic aortic aneurysm repair). In contrast, CRP plasma concentrations were elevated postoperatively in almost all patients, regardless of the type of operation. Maximum postoperative plasma levels of PCT were mostly observed on day 1 but could also be found on days 2–5, independent of the postoperative course.[53] In the case of a slow decrease or even a further increase in PCT levels during the postoperative period, a systemic inflammation or septic complication is likely.[41,43]

After severe trauma PCT is released nonspecifically with no signs of pretrauma infection/inflammation (Fig. 47.4) (our unpublished observations). An early, transient release of PCT into the circulation was observed during the first 3 days after severe trauma, and the amount of circulating PCT seemed proportional to the severity of tissue injury and hypovolemia, yet unrelated to infection. The peak PCT level was significantly higher in patients who developed MODS.[54] During the late posttraumatic period (day 7), although the CRP concentrations remained elevated in all patients the PCT concentrations were raised only in septic patients.[55]

Inhalation injury following a burn induced release of PCT correlating positively with mortality. PCT plasma levels did not correlate with the extent of skin surface area burned but was strongly correlated with pulmonary injury.[56] In contrast, Carsin et al. reported that PCT levels, which were elevated in all patients without any proven infection, correlated well with the severity of skin burn injury and were not associated with smoke inhalation injury. PCT and IL-6 peaks within 24 hours were good prognostic factors for mortality.[57]

Conclusions

The propeptide of calcitonin, PCT, comprises a new parameter in the diagnosis of infection. Serum PCT concentrations increase during severe bacterial and parasitic infections. In viral infections there is no elevation or only a mild increase. The role during fungal infections remains to be clarified. The serum concentrations of PCT increase only during severe bacterial infections accompanied by systemic signs. If bacterial infections are localized or are not accompanied by systemic signs, there is no or only a moderate change in the PCT concentration. PCT may be helpful in the differential diagnosis for generalized inflammation of infectious origin versus noninfectious origin (e.g., bacterial infection or acute rejection reaction after organ transplantation, biliary or toxic pancreatitis, in cases of bacterial

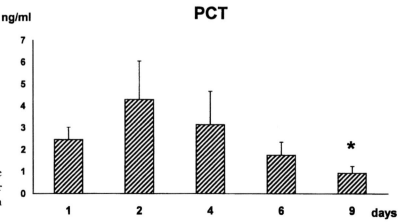

FIGURE 47.4. Time course of procalcitonin (PCT) after severe mechanical trauma. Blood was collected within 12 hours after trauma (1), on days 2–6, and on day 9 after injury. Mean values + SEM are shown ($n = 23$).

TABLE 47.1. Relation of Procalcitonin Concentrations to Inflammatory Conditions Drawn from Existing Data.

Patient condition	Procalcitonin (ng/ml)
Normal subjects	<0.5
Chronic inflammatory processes	<0.5–1.0
Viral infections	<0.5–2.0
Mild to moderate localized bacterial infections	<0.5–2.0
SIRS (multiple trauma, burns)	5–20
Severe bacterial infections, sepsis, MOF	10–1000

Data are from Meisner et al.[53]

TABLE 47.2. Neopterin Concentrations for Monitoring Activation of Cellular Immunity in Human Diseases.

Condition	Clinical application of neopterin assay
Allograft transplantation	Detects immunologic complications such as rejection and infection
	Supports the differential diagnosis
Infection	Supports the differential diagnosis (viral vs. bacterial)
	Monitors therapy (e.g., pulmonary tuberculosis)
	Predicts disease development (e.g., HIV infection)
Autoimmune disease	Supports the differential diagnosis (e.g., osteoarthritis vs. rheumatoid arthritis)
	Monitors therapy
Malignant disease	Predicts disease progression and survival

infection in patients with autoimmune disease, and in the diagnosis of bacterial or viral meningitis). During postoperative and posttraumatic SIRS, the PCT level may be elevated during the first 5 days, depending on the type of operation and the severity of the trauma. In the case of a slow decrease or even a further increase in PCT levels, a septic complication is likely. In comparison with clinical and other laboratory parameters for sepsis (e.g., fever, leukocytosis, or CRP level), PCT shows high specificity and sensitivity. CRP levels remain elevated for several days even after the septic focus has been eradicated or when a systemic inflammation is diminishing and the patient is clinically improving.[40,43] In contrast, PCT serum levels show excellent correlation with the clinical course, increasing and returning to the normal range more quickly than CRP after removal of the septic source.[40]

The question of whether routine determination of PCT in intensive care patients can provide information additional to that derived from clinical, radiologic, and microbiologic examinations remains to be clarified. Huber et al. determined the serum PCT levels of 12 consecutive ICU patients for up to 35 days after admission. In patients with septic multiple organ failure (MOF) there was a good correlation between the extent and time course of the PCT elevation with the clinical, radiologic, and microbiologic results. However, significant additional information was obtained in only one case.[58] From a practical point of view, diagnosis and monitoring of sepsis does not depend on a single parameter; they are the result of a mosaic of clinical, laboratory, and microbiologic findings. A parameter such as the PCT level could be helpful in making the clinical assessment more reliable. Table 47.1 summarizes the serum PCT concentration in relation to particular inflammatory conditions.[27]

Neopterin

The determination of neopterin concentrations in body fluids allows us to monitor the activation of cellular immunity in human diseases (Table 47.2).[59–61] Increasing neopterin concentrations sensitively indicate immunologic complications such as rejection episodes and infections in allograft recipients.[62] Neopterin concentrations correlate with the extent and activity of autoimmune disorders such as rheumatoid arthritis[63] and SLE.[64] Patients with malignant diseases have increased neopterin concentrations in urine or serum at varying frequencies: Patients with hematologic neoplasias present with the highest frequency of elevated neopterin concentration (up to 100%), and women with breast cancer have the lowest frequency (approximately 20%).[65] In cancer patients neopterin concentrations increase in parallel with the stage of the disease and are found to significantly predict disease outcome; patients with high neopterin concentrations have a higher risk for disease progression and shortened survival time. Monitoring neopterin concentrations in patients with infectious diseases was found to be clinically useful. For various infections neopterin concentrations were found to be associated with the severity of the disease, to indicate treatment response rapidly, and to be an independent predictor for the progression of disease (e.g., patients with HIV-1 infection).[66–69] In patients with septicemia neopterin concentrations allow identification of patients with a high risk of developing septic shock, multiple organ dysfunction, and death.

Biochemistry

Neopterin (Fig. 47.5) belongs to the class of pteridines that biosynthetically derive from guanosine triphosphate (GTP). GTP cyclohydrolase I cleaves the imidazole moiety of the purine GTP to synthesize 7,8-dihydroneopterin triphosphate.[61] This intermediate is converted by 6-pyruvoyl tetrahydropterin synthase to form dihydrobiopterin in the biosynthetic pathway of 5,6,7,8-tetrahydrobiopterin. Tetrahydrobiopterin is an essential cofactor of several monooxygenases, including phenylalanine-,

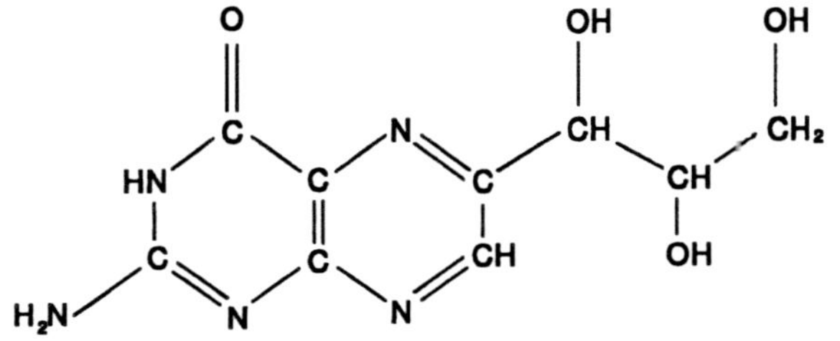

FIGURE 47.5. Neopterin (6-D-erythrotrihydroxypropyl-pterin).

tyrosine-, and tryptophan-5-hydroxylase and the nitric oxide synthases.

Interferon-γ (IFNγ) is the central stimulator for the biosynthesis of neopterin and biopterin derivatives by activating GTP cyclohydrolase I.[70] By this action tetrahydrobiopterin accumulates and only scarce amounts of neopterin derivatives are produced in most cells, such as fibroblasts or endothelial cells.[61,71] It is only in body fluids of humans and primates that relevant amounts of neopterin can be detected. Due to a relative deficiency of 6-pyruvoyl tetrahydropterin synthase in human monocytes/macrophages, activation with IFNγ leads to an accumulation of 7,8-dihydroneopterin triphosphate, which is then converted by phosphatases to neopterin and 7,8-dihydroneopterin. The latter products are detectable in cell culture supernatants and body fluids. Therefore human monocytes/macrophages appear to constitute the most relevant source of neopterin when activated with IFNγ. Data suggest that among monocytes/macrophages the dentritic cells are probably the most relevant source of neopterin production during the cell-mediated immune response (Fig. 47.6).[72] In preparations of monocytes/macrophages from peripheral blood, neopterin production was also observed upon stimulation with IFNα, but at least a 1000-fold higher dose was necessary to achieve a concentration of neopterin comparable to that induced by IFNγ.[70] Other potent inducers of macrophage activity, such as zymosan, phorbol ester, colony-stimulating factor, granulocyte/monocyte colony-stimulating factor (GM-CSF), or IFNβ, could not induce the release of significant amounts of neopterin,[73] whereas lipopolysaccharide (LPS) and tumor necrosis factor-α (TNFα) superinduce IFNγ-mediated neopterin production.[74] It has also been found that, similar to TNFα, preparations of streptococcal erythrogenic toxins are capable of amplifying neopterin production in monocytes/macrophages stimulated with IFNγ.[75]

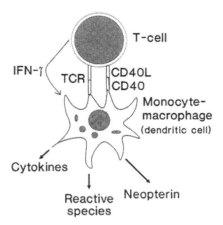

FIGURE 47.6. Formation of neopterin during the cell-mediated (Th1-type) immune response. When activated T cells interact with professional antigen-presenting cells such as monocytes/macrophages, interferon-γ (IFNγ) is released that induces formation of neopterin by the monocytes/macrophages. TCR, T cell receptor; CD40L, CD40 ligand.

Measurement of Neopterin in Biologic Fluids

Neopterin and its 7,8-dihydro form are small molecules (253 and 255 daltons, respectively) produced and released in remarkably constant proportions with aromatic neopterin/total (aromatic plus acid-oxidizable) neopterin ratios of 1:3 for urine[76] and 1:2 for serum obtained from venous blood samples. Because dihydro forms are liable, collection and storage of samples is critical and problematic for large-scale clinical handling. For daily clinical routine, only the more stable neopterin is being quantified. Easily performed serum neopterin immunoassays give neopterin concentrations averaging 5.3 ± 2.7 nM in healthy adults.[77] Because neopterin is constantly distributed in body fluids, alternative or additional measurements of neopterin concentrations in urine specimens can be performed. To take variations of urine densities into account, urinary neopterin concentrations are expressed in micromoles per mole of creatinine; measurements can be done advantageously by examining samples via high-pressure liquid chromatography.[77]

Clinical Applications of Neopterin Assays in Infectious Diseases

Distinct patterns of immune stimulation cascades are elicited during bacterial or virus infections. During acute bacterial infections a humoral [T-helper cell (Th2)-type] immune response is involved, whereas virus infections challenge primarily the cell-mediated (Th1- type) immune response.[78] Parasites and intracellularly living bacteria such as *Mycobacterium tuberculosis* typically also induce a cell-mediated immune response during the acute phase of the infection; only during the later course of the disease does a shift to Th2-type immune response seem to occur. Because of this immunologic heterogeneity, the behavior of neopterin concentrations in patients suffering from infections differs with regard to the pathogen involved.

Virus Infections

Significantly increased neopterin concentrations have been described in patients suffering from various virus infections including measles and rubella and herpes virus infections such as cytomegalovirus (CMV), Epstein-Barr virus (EBV), and varicella infections.[79-83] Patients with hepatitis A, B, and C infections have also been noted to present with increased neopterin concentrations.[84-86] In fact, increased serum neopterin concentrations are detectable in almost all patients with acute hepatitis A or B. Overall, neopterin concentrations seem to parallel the clinical presentation and the severity of infection.

In almost all of the above-mentioned studies neopterin concentrations were monitored in patients who had been referred to the hospital because of their symptomatic infections. When neopterin concentrations had already been determined during the latency period, it turned out that the increase in neopterin concentrations had begun even before the symptoms appeared or specific antibody seroconversion had become demonstrable. This was true in children with rubella infections[80] and in allograft recipients who experienced CMV infection, for example.[82] In both groups of patients an increased neopterin level was an early indicator of an ongoing virus infection that could later be confirmed serologically. Significantly increased neopterin concentrations were observed in blood donors when, despite being asymptomatic, they presented with immunoglobulin M (IgM)-CMV antibodies.[83] When antibody seroconversion takes place and the degree of viremia declines, neopterin concentrations return to normal. In most individuals with acute HIV-1 infection, neopterin levels were found to rise early, even before the onset of antibody production.[87,88] However, in contrast to other acute virus infections, after HIV-1 antibody seroconversion neopterin concentrations do not return to normal and a significant percentage of HIV-1-infected individuals have persistently increased neopterin concentrations, indicating ongoing infection and virus reproduction.[89] Neopterin concentrations in HIV-1 infection thus seem to correlate with the amount of circulating virus in the blood. During the later course of HIV-1 infection neopterin levels rise again when virus replication in the blood circulation reappears. In patients with HIV-1-related symptoms a significant inverse correlation exists between neopterin levels, $CD4^+/CD8^+$ T cell ratios, and absolute $CD4^+$ T cell number.[58,81,90]

The behavior of neopterin concentrations during retrovirus infections was confirmed in nonhuman primates. In the animal model of rhesus macaques with simian immunodeficiency virus (SIV) infection, the course of neopterin concentrations in urine and serum fully agrees with the observations made for human HIV-1 infection: Neopterin concentrations began to increase within 3–5 days after SIV inoculation,[91] and after antibody seroconversion neopterin levels declined but remained above normal in most of the animals.[91,92] Neopterin concentrations were found to be of prognostic value for the development of acquired immunodeficiency syndrome (AIDS), whereby the predictive power in homosexual men with HIV-1 infection is similar to that of $CD4^+$ T cell counts.[67] In addition, neopterin concentrations are jointly predictive with CD4 counts for disease progression[66–69] and survival.

Bacterial Infections

Acute bacterial infections are usually not associated with increased neopterin concentrations. When neopterin concentrations were compared for adult patients suffering from pneumonia or urinary tract infections, the virus infections led to significantly higher neopterin concentrations than did bacterial infections.[93] Moreover, neopterin concentrations were superior to leukocyte counts or the erythrocyte sedimentation rate for discriminating between the two types of infection, but this was true only for acute infections. Increased neopterin concentrations have been observed with protracted bacterial infections, especially of the urinary tract. The increase of neopterin in these conditions is probably due to involvement of a multitude of cytokines, such as IL-1, TNFα, and at some point also IFNγ. In patients with SLE bacterial infection was found not to influence neopterin concentrations; rather, neopterin concentrations seemed to reflect the activity of the underlying autoimmune disorder even when bacterial superinfection was proved by other means.[49] Increased neopterin concentrations were also described in patients suffering from acute rheumatic fever.[94] Here, neopterin concentrations correlated with the activity of the disease, indicating the success of therapy; high neopterin concentrations at diagnosis were associated with the development of valve lesions.

A large percentage of patients suffering from infections with intracellular bacteria present with increased neopterin concentrations. In patients with pulmonary tuberculosis, for example, neopterin concentrations correlate with the extent and activity of the disease.[95] In addition, treatment response was sensitively indicated by neopterin concentrations, which was also true in patients with HIV-1 co-infection.[96]

Parasites

Parasitic infections are associated with increased neopterin concentrations. A representative example is malaria. High neopterin concentrations have been described in patients with *Plasmodium falciparum* and *Plasmodium vivax*.[97] The highest neopterin concentrations have been observed in patients with acute onset of malaria, whereas a decline in neopterin concentrations with increasing age was observed in patients from a holoendemic area. This finding agrees well with a proposed modulation of the Th1-type (cell-mediated) immune response toward a Th2-type (humoral) immune response in chronic parasitic infections. Neopterin concentrations in cerebrospinal fluid (CSF) of patients with infectious diseases were found to be of diagnostic utility.[98] CSF neopterin indicates an intrathecal immune response and correlates with disease activity in infections such as meningitis, Lyme neuroborreliosis, or HIV-1 infection. Successful therapy of brain infections is also indicated by a rapid response of CSF neopterin concentrations. When there is no systemic involvement during intrathecal infections, neopterin concentrations in CSF are elevated, but not those in serum or urine.

Trauma and Sepsis

Sepsis in patients is accompanied by high neopterin concentrations in the urine or serum. In the first report on postoperative or posttraumatic ICU patients, a significant difference in serum neopterin concentrations was found between survivors and nonsurvivors.[99] This early report suggested a significant predictive value for neopterin in ICU patients: High levels were shown to be a strong indicator of overwhelming and finally fatal sepsis. Neopterin levels had high sensitivity and specificity, and a cutoff limit of 27.4 nM was found best to discriminate between patient groups. Remarkably, only two of the patients developing sepsis had a positive blood culture; and other clinical variables such as fever, leukopenia, or thrombocytopenia were not useful for a reliable, accurate prognosis.

Several reports confirmed and extended these results. When plasma levels of neopterin and granulocyte elastase α_1-protease inhibitor (EPI) on the one hand, and the severity of multiple organ failure on the other hand, were compared with a score for multiple organ failure,[100] the correlation of neopterin and EPI with the score was similarly strong.[101] Serum neopterin concentrations of more than 40 nM revealed a diagnostic sensitivity of 96% and specificity of 73%. The combination of neopterin with EPI gave an even better diagnostic accuracy (sensitivity 91%, specificity 99%).

In another report the relation between neopterin, phospholipase A, polymorphonuclear neutrophil (PMN) elastase, and the complement split product C3a was examined in patients with acute lung injury and sepsis.[102] A positive correlation between neopterin and phospholipase A was apparent in trauma and sepsis patients. Neopterin was not found to be markedly elevated immediately after trauma but was markedly high in patients with sepsis. ARDS was not found to exert any significant effect on neopterin concentrations.

In a larger study of patients with multiple trauma, neopterin concentrations were again found to be capable of significantly discriminating between outcome groups regarding the development of infection and early or late organ failure.[103] In another study, the same group of researchers studied patients with multiple injuries and showed a highly predictive value of neopterin concentrations for survival. The predictive value for organ failure was similar to that seen with trauma scores, and the predictive value for survival was even superior.[104] Several additional studies further underline the predictive value for disease development in patients with multiple trauma.[105–108]

Burns

Significantly increased neopterin concentrations have been described in patients with major burns,[109] correlating with the presence of bacteremia and the development of clinical sepsis. In another study[110] no significant correlation could be established between neopterin concentrations and the extent of the burned surface, although increased neopterin was found within the first 3 days after burn and persisted during the following days of observation. The presence of early endotoxinemia did not correlate with neopterin levels, but neopterin concentrations were predictive of the development of endotoxinemia in the later course of the disease.

Pancreatitis

Neopterin serum/plasma concentrations were significantly associated with the course of acute pancreatitis.[111,112] High neopterin concentrations at hospital admission were highly predictive of the development of multiple organ failure and a significant risk of death. The predictive power was similar or even better than that of CRP. Similarly, the development of pancreatic necrosis was associated with high neopterin concentrations at admission. Monitoring neopterin concentrations during follow-up of patients was found to reflect disease development and help predict its course (Fig. 47.7).

Increased Neopterin Concentrations and Deficient Cytokine Production of T cells in Patients with Sepsis

Disturbed host defense mechanisms after trauma, burns, or major surgery are deemed responsible for accelerating the

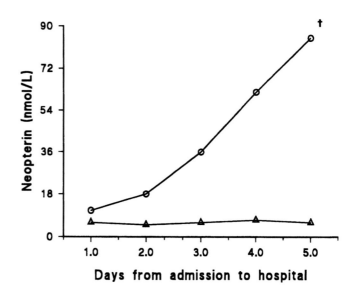

FIGURE 47.7. Course of serum neopterin concentrations in two patients with acute pancreatitis. One of them (upper curve) died from the disease (†).

septic process. Various factors augment the progressive malfunction of both humoral and cellular immune systems, such as acute-phase reactants, the complement system with its cleavage products, metabolites derived from the arachidonic acid pathway, and protein malnutrition. Therefore it seems surprising to find increased production of neopterin in patients with septicemia or sepsis syndrome who suffer from sometimes severe immunodeficiency, as increased neopterin concentrations indicate activation of cell-mediated immunity. Enhanced endogenous production of IFNγ represents a paradox, as in vitro experiments show reduced responsiveness of T cells and reduced release of cytokines such as IL-2 and IFNγ in patients with multiple trauma. Reduced responsiveness of T cells is considered responsible for increased susceptibility to whole-body inflammation, opportunistic infections, and thus the development of multiple organ failure. Hence deficient production of IFNγ by T cells is one of the most important defects of T cells caused by sepsis. The continuing increase of neopterin concentrations during the development of sepsis syndrome and MOF indicates that this model is an oversimplification.

The question arises whether cytokines other than IFNγ could be important in the increased production of neopterin in patients developing septicemia. TNFα, a polypeptide cytokine mainly produced by monocytes, macrophages, and T lymphocyte subsets, plays a central role in the development of sepsis and septic shock. Because TNFα synergistically amplifies neopterin secretion from macrophages stimulated with IFNγ,[74] it is important to understand the potential interactions between the neopterin/IFNγ/TNFα system. TNFα initiates its multiple effects on cell function by binding to specific, high-affinity cell-surface receptors. Two distinct TNFα receptors of 55–60 kDa (type I, TNFR-55) and 75–80 kDa (type II, TNFR-75) have been identified.[113] Both receptors for TNFα exist also in soluble

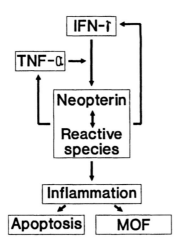

FIGURE 47.8. During cell-mediated immune reaction, interferon-γ (IFNγ) induces the production of neopterin. In parallel, the monocytes/macrophages are primed for release of various reactive species (oxidative burst). Oxidative stress develops and upregulates the release of proinflammatory cytokines such as tumor necrosis factor-α (TNFα) and IFNγ in an autocrine way. The resulting inflammation supports biochemical alterations [e.g., induction of programmed cell death (apoptosis)] on the one hand and clinical deterioration on the other, finally leading to multiple organ failure.

forms[15,114] apparently derived by proteolytic cleavage from the cell-surface forms. Close correlations between increased concentrations of sTNFRs and neopterin have been found in various diseases,[16] supporting the concept that TNFα and IFNγ may synergistically amplify their activities on target cells including the formation of neopterin (Fig. 47.8). Moreover, neopterin was found to be capable of inducing TNFα gene expression[115] and may therefore itself contribute to a proinflammatory cascade in patients with, for example, polytrauma or sepsis. Interestingly, when posttrauma patients have been treated with pentoxifylline, which is known to reduce TNFα-mediated effects, decreased neopterin concentrations were observed.[116]

In a small study the relation between neopterin and IFNγ was investigated in patients after severe multiple trauma.[117] IFNγ was found to increase in the patients, peaking on day 3 after trauma. The altitude of the peak correlated positively with the initial blood loss and the number of allogeneic packed cell transfusions received within 48 hours after trauma. In parallel with this marked IFNγ peak, a slow but steady increase of neopterin concentrations was noted. The serum and urine neopterin concentrations correlated positively with the initial IFNγ levels. The results of this study agree well with findings of a hyperdynamic sepsis model in baboons in which strong interrelations between the initial cytokine cascades after infusion of *Escherichia coli* and the neopterin production rates were found.[118]

Obviously, deficient production of IFNγ upon in vitro stimulation of T cells by soluble antigens or mitogens is associated with increased IFNγ in patients with septicemia. Similarly, in patients with HIV-1 infection, increased T cell activation in vivo is accompanied by reduced responsiveness of cells to secondary stimulation.[119,120] In these patients, immunodeficiency is also proved by the loss of in vivo skin test reactivity in patients with more advanced disease. It seems that T cells of patients with chronic infectious syndromes are exhausted by persistent stimulation, as demonstrated earlier in patients with SLE[121] and HIV-1 infection.[122] In T cells from such patients the T cell responsiveness could be restored when cells were allowed to rest in culture; the cells then responded almost normally, with proliferation and cytokine production, in response to antigenic stimulation.

Studies in patients with HIV-1 infection suggest that immunodeficiency, indicated by reduced responsiveness of in vitro stimulated T cells, is associated with a sole defect of interleukin-2 (IL-2) production, whereas IFNγ gene expression was well detectable in the cells.[123] This observation is in line with a decrease in spontaneous production of neopterin in peripheral blood mononuclear cells from patients with thermal injuries upon exogenous supplementation of cells with IL-2.[124] This effect is in contrast to the enhancement of neopterin production seen in the IL-2-treated control cells.

The finding of increased IFNγ in patients with sepsis and increasing concentrations of this cytokine contradicts the view of a shift from the Th1-type to the Th2-type immune response during disease progression. In line with the proposed shift, a decrease of Th1-type cytokines IFNγ and IL-2 but an increase of Th2-type cytokines IL-4, IL-5, and IL-10 would be expected.[125] There is evidence of increased IL-10 during sepsis. Thus it seems that there is activation of both Th compartments or a shift to the Th0 phenotype.

Increased Neopterin and Oxidative Stress

Activated cell-mediated immunity is associated with elevated concentrations of T cell-derived IFNγ, leading to the expression of proinflammatory cytokines and enhancing macrophage capacity to secrete reactive oxygen intermediates (Fig. 47.8).[73,126] In human monocytes/macrophages stimulated with IFNγ a significant relation exists between the amount of neopterin formed and the capacity to secrete reactive oxygen species such as hydrogen peroxide. Neopterin itself was found able to intensify effects of various oxidative compounds such as hydrogen peroxide and peroxynitrite. This was proven in physicochemical experiments applying chemoluminescence and in bacterial cultures and enzymatic assays.[127] The data imply that increased production of neopterin by activated monocytes/macrophages is related to oxidative stress. Thus the increased production of neopterin during infections, autoimmune disorders, and certain types of cancer[59-61] allows an indirect estimate of the degree of oxidative stress in vivo (Fig. 47.8).[128]

Oxidative stress seems to play an important role in the pathogenesis of the sepsis syndrome. It could be directly involved, inducing or supporting the development of immunodeficiency. However, oxidative stress could play an additional role in influencing redox-sensitive signal transduction pathways such as the initiation of apoptosis or gene expression of cytokines such as TNFα. In agreement with their effects on reactive species, neopterin derivatives were found to trigger apoptosis in lymphocytic and monocytic cells.[129-131] It seems that neopterin derivatives could even be directly involved in this biochemical pathway. Activated T cells are more susceptible to apoptosis than resting cells, and therefore activated Th1 cells are the first to be lost when cells are isolated from patients. Consequently, Th1-type immune responsiveness and the production of Th1-type cytokines IL-2 and IFNγ would be diminished. This conclusion is further supported by the possibility that IFNγ is capable of switching on proliferation or apoptosis in activated T lymphocytes depending on the differential expression of the α and β chains of the IFNγ receptor.[132] Thus the increased production of IFNγ and TNFα in patients could be strongly involved in the pathogenesis of immunodeficiency.[119] This would be in line with the general association between increased neopterin concentrations and the development of complications finally leading to multiple organ failure, which is a scenario similar to that in patients with other syndromes of chronic immune activation, such as parasitic and virus infections or malignant diseases.

Immune Activation and the Development of Anemia, Cachexia, and Multiple Organ Failure

As with other chronic disorders such as infections and autoimmune and malignant diseases, septicemia is commonly associated with weight loss and decreased hemoglobin concentration. Urine and serum neopterin concentrations in patients with various diseases were found to correlate inversely with hemoglobin levels and the number of red blood cells.[133] Neopterin levels were also found to correlate with, and to predict, weight loss in the patients.[134,135] It seems that such typical symptoms of chronic diseases can be much better explained as a result of chronic immune activation rather than cytokine deficiency (Fig. 47.8). TNFα is considered an important cytokine in the development of cachexia, and it strongly inhibits growth of erythroid progenitor cells in vitro. As usual, IFNγ is considered to enhance the effect of TNFα synergistically. Thus the association of high neopterin concentrations with the development of anemia and weight loss can be explained by the fact that neopterin concentrations reflect IFNγ and TNFα activity. Both cytokines seem to be critically involved in the development of these symptoms. This argument is strengthened by the fact that identical relations between high neopterin concentrations and decreased hemoglobin and increased weight loss have been found in various groups of patients, including those with HIV-1 infection or a malignant disease.

Conclusions

Sepsis and septic shock are associated with markedly elevated neopterin concentrations. Neopterin levels correlate with scores for severity of sepsis, such as the Acute Physiology and Chronic Health Evaluation (APACHE II) score and strongly predict progression to sepsis syndrome and multiple organ failure in patients with, for example, polytrauma or acute pancreatitis. There is a close association between serum and urine neopterin concentrations so long as no severe renal impairment is established in patients.[136] Thus especially in situations when daily monitoring of neopterin concentrations is desired, collection of early morning urine specimens may help patients avoid an unnecessary burden.

Because large quantities of neopterin are released by human macrophages upon stimulation with IFNγ, increased neopterin concentrations in patients with septicemia indicate enhanced production of IFNγ by activated T cells. This underscores a role of T cell activation in the pathogenesis of septic shock.

Acknowledgment. This work was supported financially by the Austrian funds Zur Förderung der wissenschaftlichen Forschung, project 10776 med., and funds from the Lorenz Böhler Gesellschaft.

References

1. Bone RC: Sepsis and its complications: the clinical problem. Crit Care Med 1994;22:S8–S11.
2. Peduzzi P, Shatney C, Sheagren J, et al: Predictors of bacteremia and gram-negative bacteremia in patients with sepsis: the Veterans Affairs Systemic Sepsis Cooperative Study Group. Arch Intern Med 1992;152:529–535.
3. Oczenski W, Fitzgerald RD, Schwarz S: Procalcitonin: a new parameter for the diagnosis of bacterial infection in the perioperative period. Eur J Anaesthesiol 1998;15:202–209.
4. Pepys MB, Baltz ML: Acute phase proteins with special reference to C-reactive protein and related proteins (pentraxins) and serum amyloid A protein. Adv Immunol 1983;34:141–212.
5. Okamura JM, Miyagi JM, Terada K, et al: Potential clinical applications of C-reactive protein. J Clin Lab Anal 1990;4:231–235.
6. Castell JV, Gomez-Lechon MJ, David M, et al: Acute phase response of human hepatocytes: regulation of acute-phase protein synthesis by interleukin-6. Hepatology 1990;12:1179–1186.
7. Povoa P, Almeida E, Moreira P, et al: C-reactive protein as an indicator of sepsis. Intensive Care Med 1998;24:1052–1056.
8. Yentis SM, Soni N, Sheldon J: C-reactive protein as an indicator of resolution of sepsis in the intensive care unit. Intensive Care Med 1995;21:602–605.
9. Waage A, Haalstensen A, Espevik T: Association between tumour necrosis factor in serum and fatal outcome in patients with meningococcal disease. Lancet 1987;1:355–357.
10. Grau GE, Taylor TE, Molyneux ME, et al: Tumour necrosis factor and disease severity in children with falciparum malaria. N Engl J Med 1989;320:1586–1591.
11. Calandra T, Baumgarner JD, Grau GE, et al: Prognostic value of tumour necrosis factor/cachectin, interleukin 1, interferon-α and interferon-γ in the serum of patients with septic shock. J Infect Dis 1990;161:982–987.
12. Damas P, Reuter A, Gysen P, et al: Tumour necrosis factor and interleukin-1 serum levels during sepsis in humans. Crit Care Med 1989;17:975–978.
13. Calandra T, Gerain J, Heumann D, et al: High circulating levels of interleukin-6 patients with septic shock: evolution during sepsis,

prognostic value, and interplay with other cytokines: the Swiss-Dutch J5 Immunoglobulin Study Group. Am J Med 1991;91:23–29.
14. Friedland JS, Porter JC, Daryanani S, et al: Plasma pro-inflammatory cytokine concentrations, Acute Physiology and Chronic Health Evaluation (APACHE) III scores and survival in patients in an intensive care unit. Crit Care Med 1996;24:1775–1781.
15. Engelmann H, Novick D, Wallach D: Two tumor-necrosis factor-binding proteins purified from human urine: evidence for immunological cross-reactivity with cell surface tumor necrosis factor receptors. J Biol Chem 1990;265:1531–1536.
16. Diez-Ruiz A, Tilz GP, Zangerle R, Baier-Bitterlich G, Wachter H, Fuchs D: Soluble receptors for tumor necrosis factor in clinical laboratory diagnosis. Eur J Haematol 1995;54:1–8.
17. Assicot M, Gendrel D, Carsin H, et al: High serum procalcitonin concentrations in patients with sepsis and infection. Lancet 1993;431:515–518.
18. Dandona P, Nix D, Wilson MF, et al: Procalcitonin increase after endotoxin injection in normal subjects. J Clin Endocrinol Metab 1994;79:1605–1608.
19. Bernard AR, Huber MB, Birnbaum RS, et al: Medullary thyroid carcinomas secrete a noncalcitonin peptide corresponding to the carboxyl-terminal region of preprocalcitonin. J Clin Endocrinol Metab 1983;56:802–807.
20. Becker KL, O'Neill W, Snider RH, et al: Hypercalcitonemia in inhalation burn injury: a response of the pulmonary neuroendocrine cell? Anat Record 1993;236:136–138.
21. Oberhoffer M, Russwurm S, Stonans I, et al: Procalcitonin m-RNA is expressed by human mononuclear cells and modulated by lipopolysaccharide and sepsis related cytokines [abstract]. Crit Care Med 1999;27(Suppl):A130.
22. Monneret G, Laroche B, Bienvenu J: Procalcitonin is not produced by circulating blood cells. Infection 1999;27:34–35.
23. Whang KT, Steinwald PM, White JC, et al: Serum calcitonin precursors in sepsis and systemic inflammation. J Clin Endocrinol Metab 1998;83:3296–3301.
24. Becker KL, Bivins LE, Radfar RH, et al: Study of calcitonin heterogeneity using a radioreceptor assay. Horm Metab Res 1978;10:457–458.
25. Zaidi M, Moonga BS, Bevis PJR, et al: Expression and function of the calcitonin gene products. Vitam Horm 1991;46:87–164.
26. Nylen ES, Whang KT, Snider RH, et al: Mortality is increased by procalcitonin and decreased by an antiserum reactive to procalcitonin in experimental sepsis. Crit Care Med 1998;26:1001–1006.
27. Meisner M: PCT, Procalcitonin: A New, Innovative Infection Parameter. Berlin; Brahms-Diagnostica, 1996.
28. Gendrel D, Assicot M, Raymond J, et al: Procalcitonin as a marker for the early diagnosis of neonatal infection. J Pediatr 1996;128:570–573.
29. Gendrel D, Raymond J, Assicot M, et al: Procalcitonin, C-reactive protein and interleukin 6 in bacterial and viral meningitis in children. Presse Med 1998;27:1135–1139.
30. Sachse C, Dressler F, Henkel E: Increased serum procalcitonin in newborn infants without infection. Clin Chem 1998;44:1343–1344.
31. Lapillone A, Basson E, Monneret G, et al: Lack of specifity of procalcitonin for sepsis diagnosis in premature infants. Lancet 1998;351:1211–1212.
32. Gerard Y, Hober D, Assicot M, et al: Procalcitonin as a marker of bacterial sepsis in patients infected with HIV-1. J Infect 1997;35:41–46.
33. Gerard Y, Hober D, Petitjean S, et al: High serum procalcitonin level in a 4-year-old liver transplant recipient with a disseminated candidiasis. Infection 1995;23:310–311.
34. De Werra I, Jaccard C, Corradin SB, et al: Cytokines, nitrite/nitrate, soluble tumor necrosis factor receptors, and procalcitonin concentrations: comparisons in patients with septic shock, cardiogenic shock, and bacterial pneumonia. Crit Care Med 1997;25:607–613.
35. Staehler M, Hammer C, Meiser B, et al: Procalcitonin: a new marker for differential diagnosis of acute rejection and bacterial infection in heart transplantation. Transplant Proc 1997;29:584–585.
36. Huber W, Schweigart U, Bottermann P: Failure of PCT to indicate severe fungal infection in two immunodeficient patients. Infection 1997;25:377–378.
37. Beaune G, Bienvenu F, Pondarre C, et al: Serum procalcitonin rise is only slight in two cases of disseminated aspergillosis. Infection 1998;26:168–169.
38. Al-Nawas B, Shah PM: Procalcitonin in acute malaria. Eur J Med Res 1997;2:206–208.
39. Smith MD, Suputtamongkol Y, Chaowagul W, et al: Elevated serum procalcitonin levels in patients with meliodosis. Clin Infect Dis 1995;20:641–645.
40. Monneret G, Labaune JM, Isaac C, et al: Procalcitonin and C-reactive protein levels in neonatal infections. Acta Paediatr 1997;86:209–212.
41. Reith HB, Lehmkul P, Beier W, et al: Procalcitonin: ein prognostischer Infektionsparameter bei der Peritonitis. Chir Gastroenterol 1995;11:47–50.
42. Al-Nawas B, Krammer I, Shah PM: Procalcitonin in diagnosis of severe infections. Eur J Med Res 1996;1:331–333.
43. Gramm HJ, Dollinger P, Beier W: Procalcitonin: ein neur Marker der inflammatorischen Wirtsantwort. Longitudinalstudien bei Patienten mit Sepsis und Peritonitis. Chir Gastroenterol 1995;11:51–54.
44. Oberhoffer M, Bögel D, Meier-Hellmann A, et al: Procalcitonin is higher in non-survivors during course of sepsis, severe sepsis, and septic shock [abstract]. Intensive Care Med 1996;22:A245.
45. Brunkenhorst FM, Forycki ZF, Wagner J: Frühe Identifizierung der biliären akuten Pankreatitis durch Procalcitonin-Immunreaktivität—vorläufige Ergebnisse. Chir Gastroenterol 1995;11:42–46.
46. Rau B, Steinbach G, Gansauge F, et al: The potential role of procalcitonin and interleukin 8 in the prediction of infected necrosis in acute pancreatitis. Gut 1997;41:832–840.
47. Eberhard OK, Langefeld I, Kuse ER, et al: Procalcitonin in the early phase after renal transplantation: will it add to diagnostic accuracy? Clin Transplant 1998;12:206–211.
48. Kunz D, Pross M, König W, et al: Diagnostic relevance of procalcitonin, IL-6 and cellular immune status in the early phase after liver transplantation. Transplant Proc 1998;30:2398–2399.
49. Eberhard OK, Haubitz M, Brunkhorst FM, et al: Usefulness of procalcitonin for differentiation between activity of systemic autoimmune disease (systemic lupus erythematosus/systemic antineutrophil cytoplasmic antibody-associated vasculitis) and invasive bacterial infection. Arthritis Rheum 1997;40:1250–1256.

50. Schwenger V, Sis J, Breitbart A, et al: CRP levels in autoimmune disease can be specified by measurement of procalcitonin. Infection 1998;26:274–276.
51. Moosig F, Csernok E, Reinhold-Keller E, et al: Elevated procalcitonin levels in active Wegener's granulomatosis. J Rheumatol 1998;25:1531–1533.
52. Becker KL, Snider RH, Silva OL, et al: Calcitonin heterogeneity in lung cancer and medullary thyroid cancer. Acta Endocrinol (kbh) 1978;89:89–99.
53. Meisner M, Tschaikowsky K, Hutzler A, et al: Postoperative plasma concentrations of procalcitonin after different types of surgery. Intensive Care Med 1998;24:680–684.
54. Mimoz O, Benoist JF, Edouard AR, et al: Procalcitonin and C-reactive protein during the early posttraumatic systemic inflammatory response syndrome. Intensive Care Med 1998;24:185–188.
55. Benoist JF, Mimoz O, Assicot M: Procalcitonin in severe trauma. Ann Biol Clin 1998;56:571–574.
56. Nylen ES, O'Neill W, Jordan MH, et al: Serum procalcitonin as an index of inhalation injury in burns. Horm Metab Res 1992;24:439–442.
57. Carsin H, Assicot M, Feger F, et al: Evolution and significance of circulating procalcitonin levels compared with IL-6, TNFα and endotoxin levels early after thermal injury. Burns 1997;23:218–224.
58. Huber W, Reichenberger J, Salmhofer H, et al: Procalcitonin—a routine parameter in intensive medicine? Intensivmed 1998;35:124–131.
59. Fuchs D, Hausen A, Reibnegger G, Werner ER, Dierich MP, Wachter H: Neopterin as a marker for activated cell-mediated immunity application in HIV-1 infection. Immunol Today 1988;9:150–155.
60. Fuchs D, Weiss G, Reibnegger G, Wachter H: The role of neopterin as a monitor of cellular immune activation in transplantation, inflammatory, infectious and malignant diseases. Crit Rev Clin Lab Sci 1992;29:307–341.
61. Wachter H, Fuchs D, Hausen A, et al: Neopterin. New York, Walter de Gruyter, 1992.
62. Reibnegger G, Aichberger C, Fuchs D, et al: Posttransplant neopterin excretion in renal allograft recipients: a reliable diagnostic aid for acute rejection and a predictive marker of long-term graft survival. Transplantation 1991;52:58–63.
63. Reibnegger G, Egg D, Fuchs D, et al: Urinary neopterin reflects clinical activity in patients with rheumatoid arthritis. Arthritis Rheum 1986;29:1063–1070.
64. Samsonov MY, Tilz GP, Egorova O, et al: Serum soluble markers of immune activation and disease activity in systemic lupus erythematosus. Lupus 1995;4:29–32.
65. Reibnegger G, Fuchs D, Fuith LC, et al: Neopterin as a marker for activated cell-mediated immunity: application in malignant disease. Cancer Detect Prevent 1991;15:483–490.
66. Fuchs D, Spira TJ, Hausen A, et al: Neopterin as predictive marker for disease progression in human immunodeficiency virus type 1 Infection. Clin Chem 1989;35:1746–1749.
67. Fahey JL, Taylor JMG, Detels R, et al: The prognostic value of cellular and serologic markers in infection with human immunodeficiency virus type 1. N Engl J Med 1990;322:166–172.
68. Moss AR, Bacchetti P, Osmond D, et al: Seropositivity for HIV-1 and the development of AIDS or AIDS related condition, three year follow up of the San Francisco General Hospital cohort. BMJ 1988;296:745–750.
69. Krämer A, Biggar RJ, Hampl H, et al: Immunologic markers of progression to acquired immunodeficiency syndrome are time-dependent and illness-specific. Am J Epidemiol 1992;136:71–80.
70. Huber C, Batchelor JR, Fuchs D, et al: Immune response-associated production of neopterin, release from macrophages primarily under control of interferon-gamma. J Exp Med 1984;160:310–316.
71. Andert SE, Griesmacher A, Zuckermann A, Müller MM: Neopterin release from human endothelial cells is triggered by inteferon-gamma. Clin Exp Immunol 1992;88:555–558.
72. Romani N, Fuchs D: Are dentritic cells a relevant source of neopterin production in clinical conditions? Pteridines (in press).
73. Nathan CF: Secretory products of macrophages. J Clin Invest 1987;79:319–326.
74. Werner-Felmayer G, Werner ER, Fuchs D, Hausen A, Reibnegger G, Wachter H: Tumour necrosis factor-alpha and lipopolysaccharide enhance interferon-induced tryptophan degradation and pteridine synthesis in human cells. Biol Chem Hoppe Seyler 1989;370:1063–1069.
75. Murr C, Baier-Bitterlich G, Fuchs D, et al: Streptococcal erythrogenic toxins induce neopterin formation in human peripheral blood mononuclear cells but not in the human myelomonocytoma cell line THP-1. Immunobiology 1996;195:224–228.
76. Fuchs D, Milstein S, Krämer A, et al: Urinary neopterin concentrations vs total neopterins for clinical utility. Clin Chem 1989;35:2305–2307.
77. Fuchs D, Werner ER, Wachter H: Soluble products of immune activation neopterin. In: Rose NR, deMacario EC, Fahey JL, Friedman H, Penn GM (eds) Manual of Clinical Laboratory Immunology. Washington DC, American Society of Microbiology, 1992;251–255.
78. Oxenius A, Karrer U, Zinkernagel RM, Hengartner H: IL-12 is not required for induction of type 1 cytokine responses in viral infections. J Immunol 1999;162:965–973.
79. Wachter H, Hausen A, Grassmayr K: Increased urinary excretion of neopterin in patients with malignant tumors and with virus diseases. Hoppe Seylers Z Physiol Chem 1979;360:1957–1960.
80. Zaknun D, Weiss G, Glatzl J, Wachter H, Fuchs D: Neopterin levels during acute rubella in children. Clin Infect Dis 1993;17:521–522.
81. Kern P, Rokos H, Dietrich M: Raised serum neopterin levels and imbalances of T-lymphocyte subsets in viral diseases, acquired immune deficiency and related lymphadenopathy syndromes. Biomed Pharmacother 1984;38:407–411.
82. Tilg H, Margreiter R, Scriba M, et al: Clinical presentation of CMV infection in solid organ transplant recipients and its impact on graft rejection and neopterin excretion. Clin Transplant 1987;1:37–43.
83. Hönlinger M, Fuchs D, Reibnegger G, Schönitzer D, Dierich MP, Wachter H: Neopterin screening and acute cytomegalovirus infections in blood donors. Clin Invest 1992;70:63.
84. Reibnegger G, Auhuber I, Fuchs D, et al: Urinary neopterin levels in acute viral hepatitis. Hepatology 1988;8:771–774.
85. Prior C, Fuchs D, Hausen A, et al: Potential of urinary neopterin excretion in differentiating chronic non-A, non-B hepatitis from fatty liver. Lancet 1987;2:1235–1237.
86. Schennach H, Schönitzer D, Fuchs D: Association between chronic hepatitis C virus infection and increased neopterin concentrations in blood donations. Clin Chem 1998;44:2225–2226.

87. Zangerle R, Schönitzer D, Fuchs D, Möst J, Dierich MP, Wachter H: Reducing HIV transmission by seronegative blood. Lancet 1992;339:130–131.
88. Gaines H, von Sydow MA, von Stedingk V, et al: Immunological changes in primary HIV-1 infection. AIDS 1990;4:995–999.
89. Fuchs D, Albert J, Asjö B, Fenyö EM, Reibnegger G, Wachter H: Association between serum neopterin concentrations and in vitro replicative capacity of HIV-1 isolates. J Infect Dis 1989;160:724–725.
90. Fuchs D, Banekovich M, Hausen A, et al: Neopterin estimation compared with the ratio of T-cell subpopulations in persons infected with human immunodeficiency virus 1. Clin Chem 1988;34:2415–2417.
91. Fendrich C, Lüke W, Stahl-Hennig C, et al: Urinary neopterin concentrations in rhesus monkeys after infection with simian immunodeficiency virus mac strain 251. AIDS 1989;3:305–307.
92. Popov J, McGraw T, Hofmann B, et al: Acute lymphoid changes and ongoing immune activation in SIV infection. J Acquir Immune Defic Syndr 1992;5:391–399.
93. Denz H, Fuchs D, Hausen A, et al: Value of urinary neopterin in the differential diagnosis of bacterial and viral infections. Klin Wochenschr 1990;68:218–222.
94. Samsonov MY, Tilz GP, Pisklakov VP, et al: Serum-soluble receptors for tumor necrosis factor-α and interleukin-2, and neopterin in acute rheumatic fever. Clin Immunol Imunopathol 1995;74:31–34.
95. Fuchs D, Hausen A, Kofler M, Kosanowski H, Reibnegger G, Wachter H: Neopterin as an index of immune response in patients with tuberculosis. Lung 1984;162:337–346.
96. Hosp M, Elliot AM, Raynes JG, et al: Neopterin, β_2-microglobulin, and acute phase proteins in HIV-1-seropositive and seronegative Zambian patients with tuberculosis. Lung 1997;175:265–275.
97. Reibnegger G, Fuchs D, Hausen A, Schmutzhard E, Werner ER, Wachter H: The dependence of cell-mediated immune activation in malaria on age and endemicity. Trans R Soc Trop Med Hyg 1987;81:729–733.
98. Hagberg L, Dotevall L, Norkrans G, Larsson M, Wachter H, Fuchs D: Cerebrospinal fluid neopterin concentrations in central nervous system infection. J Infect Dis 1993;168:1285–1288.
99. Strohmaier W, Redl H, Schlag G, Inthron D: D-Erythro-neopterin plasma levels in intensive care patients with and without septic complications. Crit Care Med 1987;15:757–760.
100. Goris RJA, Boekhorst TPA, Nuytinck JKS, Gimbrere JSF: Multiple organ failure, generalized autodestructive inflammation? Arch Surg 1985;120:1109–1115.
101. Pacher R, Redl H, Frass M, Petzl DH, Schuster E, Woloszczuk W: Relationship between neopterin and granulocyte elastase plasma levels and the severity of multiple organ failure. Crit Care Med 1989;17:221–226.
102. Kellermann W, Frentzel-Beyme R, Welte M, Jochum M: Phospholipase A in acute lung injury after trauma and sepsis its relation to the inflammatory mediators PMN-elastase, C3a, and neopterin. Klin Wochenschr 1990;67:190–195.
103. Waydhas C, Nast-Kolb D, Jochum M, et al: Inflammatory mediators, infection, sepsis, and multiple organ failure after severe trauma. Arch Surg 1992;127:460–467.
104. Nast-Kolb D, Waydhas C, Jochum M, et al: Biochemical factors as objective parameters for assessing the prognosis in polytrauma. Unfallchirurg 1992;95:59–66.
105. Holch M, Grob PJ, Fierz W, Glinz W, Geroulanos S: Immunosuppression caused by surgery and severe trauma. Helv Chir Acta 1989;56:121–124.
106. Grob P, Holch M, Fierz W, Glinz W, Geroulanos S: Immunodeficiency after major trauma and selective surgery. Pediatr Infect Dis J 1988;7:S37–S42.
107. Delogu G, Casula MA, Mancini P, Tellan G, Signore L: Serum neopterin and soluble interleukin-2 receptor for prediction of a shock state in gram-negative sepsis. J Crit Care 1995;10:64–71.
108. Pliz G, Kaab S, Kreuzer E, Werdan K: Evaluation of definitions and parameters for sepsis assessment in patients after cardiac surgery. Infection 1994;22:8–17.
109. Balogh D, Lammer H, Kornberger E, Stuffer M, Schönitzer D: Neopterin plasma levels in burn patients. Burns 1992;18:185–188.
110. Yao YM, Yu Y, Wang YP, Tian HM, Sheng ZY: Elevated serum neopterin level: its relationship to endotoxinaemia and sepsis in patients with major burns. Eur J Clin Invest 1996;26:224–230.
111. Kaufmann P, Tilz GP, Demel U, Wachter H, Kreijs JG, Fuchs D: Neopterin plasma concentrations predict the course of severe acute pancreatitis. Clin Chem Lab Med 1998;36:29–34.
112. Uomo G, Spada OA, Manes G, et al: Neopterin in acute pancreatitis. Scand J Gastroenterol 1996;17:757–760
113. Hohmann HP, Remy R, Brockhaus M, Van Loon APGM: Two different cell types have different major receptors for human tumor necrosis factor (tumor necrosis factor-α). J Biol Chem 1989;264:14927–14934.
114. Olsson I, Lantz M, Nilsson E, Peetre C, Thysell H, Grubb A: Isolation and characterization of a tumor necrosis factor binding protein from urine. Eur J Haematol 1989;42:270–275.
115. Hoffmann G, Frede S, Kenn S, et al: Neopterin-induced tumor necrosis factor-α synthesis in vascular smooth muscle cells in vitro. Int Arch Allergy Immunol 1998;116:240–245.
116. Nagy Z, Mandi Y, Gyulai ZS, Farkas G, Marton J, Balogh A: Beneficial effects of pentoxifylline in sepsis syndrome. In: Faist E (ed) Immune Consequences of Trauma, Shock and Sepsis. Bologna, Monduzzi Editor, 1997;903–908.
117. Robin B, Fuchs D, Koller W, Wachter H: Course of immune activation markers in patients after severe multiple trauma. Pteridines 1990;2:95–97.
118. Redl H, Schlag G, Bahrami S, Schade U, Ceska M, Stutz P: Plasma neutrophil-activating peptide-1/interleukin-8 and neutrophil elastase in a primate bacteremia model. J Infect Dis 1991;164:383–388.
119. Fuchs D, Malkovsky M, Reibnegger G, Werner ER, Forni G, Wachter H: Endogenous release of interferon-gamma and diminished response of peripheral blood mononuclear cells to antigenic stimulation. Immunol Lett 1989/1990;23:103–108.
120. Fuchs D, Shearer GM, Boswell RN, et al: Increased serum neopterin in patients with HIV-1 infection is correlated with reduced in vitro interleukin-2 production. Clin Exp Immunol 1990;80:44–48.
121. Huang YP, Miescher PA, Zubler RH: The interleukin-2 secretion defect in vitro in systemic lupus erythematosus is reversible in rested cultured T-cells. J Immunol 1986;137:3515–3520.
122. Lees O, Ramzaoui S, Gilbert D, et al: The impaired in vitro production of interleukin-2 in HIV infection is negatively correlated to the number of circulating $CD4^+DR^-$ T-cells and is reversed by allowing T cells to rest in culture: arguments for in vivo $CD4^+$ T-cell activation. Clin Immunol Immunopathol 1993;67:185–191.

123. Fan J, Bass HZ, Fahey JL: Elevated interferon-γ and decreased IL-2 gene expression are associated with HIV-1 infection. J Immunol 1993;151:5031–5036.
124. Teodorczyk-Injeyan JA, Cembrzynska-Nowak M, Peters WJ: Thermal injury-associated neopterin production: regulation by interleukin-2. J Burn Care Rehabil 1993;14:617–623.
125. Romagnani S: Lymphokine production by human T cells in disease states. Annu Rev Immunol 1994;12:227–257.
126. Billiau A, Dijkmans R: Interferon-gamma mechanisms of action and therapeutic potential. Biochem Pharmacol 1990;40:1433–1439.
127. Weiss G, Fuchs D, Hausen A, et al: Neopterin modulates toxicity by reactive oxygen and chloride species. FEBS Lett 1993;321:89–92.
128. Fuchs D, Baier-Bitterlich G, Wede I, Wachter H: Reactive oxygen and apoptosis. In: Sacndalios J (ed) Oxidative Stress and the Molecular Biology of Antioxidant Defences. Cold Spring Harbor, NY, Cold Spring Harbor Laboratory Press, 1997; 139–167.
129. Baier-Bitterlich G, Fuchs D, Murr C, et al: Effect of neopterin and 7,8-dihydroneopterin on tumor necrosis factor-α-induced programmed cell death. FEBS Lett 1995;364:234–238.
130. Bair-Bitterlich G, Fuchs D, Zangerle R, et al: Trans-activation of the HIV-1 promoter by 7,8-dihydroneopterin: a potential role of neopterin derivatives in AIDS progression. AIDS Res Human Retrovir 1997;13:173–178.
131. Schobersberger W, Hoffmann G, Hobisch-Hagen P, et al: Neopterin and 7,8-dihydroneopterin induce apoptosis in the rat alveolar epithelial cell line L2. FEBS Lett 1996;397:263–268.
132. Novelli F, Bernabei P, Ozmen L, et al: Switching on of the proliferation or apoptosis of activated human T lymphocytes by IFN-gamma is correlated with the differential expression of the alpha- and beta-chains of its receptor. J Immunol 1996;157:1935–1933.
133. Fuchs D, Zangerle R, Artner-Dworzak E, et al: Association between immune activation changes of iron metabolism and anemia in patients with human immunodeficiency virus (HIV-1) infection. Eur J Haematol 1993;50:90–94.
134. Denz H, Orth B, Weiss G, et al: Weight loss in patients with hematological neoplasias is associated with immune system stimulation. Clin Invest 1993;71:37–41.
135. Zangerle R, Reibnegger G, Wachter H, Fuchs D: Weight loss in HIV-1 infection is associated with immune activation. AIDS 1993;7:175–181.
136. Fuchs D, Stahl-Hennig C, Gruber A, Murr C, Hunsmann G, Wachter H: Neopterin: its clinical use in urinalysis. Kidney Int 1994;46(S47):8–11.

48
Endotoxin Antagonists

David L. Dunn

Over the last several decades our ability to prolong life and treat diseases once thought incurable has increased considerably. However, concurrent with the advent of new biotechnologic, medical, and surgical approaches to the treatment of a variety of complex disease processes has come the recognition that our abilities remain finite. In particular, infection continues to represent a substantial cause of morbidity and mortality in all groups of patients, and many of the new therapeutic modalities (e.g., cancer chemotherapy, solid organ and bone marrow transplantation, intensive care unit treatment) are associated with significantly increased rates and previously unrecognized infections.

Today, the paradigm that delineates cause and effect during serious infection no longer comprises solely the interaction of bacterial microbes with cellular and humoral components of the host defense response that results in "laudable pus." It involves a plethora of bacterial, fungal, viral, and parasitic microbes and their associated virulence factors frequently acting as both infecting organisms and triggers of the host cytokine response, in conjunction with cellular and humoral host defenses. The exaggerated host cytokine response itself has become increasingly recognized as a significant component of this paradigm, being closely associated with the occurrence of adverse effects, many of the manifestations of which appear to be integral with the clinical entity termed *sepsis syndrome*. This contention, however, has not been unequivocally substantiated in the clinical setting.

Bacterial infection and associated bacteremic episodes are common occurrences in hospitalized patients and represent a frequent cause of sepsis syndrome, a process that frequently progresses to multisystem organ failure and death. Sepsis syndrome is the thirteenth leading cause of death among patients in the United States, with as many as 400,000 cases occurring annually; surgical patients account for about 30% of these cases.[1] Although the incidence of nosocomial infection due to gram-positive microbes has superseded those caused by other organisms, gram-negative bacterial infections remain common. In particular, serious gram-negative bacterial infections at specific sites with or without associated bacteremic episodes currently account for about 35% of cases of sepsis syndrome.[2] Despite improvements in antimicrobial therapy and intensive care (e.g., aggressive fluid resuscitation, hemodynamic monitoring, and metabolic support), mortality associated with gram-negative bacterial sepsis remains at about 40%. This high mortality rate has changed little over the last several decades.[3,4]

It has been well established that gram-negative bacterial lipopolysaccharide (LPS, endotoxin), an integral component of the gram-negative bacterial outer membrane, exerts a direct toxic effect on a variety of cell types; more importantly, it triggers elaboration of a constellation of endogenous compounds that exert effects on the mammalian host during serious gram-negative bacterial infection.[5-7] Foremost among these endogenous "secondary mediators" are an array of cytokines elaborated by macrophages, monocytes, and other cell types whose secretion, in composite, appears to provoke the host septic response.[8,9] Because LPS represents such a potent and critical trigger of this response, reagents that inhibit its effects have undergone intense investigation in both the laboratory and clinical settings. Their use as adjunctive forms of therapy for sepsis syndrome due to gram-negative microbial pathogens continues to be an area of active research, with significant advances occurring.

Biochemistry and Immunology of Endotoxin

Lipopolysaccharide is an integral portion of the gram-negative bacterial cell membrane and appears to be responsible for many, if not all, of the toxic effects that occur during gram-negative bacterial sepsis. The LPS molecule is complex, with three distinct regions, each with unique pathogenic and antigenic properties: (1) O-antigen polysaccharide, a series of 30-100 repeating oligosaccharide units that comprise the major antigenic determinants for each individual strain of gram-negative bacteria; (2) a core region of a series of 10-12 saccharide residues linking the external O-antigen to the lipid A region (see below), portions of which exhibit structural similarity among some groups of bacterial genera and families (this region contains three subregions: outer, intermediate, and inner or deep core); and (3) lipid A, which is the toxic moiety of LPS

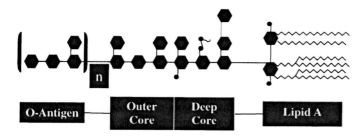

FIGURE 48.1. Biochemical and immunologic structure of gram-negative bacterial lipopolysaccharide (LPS, endotoxin). The LPS molecule has three distinct regions: (1) O-antigen polysaccharide, a series of 30–100 repeating oligosaccharide units that comprise the major antigenic determinants for each individual strain of gram-negative bacteria; (2) a core region of a series of 10–12 saccharide residues (shown as hexagons) linking the external O-antigen to the lipid A region, portions of which exhibit structural similarity among some groups of bacterial genera and families; this region contains three subregions: outer, intermediate, and inner or deep core; and (3) lipid A, which is the toxic moiety of LPS, composed of diphosphorylated diglucosamine residues containing ester and amide-linked fatty acids (jagged lines). The deep core/lipid A region may be considered a unit (i.e., DCLA) for two important reasons: (1) it encompasses the toxic moiety and (2) it is remarkably similar among even disparate species of gram-negative bacterial pathogens.

composed of diphosphorylated diglucosamine residues containing ester- and amide-linked fatty acids. (Fig. 48.1).[3,10–12] Intriguingly, whereas the O-antigen region comprises antigenic determinants unique to each strain of gram-negative microbe such that antibodies developed against it bind solely to that bacterium or its derived LPS, the deep core and lipid A (DCLA) region of LPS appears to contain cross-reactive epitopes. In fact, the latter region may be considered a unit (i.e., DCLA) for two important reasons: (1) it encompasses the toxic moiety and (2) it is remarkably similar among even disparate species of gram-negative bacterial pathogens. Not surprisingly, it is this region that has been identified as the primary target for endotoxin antagonism.

Host Response to Endotoxin

Endotoxin is a potent macrophage stimulant (directly or via activation of bioactive phospholipids such as platelet-activating factor), provoking cytokine synthesis and secretion into the internal tissue milieu and presumably thereafter into the systemic circulation by these principal target cells. Similar, but generally less potent, secretory effects have been demonstrated in experimental animal models using gram-positive bacterial organisms, toxins, or fungal microbes with or without coadministration of small amounts of endotoxin. This property of endotoxin has allowed the host cytokine response to be characterized in animal models of gram-negative bacterial infection and subsequent to the injection of gram-negative bacterial endotoxin into animals and humans; the cellular basis for this response is increasingly understood.

Lipopolysaccharide interacts with the cell membrane of macrophages, triggering secretion of a wide array of cytokines, including tumor necrosis factor-α (TNFα), interleukin-1β (IL-1β), IL-6, and IL-8. LPS-stimulated macrophages rapidly upregulate TNFα gene transcription and translation, which results in as much as a 10,000-fold increase in TNFα expression.[13,14] Unfortunately, intensive efforts to locate the putative macrophage cell surface molecule that interacts with LPS have not been successful in identifying a single entity that leads to cellular activation. Instead, a series of receptors have been identified, and it appears that several play an important role in LPS-induced macrophage activation. These receptors include CD14,[15,16] CD11b/CD18,[17] and acetyl-low density lipoprotein (acetyl-LDL);[18] but there also appear to be nonspecific interactions between LPS and the mammalian cell membrane unrelated to any specific receptor.[19] Among these entities, CD14 has sparked the most interest because endogenous LPS-binding protein (LBP) binds to LPS, which in turn engages CD14 and causes cellular activation.[20–22] Of note, CD14 receptor itself is shed from the cell surface, becoming soluble (sCD14); it appears to be responsible for binding to LPS as well.[23] LBP-facilitated LPS-mediated cellular activation via CD14 appears to be most pronounced in the presence of minute quantities of LPS, well below those observed during serious infection.[24] Therefore the relevance of this interaction to the host septic response during the sepsis syndrome remains unclear.

Subsequent to endotoxin challenge, it is well established that peak serum levels of TNFα occur within 1.5–2.0 hours and rapidly decline thereafter in animals and humans. Maximal secretion of IL-1β occurs slightly later, although it has been more difficult to measure, and elevated levels are observed inconsistently in humans, particularly during infection. IL-6 levels rise even later (>4 hours) after endotoxin injection in animals and humans, as do IL-8 levels in humans. Peak TNFα levels can occur much later (10–16 hours) after bacterial challenge in experimental models of infection, in contrast to the early peak evidenced after endotoxin injection.[25,26] These cytokines, acting in concert with the cellular and humoral branches of the immune system, are an important host defense mechanism against infection, presumably activating other cells within the local tissue milieu in the presence of invading microbes.

Subsequent to LPS-mediated release, TNFα and IL-1β mediate their effects by binding to and interacting with their specific cellular receptors. TNFα has two receptors: TNF RI (p55) and TNF RII (p75). However, the effects of TNFα appear to be manifested primarily by signal transduction through TNF receptor type I (RI), whereas TNFRII plays an integral role in T cell proliferation.[27] Similar nomenclature has been applied to the two identified IL-1 receptors, IL-1RI (p80) and IL-1RII (p68).[28] Unlike the dual roles for the two TNF receptors, only IL-1RI appears to be functional; no cellular signaling has yet been identified for IL-1RII. Of note, there is evidence that these cytokine receptors exist in both membrane-associated and soluble forms, further complicating the pattern of interaction of these cytokines with their respective receptors during gram-negative bacterial infection, bacteremia, and concurrent endotoxemia.

Concurrent with the secretion of IL-1β and TNFα during gram-negative bacterial infection and endotoxemia, a complex network of endogenous cytokine antagonists for these cytokines functions to dampen the host cytokine response. IL-1 receptor antagonist (IL-1ra) is secreted, and TNF-binding protein (TNF-BP) is shed from the cell surface (representing TNFRI); other agents tightly regulate cytokine elaboration under normal circumstances, although during severe infection an exaggerated, dysregulated cytokine response can occur.[29,30] Analysis of the relevant data increasingly supports the contention that elevated levels of a specific cytokine and its cellular receptor may not lead to adverse effects early during sepsis, whereas exaggerated cytokine secretion concurrent with secretion of the endogenous antagonist for several days may be closely correlated with deleterious consequences.[31,32]

Although it is likely that most cytokines function as intra- and intercellular regulation signals within the tissue milieu, it has been hypothesized that their widespread activation by endotoxin leads to their presence in high levels in the systemic circulation, which in turn causes unchecked activation at numerous additional tissue sites. This process has been implicated in the etiology of sepsis syndrome during gram-negative bacteremic episodes. Studies that provide support for this concept can be summarized as follows: (1) lethal endotoxin injection into experimental animals results in consistently elevated levels of TNFα and IL-1β prior to death; (2) direct injection of TNFα is associated with toxicity similar to that which occurs after endotoxin injection and eventuates in death; and (3) TNFα blockade using anti-TNFα antibodies or TNF-BP in animals during endotoxemia and/or gram-negative bacteremia is associated with diminished cytokine levels and promotes survival;[33-36] similar data regarding the role of IL-1β using IL-1ra blockade have been provided.[37,38]

Surprisingly, from a clinical prognostic standpoint, neither detection nor elevation of endotoxin, TNFα, or IL-1β levels has provided a substantial degree of correlation with standard outcome parameters: length of intensive care unit (ICU) stay, morbidity, or mortality. Perhaps the only exception concerns patients who develop meningococcal bacteremia, in whom the degree of elevation of serum TNFα was related to mortality.[39] However, a closer relation has been demonstrated between the presence of elevated IL-6 levels and these parameters.[32] In fact, inverse correlations with cytokine levels and mortality have been noted by some investigators. In one study patients who exhibited high levels of IL-1β were more likely to survive than those who exhibited low levels; IL-1ra levels were not measured in this study.[40] Also, neither the degree nor the pattern of elevation of cytokine levels has been particularly helpful for distinguishing between gram-positive, gram-negative, and fungal pathogens as causative agents of the sepsis syndrome. Thus a dichotomy exists in the clinical setting: A good correlation of outcome and elevated levels of either endotoxin or those cytokines that have been demonstrated to exert toxic effects (TNFα and IL-1β) has not been forthcoming, although it has been for those that are benign (e.g., IL-6).

A number of explanations can be put forth to explain this observation: (1) It seems likely that the transient elevations in endotoxin and either TNFα or IL-1β occur so early in the response to infection that detection is problematic; the more sustained rise in IL-6 occurs later—probably after other sentinel signs and symptoms of infection are more readily apparent—and it is more readily detected. (2) An alternative explanation is that systemic cytokine levels are not invariably reflective of the presence of elevated levels of deleterious cytokines within the tissue milieu of one or more organs affected. (3) Increasing evidence indicates that correlation with adverse effects in the clinical setting is possible only if both cytokine and soluble cytokine receptor levels are measured, and this has been undertaken only to a limited degree thus far. These issues are of critical importance when analyzing the results of extant clinical trials designing future trials in which cytokine levels might be used to satisfy entry criteria, stratify patients, or determine the timing of administration of exogenous cytokine antagonists; and assessing the need for repeated doses of a particular reagent.

Endotoxin Antagonists

In an attempt to reduce the high mortality associated with gram-negative bacterial sepsis, two principal areas of investigation have emerged: (1) development of reagents that inhibit the interaction of LPS with the putative LPS receptor(s) on the surface of the macrophage and (2) inhibition of the host cytokine response to LPS [anti-TNFα antibody, TNF-BP, IL-1ra, platelet-activating factor receptor antagonist (PAFra)]. Among the former group of reagents, several classes of compounds that serve to antagonize the effects of endotoxin have been or are being developed and characterized. They consist of agents that: (1) bind directly to LPS and thereby neutralize its effects [anti-LPS monoclonal antibodies (mAbs), naturally occurring proteins and their derivatives, e.g., bactericidal permeability inhibiting protein (BPI), *Limulus* anti-LPS factor (LALF), and certain antibiotics (polymyxin B, taurolidine)] and (2) LPS receptor antagonists [soluble CD14 receptor (sCD14), antiidiotypic, anti-DCLA mAbs] (Table 48.1). All such agents theoretically should act to interdict the interaction of LPS with cell surface receptors of a variety of cell types, including macrophages, thereby preventing the activation of intracellular signaling pathways (tyrosine kinase, protein kinase C) that lead to cytokine gene upregulation and cytokine protein synthesis and secretion.[41]

Anti-endotoxin polyclonal antibodies were initially identified as part of the host immune response to gram-negative bacterial infection and endotoxemia. Subsequent to the identification of strains of *Salmonella minnesota*, *Escherichia coli*, *Pseudomonas aeruginosa*, and other related organisms that express a truncated portion of LPS on their cell surface, active and passive immunization using these microbes or their derived LPS was

TABLE 48.1. Reagents that Antagonize the Effects of Endotoxin.

Direct LPS antagonism
  Anti-DCLA mAbs
  BPI
  LALF
  Polymyxin B
  Taurolidine

LPS receptor antagonists
  sCD14
  Anti-idiotypic, anti-DCLA mAbs

Reagents that serve to antagonize the effects of endotoxin have been or are being developed and characterized. They consist of (1) agents that bind directly to LPS and thereby directly antagonize its effects, and (2) LPS receptor antagonists. DCLA, deep core and lipid A; mAbs, monoclonal antibodies; BPI, bacterial permeability inhibiting protein; LALF, *Limulus* antilipopolysaccharide factor; LPS, lipopolysaccharide.

examined and found to exert protective capacity during experimental infection.[42,43] This effect correlated with the presence of an endogenous anti-DCLA titer, particularly of the immunoglobulin M (IgM) type, increased with patient age and correlated with favorable outcome during serious gram-negative bacterial infection.[32,44,45]

Thereafter murine and then human anti-LPS mAbs were initially described by several groups and appear to represent potent reagents, although their utility is hindered by their inability to bind to more than a single, unique strain of gram-negative bacteria or its derived LPS.[46–52] Compared to mAbs directed against the strain-specific O-antigen polysaccharide region of LPS, anti-DCLA mAbs bind with lower affinity to various types of LPS and confer less protective capacity in animal models of endotoxemia and infection (e.g., peritonitis or bacteremia).[53] Scanning electron microscopy demonstrated that anti-DCLA mAbs also bind less well to intact smooth bacteria, but that binding is enhanced by pretreating the microbes with sublethal doses of cell wall lytic antibiotic agents, perhaps exposing DCLA sites. Overall, decreased efficacy appears to be directly correlated with the extent of cross-reactivity.

The identification and characterization of three endogenous anti-LPS host defense proteins (BPI, LALF, LBP)—all of which appear to bind endotoxin and neutralize its effects in a variety of in vitro assays—have been of interest. BPI is a 55-kDa mammalian host defense protein stored in the azurophilic granules of human neutrophils and released in the presence of gram-negative bacteria. It is bactericidal and binds and neutralizes LPS derived from a wide variety of gram-negative bacteria based on its capacity to bind to lipid A.[54,55] The specificity of BPI for gram-negative bacteria results from the high affinity of this compound for the lipid A region of LPS, which involves both charge and hydrophobic interactions. The amino-terminal portion of the BPI molecule is positively charged, producing a large electrostatic attraction to the anionic sites in the core region of LPS. In addition, hydrophobic stretches in the N-terminal region of BPI interact with the lipid A moiety of LPS. Although BPI exists as an approximately 400-amino-acid protein, its bactericidal and endotoxin-neutralizing activity has been localized to the amino-terminal 200 amino acids.[56] Recombinant BPI_{23} ($rBPI_{23}$), consisting only of the 200 amino acids comprising the amino-terminus of the holoprotein, has been more effective than whole BPI against gram-negative bacteria in vitro and in vivo.[57] This finding provides additional support for the contention that molecular size may be an important factor when designing reagents that target the toxic lipid A moiety buried deep within the gram-negative outer membrane.

Limulus anti-LPS factor is a 12-kDa protein derived from amebocytes of the American horseshoe crab *Limulus polyphemus*. Purified LALF inhibits the biologic activity of LPS in vitro, including activation of human endothelial cells and murine splenocytes.[58] Preincubation of LALF with LPS in vitro reduced LPS-induced mortality in experimental models of gram-negative bacterial sepsis.[59–63] Finally, LBP is secreted as an acute-phase reactant primarily by the liver during inflammation and infection.[64,65] Unlike BPI or LALF, LBP forms a complex with LPS, which in turn binds to the CD14 receptor found on macrophages and other cell types and has the ability to augment, rather than inhibit, LPS-induced TNFα secretion by macrophages in vitro; as noted above, it probably acts similarly in vivo, albeit in the presence of small amounts of LPS.[66] Preliminary data indicate that the CD14 receptor may be shed, and the soluble form (sCD14) may act as an endotoxin antagonist as well by blocking the interaction of LPS-LBP with the cell-bound CD14 receptor, thereby inhibiting cytokine secretion.[67] In addition, mAbs directed against the CD14 receptor might also block its interaction with endotoxin and provide protection during experimental endotoxemia.[68]

The molecular biology of BPI, LALF, and LBP is of considerable interest, as each demonstrates considerable genetic sequence homology. Intriguingly, each of these proteins possesses substantial amino acid homology, and they appear to possess a common approximately 30-amino-acid region that is responsible for LPS binding (Fig. 48.2). This region possesses (1) an increased number of basic, positively charged amino acids and (2) a β-sheet conformation that may be responsible for LPS binding, as the lipid A moiety is anionically charged.[69,70] This knowledge has been used experimentally to develop and characterize novel endotoxin antagonists. For example, 27- to 30-amino-acid peptides generated based on the common regions of BPI, LALF, and LBP appear to have considerable endotoxin neutralizing capacity, to reduce cytokine levels in vitro and in vivo, and to provide in vivo protective capacity.[71] It bears mention that similar properties within the variable binding regions of anti-DCLA mAbs have been elucidated.[72]

Several additional endotoxin antagonists have been examined in experimental animal models, although their activity in the clinical setting remains to be demonstrated. They comprise (1) lipid A analogues; (2) antiidiotypic anti-endotoxin mAbs; and (3) antibiotics that have antiendotoxin characteristics. Chemical analogues of lipid A may act to abrogate the effects of lipid A and as immunostimulants.[73,74] These reagents have undergone experimental but not clinical testing. Anti-DLCA antiidiotypic mAbs have been developed in an attempt to block the

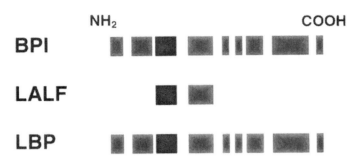

FIGURE 48.2. Molecular biology of bactericidal permeability increasing protein (BPI), *Limulus* anti-LPS factor (LALF), and lipopolysaccharide-binding protein (LBP) is of considerable interest, as each demonstrates considerable genetic sequence homology. Each of these proteins [general regions shown as rectangles: amino (NH_2) and carboxy (COOH) termini] possesses substantial amino acid homology and appears to possess a common approximately 30-amino-acid region that is responsible for LPS binding (depicted in black). This region possesses (1) an increased number of basic, positively charged amino acids and (2) a β-sheet conformation that may be responsible for LPS binding, as the lipid A moiety is anionically charged.

interaction of LPS with the macrophage cellular receptors that trigger cytokine synthesis and secretion.[75] It has been possible to demonstrate the capacity of these mAbs to bind specifically to the original anti-DCLA mAb and to inhibit TNFα-induced endotoxic activity in vitro.[76] Polymyxin B, an antibiotic that binds stoichiometrically to lipid A, represents another potent endotoxin antagonist. This compound is an amphipathic cyclic oligopeptide that contains a region that also has many basic, positively charged amino acids linked to a single fatty acid. Intriguingly, it has amino acid sequences that bear considerable homology to the endotoxin-binding regions of BPI, LALF, and LBP. Although it binds to the lipid A region of LPS with high affinity and effectively neutralizes its biologic effects, its use is limited by its systemic toxicity in vivo.

Clinical Trials

Major advances have been made in the process of conducting a number of large-scale, multicenter clinical trials in septic patients. Foremost among these advances was characterization of the host septic response in the clinical setting. This response continues to be referred to as *sepsis* (absence of organ failure) or *sepsis syndrome* (denoting sepsis plus concomitant organ failure) and is considered to be a subset of the *systemic inflammatory response syndrome* (SIRS), being distinguished from other inflammatory clinical entities (e.g., acute pancreatitis) by the presence of a source of infection. Although various investigators have used slightly different criteria, initial categorization schemes for many clinical trials defined sepsis syndrome as the presence of one or more of the following clinical parameters: (1) fever (temperature > 101°F) or hypothermia (temperature < 96°F rectal); (2) tachycardia (pulse > 90 beats/min in the absence of β-adrenergic blockade); and (3) tachypnea (respiratory rate > 20 breaths/min or the need for intubation and mechanical ventilation) or evidence of significant hemodynamic alteration [systolic blood pressure < 90 mmHg, cardiac output (CO) > 4 L/min/m^2, or systemic vascular resistance (SVR) < 800 dyne/s/cm^5] *plus* evidence of two or more of the following indicators of peripheral hypoperfusion/organ dysfunction: metabolic acidosis (arterial pH < 7.30, base deficit > 5 mmol/L, or elevated lactate > 2.5 mmol/L), hypoxia (PO_2 < 75 mmHg), acute renal or hepatic dysfunction (urine output < 30 ml/hr, serum bilirubin more than twice baseline, respectively), coagulopathy [prolonged prothrombin time, prolonged partial thromboplastin time, or decreased platelet count (less than one-half baseline or <100,000/mm^3)], or acutely altered mental status. If both tachycardia and hypotension persist after adequate fluid resuscitation and other causes (e.g., hemorrhage, myocardial infarction) of these manifestations are excluded, the designation *septic shock* appropriately continues to be applied.[1,3,77]

Subsequently, this classification scheme was simplified, although it remains unclear if it represents an advance in our understanding of the various clinical entities or merely a change in nomenclature. SIRS is now used to describe patients with two or more of the following: temperature > 38°C, heart rate > 90 beats/min, respiratory rate > 20 breaths/min, white blood cell (WBC) count > 12,000 cells/mm^3, and the presence of >10% immature band forms of neutrophils on the peripheral blood smear.[78] The term sepsis syndrome continues to be defined as SIRS resulting from an infectious process, and the term severe sepsis syndrome refers to the added presence of organ dysfunction. Septic shock continues to be redefined as the sepsis syndrome in association with hypotension that persists despite adequate fluid resuscitation. Current clinical studies indicate that about 45% of patients who develop SIRS harbor infection such that they are classified as suffering from sepsis syndrome.[79]

On the basis of a large number of experimental studies validating the concept of the ability of anti-LPS mAbs to abrogate the effects of gram-negative bacterial infection or endotoxemia, three cross-reactive anti-endotoxin mAbs that purportedly bind to the DCLA region of LPS (T88, HA-1A, E5) were developed for clinical use. Only the latter two, however, have been examined extensively in a series of clinical trials. Both HA-1A and E5 are IgM antibodies; the former has largely human components with murine antigen-binding sites (in the expectation of avoiding the human anti-mouse antibody response after administration), and the latter is murine antibody.

In four randomized, blinded, placebo-controlled studies—two using E5, two with HA-1A—routine resuscitative and supportive measures including use of fluid repletion, positive inotropic agents, and administration of appropriate antibiotics were implemented or continued, and patients were followed for 28–30 days or until death (Table 48.2).[80–83] Entry into each trial took place on the basis of a presumptive diagnosis of gram-negative bacterial sepsis, based on the presence of a high likelihood of a gram-negative bacterial infection plus specific clinical indices indicative of sepsis. The two major findings of these trials were that: (1) the current mortality of sepsis syndrome remains at about 40% and (2) despite similar initial clinical presentations, more than 60% of patients with this syndrome did not prove to

TABLE 48.2. Anti-endotoxin Monoclonal Antibody Clinical Trials.

Monoclonal antibody	Mortality due to sepsis syndrome (%)	Comment
Study 1 ($n = 468$)		
E5	40	Decreased mortality in E5-treated patients with gram-negative bacterial sepsis not in shock at entry
Placebo	41	
Study 2 ($n = 530$)		
E5	30	Enhanced resolution of organ failure in E5-treated patients with gram-negative sepsis
Placebo	26	
Study 3 ($n = 543$)		
HA-1A	39	Decreased mortality in HA-1A-treated patients with gram-negative bacteremia; a subset within this group exhibited shock at entry
Placebo	43	
Study 4 ($n = 2199$)		
HA-1A	33	None
Placebo	32	

In four randomized, blinded, placebo-controlled studies examining the efficacy of anti-endotoxin monoclonal antibodies (mAbs) to treat sepsis syndrome, two used E5 mAb, two used HA-1A mAb. Routine resuscitative and supportive measures, including use of fluid repletion, positive inotropic agents, and administration of appropriate antibiotics, were implemented or continued; and patients were followed 28–30 days or until death. Entry into each trial took place on the basis of a presumptive diagnosis of gram-negative bacterial sepsis based on a high likelihood of a gram-negative bacterial infection plus specific clinical indices indicative of sepsis. The two major findings of these trials were that: (1) the current mortality of sepsis syndrome remains at about 40% and (2) despite similar initial clinical presentation, more than 60% of patients with this syndrome did not prove to have gram-negative bacterial sepsis but were infected with gram-positive bacterial or fungal pathogens.

have gram-negative bacterial sepsis but were infected with gram-positive bacterial or fungal pathogens.

In the initial HA-1A trial, the effects of administering a single 100-mg dose of this antibody was compared to that of placebo. Among 543 patients who were treated, no significant differences were noted between HA-1A-treated patients and those who received placebo (39% vs. 43%, $p > 0.05$). In all, 197 patients (36%) demonstrated gram-negative bacteremia, and retrospective analysis demonstrated that among this subgroup 63% of patients who received HA-1A and 48% who received placebo survived 28 days ($p < 0.05$). In the subgroup of patients who developed septic shock, 33% of 54 patients receiving HA-1A died whereas 57% of 47 patients receiving placebo did so ($p < 0.05$). A large number of patients then received this reagent on a compassionate-use basis outside the confines of a structured randomized trial. A second randomized, double-blind multicenter trial was instituted to study the effects of HA-1A using only 14-day mortality as an endpoint. This trial involved 621 patients, and no salutary effect of HA-1A could be demonstrated: The mortality rates for treatment and control groups were 32% and 33%, respectively ($p = 0.864$). In fact, the mortality rates for patients without gram-negative bacteremia were higher for the treatment group than for the control group (37% vs. 41%, $p = 0.073$), which was the basis for this trial being halted.

The effect administering E5 mAb has been evaluated in two clinical trials in which 486 and 831 patients, respectively, received two 2 mg/kg/day doses on consecutive days. The first E5 trial involved 486 patients and compared the effects of two 2 mg/kg/day doses of E5 to that of placebo. In this trial, mortality was similar in the treatment and placebo groups (40% vs. 41%, $p > 0.05$). But within a subgroup of 137 treated patients (who developed gram-negative bacterial infections and evidence of sepsis but who were not in shock at the time of entry into the study) the 30-day mortality of patients receiving E5 was 30% whereas the mortality of patients receiving placebo was 43% ($p < 0.05$). The latter subgroup was then selected for examination in a second clinical trial to determine whether patients not suffering septic shock would benefit from E5 administration. The results of this study of 831 patients indicated that E5 had no effect on survival in 530 patients with documented gram-negative bacteremia, despite a trend toward improved survival in 139 patients who developed organ failure without septic shock compared to placebo. Subsequently, a number of patients also received E5 on a compassionate-use basis outside the confines of a randomized trial.

Concerns have arisen regarding the binding specificity and in vivo efficacy of these two mAbs. Analysis of experimental data has indicated HA-1A may bind in vitro not only to lipid A but also to irrelevant substances such as gram-positive bacterial and fungal antigens and to unrelated lipids.[84] Testing of both HA-1A and E5 in in vitro and in in vivo experimental animal models of gram-negative bacterial sepsis also has indicated lack of substantial biologic activity.[85,86] Therefore it appears highly likely that anti-endotoxin antibody preparations that do not exhibit suitable in vitro or in vivo activity have been tested in large-scale clinical trials. Their lack of efficacy in these trials may be due to the poor activity of these reagents coupled with the inability to identify endotoxemic patients, rather than a lack of validity of this therapeutic approach.

Sporadic attempts have been made to take advantage of the ability of polymyxin B to bind and neutralize endotoxin, despite its recognized nephrotoxicity. Thus low doses of polymyxin B have been administered systemically to septic patients; it has been immobilized to a solid fiber matrix, and ex vivo hemoperfusion has been used to remove endotoxin without systemic toxicity.[87,88] Because of the nephrotoxicity of the compound even with low doses, the former approach has not led to clinical application, and the latter has proved cumbersome. More relevant is the fact that no effect on survival has been demonstrated. In addition, the effect of taurolidine, an amino acid derivative with antiendotoxic properties, was tested in 100 patients with sepsis syndrome who were randomized to receive this agent or placebo. The frequency of gram-negative bacterial sepsis was only 12%, and no reduction in mortality was observed in patients who received this drug.[89]

When the above-mentioned anti-endotoxin mAb clinical trials are considered together with the results of clinical trials in which the effect of cytokine abrogation (e.g., anti-TNFα mAbs,

TNFR:Fc, and IL-1ra clinical trials) was studied for its impact on outcome during sepsis syndrome, some interesting data have emerged.[90-95] Specifically, although the major finding of these trials was not efficacy—as no reagent has demonstrated longevity in more than one clinical trial—tantalizing trends have been apparent in the results of each of these trials, leading to the hope that with more precise initial stratification it may be possible to select subgroups of patients who will benefit from one of these new reagents.

The reasons for lack of efficacy in these immunotherapeutic interventional trials are not clear; based on the extant data only suppositions can be offered. For example, it seems likely that the anti-LPS mAb trials may have failed owing to a lack of reagent activity plus an inability to select the subset of patients with gram-negative bacterial sepsis for targeted therapy. These two problems are surmountable, and the former should not have been an issue in the initial trials. In addition, we must realize that sepsis syndrome remains a *syndrome*, and that we have much to learn before we can successfully combat it. This didactic process must encompass much more than applying locution and definitions to clinical observations; it must include more intensive monitoring in the clinical setting to define more carefully the host cytokine response that we seek to block.

Finally, a fascinating picture is emerging concerning the molecular basis for endotoxin antagonism. Using biochemical and recombinant DNA techniques it should be possible to design a new generation of anti-LPS reagents that allow precise manipulation of molecular size and charge characteristics within the LPS-binding region to determine how best to maximize activity. It seems patent that some, but not all, of the novel compounds may provide more substantial cross-reactivity against endotoxin and have a cross-protective capacity against gram-negative endotoxemia and bacteremia; they certainly warrant further development and testing in vitro and in vivo using experimental animal models and subsequently in large-scale, multicenter clinical trials. With more precise, rapid diagnostic tests for endotoxin and even a limited number of cytokines and endogenous cytokine antagonists (e.g., IL-1β, IL-1ra, TNFα, TNF-BP, IL-6) and use of sepsis scoring systems for initial stratification, it may be possible to use more intelligently the next generation of endotoxin antagonists, perhaps in conjunction with cytokine antagonism, to reduce the mortality of sepsis syndrome.

References

1. Dunn DL: Gram-negative bacterial sepsis and sepsis syndrome. Surg Clin North Am 1994;74:621-635.
2. Anonymous: Center for Disease Control: increase in national hospital discharge survey rates for septicemia—United States, 1979-1987. JAMA 1990;263:937-938.
3. Burd RS, Cody CS, Dunn DL: Immunotherapy of Gram-Negative Bacterial Sepsis. Austin, TX, Medical Intelligence Unit, R.G. Landes, 1992.
4. Battafarano RJ, Dunn DL: Immunotherapy in critically ill patients. In: Chernow BC (ed) The Pharmalologic Approach to the Critically Ill Patient. Baltimore, Williams & Wilkins, 1994;365-378.
5. Cody CS, Dunn DL: Endotoxins in septic shock. In: Neugebauer E, Holaday J (eds) CRC Handbook of Mediators in Septic Shock. Boca Raton, FL, CRC Press, 1993;1-37.
6. Leeson MC, Fujihara Y, Morrison DC: Evidence for lipopolysaccharide as the predominant proinflammatory mediator in supernatants of antibiotic-treated bacteria. Infect Immun 1994;62:4975-4980.
7. Morrison DC: Antibiotic-mediated release of endotoxin and the pathogenesis of gram-negative sepsis. Prog Clin Biol Res 1998;397:199-207.
8. Hesse DG, Tracey KJ, Fong Y, et al: Cytokine appearance in human endotoxemia and primate bacteremia. Surg Gynecol Obstet 1988;166:147-153.
9. Fong Y, Moldawer LL, Shires GT, Lowry SF: The biologic characteristics of cytokines and their implication in surgical injury. Surg Gynecol Obstet 1990;170:363-378.
10. Rietschel ET, Kirikae T, Schade FU, et al: Bacterial endotoxin: molecular relationships of structure of activity and function. FASEB J 1994;8:217-225.
11. Raetz CR: Biochemistry of endotoxins. Annu Rev Biochem 1990;59:129-170.
12. Muller-Loennies S, Zahringer U, Seydel U, Kusumoto S, Ulmer AJ, Rietschel ET: What we don't know about the chemical and physical structure of lipopolysaccharide in relation to biological activity. Prog Clin Biol Res 1998;397:51-72.
13. Han J, Brown T, Beutler B: Endotoxin-responsive sequences control cachectin/tumor necrosis factor biosynthesis at the translational level. J Exp Med 1990;151:101-114.
14. Raetz C, Ulevitch R, Wright S, Sibley C, Ding A, Nathan C: Gram-negative endotoxin: an extraordinary lipid with profound effects on eukaryotic signal transduction. FASEB J 1991;5:2652-2660.
15. Wright SD, Ramos RA, Tobias PS, Ulevitch RJ, Mathison JC: CD14: a receptor for complexes of lipopolysaccharide (LPS) and LPS binding protein. Science 1990;249:1429-1431.
16. Ferrero E, Jiao D, Tsuberi BZ, et al: Transgenic mice expressing human CD14 are hypersensitive to lipopolysaccharide. Proc Natl Acad Sci USA 1993;90:2380-2384.
17. Wright SD, Detmers PA, Aida Y, et al: CD18 deficient cells respond to lipopolysaccharide in vitro. J Immunol 1990;144:2566-2571.
18. Hampton R, Golenbock D, Penman M, Krieger M, Raetz C: Recognition and plasma clearance of endotoxin by scavenger receptors. Nature 1991;352:342-344.
19. Morrison DC, Kirikae T, Lei MG, Chen T, Vukajlovich SW: The receptor(s) for endotoxin on mammalian cells. Prog Clin Biol Res 1994;388:3-15.
20. Tobias PS, Soldau K, Gegner JA, Mintz D, Ulevitch RJ: Lipopolysaccharide binding protein-mediated complexation of lipopolysaccharide with soluble CD14. J Biol Chem 1995;270:10482-10488.
21. Lee JD, Kato K, Tobias PS, Kirkland TN, Ulevitch RJ: Transfection of CD14 into 70Z/3 cells dramatically enhances the sensitivity to complexes of lipopolysaccharide (LPS) and LPS binding protein. J Exp Med 1992;175:1697-1705.
22. Schletter J, Brade H, Brade L, et al: Binding of lipopolysaccharide (LPS) to an 80-kilodalton membrane protein of human cells is mediated by soluble CD14 and LPS-binding protein. Infect Immun 1995;63:2576-2580.
23. Haziot A, Rong GW, Silver J, Goyert SM: Recombinant soluble CD14 mediates the activation of endothelial cells by lipopolysaccharide. J Immunol 1993;151:1500-1507.

24. Landman R, Zimmerli W, Sansano S, et al: Increased circulating soluble CD14 is associated with high mortality in gram-negative septic shock. J Infect Dis 1995;171:639–644.
25. Battafarano RJ, Burd RS, Kurrelmeyer KM, Ratz CA, Dunn DL: Inhibition of splenic macrophage tumor necrosis factor-α secretion in vivo by antilipopolysaccharide monoclonal antibodies. Arch Surg 1994;129:179–186.
26. Hack CE, Aarden LA, Thijs LG: Role of cytokines in sepsis. Adv Immunol 1997;66:101–195.
27. Banner DW, D'Arcy A, Janes W, et al: Crystal structure of the soluble human 55 kd TNF receptor-human TNF beta complex: implications for TNF receptor activation. Cell 1993;73:431–445.
28. Giri JG, Wells J, Dower SK, et al: Elevated levels of shed type II IL-1 receptor in sepsis: potential role for type II receptor in regulation of IL-1 responses. J Immunol 1994;153:5802–5809.
29. Porteu F, Nathan CF: Shedding of tumor necrosis factor receptors by activated human neutrophils. J Exp Med 1990;172:599–607.
30. Aderka D: The potential biological and clinical significance of the soluble tumor necrosis factor receptors. Cytokine Growth Factor Rev 1996;7:231–240.
31. Pruitt J, Copeland E, Moldawer L: Interleukin-1 and interleukin-1 antagonism in sepsis systemic inflammatory response syndrome and septic shock. Shock 1995;3:235–251.
32. Goldie AS, Fearon KC, Ross JA, et al: Natural cytokine antagonists and endogenous antiendotoxin core antibodies in sepsis syndrome: the Sepsis Intervention Group. JAMA 1995;274:172–177.
33. Tracey KJ, Beutler B, Lowry SF, et al: Shock and tissue injury induced by recombinant human cachectin. Science 1986;234:470–474.
34. Beutler B, Milsark IW, Cerami AC: Passive immunization against cachectin/tumor necrosis factor protects mice from lethal effects of endotoxin. Science 1985;299:867–869.
35. Tracey KJ, Fong Y, Hesse DG, et al: Anti-cachectin/TNF monoclonal antibodies prevent septic shock during lethal bacteraemia. Nature 1987;330:662–664.
36. Mohler KM, Torrance DS, Smith CA, et al: Soluble tumor necrosis factor (TNF) receptors are effective therapeutic agents in lethal endotoxemia and function simultaneously as both TNF carriers and TNF antagonists. J Immunol 1993;151:1548–1561.
37. Fischer E, Marano MA, Van Zee KJ, et al: Interleukin-1 receptor blockade improves survival and hemodynamic performance in *Escherichia coli* septic shock, but fails to alter host responses to sublethal endotoxemia. J Clin Invest 1992;89:1551–1557.
38. Ohlsson K, Bjork P, Bergenfeldt M, Hageman R, Thompson RC: Interleukin-1 receptor antagonist reduces mortality from endotoxin shock. Nature 1990;348:550–552.
39. Waage A, Halstensen A, Espevik T: Association between tumour necrosis factor in serum and fatal outcome in patients with meningococcal disease. Lancet 1987;1:355–357.
40. Cannon JG, Tompkins RG, Gelfand JA, et al: Circulating interleukin-1 and tumor necrosis factor in septic shock and experimental endotoxin fever. J Infect Dis 1990;161:79–84.
41. Shapira L, Takashiba S, Champagne C, Amar S, Van Dyke TE: Involvement of protein kinase C and protein tyrosine kinase in lipopolysaccharide-induced TNFα and IL-1β production by human monocytes. J Immunol 1994;153:1818–1824.
42. Dunn DL, Mach PA, Cerra FB: Monoclonal antibodies protect against lethal effects of gram-negative bacterial sepsis. Surg Forum 1983;34:142–144.
43. Dunn DL, Bogard WC, Cerra FB: Efficacy of type-specific and cross-reactive murine monoclonal antibodies directed against endotoxin during experimental sepsis. Surgery 1985;98:283–290.
44. McCabe WR, Kreger BE, Johns M: Type-specific and cross-reactive antibodies in gram-negative bacteremia. N Engl J Med 1972;287:261–267.
45. Zinner SH, McCabe WR: Effects of IgM and IgG antibody in patients with bacteremia due to gram-negative bacilli. J Infect Dis 1976;133:37–45.
46. Dunn DL, Bogard WC, Cerra FB: Enhanced survival during murine gram-negative bacterial sepsis by use of a murine monoclonal antibody. Arch Surg 1985;120:50–53.
47. Dunn DL, Ewald DP, Chandan N, Cerra FB: Immunotherapy of gram-negative bacterial sepsis: a single murine monoclonal antibody provides cross-genera protection. Arch Surg 1986;121:58–62.
48. Dunn DL, Priest BP, Condie RM: Protective capacity of polyclonal and monoclonal antibodies directed against endotoxin during experimental sepsis. Arch Surg 1988;123:1389–1393.
49. Kirkland TN, Colwell DE, Michalek SM, McGhee JR, Ziegler EJ: Analysis of the fine specificity and cross-reactivity of monoclonal anti-lipid A antibodies. J Immunol 1986;137:3614–3619.
50. Teng NN, Kaplan HS, Hebert JM, et al: Protection against gram-negative bacteremia and endotoxemia with human monoclonal IgM antibodies. Proc Natl Acad Sci USA 1985;82:1790–1794.
51. Mayoral JL, Dunn DL: Cross-reactive murine monoclonal antibodies directed against the core/lipid A region of endotoxin inhibit production of tumor necrosis factor. J Surg Res 1990;49:287–292.
52. Cody CS, Burd RS, Mayoral JL, Dunn DL: Protective antilipopolysaccharide monoclonal antibodies inhibit tumor necrosis factor production. J Surg Res 1992;52:314–319.
53. Dunn DL, Bogard WC, Cerra FB: Efficacy of type specific and cross-reactive murine monoclonal antibodies directed against endotoxin during experimental sepsis. Surgery 1985;98:283–290.
54. Gray BH, Haseman JR: Bactericidal activity of synthetic peptides based on the structure of the 55-kilodalton bactericidal protein from human neutrophils. Infect Immun 1994;62:2732–2739.
55. Kohn FR, Ammons WS, Horwitz A, et al: Protective effect of a recombinant amino-terminal fragment of bactericidal/permeability-increasing protein in experimental endotoxemia. J Infect Dis 1993;168:1307–1310.
56. Evans TJ, Carpenter A, Moyes D, Martin R, Cohen J: Protective effects of a recombinant amino-terminal fragment of human bactericidal/permeability-increasing protein in an animal model of gram-negative sepsis. J Infect Dis 1995;171:153–160.
57. Kelly CJ, Cech AC, Argenteanu M, et al: Role of bactericidal/permeability-increasing protein in the treatment of gram-negative pneumonia. Surgery 1993;114:140–146.
58. Aketagawa J, Miyata T, Ohtsubo S, et al: Primary structure of Limulus anticoagulant anti-lipopolysaccharide factor. J Biol Chem 1986;261:7357–7365.
59. Desch C, O'Hara P, Harlan J: Antilipopolysaccharide factor from horseshoe crab, Tachypleus tridentatus, inhibits lipopolysaccharide activation of cultured human endothelial cells. Infect Immun 1989;57:1612–1614.
60. Alpert G, Baldwin G, Thompson C, et al: Limulus antilipopolysaccharide factor protects rabbits from meningococcal endotoxin shock. J Infect Dis 1992;165:494–500.
61. Warren HS, Glennon ML, Wainwright N, et al: Binding and neutralization of endotoxin by Limulus antilipopolysaccharide factor. Infect Immun 1992;60:2506–2513.

62. Roth RI, Su D, Child AH, Wainwright NR, Levin J: Limulus antilipopolysaccharide factor prevents mortality late in the course of endotoxemia. J Infect Dis 1998;177:388–394.
63. Hoess A, Watson S, Siber GR, Liddington R: Crystal structure of an endotoxin-neutralizing protein from the horseshoe crab. Limulus anti-LPS factor, at 1.5Å resolution. EMBO J 1993;12:3351–3356.
64. Theofan G, Horwitz AH, Williams RE, et al: An amino-terminal fragment of human lipopolysaccharide-binding protein retains lipid A binding but not CD14-stimulatory activity. J Immunol 1994;152:3623–3629.
65. Gallay P, Heumann D, Le Roy D, Barras C, Glauser MP: Mode of action of anti-lipopolysaccharide-binding protein antibodies for prevention of endotoxemic shock in mice. Proc Natl Acad Sci USA 1994;91:7922–7926.
66. Han J, Bohuslav J, Jiang Y, et al: CD14 dependent mechanisms of cell activation. Prog Clin Biol Res 1998;397:157–168.
67. Haziot A, Borg GW, Lin XY, Silver J, Goyert SM: Recombinant soluble CD14 prevents mortality in mice treated with endotoxin (lipopolysaccharide). J Immunol 1995;154:6529–6532.
68. Schimke J, Mathison J, Morgiewicz J, Ulevitch RJ: Anti-CD14 mAb treatment provides therapeutic benefit after in vivo exposure to endotoxin. Proc Natl Acad Sci USA 1998;95:13875–13880.
69. Beamer LJ, Carroll SF, Eisenberg D: The BPI/LBP family of proteins: a structural analysis of conserved regions. Protein Sci 1998;7:906–914.
70. Elsbach P: The bactericidal/permeability-increasing protein (BPI) in antibacterial host defense. J Leukocyte Biol 1998;64:14–18.
71. Battafarano RJ, Dahlberg PS, Ratz CA, et al: Peptide derivatives of three distinct lipopolysaccharide binding proteins inhibit lipopolysaccharide-induced tumor necrosis factor-α secretion in vitro. Surgery 1995;118:318–324.
72. Kellogg TA, Weiss CA, Johnston JW, Wasiluk KR, Dunn DL: Antiendotoxin agents share molecular homology within their lipopolysaccharide binding domains. J Surg Res 1999;85:136–141.
73. Kim SK, Battafarano RJ, Dahlberg PS, Dunn DL: Protective effect of monophosphoryl lipid A (MPLA) during systemic candidiasis in neutropenic and normal mice. Surg Forum 1993;44:37–38.
74. Chase JJ, Kubey W, Dulek MH, et al: Effect of monophosphoryl lipid A on host resistance to bacterial infection. Infect Immun 1986;53:711–712.
75. Field SK, Morrison DC: An anti-idiotype antibody which mimics the inner-core region of lipopolysaccharide protects mice against a lethal challenge with endotoxin. Infect Immun 1994;62:3994–3999.
76. Battafarano RJ, Dahlber PS, Uknis ME, et al: A monoclonal antibody designed to mimic LPS binds to the macrophage cell surface and inhibits lipopolysaccharide-induced TNFα secretion in vitro. J Immunol (submitted).
77. Bone RC: Let's agree on terminology: definitions of sepsis. Crit Care Med 1991;19:973–976.
78. Bone RC, Balk RA, Cerra FB, et al: Definitions for sepsis and organ failure and guidelines for the use of innovative therapies in sepsis: the ACCP/SCCM Consensus Conference Committee; American College of Chest Physicians/Society of Critical Care Medicine. Chest 1992;101:1644–1655.
79. Bossink AW, Groeneveld J, Hack CE, Thijs LG: Prediction of mortality in febrile medical patients: how useful are systemic inflammatory response syndrome and sepsis criteria? Chest 1998;113:1533–1541.
80. Ziegler EJ, Fisher CJ Jr, Sprung CL, et al: Treatment of gram-negative bacteremia and septic shock with HA-1A human monoclonal antibody against endotoxin: a randomized, double-blind, placebo-controlled trial: the HA-1A Sepsis Study Group. N Engl J Med 1991;324:429–436.
81. Greenman RL, Schein RM, Martin MA, et al: A controlled clinical trial of E5 murine monoclonal IgM antibody to endotoxin in the treatment of gram-negative sepsis. JAMA 1991;266:1097–1102.
82. McCloskey RV, Straube RC, Sanders C, Smith SM, Smith CR: Treatment of septic shock with human monoclonal antibody HA-1A: a randomized, double-blind, placebo-controlled trial; CHESS Trial Study Group. Ann Intern Med 1994;121:1–5.
83. Bone RC, Balk RA, Fein AM, et al: A second large controlled clinical study of E5, a monoclonal antibody to endotoxin: results of a prospective, multicenter, randomized, controlled trial; the E5 Sepsis Study Group. Crit Care Med 1995;23:994–1005.
84. Baumgartner JD: Immunotherapy with antibodies to core lipopolysaccharide: a critical appraisal. Infect Dis Clin N Am 1991;5:915–927.
85. Warren HS, Amato SF, Fitting C, et al: Assessment of ability of murine and human anti-lipid A monoclonal antibodies to bind and neutralize lipopolysaccharide. J Exp Med 1993;177:89–97.
86. Fujihara Y, Lei MG, Morrison DC: Characterization of specific binding of a human immunoglobulin M monoclonal antibody to lipopolysaccharide and its lipid A domain. Infect Immun 1993;61:910–918.
87. Munster AM, Winchurch RA, Thupari JN, Ernst CB: Reversal of postburn immunosuppression with low-dose polymyxin B. J Trauma 1986;26:995–998.
88. Nakamura T, Suzuki Y, Shimada N, Ebihara I, Shoji H, Koide H: Hemoperfusion with polymyxin B-immobilized fiber attenuates the increased plasma levels of thrombomodulin and von Willebrand factor from patients with septic shock. Blood Purif 1998;16:179–186.
89. Willatts SM, Radford S, Leitermann M: Effect of the antiendotoxin agent, taurolidine, in the treatment of sepsis syndrome: a placebo-controlled, double-blind trial. Crit Care Med 1995;23:1033–1039.
90. Fisher CJ Jr, Opal SM, Dhainaut JF, et al: Influence of an anti-tumor necrosis factor monoclonal antibody on cytokine levels in patients with sepsis: the CB0006 Sepsis Syndrome Study Group. Crit Care Med 1993;21:318–327.
91. Abraham E, Wunderink R, Silverman H, et al: Efficacy and safety of monoclonal antibody to human tumor necrosis factor α in patients with sepsis syndrome. JAMA 1995;273:934–941.
92. Fisher CJ Jr, Slotman GJ, Opal SM, et al: Initial evaluation of human recombinant interleukin-1 receptor antagonist in the treatment of sepsis syndrome: a randomized, open-label, placebo-controlled multicenter trial; the IL-1RA Sepsis Syndrome Study Group. Crit Care Med 1994;22:12–21.
93. Fisher CJ Jr, Dhainaut JF, Opal SM, et al: Recombinant human interleukin 1 receptor antagonist in the treatment of patients with sepsis syndrome: results from a randomized, double-blind, placebo-controlled trial; phase III rhIL-1ra Sepsis Syndrome Study Group. JAMA 1994;271:1836–1843.
94. Fisher CJ Jr, Agosti JM, Opal SM, et al: Treatment of septic shock with the tumor necrosis factor receptor: Fc fusion protein; the Soluble TNF Receptor Sepsis Study Group. N Engl J Med 1996;334:1697–1702.
95. Abraham E, Glauser MP, Butler T, et al: A p55 tumor necrosis factor receptor fusion protein in the treatment of patients with severe sepsis and septic shock: a randomized controlled multicenter trial; Ro 45-2081 Study Group. JAMA 1997;277:1531–1538.

49
Blood Purification Therapy to Prevent or Treat MOF

Hiroyuki Hirasawa and Arthur E. Baue

The concept of hemodialysis and peritoneal dialysis for renal failure, which has been so successful, has been expanded into a number of techniques called blood purification. Plasmapheresis has a role in the management of refractory myasthenia gravis, Goodpasture syndrome, hemolytic uremia, and Guillain-Barré syndrome.[1] There is no doubt that removal of toxic products from the blood, such as endotoxin and mediator cytokines, could help sick, injured and septic patients. A number of clinical trials have suggested benefit for patients with systemic inflammatory response syndrome (SIRS), multiple organ dysfunction syndrome (MODS), and multiple organ failure (MOF). There are a number of clinical problems that could be helped by such techniques in addition to the removal of potassium, urea nitrogen, and creatinine for renal failure (see Chapter 36). Potential benefits include (1) removal of excess fluid contributing to heart failure, pulmonary edema, and impaired arterial and tissue oxygenation; (2) removal of humoral mediators of inflammation; (3) removal of endotoxin; (4) nutritional management; (5) correction of fluid, electrolyte, and acid-base balance; (6) support as an artificial liver (see Chapter 44).

This therapy has been reviewed in detail by one of us with colleagues in the *World Journal of Surgery*[2] and by both of us in *Current Opinion in Critical Care*.[3] We refer frequently to material from these reviews in this chapter.

Methods of Blood Purification

The new technology that allows blood purification continuously for 24 hours a day 7 days a week in critically ill patients for as long as it is needed or beneficial has been called continuous renal replacement therapy (CRRT) or continuous blood purification (CBP). This technique is believed to be easier and better than intermittent hemodialysis for intensive care unit (ICU) patients, who may be hemodynamically unstable. This approach is more physiologic with less hypotension and cerebral edema, better control of fluid overload, and better nutritional support than is intermittent hemodialysis.[2] A number of techniques can be used. Hirasawa et al. believe that the best technique for this purpose is continuous hemodiafiltration (CHDF), which can be used by ICU staff who have not been trained in hemodialysis.[2] CHDF, which is a combination of continuous hemofiltration and continuous hemodialysis with small-volume dialysate flow can remove substances of up to 30,000–40,000 molecular weight. Bleeding problems with this technique have been overcome using nafamostat mesylate, a synthetic protease inhibitor, as the anticoagulant. As described by Hirasawa et al., "CHDF is performed using a polymethylmethacrylate (PMMA) membrane hemofilter with membrane area of 1.0 m². Nafamostat mesylate, a synthetic protease inhibitor with anticoagulation properties is used as the anticoagulant. The standard blood flow, filtrate flow, and dialysate flow are 60 ml/min, 300 ml/hr, and 500 ml/hr, respectively. A special bedside console for CHDF, designed and developed by them, is applied. There were no hemorrhagic complications related to anticoagulation with nafamostat mesylate during CHDF. CHDF could be performed safely on a patient in the immediate postoperative period, or even during operation in an operating room if necessary."[2]

For endotoxin removal, polymyxin B-immobilized fibers now also are used for perfusion by blood. A flow diagram of CHDF is shown in Fig. 49.1. Cannulation is through the femoral vein with a double-lumen catheter.

Endotoxin Removal

Hemoperfusion with an immobilized polymyxin B–fiber column has been popular in Japan, where there have been numerous reports of its use in septic patients. This technique has been reviewed particularly in burn patients by Munster (see Chapter 9). Hanasawa et al.,[4] in a clinical trail in eight medical centers in Japan, found that hemodynamic parameters were a bit better using this technique for endotoxin removal. Endotoxin values and survival were not mentioned in this study. Aoki et al.[5] treated 16 patients (nonrandomized) who had septic MOF with this technique. They found a significant decrease in endotoxin levels, a decrease in the hyperdynamic circulation of sepsis, an increase in blood pressure, and a decrease in fever, with 7 of the 16 patients leaving the hospital alive. Kodama et al.[6] found a significant improvement in survival of septic patients using this

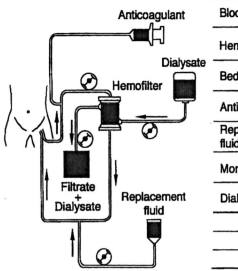

FIGURE 49.1. Flow diagram and operational conditions of CHDF.

technique of endotoxin elimination. Munster describes a series of prospective randomized trials using an endotoxin column in burn patients. Endotoxin levels decreased, but there was no effect on clinical septic complications or on the mortality rate (see Chapter 9). Thus the evidence is divided on whether endotoxin removal makes a clinical difference. There seems little doubt that endotoxin levels can be decreased, but the hypothesis has been proposed that when endotoxin is present in the blood it has perhaps already done its damage and its removal at that stage may not help the patient. More evidence will be forthcoming and will influence how widespread this technique can be used.

Removal of Humoral Mediators

It has been proposed that if excessive inflammatory mediators could be removed from the blood septic or MOF patients would benefit. There have been differences of opinion, however, as to the effect of removing such elevated concentrations of mediators and in determining if the dialysis techniques remove larger molecules. Some years ago Hirasawa et al. found that patients with SIRS, MODS, and MOF undergoing 3 days of CHDF had decreased blood levels of tumor necrosis factor (TNF), interleukin-6 (IL-6), IL-8, C3a, and lipid peroxide (Fig. 49.2). This was particularly true when the initial levels in these patients were high.[7] If the blood levels of these cytokines were low initially, CHDF had no effect on further lowering them. The authors pointed out that with low levels the level actually increased somewhat. They believed this was due to cytokine production via activation of leukocytes by the hemofilter membrane. They also believed that some level of cytokines remaining in the blood is salutary because we now know that loss of certain cytokines or their blockade is harmful in many circumstances. They also found that removal of high levels of these humoral mediators had clinical benefit for their patients. The changes in cytokine levels correlated significantly and positively with changes in the respiratory index in these patients (Fig. 49.3). Thus pulmonary function was improved. This was helpful for patients with ARDS.[8]

Bellomo et al. also found that CHF can remove cytokines from the blood of septic patients.[9] Schetz et al. challenged these data.[10] These investigators reported that the characteristics of the molecules of proinflammatory cytokines such as TNF and IL-1 could not be appropriately removed by hemofiltration, and they stated that no clinical study showed a reduction of cytokine levels with hemofiltration. Hirasawa et al.[8] said that the predominant form of TNF in the blood is a trimer with a molecular weight of 45,000–55,000, which would preclude passage through the membrane of the filter used for CRRT. On the other hand, recent work from Hirasawa's laboratory indicates that clearance of cytokines with CHDF significantly and positively correlates with the blood levels of those cytokines: the higher the blood level, the greater the clearance. This is due to the fact, they believe, that cytokines are removed with CHDF not only through convection and diffusion but also adsorption to the hemofilter membrane. Hirasawa et al.[8] believe that the difference between the results cited by Schetz et al.[10] and their own are due to Schetz's group using CHF whereas Hirasawa's group used CHDF, which they believe can remove substances more effectively and with larger molecular weights than can CHF. They also believe that the material in the hemofilter is crucial for the removal of cytokines with CHDF, as the adsorption of cytokine to the hemofilter membrane is an important mechanism of cytokine removal with CHDF. The absorbing capacity of the hemofilter membrane varies among various hemofilters made from different membranes. For this purpose, the polymethylmethacrylate (PMMA) hemofilter, which Hirasawa's group used, is best. Dr. Schetz's group did not use this filter.

Hirasawa et al. found also that there was no clearance of granulocyte elastase by the CHDF technique. The reason is that the molecular weight of granulocyte elastase is reported to be 50,000–100,000 daltons after being combined (as it does) particularly with α_1-antitrypsin.[11]

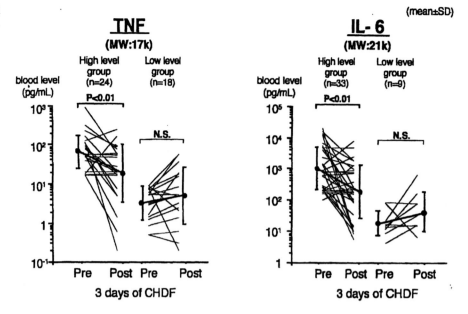

FIGURE 49.2. Changes in blood levels of TNF and IL-6 with 3 Days of CHDF with PMMA Hemofilter.

Hoffman et al. found that continuous hemofiltration in patients with sepsis eliminated certain immunomodulatory substances.[12] Membrane contact during hemofiltration did not seem to activate mediators of MODS, although certain factors such as C3a were effectively eliminated by this technique. They believe there is some promise in this. They had previously shown a correlation between the daily amount of ultrafiltrate and the survival rate. Bellomo et al. found that high-volume hemofiltration (6L/hr × 8 hours) in patients in septic shock greatly reduced the need for norepinephrine support of blood pressure.[13] Using historic controls, Hirasawa et al. believe that CHDF improved survival in MOF patients.[7]

Kline et al. reported that large-pore hemodialysis improved ventricular function in endotoxic dogs.[14] Dhainaut et al., in an editorial about that study, stated: "consequently, no clinical study has shown a reduction in cytokine levels with these techniques."[15] Either these authors do not accept the work of Hirasawa et al. and Bellomo et al., or they do not know the literature or are quibbling about techniques.[15]

Improved Tissue Oxygenation and Metabolism with CHDF

There has been considerable discussion and study of the need to increase oxygen delivery and consumption in critically ill patients. Oda et al. (with Hirasawa) found that CHDF effectively improved oxygen consumption in septic patients,[16] but it had no effect on oxygen delivery. In this study they used a combination of fluid resuscitation and catecholamines. One group was randomized to receive CHDF, and the other did not. This was an important aspect of therapy. They thought the improvement in oxygen consumption might be due to decreased interstitial edema, improvement in the microcirculation, and

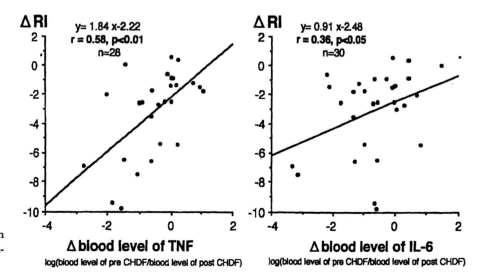

FIGURE 49.3. Correlation between changes in blood level of cytokines and changes in respiratory index (ΔRI) with 3 days of CHDF.

increased uptake of oxygen by parenchymal cells; or it might be due to removal of the humoral mediators that depress oxygen uptake by parenchymal cells. Reeves and Butt reported that continuous blood purification could be done safely in children with severe sepsis as an adjunctive therapy.[17]

Other Uses of CHDF

Some groups have used CHDF for nutritional management, particularly in patients who develop renal failure as part of MOF. This therapy can also remove any excess water given as a carrier for total parenteral nutrition (TPN) or even for enteral nutrition if it is used. Again, Hirasawa's group found that nutritional support was improved in such patients with this technique.[18] Problems of fluid, electrolytes, and acid-base balance can also be corrected by these techniques, along with removal of metabolic waste.

Conclusions

The use of renal replacement therapy or blood purification therapy in sick, septic, injured, and critically ill patients has been studied extensively in a number of clinical trials.[19,20] Its value in patients with renal and hepatic failure has been well documented. Of all the techniques available, the best and safest seems to be continuous hemodiafiltration (CHDF) with nafamostat mesilate as the anticoagulant. This technique can be used by ICU personnel without a special dialysis unit. Endotoxin removal by polymyxin B-immobilized columns dextran has been shown to reduce circulating endotoxin levels. Despite this use in burn patients, infections and mortality have not been lowered. In septic patients in the Japanese studies this technique has been more promising.[4-6] It should be evaluated prospectively and in a randomized fashion by other groups to determine how helpful and widespread its use should be.

The CHDF technique in septic or MOF patients has been found to decrease certain cytokines, particularly if they are elevated initially.[2,9] Moreover, respiratory function and tissue oxygenation (increased VO_2) have improved.[16] Other uses include nutritional support, removal of excess fluid, and correction of the acid-base balance. Again, more studies and more randomized trials are necessary to establish this technique firmly in the therapy of such patients. Certainly, some aspects of the patients are improved. The question remains: Can mortality be significantly decreased by these techniques? Because in some of the studies certain patients respond and others do not, investigators must seek the characteristics of the responders to make the therapy more precise. It may also help improve the results.

References

1. Ronco C, Brendolan A, Bellomo R: Current technology for continuous renal replacement therapies. In: Ronco C, Bellomo R (eds) Critical Care Nephrology. Dordrecht, Kluwer Academic, 1998;1269-1308.
2. Hirasawa H, Sugai T, Ohtake Y, et al: Blood purification for prevention and treatment of multiple organ failure. World J Surg 1996;20:482-486.
3. Baue AE, Hirasawa H: Editorial overview of the surgical patient. Curr Opin Crit Care 1997;3:279-285.
4. Hanasawa K, Kodama M, Aoki H, et al: New treatment of severe sepsis in septic multiple organ failure patients by extracorporeal endotoxin removal with a polmyxin B immobilized fiber column. Surg Forum 1993;44:88-89.
5. Aoki H, Kodama M, Tani T, Hanasawa K: Treatment of sepsis by extracorporeal elimination of endotoxin using polymyxin B-immobilized fiber. Am J Surg 1994;167:412-417.
6. Kodama M, Tani T, Maekawa K, et al: Endotoxin eliminating therapy in patients with severe sepsis-direct hemoperfusion using polymyxin B-immobilized fiber column. Jpn J Surg 1995;96:277-285.
7. Hirasawa H, Sugai T, Ohtake Y, et al: Continuous hemofiltration and hemodiafiltration in the management of multiple organ failure. Contrib Nephrol 1991;93:42-51.
8. Hirasawa H, Sugai T, Oda S, et al: Continuous hemodiafiltration (CHDF) removes cytokines and improves respiratory index (RI) and oxygen metabolism in patients with acute respiratory distress syndrome (ARDS). Crit Care Med 1998;26:294.
9. Bellomo R, Tipping P, Boyce N: Continuous veno-venous hemofiltration with dialysis remove cytokines from the circulation of septic patients. Crit Care Med 1993;21:522-529.
10. Schetz M, Ferdinande P, van den Berghe G, et al: Removal of pro-inflammatory cytokines with renal replacement therapy: sense or nonsense? Intensive Care Med 1995;21:169-175.
11. Hirasawa H, Sugai T, Oda S, et al: Continuous hemodiafiltration can remove humoral mediators from bloodstream of the patients with systemic inflammatory response syndrome and multiple organ failure. Blood Purif 1997;15:136-137.
12. Hoffman JN, Deppisch R, Faist E, et al: Hemofiltration in human sepsis: evidence of elimination of immunomodulatory substances. Surg Forum 1994;45:69-71.
13. Bellomo R, Baldwin I, Cole L, Ronco C: Preliminary experience with high-volume hemofiltration in human septic shock. Kidney Int 1998;54-I (Suppl 66):S182-S185.
14. Kline JA, Gordon BE, Williams C, et al: Large-pore hemodialysis in acute endotoxin shock. Crit Care Med 1999;27:588-596.
15. Dhainaut JA, Vinsonneau C, Journois D: Hemofiltration and left ventricular function in sepsis: mechanisms and clinical implications. Crit Care Med 1999;27:473-474.
16. Oda S, Hirasawa H, Isono K: Tissue oxygen metabolism and cellular injury in patients with septic multiple organ failure. J Jpn Surg Soc 1993;94:556-563.
17. Reeves JH, Butt WW: Blood filtration in children with severe sepsis: safe adjunctive therapy. Intensive Care Med 1995;21:500.
18. Hirasawa H, Sugai T, Ohtake Y, et al: Energy metabolism and nutritional support in anuric multiple organ failure patients. In: Tanaka T, Okada A (eds) Anuric Multiple Organ Failure Patients. Amsterdam, Elsevier, 1990;429-440.
19. Hirasawa H, Sugai T, Ohtake Y, et al: Continuous hemofiltration and hemodiafiltration in the management of multiple organ failure. Contrib Nephrol 1991;93:42.
20. Belomo R, Farmer M, Wright C, Parkin G, Boyce N: Treatment of sepsis-associated severe acute renal failure with continuous hemodiafiltration: clinical experience and comparison with conventional dialysis. Blood Purif 1995;13:246.

50
Antithrombin III and Tissue Factor Pathway Inhibitor: Two Physiologic Protease Inhibitors of the Coagulation System

Gerhard Dickneite and Axel Mescheder

The coagulation system represents a series of proteolytic reactions that culminate in formation of a fibrin clot. Two means of activation, the intrinsic (contact activation) pathway and the extrinsic (tissue factor) pathway, ultimately lead to the formation of thrombin (Fig. 50.1). The intrinsic pathway is activated by exposure of the contact system (factor XII, prekallikrein and high-molecular-weight kininogen) to a surface. The first reaction is proteolytic conversion of the inactive factor (F) XI to active FXIa. FXIa activates FIX, which together with its cofactor FVIIIa converts FX to FXa. FXa and the cofactor FVa represent the prothrombinase complex, which converts prothrombin (FII) to thrombin (FIIa), the central enzyme of the coagulation cascade. The extrinsic system, on the other hand, is activated when FVII comes into contact with tissue factor (TF, thromboplastin); this FVIIa–TF complex then activates FX. The FVIIa–TF complex can also activate, FIX, stressing the importance of extrinsic pathway coagulation in hemostasis. Thrombin splits off two fibrinopeptides (A and B) from fibrinogen to form clottable fibrin. Fibrin spontaneously polymerizes to form soluble fibrin, which is crosslinked by FXIIIa, leading to insoluble fibrin, which is the substrate of the blood clot.

In addition to the procoagulant factors, which promote coagulation, various mechanisms limit activation of the clotting system. The first is initiated by thrombin itself, which activates protein C to activated protein C (APC). APC inactivates the two cofactors of coagulation, FVa and FVIIIa, by proteolytic cleavage to stop the proteolytic cascade at the level of FIX and FX. Thus thrombin limits its own activation. The two other systems are specialized protease inhibitors. Antithrombin III (AT III) is a broad-acting serine protease inhibitor (SERPIN) that inhibits not only thrombin but also other coagulation proteases. Tissue factor pathway inhibitor (TFPI) is a rather specific Kunitz-type inhibitor of the FVIIa–TF complex. Figure 50.1 depicts the interaction of AT III and TFPI with the coagulation proteases. Both compounds are discussed herein.

Antithrombin III

Biochemical Characterization

The existence of an antithrombin in blood plasma that acts as a heparin cofactor was described during the 1930s by Brinkhaus et al.[1] and by Quick.[2] Abildgaard[3] and Rosenberg[4] purified AT III from plasma and characterized its interaction with heparin. AT III circulates in plasma with a concentration of 2–3 μM (150 μg/ml).[5] It is the principal inhibitor of thrombin in plasma, but the molecule is able to interact with other proteases of the coagulation/fibrinolytic system as well. In addition to acting on thrombin, AT III is an inhibitor for clotting factors IXa, Xa,[6] XIa,[7] XIIa,[8] kallikrein,[9] and plasmin.[10] Human AT III is a single-chain α_2-glycoprotein composed of 432 amino acids and having a molecular weight of 58,200 daltons as demonstrated by protein and cDNA sequencing.[11,12] It is primarily synthesized in the liver along with a signal peptide of 32 amino acids.[13] The AT III gene is located on the long arm of chromosome 1 with about 13,500 basepairs containing 7 exons.[14,15] The secreted AT III has three disulfide bridges in positions Cys^8–Cys^{128}, Cys^{21}–Cys^{95}, and Cys^{247}–Cys^{430}.[16] The molecule has four N-glycosylation sites (Asn^{96}, Asn^{135}, Asn^{155}, Asn^{192}), and the predominant form (about 90%) in human plasma carries oligosaccharide side chains in all four positions (ATα). A minor AT III fraction lacks the carbohydrate side chain at Asn^{135}; this variant is called ATβ.[17,18]

The interaction of AT III with its target protease involves a reactive bond of Arg^{393}–Ser^{394}. AT III is presented to the protease as a substrate, and the Arg–Ser bond is hydrolyzed. The protease–inhibitor complex fails to dissociate but, instead, is stabilized by forming an acylester bond between Arg^{393} and the OH side chain of the reactive serine of the protease.[19] The resulting enzyme–inhibitor complex (e.g., thrombin–antithrombin, or TAT) is irreversible; it is stable even to boiling in sodium dodecyl sulfate. The TAT complex is cleared rapidly, and its in vivo half-life is 3 minutes.[20] The complex undergoes uptake into hepatocytes, where it is degraded in the lysosomes.[20,21]

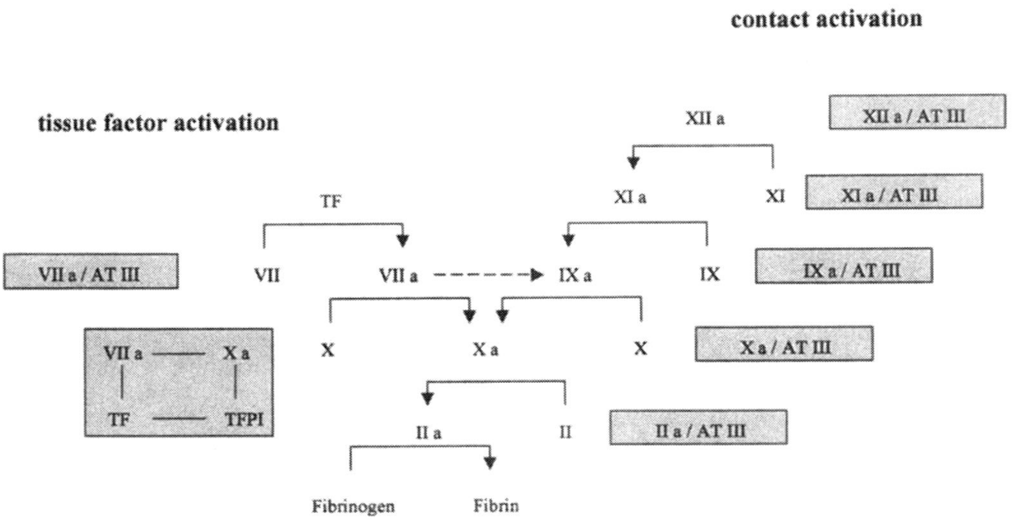

FIGURE 50.1. Inhibition of the coagulation system by antithrombin III (AT III) and tissue factor pathway inhibitor (TFPI). Active coagulation factors are designated by roman numerals to which an "a" is added for proteolytic activation. The boxes represent the individual protease–inhibitor complexes. TF, tissue factor; IIa, thrombin.

The glycosaminoglycan heparin catalyzes the inactivation of thrombin by acting as a template to which thrombin and AT III can bind to form a ternary complex.[22] Heparin accelerates the reaction of the enzyme with its inhibitor by a factor of about 1000. A pentasaccharide containing sulfated α-1,4-linked uronic acids and glucosamines was identified as the binding sequence to Arg and Lys residues on the AT III molecule.[23] Unfractionated heparin is a mixture of polysaccharides with various chain lengths ranging from 5000 to 30,000 daltons.[24] Formation of the ternary complex requires the high-molecular-weight form of heparin, which binds both AT III and thrombin. In contrast, factor Xa can be inhibited by the low-molecular-weight form of heparin (3000–9000 daltons) (LMWH), which binds to AT III but not to the target protease. After binding of the AT III–heparin complex to the protease, the affinity of heparin to AT III decreases, and heparin dissociates from the inhibitor–protease complex.

Reduced AT III plasma levels owing to genetic disorders are associated with a high rate of thrombotic disorders, such as thromboembolism. The prevalance of inherited AT III deficiencies in the normal population has been estimated to be 1 in 2000 to 1 in 5000 individuals.[25] Others have suggested an even higher prevalance: 1 in 250.[26] The genetic defect has been classified as type I or type II. Type I represents the classic deficiency with reduced levels of the circulating molecule resulting from a gene deletion (nonsense or missense mutations). During laboratory diagnosis the activity and antigen levels of AT III are found to be decreased. Type II deficiencies cover all cases with variant AT III molecules, resulting from the substitution of one amino acid by another.[27–30] Type II deficiency can be subclassified according to its disturbed function. Type II RS (reactive site) represents AT III molecules with decreased thrombin binding, whereas impaired heparin binding is designated type II HBS (heparin-binding site). In the third variant, designated type II PE (pleiotropic effects), multiple sites of the molecule are modified. Diagnostically, all type II deficiencies are characterized by decreased activity and no significant changes in antigenicity.

In contrast to the inherited AT III deficiencies, acquired forms result from insufficient synthesis due to organ failure, increased loss from plasma, or consumption coagulopathy. As the liver is the major site of AT III synthesis, hepatic diseases such as liver cirrhosis or asparaginase therapy lead to decreased AT III plasma levels. Loss of plasma AT III might be associated with burns, nephrotic syndrome, and multiple trauma. Uncontrolled activation of the coagulation system, so-called disseminated intravascular coagulation (DIC) frequently associated with severe sepsis, leads to excessive consumption of clotting factors. AT III substitution therapy appears to be the treatment of choice for both inherited and acquired disorders as is described in the next two sections.

Preclinical Studies

The pharmacologic efficacy of AT III has been intensively investigated in animal models with a focus on sepsis and DIC. (For a comprehensive review see Dickneite[31].) AT III has also been investigated in regard to other diseases associated with activation of the coagulation cascade, such as pancreatitis, trauma, preeclampsia, burns, and xenotransplantation.

The first study to demonstrate the efficacy of AT III in sepsis was a unique animal model. Mann and coworkers[32] induced a lethal, hemorrhagic syndrome in chicken embryos by injecting thromboplastin. They reported significant reduction in mortality after treatment with AT III.

Many groups have induced sepsis by administering bacterial lipopolysaccharide (LPS), which activates macrophages to secrete cytokines such as tumor necrosis factor-α (TNFα) or interleukin-1 (IL-1), which are the proinflammatory mediators that maintain the septic process. Triantaphyllopoulus[33] reported the action of AT III in a rabbit LPS sepsis model. A decrease in factors VIII and XII, prothrombin, fibrinogen, and platelet numbers followed the LPS infusion. AT III (164 U/kg body weight) was injected, resulting in plasma levels of about 4 U/ml (normal, or 100%, level is about 1 U/ml). In the placebo-treated control group, 5 of 13 rabbits died (mortality 38%) whereas all animals in the AT III group ($n = 8$) survived. AT III was shown to inhibit the LPS-induced consumption of factor XII. In a rat model of lethal endotoxemia Emerson[34] used AT III 250 U/kg given as an intravenous bolus just prior to the intravenous LPS injection. A significant long-lasting increase in survival time and prevention of fibrinogen drop was observed; the survival rate was 30% in the placebo and 80% in the AT III group. The same group reported a posttreatment study in the same rat model. AT III, given 1 hour after LPS, significantly prevented DIC and organ failure. Successful treatment of LPS-induced sepsis has also been shown for sepsis models in other species, such as dogs,[35] pigs,[36] and sheep.[37] The latter group combined AT III with α_1-protease inhibitor.

Several authors have used living bacteria to induce sepsis. Taylor et al.[38] introduced the baboon model with infused viable *Escherichia coli*. In a prophylaxis study baboons were given AT III at doses of 250 U/kg (at −60 minutes), 120 U/kg ($t = 0$), and 250 U/kg (at +180 minutes). Whereas four of five animals in the control group died, all four AT III-treated animals survived. A *Klebsiella pneumoniae* infection followed by antibiotic treatment with tobramycin (at +1 hour) in rats was used by Dickneite and Pâques.[39] AT III was administered as late as 3 or 5 hours after infection (500 U/kg IV). A significant increase in survival and prevention of fibrinogen decrease was reported. The first report about the effects of AT III on gram-positive bacterial sepsis came from Kessler et al.[40] AT III given therapeutically to guinea pigs (at +24 hours) infected with *Staphylococcus aureus* significantly increased survival and prevented DIC.

Experimental sepsis and DIC can be induced by other agents, and consequently AT III has been investigated in these models as well. Sepsis and DIC were induced by tissue factor in rabbits[31] and by lactic acid in dogs.[41] In all cases AT III efficaciously prevented consumption of coagulation factors and improved survival.

Taken together, the preclinical data unequivocally demonstrated the beneficial effect of AT III on the outcome of sepsis. AT III increased survival no matter what species of animal was used or what the inducing agent was. It was also clear that AT III has an anticoagulant effect and prevents DIC, which could be expected from its thrombin-inhibiting activity. However, evidence has accumulated during the last few years that AT III is not an anticoagulant alone. Okajima and his group[42,43] were the first to formulate the hypothesis of the antiinflammatory efficacy of AT III. According to their findings AT III induced prostacyclin release from vascular endothelium, which might be the cause for the antiinflammatory mode of action of AT III.[44] Ostrovsky et al., in a model of mesentery ischemia/reperfusion, suggested that AT III inhibits the interaction of leukocytes with endothelial cells of the vessel wall. AT III inhibited neutrophil rolling, sticking, and vascular injury. At present it is not clear if the antiinflammatory effect of AT III is due to thrombin inhibition or to interaction with a hitherto unidentified structure.

Clinical Investigations

Despite major progress in medical interventions for intensive care unit (ICU) treatment of sepsis, severe sepsis and septic shock are associated with a mortality rate as high as 55–65%.[45] Data are available to suggest that mortality is increasing along with the "graying" of the population in the developed world.[46] As treatment of this life-threatening syndrome usually is done in ICUs, it means a tremendous financial burden on health insurance. Therefore the causes of severe sepsis have come into sharp focus for clinical researchers worldwide.

Treatment strategies addressing specific cytokines involved in the pathogenesis of the syndrome have not been successful so far. In addition, counteracting the inflammatory mediator TNF did not result in a significant clinical benefit in major phase III clinical studies.

Opal et al.[47] reviewed therapeutic approaches that are currently under investigation. In addition to antiendotoxins and immunomodulators, coagulation pathway inhibitors are being developed in clinical studies. AT III, activated protein C, and tissue factor pathway inhibitor are interacting not only with the coagulation cascade but also via coagulation/inflammation cross-talk, maintaining the patency and functional capacity of the microvasculature. This prevents DIC and malperfusion, and it may support preservation of vital organ function. AT III is a serine protease inhibitor that affects multiple cellular and soluble components in the microvascular system. Thus coagulopathy may be induced owing to the deficiency of coagulation inhibitory proteins such as AT III.[48]

Balk et al.[49] suggested that the therapeutic use of AT III concentrate may produce a more positive outcome for sepsis-associated DIC, especially if treatment is started early in the course of sepsis. Fourrier and coworkers[50] investigated the clinical effect of AT III concentrate in 35 patients suffering from severe sepsis and septic shock. AT III or placebo was applied with a loading dose of 90–120 IU/kg, followed by a continuous infusion of 90–120 IU/kg/day for 4 days. The primary analysis showed a 42% (not significant, NS) reduction of 28-day all-cause mortality. These results were included in meta-analysis reported by Eisele et al.[51] In that meta-analysis the authors included additional data of a phase II clinical study on the use of AT III concentrate in patients with severe sepsis. This double-blind, placebo-controlled study indicated that administration of AT III was safe and well tolerated. There was a 39% reduction in 30-day all-cause mortality (NS), which was accompanied by a considerably shorter stay in the ICU. Patients treated with AT III exhibited a better performance in overall severity of illness and organ failure scores, which was noticeable soon after initiation of treatment. Patients treated with AT III demonstrated better resolution of preexisting organ failure and a lower incidence of new organ failure during the observation period.

The authors included this and two other double-blind, placebo-controlled phase II studies in a meta-analysis. A total of 122 patients suffering from severe sepsis confirmed the positive trend. The results of the meta-analysis demonstrated a relative 22.9% reduction (NS) in 30-day all-cause mortality in

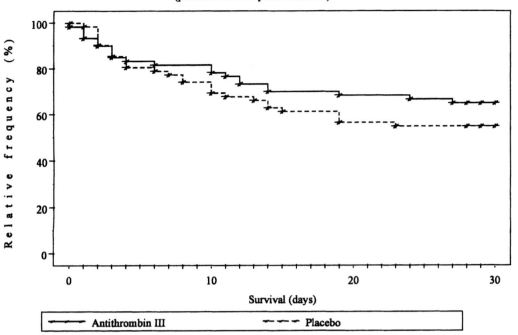

FIGURE 50.2. Survival curves of septic patients treated with AT III (solid line) or placebo (broken line). It was a Kaplan–Meier estimation (pooled over three phase II studies). Data were derived from the meta-analysis done by Eisele et al.[51]

patients treated with AT III. Figures 50.2 and 50.3 show the data of this meta-analysis, provided by Eisele et al.[51] The Kaplan–Meier graph indicates a benefit in 28-day all-cause mortality in this patient population. Figure 50.3 shows the risk ratio of the three individual studies as well as the result of the meta-analysis. To prove clinical benefit of AT III in this patient group a pivotal phase III study was recommended by the authors. Prior to the start of this phase III study a pharmacokinetic study comparing two dosage regimens (initial bolus followed by 4 days of subsequent intermittent boluses versus an initial bolus and 4 days of continuous infusion) both of which provided the patient with a total dose of 30,000 IU was performed.[52] The main efficacy variables included pharmacokinetic parameters. As shown in Fig. 50.4, plasma levels of AT III were rapidly elevated from reduced baseline levels to supranormal activity. This activity remained stable throughout the course of treatment and returned to normal after 7 days.

A worldwide, multicenter, double-blind, placebo-controlled pivotal phase III study is ongoing. It is designed to prove the clinical benefit of AT III for treatment of patients suffering from severe sepsis.

Inthorn et al.,[53] in a prospective study, investigated whether continuous long-term AT III supplementation alters the systemic inflammatory response in patients with severe sepsis. A series of 29 surgical patients with severe sepsis were randomly assigned to receive either conventional intensive care treatment or additional AT III supplementation. In addition, various cytokine levels were monitored. IL-6 plasma levels were reduced in patients treated with AT III ($p \leq 0.01$) compared to control patients. AT III supplementation prevented the continuous increase in intercellular adhesion molecule (sICAM-1) plasma concentration observed in control patients and led to a significant fall in soluble sE-selectin and C-reactive protein (CRP) concentration ($p \leq 0.01$). This reduction corresponded to a downregulation of body temperature over time ($p \leq 0.01$). No AT III effect on IL-8, polymorphonuclear neutrophil (PMN) elastase concentration, or total leukocyte count was detected. The authors concluded that long-term AT III supplementation attenuates the systemic inflammatory response in patients with severe sepsis. The downregulation of IL-6 may also explain the fall in endothelium-derived adhesion molecules and may represent the molecular basis by which AT III exerts its beneficial effects on organ function.

Baudo et al.[54] reported data on the efficacy of AT III therapy in terms of mortality in a selected group of patients admitted to the ICU. A series of 120 patients with an AT III concentration < 70% were included in a double-blind multicenter study. They were randomized to receive AT III (total dose 24,000 units) or placebo treatment. Of the 120 patients, 56 had septic shock. AT III concentrations in the serum group remained constant throughout the treatment period (range 97–102%). There was no difference in overall survival between the two groups: 50% and 46% for AT III and placebo, respectively. A Cox analysis was carried out after adjustment because the two groups were not balanced. Treatment with AT III decreased the risk of death with an odds ratio of 0.56. Septic shock and the baseline multiple organ failure score were negatively associated with survival, and the plasma activity level was positively associated with survival odds ratio of 0.97 for each 1% increase in the AT III plasma concentration at baseline. The authors concluded

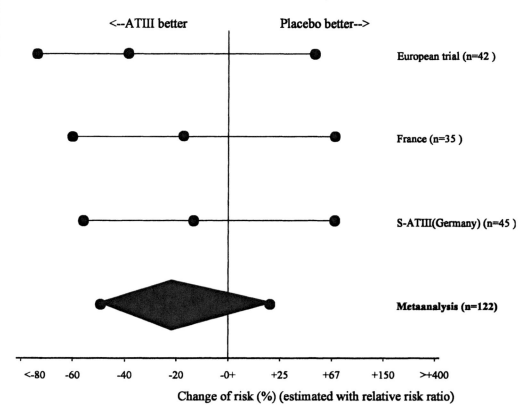

FIGURE 50.3. Risk assessment of 28-day all-course mortality. The panel comprises three sepsis trials that were pooled in a meta-analysis.[51] The positive trend in the pooled data was not statistically significant.

that replacement therapy may reduce mortality in the subgroup of septic shock patients only.

Tissue Factor Pathway Inhibitor

Biochemical Characterization

Tissue factor pathway inhibitor (TFPI) is a lipoprotein-associated potent direct inhibitor of the FVIIa–TF complex in association with FXa.[55] Historically, TFPI has been referred to as antithromboplastin.[56] More recent names are extrinsic pathway inhibitor (EPI) and lipoprotein-associated coagulation inhibitor (LACI). At the 1991 conference of the International Society of Thrombosis and Haemostasis investigators decided on the name tissue factor pathway inhibitor.

The molecule contains 276 amino acid residues and is secreted along with a 24/28AS-residue signal peptide. The TFPI gene contains nine exons[57,58] TFPI is a Kunitz-type inhibitor with three tandem domains. Two of the Kunitz domains bind to FVIIa or FXa, respectively; the function of the third domain is unknown. Inhibition of the FVIIa–TF complex by TFPI is rather complicated and depends on binding TFPI to FXa; thus a quarternary complex of FVIIa–TF–FXa–TFPI is formed (Fig. 50.1). The first step in this series of events is formation of a stoichiometric complex between TFPI and FXa, a reaction that does not require calcium ions. The second Kunitz domain has been identified as the structure that interacts with FXa.[59] To inhibit the FVIIa–TF complex, the first Kunitz domain of TFPI and the amino terminal γ-carboxyglutaminic acid domain of FXa must both bind to FVIIa. The resulting complex is thus no longer able to initiate the extrinsic pathway of coagulation. TFPI is a potent trypsin inhibitor; it modestly inhibits plasmin and chymotrypsin.

The molecule is located in three compartments: (1) circulating in plasma; (2) sequestered to platelets; and (3) bound to endothelial cells.[60] In plasma TFPI circulates bound to lipoprotein. There is some variation concerning the molecular weight, the major form being 34,000 daltons in the TFPI–LDL (low density lipoprotein) complex. In high density lipoprotein (HDL) the 40,000-dalton form dominates, and in very low density lipoprotein (VLDL) both 34,000- and 40,000-dalton variants of TFPI exist. About 10% of the TFPI in blood is associated with platelets, which release the inhibitor after stimulation with thrombin.[61] Infusion of heparin leads to a dramatic increase in circulating TFPI.[62,63] The source of the heparin-releasable TFPI is thought to be endothelium, where TFPI might be bound to glucosaminoglycans. Heparin thus exerts its anticoagulant effect not only by increasing the affinity of AT III to thrombin but also by releasing TFPI, thereby inhibiting the extrinsic coagulation pathway. TFPI plasma concentrations in normal individuals are approximately 100 ng/ml (2.5 nmol/L).[64]

Preclinical Studies

As already stated above, the rationale for using coagulation inhibitors as therapy for sepsis is that septic disorders are

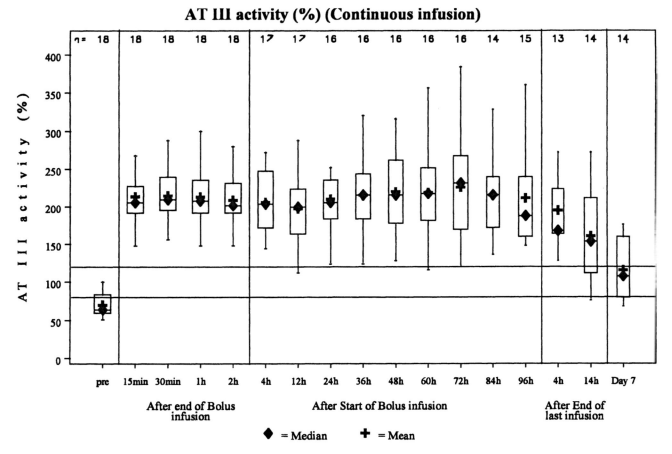

FIGURE 50.4. AT III plasma levels in patients with severe sepsis treated with a continuous infusion of AT III concentrate. A total of 30,000 units/patient was infused over a period of 4 days.

frequently associated with DIC. As TF is the initiator of the extrinsic pathway, infusion of soluble TF is associated with DIC, as shown in experimental models.[65,66] Moreover, administration of endotoxin was shown to induce expression of TF on the surface of monocytes and endothelial cells.[67,68] First attempts to inhibit the extrinsic coagulation pathway came from experiments with monoclonal antibodies (mAbs) against TF in rabbits and baboons.[69,70] Inhibition of DIC by an mAb against FVII/FVIIa in experimental rabbit septic shock was reported by Warr et al.[69]

The TFPI has been investigated in animal models (e.g., rabbits, pigs, baboons). The molecule was demonstrated to inhibit TF-induced DIC in rabbits.[65] Haskel et al.[71] demonstrated that arterial reocclusion after thrombolysis was prevented by TFPI. Bregengard and coworkers[72] used the recombinant two-domain TFPI analogue (2D-TFPI) to prevent DIC in rabbits. DIC was induced by two injections of *Escherichia coli* LPS 24 hours apart. 2D-TFPI (0.31–3.0 mg/kg) was administered together with the second LPS dose and significantly prevented a decrease in fibrinogen, factor VIII, and platelets as well as deposition of fibrin in the kidneys. Several papers from Taylor's group dealt with the effect of TFPI on lethal baboon sepsis. In this model an intravenous *E. coli* infusion led to death (80–100%) due to septic shock after 30–40 hours. Creasey et al.[73] demonstrated that administration of TFPI 4 mg/kg (recombinant, expressed in hepatoma cells) 30 minutes after LPS resulted in permanent survivors (>7 days). Concurrently, the decrease in fibrinogen and the increase in fibrin degradation products, as well as the increase in prothrombin time (PT) and the activated thromboplastin time (aPTT), were prevented. The authors reported a terminal half-life of 2 hours for TFPI. There was some prolongation of survival time even when TFPI was given 4 hours after *E. coli* infusion. In the same model the nonglycosylated TFPI containing an additional alanine residue at the amino-terminus expressed in *E. coli* (ala-TFPI) was investigated.[74] Treatment with ala-TFPI 2.7 or 7.4 mg/kg starting at 30 minutes after *E. coli* resulted in improvement of the survival rate and prevention of DIC compared to those in the controls. Moreover, TFPI was shown to decrease IL-6 levels.

Camerota et al.[75] investigated a combination of TFPI and antibiotics in a rabbit peritonitis model induced by intraperitoneal instillation of *E. coli* mixed with hemoglobin and mucin. A 24-hour infusion of ala-TFPI, starting 4 hours after induction of the peritonitis, significantly increased survival. Goldfarb et al.[76] described the effect of TFPI in a pig *E. coli*/fibrin peritonitis model. A rec. TFPI dose of 1 mg/kg bolus was followed by a 48-hour infusion of 10 μg/kg/min (starting 15 minutes before clot implantation). In this model TFPI significantly decreased TNF and IL-8. The survival rate increased nonsignificantly from 25% in the control group to 42% in the TFPI-treated pigs.

As with AT III, the mode of action of TFPI is not ultimately understood. Preclinical studies with both coagulation inhibitors clearly favor an anti-DIC effect. Whereas with AT III prevention of leukocyte adherence and margination was described,[44] this effect has not yet been clearly demonstrated for TFPI.[77] However, Park et al.[78] reported that TFPI binds to LPS, thereby preventing the interaction of LPS with its cellular receptor CD14. Thus TFPI might act via neutralization of endotoxin. The rationale for the dosing of TFPI is not clear. Circulating TFPI levels, in contrast to AT III, are elevated during sepsis up to about twice normal, as shown in humans[79] and monkeys.[80]

Clinical Investigations

Tissue factor pathway inhibitor appears to be the major physiologic inhibitor of TF-induced coagulation,[81] controlling the activation of blood coagulation while antithrombin regulates additionally the final stage. Both proteins inhibit the intermediate stage of activation. Subnormal levels of TFPI increase the risk of DIC in septic conditions and the risk of occlusive thrombi from damaged vascular intima or fissured arteriosclerotic plaques.[82]

Johnson et al.[83] described rTFPI-mediated inhibition of IL-8 synthesis induced by coagulation and endotoxin in human whole blood cultures. Their findings might indicate an inhibiting effect not only on intravascular coagulation but also on the inflammatory response. In the clinical situation of sepsis, plasma TFPI levels are generally normal or increased (twofold increase, about 0.2 µg/ml). Despite this fact, the application of exogenous TFPI reaching plasma levels of 1–2 µg/ml may effectively reduce FVIIa–TF complex activity,[84] which may be indicative of a relative deficiency. Shimura and coworkers[85] noted that during the clinical course of DIC plasma TF antigen was increased first, and an increase of the plasma TFPI level followed the increase in plasma TF level. The authors concluded that plasma TFPI is released from vascular endothelial cells and may reflect vascular endothelial cell injury. Endothelial and monocyte generation of tissue factor is activated by bacterial products and endotoxin. Activation of TF is counteracted by TFPI. The potential for TFPI substitution to inhibit activation of the coagulation cascade during sepsis requires further study.[86]

Kamikubo et al.[87] reported data on the possible interaction of h-rTFPI, heparin, and AT III. In the presence of heparin, AT III effectively inhibited factor Xa, resulting in complete abrogation of complex formation between h-rTFPI and Xa. In addition, AT III induced dissociation of the preformed h-rTFPI–Xa complex, indicating interference with the catabolism of TFPI mediated via Xa.

Holst et al.[88] investigated the effect of protamine sulfate on plasma TFPI released by intravenous and subcutaneous unfractionated and low-molecular-weight heparin (LMWH) in an open, nonrandomized study of 10 healthy volunteers. TFPI was released by intravenous application of unfractionated heparin, and LMWH, as well as by subcutaneous LMWH. TFPI remained in the circulation only for as long as heparin was present and showed a pharmacokinetic profile comparable to that of unfractionated heparin.

Conclusions and Outlook

Despite large clinical intervention studies of septic shock, treatment of this severe disease is still associated with a high mortality rate and remains a clinical challenge. Until now, treatment with antiendotoxic agents (e.g., anti-LPS antibodies) and nonspecific (steroids, nonsteroidal antiinflammatory drugs) or specific antiinflammatory agents (anti-TNF, anti-IL-1) have not generated clear-cut proof of benefit in clinical studies. The discouraging results led to a change in paradigm: Anticoagulation therapy, which offers a dual mechanism of action, became the focus of interest. The dual mechanism implies not only classic inhibition of clotting but also modulation of the inflammatory system. Concerning the latter, especially interactions between leukocytes and vascular endothelium are under investigation. All three principal physiologic anticoagulation agents (AT III, TFPI, APC) are now subject to international multicenter studies in patients with severe sepsis. During the next few years well designed phase III clinical studies will prove whether coagulation inhibitors are a viable therapeutic option for the treatment of severe septic disorders.

References

1. Brinkhous KM, Smith HP, Warner ED, et al: The inhibition of blood clotting: an unidentified substance which acts in conjunction with heparin to prevent the conversion of prothrombin to thrombin. Am J Physiol 1939;125:683–687.
2. Quick AJ: The normal antithrombin of the blood and its relation to heparin. Am J Physiol 1938;123:712–719.
3. Abildgaard U: Binding of thrombin to antithrombin III. Scand J Clin Lab Invest 1969;24:23–27.
4. Rosenberg RD, Damus PS: The purification and mechanism of action of human antithrombin-heparin cofactor. J Biol Chem 1973;248:6490–6506.
5. Conrad J, Brosstad F, Larsen ML, et al: Molar antithrombin concentration in normal human plasma. Haemostasis 1983;13:363–368.
6. Kurachi K, Fujikawa K, Schmer G, et al: Inhibition of bovine factor IXa and factor Xαβ by antithrombin III. Biochemistry 1976;15:373–377.
7. Scott CF, Colman RW: Factors influencing the acceleration of human factor XIa inactivation by antithrombin III. Blood 1989;73:1873–1879.
8. Stead N, Kaplan AP, Rosenberg RD: Inhibition of activated factor XII by antithrombin-heparin cofactor. J Biol Chem 1976;251:6481–6488.
9. Lahiri B, Rosenberg RD, Talamo RC, et al: Antithrombin III: an inhibitor of human plasma kallikrein. Fed Proc 1974;33:642a.
10. Highsmith RF, Rosenberg RD: The inhibition of human plasmin by human antithrombin-heparin cofactor. J Biol Chem 1974;249:4335–4338.
11. Petersen TE, Dudek-Wojciechowska G, Sottrup-Jensen L, et al: Primary structure of antithrombin III (heparin cofactor): partial

homology between α₁-antitrypsin and antithrombin III. In: Collen D, Wiman B, Verstraete M (eds) The Physiological Inhibitors of Coagulation and Fibrinolysis. Amsterdam, Elsevier, 1979;43-54.

12. Chandra T, Stackhouse R, Kidd VJ, et al: Isolation and sequence characterization of a cDNA clone of human antithrombin III. Proc Natl Acad Sci USA 1983;80:1845-1848.

13. Lane DA, Casor R: Antithrombin: structure, genomic organization, function and inherited deficiency. Baillieres Clin Haematol 1989;2:961-998.

14. Blajchman A, Richard CA, Francoise Fernandez-Rachubinski, et al: Molecular basis of inherited human antithrombin deficiency. Blood 1992;80:2159-2171.

15. Bock SC, Prochownik EV: Molecular genetic survey of 16 kindreds with hereditary antithrombin III deficiency. Blood 1987;70:1273.

16. Sun XJ, Chang JY: Heparin binding domain of human antithrombin III inferred from the sequential reduction of its three disulfide linkages: an efficient method for structural analysis of partially reduced proteins. J Biol Chem 1989;264:11288-11296.

17. Peterson CB, Blackburn MN: Isolation and characterization of an antithrombin III variant with reduced carbohydrate content and enhanced heparin binding. J Biol Chem 1985;260:610-615.

18. Brennan SO, George PM, Jordan RE: Physiological variant of antithrombin-III lacks carbohydrate sidechain at Asn 135. FEBS Lett 1987;219:431-439.

19. Björk I, Jackson CM, Jörnval H, et al: The active site of antithrombin: release of the same proteolytically cleaved form of the inhibitor from complexes with factor IXa, factor Xa, and thrombin. J Biol Chem 1982;257:2406-2413.

20. Pizzo SV: The physiologic role of antithrombin III as an anticoagulant. Semin Hematol 1994;31:4-7.

21. Shifman MA, Pizzo SV: The in vivo metabolism of antithrombin III and antithrombin III complexes. J Biol Chem 1982;257:3243-3328.

22. Hirsh J, Dalen JE, Deykin D, et al: Heparin: mechanism of action, pharmacokinetics, dosing, considerations, monitoring, efficacy, and safety. Chest 1992;102:337S-351S.

23. Casu B: Heparin structure. Haemostasis 1990;20:62-73.

24. Verstraete M: Heparin and thrombosis: a seventy year long story. Haemostasis 1990;20:4-11.

25. Thaler E, Lechner K: Antithrombin III deficiency and thromboembolism. Clin Haematol 1981;10:369.

26. Tait RC, Walker ID, Perry DJ, et al: Prevalence of antithrombin III deficiency subtypes in 4000 healthy blood donors. Thromb Haemost 1991;65:839.

27. De Stefano V, Finazzi G, Mannucci PM: Inherited thrombophilia: pathogenesis, clinical syndromes and management. Blood 1996; 87:3531-3544.

28. Demers C, Ginsberg JS, Hirsch J, et al: Thrombosis in antithrombin-III-deficient persons. Ann Intern Med 1992;116:754-761.

29. Sheffield W, Wu Ye L, Blajchman MA: Antithrombin: structure and function. Mol Basis of Thromb Haemost 1995;355-377.

30. Blajchman MA: An overview of the mechanism of action of antithrombin and its inherited deficiency states. Blood Coag Fibrinol 1994;5(1):S5-S11.

31. Dickneite G: Antithrombin III in animal models of sepsis and organ failure. Semin Thromb Haemost 1998;24:61-69.

32. Mann LT, Jensenius JC, Simonsen M, et al: Antithrombin III: protection against death after injection of thromboplastin. Science 1969;166:517-518.

33. Triantaphyllopoulus DC: Effects of human antithrombin III on mortality and blood coagulation induced in rabbits by endotoxin. Thromb Haemost 1984;51:232-235.

34. Emerson TE: Protection against disseminated intravascular coagulation and death by antithrombin III in the Escherichia coli endotoxemic rat. Circ Shock 1987;21:1-13.

35. Hauptmann JG, Hassouna HI, Bell TG, et al: Efficacy of antithrombin III in endotoxin-induced disseminated intravascular coagulation. Circ Shock 1988;25:111-122.

36. Dickneite G, Leithäuser B: Influence of antithrombin III on coagulation and inflammation in porcine septic shock. Arterioscl Thromb Vasc Biol 1999;19:1566-1572.

37. Redens TB, Leach WJ, Bogdanoff DA, et al: Synergistic protection from lung damage by combining antithrombin III and alpha-1-proteinase inhibitor in the E. coli endotoxic sheep pulmonary dysfunction model. Circ Shock 1988;26:15-26.

38. Taylor FB, Emerson TE, Jordan R, et al: Antithrombin III prevents the lethal effects of Escherichia coli infusion in baboons. Circ Shock 1988;26:227-235.

39. Dickneite G, Pâques EP: Reduction of mortality with antithrombin III in septicemic rats: a study of Klebsiella pneumoniae induced sepsis. Thromb Haemost 1993;2:98-102.

40. Kessler CM, Tang Zch, Jacobs HM, et al: The suprapharmacologic dosing of antithrombin concentrate for Staphylococcus aureus-induced disseminated intravascular coagulation in guinea pigs: substantial reduction in mortality and morbidity. Blood 1997;89:4393-4401.

41. Mammen EF, Miyakawa T, Phillips TF: Human antithrombin concentrates and experimental disseminated intravascular coagulation. Semin Thromb Haemost 1985;11:373-383.

42. Uchiba M, Okajima K, Murakami K, et al: Effects of antithrombin III (AT III) and TRP49-modified AT III on plasma levels of 6-keto-PGF₁α in rats. Thromb Res 1995;80:201-208.

43. Uchiba M, Okajima K, Murakami K: Effects of various doses of antithrombin III on endotoxin-induced endothelial cell injury and coagulation abnormalities in rats. Thromb Res 1998;89: 233-241.

44. Ostrovsky L, Woodman RC, Payne D, et al: Antithrombin III prevents and rapidly reverses leukocyte recruitment in ischemia reperfusion. Circulation 1997;96:2302-2310.

45. Rangel-Frausto MS, Pittet D, Costigan M, et al: The natural history of the systemic inflammatory response syndrome (SIRS): a prospective study. JAMA 1995;273:117-123.

46. Linde-Zwirble WT, Angus DC, Carcillo J, et al: Age-specific incidence and outcome of sepsis in the US. Crit Care Med 1999;27:A33.

47. Opal S: New treatment in sepsis. Biomed Prog 1998;11:52-56.

48. Wheeler AP, Bernard GR: Treating patients with severe sepsis. N Engl J Med 1999;340:207-214.

49. Balk R, Emerson T, Fourrier F, et al: Therapeutic use of antithrombin concentrate in sepsis. Semin Thromb Haemost 1998;24:183-194.

50. Fourrier F, Chopin C, Huart J, et al: Double-blind, placebo-controlled trial of antithrombin III concentrates in septic shock with disseminated intravascular coagulation. Chest 1993;104: 882-888.

51. Eisele B, Lamy M, Thijs LG, et al: Anithrombin III in patients with severe sepsis: a randomized, placebo-controlled, double-blind multicenter trial plus a meta-analysis on all randomized, placebo-controlled, double-blind trials with antithrombin III in severe sepsis. Intensive Care Med 1998;24:663-672.

52. Thijs LG, Eisele B, Keinecke H-O, et al: Antithrombin III in patients with severe sepsis: a dosage regimen finding and pharmacokinetic study. Intensive Care Med 1997;23:S55.

53. Inthorn D, Hoffmann JN, Hartl WH, et al: Effect of antithrombin III supplementation on inflammatory response in patients with severe sepsis. Shock 1998;10:90–96.
54. Baudo F, Caimi TM, de Cataldo F, et al: Antithrombin III (AT III) replacement therapy in patients with sepsis and/or postsurgical complications: a controlled double-blind, randomized, multicenter study. Intensive Care Med 1998;24:336–342.
55. Broze GJ: The role of tissue factor pathway inhibitor in a revised coagulation cascade. Semin Hematol 1992;29:159–169.
56. Schneider CI: The active principle of placental toxin: thromboplastin; its inactivator in blood: antithromboplastin. Am J Physiol 1947;149:123–129.
57. Van der Logt CPE, Reitsma PH, et al: Intron-exon organization of the human gene coding for the lipoprotein-associated coagulation inhibitor: the factor Xa dependent inhibitor of the extrinsic pathway of coagulation. Biochemistry 1991;30:1571–1577.
58. Girard TJ, Eddy R, Wesselschmidt R: Structure of the human lipoprotein-associated coagulation inhibitor gene: intron/exon gene organization and localization of the gene to chromosome 2. J Biol Chem 1991;266:5036–5041.
59. Girard TJ, Warren LA, Novotny WF: Nature 1989;338:518–520.
60. Novotny WF: Tissue factor pathway inhibitor. Semin Thromb Haemost 1994;20:101–108.
61. Novotny WF, Girard TJ, Miletich JP: Platelets secrete a coagulation inhibitor functionally and antigenically similar to the lipoprotein-associated coagulation inhibitor. Blood 1988;72:2020–2025.
62. Sandset PM, Abildgaard U, Larsen ML: Heparin induces release of extrinsic coagulation pathway inhibitor (EPI). Thromb Res 1988;50:803–813.
63. Hansen JB, Sandset PM, Huseby KR, et al: Depletion of intravascular pools of tissue factor pathway (TFPI) during repeated or continuous intravenous infusion of heparin in man. Thromb Haemost 1996;76:703–709.
64. Warr TA, Warn-Cramer BJ, Rao LVM: Human plasma extrinsic pathway inhibitor activity. I. Standardization of assay and evaluation of physiologic variables. Blood 1989;74:201–206.
65. Day KC, Hoffman LC, Palmier MO, et al: Recombinant lipoprotein-associated coagulation inhibitor inhibits tissue thromboplastin-induced intravascular coagulation in the rabbit. Blood 1990;76:1538–1545.
66. Kouz J: Influence of recombinant hirudin on tissue-factor-induced activation of coagulation in rabbits. Haemostasis 1996; 26:179–186.
67. Brozna JP: Cellular regulation of tissue factor. Blood Coag Fibrinol 1990;1:415–426.
68. Nawroth P, Kisiel W, Stern D: The role of endothelium in the homeostatic balance of haemostasis. Clin Haematol 1985;14: 531–546.
69. Warr TA, Rao LV, Rapaport SI: Disseminated intravascular coagulation in rabbits induced by administration of endotoxin or tissue factor: effect of anti-tissue factor antibodies and measurement of plasma extrinsic pathway inhibitor activity. Blood 1990;75: 1481–1489.
70. Taylor FB, Chang A, Ruf W: Lethal E. coli septic shock is prevented by blocking tissue factor with monoclonal antibody. Circ Shock 1991;33:127–133.
71. Haskel EJ, Torr SR, Day KC: Prevention of arterial reocclusion after thrombolysis with recombinant lipoprotein-associated coagulation inhibitor. Circulation 1991;84:821–827.
72. Bregengard C, Nordfang O, Wildgoose P, et al: The effect of two-domain tissue factor pathway inhibitor on endotoxin-induced disseminated intravascular coagulation in rabbits. Blood Coag Fibrinol 1993;4:669–706.
73. Creasey AA, Chang ACK, Feigen L, et al: Tissue factor pathway inhibitor reduces mortality from Escherichia coli septic shock. J Clin Invest 1993;91:2850–2860.
74. Carr C, Bild GS, Chang ACK, et al: Recombinant E. coli-derived tissue factor pathway inhibitor reduces coagulopathic and lethal effects in the baboon gram-negative model of septic shock. Circ Shock 1995;44:126–137.
75. Camerota AJ, Creasey AA, Patla V: Delayed treatment with recombinant human tissue factor pathway inhibitor improves survival in rabbits with gram-negative peritonitis. J Infect Dis 1998;177:668–676.
76. Goldfarb RD, Glock D, Johnson K, et al: Randomized, blinded, placebo-controlled trial of tissue factor pathway inhibitor in porcine septic shock. Shock 1998;4:258–264.
77. Randolph MM, White GL, Kosanke SD, et al: Attenuation of tissue thrombosis and hemorrhage by ala-TFPI does not account for its protection against E. coli. Thromb Haemost 1998;79: 1048–1053.
78. Park CT, Creasey AA, Wright SD: Tissue factor pathway inhibitor blocks cellular effects of endotoxin by binding to endotoxin and interfering with transfer of CD14. Blood 1997; 89:4268–4274.
79. Novotny WF, Brown SG, Miletich JP, et al: Plasma antigen levels of the lipoprotein associated coagulation inhibitor in patient samples. Blood 1991;78:387–393.
80. Sabharwal AK, Bajaj SP, Ameri A, et al: Tissue factor pathway inhibitor and von Willebrand factor antigen levels in adult respiratory distress syndrome and in a primate model of sepsis. Am J Respir J Crit Care Med 1995;151:758–767.
81. Bajaj MS, Bajaj SP: Tissue factor pathway inhibitor: potential therapeutic applications. Thromb Haemost 1997;78: 471–477.
82. Abildgaard U: Relative roles of tissue factor pathway inhibitor and antithrombin in the control of thrombogenesis. Blood Coag Fibrinol 1995;6:S45–S49.
83. Johnson K, Aarden L, Choi Y, et al: The proinflammatory cytokine response to coagulation and endotoxin in whole blood. Blood 1996;87:5051–5060.
84. Girard TJ: Tissue factor pathway inhibitor. In: Sasahara A, Loscalzo J (eds) Novel Therapeutic Agents in Thrombosis and Thrombolysis. New York, Marcel Dekker, 1997;225–260.
85. Shimura M, Wada H, Waikta Y, et al: Plasma tissue factor and tissue factor pathway inhibitor levels in patients with disseminated intravascular coagulation. Am J Hematol 1996; 52:165–170.
86. Fourrier F, Jourdain M, Tournois A, et al: Coagulation inhibitor substitution during sepsis. Intensive Care Med 1995;21: S264–S268.
87. Kamikubo Y, Hamuro T, Takemoto S, et al: A kinetic analysis of the interaction of human recombinant tissue factor pathway inhibitor with factor Xa utilizing an immunoassay and the effect of antithrombin III/heparin on the complex formation. Thromb Res 1998;89:179–186.
88. Holst J, Lindblad B, Bergquist D, et al: The effect of protamine sulphate on plasma tissue factor pathway inhibitor released by intravenous and subcutaneous unfractionated and low molecular weight heparin in man. Thromb Res 1997; 86:343–348.

51
Rationale for Glucocorticoid Treatment in Septic Shock and Unresolving ARDS

G. Umberto Meduri

There is renewed interest on the topic of glucocorticoid therapy in patients with septic shock and acute respiratory distress syndrome (ARDS). Four small double-blind, randomized trials evaluating prolonged glucocorticoid (GC) therapy in patients with septic shock or unresolving ARDS (sepsis-induced) have been completed.[1-4] In all four, prolonged GC treatment was associated with rapid, significant clinical improvement. In two of them, survival was an endpoint, and both reported a significant reduction in mortality.[1,4] Such significant results probably reflect a medium to large beneficial effect of therapy, although there is some concern that the small sample size may be insufficient to evaluate an outcome benefit confidently. The findings of these studies are in apparent contradiction with the results of previous randomized, multicenter trials investigating massive doses of GC therapy in sepsis and ARDS.[5-10] Two meta-analyses carefully reviewed these older trials for their adherence to principles of methodologic quality and concluded that the available evidence does not support the use of GCs in patients with sepsis or septic shock, and that treatment may be associated with increased mortality due to secondary infections.[11,12] However, the evidence reviewed in these meta-analyses pertained exclusively to studies investigating a short course of massive doses of GC during early sepsis and septic shock, and the conclusions may apply only to this restricted administration of GC treatment.

It is likely that the positive findings of the more recent randomized studies will encourage a critical reevaluation and stimulate additional investigation of GCs as an inexpensive, safe form of immunomodulation. When comparing the GC trials of the past to the recent trials, three major differences are apparent: (1) timing of administration: in the recent trials treatment was initiated 2–10 days after disease onset in patients who failed to improve, thus probably selecting a more uniformly sicker patient population; (2) dosage: in the past trials the daily GC doses employed were 5–140 times higher than those used in the recent trials; and (3) duration of administration: in the past trials treatment consisted of administering one to four doses every 6 hours, whereas the strategy of the recent trial was to achieve disease resolution and to prolong treatment as long as was necessary (5–32 days).

This chapter reviews the clinical and basic science information gained during the 1990s about the cellular mechanisms involved in activation of the host defense response and its regulation by GCs, attempting to elucidate how changes in dosage and duration of GC administration are associated with such disparate results. Three selected areas are discussed: (1) host defense response and endogenous GC production; (2) exaggerated host defense response and ensuing GC resistance; and (3) the importance of extended GC treatment—an important and previously neglected critical variable in therapeutic outcome—in disease resolution.

Host Defense Response to Insults

The host defense response to insults is similar despite the tissue involved. It consists of an interactive network of simultaneously activated pathways that work in an integrated fashion to increase the host's chance of survival. It is now recognized that when inflammatory signals reach the cell surface they initiate a series of events leading to activation of cytoplasmic transcription factors: DNA-binding proteins that regulate the transcription of target genes into messenger RNA. Important transcription factors associated with the host defense response include nuclear factor-κB (NF-κB), NF-IL-6, activator protein-1 (AP-1), the glucocorticoid receptor complex, and the heat shock transcription factor (HSF).[13] NF-κB is recognized as the transcription factor critical for maximal expression of multiple cytokines. In unstimulated cells NF-κB is found in cytoplasm bound to the inhibitory protein IκB (Fig. 51.1). When cells are stimulated by inflammatory signals, specific kinases phosphorylate IκB and cause its rapid degradation. The activated form of NF-κB then moves rapidly to the nucleus, initiating mRNA transcription of proinflammatory cytokines: tumor necrosis factor-α (TNFα), interleukins (IL-1β, IL-2, IL-6), chemokines (e.g., IL-8), cell adhesion molecules (e.g., intercellular adhesion molecule-1, E-selectin), and inflammation-associated enzymes [cyclooxygenase (COX), phospholipase A_2 (PLA_2), inducible nitric oxide (iNOS)].[18]

Cellular responses in host defense response are regulated by a complex interaction among cytokines with final effects on the

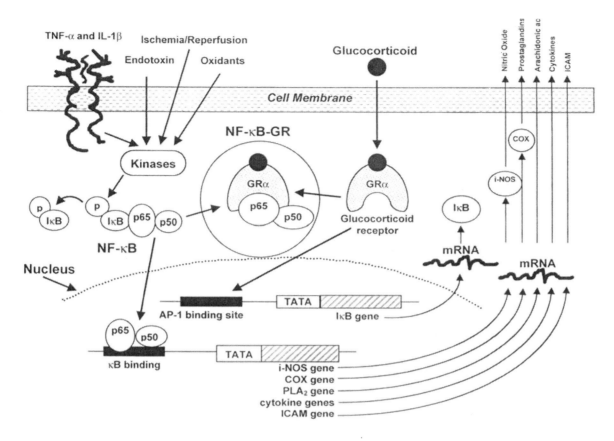

FIGURE 51.1. Interaction between NF-κB and the activated glucocorticoid (GC) receptor. When cells are stimulated by inflammatory signals, specific kinases phosphorylate the inhibitory protein IκB and causes its rapid degradation. The activated form of NF-κB then moves to the nucleus, initiating the transcription of mRNA of proinflammatory cytokines, chemokines, cell adhesion molecules, and inflammation-associated enzymes (cyclooxygenase, phospholipase A_2, inducible nitric oxide). Cortisol or exogenous GCs freely cross into the cytoplasm and bind to their specific GC receptors (GR). Activated GRs inhibit the transactivational effects of NF-κB via a dual mechanism by: (1) physically interacting with the p65 subunit; and (2) inducing the IκB inhibitory protein, which traps NF-κB in inactive cytoplasmic complexes catabolized by the ubiquitin–proteasome pathway.[14–16] (Modified from Barnes and Adcock,[17] with permission.)

surrounding microenvironment not directly induced by the initiating insult. In this regard, cytokines have concentration-dependent biologic effects.[19] At low concentration they regulate homeostasis, and at progressively higher concentrations they mediate proportionally stronger local and then systemic responses. Among a broad spectrum of proximal mediators, cytokines of the IL-1 and TNF family appear uniquely important in initiating all key aspects of the host defense response.[20,21] TNFα and IL-1β stimulate their own and each other's secretion, and both promote the release of IL-6 (NF-IL-6 the transcription factor responsible for IL-6 gene activation after IL-1 stimulation). The cell most commonly associated with initiating the host defense response cascade is the tissue macrophage or the blood monocyte.[20] The biologic actions of cytokines during the host defense response are pleiotropic and redundant, each factor exerting multiple effects on different target cells (also a source of cytokines), and different factors acting on the same cell to induce similar effects. Once released, TNFα and IL-1β act on epithelial cells, stromal cells (fibroblasts and endothelial), the extracellular matrix (ECM), and recruited circulating cells (neutrophils, platelets, lymphocytes) to cause secondary waves of cytokine release, with amplification of the host defense response.[20] The effects of individual cytokines on acute-phase proteins[22] and nitric oxide production have been reviewed elsewhere.[23]

Cytokines TNFα and IL-1β are the proximal mediators of all key aspects of the host defense response, including inflammation,[24] coagulation (intravascular clotting and extravascular fibrin deposition),[25] tissue repair,[26–28] modulation of the immune response,[29] and activation of the hypothalamic–pituitary–adrenal (HPA) axis with production of GCs.[30,31] These five pathways of the host defense response (Table 51.1) are activated simultaneously (slight delay for activation of the HPA axis) and work in synergy to eliminate or control the noxious offenders.[32] Activation of the sympathetic system to release catecholamines and increased hepatic production of acute-phase reactants are an integral part of the host defense response and are under the influence of GCs. During stress the epinephrine response parallels HPA axis stimulation.[13] GCs and ACTH affect several key regulatory enzymes in catecholamine biosynthesis and

TABLE 51.1. Components of the Host Defense Response.

Inflammation
  Vasodilation and stasis
  Increased expression of adhesion molecules
  Increased permeability of the microvasculature with exudative edema
  Leukocyte extravasation[a]
  Release of leukocyte products potentially causing tissue damage

Coagulation
  Activation of coagulation
  Inhibition of fibrinolysis
  Intravascular clotting
  Extravascular fibrin deposition

Tissue repair
  Angiogenesis
  Epithelial growth
  Fibroblast migration and proliferation
  Deposition of extracellular matrix and remodeling

Modulation of the immune response
  Fever
  Induction of heat-shock proteins
  Release of neutrophils from the bone marrow
  Priming of phagocytic cells
  T cell proliferation
  Antibody production

Activation of the hypothalamic–pituitary–adrenal axis
  Release of ACTH with cortisol production
  ACTH and cortisol modulation of the sympathetic nervous system
  Cortisol modulation of acute-phase protein production by the liver[b]

[a]Initially polymorphonuclear cells and later monocytes.
[b]Elevated levels of circulating glucocorticoids synergize with IL-6 in inducing hepatic synthesis and secretion of "acute-phase" reactants such as fibrinogen, protease inhibitors, complement C3, ceruloplasmin, haptoglobin, and C-reactive protein.

influence the number and functional state of adrenergic receptors.[13] Catecholamine–GC interactions play an important role in the maintenance of vascular tone,[13] and glucocorticoids influence several key regulatory systems important for maintaining blood pressure (Fig. 51.2).[34] Acute-phase reactants are essential in many aspects of the host defense: Fibrinogen influences coagulation and tissue repair; complement C3 affects opsonization; C-reactive protein inhibits neutrophil chemotaxis; and protease inhibitors limit tissue damage during inflammation. Production of these reactants is enhanced by GCs.[20,22,35]

The host defense response is essentially a protective response of tissues that serves to destroy, dilute, or wall off injurious agents[36] and to repair any consequent tissue damage. Repair consists of replacing injured tissue by regenerating native parenchymal cells and filling defects with fibroblastic tissue. However, if unchecked and unregulated, a protracted and exaggerated release of "inflammatory" mediators leads to deterioration of organ function rather than restoration of homeostasis.[37–39] In the absence of inhibitory signals, the continued production of host defense response mediators sustains inflammation with tissue injury, intra- and extravascular coagulation, and proliferation of mesenchymal cells (fibroproliferation) with deposition of ECM, resulting in fibrosis (Fig. 51.3).[41]

Activation of the HPA Axis and Control of the Host Defense Response

Generation of inflammatory cytokines during the host defense response is normally strongly controlled by a number of homeostatic regulatory mechanisms including shedding of specific cytokine receptors on host cells, synthesis of endogenously generated cytokine antagonists, synthesis of antiinflammatory cytokines, downregulation, and most importantly activation of the HPA axis with production of GCs.[21] The discovery of GC receptors (GRs) has led to the gradual realization that a single, basic molecular mechanism initiates most GC actions.[42] Munck et al., in a landmark review, proposed that physiologically the function of stress-induced

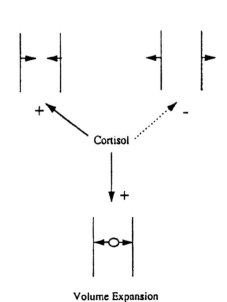

Vasoconstrictor Systems
  Catecholamines
  Arginine vasopressin
  Angiotensin II
  Endothelin

Vasodilatory Systems
  Kallikrein system
  Prostacyclin system
  NO synthase
  Inflammatory mediators

FIGURE 51.2. Effect of cortisol on arterial blood pressure. Cortisol potentiates the effects of vasoconstrictor systems, inhibits vasodilatory systems, and through its mineralocorticoid properties retains salt and increases blood volume. TNFα and IL-1, both of which are inhibited by cortisol, represent major vasodilatory stimulants during the inflammatory stress of sepsis, septic shock, and ARDS. (From Meduri and Chrousos,[33] with permission.)

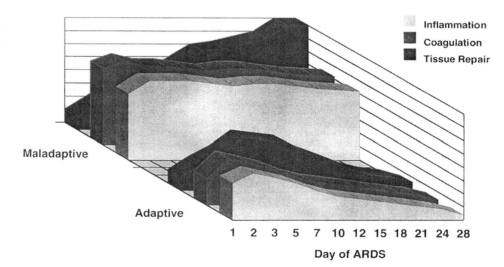

FIGURE 51.3. Inflammation, coagulation, and tissue repair in patients with adaptive and maladaptive host defense responses. (Data obtained from Meduri).[40]

increases in GC levels is to protect against the host normal defense reactions that are activated by stress but not to protect against the source of stress per se. They also proposed that GCs accomplish this function by turning off those normal defense reactions, thereby preventing them from overshooting and ultimately threatening homeostasis.[42] This influence is assumed to be sufficiently delayed in relation to the initial stress stimulus to allow the appropriate defense mechanisms to become activated.[42,43] However, this protective mechanism is not always effective, as demonstrated by the exaggerated and autodestructive host reaction seen in nonsurvivors of sepsis or ARDS.

Peripherally generated TNFα, IL-1β, and IL-6 activate the HPA axis independently at some or all of its levels [hypothalamic corticotropin-releasing hormone (CRH) neurons, pituitary corticotrophs, and the adrenal cortex], and in combination their effects are synergistic.[30,31] The HPA axis responds in a graded manner to greater intensities of stress with increased production of ACTH and GCs. ACTH is the predominant but not the only regulator of GC secretion. Other factors, including angiotensin and vasopressin, also influence adrenal GC secretion.[44] GCs are secreted directly into the circulation immediately after their synthesis. Cortisol, the major human GC, circulates bound (95%) to a corticosteroid-binding globulin (CBG) synthesized primarily by the liver, thereby providing a large reservoir that is released at sites of inflammation or tissue remodeling.[45]

Glucocorticoids exert most of their effects through specific, ubiquitously distributed intracellular (3000–100,000 per cell) GRs. GR activation and translocation have been studied extensively, and the molecular mechanisms involved in these processes have been reviewed.[13,46] The response of a single cell exposed to GCs is the result of the interplay between the following: (1) concentration of the free hormone; (2) relative potency of the hormone (influenced by biologic activity, affinity for the GR, and ability to retain the GR in the nucleus); and (3) ability of the cell to receive and transduce the hormonal signal.[14] Because the GR ultimately controls pertinent gene expression, anything that affects its binding affinity, transportation to the nucleus, number, conformation, or possible interaction with other relevant transcription factors can affect the response of the cells to GCs and, from the clinical point of view, the response of the individual to GC administration during intense inflammation. Thus to be responsive to GCs, a system must fulfill the following criteria: (1) sufficient amounts of GC must be made available; (2) GRs must be present and responsive; and (3) target genes of interest must be active and GC-regulatable. If one of these factors is defective, the system does not respond properly.

Glucocorticoids modulate the host defense response at virtually all levels, protecting the host from immune system overreaction.[32,47,48] Many of the antiinflammatory activities of GCs are exerted by GR-mediated blockade of the activity of transcription factors NF-κB and AP-1. Activated GRs inhibit the transactivational effects of NF-κB via a dual mechanism, by (1) physically interacting with the p65 subunit and (2) inducing the IκB inhibitory protein, which traps NF-κB in inactive cytoplasmic complexes catabolized by the ubiquitin–proteasome pathway (Fig. 51.1).[14–16] By these mechanisms, activated GRs inhibit the transcription of several cytokines,[46,49] inflammation-associated enzymes,[46,50] and adhesion molecules (Table 51.2).[46] GCs also have an inhibitory effect on fibrogenesis,[51] and act in synergy with interleukin-1 (IL-1) receptor antagonist,[52] and the antiinflammatory cytokines IL-4, IL-10, and IL-13.[53]

Exaggerated Host Defense Response and Associated Glucocorticoid Inadequacy/Resistance

Increased activation of NF-κB has been demonstrated in the peripheral monocytes of patients with sepsis and in the alveolar macrophages of patients with established ARDS.[54–56] During an observation period of 14 days, nonsurvivors of sepsis had significantly higher NF-κB activity ($p < 0.001$) in their peripheral mononuclear cells than did survivors.[56] In agreement, several studies have reported that nonsurvivors of sepsis[57–63] and ARDS[63–68] exhibit exaggerated and protracted elevation of

TABLE 51.2. Effect of Glucocorticoids on Gene Transcription.

Increased transcription
 Lipocortin-1
 β_2-Adrenoceptor
 Endonucleases
 Secretory leukocyte protease inhibitor
 Inhibitory protein IκB

Decreased transcription
 Cytokines (TNFα, IL-1, IL-2, IL-3, IL-4, IL-5, IL-6, IL-8, IL-11, IL-12, IL-13, GM-CSF, RANTES, MIP-1α)
 Inducible nitric oxide synthase (iNOS)
 Inducible cyclooxygenase (COX-2)
 Inducible phospholipase A$_2$ (cPLA$_2$)
 Endothelin-1
 NK1-receptors
 Adhesion molecules (ICAM-1, E selectin)

From Barnes and Adcock,[17] with permission.
TNF, tumor necrosis factor; IL, interleukin; GM-CSF, granulocyte/macrophage colony-stimulating factor; RANTES, regulated upon activation, normal T cell expressed and secreted; MIP-1α, macrophage inflammatory protein-1α.

circulating proinflammatory cytokine levels. In patients with sepsis-induced ARDS we found that elevated proinflammatory cytokine levels on day 1 predicted a persistent elevation over time[63] (Fig. 51.4), suggesting that loss of autoregulation is an early event in the course of lethal sepsis.

Glucocorticoid protection is not always effective, as demonstrated by the exaggerated and protracted elevation of circulating inflammatory cytokines seen in nonsurvivors of sepsis and ARDS, who usually have elevated (albeit ineffective) levels of circulating ACTH and cortisol,[69] furthermore, the degree of cortisolemia frequently correlates with the severity of the illness and the mortality rate,[70–72] and it is associated with an altered response of the HPA axis to suppression by dexamethasone and stimulation by CRH and ACTH.[61] Cortisol elevation is achieved by several mechanisms, including: (1) activation of the HPA axis; (2) GC resistance due to alterations in GR binding; (3) failure of pituitary and hypothalamus GC negative feedback; (4) decreased binding to CBG;[73–75] and (5) decreased cortisol extraction from the blood.[69,70] In critically ill patients, dexamethasone infusion at a dose that easily suppresses ACTH and cortisol secretions in normal subjects is minimally effective,[71,73] with pre- and postinfusion cortisol and ACTH levels remaining significantly higher in nonsurvivors.[71] In addition, the negative feedback of endogenous GC is clearly altered, and stimulation with CRH causes a significant increase (7–450%) in ACTH response despite cortisol levels sufficient to abolish a CRH-induced ACTH surge in normal subjects.[71] Following CRH stimulation, nonsurvivors have a smaller increase in cortisol levels despite a percentage increase in ACTH production similar to that in survivors.[71] Other studies have also found a lower cortisol response to ACTH in nonsurvivors of septic shock.[76–78]

Unquestionably, the elevation of GC secretion in nonsurvivors is inadequate to meet the needs of the concurrent host

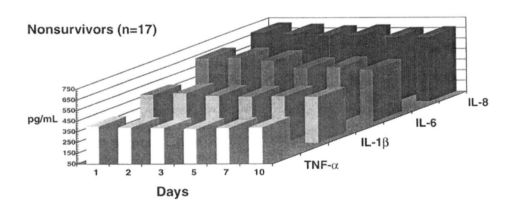

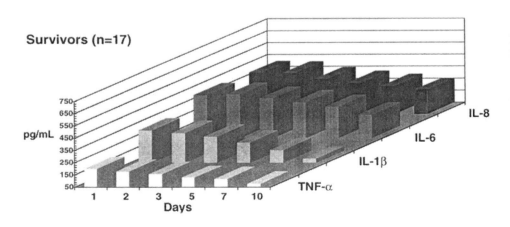

FIGURE 51.4. Plasma inflammatory cytokine levels over time in survivors and nonsurvivors. Plasma TNFα, IL-1β, IL-6, and IL-8 levels from days 1 to 10 of sepsis-induced ARDS. On day 1 of ARDS, nonsurvivors ($n = 17$) had significantly higher ($p < 0.001$) TNFα, IL-1β, IL-6, and IL-8 levels. Over time, nonsurvivors had persistent elevation, whereas survivors ($n = 17$) had a rapid decline. These findings indicate that loss of autoregulation is an early phenomenon. (Data obtained from Headley et al.[37] and Meduri et al.[63])

defense response and its adverse systemic effects. This could be due to tissue resistance to GCs, inadequacy of the level and duration of endogenous GC elevation to suppress a host defense response gone awry, or both.[33] GC resistance from altered GR function may be partially responsible for the changes in the HPA axis of critically ill patients and could result in an augmented ACTH response to CRH.[71] Two groups of investigators have recognized that cytokines can cause concentration-dependent resistance to GCs by reducing the GR binding affinity for cortisol.[79,80] Although the exact mechanisms have not been clarified, researchers have postulated that an excess of cytokine-induced transcription factors, such as NF-κB and AP-1, may form complexes with activated GRs, preventing GR interaction with DNA and the expression of GC-responsive element (GRE)-mediated antiinflammatory activity.[14] Such inhibition of cortisol binding to GRs was demonstrated in T cells incubated with a combination of IL-2 and IL-4;[80] IL-1, IL-6, and interferon-γ (IFNγ);[79] or IL-13.[81] GC resistance was induced in a cytokine concentration-dependent fashion and was reversed by the removal of cytokines.[80]

This line of evidence is reinforced by the results of experimental studies.[82-84] In a sheep model of sepsis-induced ARDS, maximal binding capacity of GRs decreased continuously after endotoxin infusion, and there was a marked elevation of cortisol levels.[82] The reduced GR binding correlated negatively ($r = -0.87$, $p < 0.01$) with PLA$_2$ (the rate-limiting enzyme in eicosanoid metabolism) activity. In a rat model of septic shock, GR blockade by mifepristone (RU486) exacerbated the physiologic and pathologic changes induced by endotoxemia.[83] PLA$_2$ activity in rats with 80% GR blockade was more marked than in those with 50% GR blockade.[83] Monocytes of patients with sepsis develop near-total GC resistance in vitro by adding cytokines, especially IL-2.[85] The reduction in GC responsiveness therefore appears to become greater as the intensity of the inflammatory response increases. In addition, this inflammatory cytokine-induced GC resistance could be increased by stimulation of the natural non-GC binding isoform of the GR (GRβ), an isoform that has dominant negative effects on the classic GR (GRα).[14,86]

Experimental and Clinical Evidence to Support Prolonged Glucocorticoid Treatment for Sepsis and ARDS

A significant body of experimental literature has provided clear, although unappreciated, evidence that the dosage and duration of GC administration influence the treatment response and outcome in septic shock and in ARDS.[87-98] In 1956 Levitin and collaborators demonstrated that when exogenous GCs are given by different routes of administration, protection from endotoxin correlated with the blood levels and rates of disappearance from the circulation.[87] In 1963 Lillehei et al. showed that dogs injected with a lethal dose of endotoxin maintained aortic and renal pressure during an infusion of hydrocortisone (50 mg/kg), and the protective effects rapidly disappeared with discontinuation of administration.[89] Pitcairn et al. found that when male Sprague-Dawley rats were injected with a lethal dose of *Escherichia coli*, concomitant administration of dexamethasone, with or without antibiotics, dramatically improved survival at 8 hours. However, as circulating dexamethasone levels decreased over time, the early benefits were lost and mortality increased by 20 hours.[90] During the late 1970s Hinshaw and collaborators reported a series of experimental studies evaluating the response to methylprednisolone (30 mg/kg) initiated at various times from initiation of a 2- to 5-hour *E. coli* infusion. These investigators recognized early in their work that the half-life of methylprednisolone is only 3-4 hours, and that the early beneficial response to a 30 mg/kg bolus could be sustained only if therapeutic levels were maintained with a continuous infusion of methylprednisolone.[91-93] With a continuous infusion, outcome was improved, even when initiation of methylprednisolone treatment was delayed by a few hours.[99] In 1982 Greisman reported on a study designed to investigate prospectively the impact that dosage and duration of administration have on the efficacy of methylprednisolone to prevent murine gram-negative mortality not preventable by antibiotics alone.[94] Outbred mice were injected intraperitoneally with one LD$_{90-100}$ dose of *Escherichia coli*, *Proteus mirabilis*, or *Klebsiella pneumoniae*. Standardized models were created by selecting a time delay in initiating antibiotic therapy that resulted in 50-70% mortality. In these models, methylprednisolone was tested at three different concentrations and either as single or repeated injections at 4-hour intervals. A methylprednisolone dose of 30 mg/kg provided superior protection to either 10 mg/kg or 60 mg/kg, as single or multiple injections. More importantly, they observed a significant incremental reduction in mortality with repetitive administration.[94] Similarly, in a rat model of butylated hydroxytoluene-induced acute lung injury, GC administration was shown to be effective in decreasing lung collagen and edema formation so long as treatment was prolonged; withdrawal rapidly negated the positive effects of therapy.[96-98]

Two randomized studies evaluating massive doses of methylprednisolone in septic shock provided useful data for evaluating the impact of treatment duration on the physiologic response[5,6] and outcome in patients with septic shock.[6] Lucas and Ledgerwood[5] observed a significant increase in mean arterial blood pressure during the 48 hours of dexamethasone (6 mg/kg) infusion, but this positive response disappeared when GC therapy was discontinued. Sprung and collaborators[6] reported significant benefits early in the course of treatment. Reversal of shock, defined by strict criteria, was significantly more frequent in treated patients (58% vs. 38%, $p < 0.05$), and the difference was more striking in those treated within 4 hours of developing shock (73% vs. 20%, $p < 0.05$) or in those who survived more than 12 hours (71% vs. 14%, $p < 0.05$). At 133 hours after treatment mortality was 40% versus 69% ($p < 0.05$). The differences in reversal of shock and mortality disappeared later in the course of the study, leading the authors to speculate whether continuation of treatment might have sustained this initial improvement. Because the rate of methylprednisolone elimination is significantly affected by the presence of shock (half-life 9–20 hours) the pharmacologic effect of GC treatment may have extended beyond 72 hours, providing an explanation for the above findings.

Clinical studies evaluating physiologic and biologic markers of inflammation over time in patients with sepsis, septic shock, and ARDS have shown that prolonged GC treatment is essential to achieve a significant, sustained reduction in the circulatory levels of inflammatory mediators, including TNFα, IL-1β, IL-6, IL-8, and PLA$_2$[100,101] and a decrease in collagen synthesis.[102] Three clinical studies demonstrated that premature discontinuation of prolonged GC administration in septic shock[101] and in unresolving ARDS[103,104] was associated with physiologic deterioration that resolved with reinstitution of treatment. In the septic shock study, the clinical deterioration upon premature discontinuation of GC treatment was also accompanied by a rebound elevation of PLA$_2$ and C-reactive protein levels, which decreased with reinstitution of therapy.[101]

Studies suggest that premature discontinuation of GC therapy may not only lead to loss of early treatment benefits but may in fact be harmful. Indeed, in another study the cytokine response to lipopolysaccharide challenge in humans was significantly enhanced by a prior (12–144 hours) short course of GCs.[105] This observation may explain the differences in infection-related mortality between studies utilizing a short course (24 hours)[106] versus a prolonged course of methylprednisolone treatment.[4,37]

Rationale for Prolonged Glucocorticoid Administration

Studies indicate that excessive inflammatory activity in patients with sepsis, septic shock, or ARDS may induce noncompensated GC resistance in target organs, thereby negating the beneficial suppressive influence of an inadequately secreted endogenous cortisol on the dysregulated host defense response. Prolonged treatment with increased doses of exogenous GCs may be necessary to compensate adequately for the inability of target organs to respond to endogenous cortisol and for the inability of the host to produce appropriately elevated levels of GCs. If the proposed pathophysiologic construct is correct, prolonged GC therapy may be useful, not as an antiinflammatory treatment per se but as hormonal supplementation to compensate for the host's inability to produce appropriately elevated levels of cortisol or for the inability of target organs to respond to endogenous cortisol. Adequate hormonal supplementation should modify the intracellular balance among activated transcription factors (e.g., NF-κB, AP-1, GR), thus converting an initially dysregulated (maladaptive) host defense response to a regulated (adaptive) one. In this context, GC treatment is directed at the core pathogenetic mechanism of sepsis and should affect all pathways of the host defense response. GR-mediated blockade or NF-κB transcriptional activity should decrease (not suppress) the synthesis of proximal and distal mediators of the host defense response; and if this beneficial response is sustained over time, patients should experience a reversal of physiologic and clinical abnormalities. Alternative modalities to block NF-κB are being investigated.[107]

For patients with sepsis or ARDS, there is no direct evidence demonstrating that GC treatment induces a reduction in intracellular activation of transcription factors NF-κB or AP-1. Indirect evidence for such action, however, is provided by clinical studies that have monitored, before and during prolonged GC administration, the blood concentration of several mediators transcribed by NF-κB. In these studies treatment was associated with a rapid, significant reduction in plasma levels of inflammatory mediators (TNFα, IL-1β, IL-6, IL-8, PLA$_2$),[100,101] adhesion molecules,[108] and markers of collagen synthesis.[102] So long as treatment was continued, the concentrations of these biologic markers continued to decrease, and physiologic and clinical variables improved in parallel. In a randomized study of patients with sepsis-induced unresolving ARDS,[109] this beneficial biologic and physiologic response was observed only in patients randomized to prolonged methylprednisolone administration, whereas no change was observed in those receiving placebo. In three clinical studies premature discontinuation of prolonged GC administration to patients with septic shock[101] or unresolving ARDS[103,104] was associated with physiologic deterioration that improved with reinstitution of treatment. In the septic shock study, the clinical deterioration upon premature discontinuation of GC treatment was accompanied by a rebound elevation of PLA$_2$, and C-reactive protein levels, which decreased with reinstitution of therapy.[101] Finally, two reports provided indirect evidence to support the concept of endogenous GC resistance in patients with sepsis or unresolving ARDS. In a study of patients with septic shock, plasma cortisol levels decreased during hydrocortisone infusion and returned toward pretreatment values after discontinuing therapy.[101] Similarly, in patients with unresolving ARDS we have found that prolonged GC administration was associated with a significant reduction in ACTH and cortisol levels, in parallel with a reduction in circulating inflammatory cytokine levels (personal unpublished data).

Conclusions

Evidence indicates that in patients with septic shock or ARDS excessive activation of the host defense response may induce noncompensated GC resistance in target organs, a condition potentially responsive to exogenous GC supplementation. Patients with a dysregulated host defense response have persistent immune cell activation of NF-κB (a critical transcription factor for the maximal expression of multiple cytokines) and protracted elevation of inflammatory cytokine levels over time. In both uncontrolled and controlled studies, prolonged GC treatment of patients with septic shock or unresolving ARDS was associated with a rapid, significant, sustained reduction in circulating levels of these markers of disease activity and progressive physiologic improvement. No other treatment intervention for sepsis or ARDS has yet provided this level of evidence. Although the results of four recent randomized studies are encouraging, pharmacokinetic and pharmacodynamic studies of exogenous GCs in sepsis and ARDS are not yet available to guide optimal drug administration, and today's treatment dosing is essentially empiric. Additional research is necessary to advance our understanding on the complex mechanisms that influence endogenous and exogenous GC activities at the cellular level during acute, life-threatening inflammation.

Acknowledgments. Partial support was provided by the Baptist Memorial Health Care Foundation and The Assisi Foundation of Memphis. I am indebted to Vivian Gomez for assistance in preparing the manuscript and the figures.

References

1. Bollaert PE, Charpentier C, Levy B, Debouverie M, Audibert G, Larcan A: Reversal of late septic shock with supraphysiological doses of hydrocortisone. Crit Care Med 1998; 26:645–650.
2. Briegel J, Haller M, Forst H, et al: Effect of hydrocortisone on reversal of hyperdynamic septic shock: a randomized, double-blind, placebo-controlled, single-center study. Crit Care Med 1999 (in press).
3. Chawla K, Kupfer Y, Goldman I, Tessler S: Hydrocortisone reverses refractory septic shock [abstract]. Crit Care Med 1999;27:A33.
4. Meduri GU, Headley AS, Golden E, et al: Prolonged methylprednisolone treatment improves lung function and outcome in patients with unresolving acute respiratory distress syndrome: results of a randomized, double-blind, placebo-controlled trial. AM J Respir Crit Care Med 1997;155:A391.
5. Lucas CE, Ledgerwood AM: The cardiopulmonary response to massive doses of steroids in patients with septic shock. Arch Surg 1984;119:537–541.
6. Sprung CL, Caralis PV, Marcial EH, et al: The effects of high-dose corticosteroids in patients with septic shock. N Engl J Med 1984;311:1137–1143.
7. Bone RC, Fisher CJ, Clemmer TP, et al: A controlled trial of high-dose methylprednisolone in the treatment of severe sepsis and septic shock. N Engl J Med 1987;317:653–658.
8. Hinshaw L, Peduzzi P, Young E, et al: Effect of high-dose glucocorticoid therapy on mortality in patients with clinical signs of systemic sepsis. N Engl J Med 1987;317:659–665.
9. Luce JM, Montgomery AB, Marks JD, Turner J, Metz CA, Murray JF: Ineffectiveness of high-dose methylprednisolone in preventing parenchymal lung injury and improving mortality in patients with septic shock. Am Rev Respir Dis 1988;138:62–68.
10. Bernard GR, Luce JM, Sprung CL, et al: High-dose corticosteroids in patients with the adult respiratory distress syndrome. N Engl J Med 1987;317:1565–1570.
11. Lefering R, Neugebauer EAM: Steroid controversy in sepsis and septic shock: a meta-analysis. Crit Care Med 1995;23:1294–1303.
12. Cronin L, Cook DJ, Carlet J, et al: Corticosteroid treatment for sepsis: a critical appraisal and meta-analysis of the literature. Crit Care Med 1995;23:1430–1439.
13. Udelsman R, Holbrook NJ: Endocrine and molecular responses to surgical stress. Curr Probl Surg 1994;31:653–720.
14. Bamberger CM, Shulte HM, Chrousos GP: Molecular determinants of glucocorticoid receptor function and tissue sensitivity to glucocorticoids. Endoc Rev 1996;17:245–261.
15. Scheinman RI, Cogswell PC, Lofquist AK, Baldwin AS: Role of transcriptional activation of IκBa in medication of immunosuppression by glucocorticoids. Science 1995;270:283–290.
16. Wissink S, Van Heerde EC, Van der Burg B, Van der Saag PT: A dual mechanism mediates repression of NF-κB activity of glucocorticoids. Mol Endocrinol 1998;12:355–363.
17. Barnes PJ, Adcock IM: Glucocorticoids receptors. In: Crystal RG, West JB, Weibel ER, Barnes PJ (eds) The Lung Scientific Foundations, 2nd ed. Philadelphia, Lippincott-Raven, 1997;37–55.
18. Barnes PJ, Karin M: Nuclear factor-κB: a pivotal transcription factor in chronic inflammatory diseases. N Engl J Med 1997;336:1066–1071.
19. Cerami A: Inflammatory cytokines. Clin Immunol Immunopathol 1992;62:S3–S10.
20. Baumann H, Gauldie J: The acute phase response. Immunol Today 1994;15:74–80.
21. Heumann D, Glauser MP: Pathogenesis of sepsis. Sci & Med 1994;1:28–37.
22. Pannen BHJ, Robotham JL: The acute-phase response. New Horiz 1995;3:183–197.
23. Albina JE, Reichner JS: Nitric oxide in inflammation and immunity. New Horiz 1995;3:46–64.
24. Strieter RM, Lukacs NW, Standiford TJ, Kunkel SL: Cytokines and lung inflammation: mechanisms of neutrophil recruitment to the lung. Thorax 1993;48:765–769.
25. Van Der Poll T, Buller HR, Cate HT, et al: Activation of coagulation after administration of tumor necrosis factor to normal subjects. N Engl J Med 1990;322:1622–1627.
26. Elias JA, Freundlich B, Kern JA, Rosenbloom J: Cytokine networks in the regulation of inflammation and fibrosis in the lung. Chest 1990;97:1439–1445.
27. King RJ, Jones MB, Minoo P: Regulation of lung cell proliferation by polypeptide growth factors. Am J Physiol 1989;257: L23–L38.
28. Postlethwaite AE, Seyer JM: Stimulation of fibroblast chemotaxis by human recombinant tumor necrosis factor α (TNF-α) and a synthetic TNF-α 31-68 peptide. J Exp Med 1990;172:1749–1756.
29. Meduri GU, Estes RJ: Pathogenesis of ventilator-associated pneumonia: the lower respiratory tract. Intensive Care Med 1995;21:452–461.
30. Perlstein RS, Whitnall MH, Abrams JS, Mougey EH, Neta R: Synergistic roles of interleukin-6, interleukin-1, and tumor necrosis factor in the adrenocorticotropin response to bacterial lipopolysaccharide in vivo. Endocrinology 1993;132:946–952.
31. Hermus ARMM, Sweep CGJ: Cytokines and the hypothalamic-pituitary-adrenal axis. J Steroid Biochem Mol Biol 1990;37: 867–871.
32. Meduri GU: The role of the host defense response in the progression and outcome of ARDS: pathophysiological correlations and response to glucocorticoid treatment. Eur Respir J 1996;9:2650–2670.
33. Meduri GU, Chrousos GP: Duration of glucocorticoid treatment and outcome in sepsis: is the right drug used the wrong way? Chest 1998;114:355–360.
34. Magiakou MA, Mastorakos G, Zachman K, Chrousos GP: Blood pressure in children and adolescents with Cushing syndrome before and after surgical cure. J Clin Endocrinol Metab 1997;82:1734–1738.
35. Fischer JE, Hasselgren PO: Cytokines and glucocorticoids in the regulation of the "hepato-skeletal muscle axis" in sepsis. Am J Surg 1991;161:266–271.

36. Gallin JK, Goldstein IM, Snyderman R: Overview. In: Gallin JI, Goldstein IM, Snyderman R (eds) Inflammation: Basic Principles and Clinical Correlates. New York, Raven, 1988;1–3.
37. Headley AS, Tolley E, Meduri GU: Infections and the inflammatory response in acute respiratory distress syndrome. Chest 1997;111:1306–1321.
38. Christou NV: Host defense mechanisms of surgical patients: friend or foe? Arch Surg 1996;131:1136–1139.
39. Guirao X, Lowry SF: Biologic control of injury and inflammation: much more than too little or too late. World J Surg 1996;20:437–446.
40. Meduri GU: Host defense response and outcome in ARDS. Chest 1997;112:1154–1158.
41. Kovacs EJ, Dipietro LA: Fibrogenic cytokines and connective tissue production. FASEB J 1994;8:854–861.
42. Munck A, Guyre PM, Holbrook NJ: Physiological functions of glucocorticoids in stress and their relation to pharmacological actions. Endocr Rev 1984;5:25–44.
43. Zuckerman SH, Shellhaas J, Butler LD: Differential regulation of lipopolysaccharide-induced interleukin 1 and tumor necrosis factor synthesis: effects of endogenous and exogenous glucocorticoids and the role of the pituitary-adrenal axis. Eur J Immunol 1989;19:301–305.
44. Vermes I, Beishuizen A, Hampsink RM, Haanen C: Dissociation of plasma adrenocorticotropin and cortisol levels in critically ill patients: possible role of endothelin and atrial natriuretic hormone. J Clin Endocrinol Metab 1995;80:1238–1242.
45. Hammond GL: Potential functions of plasma steroid-binding proteins. Trends Endocrinol Metab 1995;6:298–304.
46. Barnes PJ, Greening AP, Crompton GK: Glucocorticoid resistance in asthma. Am J Respir Crit Care Med 1995;152:S125–S142.
47. Chrousos GP: The hypothalamic-pituitary-adrenal axis and immune-mediated inflammation. N Engl J Med 1995;332:1351–1362.
48. Elenkov IJ, Papanicolaou DA, Wilder RL, Chrousos GP: Modulatory effects of glucocorticoids and catecholamines on human interleukin-12 and interleukin-10 production: clinical implications. Proc Assoc Am Physicians 1996;108:1–8.
49. Detera-Wadleigh SD, Karl M: The glucocorticoid receptor gene. Ann Intern Med 1993;119:1113–1124.
50. Pruzanski W, Vadas P: Phospholipase A_2: a mediator between proximal and distal effectors of inflammation. Immunol Today 1991;12:143–146.
51. Meduri GU, Belenchia JM, Estes RJ, Wunderink RG, El Torky M, Leeper KV Jr: Fibroproliferative phase of ARDS: clinical findings and effects of corticosteroids. Chest 1991;100:943–952.
52. Santos AA, Scheltinga MR, Lynch E, et al: Elaboration of interleukin 1-receptor antagonist is not attenuated by glucocorticoids after endotoxemia. Arch Surg 1993;128:138–144.
53. Hart PH, Whitty GA, Burgess DR, Croatto M, Hamilton JA: Augmentation of glucocorticoid action on human monocytes by interleukin-4. Lymphokine Res 1990;9:147–153.
54. Schwartz MD, Moore EE, Moore FA, et al: Nuclear factor-κB is activated in alveolar macrophages from patients with acute respiratory distress syndrome. Crit Care Med 1996;24:1285–1292.
55. Maus U, Pavlidis T, Rosseau S, Seeger W, Lohmeyer J: Increased proinflammatory cytokine gene expression in alveolar macrophages is associated with changes in NF-κB DNA binding activity in septic ARDS [abstract]. AJRCCM 1998;157:A459.
56. Böhrer H, Qiu F, Zimmermann T, et al: Role of NFκB in the mortality of sepsis. J Clin Invest 1997;100:972–984.
57. Damas P, Ledoux D, Nys M, et al: Cytokine serum level during severe sepsis in human IL-6 as a marker of severity. Ann Surg 1992;215:356–362.
58. Calandra T, Gerain J, Heumann D, Baumgartner JD, Glauser MP, Swiss-Dutch J5 Immunoglobulin Study Group: High circulating levels of interleukin-6 in patients with septic shock: evolution during sepsis, prognostic value, and interplay with other cytokines. Am J Med 1991;91:23–29.
59. Calandra T, Baumgartner JD, Grau GE, et al: Prognostic values of tumor necrosis factor/cachectin, interleukin-1, interferon-α, and interferon-γ in the serum of patients with septic shock. J Infect Dis 1990;161:982–987.
60. Pinski MR, Vincent JL, Deviere J, Alegre M, Kahn RJ, Dupont E: Serum cytokine levels in human septic shock: relation to multiple-system organ failure and mortality. Chest 1993;103:565–575.
61. Sullivan JS, Kilpatrick L, Costarino AT, Lee SC, Harris MC: Correlation of plasma cytokine elevations with mortality rate in children with sepsis. J Pediatr 1992;120:510–515.
62. Dofferhoff ASM, De Jong HJ, Bom VJJ, et al: Complement activation and the production of inflammatory mediators during the treatment of severe sepsis in humans. Scand J Infect Dis 1992;24:197–204.
63. Meduri GU, Headley S, Kohler G, et al: Persistent elevation of inflammatory cytokines predicts a poor outcome in ARDS: plasma IL-1β and IL-6 are consistent and efficient predictors of outcome over time. Chest 1995;107:1062–1073.
64. Roumen RMH, Hendriks T, van der Ven-Jongekrijg J, et al: Cytokine patterns in patients after major vascular surgery, hemorrhagic shock, and severe blunt trauma: relation with subsequent adult respiratory distress syndrome and multiple organ failure. Ann Surg 1993;218:769–776.
65. Romaschin AD, DeMajo WC, Winton T, et al: Systemic phospholipase A_2 and cachectin levels in adult respiratory distress syndrome and multiple-organ failure. Clin Biochem 1992;25:55–60.
66. Groeneveld ABJ, Raijmakers PGH, Hack CE, Thijs LG: Interleukin 8-related neutrophil elastase and the severity of the adult respiratory distress syndrome. Cytokine 1995;7:746–752.
67. Meduri GU, Kohler G, Headley S, Tolley E, Stentz F, Postlethwaite A: Inflammatory cytokines in the BAL of patients with ARDS: persistent elevation over time predicts poor outcome. Chest 1995;108:1303–1314.
68. Baughman RP, Gunther KL, Rashkin MC, Keeton DA, Pattishall EN: Changes in the inflammatory response of the lung during acute respiratory distress syndrome: prognostic indicators. Am J Respir Crit Care Med 1996;154:76–81.
69. Melby JC, Egdahl RH, Spink WW: Secretion and metabolism of cortisol after injection of endotoxin. J Lab Clin Med 1960;56:50–62.
70. Melby JC, Spink WW: Comparative studies on adrenalcortical function and cortisol metabolism in healthy adults and in patients with shock due to infection. J Clin Invest 1958;37:1791–1798.
71. Reincke M, Allolio B, Wurth G, Winkelmann W: The hypothalamic-pituitary-adrenal axis in critical illness: response to dexamethasone and corticotropin-releasing hormone. J Clin Endocrinol Metab 1993;77:151–156.
72. Briegel J, Forst H, Hellinger H, Haller M: Contribution of cortisol deficiency to septic shock. Lancet 1991;338:507–508.

73. Perrot D, Bonneton A, Dechaud H, Motin J, Pugeat M: Hypercortisolism in septic shock is not suppressible by dexamethasone infusion. Crit Care Med 1993;21:396–401.
74. Savu L, Zouaghi H, Carli A, Nunez EA: Serum depletion of corticosteroid binding activities: an early marker of human septic shock. Biochem Biophys Res Commun 1981;102:411–419.
75. Pugeat M, Bonneton A, Perrot D, et al: Decreased immunoreactivity and binding activity of corticosteroid-binding globulin in serum in septic shock. Clin Chem 1989;35:1675–1679.
76. Rothwell PM, Udwadia ZF, Lawler PG: Cortisol response to corticotropin and survival in septic shock. Lancet 1991;337:1230–1231.
77. Sibbald WJ, Short A, Cohen MP, Wilson RF: Variations in adrenocortical responsiveness during severe bacterial infections: unrecognized adrenocortical insufficiency in severe bacterial infections. Ann Surg 1977;186:29–33.
78. Soni A, Pepper GM, Wyrwinski PM, et al: Adrenal insufficiency occurring during septic shock: incidence, outcome, and relationship to peripheral cytokine levels. Am J Med 1995;98:266–271.
79. Almawi WY, Lipman ML, Stevens AC, Zanker B, Hadro Et, Strom TB: Abrogation of glucocorticosteroid-mediated inhibition of T cell proliferation by the synergistic action of IL-1, IL-6, and IFN-γ. J Immunol 1991;146:3523–3527.
80. Kam JC, Szefler SJ, Surs W, Sher ER, Leung DYM: Combination IL-2 and IL-4 reduces glucocorticoid receptor-binding affinity and T cell response to glucocorticoids. J Immunol 1993;151:3460–3466.
81. Spahn JD, Szefler SJ, Surs W, Doherty DE, Nimmagadda SR, Leung DYM: Induction of diminished monocyte glucocorticoid receptor-binding affinity. J Immunol 1996;157:2654–2659.
82. Liu LY, Sun B, Tian Y, Lu BZ, Wang J: Changes of pulmonary glucocorticoid receptor and phospholipase A_2 in sheep with acute lung injury after high dose endotoxin infusion. Am Rev Respir Dis 1993;148:878–881.
83. Fan J, Gong X, Wu J, Zhang Y, Xu R: Effect of glucocorticoid receptor (GR) blockade on endotoxemia in rats. Circulatory shock 1994;42:76–82.
84. Molijn GJ, Spek JJ, van Uffelen JC, et al: Differential adaptation of glucocorticoid sensitivity of peripheral blood mononuclear leukocytes in patients with sepsis or septic shock. J Clin Endocrinol Metab 1995;80:1799–1803.
85. Molijn GJ, Spek JJ, Van Uffelen JC, et al: Differential adaptation of glucocorticoid sensitivity of peripheral blood mononuclear leukocytes in patients with sepsis or septic shock. J Clin Endocrinol Metab 1995;80:1799–1803.
86. Leung DYM, Hamid Q, Vottero A, et al: Association of glucocorticoid insensitivity with increased expression of glucocorticoid receptor β. J Exp Med 1997;186:1567–1574.
87. Levitin H, Kendrick MI, Kass EH: Effect of route of administration on protective action of corticosterone and cortisol against endotoxin. Proc Soc Exp Biol Med 1956;93:306–309.
88. Weil MH, Allen KS: The effect of steroids on shock due to endotoxin. In: Mills LC Inflammation and Diseases of Connective Tissue. A Hahneman Symposium Saundars, Philadelphia 1961:768–778.
89. Lillehei RC, Longerbeam JK, Bloch JH: Physiology and therapy of bacteremic shock. Am J Cardiol 1963;12:599–613.
90. Pitcairn M, Schuler J, Erve PR, Holtzman S, Schumer W: Glucocorticoid and antibiotic effect on experimental gram-negative bacteremic shock. Arch Surg 1975;110:1012–1015.
91. Hinshaw LB, Coalson JJ, Benjamin BA, et al: *Escherichia coli* shock in the baboon and the response to adrenocorticosteroid treatment. Surg Gynecol Obstet 1978;147:545–557.
92. Hinshaw LB, Keller BK, Archer LT, Flournoy DJ, White GL, Philips RW: Recovery from lethal *Escherichia coli* shocks in dogs. Surg Gynecol Obstet 1979;149:545–553.
93. Hinshaw LB, Archer LT, Beller-Todd BK, et al: Survival of primates in LD_{100} septic shock following steroid/antibiotic therapy. J Surg Res 1980;28:151–170.
94. Greisman SE: Experimental gram-negative bacterial sepsis: optimal methylprednisolone requirements for prevention of mortality not preventable by antibiotics alone. Proc Soc Exp Biol Med 1982;170:436–442.
95. Jones RL, King EG: The effects of methylprednisolone on oxygenation in experimental hypoxemic respiratory failure. J Trauma 1975;15:297–303.
96. Hesterberg TW, Last JA: Ozone-induced acute pulmonary fibrosis in rats: prevention of increased rates of collagen synthesis by methylprednisolone. Am Rev Respir Dis 1981;123:47–52.
97. Hakkinen PJ, Schmoyer RL, Witschi HP: Potentiation of butylated-hydroxytoluene-induced acute lung damage by oxygen: effects of prednisolone and indomethacin. Am Rev Respir Dis 1983;128:648–651.
98. Kehrer JP, Klein-Szanto AJP, Sorensen EMB, Pearlman R, Rosner MH: Enhanced acute lung damage following corticosteroid treatment. Am Rev Respir Dis 1984;130:256–261.
99. Hinshaw LB, Archer LT, Beller-Todd BK, Benjamin B, Flournoy DJ, Passey R: Survival of primates in lethal septic shock following delayed treatment with steroid. Circulatory Shock 1981;8:291–300.
100. Meduri GU, Headley S, Tolley E, Shelby M, Stentz F, Postlethwaite A: Plasma and BAL cytokine response to corticosteroid rescue treatment in ARDS. Chest 1995;108:1315–1325.
101. Briegel J, Kellermann W, Forst H, et al: Low-dose hydrocortisone infusion attenuates the systemic inflammatory response syndrome. Clin Invest 1994;72:782–787.
102. Meduri GU, Headley EA, Tolley A, Chin A, Stentz F, Postlethwaite A: Plasma and BAL procollagen type I & III levels during ARDS and in response to prolonged methylprednisolone treatment [abstract]. Am J Resp Crit Care Med 1998;157:A460.
103. Ashbaugh DG, Maier RV: Idiopathic pulmonary fibrosis in adult respiratory distress syndrome: diagnosis and treatment. Arch Surg 1985;120:530–535.
104. Hooper RG, Kearl RA: Established ARDS treated with a sustained course of adrenocortical steroids. Chest 1990;97:138–143.
105. Barber AE, Coyle SM, Marano MA, et al: Glucocorticoid therapy alters hormonal and cytokine responses to endotoxin in man. J Immunol 1993;150:1999–2006.
106. Bone RC, Fisher CJ Jr, Clemmer TP, Slotman GJ, Metz CA: Methylprednisolone severe sepsis study group: early methylprednisolone treatment for septic syndrome and the adult respiratory distress syndrome. Chest 1987;92:1032–1036.
107. Christman JW, Lancaster LH, Blackwell TS: Nuclear factor κB: a pivotal role in the systemic inflammatory response syndrome and new target for therapy. Intensive Care Med 1998;24:1131–1138.
108. Meduri GU: Levels of evidence for the pharmacological effectiveness of prolonged methylprednisolone treatment in unresolving acute respiratory distress syndrome. Chest 1999;116:116–118.
109. Meduri GU, Headley S, Carson S, Umberger R, Kelso T, Tolley E: Prolonged methylprednisolone treatment improves lung function and outcome of unresolving ARDS: a randomized, double-blind, placebo-controlled trial. JAMA 1998;280:159–165.

52
Pathophysiologic and Clinical Importance of Stress-Induced Th1/Th2 T Cell Shifts

Siegfried Zedler and Eugen Faist

The fact that T cells can differentiate and become polarized to produce a certain limited spectrum of cytokines and mediate only a subset of potential T cell functions during cell–cell interactions continues to be an area of intense investigation. The mechanisms by which T-helper (Th) cells mobilize various effector reactions remained unclear until 1986 when Mosmann and Coffman started a conceptual revolution in immunology by dividing murine T cell clones, or Th cells, into the now familiar two subpopulations, Th1 and Th2 based on their restricted and stereotyped profile of cytokine secretion.[1] These same two subsets can be generated from ex vivo populations when cultured under appropriate conditions;[2] they can also be recovered from immunized animals[3] and from patients suffering from a variety of diseases.[4]

Th1 and Th2 Cell Characteristics

The T cells are able to synthesize and secrete various patterns of cytokines, depending on their stage of differentiation and on whether they have polarized to produce restricted patterns. Th1 and Th2 patterns of cytokine secretion correspond to activated effector phenotypes generated during both cell-mediated and humoral immune responses. They do not exist among naive T cells or possibly even among long-term memory cells. Naive T cells and uncommitted, resting memory T cells produce principally or entirely interleukin-2 (IL-2),[5] which they use for their own growth. The differentiation of resting T cells into Th1/Th2 effector phenotypes may proceed through an intermediate state of expressing a broad range of potent cytokines upon restimulation. At this and later points in their development and in the absence of clearly polarizing signals, CD4$^+$ Th cell subsets with a less differentiated cytokine profile than Th1 and Th2, designated Th0, usually arise.[6] Th0 cells may dominate the earliest stages of some responses and mediate intermediate effector functions, depending on the ratio of cytokines produced and the nature of the responding cells.[7] Alternatively, T cells can be restricted to producing one of two highly polarized patterns of cytokine secretion, which have biologic relevance, as it has been demonstrated that different Th cell subsets have different functions. Th1 cells secrete IL-2, interferon-γ (IFN-γ), and lymphotoxin (tumor necrosis factor-β, or TNFβ) and are responsible for the production of opsonizing and complement-fixing antibodies of the immunoglobulin G2a (IgG2a) class, macrophage activation, and delayed-type hypersensitivity (DTH) reactions. On the other hand, Th2 cells, producing cytokines such as IL-4, IL-5, IL-6, IL-10, and IL-13, were originally defined as predominant helpers of B cell responses, including IgE and IgG1 isotype switching and mucosal immunity, through production of mast cell and eosinophil growth and differentiation and facilitation to IgA synthesis. Moreover, several macrophage functions are inhibited by Th2-derived IL-4, IL-10, and IL-13.[1] de Waal Malefyt et al.[8] showed that IL-13 was produced by human T cell clones by Th1, Th2, and Th0 cells, suggesting that IL-13 is not a typical Th2 cytokine. In peripheral human T cells, IL-13 is secreted by both human CD45RA$^+$ naive T cells and CD45R0$^+$ memory T cells. Its production was increased by IL-4 and decreased by IL-12, in contrast to IL-4, which is produced only by CD45R0$^+$ T cells.[9] Furthermore, IL-13 was co-expressed with IL-4 but not IFNγ in individual CD45R0$^+$ cells, although IL-13 and IL-4 were produced with different kinetics. The authors suggested that IL-13, together with the long-lasting production, may have IL-4-like functions in situations where T cell-derived IL-4 is still absent or where its production has already been downregulated.

Although there are many well documented Th1 and Th2 responses, they are not the only cytokine patterns possible; cells producing high levels of transforming growth factor-β (TGF-β) have been termed Th3.[10] Using TGFβ and anti-IFNγ to inhibit Th2 and Th1 differentiation, it is possible to keep CD4$^+$ T cells in a proliferating, IL-2-secreting state. Subsequent restimulation of such cells in the presence of IL-4 or TGFβ results in the generation of Th2- or Th1-like cytokine secretion patterns, respectively.[11] T cell subsets were originally described for Th cells that bear the cell surface marker CD4. These cells recognize and respond to antigenic peptides that have been processed for presentation by class II molecules of the major histocompatibility complex (MHC). Cytokine secretion is not confined to CD4$^+$ T cells, however, and it has been shown that analogous, but not identical, CD8-bearing cytotoxic T cells that recognize peptides presented by class I MHC molecules[12] are also susceptible to polarization, as are the minor T cell subsets bearing the γδ rather than the αβ type of the CD8 receptor.[13] Although such polarized populations of Th1- and Th2-type cells were originally difficult to observe in human systems, it is now clear that they can be isolated from peripheral blood during chronic infectious diseases and allergy.[14,15] Human Th1 and Th2 cells show functional properties comparable to murine Th1 and Th2 cells,[7] although in humans the expression of some cytokines (e.g., IL-2, IL-6, IL-10, IL-13) is not as tightly restricted to a single subset as it is in mouse T cells. Several other proteins are secreted both by Th1 and Th2 cells, including IL-3, TNFα, granulocyte/macrophage colony-stimulating factor (GM-CSF), and members of the chemokine families. Human Th1-like and Th2-like cells also differ in their cytolytic potential, mode of help for B cell antibody synthesis, and ability to activate monocytic cells.[4,7]

Mechanism of Th1 and Th2 Cell Development

Given the different consequences of immune responses dominated by Th1 or Th2 subsets, knowledge of the mechanisms determining the development of these cells becomes central to understanding immune regulation. In the murine system, the general consensus is that Th1 and Th2 cells arise from common naive precursors, which secrete large amounts of IL-2 but little IL-4 or IFNγ. The most definitive studies highlight a primary role for cytokines themselves in the maturation of naive Th cells into Th1 or Th2 cells.[16,17] IFNγ promotes differentiation of Th1 cells both in vitro and in vivo.[18] Interestingly, IL-12, a powerful inducer of IFNγ that can be derived from antigen-presenting cells (APCs) such as macrophages and dendritic cells, also promotes Th1 differentiation.[17] Additional cofactors such as IL-1α, TNFα, and IL-18 further support the generation of type 1 responses.[19,20] The IL-12 present and the type 1 subsets generated in turn inhibit differentiation toward the type 2 direction by producing IFNγ.[21] In contrast, IL-4 is the most important factor in determining the maturation of naive Th cells into Th2 cells.[22] In humans, only secondary responses to common environmental antigens can be assessed. Nevertheless, experiments by Romagnani[23] supported the view that cytokines produced by "natural immunity" cells such as macrophages and natural killer (NK) cells, play a critical regulatory role in determining the development of Th cells into one or another cytokine profile. Before the Th1-promoting role of IL-12 was discovered, it was reported that the addition of IFNα, TGFβ, IL-12, or IL-1 receptor antagonist (IL-1ra) promoted differentiation of allergen-specific T cells into the Th0/Th1 phenotype instead of the Th2/Th0 phenotype. In contrast, the addition of IL-4 or anti-IL-12 antibody (or both) resulted in differentiation of antigen-specific T cells into Th0/Th2 cells instead of Th1 cells.[24,25] Moreover, Romagnani's group[26] found that IL-12 induces stable priming for IFNγ production during differentiation of human Th cells and transient IFNγ production in established Th2 clones. In summary, these data indicate that IL-12 and even IFNγ, IFNα (which in turn induces IFNγ production by both T cells and NK cells), and TGFβ favor the development of Th1 cells.[27] Potential sources of IL-4 required by human T cells to develop into IL-4-producing Th2 cells are not as clear. None of the traditional APCs makes IL-4, thereby providing no candidates to deliver high concentrations of this cytokine to responding T cells. It has been shown that stored IL-4 can be released by human bone marrow non-T, non-B cells belonging to the mast cell/basophil lineage in response to Fc receptor triggering[28] and by mast cells,[29] basophils,[30] and eosinophils.[31] Because cross-linking of Fc receptors prior to a specific immune response that had produced specific IgG and IgE antibodies is required, it is unlikely that IL-4 production of these cells accounts for the development of the Th2 profile during the primary response.[7] Their production of IL-4 could potentially play a role only late in the immune response.

Another source of IL-4 is a unique minor subset of T cells, the CD4+NK1.1+ cells, which are known to release IL-4 spontaneously.[32] However, it is not yet clear what conditions would preferentially activate them to make IL-4. On the other hand, despite the presence of anti-IL-4 antibodies, human naive CD45RA+ peripheral blood cells themselves are capable of producing small amounts of IL-4 in the absence of any preexisting source of this protein.[33] The inducing effect of IL-4 dominates over other cytokines so that if a necessary threshold is reached differentiation of the Th cell into the Th2 phenotype occurs.[34]

Thus there is increasing evidence suggesting that maturation of naive human T cells toward a Th2 profile is the basic type of a specific effector response, which mainly depends on the levels and kinetics of autocrine IL-4 production at priming.[27] Moreover, Rincon et al. have shown that IL-6 derived from APCs can polarize naive Th cells to effector Th2 cells by inducing the initial production of IL-4 in CD4+ T cells.[35] Prostaglandin E$_2$ (PGE$_2$) has also been suggested to favor the development of Th2 responses by inhibiting both the synthesis of IL-12 by dendritic cells and the production of IFNγ by T cells.[34] On the contrary, it seems that priming naive T cells to secrete IFNγ results from stimulation of "natural immunity" and consequent release of IL-12 and IFNα/β by different pathogens.[27]

CD8+ T cells were previously viewed as being CD4+-dependent IFNγ and TNFα-secreting cytotoxic T cells (Tc), whereas CD4+ T cells were seen as being the major immune regulatory cell. A number of groups have shown that CD8+ effector T cells from rats, mice, and humans are also capable of secreting large amounts of cytokines and can do so in a polarized fashion.[36,37] CD4+ and CD8+ subsets can differentiate under similar conditions; IL-12 and IFNγ encourage CD8+ precursors to develop into Th1-like cells, whereas IL-4 induces generation of the Th2-like phenotype. The Th1-like CD8+ subpopulation was postulated to be a "cytotoxic" type, in contrast to the Th2-like CD8+ subpopulation, which was postulated to be a "suppressor" type.[38,39] Nevertheless, even the Th2-like CD8+ subset has been shown to exert cytolytic activity,[40] and the whole CD8[+] population has been defined as being T cytotoxic (Tc), including the Tc1 (i.e., Th1-like CD8[+]) and Tc2 (i.e., Th2-like CD8[+]) subpopulations.[41] Once committed, neither of the CD8[+] Tc subsets can be converted to the other cytokine secretion profile.[42]

The presence or absence of their characteristic cytokines during cell killing does not appear to affect cytotoxicity, and both Tc1 and Tc2 cells kill mainly by a Ca^{2+}/perforin-dependent mechanism and to a lesser extent via Fas.[41] As mentioned above, the CD8[+] subset currently defined as "suppressor" shows cytolytic activity, independent on its phenotypic (CD28-CD11b[+]) or cytokine (Th2-like) identification, so the classic split between the terms cytotoxic and suppressor seems to be no longer useful in a general sense.[43] Cytokines released by both Th1 cells Th1-like CD8[+] cells suppress the activity of Th2 cells, whereas proteins secreted by both Th2 cells and Th2-like CD8[+] cells can suppress the activity of Th1 cells.[39] de Panfilis[44] proposed that the term "suppressor" CD8[+] T cell be avoided, and they reminded us that suppression is a phenomenon regarding the reciprocal control of four T cell subsets (Th1, Th2, Th1-like CD8[+], Th2-like CD8[+]), which regulate one another secondarily to the differential production of cytokines by subsets of CD4[+] or CD8[+] T cells. Tc2 cells represent a relatively recent discovery, and less is known about how these cells fit into the classic type 1/type 2 network. Because CD8[+] T cells often secrete a Th1-like cytokine pattern, it was difficult to identify Tc2 cells previously. This may have been due to the strong bias of CD8[+] cells toward differentiation into IFNγ producers. Indeed, during initial priming, CD8[+] T cells require a higher dose of IL-4 than do their CD4[+] counterparts to become IL-4-producing cells.[41] Polarized CD8[+] T cells are not just in vitro phenomenon; they have also been isolated in a variety of human and murine disease states. CD8[+] Tc1 cells have been isolated from patients with tuberculoid leprosy,[38] and Tc2-like cells were found in patients with lepromatous leprosy and in those human immunodeficiency virus (HIV) infections with high IgE levels.[45,46] A summary of the α/β T cell subsets are outlined in Table 52.1.

Clinical Effects of Cytokines

In the sequelae of massive traumatic stress, substantial impairment of immunologic reactivity has been demonstrated to correlate clinically with increased susceptibility to serious infection, sepsis, septic shock, and multiple organ dysfunction. As a consequence of an initial infection or trauma, hyperinflammatory activation (SIRS) of the immune system may follow with overshooting release of proinflammatory mediators and an antiinflammatory response characterized by paralysis of immune competence; this state is called the compensatory antiinflammatory response syndrome (CARS). The numerous counterregulatory mechanisms include specific cytokine inhibitors (soluble TNF receptor, IL-1 receptor antagonist), and antiinflammatory cytokines such as IL-4, IL-10, IL-13, and TGFβ. CARS manifests as systemic immune dysfunction and anergy, and it causes increased susceptibility to infections, even by organisms not normally pathogenic in the uncompromised host.

The term systemic inflammatory response syndrome (SIRS) is applied to a generalized inflammatory process, irrespective of cause; it is characterized by the presence of such clinical criteria as abnormal body temperature, tachycardia, tachypnea, and leukocytosis or leukopenia. Although a localized, appropriate inflammatory response is of benefit in combating infection and promoting healing, an excessive response predisposes to sepsis or further tissue damage. The failure of therapeutic trials has revealed a diagnostic dilemma. Knowing that anticytokine strategies yield beneficial effects, we do not know in which predominant state of immune function—hyperinflammation, immunosuppression, or both alternating (mixed antagonistic response syndrome, or MARS)—the patient is at the time of drug administration. Diagnostic tests are needed to establish the state of the patients' immune system by differentiating SIRS from the immunosuppression associated with CARS. Novel methodology for the investigation, which has focused on surface markers and intracellular protein detection by flow cytometry at the single cell level,[48,49] provides a powerful diagnostic tool for determining a shift of functionality in T cell subsets by their individual cytokine profiles.

TABLE 52.1. Summary of α/β T Cell Subsets as Defined by Surface Marker Expression, Cytokine Profiles, and Function.

Surface markers	Th1 CD4	Th2 CD4	Tc1 CD8	Tc2 CD8	Th3 CD4/CD8	Tr1 CD4
Cytokine profile						
IFNγ	+++	−	+++	−	−/−	+
IL-2	+++	−	+++	−	−/−	−
IL-4	−	+++	−	+++	−/+	−
IL-5	−	+++	−	+++	−/−	++
IL-6	−	+++	−	+++	−/−	−
IL-10	−	+++	−	+++	−/+	++−
IL-13	−	+++	−	+++	−/−	−
TGFβ	++	++	++	++	+++/+++	+
Function	DTH, CMI	B cell help	Immunity to viruses	Immune suppression	Suppression through TGFβ	Suppression of Th1 responses

Modified from Thomas and Kemeny,[47] with permission.
IFN, interferon; IL, interleukin; TGF, transforming growth factor; DTH, delayed-type hypersensitivity; CMI, cell-mediates immunity.

We have used this valuable technology to determine the functional potential of $CD4^+$ and $CD8^+$ T cell subsets as mediators of de novo synthesis and to evaluate the participation of these subsets in the immune response at distinct times after major burns.[50,51] Severe injury, hemorrhage, or trauma leads to profound depression of both humoral and cell-mediated immunity. Particularly, thermal injury impairs host defense mechanisms against invading microorganisms; and the immunosuppression that occurs after burn trauma results in increased susceptibility to infection. Employing flow cytometry, we determined that both the $CD4^+$ and $CD8^+$ lymphocyte subsets participated in the IL-4 response. In controls, more $CD4^+$ T cells synthesized and accumulated IL-4 than did $CD8^+$ T cells, whereas the reverse was true for burned patients during their posttraumatic course. When discriminating the study population for survivors versus nonsurvivors (Fig. 52.1), we found that the number of IL-4-producing $CD8^+$ cells significantly unregulated and correlated with the mortality rate. Moreover, intracellular IL-4 was highly correlated with soluble IL-4 assayed by the enzyme-linked immunosorbent assay (ELISA) in the supernatant phase of cultured lymphocytes. As demonstrated in Fig. 52.2 the ionomycin and phorbol myristate acetate (PMA)-induced IL-4 synthesis of peripheral blood cells was dramatically unregulated during the first week following major burn injury.

On the other hand, $CD4^+$ and $CD8^+$ cells of healthy volunteers produced appreciable levels of IFNγ upon treatment with ionomycin and PMA, but the $CD8^+$ subset secreted twice as much IFNγ as the matched $CD4^+$ subset. Similar to what was observed in controls, more $CD8^+$ cells produce IFNγ than $CD4^+$ cells following injury, but only the IFNγ response in the $CD8^+$ subset was correlated with the survival rate. When assessing the percentage of IFNγ-producing $CD8^+$ cells in survivors (Fig. 52.3), up to 70% higher cell numbers were

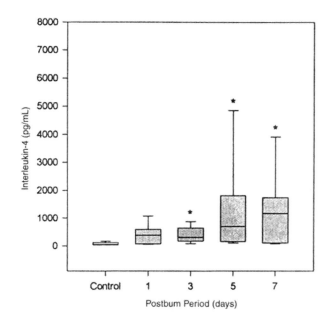

FIGURE 52.2. Changes in the ex vivo capacity of peripheral blood mononuclear cells (PBMCs) to release IL-4 in response to ionomycin and phorbol myristate acetate (PMA) during a 24-hour period after they were harvested on consecutive days after burn injury compared to controls. Patients' PBMCs had excessively enhanced IL-4 production.

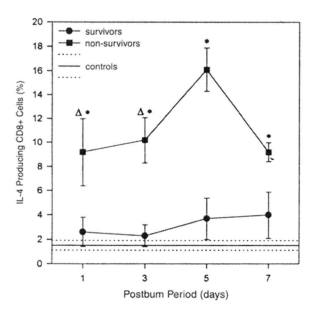

FIGURE 52.1. Differential IL-4 synthesis in $CD8^+$ cells following burns compared to controls. The frequency of $CD8^+$ IL-4-producing cells in nonsurvivors was significantly higher than in controls, although the response of survivors was within the range of the controls (*$p < 0.05$ vs. control; $^\Delta p < 0.05$ vs. survivors).

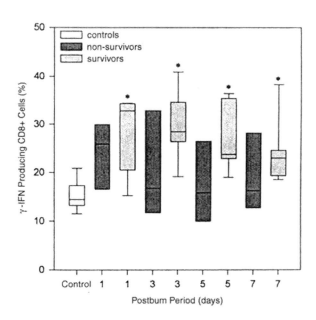

FIGURE 52.3. Differential IFNγ production in $CD8^+$ cells following burns compared with controls. The proportion of $CD8^+$ IFNγ-producing cells in survivors was significantly higher than in controls. There were no significant differences when the patients' groups were compared with one another.

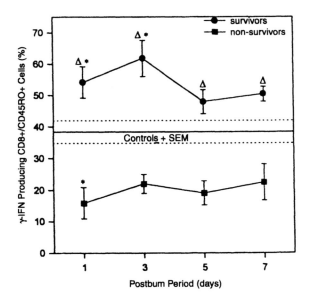

FIGURE 52.4. Differential IFNγ production in the CD8$^+$ memory/effector cell subset (CD8$^+$/CD45RO$^+$) following burn trauma. The nonsurviving group showed a significant decrease of IFNγ synthesis compared to survivors ($^\Delta p < 0.05$ vs. survivors), whereas IFNγ synthesis in survivors was significantly higher than in controls on days 1 and 3 after burn ($^* p < 0.05$ vs. control).

detected compared with those of the controls, whereas IFNγ synthesis in nonsurvivors was within the control range. In both populations (survivors and nonsurvivors) within the putative naive CD8$^+$/CD45RA$^+$ subset significantly enhanced cell numbers capable of producing IFNγ were detected compared to those in controls. In contrast, the memory/effector CD8$^+$/CD45RO$^+$ subset in nonsurvivors showed a significant decrease of IFNγ synthesis compared to that in survivors, whereas IFNγ synthesis in survivors was significantly above the control level on days 1 and 3 after burn (Fig. 52.4).

Laboratory Differentiation of CARS Components

The last decade has predominantly focused on treatment of injured and operated patients with innovative antiinflammatory agents with, retrospectively, no exhaustive knowledge that the patients were truly in an exclusive proinflammatory state.[52] There was hope for the "magic bullet" that would improve the outcome of patients with SIRS. Enrolling all patients who fit these entry criteria does not cause inclusion of only those patients in a proinflammatory state. This led to a heterogeneous population of patients and predictable results. All studies have been negative, harmful, or ambiguous. The purpose of our present study was to try to develop a new set of tests to avoid the aforementioned catastrophe. With these tests we believe we can differentiate the immunosuppression of CARS and possibly save SIRS or septic patients with CARS from inappropriate treatment. In addition, the objective of the diagnostic tests was to identify and enumerate T cell subpopulations in patients with major burn injury based on their IL-4 and IFNγ secretion profiles via multiparameter flow cytometry. This new method provides a highly specific, sensitive assessment of surface antigens and intracellular cytokines simultaneously and has the capacity for rapid analysis of the large number of cells required to make statistically significant determinations.

In our opinion, determination of soluble cytokines in the supernatants of peripheral blood mononuclear cell (PBMC) cultures alone does not represent an adequate or precise method to prove supposed changes in T cell reactivity, as PBMCs do not consist exclusively of T cells. Other mononuclear leukocytes, such as B cells, NK cells, and monocytes, can also potentially be induced to secrete cytokines in response to the same stimuli. Also, the proportions of the various cell types may vary after trauma, especially from patient to patient, depending on the severity of the injury.

To overcome this problem, our approach was designed to correlate IL-4 and IFNγ de novo synthesis profiles of polyclonally activated PBMCs with corresponding extracellular proteins. Previous studies from our laboratory indicated progressive deterioration of the capacity of PBMCs to respond to mitogens after severe burn sepsis and mechanical injury.[53] This led us to speculate that diminished IL-2 and IFNγ production might be due to elevated IL-4 levels. Our data clearly demonstrate that major burns induce a shift of cytokine response to a predominantly immunosuppressive Th2 phenotype. Hence high intracellular IL-4 levels predominantly from the CD8$^+$ lymphocytes and diminished percentages of IFNγ producing cells within the memory/effector (CD8$^+$/CD45RO$^+$) subset correlate with poor clinical outcome. In our opinion, intracellular cytokine detection clearly has the potential to become a new practical standard assay for screening high risk patients. This research should help us define CARS and the immunosuppression associated with it. In addition to this approach, what further defines CARS is a decrease in HLA-DR expression on monocytes.[54] Thus CARS can now be diagnostically defined by anergy,[55] a shift to Th2 cells demonstrating a CD8$^+$ phenotype, increased IL-4, and decreased HLA-DR. This series of findings probably contraindicates antiinflammatory therapy in septic patients.

Conclusions

It must be the principal goal of modern immunotherapy to prevent conversion from a state of systemic inflammatory response in an immunocompromised host to a state of bacterial sepsis and septic shock. Furthermore, it is our understanding that any immunomodulatory intervention should occur at the earliest possible time after tissue destruction, with or without a bacterial component, to prevent life-threatening bacterial infections. The desirable stage-specific pharmacologic aim is therefore to provide prophylaxis against the development of hyperinflammation to protect lymphocytes, macrophages, granulocytes, and the endothelial cell system from hyperactivation and cell exhaustion, that is, to provide therapeutic restoration of immune competence.

Despite all the progress that has been made in understanding globally the mechanisms of host defense dysfunction during trauma, shock, and sepsis, the precondition required for employing immunotherapeutic interventions effectively in surgical patients in the near future depends on our ability to measure the activation state of host defenses accurately, to clearly comprehend the interactions of the various components of the immune system during health and disease, and to identify more rapidly and precisely the pathogens and microbial toxins present.[56]

References

1. Mosmann TR, Coffman RL: Th1 and Th2 cells: different patterns of lymphokine secretion lead to different functional properties. Annu Rev Immunol 1989;7:145–173.
2. Swain SL, Croft M, Dubey C, et al: From naive to memory T cells. Immunol Rev 1996;150:143–167.
3. Sher A, Coffman RL: Regulation of immunity to parasites by T cells and T cell-derived cytokines. Annu Rev Immunol 1992;10:385–409.
4. Romagnani S: Lymphokine production by human T cells in disease states. Annu Rev Immunol 1994;12:227–257.
5. Swain SL, Weinberg AD, English M: CD4+ T cell subsets: lymphokine secretion of memory cells and of effector cells that develop from precursors in vitro. J Immunol 1990;144:1788–1799.
6. Street NE, Schumacher JH, Fong TA, et al: Heterogeneity of mouse helper T cells: evidence from bulk cultures and limiting dilution cloning for precursors of Th1 and Th2 cells. J Immunol 1990;144:1629–1639.
7. Romagnani S: Biology of human TH1 and TH2 cells. J Clin Immunol 1995;15:121–129.
8. De Waal Malefyt R, Abrams JS, Zurawski SM, et al: Differential regulation of IL-13 and IL-4 production by human CD8+ and CD4+ Th0, Th1 and Th2 T cell clones and EBV-transformed B cells. Int Immunol 1995;7:1405–1416.
9. Jung T, Wijdenes J, Neumann C, de Vries JE, Yssel H: Interleukin-13 is produced by activated human CD45RA+ and CD45RO+ T cells: modulation by interleukin-4 and interleukin-12. Eur J Immunol 1996;26:571–577.
10. Chen Y, Kuchroo VK, Inobe J, Hafler DA, Weiner HL: Regulatory T cell clones induced by oral tolerance: suppression of autoimmune encephalomyelitis. Science 1994;265:1237–1240.
11. Sad S, Mosmann TR: Single IL-2-secreting precursor CD4 T cell can develop into either Th1 or Th2 cytokine secretion phenotype. J Immunol 1994;153:3514–3522.
12. Croft M, Carter L, Swain SL, Dutton RW: Generation of polarized antigen-specific CD8 effector populations: reciprocal action of interleukin (IL)-4 and IL-12 in promoting type 2 versus type 1 cytokine profiles. J Exp Med 1994;180:1715–1728.
13. Ferrick DA, Schrenzel MD, Mulvania T, Hsieh B, Ferlin WG, Lepper H: Differential production of interferon-gamma and interleukin-4 in response to Th1- and Th2-stimulating pathogens by gamma delta T cells in vivo. Nature 1995;373:255–257.
14. Romagnani S: Human TH1 and TH2 subsets: doubt no more. Immunol Today 1991;12:256–257.
15. Parronchi P, Macchia D, Piccinni MP, et al: Allergen- and bacteria antigen-specific T-cell clones established from atopic donors show a different profile of cytokine production. Proc Natl Acad Sci USA 1991;88:4538–4542.
16. Swain SL: IL4 dictates T-cell differentiation. Res Immunol 1993;144:616–620.
17. Hsieh CS, Macatonia SE, Tripp CS, Wolf SF, A OG, Murphy KM: Development of TH1 CD4+ T cells through IL-12 produced by Listeria-induced macrophages. Science 1993;260:547–549.
18. Heinzel FP, Sadick MD, Holaday BJ, Coffman RL, Locksley RM: Reciprocal expression of interferon gamma or interleukin 4 during the resolution or progression of murine leishmaniasis: evidence for expansion of distinct helper T cell subsets. J Exp Med 1989;169:59–72.
19. Shibuya K, Robinson D, Zonin F: IL-1alpha and TNFalpha are required for IL-12-induced development of Th1 cells producing high levels of IFN gamma in BALB/c but not C57BL/6 mice. J Immunol 1998;160:1708–1716.
20. Robinson D, Shibuya K, Mui A: IGIF does not drive Th1 development but synergizes with IL-12 for interferon-gamma production and activates IRAK and NFkappaB. Immunity 1997;7:571–581.
21. Seder RA, Gazzinelli R, Sher A, Paul WE: Interleukin-12 acts directly on CD4 T-cells to enhance priming for interferon-gamma production and diminishes interleukin-4 inhibition of such priming. Proc Natl Acad Sci USA 1993;90:10188–10192.
22. Seder RA, Paul WE, Davis MM, Fazekas de St. Groth B: The presence of interleukin 4 during in vitro priming determines the lymphokine-producing potential of CD4+ T cells from T cell receptor transgenic mice. J Exp Med 1992;176:1091–1098.
23. Romagnani S: Induction of TH1 and TH2 responses: a key role for the 'natural' immune response? Immunol Today 1992;13:379–381.
24. Maggi E, Parronchi P, Manetti R, et al: Reciprocal regulatory effects of IFN-gamma and IL-4 on the in vitro development of human Th1 and Th2 clones. J Immunol 1992;148:2142–2147.
25. Manetti R, Parronchi P, Giudizi MG, et al: Natural killer cell stimulatory factor (interleukin 12 [IL-12]) induces T helper type 1 (Th1)-specific immune responses and inhibits the development of IL-4 producing Th cells. J Exp Med 1993;177:1199–1204.
26. Manetti R, Gerosa F, Giudizi MG, et al: Interleukin 12 induces stable priming for interferon gamma (IFN-gamma) production during differentiation of human T helper (Th) cells and transient IFN-gamma production in established Th2 cell clones. J Exp Med 1994;179:1273–1283.
27. Romagnani S, Parronchi P, De MM, et al: An update on human Th1 and Th2 cells. Int Arch Allergy Immunol 1997;113:153–156.
28. Piccinni MP, Macchia D, Parronchi P, et al: Human bone marrow non-B non-T cells produce interleukin 4 in response to crosslinkage of Fc epsilon and Fc gamma receptors. Proc Natl Acad Sci USA 1991;88:8656–8660.
29. Bradding P, Feather IH, Howarth PH, et al: Interleukin 4 is localized to and released by human mast cells. J Exp Med 1992;176:1381–1386.
30. Brunner T, Heusser CH, Dahinden CA: Human peripheral blood basophils primed by interleukin 3 (IL-3) produce IL-4 in response to immunoglobulin E receptor stimulation. J Exp Med 1993;177:605–611.
31. Moqbel R, Ying S, Barkans J, et al: Identification of messenger RNA for IL-4 in human eosinophils with granule localization and release of the translated product. J Immunol 1995;155:4939–4947.
32. Yoshimoto T, Paul WE: CD4pos, NK1.1pos T cells promptly produce interleukin 4 in response to in vivo challenge with anti-CD3. J Exp Med 1994;179:1285–1295.
33. Kalinski P, Hilkens CM, Wierenga EA, et al: Functional maturation of human naive T helper cells in the absence of accessory cells:

34. Romagnani S: The Th1/Th2 paradigm. Immunol Today 1997;18:263–266.
35. Rincon M, Anguita J, Nakamura T, Fikrig E, Flavell RA: Interleukin (IL)-6 directs the differentiation of IL-4-producing CD4$^+$ T cells. J Exp Med 1997;185:461–469.
36. Paliard X, de Waal Malefijt R, Yssel H, et al: Simultaneous production of IL-2, IL-4, and IFN-gamma by activated human CD4$^+$ and CD8$^+$ T cell clones. J Immunol 1988;141:849–855.
37. Horvat B, Loukides JA, Anandan L, Brewer E, Flood PM: Production of interleukin 2 and interleukin 4 by immune CD4-CD8$^+$ and their role in the generation of antigen-specific cytotoxic T cells. Eur J Immunol 1991;21:1863–1871.
38. Salgame P, Abrams JS, Clayberger C, et al: Differing lymphokine profiles of functional subsets of human CD4 and CD8 T cell clones. Science 1991;254:279–282.
39. Kemeny DM, Noble A, Holmes BJ, Diaz-Sanchez D: Immune regulation: a new role for the CD8$^+$ T cell. Immunol Today 1994;15:107–110.
40. Carter LL, Dutton RW: Relative perforin- and Fas-mediated lysis in T1 and T2 CD8 effector populations. J Immunol 1995;155:1028–1031.
41. Mosmann TR, Sad S: The expanding universe of T cell subsets: Th1, Th2 and more. Immunol Today 1996;17:138–146.
42. Sad S, Marcotte R, Mosmann TR: Cytokine-induced differentiation of precursor mouse CD8$^+$ T cells into cytotoxic CD8$^+$ T cells secreting Th1 or Th2 cytokines. Immunity 1995;2:271–279.
43. Seder RA, Le Gros GG: The functional role of CD8$^+$ T helper type 2 cells. J Exp Med 1995;181:5–7.
44. De Panfilis G: Do T 'suppressor' cells exist? Int J Immunopathol Pharmacol 1997;10:107–109.
45. Coyle AJ, Erard F, Bertrand C, Walti S, Pircher H, Le Gros G: Virus-specific CD8$^+$ cells can switch to interleukin 5 production and induce airway eosinophilia. J Exp Med 1995;181:1229–1233.
46. Romagnani S, Maggi E, Del Prete G: An alternative view of the Th1/Th2 switch hypothesis in HIV infection. AIDS Res Hum Retroviruses 1994;10(5):iii–ix.
47. Thomas MJ, Kemeny DM: Novel CD4 and CD8 T-cell subsets. Allergy 1998;53:1122–1132.
48. Jung T, Schauer U, Heusser C, Neumann C, Rieger C: Detection of intracellular cytokines by flow cytometry. J Immunol Methods 1993;159:197–207.
49. Sander B, Andersson J, Andersson U: Assessment of cytokines by immunofluorescence and the paraformaldehyde-saponin procedure. Immunol Rev 1991;119:65–93.
50. Zedler S, Faist E, Ostermeier B, von Donnersmarck GH, Schildberg FW: Postburn constitutional changes in T-cell reactivity occur in CD8$^+$ rather than in CD4$^+$ cells. J Trauma 1997;42:872–880; discussion 880–881.
51. Zedler S, Bone RC, Baue AE, v. Donnersmarck GH, Faist E: T-cell reactivity and its predictive role in immunosuppression after burns. Crit Care Med 1999;27:66–72.
52. Bone RC: Why sepsis trials fail. JAMA 1996;276:565–566.
53. Faist E, Schinkel C, Zimmer S, Kremer JP, Von Donnersmarck GH, Schildberg FW: Inadequate interleukin-2 synthesis and interleukin-2 messenger expression following thermal and mechanical trauma in humans is caused by defective transmembrane signalling. J Trauma 1993;34:846–853; discussion 853–854.
54. Kox WJ, Bone RC, Krausch D, et al: Interferon gamma-1β in the treatment of compensatory anti-inflammatory response syndrome: a new approach: proof of principle. Arch Intern Med 1997;157:389–393.
55. Christou NV: Host-defence mechanisms in surgical patients: a correlative study of the delayed hypersensitivity skin-test response, granulocyte function and sepsis. Can J Surg 1985;28:39–46, 49.
56. Dunn D: Immunomodulation. In: Maekins JL (ed) Surgical Infections. New York, Scientific American, 1994;475–491.

53
Pathophysiologic and Clinical Role of Interferon-γ and Its Release Triggering Cytokines IL-12 and IL-18

Eugen Faist, C. Schinkel, and C. Kim

This chapter reviews the pathophysiologic aspects of interferon-γ, a most potent macrophage activating factor, and its two functionally related mediators—IL-12 and IL-18. In addition, the clinical impact of these cytokines as potentially useful therapeutic molecules will be discussed.

Interferon-γ

Interferon-γ (IFNγ), also called immune or type 2 interferon, is a homodimeric glycoprotein containing approximately 21- to 24-kDa subunits. IFNγ is produced by naive T-helper (Th) cells (Th0) and Th1 CD4$^+$ T cells and by nearly all CD8$^+$ T cells. Transcription is directly initiated as a consequence of antigen activation and is enhanced by interleukin-2 (IL-2), IL-12, and IL-18. IFNγ is also produced by natural killer (NK) cells, which are the principal source of this cytokine in T cell-deficient mice.

As its name implies, IFNγ shares many activities with type 1 interferons (IFNα, IFNβ). Specifically, IFNγ induces an antiviral state, and it acts antiproliferatively. IFNγ binds to a unique cell surface receptor, different from but structurally related to that utilized by type 1 interferons. Importantly, IFNγ has several properties related to immunoregulation that separate it functionally from type 1 interferons.[1,2]

1. IFNγ is a potent activator of mononuclear phagocytes. It directly induces synthesis of enzymes that mediate the respiratory burst, allowing macrophages to kill phagocytic microbes. Along with second signals, such as lipopolysaccharide (LPS) and perhaps tumor necrosis factor (TNF), it allows macrophages to kill tumor cells. Cytokines that cause such functional changes in mononuclear phagocytes have been called macrophage-activating factors (MAFs). IFNγ is the principal MAF and provides the means by which T cells activate macrophages.

2. IFNγ increases class I major histocompatibility complex (MCH-I) molecule expression and causes a wide variety of cell types to express MHC-II molecules. Thus IFNγ amplifies the cognitive phase of the immune response by promoting activation of class II-restricted CD4$^+$ Th cells. In vivo IFNγ can enhance both cellular and humoral immune responses through these actions during the cognitive phase.

3. IFNγ acts directly on T and B lymphocytes to promote their differentiation. IFNγ promotes differentiation of naive CD4$^+$ T cells to the Th1 subset and inhibits the proliferation of Th2 cells. IFNγ is one of the cytokines required for maturation of CD8$^+$ cytotoxic lymphocytes. It was found that IFNγ enhances B cell antigen-presenting activity,[3] promotes switching to the immunoglobulin (Ig) IgG2a and IgG3 subclasses, and inhibits switching to IgG1 and IgE.[4]

4. Additional functional properties of IFNγ include polymorphonuclear neutrophil (PMN) activation via upregulation of their respiratory burst capacity, stimulation of the cytolytic activity of NK cells, and activation of vascular endothelial cells.[5]

Clinical testing of human recombinant IFNγ (hrIFNγ) in cancer patients was initiated in 1984. Jaffe and Sherwin[6] and others[7,8] have carried out a number of clinical trials with hrIFNγ in patients with various hematologic and nonhematologic malignancies, including metastatic renal cell carcinoma and chronic myeloid leukemia. Overall, these trials could demonstrate antitumoricidal activity for hrIFNγ characterized by no unusual or severe toxicities.

From a patient's perspective, acute signs of IFN toxicity include fever, chills, malaise, and arthralgias; the chronic constitutional effects are fatigue, anorexia, weight loss, and depression. The symptoms of acute toxicity primarily occur on the first or second day of administration and are rarely difficult to manage thereafter. The chronic side effects are more troublesome and may become dose-limiting. Myelosuppression and hepatotoxicity represent serious side effects but occur infrequently.[9]

Evidence of enhanced macrophage oxidant production (HLA-DR and Fc receptor expression) following hrIFNγ therapy has led to trials of rIFNγ in infectious diseases in which there is an apparent defect in macrophage function. Clinical trials of the treatment of patients with leprosy, visceral leishmaniasis, and chronic granulomatous disease revealed that IFNγ can contribute to a successful therapy of these chronic diseases.[10–12]

Interest has focused on the use of rIFNγ in patients sustaining acute traumatic injury. The rationale for this application has been based on in vitro investigations. Following severe injury, depressed cell-mediated immune response parameters such as decreased HLA-DR receptor expression, decreased IFNγ release, and increased prostaglandin E_2 (PGE_2) production up to 21 days following injury could be demonstrated.[13] PGE_2 has been shown to inhibit IFNγ induction and to suppress IL-2-producing Th cells.[14]

In an in vitro study we demonstrated that IFNγ represents a potent cofactor for the consistent induction of LPS-driven pro- and antiinflammatory mediator synthesis. We were investigating the in vitro cytokine release in whole blood cultures of 19 patients undergoing open cardiac surgery under extracorporeal circulation. Whole blood was incubated for 12 hours under continuous rotation with LPS (1 μg/ml) with or without hrIFNγ (10 ng/ml). No release-enhancing effect of recombinant IFNγ was found for IL-1β, TNF receptors 55 and R75, or neopterin, whereas inductive capacity for mediator release could be demonstrated for TNFα, IL-12, IL-1 receptor antagonist (IL-1ra), PGE_2, and IL-6. Except for IL-6 we showed a significantly more powerful impact of IFNγ on mediator production in in vivo preactivated cells from traumatized individuals compared to cells taken from a homeostatic environment. A stunning finding from this study was that IFNγ can induce production of its own promoting cytokine IL-12 apparently within a positive feedback mechanism (Fig. 53.1).

Other studies have demonstrated that exogenous IL-12 can restore Th1 cytokine production and resistance to infection under traumatic stress.[15,16] Furthermore, it must be emphasized that IFNγ not only has proinflammatory properties, as proposed in several reports,[17–19] it has more pluripotent immunoregulatory properties, as demonstrated by us with the enhancement of PGE_2 and IL-1ra antiinflammatory mediator release in an ex vivo whole blood model. From that study we concluded that in vitro administration of hrIFNγ results in crucial amplification of many of the important mediators involved during the acute-phase response following major trauma.

The role of IFNγ in terms of its potential clinical significance was investigated in several studies by Polk's group.[20–22] They showed that patients who developed major infections after trauma had significantly lower monocyte HLA-DR expression for up to 4 weeks after injury. In parallel with suppressed monocyte HLA-DR antigen expression, there was profound depression of IFNγ production after mitogen stimulation. Polk et al. demonstrated that IFNγ was able to restore HLA-DR expression on monocytes/macrophages (Mφ) in severely injured patients.[23] Based on these findings, several trials with patients following major mechanical and burn trauma have been conducted to assess the efficacy of IFNγ to reduce infection and death.[24,25] One preliminary trial indicated the IFNγ reverses trauma-induced diminution of macrophage/monocyte expression of MHC-II HLA-DR antigen; however, no difference in the incidence of infection or mortality rates was noted between the treatment arms of this study. Comparable infection rates were seen with or without IFNγ therapy, although the patients treated with IFNγ experienced fewer deaths related to infection. These findings corroborate results from a number of experimental studies that showed that IFNγ administration in animals and patients with surgical infections is associated with improved outcome, decreased translocation following transfusion and thermal injury, and reduced susceptibility to sepsis following hemorrhagic shock.[17,26,27]

Wasserman et al. reported the results of a European phase III multicenter trial on the prevention of severe burn-related infections with hrIFNγ. They found no protection for the

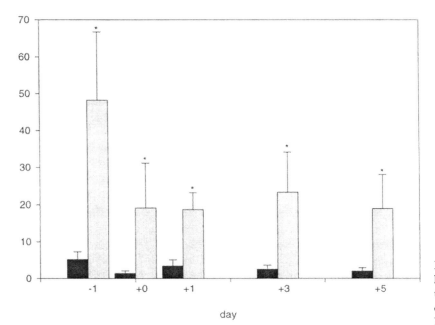

FIGURE 53.1. Perioperative effects of IFNγ (10 ng/ml) on lipopolysaccharide (LPS) (1 μg/ml)-induced IL-12 synthesis in whole blood. IFNγ is shown to induce significantly the release of its own promoter protein. *$p < 0.05$ LPS versus LPS/IFNγ.

IFNγ-treated patients from infections or decreased infection-associated mortality.[28]

Interferon-γ is also known to prime the Mϕ for subsequent inflammatory stimuli, resulting in production of cytokines and cytokine receptors.[29,30] IFNγ stimulates production of TNF and IL-1 in response to endotoxin and other inflammatory stimuli.[31,32] Thus it has been shown that under certain conditions IFNγ mediates the lethality of endotoxin and TNFα via its overwhelming inductive capacity for TNFα release in LPS-activated Mϕ.[19,33] Thus profound attention must be paid to the appropriate timing of rhIFNγ therapy, as its undue administration (e.g., during a state of unrecognized septic inflammation) might result in a deleterious uncontrollable runaway acute-phase reaction.

In a small clinical trial that included nine septic patients, Volk's group reported restoration of HLA-DR expression and ex vivo LPS-induced TNFα secretion in eight of the nine patients.[34] Additional larger clinical trials must prove if hrIFNγ treatment in a carefully selected population group might represent a successful approach to enhancing survival in critically ill patients. Volk et al. suggested that these parameters indicate that infection-induced anergy or immune paralysis can be overcome with IFNγ.

We and others have proposed that IFNγ might exert its most profound effect perhaps in combination with other biologic response modifiers [e.g., granulocyte colony-stimulating factor (G-CSF)], provided that we can identify patients who are optimal responders.[35,36] It is of crucial importance to determine rapidly the immune and inflammatory status of patients with CARS or SIRS and to establish more precisely the quantitative and qualitative amounts needed for their immunomodulatory therapy. Thus far it seems that we have not been able to identify these individuals adequately in the setting of trauma or thermal injury. The precondition for effective titration of hrIFNγ consists in a pragmatic pattern of biochemical parameters for on-line screening of the critically ill compromised host.

In conclusion, IFNγ has important amplifying, but highly differentiated, properties for acute-phase regulation and the immune response in traumatized and infected individuals. Despite the more or less disappointing results of clinical studies of trauma and sepsis using hrIFNγ, we should continue to include this substance in our reflections about therapeutic regimens to overcome perioperative and posttraumatic immune disorders.

Interleukin-12

In 1989 Kobayashi et al. identified a natural killer cell stimulatory factor (NKSF) in cell-free supernatants of a phorbol diester-stimulated Epstein-Barr virus (EBV)-transformed human B lymphoblastoid cell line.[37] NKSF, later named IL-12, induces IFNγ production in peripheral blood lymphocytes (PBLs), enhances the cytotoxicity of NK cells, and stimulates proliferation of PBLs. Another name for IL-12 was cytotoxic lymphocyte maturation factor (CLMF), described in 1990 by Stern et al.;[38] this protein, synergistically with IL-2, activates cytotoxic lymphocytes and lymphokine-activated killer (LAK) cells. Purified NKSF and CLMF were found to be disulfide-linked heterodimeric proteins composed of 35- and 40-kDa subunits (p35 and p40). Gene cloning for these subunits revealed that NKSF and CLMF were identical.[39,40] Whereas the heavy chain p40 shows homology with the extracellular domain of soluble IL-6R, p35 shares sequence homology with IL-6 and G-CSF. Therefore it has been postulated that the IL-12 heterodimer might be analogous to a secreted cytokine–soluble receptor complex.[37] Only the p70 heterodimer is biologically active, even though all IL-12 releasing cells synthesize 10- to 100-fold higher amounts of free p40 chains.[41] IL-12 is secreted from a variety of antigen-presenting cells, including Mϕ, B cells, dendritic cells, neutrophils, Langerhans cells, and keratinocytes, although Mϕ appear to be the major source of the protein. IL-12 release is stimulated by bacteria, bacterial products, and intracellular parasites.[42] Granulocyte/monocyte colony-stimulating factor (GM-CSF) and IFNγ enhance release of IL-12,[43] whereas IL-10 is a major inhibitor of IL-12 production.[44] Among the most important biologic activities of IL-12 are the induction of cytokine production, proliferation, and cytotoxicity in T and NK cells. Within 3–4 hours after contact with bacteria or bacterial products, such as endotoxin, phagocytes synthesize IL-12, which then immediately induces rapid release of IFNγ by NK cells and later by T cells. IL-12 induces the production of IFNγ and other cytokines (i.e., GM-CSF). It influences phagocytic cells by induction of the "oxidative burst" and nitric oxide (NO) release. Thus IL-12 acts as a proinflammatory cytokine during infection. A positive feedback mechanism has been observed for IL-12 and IFNγ which is being controlled by negative regulators such as IL-10, IL-4, IL-13, and transforming growth factor-β (TGFβ).[45] The release of IL-12 with consecutive synthesis of cytokines, especially IFNγ, during the early phase of infection determines the development of the immune response and the differentiation of T cells. IL-12 acts as major inducer of Th1 responses and inhibits IL-4-producing T cells.[46,47]

The existence of Th subtypes that differ in their cytokine secretion patterns and effector functions was originally described by Mosmann et al. in 1986.[48] Because important immunoregulatory cytokines are also produced by non-T cells, including Mϕ, NK cells, and B cells, the different Th responses and cytokine profiles have been redefined as "type 1" and "type 2."[49] A type 1 response is a strong cellular immune response with normal or increased levels of IL-2, IL-12, and IFNγ; and a type 2 response is a reduced or undetectable cellular response accompanied by an increase in IL-4, IL-5, IL-6, IL-10, and IL-13 as well as by enhanced B cell activity. Several studies have shown that the balance or imbalance between the two subtypes determines the susceptibility to infectious disease, its expression, and its prognosis. Polarization toward the type 2 response to represent one of the crucial contributing factors to posttraumatic impairment of immunologic reactivity has been suggested with its consecutive clinical correlate of increased susceptibility to infection.[50,51]

In an immunomechanistic study with patients who had sustained severe burn trauma or major multiple injuries, we found evidence that early after trauma a constitutional change occurred on the type 1 and type 2 axes.[52] Peripheral blood mononuclear cells (PBMCs) of patients and healthy volunteers were isolated on consecutive days after injury and Mϕ-depleted cells were incubated with phytohemagglutinin (PHA) mitogen with or without addition of phorbol ester (PMA). Furthermore, the impact of IL-12 as the pivotal type 1 response inducing cytokine on mediator protein release of PHA- or PHA/PMA-stimulated cells was investigated. The results are depicted in Fig. 53.2. The release patterns of the type 2 cytokines IL-4, IL-10, and IL-13 and of IFNγ and IL-2 showed similar profiles in PHA/PMA cultures, with peak values on days 1 and 3. Thereafter a continuous decrease in protein synthesis became apparent, reaching normal levels within the end of the observation period. Supernatants of solely mitogen-stimulated cell cultures contained significantly lower concentrations of IFNγ and higher amounts of IL-4 and IL-13 than the controls. Analysis of cytokine mRNA expression revealed a close correlation between mRNA expression signal intensity and the quantity of proteins released, indicating that the major regulatory site is located on the pretranscriptional/transcriptional level. These findings corroborated the results of earlier studies, indicating that severe injury causes an imbalance of cytokine responses within the two subtypes toward the type 2 side. Although the CARS theory indicates that the counterregulatory response occurs in a delayed fashion after initial posttraumatic hyperinflammation,[53] we clearly observed peak levels especially of type 2 cytokine release immediately after injury. Therefore we hypothesized that antiinflammatory cellular reactions do not appear secondarily in a compensatory manner but, rather, parallel to the initial inflammatory reaction in a more complementary fashion.

Addition of rhIL-12 led to a marked increase in IFNγ release in patients' cell culture supernatants, whereas the production of IL-2, IL-4, and IL-13 remained unaffected. Exogenously administered to PBMC cultures, rhIL-12 induced a strong increase in IFNγ synthesis, a fact that has been known to be one of the essential characteristics of IL-12.[54] We observed that the impact of IL-12 on IFNγ release is much more pronounced in patients' cell cultures than in control cultures. The responsiveness of patients' cells to IL-12 was significantly increased compared to that of cells obtained from a homeostatic environment; this may be due to synergism with other cytokines secreted under stress or an increase of receptor expression. A synergistic effect of IL-12 with IL-2[37] and TNFα[55] has been reported. IL-12 mediates the provision of high amounts of IFNγ during infectious or inflammatory diseases.

Interestingly, with the addition of IL-12 to the culture medium, the release of the antiinflammatory mediator IL-10 was significantly elevated in cells from healthy and traumatized individuals compared to those in control cultures. As described earlier, IL-10 inhibits some of the activities of IL-12;[44] therefore induction of IL-10 synthesis by IL-12 might represent an autoregulatory mechanism. Morris et al. showed in 1994 that injection of IL-12 in mice led to a 46-fold increase in IL-10 mRNA expression in splenocytes and to an increase of the number of IL-10 releasing splenocytes.[56] Goebel and colleagues demonstrated that IL-12 treatment of burned mice results in elevated levels of IFNγ and TNFα, but at the same time it does not decrease elevated IL-10 levels. A balance between pro- and antiinflammatory mediators seems to be maintained during infection and stress via IL-10.[57]

Murine studies of O'Sullivan et al. also demonstrated that application of exogenous IL-12 can restore Th1 cytokine production under conditions of traumatic stress.[50] A clinical multicenter trial might further elucidate the role of IL-12. Undoubtedly, IL-12 is a forceful regulatory weapon for counterregulation of trauma-induced paralytic immune aberrations.

Interleukin-18

Initially described in 1989 as IFNγ-inducing factor (IGIF), IL-18 is a novel proinflammatory cytokine that has various biologic properties. Nakamura and colleagues observed endotoxin-mediated serum activity inducing IFNγ release from mouse spleen cells.[58] The serum activity did not directly induce IFNγ but, rather, acted as a co-stimulant together with IL-2 or mitogens. Addition of neutralizing antibodies to IL-1, IL-4, IL-5, IL-6, or TNF proved that it was a distinct factor. Six years later the same scientists demonstrated the presence of this endotoxin-induced co-stimulant for IFNγ in mouse livers that had been preconditioned with *Propionibacterium acnes*.[59] In this model, excessive proliferation of Kupffer cells is induced in the presence of the bacteria, and a low dose of LPS becomes lethal in preconditioned animals. Neutralizing antibodies to IGIF were shown to prevent the fulminant hepatitis completely.

The IGIF is a nonglycosylated protein with a molecular mass of 19 kDa. IGIF/IL-18 is primarily produced by activated Kupffer cells and Mϕ but also by keratinocytes after allergen contact and cells of the adrenal gland and neurohypophysis during cold stress. Because of its remarkable relatedness in the protein folding pattern and the amino acid sequence with IL-1β, IGIF was also named IL-1γ.[60] Yet whether IGIF can be considered a member of the IL-1 family is doubtful.[61] The IL-1 family members IL-1β, IL-1α, and IL-1ra are defined by their binding to the same receptor type, the IL-1 receptor type I (IL-1RI) and the IL-1R type II decoy receptor. IGIF does not fulfill this essential criterion; consequently, the protein was named IL-18 rather than IL-1γ. It is still remarkable that proIL-18, the inactive propeptide, is activated by the IL-1β converting enzyme (ICE, caspase 1) and represents the natural ligand for the IL-1R related protein (IL-1Rrp).[62]

Interleukin-18 has pleiotropic biologic activities. It is notable that IL-18 itself cannot induce IFNγ production from T lymphocytes but depends on a second stimulus (e.g., IL-2, IL-12, mitogens).[63] Nevertheless, it is essential for IFNγ production induced by microbial agents. Fantuzzi et al. demonstrated in 1998 that in vitro LPS and zymosan-induced IFNγ production from murine spleen cells is strongly reduced in the presence of neutralizing antibodies to murine IL-18.[64] Other activities of IL-18, such as induction of TNFα, IL-1β, several chemokines

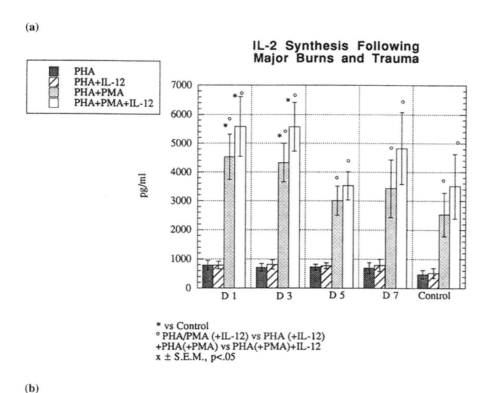

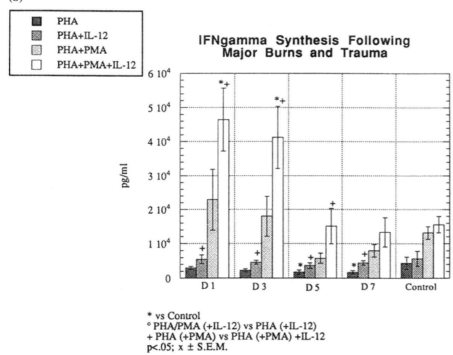

FIGURE 53.2. Posttraumatic (major burns and trauma) IL-2 (a) and IFNγ (b) release in monocyte-depleted peripheral blood mononuclear cell (PBMC) cultures after 20 hours of incubation with PHA, PHA IL-12, PHA/PMA, and PHA/PMA/IL-12. IL-12 is shown to induce significant enhancement of IFNγ in PHA/PMA-stimulated cell cultures on D1–D5. PHA, phytohemagglutin; PMA, phorbol myristate acetate.

(i.e., IL-8), Fas ligand, and nuclear translocation factor κB (NF-κB),[62] rank this cytokine with other proinflammatory cytokines. In addition, IL-18 facilitates the release of GM-CSF by T cells[65] and downregulates IL-10 release.

As a principal inducer of the type 1 response, IL-12 is a strong stimulant for the release of IFNγ from T cells. Hence an obvious question was whether IFNγ release induced by IL-18 is mediated by IL-12. Okamura et al. reported in 1995 that

IL-18 induced larger amounts of IFNγ secreted by murine Th1 cells than did IL-12.[59] The addition of neutralizing murine anti-IL-12 antibody to the culture did not inhibit the IL-18-induced IFNγ release, nor did anti-IL-18 antibody change the IL-12 induced release of this mediator. In conclusion, the two cytokines act independently of one another, although a synergistic effect on IFNγ production does exist. One underlying mechanism for this effect might be the finding that IL-12 induces the IL-18 receptor (IL-18r) on purified naive T cells stimulated with anti-CD3 plus anti-CD28.[65] IL-2, on the other hand, decreases the expression of IL-18r. Whereas IL-18 synergizes with IL-12 in Th1 cell activation, IL-18 has no effect on Th2 cells for their IL-4 production following antigen stimulation. IL-18 does exert one effect not seen with IL-12: It augments IL-2 production following antigen or anti-CD3 treatment of Th1 cells.[67] Robinson and colleagues determined that IL-18 does not induce Th1 differentiation as does IL-12; but they confirmed the synergy of the two cytokines and showed that it could activate the IL-1 receptor associated kinase (IRAK), as well as NFκB.[68]

Elevated levels of circulating IL-18 were found in patients with various leukemias.[69] Using a specific enzyme-linked immunosorbent assay (ELISA) for human mature IL-18, healthy subjects exhibited plasma IL-18 levels between 50 and 150 pg/ml. Conti et al. detected newly synthesized IL-18 mRNA in the adrenal gland of reserpine-treated rats and found that acute cold stress strongly induced IL-18 gene expression.[70] Few investigations have concerned IL-18 plasma levels during infection, sepsis, or shock. In a study scrutinizing the presence of IL-18 in human sepsis, Oberholzer et al. collected blood from 20 patients with severe sepsis [Acute Physiology and Chronic Health Evaluation (APACHE II) 20.9 ± 1.8] on consecutive days after diagnosis and compared the IL-18 levels to those found in patients with multiple injury ($n = 30$) [Injury Severity Score (ISS) 39.5 ± 4.2] and healthy humans ($n = 36$).[71] IL-18 was significantly increased in patients with sepsis throughout the study period (530 ± 664 pg/ml) compared to that in severeley injured patients (181 ± 13 pg/ml) and healthy controls (188 ± 10 pg/ml). Patients who died from septic shock had a significantly enhanced level of circulating IL-18 (787 ± 133 pg/ml) compared to that in survivors (599 ± 38 pg/ml).[71] The role of IL-18 must be clarified by further clinical studies to evaluate the potential of this new mediator as a diagnostic and therapeutic agent under various pathophysiologic conditions.

Conclusions

Despite a wide array of available and promising in vitro data, the clinical/therapeutic role of IFNγ must still be elucidated. There are still no realizable clinical data available for IL-12 up to now. Clinical studies in well defined patient groups are urgently needed for IFNγ-like cytokines (GM-CSF) and for IFNγ-inducing cytokines to understand its potentially valuable role for counteracting the lack of immunologic reactivity in patients under conditions of traumatic and chronic infectious stress.

References

1. Farrar MA, Schreiber RD: The molecular cell biology of interferon-gamma and its receptor. Annu Rev Immunol 1993;11:571–611.
2. Williams JG, Jurkovich GJ, Maier RV: Current research review: interferon-γ: a key immunoregulatory lymphokine. J Surg Res 1993;54:79–93.
3. Hawrylovicz CM, Unanue EJ: Regulation of antigen presentation. I. IFN-gamma induces antigen presenting properties on B cells. J Immunol 1988;141:4083–4088.
4. Snapper CM, Peschel C, Paul WE: IFN-gamma stimulates IgG2a secretion by murine B cells stimulated with bacteria lipopolysaccharide. J Immunol 1988;140:2121–2127.
5. Young HA, Hardy KJ: Role of interferon-γ in immune cell regulation. J Leukocyte Biol 1995;58:373–381.
6. Jaffe HS, Sherwin SA: The early clinical trials of recombinant human interferon-gamma. In: Freedman R, Merigan T, Sreevalson T (eds) Interferons as Cell Growth Inhibitors and Antitumor Factors. New York, Liss, 1986.
7. Quesada JR, Kurzrock R, Sherwin SA, Gutterman JU: Phase II studies of recombinant human interferon gamma in metastatic renal cell carcinoma. J Biol Response Mod 1987;6:20.
8. Kurzrock R, Talpaz M, Knatarjian H, et al: Therapy of chronic myelogenous leukemia with recombinant interferon-gamma. Blood 1987;70:943.
9. Borden EC, Parkinson D: Interferons: effectiveness, toxicities, and costs. Ann Intern Med 1996;125:614–615.
10. Badaro R, Falcoff E, Badaro FS, et al: Treatment of visceral leishmaniasis with pentavalent antimony and interferon-gamma. N Engl J Med 1990;322:16.
11. Nathan CR, Kaplan G, Levis WR, et al: Local and systemic effects of low doses of recombinant interferon-gamma after intradermal injection in patients with lepromatous leprosy. N Engl J Med 1986;315:6.
12. Gallin JI, Malech HL, Weening RS, et al: A controlled trial of interferon gamma to prevent infection in chronic granulomatous disease. N Engl J Med 1991;324:509.
13. Faist E, Mewes A, Straser T, et al: Alteration of monocyte function following major injury. Arch Surg 1988;123:287.
14. Vervliet G, Deckmyn H, Carton H, Billiau A: Influence of prostaglandin E$_2$ and indomethacin on interferon gamma production by peripheral blood leukocytes of multiple sclerosis patients and healthy donors. J Clin Immunol 1985;5:102.
15. Faist E, Wichmann M, Kim C: Immunosuppression and immunomodulation in surgical patients. Curr Opin Crit Care 1997;3:293–298.
16. Heinzel FP, Rerko RM, Ling P, Hakimi J, Schoenhaut D: Interleukin 12 is produced in vivo during endotoxemia and stimulates synthesis of gamma interferon. Infect Immun 1994;62:4244–4249.
17. Ertel W, Morrison MH, Ayala A, Dean RE, Chaudry ICH: Interferon-γ attenuates hemorrhage-induced suppression of macrophage and splenocyte functions and decreases susceptibility to sepsis. Surgery 1992;111:177–187.
18. Doherty GM, Lange JR, Langstein HN, Alexander HR, Buresh CM, Norton JA: Evidence of IFNγ as a mediator of the lethality of

endotoxin and tumor necrosis factor-α. J Immunol 1992;149: 1666–1670.
19. Jurkovich GJ, Mileski WJ, Maier RV, et al: Interferon-gamma increases sensitivity to endotoxin. J Surg Res 1991;51:197–203.
20. Polk HC, Wellhausen SR, Regan MP, et al: A systematic study of host defense processes in badly injured patients. Ann Surg 1986;204:282.
21. Livingston D, Appel S, Wellhausen S, Sonnenfeld G, Polk H: Depressed interferon gamma production and monocyte HLA-DR expression after severe injury. Arch Surg 1988;1234:1309.
22. Hershman MJ, Appel SH, Wellhausen SR, Sonnenfeld G, Polk HC: Interferon-gamma increases HLA-DR expression on monocytes in severely injured patients. J Interferon Res 1987;7:695.
23. Livingston DH, Malangoni MH: Interferon-gamma restores immune competence after hemorrhagic shock. J Surg Res 1988;45:37.
24. Dries DJ, Jurkovich GJ, Maier RV, et al: Effect of interferon-gamma on infection-related death in patients with severe injuries. Arch Surg 1994;129:1031–1041.
25. Mock CN, Dries DJ, Jurkovich GJ, et al: Assessment of two clinical trials: interferon-gamma therapy in injury. Shock 1996;5:235–240.
26. Gennari R, Alexander W, Eaves-Pyles T: IFN-gamma decreases translocation and improves survival following transfusion and thermal injury. J Surg Res 1994;56:530–536.
27. Polk HC, Cheadle WG, Livingston DH, et al: A randomized prospective clinical trial to determine the efficacy of interferon-γ in severely injured patients. Am J Surg 1992;163:91–196.
28. Wasserman D, Ioannovich JD, Hinzmann RD, Deichsel G, Steinmann GG: Interferon-γ in the prevention of severe burn-related infections: a European phase III multicenter trial. Crit Care Med 1998;26:434–439.
29. DeMaeyer-Guinyaad J, DeMayer E: Immunomodulation by interferons: recent developments. Interferon 1985;6:69.
30. Mogensen S, Vrelizer J: The interferon-macrophage alliance. Interferon 1987;8:55.
31. Arenzana-Siesdedos F, Virelizier JL: Interferons as macrophage-activating factors. II. Enhanced secretion of interleukin 1 by lipopolysaccharide-stimulated human monocytes. Eur J Imunol 1983;13:437.
32. Nedwin GE, Svedersky LP, Bringman TS, Palladino MA, Goeddel DV: Effect of interleukin-2, interferon-gamma and mitogens on the production of tumor necrosis factors alpha and beta. J Immunol 1985;4:2492.
33. Silva AT, Cohen J: Role of interferon-gamma in experimental gram-negative sepsis. J Infect Dis 1992;166:331–335.
34. Döcke WD, Randow F, Syrbe U, et al: Monocyte deactivation in septic patients: restoration by IFN-gamma treatment. Nat Med 1997;3:678–681.
35. Baue AE: Multiple organ failure, multiple organ dysfunction syndrome, and systemic inflammatory response syndrome. Arch Surg 1997;132:703–707.
36. Dries DJ: Interferon: therapy for infectious complications of injury: a called third strike [editorial]? Crit Care Med 1998;26:419–420.
37. Kobayashi M, Fitz L, Ryan M, et al: Identification and purification of natural killer cell stimulatory factor (NKSF), a cytokine with multiple biologic effects on human lymphocytes. J Exp Med 1989;70:827–846.
38. Stern A, Podlaski F, Hulmes J: Purification to homogenity and partial characterization of cytotoxic lymphocyte maturation factor from human B lymphoblastoid cells. Proc Natl Acad Sci USA 1990;87:6808–6812.
39. Wolf SF, Temple PA, Kobayashi M, et al: Cloning of cDNA for natural killer cell stimulatory factor, a heterodimeric cytokine with multiple biologic effects on T and natural killer cells. J Immunol 1991;145:3074–3081.
40. Gately M, Wolitzky A, Quinn P: Regulation of human cytolytic lymphocyte responses by interleukin-12. Cell Immunol 1992; 143:127–142.
41. D'Andrea A, Rengaraju M, Valiante N: Production of natural killer cell stimulatory factor (NKSF/IL-12) by peripheral blood mononuclear cells. J Exp Med 1992;176:1387–1398.
42. Trinchieri G, Wysocka M, D'Andrea A, et al: Natural killer cell stimulatory factor (NKSF) or interleukin-12 is a key regulator of immune response and inflammation. Prog Growth Factor Res 1992;4:355–368.
43. Hvjek E, Lischner H, Hyslop T: Cytokine patterns during progression to AIDS in children with perinatal HIV infection. J Immunol 1995;155:4060–4071.
44. D'Andrea A, Aste-Amezaga M, Valiant N: Interleukin-10 inhibits human lymphocyte IFNγ production by suppressing natural killer cell stimulatory factor/interleukin-12 synthesis in accessory cells. J Exp Med 1993;178:1041–1048.
45. D'Andrea A, Ma X, Aste-Amezaga M: Stimulatory and inhibitory effects of IL-4 and IL-13 on production of cytokines by peripheral blood mononuclear cells: priming for IL-12 and TNF-α production. J Exp Med 1995;181:537–546.
46. Trinchieri G: Interleukin-12 and its role in the generation of TH1 cells. Immunol Today 1993;14:335–338.
47. Scott P: IL-12: initiation cytokine for cell-mediated immunity. Science 1993;260:496–497.
48. Mosmann T, Cherwinski H, Bond M: Two types of murine helper T-cell clone. J Immunol 1986;136:2348–2357.
49. Clerici M, Shearer GM: The Th1-Th2 hypothesis of HIV infection: new insights. Immunol Today 1994;15:575–581.
50. O'Sullivan ST, Lederer JA, Horgan AF, et al: Major injury leads to predominance of the T helper 2 lymphocyte phenotype and diminished interleukin-12 production associated with decreased resistance to infection. Ann Surg 1995;222:482–492.
51. Zedler S, Faist E, Ostermeier B, von Donnersmarck GH, Schildberg FW: Postburn constitutional changes in T-cell reactivity occur in $CD8^+$ rather than in $CD4^+$ cells. J Trauma 1997;42: 872–880; discussion 880–881.
52. Kim C, Kremer JP, von Donnersmarck GH, et al: The profile of T helper 1/TH2 responses post-major trauma. Surg Forum 1997;48:92–95.
53. Bone R: Sir Isaac Newton, sepsis, SIRS, and CARS. Crit Care Med 1996;24:1125–1128.
54. Chan S, Perussia B, Gupta J: Induction of IFNγ production by NK cell stimulatory factor (NKSF): characterization of the responder cells and synergy with other inducers. J Exp Med 1991;173: 869–879.
55. Tripp C, Wolf S, Unanue E: Interleukin-12 and tumor necrosis factor α are costimulators of interferon γ production by natural killer cells in severe combined immunodeficiency mice with listeriosis, and interleukin-10 is a physiologic antagonist. Proc Natl Acad Sci USA 1993;90:3725–3729.
56. Morris SC, Madden KB, Adamovicz JJ, et al: Effects of IL-12 on in vivo cytokine gene expression and Iγ isotope selection. J Immunol 1994;152(13):1047–1056.
57. Goebel A, Kavanagh E, Saporoschetz J, et al: Interleukin-10 production is preserved by interleukin-12 therapy that restores resistance to infection after injury. In: Proceedings for the 53rd

Annual Sessions of the 1998 Clinical Congress, October 25–30, Orlando, vol 49, 1998;82–84.
58. Nakamura K, Okamura H, Wada M, Nagata K, Tamura T: Endotoxin-induced serum factor that stimulates gamma interferon production. Infect Immun 1989;57:590–595.
59. Okamura H, Tsutsui H, Komatsu T, et al: Cloning of a new cytokine that induces interferon-γ. Nature 1995;373:88–91.
60. Bazan JF, Timans JC, Kaselein RA: A newly defined interleukin-1? Nature 1996;379:591.
61. Dinarello CA, Novick D, Puren AJ, et al: Overview of interleukin-18: more than an interferon-γ inducing factor. J Leukocyte Biol 1998;63(6):658–664..
62. Torigoe K, Ushio S, Okura T, et al: Purification and characterization of the human interleukin-18 receptor. J Biol Chem 1997;272:25737–25742.
63. Kohno K, Kataoka J, Ohtuski T, et al: IFNγ-inducing factor (IGIF) is a co-stimulatory factor on the activation of Th1 but not Th2 cells and exerts its effect independently of IL-12. J Immunol 1997;158:1541–1550.
64. Fantuzzi G, Puren AJ, Harding MU, Livingston DJ, Dinarello CA: Interleukin-18 regulation of interferon gamma production and cell proliferation as shown in interleukin-1beta-converting enzyme (caspase-1)-deficient mice. Blood 1998;15:2118-2125.
65. Udagawa N, Horwood NJ, Elliot J, et al: Interleukin-18 is produced by osteoblasts and acts via granulocyte macrophage colony-stimulating factor and not via interferon-γ to inhibit osteoclast formation. J Exp Med 1997;185:1005–1012.
66. Ahn HJ, Maruo S, Tomura M, et al: A mechanism underlying synergy between IL-12 and IFN-gamma-inducing factor in enhanced production of IFN-gamma. J Immunol 1997;159:2125–2131.
67. Murphy KM: T lymphocyte differentiation in the periphery. Curr Opin Immunol 1998;10:226–232.
68. Robinson D, Shibuya K, Mui A, et al: IGIF does not drive TH1 development but synergizers with IL-12 for interferon gamma production and activates IRAK and NF-kappa B. Immunity 1997;7:571–581.
69. Taniguchi M, Nagaoka K, Kunikata T, et al: Characterization of anti-human interleukin-18 (IL-18)/interferon inducing factor (IGIF) monoclonal antibodies and their application in the measurement of human IL-18 ELISA. J Immunol Methods 1997;206:107–113.
70. Conti B, Jahng JW, Tinti C, Son JH, Joh TH: Induction of interferon-γ inducing factor in the adrenal cortex. J Biol Chem 1997;272:2035–2037.
71. Oberholzer A, Steckholzer K, Haneki O, et al: Increased circulating levels of interleukin-18 during severe sepsis in humans. In: Proceedings for the 53rd Annual Sessions of the 1998 Clinical Congress, October 25–30, Orlando, vol 49, 1998;88–90.

54
Interleukin-11: Potential Therapeutic Activity in Systemic Inflammatory States

Steven M. Opal and James C. Keith, Jr.

Interleukin-11 (IL-11) is a multifunctional, immunoregulatory cytokine with several unique attributes that has therapeutic potential in a number of systemic inflammatory states. Like many other pleiotropic cytokines, IL-11 has myriad biologic activities that could be beneficial in the treatment of selected patient populations. IL-11 functions as a growth factor, cytoprotective molecule, antiinflammatory cytokine, regulator of enzymatic activity, and cell maturation factor depending on the target tissue.[1,2] It has also received regulatory approval as a platelet restorative agent following cytoreductive chemotherapy.[3] The numerous physiologic activities of IL-11 offer an opportunity to explore many other potential therapeutic indications for this cytokine in clinical medicine. Systemic inflammatory syndromes such as septic shock, inflammatory bowel disease, inflammatory arthritis, preeclampsia, ischemia/reperfusion injury, chemotherapy- and radiation-induced mucositis, and a variety of other hematologic and immunologic disorders may be amenable to IL-11 therapy.[1,3,4] This chapter focuses on those attributes of IL-11 that make it an attractive candidate for treatment of systemic inflammatory disorders including septic shock.

Molecular Biology of IL-11

The human IL-11 gene, which is located on the long arm of human chromosome 19 (19q, 13.3–13.4), contains five exons and four introns. The 5' noncoding region upstream from the coding sequence contains several potential binding sites for regulatory elements, including an AP-1 site, a CTF/NF-1 site, SP-1, EF/C phorbol ester-inducible elements, and an interferon-responsive element IFN/1 in close proximity to the IL-11 gene. The 3' untranslated end of the human IL-11 gene has several AUUUA repetitive sequences that may be involved in the control of mRNA stability and an IL-1-responsive element. There are also *Alu* repeats in the 3' noncoding region of the IL-11 gene.[2,5]

Two polyadenylation sites at the 3' noncoding region of the gene give rise to a prominent 2.5-kb RNA transcript and a minor 1.5 kb RNA transcript. Both transcripts generate to the identical translated IL-11 proteins as the transcripts differ only in the length of the 3' noncoding region based on alternate polyadenylation site usage. The human IL-11 gene codes for a 199-amino-acid protein that contains a 21-amino-acid leader sequence at its amino-terminus. This signal peptide is cleaved during the process of release of the final extracellular cytokine product.[2] The circulating form of IL-11 in humans is a 178-amino-acid protein. The current form of recombinant human IL-11 (rhIL-11) is generated from an *Escherichia coli* system that produces a 177-amino-acid protein. Recombinant human IL-11 is identical to the natural human product except for the absence of a single proline moiety at the amino-terminus of IL-11. This amino acid deletion does not affect the biologic activity of the rIL-11 molecule. IL-11 is produced in low levels constitutively in a variety of tissues. Circulating blood levels of IL-11 have been measured in patients with thrombocytopenia,[3] disseminated intravascular coagulation (DIC),[6] and rheumatoid arthritis;[7] but the cytokine is otherwise not readily measurable in the circulation of patients under resting conditions.[3]

Interleukin-11 has many unusual features in human cytokine biology, and no primary structural homologies with other cytokines have thus far been identified. The cytokine has a 4α helical bundle topology that is similar in tertiary structure to that of several other cytokines [e.g., IL-2, IL-4, and granulocyte colony-stimulating factor (G-CSF)] and human growth hormone. The protein lacks cysteine residues, and so there are no disulfide bridges; there are also no asparagine-linked glycosylation sites. The protein contains an unusually large number of proline and leucine residues as well as basic amino acids resulting in an apparent isoelectric point of approximately 11.7.[3,8] The carboxy-terminal end of the molecule appears to be the principal site of binding to its α receptor and is essential for biologic activity of the cytokine.[9,10] IL-11 synthesis in tissue culture systems demonstrate that IL-1, transforming growth factor-β (TGFβ), retinoic acid, phorbol myristate acetate (PMA), and a variety of respiratory viruses induce IL-11 synthesis.[3] Signals for IL-11 synthesis in vivo are not well understood. The only known stimulus for generation of systemic levels of IL-11 in humans is the presence of severe thrombocytopenia. A reciprocal relation exists between platelet counts and endogenous IL-11 synthesis following myelosuppressive chemotherapy.[11]

Molecular Biology of the IL-11α Receptor

Interleukin-11 belongs to a family of cytokines that utilize the gp130 receptor signal complex on target cells as part of their cellular signal transducing unit. IL-11 first binds to its specific cytokine receptor, known as IL-11 receptor α, prior to its interaction with the gp130 receptor complex. Current evidence indicates that the IL-11 ligand and the α receptor dimerize before interacting with the gp130 signal transducing unit.[12,13] The precise stoichiometry of this reaction remains uncertain at the present time for IL-11. Another gp130 receptor ligand, IL-6, forms a hexamer consisting of a dimer of IL-6 with its IL-6 receptor and a homodimer of the gp130 cellular receptor. Other members of the gp130 receptor ligand family form a hexameric structure with a heterodimeric intracellular signaling complex. Leukemia inhibitory factor (LIF) forms a hexamer with its receptor in a dimeric form complexed with one gp130 protein and a unique LIF receptor β subunit. A heterodimer then forms between the β receptor and the intracellular domain of the gp130 receptor. This hexameric unit results in signal activation for LIF.[13]

It is not clear if IL-11 forms a pentameric structure with two IL-11/IL-11 receptor α subunits in contact with a single gp130 molecule, or a hexameric complex exists with an unidentified β receptor subunit for IL-11.[3,13] The α receptor for IL-11 exists as a membrane-associated protein or as a soluble protein. Both the soluble and membrane-bound forms of the IL-11 α receptor are biologically active, although it appears that the membrane-bound protein has greater physiologic activity.[14,15] The soluble α receptor may substitute for the absence of membrane-bound IL-11 receptor α on cells that have the ubiquitous gp130 receptor on their cell membrane but lack membrane-associated IL-11 receptor α. The soluble α receptor may even function as an IL-11 antagonist under receptor site limiting conditions in which there are limited numbers of gp130 receptors in contact with small numbers of membrane-bound IL-11 α receptors and excess numbers of soluble IL-11 receptors.[15]

The chain of the IL-11 receptor α protein has recently been cloned and characterized.[12] The protein consists of an extracellular domain with two N-glycosylation sites and a transmembrane and intracellular domain. A transcript has been identified that consists of the soluble extracellular domain of the α receptor for IL-11. The gene for the IL-11 α receptor has been localized to the short arm of human chromosome 9 at position 9p13. The gene consists of a large sequence of DNA of approximately 10 kb and contains 13 distinct exons. The resulting translated protein has 24% amino acid sequence homology with the IL-6 receptor α chain and 22% sequence homology with the ciliary neutrophic factor (CNTF) receptor α chain.[12]

The IL-11 α receptor shares structural similarities with the hematopoietin receptor family, including proline residues spaced at 100 amino acids between subdomains and a region with a four-cysteine residue and a single tryptophan residue motif. The IL-11 receptor alone binds with low affinity to IL-11 [dissociation constant (Kd)] of approximately 20 nmol/ml] and is insufficient to transduce a physiologic signal in target tissues. The generation of high-affinity receptor for IL-11 biologic activity requires co-expression of the IL-11 α receptor along with gp130. In this multicomponent complex, the Kd is approximately 0.5 nmol/ml.[12,13] The murine IL-11 receptor has two distinct gene loci, but only a single gene locus has been identified for the human IL-11 α receptor.[16]

Using the reverse transcriptase polymerase chain reaction (PCR) for mRNA of the IL-11 α receptor, it has been shown that receptor expression is detectable at a low level in multiple tissues. The gene for IL-11 α receptor is detected at an early stage of embryogenesis in the murine system and is found in the developing brain, bone, and cartilage.[3] It has been shown that IL-11 activity is essential during embryogenesis, as the IL-11 α receptor knockout female mouse is infertile. Infertility is found to be the result of defective generation of decidual cells at a critical phase of embryo implantation into the female uterine lining.[17]

The signaling events that occur following interaction of IL-11 with its α receptor and gp130 are not completely understood at the present time. It is known that IL-11 binding activates synthesis of cytoplasmic tyrosine kinases of the JAK/TYK family and serine-threonine kinases in the MAP kinase family. Phosphorylation of STAT3 is known to occur, resulting in signal transduction and transcription of IL-11-responsive genes.[1-3]

Mechanism of Action of IL-11

Monocyte/Macrophage Cell Lines

Trepicchio and colleagues at the Genetics Institute have demonstrated that one of the principal functions of IL-11 is downregulation of the proinflammatory cytokine response in macrophages.[18] IL-11 reduces the rate of nuclear translocation of NFκB, a principal transcriptional activator for proinflammatory cytokine genes including IL-1, tumor necrosis factor-α (TNFα), and IL-12.[19] NFκB also promotes synthesis of nitric oxide (NO) via activation of inducible nitric oxide synthase (iNOS). IL-11 impedes the nuclear translocation of NFκB through the ability of IL-11 to upregulate synthesis of the cytoplasmic inhibitor IκB. It has been demonstrated that both IκBα and IκBβ genes are activated following exposure to IL-11.[19] It results in the generation of increased levels of IκB in the cytoplasm of mononuclear cells. IκB binds to components of the NFκB complex and inhibits translocation of active forms of NFκB (p50:p65 heterodimers) into the nucleus of mononuclear cells. IκB is phosphorylated and degraded by a series of kinase reactions that follow cellular activation by lipopolysaccharide (LPS), TNF, and a variety of other cell stimuli. The constant degradation of IκB is counterbalanced by the increased synthesis rate of IκB by IL-11. In this fashion, high endogenous levels of cytoplasmic IκB are maintained, thereby limiting NFκB nuclear translocation (Fig. 54.1).

This activity may account for the observation that IL-11 in vitro and in vivo attenuates the synthesis of IL-1, TNF, and the p40 subunit of IL-12 from monocyte/macrophage cell lines after stimulation with LPS and a number of other inflammatory

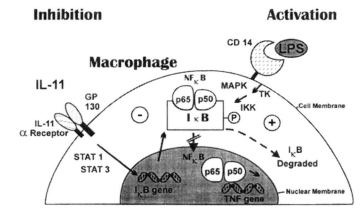

FIGURE 54.1. Pathways of interleukin-11 (IL-11) attenuation of the inflammatory response in monocyte/macrophage cell lines. Activation proceeds following a stimulus with lipopolysaccharide (LPS) through its interaction with CD14 with subsequent activation of macrophages. It goes through a series of kinases including tyrosine kinase (TK), mitogen-activated protein kinases (MAPK), and IκB kinase (IKK). This series of kinases results in phosphorylation of IκB with its subsequent degradation, which allows NFκB to translocate to the nucleus with activation of proinflammatory cytokines. IL-11 interacts with its α receptor and GP130 to activate signal transduction and transcription (STAT1 and STAT3). This interaction results in activation of IκB genes with increased synthesis of IκB, which tends to hold NFκB in the cytoplasm and to attenuate proinflammatory cytokine responses. (Adapted from Trepicchio et al.[19])

stimuli.[18,20] IL-11 mediates these antiinflammatory effects directly and without activation of other antiinflammatory cytokines such as IL-10 and TGFβ. IL-11 has no effect on the cell surface expression of major histocompatibility complex class II (MHC-II) molecules, accessory molecules such as B7.2, or membrane-bound CD14.[18] In this respect, IL-11 is not as suppressive a monocyte modulator as the antiinflammatory cytokine IL-10.[21]

Lymphocytes

Evidence indicates that IL-11 functions in many respects as a T-helper subtype 2 (Th2)-type cytokine and assists in polarization of the CD4 T lymphocyte responses toward a humoral immune response.[22] IL-11 has been shown to diminish IL-2 and interferon-γ (IFNγ) production, whereas IL-4 levels are increased. IL-11 reduces cellular proliferation in mixed lymphocyte cultures but does not affect the generation of cytotoxic T lymphocytes. IL-11 does not induce synthesis of the principal Th2-type cytokine IL-10.[21] Therefore IL-11 mediates its effects on lymphokines directly and not through induction of IL-10 synthesis. The molecular events that regulate lymphocyte activity following exposure to IL-11 is an area of active investigation at the present time.

Effects of IL-11 on Epithelial Cells

Interleukin-11 has a number of salutary effects on epithelial cell physiology that may prove to be of considerable therapeutic value in clinical medicine. IL-11 has been shown to be remarkably cytoprotective to epithelial membranes following a variety of injurious agents, including chemotherapeutic drugs, ionizing radiation, toxins, chemical injury, and oxidant stress.[23-26] It has been shown that the IL-11 α receptor is expressed on the cell surface of epithelial cells, and mRNA for the receptor has been detected in a variety of epithelial cell lines.[3] IL-11 prevents apoptosis and protects clonogenic stem cells from impairment of their reproductive capacity following radiation injury.[27,28] These stem cells within the intestinal crypts have the capacity to repopulate epithelial surfaces following irradiation or chemotherapy and maintain mucosal integrity.[29]

In epithelial cell tissue culture, IL-11 results in cell cycle arrest through prolongation of the G_1–S phase of the cellular growth cycle. This is mediated at least in part through IL-11-induced inhibition of pRb phosphorylation. This phosphorylation reaction is an important initiation event in cell cycling.[30] IL-11 also has a trophic effect on gastrointestinal mucosa; IL-11 administration to rats undergoing massive small bowel resection had faster recovery of small bowel mucosa, weight gain, villous height, and crypt cell mitotic indices than did the control animals.[31] The effects of IL-11 on attenuation of proinflammatory cytokines may also have beneficial effects on gastrointestinal membrane physiology during systemic inflammatory states.[24] TNFα induces necrosis of the gastrointestinal tract and IFNγ has been shown to increase mucosal permeability by altering tight junction integrity of the gastrointestinal mucosa. Reduction of TNFα and IFNγ levels by IL-11 may preserve gastrointestinal membrane integrity in the presence of systemic inflammation.[3,22,32]

Effects of IL-11 in Hematopoietic Cells

Interleukin-11 is best known as a platelet restorative agent following cytoreductive chemotherapy.[1,3] The hematologic effects and other immunologic activities[33-36] of IL-11 are summarized in Table 54.1. IL-11 was first isolated as a hematopoietic growth factor from the bone marrow microenvironment.[2] Recombinant IL-11 stimulates thrombopoiesis and increases platelet counts in normal animals. In myelosuppressed animals or after bone marrow transplantation, rhIL-11 stimulates myelopoiesis, thrombopoiesis, and erythropoiesis.[1-3,37]

The extent to which each differentiated cell line in the hematopoietic system is activated depends on the animal model studied. IL-11 works in concert with other bone marrow growth factors [e.g., IL-3, stem cell factor (SCF), granulocyte/monocyte colony-stimulating factor (GM-CSF)] to induce synthesis of hematopoietic cells.[3] Interestingly, IL-11 α receptor knockout mice exhibit normal hematopoiesis.[14] This finding indicates that IL-11 is not essential for hematopoietic maturation, at least in the murine system. IL-11 works during the early phases of platelet production and stimulates committed stem cell differentiation toward megakaryocytopoiesis.

This important physiologic effect of IL-11 has been utilized to assist bone marrow recovery in patients following cytoreductive chemotherapy. IL-11 is now approved as a platelet restorative agent following chemotherapy-induced myelosuppression.[38]

TABLE 54.1. Effects of IL-11 in Experimental Systems.

Hematopoietic cells
  Stimulates stem cells in combination with IL-3 and stem cell factor[2]
  Stimulates megakaryocytopoiesis and thrombopoiesis combination with IL-3[2]
  Stimulates myelopoiesis in combination with M-CSF, G-CSF, and GM-CSF[3]
  Stimulates erythropoiesis in combination with SCF and erythropoietin[1,2]

Immune cells
  Attenuates TNF, IL-1, and IL-12 production by macrophages[18]
  Supports a Th-2 type response in CD4 cells[22]
  Decreases IFNγ and IL-2 production and increases IL-4 production[22]
  Supports antigen-specific B cell responses with differentiation to plasma cells[2]
  Supports plasmacytoma growth in the murine system but not in the human system[3]

Epithelial cells
  Protects clonogenic stem cells following irradiation[28]
  Increases mitotic index of crypt epithelial cells after irradiation or chemotherapy[24]
  Supports normal villous height following chemotherapy[33]
  Lengthens G_1–S phase growth cycle[30]
  Reduces apoptosis of epithelial cells after irradiation and chemotherapy[27]
  Trophic effect of epithelial tissue following small bowel resection[31]

Other cells and tissues
  Osteoclast activator[3]
  Neuronal growth factor in the hippocampus[1]
  Supports spermatogenesis[3] (recovery after chemotherapy)
  Adipogenesis inhibition[2]
  Support decidua formation after embryo implantation[17]
  Supports the hepatic acute-phase protein response[2]
  Inhibits natriuresis (sodium retention)[3]
  Inhibits nitric oxide synthesis by endothelial cells[20]
  Synthesis of tissue inhibitor of metalloproteinase-1[34,35]
  Stimulates synthesis of heme oxygenase[36]

IL, interleukin; G-, M-, GM-CSF, granulocyte-, macrophage-, granulocyte/macrophage colony-stimulating factors, respectively; TNF, tumor necrosis factor; Th, T-helper lymphocyte; IFNγ, interferon-γ; SCF, stem cell factor.

Physiologic Effects of IL-11 at the Cellular Level

Table 54.1 summarizes the myriad biologic activities observed following administration of IL-11 in a variety of experimental systems. IL-11 is truly a multifunctional cytokine that affects the structure and function of a multitude of cells in the hematopoietic and nonhematopoietic systems. The physiologic effects of IL-11 in vivo may differ depending on the tissue receptor density and tissue sensitivity to IL-11, the cytokine and hormonal status of the target tissue, and the physiologic state of the host.

Preclinical Experience with IL-11 in Models of Localized Inflammation

In addition to extensive preclinical evidence of efficacy as a hematopoietic factor and platelet restorative factor after chemotherapy or radiation-induced myelosuppression, IL-11 has been shown to have beneficial effects in a variety of models of localized or systemic inflammation. IL-11 has been shown to attenuate local inflammatory responses following a number of chemical toxin, microbial, or immune-mediated inflammatory processes. IL-11 diminishes the gastrointestinal inflammation following acetic acid injury to the colonic mucosa in the experimental rat system.[39] It has also been shown to attenuate the histologic damage and inflammatory cell infiltrates following exposure of rat mucosa to Clostridium difficile toxin A.[26] Transgenic rats expressing human HLA-B27 and β_2-microglobulin develop a spontaneous inflammatory colitis similar to Crohn's disease.[24] These inflammatory infiltrates are markedly attenuated following IL-11 treatment. The histopathology and resulting diarrhea in these transgenic animals are significantly improved by administration of recombinant human IL-11.

Interleukin-11 has been studied extensively in a variety of animal models following radiation- or chemotherapy-induced epithelial cell injury. IL-11 has been shown to limit the mucositis associated with chemotherapy,[25] preserve gut function,[21–24] and improve survival in a number of animal models following intestinal injury.[3,22–24] It may also have a role in limiting pulmonary injury following irradiation. IL-11 has been shown to reduce local production of TNFα following radiation-induced injury in mice.[40] This activity of IL-11 may prove to be therapeutically useful in the prevention of radiation pneumonitis and other forms of pulmonary inflammation in clinical medicine.

Interleukin-11 has been shown to have a role in controlling the inflammatory response in joint tissues of patients with rheumatoid arthritis.[7] Joint fluid levels of IL-11 are measurable in many patients with rheumatoid arthritis and are found in concentrations that exceed levels found in the serum of normal subjects. Administration of an anti-IL-11 antibody increases TNF production in synovial membrane cells, indicating that endogenous IL-11 limits TNF production in inflammatory arthritis. The administration of IL-11 along with its soluble receptor was able to reduce the amount of TNF found in synovial membrane cells from rheumatoid arthritis patients.[7]

Preclinical Studies of IL-11 in Systemic Inflammatory States

Considerable experimental evidence exists that supports the potential clinical utility of IL-11 in systemic inflammatory states. IL-11 has been shown to have antiinflammatory properties that attenuate the proinflammatory response of both monocyte- and lymphocyte-derived cytokines. Importantly, IL-11 attenuates the synthesis of TNFα, IL-1, IL-12, and INFγ, but it does not ablate the host's ability to generate these essential inflammatory molecules.[33] Complete inhibition of these host inflammatory cytokines has been shown to be detrimental in some experimental models of systemic bacterial infection.[41]

The remarkable capacity of IL-11 to maintain mucous membrane integrity following a variety of noxious stimuli is a highly desirable attribute. Maintenance of the gastrointestinal and respiratory epithelial barrier limits translocation of endotoxin and intact bacterial pathogens. IL-11 may prove to be of particular value to critically ill patients with systemic inflammatory states. It also supports B cell responses and plasma cell differentiation and immunoglobulin synthesis. IL-11 is a hematopoietic growth factor and stimulates hepatic acute-phase protein synthesis. All of these physiologic effects may benefit the host in the presence of systemic bacterial infection.

Interleukin-11 has been shown to attenuate the hemodynamic sequelae of endotoxin challenge in a rabbit model.[17] It has also been shown to induce survival benefit in mice following staphylococcal superantigen-induced shock.[42] IL-11 is beneficial in a number of models of radiation- and chemotherapy-induced neutropenia and gastrointestinal injury complicated by systemic sepsis.[22,24-26] IL-11 provides a significant survival benefit to neutropenic rats in the presence of bacterial sepsis with *Pseudomonas aeruginosa*.[33] IL-11 is beneficial alone, in combination with antimicrobial agents, or in combination with other hematopoietic growth factors such as G-CSF.[50]

Evidence indicates that IL-11 does not exacerbate systemic infection with *Listeria monocytogenes* in a murine model of bacterial sepsis.[43] These studies report that IL-11 attenuates host inflammatory mediators but does not ablate these responses and puts the host at risk for opportunistic bacterial infections such as *Listeria monocytogenes* sepsis.

Clinical Experience with IL-11

Interleukin-11 was approved for treatment of chemotherapy-induced thrombocytopenia in 1997. The pharmacology and pharmacokinetics have been studied in patients and normal volunteers.[1,3,44,45] rh-IL-11 has been well tolerated in humans at doses up to 50 µg/kg given subcutaneously or intravenously.[38,44,46] IL-11 given subcutaneously has linear pharmacokinetics in the dose range of 10–75 µg/kg. The terminal half-life of IL-11 after subcutaneous administration is up to 8 hours, and drug accumulation after repeated dosing has not been observed. Bioavailability of IL-11 in humans has been reported at 65–85%. Drug metabolism and excretion occurs predominantly through renal filtration and metabolism. Drug clearance is reduced by about 55% in patients requiring hemodialysis.[47]

The most common adverse event is hemodilution, which is most likely caused by renal volume retention.[3,45,47,48] In a normal volunteer study, it was demonstrated that concurrent diuretic therapy could abolish IL-11-induced volume expansion.[45] Clinical adverse events with lesser frequency have included a mild injection site reaction and atrial dysrhythmia.

Current Status of Clinical Trials with rhIL-11

Currently, rhIL-11 is being evaluated in clinical trials for a variety of indications, including chemotherapy-induced oral and gastrointestinal mucositis, rheumatoid arthritis, and psoriasis. Trials are also continuing in Crohn's disease.[45] In addition to these current clinical trials, IL-11 may prove useful for management of ischemia/reperfusion injury of the gastrointestinal tract, prevention of bacterial sepsis in the neutropenic patient, and septic shock. The results of the current series of clinical trials will determine the future directions of IL-11 as a therapeutic agent in a wide variety of systemic inflammatory states.

References

1. Leng SX, Elias JA: Interleukin-11. Int J Biochem Cell Biol 1997;29:1059–1062.
2. Du XX, Williams DA: Interleukin-11: a multifunctional growth factor derived from the hematopoietic micro-environment. Blood 1994;83:2023–2030.
3. Dorner AJ, Goldman SJ, Keith JC Jr: Interleukin-11: biological activity and clinical studies. Biodrugs 1997;8:418–429.
4. Sach GP, Studena K, Sargent K, et al: Normal pregnancy and preeclampsia both produce inflammatory changes in peripheral blood leukocytes akin to those of sepsis. Am J Obstet Gynecol 1998;179:80–86.
5. Paul S, Bennett F, Calvetti J, et al: Molecular cloning of a cDNA encoding interleukin-11, a stromal cell-derived lymphopoietic and hematopoietic cytokine. Proc Natl Acad Sci USA 1990;84:7512–7516.
6. Endo S, Inada K, Arakawa N, et al: Interleukin-11 levels in patients with disseminated intravascular coagulation. Res Commun Mol Pathol Pharmacol 1996;91:253–256.
7. Hermann JA, Hall MA, Maini RN, et al: Important immunoregulatory role of interleukin-11 in the inflammatory process in rheumatoid arthritis. Arthritis Rheum 1998;41:1388–1397.
8. McKinley D, Wu Q, Yang-Fang T, et al: Genomic sequence and chromosomal location of human interleukin-11 gene (IL-11). Genomics 1992;13:814–819.
9. Czupryn M, Bennett F, Dube J, et al: Alanine-scanning mutogenesis of human interleukin-11: identification of regions important for biologic activity. Ann NY Acad Sci 1995;762:152–164.
10. Miyadai K, Ohsumi J, Yoshimura C, et al: Importance of the carboxy-terminus of human interleukin-11 in conserving its biological activity. Biosci Biotechnol Biochem 1996;60:541–542.
11. Chang M, Suen Y, Meng G, et al: Differential mechanisms in the regulation of endogenous levels of thrombopoietin and interleukin-11 during thrombocytopenia: insight into the regulation of platelet production. Blood 1996;88:3354–3362.
12. Van Leuven F, Stas L, Hilliker C, et al: Molecular cloning and characterization of the human interleukin-11 receptor α-chain gene, IL-11ra, located on chromosome 9p13. Genomics 1996;31:65–70.
13. Neddermann P, Graziani R, Ciliberto G, et al: Functional expression of soluble interleukin-11 (IL-11) receptor alpha and stoichiometry of in vitro IL-11 receptor complexes with gp130. J Biol Chem 1996;271:30986–30991.
14. Nandurkar HH, Robb L, Tarlinton D, et al: Adult mice with targeted mutation of the interleukin-11 receptor (IL-11RA) display normal hematopoiesis. Blood 1997;90:2148–2159.
15. Curtis DJ, Hilton DJ, Roberts B, et al: Recombinant soluble interleukin-11 (IL-11) receptor-α-chain can act as an IL-11 antagonist. Blood 1997;90:4403–4412.
16. Bilinski P, Hall MA, Neuaus H, et al: Two differentially expressed interleukin-11 receptor genes in the mouse genome. Biochem J 1996;320:359–363.
17. Robb L, Li R, Nandurkar HH, et al: Infertility in female mice lacking the receptor for interleukin-11 is due to defective uterine response to implantation. Nat Med 1998;4:303–308.

18. Trepicchio WI, Bozza M, Pedneault G, et al: Recombinant human IL-11 attenuates the inflammatory response through down-regulation of pro-inflammatory cytokine release and nitric oxide production. J Immunol 1996;157:3627–3634.
19. Trepicchio WL, Wang L, Bozza M, et al: Interleukin-11 regulates macrophage effector function through the inhibition of nuclear factor-κB. J Immunol 1997;159:5661–5669.
20. Misra BR, Ferranti TJ, Donelly LH, et al: Recombinant interleukin-11 prevents hypotension in lipopolysaccharide-treated anaesthesized rabbits. J Endo Res 1996;3:297–305.
21. Opal SM, Wherry J, Grint P: Interleukin-10: potential benefits and possible risks in clinical infectious diseases. Clin Infect Dis 1998;27:1497–1507.
22. Hill GR, Cooke KR, Teshima T, et al: Interleukin-11 promotes T cell polarization and prevents acute graft-vs-host disease after allogeneic bone marrow transplantation. J Clin Invest 1998;201:115–123.
23. Du XX, Doerschuk CM, Orazi A, et al: A bone-marrow-stromal-derived growth factor, interleukin-11 stimulates recovery of small intestinal mucosal cells after cytoablative therapy. Blood 1994;83:33–37.
24. Keith JC Jr, Albert L, Sonis ST, et al: IL-11, a pleiotropic cytokine: exciting new effects of IL-11 on gastrointestinal mucosal biology. Stem Cells 1994;12:79–90.
25. Sonis S, Clark J: Prevention and management of oral mucositis induced by antineoplastic therapy. Oncology 1991;5:11–18.
26. Castagliuolo I, Kelly CP, Qui BS, et al: Interleukin-11 inhibits Clostridium difficile toxin A enterotoxicity in rat ileum. Am J Physiol 1997;273:G333–G341.
27. Orazi A, Du XX, Yang Z, et al: Interleukin-11 prevents apoptosis and accelerates recovery of small intestinal mucosa in mice treated with combined chemotherapy and radiation. Lab Invest 1996;75:33–40.
28. Potten CS: Interleukin-11 protects the clonogenic stem cells in murine small intestinal crypts from impairment of their reproductive capacity by radiation. Int J Cancer 1995;62:356–361.
29. Booth C, Potten CS: Effects of interleukin-11 on the growth of intestinal epithelial cells in vitro. Cell Prolif 1995; 29:581–594.
30. Peterson RL, Bozza MM, Dorner AJ: Interleukin-11 induces intestinal epithelial growth arrest through effects on retinoblastoma protein phosphorylation. Am J Pathol 1996;149:895–905.
31. Liu Q, Du XX, Schindel DT, et al: Trophic effects of interleukin-11 in rats with experimental short bowel syndrome. J Pediatr Surg 1996;31:1057–1060.
32. Adams RB, Planchon SM, Roche JK: IFNγ modulation of epithelial barrier function. J Immunol 1993;150:2356–2363.
33. Opal SM, Jhung J, Keith JC Jr, et al: Human recombinant interleukin-11 in the treatment of immunocompromised animals with experimental Pseudomonas aeruginosa sepsis. J Infect Dis 1998;178:1205–1208.
34. Maier R, Genu V, Llotz M: Interleukin-11, an inducible cytokine in human articular chondrocytes and synovial sites stimulates the production of tissue inhibitor metalloproteinases. J Biol Chem 1993;268:21527–21532.
35. Roeb E, Graveve L, Hoffman R, et al: Regulation of tissue inhibitor of metalloproteinases-1 gene expression by cytokines and dexamethasone and reat hepatocyte primary cultures. Hepatology 1993;18:1437–1442.
36. Willis D, Moore AR, Frederick R, et al: Heme oxygenase: a novel target for the modulation of the inflammatory response. Nat Med 1996;2:87–90.
37. Du XX, Neben T, Goldman S, et al: Effects of recombinant human interleukin-11 on hematopoietic reconstitution in transplant mice: acceleration of recovery of peripheral blood neutrophils and platelets. Blood 1993;81:27–34.
38. Tepler I, Elias L, Smith JW, et al: A randomized, placebo-controlled trial of recombinant human interleukin-11 in cancer patients with severe thrombocytopenia due to chemotherapy. Blood 1996;87:3607–3614.
39. Albert LM, Ferranti FJ, Erickson JE, et al: Dose response and schedule studies of recombinant human interleukin-11 in acetic acid-induced colonic injury in rats [abstract]. Gastroenterology 1995;109(Suppl 4):A316.
40. Redlich CA, Gao X, Rocxwell S, et al: Interleukin-11 enhances survival and decreases TNF production after radiation-induced thoracic injury. J Immunol 1996;157:1705–1710.
41. Opal SM, Cross AS, Jhung JW, et al: Potential hazards of combination immunotherapy in the treatment of experimental septic shock. J Infect Dis 1996;173:1415–1421.
42. Barton BE, Shortall J, Jackson JV: Interleukins-6 and -11 protect mice from mortality in a staphylococcal enterotoxin-induced toxic shock model. Infect Immun 1996;64:714–718.
43. Opal SM, Keith JC Jr, Palardy JE, et al: Human recombinant interleukin-11 has anti-inflammatory activity but does not exacerbate systemic Listeria infection. ICAAC Abstr 1998;306, abstract G-79.
44. Gordon MS, McCaskill-Stevens WJ, Battiato LA, et al: A phase 1 trial of recombinant human interleukin-11 (neumega rhIL-11 growth factor) in women with breast cancer receiving chemotherapy. Blood 1996;87:3615–3624.
45. Dykstra K, Rogge H, Stone A, et al: Effect of diuretic treatment on rhIL-11 induced salt and water retention. Blood 1996;88 (Suppl 1):346a.
46. Aoyama K, Uchida T, Takanuki F, et al: Pharmacokinetics of recombinant human interleukin-11 (rhIL-11) in healthy male subjects. Br J Clin Pharmacol 1997;43:571–578.
47. Hutabarat R, Dykstra F, Patterson D, et al: Pharmacokinetic study of rhIL-11 in subjects with renal failure and normal volunteers. Pharm Res 1997;14:S-606.
48. Ault K, Mitchell I, Knowles C, et al: Recombinant interleukin-11 (Neumega™ rhIL-11 growth factor) increases platelet volume and decreases sodium excretion in normal human subjects [abstract]. Blood 1994;84(Suppl 10):376A.
49. Bank S, Sninsky C, Robinson M, et al: Safety and activity evaluation of rhIL-11 in subjects with active Crohn's disease [abstract]. Gastroenterology 1997;112(Suppl 1), abstract A883.
50. Opal SM, Jhung J, Keith JC Jr., Goldman SJ, Palardy JE, Parejo N: The additive effects of recombinant human interleukin-11 and granulocyte-colony stimulating factor in experimental gram-negative sepsis. Blood 1999;93:1–7.

55
Minimal Surgical Procedures to Decrease the Stress Response and New Potential Therapeutic Agents

Arthur E. Baue

The frequency and popularity of so-called minimal operations attest to their acceptance by patients, surgeons, and other physicians. Certainly patients have less pain, leave the hospital much sooner, and recover more rapidly. There is also a well documented decrease in the neuroendocrine stress response to injury, which should lead to decreased systemic inflammatory reaction syndrome (SIRS) and less multiple organ dysfunction syndrome (MODS) and multiple organ failure (MOF). The reasons for this response, the effects of minimal procedures, and the results are reviewed.

Minimal Surgical Procedures to Reduce the Stress Response

Hans Christian Jacobaeus, a Swedish physician, suggested that a cystoscope could be placed into the pleural cavity to help with the diagnosis and treatment or lysis of adhesions in patients with pulmonary tuberculosis. He first used this procedure in 1901 and reported it in the German literature in 1910.[1] Some years later he described the cauterization of adhesions for pneumothorax treatment of tuberculosis[2] and the importance of thoracoscopy for surgery of the chest[3]. This method was used commonly until antibiotic therapy became prevalent, after which operative thoracoscopy all but disappeared in North America.

The next development was in the field of obstetrics and gynecology in which laparoscopic sterilization was first performed in 1941 in the United States.[4] The equipment available at that time was primitive by today's standards, using a low-flow, volume-driven insufflator; the range of operative instruments was limited, and there was no videoscopic capability. The possibility of treating an ectopic pregnancy with a laparoscopic technique was described during the late 1970s.[5]

A form of peritoneoscopy was carried out during the 1950s and 1960s in which an instrument similar to a cystoscope was inserted into the peritoneal cavity to have a look at the liver, gallbladder, and other abdominal organs. Biopsy could be done with such instrumentation in exactly the same way as with a urethroscope or a cystoscope. Visualization of the pleural space using an instrument such as a mediastinoscope was also carried out and allowed pleural biopsy.

The development of a charge coupling device, which is a light-sensitive silicon chip, led to the development of miniaturized video cameras. Such a video camera, when attached to a fiberoptic telescope, provided a well defined, magnified image on a television or video monitor. This allowed the operating surgeon to work with an assistant or several assistants to hold the thoracoscope for visualization while several other small incisions were made to perform an operation. This led to a great surge in procedures performed by such techniques, including laparoscopic cholecystectomy, which became extremely popular. This technique was associated with initial complications, as the learning curve was steep. Surgeons performing this procedure today have learned to use it appropriately and so prevent complications, and the results have been excellent. This new technology also led to rapid increases in utilization of laparoscopic techniques in obstetrics and gynecology, particularly with laparoscopy assisted hysterectomy and other adnexal procedures.[6]

This era was followed by a proliferation of thoracoscopic procedures, gynecologic procedures, obstetric procedures, and general surgical procedures in the peritoneal cavity. Laparoscopic techniques were adopted to assist in colon surgery with some positive results. Laparoscopic appendectomy was carried out, as were laparoscopic splenectomy, laparoscopic hernia repair, and other techniques. Today, minimal cardiac surgical procedures are being carried out using direct bypass grafts without cardiopulmonary bypass with the assistance of video-assisted thoracoscopic capability.

Video-Assisted Techniques in the Chest

Video-assisted techniques via the thoracoscopic approach using several small incisions have now been used for lung biopsy, thoracic sympathectomy, lobectomy on occasion, evaluation of penetrating thoracoabdominal trauma, evaluation and resection of indeterminant solitary pulmonary nodules, primary treatment of spontaneous pneumothorax by ligation of blebs, wedge resection of peripheral lung cancers in high risk patients, esophageal myotomy and other esophageal procedures, volume reduction procedures for patients with emphysema, and treatment of chylothorax, among other procedures.[7] Computed tomography (CT)-guided localization of pulmonary nodules with methylene blue injections facilitate thoracoscopic resection.

The safety and versatility of video-thoracoscopy offered a minimally invasive procedure with acceptable risk for patients previously inoperable by standard thoracotomy, which was borne out in subsequent reports. A comparative study of video-assisted thoracic surgery (VATS) and muscle-sparing open thoracotomies by Landreneau et al. showed that VATS reduced postoperative pain, improved early shoulder girdle function, and shortened hospital stay for selected patients who required pulmonary resection of peripheral lung lesions.[8]

Decreased Metabolic Stress Response with Minimum Surgical Procedures

Glaser et al. compared the general stress response to conventional and laparoscopic cholecystectomy and found that with conventional cholecystectomy there were higher epinephrine, glucose, interleukin-1β (IL-1β), and IL-6 levels but there was no difference in ACTH, cortisol, or IL-8 levels.[9] Conventional cholecystectomy also had greater analgesia demands and much higher pain scores, although Ortega et al. found that the adrenal cortical, adrenal medullary, thyroid, pituitary, and glucose homeostatic axes responses were similar or identical in both groups.[10] The abdominal wall lift technique to provide access to the peritoneal cavity, compared with carbon dioxide insufflation, was associated with a greatly decreased neuroendocrine response and better preservation of renal function.[11] Ellstrom et al. found indications of serious tissue trauma during both laparoscopic and abdominal hysterectomy, but the laparoscopy patients had less pain and a shorter hospital stay.[12] Ellstrom et al. also compared abdominal and laparoscopic hysterectomy. Their results suggested no difference in IL-6, cortisol, C-reactive peptide, polymorphonuclear neutrophil (PMN) elastase, and other parameters. It must be noted that for their abdominal approach they used a Pfannenstiel incision, no diathermy, and propofol-fentanyl in contrast to their laparoscopic technique. When diathermy was used extensively and clearly, there was much more tissue injury. Squirrell et al. found that laparoscopic cholecystectomy was associated with less tissue destruction and pain than a small-incision procedure.[13] Elective laparoscopic cholecystectomy was found by Glerup et al. to nearly abolish the postoperative hepatic catabolic stress response.[14] Superior nitrogen balance after a laparoscopy-assisted colectomy was found by Senagore et al.[15] Schauer et al. found significantly less pulmonary impairment after laparoscopic cholecystectomy compared to the conventional operation.[16] Freund et al. found that laparoscopic cholecystectomy significantly reduced 30-day wound infection and 6-month mortality in a comparative study in Israel.[7] Laparoscopy-assisted colon resections were found by Zucker et al. to provide faster return of gastrointestinal (GI) function (earlier time to pass flatus, resumption of oral intake, and first bowel movement), shorter hospital stay, and decreased operation-related infectious complications.[18] Kehlet et al. reviewed the impact of laparoscopic surgery on stress responses and found that laparoscopic surgery reduced the inflammatory response (C-reactive protein, IL-6), reduced the immunomodulatory response, improved pulmonary function with less hypoxemia,[19] and reduced the risk of infectious complications.

The immune response during minimal procedures has been evaluated extensively. Trus et al. found that laparoscopy was associated with less immunosuppression than laparotomy. Cell-mediated immunity was much less impaired.[20] Vallina and Velasco found some attenuation of immune functions after laparoscopic cholecystectomy, which was much less than with an open procedure.[21] Redman et al. found that immune function in patients undergoing laparoscopic cholecystectomy was preserved during the postoperative period.[22] This was the conclusion of Bessler et al. after colon resection.[23] Kloosterman et al. found that laparoscopic cholecystectomy significantly improved parameters reflecting immunocompetence, another argument in support of this procedure. Laparoscopic procedures did not increase the number of white blood cells or the IL-6 level, and phytohemagglutinin stimulation was normal.[24] Iwanaka et al. found that minimally invasive operations optimized macrophage viability and decreased cytotoxic cytokine production, which provides evidence for the physiologic benefits of minimally invasive techniques.[25] Decker et al. found that a shift in type I type II, T-helper cell balance was favorably affected by a laparoscopic technique, which was a much less stressful procedure.[26] Gitzelmann et al. also found that a minimal surgical procedure reduces postoperative impairment of the cell-mediated immune response.[27] The systemic immune response to laparoscopic cholecystectomy was reviewed by Vittimberga et al., who concluded that, "The body's response to laparoscopy is one of lesser immune activation as opposed to immunosuppression in standard operations."[28]

Clinical Results

Even though immune functions are preserved and the stress response is less with a laparoscopic cholecystectomy, does it mean that patients are better off and the results are better, with lower morbidity and mortality? This subject was addressed by Sarli et al., who used a matched case-control approach. They found that the total rate of complications in the open cholecystectomy group was 16% compared with 5% in the laparoscopic group ($p < 0.003$). The complications in the laparoscopic group were also much less of a problem. The complication rate associated with laparoscopic procedures significantly decreases with experience.[29] Thus with confidence one can say that symptomatic cholelithiasis is best treated with decreased morbidity and perhaps mortality using a laparoscopic approach. Laparoscopic cholecystectomy was evaluated in the geriatric population by Behrman et al., who found a 14% incidence of cardiopulmonary complications in those having a laparoscopic procedure in contrast to 43% of those having an open procedure.

In addition, the complications in the laparoscopic group were not serious or significant.[30]

Inguinal hernias can be repaired by laparoscopic techniques, but for such minor procedures laparoscopic repair may not be that much better. Hernia repair with regional anesthesia is also satisfactory and allows the patient to go home later the same day. Two separate prospective randomized trials reported opposite results. Schrenk et al. found no benefit from laparoscopic hernia repair compared with a Shouldice repair,[31] whereas Kozol et al. from the Veterans administration system found significantly less postoperative pain with laparoscopic repair.[32] All patients in these studies had general anesthesia for comparability. It seems clear-cut, not only from general clinical experience but from excellent comparative studies, that laparoscopic procedures are associated with decreased morbidity and perhaps decreased mortality. Their use should decrease the incidence of SIRS, MODS, and MOF.

Perioperative Anesthetic and Drug Therapy to Decrease the Stress Response

Epidural or spinal anesthesia and agents such as fentanyl and morphine may decrease the response to injury by decreasing the cortisol, cyclic adenosine monophospate (cAMP), and glucose responses.[33] Epidural analgesia also prevents sensitization of the spinal cord by pain. This effect may be enough to decrease morbidity.[34] In one study a combination of prednisolone, epidural analgesia, and indomethacin decreased the stress response in patients having colon operations. In that experience there was decreased pain, decreased hyperthemia, better pulmonary function, less pronounced fatigue, less prostaglandin E_2 (PGE_2), IL-6, and C-reactive protein. Thus a combined neural and hormonal blockade inhibited the global stress response to operation.[35] The combined use of thoracic epidural analgesia and blockage of glucagon, and cortisol by somatostatin, and etomidate prevented the hepatic and catabolic effects after cholecystectomy.[36] This finding helps define the mechanisms of injury more than it does therapy. The physiologic response to stress can be attenuated by deep anesthesia with sufentanil and postoperative analgesia with high doses of opioids in high risk neonates undergoing cardiac surgery.[37] Thoracic epidural anesthesia also improved the outcome after breast surgery.[38] There was earlier hospital discharge and decreased nausea and vomiting.

Epidural anesthesia appears to attenuate the hormonal response to stress by blocking afferent pain stimuli that may elicit a subconscious sympathetic response even in a patient under general anesthesia.[39] During resection of esophageal cancers thoracic epidural analgesia was found to decrease the need for ventilatory support and the ventilatory complications, particularly fatal respiratory complications.[40] Fentanyl prevented the cortisol response to abdominal operations but did not affect the patients, hyperglycemic response. On the other hand, an epidural anesthetic produced a smaller effect on cortisol but prevented the hyperglycemic response.[41] Awake epidural anesthesia was associated with improved natural killer (NK) cell cytotoxicity and a decreased stress response.[42] With general endotracheal anesthesia there were decreased NK cells and increased plasma epinephrine and cortisol, whereas with awake epidural anesthesia there was no change in NK cells and much less change in epinephrine and cortisol. Thus cancer patients may have improved killing of embolized tumor cells during operation performed under epidural anesthesia, but this hypothesis has not yet been documented.[42] Morphine in large doses abolishes the initial endocrine and metabolic changes seen during open-heart surgery.[43]

During stressful intensive care unit (ICU) procedures Cohen et al. found that propofol at doses administered in this study significantly reduced the hemodynamic and metabolic stresses caused, for example, by chest physical therapy.[44] Schulze et al. found that a single high dose of a glucocorticoid-prednisolone before colonic surgery seemed to improve postoperative pulmonary function and mobilization and to reduce the plasma cascade activators of the inflammatory response and immunofunction without detrimental effects on wound healing.[45] Chambrier et al. found that ibuprofen, given during the perioperative period, reduced the endocrine response and cytokine release in patients having major surgical operations.[46]

Lamotrigine is a new orally administered antiepileptic drug that has an analgesic effect in some acute and chronic painful conditions. This drug was given to patients having a transurethral prostatectomy with spinal anesthesia, and the observers found that there was a reduction in total analgesic requirement postoperatively.[47]

Ketorolac tromethamine (Toradol) is a new commercially available nonsteroidal antiinflammatory agent that produces minimal tissue irritation so it can be given intramuscularly.[48] It was administered to postoperative patients for analgesia in combination with patient-controlled intravenous narcotic analgesia, and it significantly decreased narcotic requirements.[48]

Normothermia

It is well established that even mild hypothermia during an operative procedure is deleterious. Normothermia should be maintained during major surgery, as it has been found to reduce the incidence of morbid cardiac events,[49] reduce the incidence of surgical wound infections, and shorten hospitalization.[50] Trauma patients should be rewarmed rapidly, which improves survival.[51]

Cardiopulmonary Bypass for Cardiac Operations: An Inflammatory Event

There has been considerable work done on the effects of cardiopulmonary bypass and its initiation of an inflammatory response. Whether the latter is due to blood being exposed to foreign surfaces, to the pumping, or to other abnormalities cannot be fully established, but there is no doubt that it occurs and can be deleterious, particularly in high risk patients. Tumor necrosis factor-α (TNFα) activation and other factors are also involved.

Major efforts to control this inflammatory process have been carried out. Westhuyzen et al. used preoperative supplementation with α-tocopherol and ascorbic acid to try to reduce myocardial injury in patients undergoing cardiac operations. It decreased the depletion of antioxidants in plasma but had no clinical effect.[52] Intravenous triiodothyronine (T_3) has been found by a number of investigators to improve myocardial function and reduce morbidity after coronary artery bypass surgery.[53] Chiba et al. used depletion of leukocytes and platelets to reduce cardiac dysfunction after cardiopulmonary bypass and found it to be effective.[54]

Gott et al. modified the risks of extracorporeal circulation in a trial using four antiinflammatory strategies. They used leukocyte reduction and leukocyte filtration for all blood products in all patients. Aprotinin was given to high risk patients and patients having reoperations for coronary disease. All patients except diabetics received preoperative corticosteroids (methylprednisolone). The authors found that, as they stated, "these pharmacologic and mechanical strategies significantly attenuated the inflammatory responses to extracorporeal circulation."[55] This also improved patient outcome, and the increased cost was offset by the significantly reduced risk. Thus there seems little doubt that reduction of the inflammatory response during cardiac procedures with cardiopulmonary bypass is helpful.

Another way to alter this situation is to carry out myocardial revascularization without cardiopulmonary bypass. This technique has been studied by Brasil et al. who found that patients undergoing revascularization without cardiopulmonary bypass had no evidence of TNFα in their serum, there was less hypotension, they required fewer inotropic agents, and they had a lower heart rate. There was decreased postoperative bleeding, decreased orotracheal intubation time, and less pronounced leukocytosis.[56] Thus elimination of cardiopulmonary bypass decreases the inflammatory response to the operation. Gu et al. also found that patients undergoing minimally invasive coronary artery bypass grafting had a greater reduction in the inflammatory response, postoperative morbidity, and hospital stay compared with patients who had conventional grafting with cardiopulmonary bypass.[57]

Clinical Trials of Other New and Potential Therapeutic Agents

This section covers therapies that are being evaluated in patients but have not yet become established or come into common use. Some are exciting and may in the future become part of our regular or standard therapy, and others may disappear. Some may be controversial in that they are championed by one group of clinical investigators, but their positive results have not been confirmed by others. Many will help some but not all patients and so will not make a significant overall difference. The major reason for this is that they do not provide specific treatment for a disease or an abnormality. They primarily attenuate the inflammatory response or improve one aspect of a complex pathophysiologic state. Perhaps they should be used in combination with other agents in a multiagent therapy (see Chapter 55).

Although some therapies presently being evaluated in experimental animals may eventually be found to be worthwhile clinically, I do not describe them here because (1) there are so many such studies underway; and (2) they are probably a long way from being tested clinically if ever. There is a tendency for some investigators to overstate the importance of their results in animals and to suggest potential clinical relevance based on a study of 20 rats. An example of such "a promissory note"[58] was found in an abstract of a recent publication: "These biologic effects suggest . . . as a promising candidate for the treatment of sepsis in humans."

There are a number of clinical trials underway. Three trial phases are required by the U.S. Food and Drug Administration (FDA) for approval and general use of a drug. After preliminary and often extensive animals trials, a phase I trial is undertaken in which the agent is given to normal humans to determine toxicity. A phase II trial is one in which the agent is given to patients who have the target problem, such as sepsis or septic shock. This trial determines whether the agent harms such patients. A phase III trial is a prospective randomized, placebo-controlled trial with a specific endpoint, such as a 28-day mortality. Many have argued that mortality at 28 days is too rigorous and other endpoints should be used, such as improvement in the patient's condition or a better MODS score. However, as Buckman has said, "What good is it if a patient improves, but in the end dies anyway". Table 55.1 lists agents that have undergone extensive animal experimentation with often exciting results. They are now either being considered for clinical trials or such trials are underway. I do not review them all, but they are agents with which you may be familiar or are involved in studying. I comment on some of the agents for which some clinical results are known but they are not established therapy in general use (Table 55.2).

Various exciting approaches to treatment of extremely ill patients are described in other chapters. I have also reviewed various agents that could be helpful in a multiagent therapy approach and in therapies that seem beneficial in preventing or treating MOF (see Chapter 67). Some of them could have been included in this chapter. I recommend that those who are interested also read Chapter 67.

Lisophylline is a synthetic small-molecule methylxanthine that is presently being studied in a phase III trial in septic patients. It seems to help high risk bone marrow transplant patients in the inflammatory response to high dose IL-2 therapy for malignancies.[59] Whether it is effective by itself in septic patients remains to be seen.

PGG-glucan (betafectin) is a soluble glucose polymer (beta 1-3 polyglucose) that stimulates and enhances specific humoral and cellular responses to challenge by infectious organisms. It has been studied now in phase I and II trials by several investigators. Babineau et al. found that PGG-glucan was generally safe and well tolerated, and they thought it would decrease postoperative infection rates.[60,61] de Felippe et al. treated severe trauma patients with glucan when they entered the ICU without

TABLE 55.1. Proposals for Clinical Trials or Trials that are Underway.

Tetravalent guanyl hydrazone to limit cytokine excess—pending
Tissue factor pathway inhibitor—pending
NO scavengers: pyridoxylated hemoglobin (see Chapter 63)
Iron chealtors: perfusol and DTPA iron III—phase I–II
Pentoxifylline
Lisofylline—phase III
PGG-glucan (beta fectin)—phase III
Reconstituted high density lipoprotein: rHDL (see Chapter 46)
High-affinity endotoxin binding substances (see Chapter 46)
Lipid, A antagonist (E5531): an NCE component LPS binding (see Chapter 46)
$rBPI_{21}$ (Neuprex): binds endotoxin and has antibacterial activity (see Chapter 46)—phase III for meningococcemia
PMX-622: polymyxin B and dextran 70 (see—phase II)
Synthetic antiendotoxin peptides (see Chapter 46)
Interferon-γ (IFNγ) in patients with immunoparalysis (see Chapter 52)
Liposomal prostaglandin E_1 (PGE_1) for ARDS (see Chapter 35)—phase III
Somatostatin for ARDS (see Chapter 35)
Humanized CD11/CD18 monoclonal antibody (mAb)
rhGM-CSF in burn patients (see Chapters 32, 64)
IL-11 (see Chapter 54)
rhG-CSF: Filgastin
IL-10 (see Chapter 53)
Anti-CD14 mAbs
Tyrosine kinase inhibitors
NF-κB inhibition—pending
Trilazed mesylate (Freedox), a membrane stabilizer—phase III
Anti-LFA-1 and anti-I Can-1-mAbs to protect the kidneys
More powerful endotoxin mAbs (see Chapter 46)
PGE_1 to inhibit platelet decrease after massive blood transfusion
Platelet-activating factor receptor antagonists in pancreatitis (see Chapter 21)
Recombinanat activated protein C (rhAPC)—phase III beginning
PHP Hgb: pyridoxylated hemoglobin (see Chapter 64)
Neupogen (G-CSF) (see Chapter 64)
Ceramide pathway inhibitor
Selective cyclooxygenase (COX-2) inhibitors—Melissa and Select trials
Ketoconazole: to prevent ARDS
Proteinase inhibtors: aprotinin or trasylol (evaluated in the past for clinical pancreatitis), nafamostat mesylate, gabexate mesylate, ulinastatin—pending

infection.[62] The authors randomized the trial and found that the incidence of pneumonia was decreased in the treated group, as was overall sepsis. Thus they found a decrease in nosocomial infections. This substance should be subjected to a randomized multiinstitutional phase III trial to determine if it really is that effective prophylactically.

Plasma C1-inhibitor is the major inhibitor of both the classic pathway of the complement system and contact activation.

TABLE 55.2. Agents Evaluated Clinically.

Pentoxifylline
Clonidine
Antioxidants such as N-acetylcysteine
Enalaprilat
β-Glucan
Lisophylline
Tirilazad mesylate
Ketoconazole
Allopurinol

A relative deficiency of C1-INH has been proposed as an important contributor to the development of shock and organ failure. It has been used now in a small number of patients. This therapy resulted in a decrease in daily fluid balance with a tendency toward higher arterial/inspired oxygen ratios. Thus the edema of injuries seemed to be alleviated.[63] More work needs to be done with this substance.

A preoperative α_2-adrenergic receptor agonist, clonidine, prevented deterioration of renal function after cardiac surgery in a randomized control trial by Kulka et al. It was thought that this result might be due to clonidine-induced reduction in the sympathetic nervous system response to cardiac surgery.[64]

N-Acetylcysteine (NAC), an antioxidant, improves oxygen extraction capabilities and cardiac function during sepsis in experimental studies.[65] It has been widely used clinically in the successful treatment of the free-radical-mediated condition of acetaminophen toxicity.[66] This seems to be a highly specific effect and a highly specific condition. In a clinical trial NAC increased gastric intramucosal pH, which in effect was related to improved survival in this study.[67] However, in another clinical trial, treatment with NAC depressed cardiac function.[68] Suter et al. found that intravenous NAC for 72 hours improved oxygenation and reduced the need for ventilatory support but did not reduce the development of ARDS or mortality.[69] Thus whether NAC will be useful clinically in the future and in what circumstances remains to be established.

An angiotensin-converting enzyme inhibitor, enalaprilat, was given to critically ill patients and was found to improve gut perfusion, as measured by gastric tonometry. This effect seems to be independent of changes in systemic perfusion. This agent could be an adjunct in the treatment of injured patients.[70] Anticatabolic and anabolic strategies in critical illness have been reviewed by Chang et al. In the first group of anticatabolic agents are nutrients and nutrient metabolites (i.e., proteins, specific amino acids, glutamine, arginine, and branched-chain amino acids, especially leucine). Anabolic strategies include anabolic hormones (i.e., growth hormone, testosterone, and the testosterone analogue oxandrolone). In certain circumstances, these agents seem to be helpful. The pros and cons are discussed in a review article.[71] The amino acid glutamine also functions as an antioxidant. Patients receiving daily antioxidant infusions that include glutamine seem to have less lipid peroxidation or, in other words, less oxygen radical damage.[72]

Pentoxifylline is a xanthine derivative approved by the FDA in the United States for the treatment of patients who have intermittent claudication due to occlusive vascular disease. According to Hotchkiss and Karl, the clinical efficacy of this agent is thought to result primarily from improved flexibility of erythrocytes and reduced blood viscosity.[73] This agent also has a number of effects on the inflammatory cascade and various other activities. It has been studied in a placebo-controlled clinical study of severe sepsis by Zable et al.[74] Such patients seemed to be somewhat improved, particularly in some aspects of cardiovascular function. However, the authors recommend a multicenter trial before further use. Schröder et al. evaluated the therapeutic effect of pentoxifylline on cardiopulmonary, renal, and hepatic dysfunction in patients with sepsis. In this randomized trial, pulmonary dysfunction was significantly improved during the second week after treatment, but it did not result in improved survival.[75] Staubach et al. found that pentoxifylline beneficially influenced cardiopulmonary dysfunction in patients with sepsis without adverse effects; again, however, mortality was not decreased.[76] Bacher et al. also found that pentoxifylline, given to septic patients, resulted in significant improvement in hemodynamic performance compared to critically ill nonseptic patients.[77] Hoffman et al. found that pentoxifylline decreased the incidence of MOF in patients after major cardio-thoracic surgery, but again there were no differences in mortality.[78] Pentoxyfylline in other patients undergoing coronary artery bypass surgery was found by Kleinschmidt et al. to have no effect whatsoever on mononuclear cell or gene cytokine expression.[79] Thus pentoxifylline is an interesting agent with a number of effects. Studies are needed in injured, operated, septic patients to determine when it will be helpful, where it will be helpful, and in what doses. It certainly has some promise of being an adjunctive measure if the answer to these questions can be determined. Hotchkiss and Karl warn that this agent may increase the frequency of infections.[73]

Ketoconazole is a thromboxane A_2 synthetase inhibitor given to patients within the first 24 hours after a diagnosis of sepsis and arrival in the ICU to determine whether the frequency of ARDS might be affected. It resulted in a significant reduction in the frequency of ARDS compared with the placebo group (64% vs.15%). The mortality was also reduced from 39% in the placebo group to 15% in the test group. The drug was given in the gastrointestinal tract.[80] Thus ARDS may be decreased, and these interesting results need to be confirmed by other studies and other groups.

The finding of opiate receptors and endogeneous opioid peptides (endorphins) suggested their involvement in shock.[81] The opioid antagonist naloxone has been tried in many clinical situations. A meta-analysis of nalaxone as therapy for shock in patients indicated that it improved blood pressure, but the mortality rate was not affected.[82]

Other recent clinical trials are of interest. In a phase III trial of a nonselective nitric oxide synthase (NOS) inhibitor in patients with septic shock, the NOS inhibitor increased mortality.[83] A phase II trial of recombinant human activated protein in septic patients produced a trend toward decreased mortality.[84] Clenbuterol, a β-adrenoreceptor agonist, produced better inspiratory force, muscle strength, and 6-minute walking distance after cardiac surgery in elderly patients.[85] A phase III trial of liposomal PGE_1 in patients with ARDS indicated that the agent was well tolerated but did not decrease mortality and did not increase time off a ventilator.[86] However, when anticytokine therapy was used for a true specific inflammatory disease such as rheumatoid arthritis, it helped.[87] Other drugs, agents, and substances will be brought to clinical trial, but how many, if any, of these agents will come into general use remains to be established. For certain specific problems they may help, such as N-acetylcysteine in acetaminophen poisoning.[66]

References

1. Churchill ED: Surgeons to Soldiers. Philadelphia, Lippincott 1972.
2. Schultz SG: Homeostasis, Humpty-Dumpty and integrative biology. News Physiol Sci 1996;11:238–246.
3. Vogel S: Academically correct biological science. Am Scientist 1998;Nov/Dec:504–506.
4. Power FH, Barnes AC: Sterilization by means of peritoneoscopic fulguration: a preliminary report. Am J Obset Gynecol 1941; 41:1093.
5. Bruhat MA, Manhes H, Mage G, Pouly JL: Treatment of ectopic pregnancy by means of laparoscopy. Fertil Steril 1980;33:411–414.
6. Rock JA, Warshaw JR: The history and future of operative laprascopy. Am J Obset Gynecol 1994;170:7–11.
7. Kaiser LR: Video-assisted thoracic surgery: current state of the art. Ann Surg 1994;220:720–734.
8. Landreneau RJ, Hazelrigg SR, Mack MJ, et al: Differences in postoperative pain, shoulder function and morbidity between video-assisted thoracic surgery and muscle-sparing open thoracotomies. Ann Thorac Surg (in press).
9. Glaser F, Sannwald GA, Buhr HJ, et al: General stress response to convnentional and laparoscopic cholecystecomy. Ann Surg 1995; 221:372–380.
10. Ortega AE, Peters JH, Incarbone R, et al: A prospective randomized comparison of the metabolic and stress hormonal responses of laproscopic and open cholecystectomy. J Am Coll Surg 1996; 183:249–256.
11. Koivulsalo AM, Kellokumpu I, Scheinin M, et al: Randomized comparison of the neuroendocrine response to laproscopic cholecystectomy using either conventional or abdominal wall lift techniques. Br J Surg 1996;83;1532–1536.
12. Ellstrom M, Bengtsson A, Tylman M, et al: Evaluation of tissue trauma after laparoscopic and abdominal hysterectomy: measurements of neutrophil activation and release of interleukin-6, cortisol, and C-reative protein. J Am Coll Surg 1996;182:423–430.
13. Squirrell DM, Majeed AW, Troy G, et al: A randomized, prospective, blinded comparison of postoperative pain, metabolic response, and perceived health after laparoscopic and small incision cholecystectomy. Surgery 1998;123:485–495.
14. Glerup H, Heindroff H, Flyvbjerg A, et al: Elective laparoscopic cholecystectomy nearly abolishes the postoperative hepatic catabolic stress response. Ann Surg 1995;221:214–219.
15. Senagore AJ, Kilbride MJ, Luchtefeld MA, et al: Superior nitrogen balance after laparoscopic-assisted colectomy. Ann Surg 1995; 221:171–175.
16. Schauer PR, Luna L, Schauer PH, et al: Pulmonary function after laproscopic cholecystectomy in high risk patients. Surgery (in press).
17. Freund HR, Simchen E, Zister Y, Durst AL: Laproscopic cholecystectomy significantly reduces 30-day wound infection rate and 6-months' mortality: a prospective study of open vs. laproscopic cholecystectomy. Arch Surg (in press).
18. Zucker KA, Curet MJ, Pitcher DE, et al: Prospective randomized trial comparing laparoscopic assisted versus open colon resection. Ann Surg (in press).
19. Kehlet H, Jorgen Nieslen H: Impact of laparoscopic surgery on stress responses, immunofunction, and risk of infectious complications. Soc Crit Care Med 1998;6:80–88.
20. Trus TL, Laycock WS, Branum GD, Hunter JG: Laparoscopy if associated with less immuno-suppression than laparotomy. Arch Surg (in press).

21. Vallina VL, Velasco JM: The influence of laparoscopy on lymphocyte subpopulations in the surgical patient. Surg Endosc 1996;10:481–484.
22. Redmond HP, Watson RWG, Houghton T, et al: Immune function in patients undergoing open vs. laparoscopic cholecystectomy. Arch Surg 1994;129:1240–1246.
23. Bessler M, Whelan RL, Halverson A, et al: Is immune function better preserved after laparoscopic versus open colon resection? Surg Endosc 1994;8:881–883.
24. Kloosterman T, von Blomberg ME, Borgstein P, et al: Unimpaired immune functions after laparoscopic cholecystectomy. Surgery 1994;115:424–428.
25. Iwanaka T, Arkovitz MS, Arya G, Ziegler MM: Evaluation of operative stress and peritoneal macrophage function in minimally invasive operations. J Am Coll Surg 1997;184:357–363.
26. Decker D, Schöndorf BE, Bidlingmaier F, et al: Surgical stress induces a shift in the type-1/type-2 T-helper cell balance, suggesting down-regulation of antibody-mediated immunity commensurate to the trauma. Surgery 1995;119:316–325.
27. Gitzelman CA, Mendoza-Sagaon M, Ahmad SA, et al: Cell-mediated immune response: laparoscopy versus laparatomy. Surg Forum 1998;27:148–150.
28. Vittimberga FJ, Foley DP, Meyers WC, Callery MP: Laparoscopic surgery and the systemic immune response. Ann Surg 1998;227:326–334.
29. Sali L, Pietra N, Sansebastiano G, et al: Reduce postoperative morbidity after elective laparoscopic cholecystectomy; stratified matched case-control study. World J Surg 1997;21:872–879.
30. Behrman SW, Melvin WC, Babb ME, et al: Laparoscopic cholecystectomy in the geriatric population. Am Surg 1996;62:386–390.
31. Schrenk P, Woisetschläger R, Rieger R, Wayand W: Prospective randomized trial comparing postoperative pain and return to physical activity after transabdominal prepertional, total preperitoneal or Shaouldice technique for inguinal hernia repair. Br J Surg 1996;83:1563–1556.
32. Kozol R, Lange PM, Kosir M, et al: A prospective, randomized study of open vs laparoscopic inguinal hernia repair: an assessment of postoperative pain. Arch Surg 1997;132;292–295.
33. Smeets HJ, Kievitz J, Dulfer FT: Endocrine-metabolic response to abdominal aortic surgery; a randomized trial of general anaesthesia versus general plus epidural anaesthesia. World J Surg 1993;17:601–607.
34. Dickenson AH: NMDA receptor antagonists a analgesics. In: Fields HL, Lienbeskind JC (eds) Progress in Pain Research and management, Vol 1. Seattle, WA, International Association for the study of pain 1994;173–187.
35. Schulze S, Sommer P, Bigler D, et al: Effect on combined prednisolone, epidural analgesia, and indomethacin on the systemic response after colonic surgery. Arch Surg 1992;127:325–331.
36. Heindorff H, Schulze S, Mogensen T, et al: Hormonal and neural blockade prevents the postoperative increase in amino acid clearance and urea synthesis. Surgery 1992;111:543–550.
37. Moore R, Yang S, McNicholas R, et al: Hemodynamics and anesthetic effects of sufentanil as the sole anesthetic for pediatric cardiovascular surgery. Anesthesiology 1985;62;725.
38. Lynch EP, Welch KJ, Carabuena JM, Eberlein TJ: Thoracic epidural anesthesia improves outcome after breast surgery. Ann Surg 1995;222:663–669.
39. Dubner R, Ruda MA: Activity-dependent neuronal plasticity following tissue injury and inflammation. Trends Neurosci 1992;15:92–103.
40. Watson A, Allen PR: Influence of thoracic epidural analgesia on outcome after resection for esophageal cancer. Surgery 1994;115:429–432.
41. St. Haxholdt O, Kehely H, Dyrberg V: Effect of fentanyl on the cortisol and hyperglycemic response to abdominal surgery. Acta Anaesthesiol Scand 1981;25:434–436.
42. Koltun WA, Bloomer MM, Tilberg AF, et al: Awake epidural anesthesia is associated with improved natural killer cell cytotoxicity and a reduced stress response. Am J Surg 1996;171:68–73.
43. Brandt EG, Kehlet V, Aronson GT: Large doses of morphine in cardiac surgery. Acta Anaesthesiol Scand 1978;22:400–407.
44. Cohen D, Horluchi K, Kemper M, Weissman C: Modulating effects of propofol on metabolic and cardiopulmanory responses to stressful intensive care unit procedures. Crit Care Med 1996;24:612–617.
45. Schulze S, Andersen J, Overgaard H, et al: Effect of prednisolone on the systemic response and wound healing after colonic surgery. Arch Surg 1997;132:129–135.
46. Chambrier C, Chassard D, Bienvenu J, et al: Cytokine and hormonal changes after cholecystectomy: effect of ibuprofen pretreatment. Ann Surg 1996;224:178–182.
47. Bonicalzi V, Canavero S, Cerutti F, et al: Lamotrigine reduces total postoperative analgesic requirement: a randomized double-blind, placebo-controlled pilot study. Surgery 1997;122:567–570.
48. Cataldo P, Sengore AJ, Kilbride MJ: Ketorolac and patient controlled analgesia in the treatment of postoperative pain. Surg Gynecol Obstet 1993;176:435–438.
49. Frank SM, Fleisher LA, Breslow MJ, et al: Perioperative maintenance of normotherima reduces the incidence of morbid cardiac events. JAMA 1997;277:1127–1134.
50. Kurz A, Sessler DI, Lenhardt R: Perioperative normotherima to reduce the incidence of a surgical wound infection and shorten hospitalization. N Engl J Med 1996;334:1209–1216.
51. Gentilello LM, Jurkovich GJ, Stark MS, et al: Hypothermia in critically injured trauma victims: is it protective or harmful? Ann Surg (in press).
52. Westhuyzen J, Cochrane AD, Tesar PJ, et al: Effect of preoperative supplementation with α-tocopheral and ascorbic acid on mycocardial injury in patients undergoing cardiac operations. J Thorac Cardiovasc Surg 1997;113:942–948.
53. Mullis-Jansson SL, Argenziano M, Corwin SJ, et al: Intravenous T_3 improves myocardial function and reduces morbidity after coronary bypass surgery: results of a double-blind randomized trial. J Thorac Cardiovasc Surg 1999;1M:1128–1135.
54. Chiba Y, Morioka K, Muraoka R, et al: Effects of depletion of leukocytees and platelets on cardiac dysfunction after cardiopulmonary bypass. Ann Thorac Surg 1998;65:107–114.
55. Gott JP, Cooper WA, Schmidt FE, et al: Modifying risk for extracorporeal circulation: trial of four antiinflammatory strategies. Ann Thorac Surg 1998;66:747–754.
56. Brasil LA, Gomes WJ, Salomão EC, Buffolo E: Inflammatory response after myocardial revascularization with or without cardiopulmonary bypass. Ann Thorac Surg 1998;66:56–59.
57. Gu YJ, Mariani MA, Van Oeveren W, et al: Reduction of the inflammatory response in patients undergoing minimally invasive coronary artery bypass grafting. Ann Thorac Surg 1998;65:420–424.
58. Baue AE: The promissory note in scientific research. Am J Surg 1998;175:2–3.

59. Kammula US, White DF, Rosenberg SA: Trends in the safety of high dose bolus interleukin-2 in patients with metastatic cancer. Cancer 1998;83:797–785.
60. Babineau TJ, Marcello P, Swails W, et al: Randomized phase I/II trial of a macrophage-specific immunomodulator (PCG-glucan) in high-risk surgical patients. Ann Surg 1994;220:601–609.
61. Babineau TJ, Hackford A, Kenler A, et al: A phase II multicenter, double-blind, randomized, placebo-controlled study of three dosage of an immunomodulator (PCG-glucan) in high risk surgical patients. Arch Surg 1994;129:1204–1210.
62. De Felippe J, da Rocha e Silva M, Maciel FMB, de Macedo Soares A, Mendes NF: Infection prevention in patients with severe multiple trauma with the immunomodulator beta1-3 polyglucose (glucan). Surg Gynecol Obset 1993;177:383–388.
63. Vangerow B, Marx G, Leuwer M, Rueckoldt H: C1-inhibitor substitution as ultima ratio therapy in septic shock: experience with 15 patients. Crit Care Med 1998;2:19.
64. Kulka PJ, Tryba M, Zenz M: Preoperative α_2-adrenergic receptor agoinsts prevent the deterioration of renal function after cardiac surgery: results of a randomized controlled trial. Crit Care Med 1996;24:947–952.
65. Bakker J, Zhang H, Depierreux M, et al: Effects of N-acetylcysteine in endotoxic shock. J Crit Care 1994;9:236–43.
66. Flannagan RJ, Meredith TJ: Use of N-acetyl cystein in clinical toxicology. Am J Med 1991;91:131–139.
67. Reinhart K, Spies CD, Meier Hellman A, et al: N-acetylcysteine preserves oxygen consumption and gastric mucosal pH during hyperoxic ventilation. Am J Respir Crit Care Med 199;151:773–779.
68. Peak SL, Moran JL, Leppard PI: N-acetyl cysteine depresses cardiac performance in patients with septic shock. Crit Care Med 1996;24:1302–1310.
69. Suter PM, Domenighetti G, Schaller M-D, et al: Acetylcysteine enhances recovery from acute lung injury in man, a randomized, double-blind, placebo-controlled clinical study. Chest 1994;105:190–194.
70. Kincaid EH, Miller PR, Meredith JW, Chang MC: Enalaprilat improves gut perfusion in critically injured patients. Shock 1998;9:79–83.
71. Chang DW, DeSanti L, Demling RH: Anticatabolic and anabolic strategies in critical illness: a review of current treatment modalities. Shock 1998;10:155–160.
72. Smolle KH, Khoschsorur G, Wonish W, Tatzber F: Lipid peroxidation parameters and antioxidant status of critically ill intensive care unit patients. Crit Care 1998;2:12.
73. Hotchkiss RS, Karl IE: Pentoxifylline and modulation of the inflammatory response. Crit care Med 1998;26:427–428.
74. Zabel P, Staubach KH, Stüber F, Schröder J: Placebo-controlled clinical study with pentoxifylline in severe sepsis. Shock (in press).
75. Schröder J, Stauback KH, Stüber F, Zabel P: Pentoxifyllin als adjuvante Therapie der Multiorgandysfunktion [Adjuvant therapy in multiple organ dysfunction with pentoxyfylline]. Langenbecks Arch Chir 1998;1:461–465.
76. Staubach KH, Schröder J, Stüber F, et al: Effect of pentoxifylline in severe sepsis: results of a randomized, double-blind, placebo-controlled study. Arch Surg 1998;133:94–100.
77. Bacher A, Mayer N, Klimscha W, et al: Effects of pentoxifylline on hemodynamics and oxygenation in septic and nonseptic patients. Crit Care Med 1997;25:795–800.
78. Hoffmann H, Markewitz A, Kreuzer E, et al: Pentoxifylline decreases the incidence of multiple organ failure in patients after major cardio-thoracic surgery. Shock 1998;9:235–240.
79. Kleinschmidt S, Wanner GA, Bussmann D, et al: Proinflammatory cytokine gene expression in whole blood from patients undergoing coronary artery bypass surgery and its modulation by pentoxifylline. Shock 1998;9:112–20.
80. Yu M, Tomasa G: A double-blind, prospective, randomized trial of ketoconazole, a thromboxane synthetase inhibitor, in the prophylaxis of the adult respiratory distress syndrome. Crit Care Med 1993;21:1635–1642.
81. Hughes J: Isolation of an endogenous compound from the brain with pharmacological properties similar to morphine. Brain Res 1975;88:295–308.
82. Boeuf B, Gauvin F, Guerguerian AM, et al: Therapy of shock with naloxone: a meta-analysis. Crit Care Med 1998;26:1910–1916.
83. Grover R, Lopez A, Lorente J, et al: Multi-center, randomized, placebo-controlled, double blind study of the nitric oxide synthase inhibitor 546C88: effect on survival in patients with septic shock. Crit Care Med 1999;27:A33.
84. Bernard GR, Hartman DL, Helterbrand JD, et al: Lilly Research laboratories: recombinant human activated protein C (rhAPC) produces a trend toward improvement in morbidity and 28 day survival in patients with severe sepsis. Crit Care Med 1999;27:A33.
85. Godje O, Gulbins H, Hilge R, et al: Prevention of respiratory muscle wastage and improvement of physical fitness by clenbuterol in patients after cardiac operations in the 8th decade of life. Crit Care Med 1999;27:A38.
86. Vincent JL, Brase R, Dhainaut JF, et al: a multicenter double-blind, placebo-controlled study of liposomal prostaglandin E1 (TLC C-53) in patients with acute respiratory distress syndrome. Crit Care med 1999;27:A164.
87. O'Dell JR: Anticytokine therapy: a new era in the treatment of rheumatoid arthritis? N Engl J Med 1999;340:310–312.

56
Wound Healing: Physiology, Clinical Progress, Growth Factors, and the Secret of the Fetus

David T. Efron, Maria B. Witte, and Adrian Barbul

Wound healing is an organized cascade of cellular and biochemical events that occur in a timely, predictable, limited fashion. An important feature of normal wound healing is its regulated transition from an exuberant cellular, mainly inflammatory response to a quiescent, acellular, remodeling phase. Progression through the phases of healing is governed by various growth factors and cytokines produced locally and systemically in response to the injury.

It is important to note that the populations of cells that participate in the timely healing of wounds are of the same types that are implicated in causing and participating in global inflammatory responses such as the systemic inflammatory response syndrome (SIRS). As such, altered, prolonged, delayed, or imbalanced production of cytokines and growth factors can disrupt or delay the wound healing process.

When wounds fail, the process may be characterized as globally impaired, as observed with diabetes or chronic steroid use, or delayed, as noted with infections or malnutrition. In the first instance, the wound never achieves the mechanical characteristics of a normally healed wound; with delayed healing, some mechanical integrity is achieved but belatedly. Clinically, acute wound failure and chronic wounds are two pathophysiologically distinct entities requiring different therapeutic strategies. A better understanding of the pathophysiology of wound healing inevitably helps in the prevention and treatment of wound failure.

Mature Wound Healing

Phases of Healing

Normal wound healing follows a predictable pattern that can be divided into well defined phases. An approximate timeline of these events is depicted in Fig. 56.1. Hemostasis and subsequent inflammation represent the earliest responses to injury. With platelet degranulation and fibrin clot formation there is release of chemotactic compounds that give rise to the characteristic inflammatory infiltrate consisting of neutrophils and subsequently macrophages and lymphocytes. Inflammatory cells serve multiple roles and prepare the wound for the next phases of fibroplasia and angiogenesis. The proliferative phase is characterized by fibroblast and endothelial cell migration and proliferation, thus reestablishing the tissue integrity of the defect. The remodeling of the wound is the longest phase and results in scar reorganization and strength acquisition.

Wound Cells

The cascade of wound healing always starts with an injury leading to activation of the coagulation system. The clot formation stops bleeding and degranulates platelets, leading to the first significant release of cytokines and growth factors. The platelet α granules contain multiple factors, such as platelet-activating factor, platelet-derived growth factor (PDGF), thromboxane, prostaglandins, serotonin, and adenosine dinucleotide.[1] The fibrin clot serves as the scaffolding for subsequent cellular infiltration.[2]

Cellular infiltration after injury follows a characteristic predetermined sequence (Fig. 56.1). The first to appear are neutrophils. Although traditionally held to be nonessential for wound healing in the absence of infection,[3] studies suggest that leukocytes are a major source of cytokines early during inflammation, especially tumor necrosis factor-α (TNFα).[4] Neutrophils thus may have a potential role in subsequent angiogenesis and collagen synthesis. Neutrophils also release proteases such as collagenases and participate in matrix and ground substance degradation during the early phase of wound healing.[5]

Different subpopulations of polymorphonuclear leukocytes (PMNs), albeit low in numbers, may have distinct functions. A recently established leukocyte subpopulation are the fibrocytes. These fibroblast-like cells have some leukocyte-specific features: They are found at the site of injury shortly after trauma, they synthesize matrix (collagen types I and III), and they display the spindle shape of fibroblasts. The fibrocytes also express leukocyte-associated antigenic structures such as CD34 and can act as antigen-presenting cells during T cell proliferation.[6-8]

Eosinophilic neutrophils are part of the cellular infiltrate after skin wounding; although their role is not known, in hamsters

PHASES OF HEALING

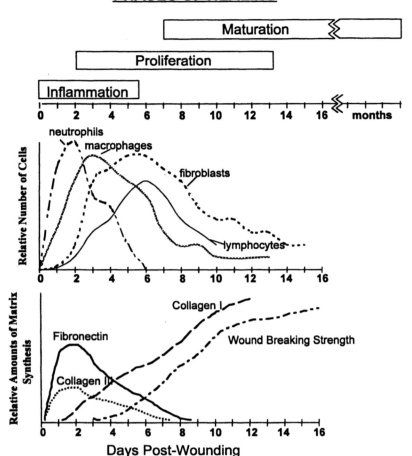

FIGURE 56.1. Time line of the phases of healing coincidental with cellular infiltration and matrix deposition. (Adapted from Witte and Barbul,[1] with permission.)

eosinophil depletion using an anti-interleukin-5 (IL-5) antibody significantly accelerated wound closure.[9]

Mast cells are known to participate in inflammation. Recent work suggests that mast cells may have a role in wound healing as a major source of cytokines, such as fibroblast growth factor (FGF), IL-1, IL-3, IL-4, PDGF, TNFβ, and tumor growth factor-β (TGFβ) as well as heparin, histamine, leukotrienes, and other factors.[10] Mast cells can regulate vascular tone and permeability, coagulation, and chemoattraction of other cells during the early phase of wound healing. In vitro work has shown that mast cells stimulate fibroblast proliferation probably via histamine release.[11] Mast cell-derived TGFβ, FGF, and IL-4 are potent stimulators of extracellular matrix synthesis.[12,13] The exact contribution of mast cell-derived cytokines to wound healing remains to be fully elucidated.

Macrophages, the most important element in the early cascade of healing, comprise the second line of inflammatory cells that invade the wound. Macrophages carry out multiple functions (Fig. 56.2) and are essential to successful healing.[14] Macrophages supplement and complete the phagocytosis begun by neutrophils and participate in microbial stasis via oxygen radical synthesis and nitric oxide production. Macrophages are also directly involved in activation and recruitment of other cells via mediators such as cytokines and growth factors and by cell-cell interaction and intercellular adhesion molecules (ICAMs). By releasing such mediators as TGFβ, vascular endothelial growth factor (VEGF), insulin-like growth factor (IGF), and epithelial growth factor (EGF), macrophages regulate cell proliferation, matrix synthesis, and angiogenesis.[15] Macrophages are also a major source of lactate, which stimulates angiogenesis and collagen synthesis.[16]

Another constant cell population that invades the wound are lymphocytes, which are less numerous than macrophages. T lymphocytes are essential to wound healing, although their role is not fully defined. Depletion of wound T lymphocytes decreases wound strength and collagen content.[7] Selective depletion of the CD8$^+$ suppressor subset of T lymphocytes enhances wound healing; depletion of the CD4$^+$ helper subset has no effect.[18] As a result of these findings, a noncharacterized subpopulation of wound healing-enhancing T lymphocytes was postulated to exist.

Congenitally athymic nude mice, which have an impaired T cell system, and thymectomized adult rats both demonstrate better breaking strength and increased wound collagen deposition than normal animals.[19,20] Although the thymus appears to exert a downregulating effect on wound healing, administration of IL-2 or thymosin-α_1, both potent stimulators of lymphocyte proliferation and differentiation, improves wound healing.[21,22]

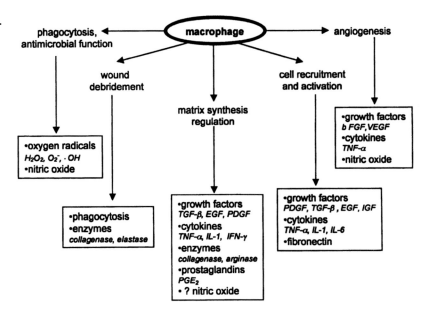

FIGURE 56.2. Various functions of wound macrophages. (Adapted from Witte and Barbul,[1] with permission.)

Lymphocytes can exert a direct downregulating effect on fibroblast collagen synthesis by cell-associated interferon-γ (IFNγ), TNFα, and IL-1a.[23] This effect is abrogated if the cells are physically separated, demonstrating that extracellular matrix synthesis is regulated not only via soluble factors but also via direct cell–cell contact between lymphocytes and fibroblasts.

Fibroblasts and endothelial cells are the last cell populations to infiltrate the healing wound. The strongest chemotactic factor for fibroblasts is PDGF.[24,25] Recruited fibroblasts must become activated from a quiescent state prior to participation in healing. This activation is partially induced by the cytokines released from macrophages. The primary functions of wound fibroblasts are matrix synthesis and remodeling. Fibroblasts isolated from wounds differ significantly from nonwound fibroblasts in that they have higher contractile and matrix-synthesizing capacity.[26] The contractile property of fibroblasts is due to their expression of smooth muscle α-actin, which is organized into stress fibers within the cell; smooth muscle α-actin can be induced in vitro by TGFβ[27] or by the addition of wound fluid to cultured fibroblasts.[26] This contractile phenotype is not permanent, as myofibroblasts undergo apoptosis during the repair process.[28]

Wound-derived fibroblasts also synthesize more collagen than non-wound-derived fibroblasts.[26] The mechanism that induces high collagen production is not well understood. The cytokine-rich wound environment plays a significant role as exposure of fibroblasts to wound fluid induces increased collagen synthesis.[29] Additionally, lactate accumulates in wound fluid over time (10–15 mM), and it regulates collagen synthesis through a mechanism involving ADP-ribosylation.[30,31]

Wound fibroblasts have been shown to produce nitric oxide (NO), which in turn influences their collagen metabolism.[32] Normal dermal fibroblasts do not produce NO spontaneously. Upon exposure to wound fluid, dermal fibroblasts can be induced to synthesize NO,[33] which may be at least partially responsible for the switch to a wound fibroblast phenotype.

Similarly, induction of NO synthesis in epithelial cells and keratinocytes correlates with a switch in phenotype.[34,35]

In vivo administration of NO donors and direct in vivo transfection of the inducible nitric oxide synthase (iNOS) gene enhances wound strength and collagen deposition under experimental conditions.[36,37] iNOS knockout mice exhibit delayed healing of excisional wounds, an effect reversible by in vivo transfection of the iNOS gene.[38] These data provide further support for a significant role of NO in wound healing, although the exact mechanism of action remains to be defined fully.

Hand in hand with the proliferation of fibroblasts, there is extensive proliferation of endothelial cells. These cells participate in the formation of new capillaries (angiogenesis), which is essential to successful wound healing. Endothelial cells originate from intact venules close to the wound. Their replication, migration, and new tubule formation is under the influence of cytokines and growth factors such as TNFα, TGFβ, and VEGF. The major source of VEGF is macrophages,[39] although many other cells produce it as well; VEGF receptors are located specifically on endothelial cells.[40] The angiogenic effects of lactate and hypoxia are probably mediated through an ADP-ribosylation process that leads to enhanced VEGF synthesis.[23] NO also stimulates angiogenesis.[41]

Wound Matrix

Wound strength and mechanical integrity in the fresh wound are determined by both the amount and quality of newly deposited collagen. The deposition of matrix at the wound site follows a characteristic pattern: Fibronectin and collagen type III constitute the early matrix scaffolding; glycosaminoglycans and proteoglycans represent the next significant matrix components, and collagen type I is the final matrix.

Collagen synthesis is a highly controlled metabolic process. Several posttranslational steps including hydroxylation and

TABLE 56.1. Potential Therapeutic Modalities for Wound Regulation.

Target	Effector	Result	Reference
Collagen synthesis	Collagenase inhibitor (GM6001)	Increased wound strength; reduced inflammation	44
	L-Arginine	Increased collagen formation; increased wound strength; enhanced immune function	45–47
	NO donors	Increased collagen formation; increased wound strength	36
Cytokine neutralization	TNFα (TNF-binding protein)	Increased skin and GI wound strength	48,49
Cytokine gene transfer	TGFβ, iNOS	Increased wound collagen and breaking strength	37,50
Antisense technology	TGFβ, thrombospondin	Decreased scarring; decreased reepithelialization and dermal reorganization	51–54
Dressings	Hyaluronic acid	Increased healing rate	55,56
	Growth factors (PDGF, FGF, EGF, PDWHF, GM-CSF)	Generally increased incidence and rates of healing	57–70
Adhesion modulation	Hyaluronic acid	Decreased postoperative adhesion formation	71,72
Bioartificial tissue	Artificial skin composite of ECM and epidermal graft or keratinocytes	Ready-made tissue cover of wound	57

NO, nitric oxide; TNF, tumor necrosis factor; iNOS, inducible nitric oxide synthase; TGF, tumor growth factor; PDGF, platelet-derived growth factor; FGF, fibroblast growth factor; EGF, epithelial growth factor; GM-CSF, granulocyte/macrophage colony-stimulating factor; ECM, extracellular matrix; GI, gastrointestinal; PDWHF, platelet derived wound healing factor.

glycosylation of proline and lysine residues, as well as the formation of interchain and intrachain disulfide bonds are required to achieve the classic triple helix structure of the collagen molecule. After several weeks the amount of collagen in the wound levels off, although gain in tensile strength continues for many weeks more. Fibril formation and fibril crosslinking result in decreased solubility, increased strength, and increased resistance to enzymatic degradation of the collagen matrix.

There is a constant turnover of collagen in the extracellular matrix with replacement of early wound collagen and during normal tissue homeostasis. Collagenolysis is carried out by tissue metalloproteases, specifically collagenases. Both collagen synthesis and lysis are strictly controlled by cytokines and growth factors. Some factors act on both arms of the pathway. For example, TGFβ increases new collagen transcription and decreases collagen breakdown by stimulating synthesis of tissue inhibitors of metalloprotease (TIMP).[42] This balance of collagen deposition and degradation is the ultimate determinant of wound strength and integrity.

Collagen synthesis and posttranslational modifications are highly dependent on systemic factors, such as adequate oxygen supply, the presence of sufficient nutritional cofactors (e.g., vitamins, trace metals), and a favorable environment (lack of steroids, radiation-induced damage, and infection). Measures should be taken to reverse the systemic effect of these factors to optimize healing. Some examples include the administration of vitamin A to patients with hydrocortisone treatment, revascularization in patients with limb ischemia, establishment of adequate nutrition in case of malnutrition, or treatment of infection before wounding. All are important if not essential adjuncts to wound care. Clinically, enhancing the oxygen supply improves wound healing; and although there are no prospective randomized clinical trials, there is evidence that hyperbaric oxygen therapy is of some benefit to patients with peripheral vascular disease and diabetes.[43]

Although sufficient collagen deposition is vital for successful wound healing, it is noteworthy that few clinically therapeutic options exist that modulate collagen synthesis (Table 56.1). Experimentally and in healthy human volunteers, the administration of supplemental arginine leads to enhanced wound collagen accumulation, most likely secondary to increased synthesis.[45,46,73] Another approach is to intervene during the collagen remodeling phase. Administration of a collagenase inhibitor (GM6001) significantly enhances wound-breaking strength in rats without affecting scar collagen content.[44] Surprisingly, the collagenase inhibitor decreased the inflammatory response and angiogenesis and altered the postinjury cytokine profile of TNFα and TGFβ.

As mentioned above, matrix accumulation ceases a few weeks after wounding, but the process of matrix remodeling continues for several months. Even after remodeling, the organization and wound strength of the healing scar never reaches that of unwounded tissue.[74] Newly formed granulation tissue is replaced gradually by the mature scar, which is avascular and acellular. The resolution of inflammation and cellular infiltration after wounding is not well understood, although apoptosis plays a role.[75,76]

Growth Factors

Growth factors are polypeptides that regulate, directly or indirectly, all phases of wound healing. The physiologic and therapeutic role of growth factors is continually being expanded and refined. Growth factors act via autocrine, paracrine, or endocrine mechanisms and are generally present in nanogram concentrations in the wound environment.[24]

TABLE 56.2. Summary of Growth Factor Therapy in Human Wounds.

Growth factor and wound type	Study	Benefit	Design/dose	Reference
PDGF BB				
Pressure ulcers	Phase I/II	Dose-dependent improvement	Placebo vs. 0.01, 0.1, and 1.0 mg/cm^2	58
Pressure ulcers	Phase I/II	Significantly reduced size	100 or 300 mg/ml	59
Diabetic neuropathic ulcers	Double-blind, prospective, randomized	Significant vs. placebo		60
Diabetic neuropathic ulcers	Phase III	Increased incidence of wound closure; decreased time to closure	Placebo vs. 30 and 100 g/g	68
Pressure ulcers	Double-blind, prospective, randomized	Increased incidence of complete healing	Placebo vs. 100 and 300 g/g qd and bid	69
EGF				
Venous ulcers	Double-blind, prospective	NS	Placebo vs. 10 mg/ml	61
Skin graft donor site	Double-blind, prospective, randomized	Healing shortened by 1.5 days	EGF 10 mg/ml in sulfadiazine vs. sulfadiazine	62
Skin graft donor site	Double-blind, prospective, randomized	NS		63
Basic FGF				
Diabetic neuropathic ulcers	Double-blind, prospective, randomized	NS	bFGF vs. placebo	64
PDWHF				
Various ulcers	Randomized, prospective	Significantly better	PDWHF vs. placebo	65
Diabetic neuropathic ulcers	Double-blind, prospective, randomized	80% vs. 20% closure	PDWHF vs. saline	66
Various ulcers	Double-blind, prospective, randomized	NS	PDWHF vs. placebo	67
rhuGM-CSF				
Venous ulcers	Double-blind, prospective, randomized	Dose-dependent increased rate of healing	Placebo vs. 200 and 400 g/wound/week	70

See Table 56.1 for other abbreviations.

Growth factors act differentially depending on the local concentration. For example, TGFβ acts as a proliferative agent at low concentrations but suppresses fibroblast proliferation at higher concentrations.[77] Growth factors have divergent actions on different cells: They can be chemoattractive to one cell type yet stimulate replication of a different cell type. Little is known about the ratio of growth factor concentrations, which may be as important as the absolute concentration of individual growth factors.

Growth factors act on cells via surface receptor binding. Various types have been described, such as ion channels, G-protein-linked receptors, or enzyme-linked receptors. The response elicited in the cell is usually one of phosphorylation or dephosphorylation of second messenger molecules through the action of phosphatases or kinases, resulting in activation or deactivation of proteins in the cytosol or nucleus of the target cell. Phosphorylation of nuclear proteins is followed by initiation of the transcription of target genes.[78] The signal is stopped by internalization of the receptor-ligand complex.

One hypothesis for the chronicity of nonhealing wounds invokes a paucity of growth factors in the wound environment.[79,80] Enhanced bacterial degradation, entrapment in fibrin clots, or decreased overall synthesis are factors that contribute to the diminished growth factor concentration in chronic wounds. Interestingly, most current formulations for clinical application of growth factors to chronic wounds deliver concentrations approximately 10^3 higher than those observed physiologically.

The most significant randomized human studies of growth factors in wound healing are summarized in Table 56.2. The results obtained thus far support the clinical application of growth factors in wound care centers as part of studies or a whole-team approach to problem wounds.

Fetal Wound Healing

In 1971 Burrington noted that fetal lambs achieved scarless healing of linear incisional wounds created in utero.[81] Since that time there has been an accumulation of clinical and experimental data suggesting that fetuses and neonates heal faster and with less scarring than adults. Although early fetal healing is clearly characterized by the absence of scarring and a healing process more akin to regeneration of the injured tissue, there is a phase of transition during gestational life when a more adult-like

TABLE 56.3. Unique Characteristics of Fetal Healing.

Sterile, fluid environment (amniotic fluid) rich in growth factors
Markedly decreased wound oxygen tension
Markedly decreased inflammatory response
Enhanced hyaluronic acid component of the extracellular matrix
More rapid wound cellular proliferation, extracellular matrix deposition, epithelialization, and wound closure
Decreased angiogenesis

healing pattern emerges, one characterized by scar formation albeit reduced. In nonhuman primates this "transition wound" occurs at the beginning of the third trimester.[82] During this period healing is characterized by scarless wound healing but with loss of the ability to regenerate skin appendages. Classic adult healing with scar formation is present later during gestation, although overall healing continues to be faster than in adults.

Understanding how fetal wounds are able to achieve integrity without evidence of scarring may allow manipulation to minimize or eliminate harmful fibrosis in adults. Several aspects of the healing fetal wound are different from that of the adult (Table 56.3). One strikingly obvious difference between fetal and mature postnatal healing is the wound environment. The fetal wound is bathed in a warm, sterile, protected fluid environment, whereas the adult wound is not. Several elegant experiments, however, have demonstrated that scarless healing may occur outside the amniotic fluid environment and that scars do occur in utero.[83–86] The oxygen content of fetal (PO_2 16–20 mmHg) and adult (PO_2 45–60 mmHg) wounds are markedly different.[84,87] Clearly, hypoxia does not have the same detrimental effects on fetal healing as it does in the adult wounds.

There are also major qualitative and quantitative differences between the fetus and the adult organism regarding the inflammatory phase. The early fetus is neutropenic,[88] and there is a paucity of identifiable PMNs in the early fetal wound.[89] Macrophage infiltration of fetal wounds is also reduced.[90] The extent of the inflammatory response correlates directly with the amount of scar formation in all healing wounds, and reduced fetal inflammation may partially explain the observed reduced scarring. In turn, the diminished fetal inflammatory response is due to the immaturity of the fetal immune system, the sterile environment in which the fetus resides, and the differential control and production of cytokines and growth factors in fetal tissues.

Differences in the healing response may be secondary to different growth factor responses. Although PDGF is equally present in the fetus and adult,[91] TGFβ, which stimulates fibroplasia, is nearly absent in the fetal wound environment. Exogenous addition of TGFβ to fetal wounds that would otherwise heal without scar results in scarring.[84,92]

The TGFβ family consists of three isoforms (β1, β2 and β3) that are structurally related but play different roles in the healing wound. The blocking of TGFβ1 or TGFβ2 using neutralizing antibodies considerably reduces scar formation in adult wounds.[93] Exogenous addition of TGFβ3 downregulates wound TGFβ1 and TGFβ2 levels and results in a reduction in scarring. These data imply that the balance between the concentration or activity of the isoforms is important for regulating scar production. It is unclear whether the alterations in TGFβ isoform expression cause an alteration in the inflammatory response, which then is reflected in the subsequent scar formation.

Another recognized difference between fetal and adult wounds is in the extracellular environment. The fetal wound is characterized by excessive and extended hyaluronic acid production. Repeated alternating units of N-acetylglucosamine and glucuronic acid make up hyaluronic acid, a high-molecular-weight glycosaminoglycan that is produced primarily by fibroblasts. Although both fetal and adult wounds demonstrate early hyaluronic acid production, it is sustained only in the fetal wound. Components of amniotic fluid, most specifically fetal urine, have a unique ability to stimulate hyaluronic acid production, which has been implicated in scarless healing.[94]

In vivo analysis in multiple animal models show that fetal wounds produce collagen in amounts similar to those in adult wounds. The final collagen content of the fetal wound matches that of uninjured skin. Fetal fibroblasts produce more collagen than adult fibroblasts, and the increased level of hyaluronic acid may aid in the higher organization of collagen.[95] Hyaluronic acid has been used topically to enhance healing (Table 56.1) or inhibit postoperative adhesion formation.[71,72]

As our understanding of the pathophysiology of wound healing increases we are better able to facilitate the healing of both simple and complicated wounds. The secrets behind fetal tissue regeneration lie within a complex combination of cytokine and growth factor regulation as well as tissue differentiation and maturity, the unmasking of which is far from complete.

References

1. Witte MB, Barbul A: General principles of wound healing. Surg Clin North Am 1997;77:509–528.
2. Kurkinen M, Vaheri A, Roberts PJ, et al: Sequential appearance of fibronectin and collagen in experimental granulation tissue. Lab Invest 1980;43:47–51.
3. Simpson DM, Ross R: The neutrophilic leukocyte in wound repair. a study with antineutrophil serum. J Clin Invest 1972;51:2009–2023.
4. Feiken E, Romer J, Eriksen J, et al: Neutrophils express tumor necrosis factor-alpha during mouse skin wound healing. J Invest Dermatol 1995;105:120–123.
5. Welgus HG, Senior RM, Parks WC, et al: Neutral proteinase expression by human mononuclear phagocytes: a prominent role of cellular differentiation. Matrix 1992;1(Suppl)1:363–367.
6. Bucala R, Spiegel LA, Chesney J, et al: Circulating fibrocytes define a new leukocyte subpopulation that mediates tissue repair. Mol Med 1994;1:71–81.
7. Chesney J, Bacher M, Bender A, et al: The peripheral blood fibrocyte is a potent antigen-presenting cell capable of priming naive T cells in situ. Proc Natl Acad Sci USA 1997;94:6307–6312.

8. Chesney J, Metz C, Stavitsky AB, et al: Regulated production of type I collagen and inflammatory cytokines by peripheral blood fibrocytes. J Immunol 1998;160:419–425.
9. Yang J, Torio A, Donoff RB, et al: Depletion of eosinophil infiltration by anti-IL-5 monoclonal antibody (TRFK-5) accelerates open skin wound epithelial closure. Am J Pathol 1997;151:813–819.
10. Gottwald T, Coerper S, Schäffer M, et al: The mast cell-nerve axis in wound healing: a hypothesis. Wound Repair Regen 1998;6:8–20.
11. Kupietzky A, Levi SF: The role of mast cell-derived histamine in the closure of an in vitro wound. Inflamm Res 1996;45:176–180.
12. Postlethwaite AE, Holness MA, Katai H, et al: Human fibroblasts synthesize elevated levels of extracellular matrix proteins in response to interleukin 4. J Clin Invest 1992;90:1479–1485.
13. Levi SF, Rubinchik E: Activated mast cells are fibrogenic for 3T3 fibroblasts. J Invest Dermatol 1995;104:999–1003.
14. Leibovich SJ, Ross R: The role of the macrophage in wound repair: a study with hydrocortisone and antimacrophage serum. Am J Pathol 1975;78:71–100.
15. DiPietro LA: Wound healing: the role of the macrophage and other immune cells. Shock 1995;4:233–240.
16. Zabel DD, Feng JJ, Scheuenstuhl H, et al: Lactate stimulation of macrophage-derived angiogenic activity is associated with inhibition of poly(ADP-ribose) synthesis. Lab Invest 1996;74:644–649.
17. Efron JE, Frankel HL, Lazarou SA, et al: Wound healing and T-lymphocytes. J Surg Res 1990;48:460–463.
18. Barbul A, Breslin RJ, Woodyard JP, et al: The effect of in vivo T helper and T suppressor lymphocyte depletion on wound healing. Ann Surg 1989;209:479–483.
19. Barbul A, Shawe T, Rotter SM, et al: Wound healing in nude mice: a study on the regulatory role of lymphocytes in fibroplasia. Surgery 1989;105:764–769.
20. Barbul A, Sisto D, Rettura G, et al: Thymic inhibition of wound healing: abrogation by adult thymectomy. J Surg Res 1982;32:338–342.
21. Barbul A, Knud HJ, Wasserkrug HL, et al: Interleukin 2 enhances wound healing in rats. J Surg Res 1986;40:315–319.
22. Malinda KM, Sidhu GS, Banaudha KK, et al: Thymosin alpha 1 stimulates endothelial cell migration, angiogenesis, and wound healing. J Immunol 1998;160:1001–1006.
23. Rezzonico R, Burger D, Dayer JM: Direct contact between T lymphocytes and human dermal fibroblasts or synoviocytes down-regulates types I and III collagen production via cell-associated cytokines. J Biol Chem 1998;273:18720–18728.
24. Grotendorst GR: Chemoattractants and growth factors. In: Cohen K, Diegelmann RF, Lindblad WJ (eds) Wound Healing, Biochemical and Clinical Aspects. Philadelphia, Saunders, 1992; 237–247.
25. Bonner JC, Osornio-Vargas AR, et al: Differential proliferation of rat lung fibroblasts induced by the platelet-derived growth factor-AA, -AB, and -BB isoforms secreted by rat alveolar macrophages. Am J Respir Cell Mol Biol 1991;5:539–547.
26. Regan MC, Kirk SJ, Wasserkrug HL, et al: The wound environment as a regulator of fibroblast phenotype. J Surg Res 1991;50:442–448.
27. Serini G, Gabbiani G: Modulation of a-smooth muscle actin expression in fibroblasts by transforming growth factor-b isoforms: an in vivo and in vitro study. Wound Repair Regen 1996;4:278–287.
28. Desmouliere A, Redard M, Darby I, et al: Apoptosis mediates the decrease in cellularity during the transition between granulation tissue and scar. Am J Pathol 1995;146:56–66.
29. Pricolo VE, Caldwell MD, Mastrofrancesco B, et al: Modulatory activities of wound fluid on fibroblast proliferation and collagen synthesis. J Surg Res 1990;48:534–538.
30. Hunt TK, Pai MP: The effect of varying ambient oxygen tensions on wound metabolism and collagen synthesis. 1972;135:561–567.
31. Hussain MZ, Ghani QP, Hunt TK: Inhibition of prolyl hydroxylase by poly(ADP-ribose) and phosphoribosyl-AMP: possible role of ADP-ribosylation in intracellular prolyl hydroxylase regulation. J Biol Chem 1989;264:7850–7855.
32. Schaffer MR, Efron PA, Thornton FJ, et al: Nitric oxide, an autocrine regulator of wound fibroblast synthetic function. J Immunol 1997;158:2375–2381.
33. Witte MB, Efron DT, Kiyama T, et al: Wound fluid regulates nitric oxide expression in fibroblasts. Surg Forum 1998;49:623–624.
34. Paulsen SM, Wurster SH, Nanney LB: Expression of inducible nitric oxide syntase in human burn wounds. Wound Repair Regen 1998;6:142–148.
35. Noiri E, Peresleni T, Srivastava N, et al: Nitric oxide is necessary for a switch from stationary to locomoting phenotype in epithelial cells. Am J Physiol 1996;270:C794–C802.
36. Witte MB, Thornton FJ, Kiyama T, et al: Nitric oxide enhances wound collagen deposition in diabetic rats. Surg Forum 1997;48:665–667.
37. Thornton FJ, Schaffer MR, Witte MB, et al: Enhanced collagen accumulation following direct transfection of the inducible nitric oxide synthase gene in cutaneous wounds. Biochem Biophys Res Commun 1998;246:654–659.
38. Yamasaki K, Edington HDJ, McClosky C, et al: Reversal of impaired wound repair in iNOS-deficient mice by topical adenoviral-mediated gene transfer. J Clin Invest 1998;101:967–971.
39. Xiong M, Elson G, Legarda D, et al: Production of vascular endothelial growth factor by murine macrophages: regulation by hypoxia, lactate, and the inducible nitric oxide synthase pathway. Am J Pathol 1998;153:587–598.
40. Ferrara N, Davis-Smith T: The biology of vascular endothelial growth factor. Endocr Rev 1997;18:4–25.
41. Murohara T, Asahara T, Silver M, et al: Nitric oxide synthase modulates angiogenesis in response to tissue ischemia. J Clin Invest 1998;101:2567–2578.
42. Zhou LJ, Ono I, Kaneko F: Role of transforming growth factor-beta 1 in fibroblasts derived from normal and hypertrophic scarred skin. Arch Dermatol Res 1997;289:645–652.
43. Faglia E, Favales F, Aldeghi A, et al: Adjunctive systemic hyperbaric oxygen therapy in treatment of severely ischemic diabetic foot ulcer: a randomized study. Diabetes Care 1996;19:1338–1343.
44. Witte MB, Thornton FJ, Kiyama T, et al: Metalloproteinase inhibitors and wound healing: a novel enhancer of wound strength. Surgery 1998;124:464–470.
45. Barbul A, Lazarou S, Efron DT, et al: Arginine enhances wound healing and lymphocyte immune responses in humans. Surgery 1990;108:331–337.
46. Kirk SJ, Hurson M, Regan MC, et al: Arginine stimulates wound healing and immune function in aged humans. Surgery 1993;114:155–160.

47. Hurson M, Regan MC, Kirk SJ, et al: Metabolic effects of arginine in a healthy elderly population. JPEN 1995;19:227–230. Erratum. JPEN 1995;19:329.
48. Maish GO, Shumate ML, Ehrlich HP, et al: Tumor necrosis factor binding protein improves incisional wound healing in sepsis. J Surg Res 1998;78:108–117.
49. Regan MC, Kirk SJ, Hurson M, et al: Tumor necrosis factor-alpha inhibits in vivo collagen synthesis. Surgery 1993;113:173–177.
50. Benn SI, Whitsitt JS, Broadley KN, et al: Particle-mediated gene transfer with transforming growth factor-beta1 cDNAs enhances wound repair in rat skin. J Clin Invest 1996;98:2894–2902.
51. Choi BM, Kwak HJ, Jun CD, et al: Control of scarring in adult wounds using antisense transforming growth factor-beta1 oligodeoxynucleotides. Immunol Cell Biol 1996;74:144–150.
52. Chung HT, Choi BM, Jun CD, et al: Antisense transforming growth factor-beta1 in wound healing. Antisense Nucleic Acid Drug Dev 1997;7:257–261.
53. Kim HM, Choi DH, Lee YM: Inhibition of wound-induced expression of transforming growth factor-beta1 mRNA by its antisense oligonucleotides. Pharmacol Res 1998;37:289–293.
54. DiPietro LA, Nissen NN, Gamelli RL, et al: Thrombospondin 1 synthesis and function in wound repair. Am J Pathol 1996;148:1851–1860.
55. Ortonne JP: A controlled study of the activity of hyaluronic acid in the treatment of venous leg ulcers. J Dermatol Treat 1996;7:75–81.
56. Murashita T, Nakayama Y, Hirano T, et al: Acceleration of granulation tissue ingrowth by hyaluronic acid in artificial skin. Br J Plast Surg 1996;49:58–63.
57. Stocum DL: Regenerative biology and engineering: strategies for tissue restoration. Wound Repair Regen 1998;6:276–290.
58. Robson MC, Phillips LG, Thomason A, et al: Platelet-derived growth factor-BB for the treatment of chronic pressure ulcers. Lancet 1992;339:23–25.
59. Mustoe TA, Cutler NR, Allman RM, et al: A phase II study to evaluate recombinant platelet-derived growth factor-BB in the treatment of stage 3 and 4 pressure ulcers. Arch Surg 1994;129:213–219.
60. Steed DL, Webster MW: Topical recombinant human pltelet-derived growth factor (rhPDGF-B) accelerates healing of diabetic neurotrophic foot ulcers. J Vasc Surg 1995;21:71–81.
61. Falanga V, Eaglstein WH, Bucalo B: Topical use of human recombinant epidermal growth factor (h-EGF) in venous ulcers. J Dermatol Surg Oncol 1992;18:614–616.
62. Brown GL, Nanney LB, Griffen J, et al: Enhancement of wound healing by topical treatment with epidermal growth factor. N Engl J Med 1989;321:76–79.
63. Cohen IK, Crossland MC, Garrett A, et al: Topical application of epidermal growth factor onto partial-thickness wounds in human volunteers does not enhance reepithelialization. Plast Reconstr Surg 1995;96:251–254.
64. Richard JL, Parer RC, Daures JP, et al: Effect of topical basic fibroblast growth factor on the healing of chronic diabetic neuropathic ulcer of the foot: a pilot, randomized, double-blind, placebo-controlled study. Diabetes Care 1995;18:64–69.
65. Knighton DR, Ciresi K, Fiegel VD, et al: Stimulation of repair in chronic, nonhealing, cutaneous ulcers using platelet-derived wound healing formula. Surg Gynecol Obstet 1990; 170:56–65.
66. Steed DL, Goslen JB, Holloway GA, et al: Randomized prospective double-blind trial in healing chronic diabetic foot ulcers: CT-102 activated platelet supernatant, topical versus placebo. Diabetes Care 1992;15:1598–1604.
67. Krupski WC, Reilly LM, Perez S, et al: A prospective randomized trial of autologous platelet-derived wound healing factors for treatment of chronic nonhealing wounds: a preliminary report. J Vasc Surg 1991;14:526–532.
68. Weiman TJ, Smeill JM, Su Y: Efficacy and safety of a topical gel formulation of recombinant human platelet-derived growth factor-BB (becaplermin) in patients with chronic neuropathic diabetic ulcers: a phase III randomized placebo-controlled double-blind study. Diabetes Care 1998;21:822–827.
69. Rees RS, Robson MC, Smeill JM, et al: A randomized, double-blind, placebo-controlled study of becapleramin (recombinant human platelet-derived growth factor-BB) gel in the treatment of pressure ulcers. Wound Repair Regen 1998;6:A246.
70. Marques Da Costa R, Jesus FMR, Aniceto C, et al: Randomized, double-blind, placebo-controlled, dose-ranging study of granulocyte-macrophage colony stimulating factor in patients with chronic venous leg ulcers. Wound Repair Regen 1999;7:17–25.
71. Seeger JM, Kaelin LD, Staples EM, et al: Prevention of postoperative pericardial adhesions using tissue-protective solutions. J Surg Res 1997;68:63–66.
72. Burns JW, Colt MJ, Burgees LS, et al: Preclinical evaluation of Seprafilm bioresorbable membrane. Eur J Surg Suppl 1997; 577:40–48.
73. Barbul A: Arginine: biochemistry, physiology and therapeutic implications. JPEN J Parent Enteral Nutr 1986;10:227–238.
74. Levenson SM, Geever EF, Crowley LV, et al: The healing of rat skin wounds. Ann Surg 1965;161:293–308.
75. Belligan GJ, Caldwell H, Howie SEM, et al: In vivo fate of the inflammatory macrophage during the resolution of inflammation. J Immunol 1996;157:2577–2585.
76. Savill J: Apoptosis in resolution of inflammation. J Leukoc Biol 1997;61:375–380.
77. Popik W, Inglot AD: Combined action of interferons and transforming growth factor beta on the proliferation of human fibroblasts. Arch Immunol Ther Exp 1991;39:19–26.
78. Jans DA, Hassan G: Nuclear targeting by growth factors, cytokines, and their receptors: a role in signaling? Bioessays 1998;20:400–411.
79. Barone EJ, Yager DR, Pozez AL, et al: Interleukin-1alpha and collagenase activity are elevated in chronic wounds. Plast Reconstr Surg 1998;102:1023–1027.
80. Yager DR, Zhang LY, Liang HX, et al: Wound fluids from human pressure ulcers contain elevated matrix metalloproteinase levels and activity compared to surgical wound fluids. J Invest Dermatol 1996;107:743–748.
81. Burrington JD: Wound healing in the fetal lamb. J Pediatr Surg 1971;6:523–528.
82. Lorenz PH, Whitby DJ, Longaker MT, et al: Fetal wound healing: the ontogeny of scar formation in the non-human primate. Ann Surg 1993;217:391–396.
83. Longaker MT, Whitby DJ, Ferguson MWJ, et al: Adult skin wounds in the fetal environment heal with scar formation. Ann Surg 1994;219:65–72.
84. Adzick NS, Lorenz HP: Cells, matrix, growth factors, and the surgeon. Ann Surg 1993;220:10–18.
85. Lorenz HP, Longaker MT, Perkocha LA, et al: Scarless wound repair: a human fetal skin model. Development 1992;114:253–259.

86. Lorenz HP, Longaker MT, Whitby DJ, et al: Scarless fetal skin repair is intrinsic to the fetal fibroblast. Surg Forum 1992;43:696–697.
87. Bleacher JC, Adolph VR, Dillon PW, et al: Fetal tissue repair and wound healing. Dermatol Clin 1993;11:677–683.
88. Cates K, Rowe J, Ballow M: The premature infant as a compromised host. Curr Probl Pediatr 1983;13:6–13.
89. Adzick NS, Harrison MR, Glick PL, et al: Comparison of fetal, newborn and adult rabbit wound healing by histologic, enzyme-histochemical and hydroxyproline determinations. J Pediatr Surg 1991;20:315–319.
90. Ferguson MWJ, Howarth GF: Marsupial models of scarless fetal wound healing. In: Adzick NS, Longaker MT (eds) Fetal Wound Healing. New York, Elsevier, 1992;95–124.
91. Whitby DJ, Ferguson MW: Immunohistochemical localization of growth factors in fetal wound healing. Dev Biol 1991;147:207–215.
92. Krummel TM, Michna BA, Thomas BL, et al: TGF-β induces fibrosis in a fetal wound model. J Pediatr Surg 1988;23:647–652.
93. Shah M, Foreman DM, Ferguson MWJ: Neutralizing antibody to TGF-β1,2 reduces cutaneous scarring in adult rodents. J Cell Sci 1994;107:1137.
94. Longaker MT, Adzick NS: The biology of fetal wound healing: a review. Plast Reconstr Surg 1990;87:788–798.
95. Thomas BL, Krummel TM, Melany M, et al: Collagen synthesis and type expression by fetal fibroblasts in vitro. Surg Forum 1988;39:642.

57
Problems with Magic Bullets: Future Trials and Multiagent Therapy

Arthur E. Baue

Although nobody really believes it, let us pretend that inflammation really exists as an entity among biologic mechanisms.... The end result [of inflammation] is not defense; it is an agitated, committee-directed harem-scarum effort to make war.
—Lewis Thomas.[1]

The explosion of knowledge about mediators of inflammation, injury, and infection has been impressive. These topics are described in other chapters in this book and are summarized in Table 57.1. Antagonists to all of these substances have been produced as monoclonal antibodies, receptor antagonists, or other enzymes or blocking agents; and many have been tried clinically. Many of these agents and the clinical trials have been reviewed by Neugebauer et al.[2] The frequency of infection, sepsis, injury, or inflammation in producing multiple organ failure led to clinical trials of these so-called magic bullets for the treatment of patients with sepsis and after injury. These trials have had limited success or negative results, despite considerable evidence of the efficacy or protection by such agents in experimental animals and in studies of human volunteers. I believe the major reasons for these negative results have been (1) the use of general entry criteria for the trials rather than the treatment of specific diseases or injuries and (2) the redundancy and overlap of these complex, interacting substances. Thus the "magic bullet" approach has failed because it oversimplifies a complex biologic system.[3]

The results of another negative randomized double-blind placebo controlled multicenter phase III trial have now been published indicating that platelet-activating factor receptor antagonists in patients with severe gram-negative bacterial sepsis did not improve the mortality rate.[4] This report was accompanied by an editorial "The Siren Song of Confirmatory Sepsis Trials" on selection bias and sampling error.[5] Perhaps it is simply that a single nonspecific agent does not do anything in the treatment of infected patients.

Remote Organ Damage

An overwhelming inflammatory process initiated by a disease or injury may jeopardize the patient. Such a life-threatening process is produced by a multitude of mediators that are activated nonspecifically by a host of abnormalities ranging from trauma to infection to myocardial infarction and to a low cardiac output in patients who have undergone an operation for cardiac disease.

Damage to a remote organ such as the lung occurs with ischemia/reperfusion injury of the lower extremities or the gastrointestinal tract. It may also occur with infections such as peritonitis. The response to injury, infection, ischemia, and inflammation is a complex, multimediated, overlapping, redundant system. Many experimental and clinical models indicate the virulence of such an uncontrolled response and the problems produced by mediators. Such an autodestructive phenomenon was suggested by Ehrlich and Morganroth in 1901 when they described the possibility of an autoimmune response they called a potential "horror autotoxicus."[6] I have referred to overwhelming inflammation as a modern horror autotoxicus.[7] Thus overwhelming inflammation can jeopardize a patient, no matter what its cause, but there is no single mediator that causes most or all of the trouble.

An inflammatory response is also a major defense for the host. It helps to heal wounds, control infection, and support the individual during stress. Inflammation is necessary for survival. If it is necessary but becomes excessive with severe illness, can we control the excess without interfering with what is needed? Natural reactions and substances produced by patients for controlling an excessive inflammatory response are being identified and evaluated. They include the antiinflammatory cytokinases, natural receptor antagonists, and bacterial permeability increasing BPIP protein to bind endotoxin. All biologic reactions have such feedback loops or control mechanisms. These substances have been or will be evaluated in patients. The importance of the stage at which a patient is in the proinflammatory state or the later antiinflammatory state is emphasized.

Can We Modulate Inflammation?

Can we fool Mother Nature by blocking, stimulating, or replacing the substances and abnormalities of an inflammatory response? So far the many clinical trials based on legitimate, important, basic research on proven substances to control sepsis

TABLE 57.1. Mediators of Injury, Inflammation, and Infection.

Platelet-activating factors
Endotoxin
Interleukins
Tumor necrosis factor
Cyclooxygenase metabolites
Bradykinin
Endorphins
Adhesion molecules
Nitric oxide
White blood cell products/elastase
Superoxide radicals
Complement

The explosion of knowledge about mediators of inflammation, injury, and infection has been impressive. These mediators are described in other chapters in this book and are summarized here. Antagonists to all of these substances have been produced as monoclonal antibodies, receptor anatagonists, or other enzymes or blocking agents; many have been tried clinically. Many of these agents and the trials have been reviewed by Neugebauer et al.[2]

or an excessive inflammatory response have all been negative. The endpoint in most if not all of these studies was mortality within 28 days. These trials included HA-1A monoclonal antibodies to endotoxin, J-5 monoclonal antibodies to entotoxin, antitumor necrosis factor (TNF) antibodies, an interleukin-1 (IL-1) receptor antagonist, soluble TNF receptors, a TNF receptor–fusion protein, platelet-activating factor antagonists, a bradykinin antagonist, taurolidine, antithrombin III concentrate, and interferon-γ (IFNγ). Dellinger[8] has reviewed these trials, questioning whether new trials based on post hoc analysis of a previous trial can be successful. Previous attempts have not succeeded.

Danner et al.,[9] Natanson et al.,[10] Suffredini et al.,[11] and Eichacker et al.[12] from the National Institutes of Health each presented papers at a recent shock forum in Vienna, Austria. They suggested that the therapeutic premise of benefit from inhibiting endotoxin or host inflammatory mediators in patients with sepsis or septic shock may be flawed and that inhibition of neutrophils by monoclonal antibodies to adhesion molecules may be deleterious. Inhibition of nitric oxide may produce more harm than good. Antiendotoxin strategies may work only if used before the insult. A monoclonal antibody to TNF protects against an injection of endotoxin (intravascular insult),[13] but anti-TNF monoclonal antibodies increase the mortality associated with peritonitis in animals (intraperitoneal infection).[14] IL-1 receptor antagonist (IL-1ra) and IL-1 in small doses protected animals from *Klebsiella pneumoniae*, whereas larger doses of IL-1ra increased lethality.[15] TNF and IL-1 are thought to produce many of the systemic manifestations of inflammation, but they are also necessary in certain circumstances. Cannon et al.[16] concluded that "the association of mortality for burned patients with low circulating IL-1β indicates that it is an essential mediator of host defense." Luger et al.[17] found that decreased serum IL-1 levels predicted death in patients with sepsis. Many other examples of such biologic conundrums exist. Thus the complexity and heterogeneity of the underlying disease processes and their life-threatening manifestations, the contradictory underlying pathologic processes, and the complex and redundant mediator–inflammatory system indicate that we have much to learn.

Suggestions for Future Studies

One recommendation is to use alternative or surrogate endpoints, such as a reduction in the severity of illness score, decreased intensive care unit (ICU) time, decreased time on a ventilator, and other evidence of clinical improvement. This is all well and good, but if the clinically improved patients die as frequently as the controls what have we accomplished?

Another recommendation was to perform randomized trials only in patients at high risk of dying, such as with a high Acute Physiology and Chronic Health Evaluation (APACHE III) score. Some believe that rapid identification of circulating endotoxin, gram-negative bacteremia, and other evidence of infection can help. I believe there is an even more important recommendation: to emphasize treating specific diseases in these trials, rather than just the inflammatory manifestations. The patient who has undergone multiple forms of trauma is different from the patient with a perforated ulcer or a perforated colon with peritonitis; and both are different from the patient with a urinary tract infection, pancreatitis, necrotizing pneumonia, or end-stage chronic obstructive pulmonary disease with pneumonia. The criticisms of my recommendation are that trials based on specific problems or diseases take longer and it is more difficult to accumulate a sufficient number of patients. This is true, but the present approach is not working. Most previous and successful "magic bullets," such as penicillin and smallpox vaccination, were slow in development, and all treated or prevented specific diseases (e.g., the poliomyelitis vaccine). On the other hand, nonspecific remedies, such as aspirin and nonsteroidal antiinflammatory agents, help patients feel better, but they do not cure or treat the disease. Another proposal is to consider multiagent therapy.

Multiple Therapeutic Agents for Other Diseases

There are many human diseases for which multiple agents are required for appropriate therapy. They include antituberculous therapy for tuberculosis, immunosuppression for transplanted organs, inotropes and diuretics for heart failure, multiple antibiotics for polymicrobial peritonitis, cancer chemotherapy, and support of the gastrointestinal tract. A review of several of these disease processes illustrates the difficulties and the evolution that occurred in therapy with multiple agents.

The development of chemotherapy for tuberculosis and its evolution over the years serves as an example of the problems even when dealing with a specific disease and one organism—which may be typical or atypical and may develop resistance to antibiotics. Waksman and colleagues isolated streptomycin in 1994.[18] It was found to be effective against tuberculosis in a small trial in 1945,[19] followed by a large national trial in 1947, with impressive clinical results.[20] It was immediately evident, however, that there was a high incidence of relapse and development of resistant organisms.[21] To counteract this effect, p-aminosalicylic acid (PAS), a drug that had mild tuberculostatic activity, was used in combination with streptomycin in a trial in 1948–1949.[22] PAS extended the time during which streptomycin could be administered without the bacteria developing resistance.

In 1950 a specific program by industry led to the development of a synthetic antituberculous agent called isonicotinic acid hydrazide (INH), or isoniazid. It was highly effective in vitro and was strikingly successful in patients in 1952.[23] It ushered in the modern era of chemotherapy. Other drugs were then developed.

The present recommended basic treatment for previously untreated patients with pulmonary tuberculosis is initial therapy with isoniazid, rifampin, and pyrazinamide given daily for 2 months followed by 4 months of isoniazid and rifampin.[24] Ethambutol can be added during the initial 2 months if there is any suspicion of resistance or if the patient is thought to be infected with human immunodeficiency virus (HIV).

Thus there has been a steady and continuing evolution of appropriate multiagent chemotherapy for tuberculosis. We are reminded, however, that tuberculosis is a single disease that primarily involves the lungs initially even though there are variations in the organism (e.g., from typical to atypical to resistant). Much of the development of successful treatment of tuberculosis was done by in vitro studies of the organism in culture and then trial and error clinically.[25,26] Also, each of the agents used in combination was effective for some time when used singly.

The development of cancer chemotherapy is another example of the complexities and difficulty of treating the manifestations and causes of human disease. Cancer chemotherapy was initially modeled after the multiagent treatment of tuberculosis. Paul Ehrlich coined the word "chemotherapy" at the turn of the century. He used rodent models of infectious diseases to develop antibiotics, which led Clowes at Roswell Park Memorial Institute during the early 1900s to develop inbred rodent lines to carry transplanted tumors to screen for potential anticancer drugs.[27]

The first modern chemotherapeutic agents were a product of a secret gas program in both World Wars. There was an explosion in Bari Harbor during World War II, and seamen were exposed to mustard gas, which caused bone marrow and lymphoid suppression.[28] This led to trials in patients with hematopoietic neoplasms such as Hodgkin's disease and lymphocytic lymphomas. Chemotherapy was first attempted at the Yale Cancer Center in 1943. Because of the secret nature of the wartime gas program, these results were not published until 1946.[29] Initially, there was great excitement because of regression of the neoplasms, but it was followed by discouragement because the tumors always grew back.

Farber then observed that folic acid accelerated leukemia, so folic acid antagonists were developed.[30] Early therapy for childhood leukemias and Hodgkin's disease was with combination chemotherapy. There was then a long period of trial and error, observation of chemotherapy failures, and many other problems. DeVita stated that, with some exceptions (choriocarcinoma and Burkitt's lymphoma), single drugs and standard doses do not cure cancer.[31] During the early years of chemotherapy, drug combinations were developed based on known biochemical actions of available anticancer drugs rather than on their clinical effectiveness. They were largely ineffective. DeVita stated that the era of effective combination chemotherapy began when an array of active drugs from different classes became available for use in combination for the treatment of leukemias and lymphomas.[31] He concluded that for multiagent cancer chemotherapy only drugs known to be partially effective against the same tumor when used alone should be selected for use in combination. The least toxic drugs should be used given in an optimal dose and schedule. The principle of cancer chemotherapy has been based on clinical trials designed and dominated by the use of alternating cycles of combination chemotherapy.[32]

The response to chemotherapy is affected by the biology of the tumors' growth, and all cancers are different. They respond to different agents. What is effective against one malignancy may do nothing for another. Malignancy is not a common denominator for therapy. Some tumors are hormone-dependent, some respond to radiation therapy, some respond to chemotherapy and various combinations, some respond to both, and some respond to operation with or without adjuvants. Staging and grade also have a lot to do with this. It is apparent now that permanent cure of malignancy is unusual, and the malignant setting in patients is important in terms of oncogeny influence, genetic mutations, and other factors.

The lessons learned from the treatment of tuberculosis and cancer indicate that specific diseases must be treated by a combination of agents, each of which has been shown to be effective individually in some way, shape, or form. In addition, these processes of infection and neoplasia are chronic; they are not immediate, acute, life-threatening problems. Treatment can be carried out over many weeks. There are many dissimilarities between the use of multiple chemotherapy for these diseases and the possibility of using agents for the control of acute inflammation and of acute, life-threatening systemic inflammatory response syndrome (SIRS), multiple organ dysfunction syndrome (MODs), and multiple organ failure (MOF).

Experimental Studies of Multiple Agents for Inflammation

Therapy for excessive inflammation could require control or replenishment of a number of agents shown in Table 57.2. Several years ago, Redl and Schlag hosted a shock conference in Vienna during which a number of speakers presented models for the use of multiple agents or multiple-component therapy for the treatment of sepsis and septic shock in critically ill surgical patients. Aasen and colleagues from Oslo, Norway, presented a study conducted in a pig model receiving endotoxin. They used a combination of three protease inhibitors (C1 inhibitor, antithrombin III, aprotinin) together with methylprednisolone,

TABLE 57.2. Therapy for Excessive Inflammation to Control Proinflammatory Mediators.

Endotoxin
Proinflammatory cytokines
Bradykinin
Proteinases
Oxygen radicals
Coagulation activation
Adhesion molecule expression
Complement activation
Cyclooxygenase and lipoxygenase activation
Histamine stimulation

naloxone, ketanserin, and promethazine.[33] This "cocktail" protected the animal against endotoxin-induced changes in the plasma enzyme cascade systems. At the same meeting Opal and colleagues from Brown University used an established infection model of *Pseudomonas* sepsis and treated the animals with a combination of a J-5 antisera, an opsonophagocytic monoclonal antibody (mAb), and an anti-TNF mAb.[34] They found that it provided significantly greater protection than single-component therapy.

Faist presented a hypothesis for a combined therapeutic strategy that included (1) global short-term (<72 hours) down-regulation of inflammatory monocyte activity and polymorphonuclear neutrophils (PMNs) by drugs such as pentoxifylline and IL-10 or IL-13; (2) prevention of excessive monocyte/macrophage stimulation by neutralization of circulating endotoxins with high-dose polyvalent receptors; and (3) upregulation of cell-mediated specific immune performance to overcome posttraumatic immune paralysis by administration of substances such as thymokinetic hormones [e.g., IFNγ and granulocyte colony-stimulating factor (G-CSF)].[35] This combination reflects a highly balanced view. At that conference Fischer suggested that a combination of agents could be helpful and should be evaluated.[36] He listed BPIP for its antiendotoxin effects, IL-1ra for its anticytokine effects, antithrombin III to protect against the coagulation cascade, and a complement inhibitor to decrease the complement cascade.

There have been more recent studies that may alter these hypotheses and proposals. For example, Mannick et al. found that a monoclonal antibody to IL-10 restored resistance to a septic challenge in an animal model.[37] Dalton et al. found that combined administration of IL-1ra and soluble tumor necrosis factor receptor (sTNF-r) decreased mortality and organ dysfunction in animals after hemorrhagic shock.[38]

Clinical Studies of Multiple Therapeutic Agents

Knox et al. used a combined chemotherapeutic regimen in burn patients in which they gave antioxidants, including vitamins C and E and glutamine, with an endotoxin binder (parenteral polymyxin B), a cyclo/lipoxygenase inhibitor (ibuprofen), and reconstituted human growth hormone.[39] They believe that this combination lowered the mortality rate based on a comparison with historical controls.

Kirton et al. use a three-arm strategy in trauma patients.[40] First, they block free radical production; next they provide scavengers; and then they bolster the patients' natural defenses by infusing mannitol, folate, hydrocortisone, selenium, lidocaine, polymyxin B, vitamin C, and Zantac. This phase is followed by a maintenance infusion of these substances and a gut formula given enterally containing glutamine, acetylcysteine, and vitamins A and E. In addition, they try to normalize gastric pH (pHi) by circulatory support. They believe that they have been able to maintain the same mortality rate with this regimen despite increased severity of injury in the trauma patients treated. They also used historical controls.

Gott et al. studied risk reduction with cardiopulmonary bypass in patients.[41] They found that pharmacologic and mechanical strategies to blunt the inflammatory response to cardiopulmonary bypass improved patient outcome significantly and were highly cost-effective. They used methylprednisolone, aprotinin, leukocyte filtration, and heparin-bonded circuitry.

A review of the randomized trials of agents evaluated for sepsis or SIRS (potential magic bullets) shows that there was some benefit for patients in some of the trials even though the 28-day mortality rate was not improved. I review only several examples here, although there are many others.

Supplementation of antithrombin III (AT III) in patients with severe sepsis did not improve overall mortality, although treated patients required fewer days of ventilatory support, spent less time in the ICU, and had decreased organ failure.[42] In another study, AT III resolved disseminated intravascular coagulation. The oxygenation index (PaO_2/FiO_2 ratio) improved, and pulmonary hypertension decreased.[43] There was also a decreased rise in serum bilirubin and decreased need for renal support therapy. Thus it is possible that several such agents could, when combined, provide overall benefits for patients. These treatments, however, are costly. What will be the result?

Potential hazards of combination immunotherapy were described by Opal et al., who gave a combination of anticytokines, aTNF-binding protein, and a recombinant human IL-1ra to a *Pseudomonas aeruginosa* model in neutropenic rats. This regimen resulted in death of all animals due to disseminated microabscesses.[44]

There are many difficulties when evaluating a multiagent therapeutic trial, particularly when we are dealing with injury, operation, sepsis, and inflammation and not a specific disease process. Whether anyone will ever be able to demonstrate the worthwhileness of a multiagent therapeutic approach remains to be determined. Certainly single agents that block various individual mediators have not been the answer.

Ideal Combinations of Agents

Because of the many mediators, each of which seems to have a role in the pathogenesis of excessive inflammation, it makes scientific sense to use multiple agents. If we tried to put together

TABLE 57.3. Agents Requiring Replenishment.

Antiinflammatory mediators
Antioxidants
Immunostimulators

an ideal combination of agents for excessive inflammation, what would be the components? Certainly, early on in the disease process some attempts to block proinflammatory mediators (Table 57.2) should be worthwhile. Soon thereafter supplemental antiinflammatory mediators seem necessary (Table 57.3).

Included should be control of the many enzyme cascades that are activated by shock, trauma, or infection (Table 57.4). How many of these it is necessary or important (or even possible) to block is not known. How do we begin to formulate such an approach? What is the timing? What is the cost? If the multiagent cocktail becomes beneficial, what ingredients are critical? Some may be ineffective.

What is the model on which to test such approaches? One example is the sheep model developed by Dwenger et al.[45] The models were reviewed by Redl et al.[46] A baboon model in the final development stage could be helpful for multiagent testing.[46] Would that fill the bill? Perhaps so, or do we also need new "multiple models" to cope with a "two- or multiple-hit" theory as suggested.[47] In any case, it is difficult to prepare a sufficient multidimensional protocol for such a study. We are told that the Food and Drug Administration (FDA) in the United States would probably not approve a multiagent

TABLE 57.4. Control of Enzyme Cascades Activated by Shock, Trauma, and Infection.

Control of proinflammatory mediators
  Scavenging of inducers
  Endotoxin, recombinant bacterial permeability inhibitor$_{21}$ (rBPI$_{21}$)
  Proinflammatory mediator blockade
  Interleukin-1 receptor antagonist (IL-1ra)
  Soluble tumor necrosis factor receptor (sTNFr)
  Anti-TNF monoclonal antibody (mAb): to restore function

Supplementation of antiinflammatory agents
  IL-10: to reduce inflammation
  IL-12, IL-13
  Anti-IL-10 mAb to restore immune function
  Recombinant high density lipoprotein (rHDL)
  Antioxidants
  Protease inhibitors
  Tissue factor pathway inhibitor

Cascade control
  Coagulation: antithrombin III (AT III)
  Complement inhibitor
  Cyclooxygenase and lipoxygenase inhibition: ibuprofen
  Histamine antagonist
  Bradykinin antagonist

Control of other factors
  Platelet-activating factor (PAF) antagonist
  Immunomodulators: drugs, diet
  Antiadhesion agents

TABLE 57.5. Individual Therapies.

Pentoxifylline
AT III in septic patients
Enteral immunonutrition
High DO$_2$ and VO$_2$ in sick patients
Nitric oxide synthase with severe sepsis
G-CSF in septic patients
Omeprazole suspension
In-line heat moisture-exchange filter and heated wire
  humidifiers in patients on ventilators

Each therapy modality provides some improvement in sick patients in an ICU but may not by itself change the mortality rate.
AT III, antithrombin III; DO$_2$, VO$_2$, delivery and utilization of oxygen; G-CSF, granulocyte colony-stimulating factor.

approach. However, all of the agents used by Demling's group,[39] and Kirton et al.[40] are already approved prescription drugs or are over-the-counter drugs. Does that allow them to be used in a multiagent cocktail without informed consent? I know of no opinion regarding that possibility. Perhaps a trial in Europe would help. In the meanwhile, we may learn more from the use of multiple agents in animal studies.

Other therapeutic contributions make good sense clinically, but the evidence is divided over the worthiness of the effort (Table 57.5). They may help in some patients. Some of them are also controversial, with some trials indicating clinical improvement and others failing to document such changes (Table 57.6). Some may improve a patient's condition but not decrease mortality. None has been accepted universally. All of the protocols have active supporters and some distractors. For example, in a randomized trial of early enteral nutrition in patients having major operations Heslin et al.[48] found no benefit, whereas Braga et al. in a randomized trial after abdominal surgery[49] and Bryg and Beale in a meta-analysis found that enriched enteral nutrition decreased the severity of infection, length of hospital stay, and days on a ventilator—but there was no change in mortality.[50] Immediate postoperative enteral feeding may decrease mobility and impair respiratory mechanics. In general, most believe that early immune-enhanced enteral feeding is worthwhile when tolerated by the patient.

Measurement of gastric intramucosal pH (pHi) has been found to be helpful in resuscitation and patient care, but it is cumbersome to use and has not been universally adopted. Those who have used this monitoring technique have found it helpful for improving blood flow to the gut (perhaps microcirculatory flow) and outcome. Increasing the pHi to normal has been associated with decreased mortality.[51,52] The use of air in the balloon rather than saline has made the technique much easier (see Chapter 25).

Another example is the result of a randomized phase III trial of inhaled nitric oxide (NO) for patients with acute respiratory distress syndrome (ARDS). Dellinger et al. found that NO was well tolerated and produced a significant improvement in oxygenation (PaO$_2$) (>20%) in 60% of patients, but there was no change in overall mortality or in the number of days alive

TABLE 57.6. Therapy That Is Controversial When Used in All ICU Patients but Is Sometimes Useful in Certain Situations.

Therapy	Purpose
Selective gut decontamination	Acute liver failure, burns, pancreatitis
Inhaled NO	Certain patients with ARDS
Intraoperative maintenance of tissue perfusion	Prevents ARDS in surgical patients
Protective ventilation strategy	Improved weaning
Avoiding ranitidine	May increase infections
Lexipafant (PAF antagonist)	Acute pancreatitis
Venovenous hemofiltration	Septic patients
Inhaled NO	Patients with ARDS after pulmonary resection
ECMO	End-stage ARDS
rhGH	Short bowel syndrome
rhG-CSF	Septic patients with neutropenia
Partial liquid ventilation	Trauma patients
N-Acetylcysteine	Acute lung injury
Avoid hypothermia	Decreases mortality with trauma, and wound infections after abdominal operations
rBPI	After liver resection
Enalaprilat	Improves gut perfusion in injured patients
Selenium	Improves clinical outcome and decreases acute renal failure
PGE_1	May decrease mortality in trauma patients
Plasma C1 INH (complement inhibitor)	Patients seem improved
Ventilation with (1) prone position, (2) kinetic therapy bed, (3) rotational therapy	Alleviates ARDS
Lysophyline	Protects with IL-2 therapy and after bone marrow transplants
Hypertonic 7.5% saline and/or 6% dextran 70	Resuscitation particularly with head injury patients

No, nitric oxide; PAF, platelet-activating factor; ECMO, extracorporeal membrane oxygenation; rhGH, recombinant human growth hormone; rhG-CSF, recombinant human granulocyte colony-stimulating factor; PGE_1, prostaglandin E_1; ARDS, acute respiratory distress syndrome; IL-2, interleukin-2; rBPI recombinant bacterial permeability inhibitor.

and off mechanical ventilation.[53] The same results were also seen in surgical patients. One editorialist group described it as a negative study,[54] whereas Zapol described the results as potentially positive.[55] He urged the use of NO in patients with ventilatory failure alone (no other problems). This raises the question as to whether ARDS is truly a syndrome—it is not a disease. Perhaps some diseases that produce respiratory failure are susceptible to inhaled NO and others are not. It is worth a try.

Mathisen et al. have reported the early use of inhaled NO in patients developing ARDS after lung resection (a more homogeneous group).[56] Previously the mortality in their experience was 85.7%. With NO, the PaO_2/FiO_2 ratio and chest radiographs improved progressively in all patients. Seven of the ten patients survived. The three who died had sepsis, and none died of ARDS. Patients with ARDS who require ventilator support seem to benefit from rotational kinetic therapy and positioning in a prone position from time to time. Other ventilator strategies that seem to help include inverse-ratio ventilation and permissive hypercapnia.

Patients who achieve adequate or high oxygen transport (DO_2) and oxygen consumption (VO_2) after an injury or operation or with an illness are said to be more likely to survive.[57] Some believe that if a treatment can drive oxygen transport and oxygen consumption to supernormal values, the chances of survival are increased. Others have found evidence to the contrary. All in all, if one is sick it is better to have high DO_2 and VO_2 unless it is artificially increased by catecholamines.[58] It has been known for many years that patients after injury, after operation, or with sepsis must be able to increase the cardiac index to survive.

Hypertonic solutions (saline-dextran) have been found to be of great benefit in animal experiments[59] and of some benefit in clinical trials. However, the benefit has not been enough to recommend that they be used commonly or routinely.[60] The same is true for synthetic colloids such as pentastarch, which is safe and efficient and reduces intravenous volumes required for resuscitation.[61] One situation where hypertonic solutions may be of value is in patients with head injury.[62] Such solutions do not increase intracranial pressure and, in fact, tend to decrease it. Whether the use of hypertonic solutions for resuscitating trauma patients would result in a more rapid increase in microcirculatory blood flow and improve their overall situation has not been established.[63]

Thangathurai et al. maintained intraoperative tissue perfusion by nitroglycerin and fluids in high risk patients.[64] None of 155 such patients developed ARDS. This is a promising, physiologic approach to patient care and requires verification.

Pentoxifylline has a number of admirable qualities demonstrated in experimental animals, such as restoring cardiac performance and tissue perfusion and decreasing susceptibility to sepsis. Thus it should be worthwhile clinically. Two clinical trials have suggested some hemodynamic improvement, such as increased DO_2 and VO_2.[65,66] Whether these changes are enough for this agent to be used more widely remains to be determined.

Some have found selective gut decontamination to be worthwhile in general ICU patients, whereas others have found no benefit in trauma ICU patients. Sun et al., in an meta-analysis, suggested that the possibility that this therapy reduces mortality is significantly better in patients with a high mortality risk at study entry.[67] Selective gut decontamination seems to be therapy in search of the right patient. When this modality was used in patients with specific disease processes, such as acute pancreatitis where gut bacteria may play a role, there was reduced mortality and general improvement.[68] Baxby et al. reviewed the 13-year history of selected decontamination in 46 trials. They recommended treating specific problems: patients with liver disease or burns and medical patients after some days in the ICU on mechanical ventilation.[69]

Extracorporeal membrane oxygenation (ECMO) has allowed survival of some patients with severe respiratory failure who were not improved by other means. These patients would certainly have died otherwise.[70]

Hirasawa et al. continue to use hemodiafiltration in ICU patients.[71] They found decreased cytokine mediators and an improved respiratory index and tissue oxygenation in patients with ARDS who received this treatment. Honore et al. also reported benefit from this therapy.[72]

There are many other experiences and therapies that could be cited and may be worthwhile. In this survey, I have given some examples and have not tried to be exhaustive in reviewing them. Are these studies then negative or positive? Some help is provided but not enough to decrease the death rate in the treated patient. I now favor another interpretation. In complex clinical situations and in very sick patients, adjunctive or supplementary therapy may help the patient but it requires more than a single intervention to improve mortality. It is also possible that such an intervention is helpful in a certain group of patients but not in others. If you spread too wide a net for entry into a study, the results may be negative because of so many different disease processes in sick patients in the study.

Conclusions and Recommendations

I recommend that we study what agent or agents help with certain clinical problems, situations, or diseases, such as burns, pancreatitis, multiple trauma, peritonitis, and ventilator-associated pneumonia. In addition, we must distinguish septic shock with gram-negative organisms from that with gram-positive organisms and fungus infections. We must distinguish ARDS patients with chronic obstructive pulmonary disease from patients with ARDS after thoracic surgery, patients after chest trauma, and other medical patients with ARDS. There are many questions that arise and must be answered. Treating sick patients by nonspecific therapy for their disease or diseases has not helped. We have learned that lesson.

References

1. Thomas L: Adaptive Aspects of Inflammation Symposium of the International Inflammation Club. Kalamazoo, Upjohn, 1970.
2. Neugebauer E, Rixen D, Raum M, Schafer U: Thirty years of antimediator treatment in sepsis and septic shock: what have we learned? Langenbecks Arch Surg 1998;383:26–34.
3. Baue AE: Multiple organ failure, multiple organ dysfunction syndrome and systemic inflammatory response syndrome: Why no magic bullets? Arch Surg 1997;132:703–707.
4. Dhainaut J, Tenaillon A, Hemmer M, et al: Confirmatory platelet-activating factor receptor antagonist trial in patients with severe gram-negative bacterial sepsis: a phase III, randomized, double-blind, placebo-controlled, multicenter trial. Crit Care Med 1998;26:1963–1972.
5. Natanson C, Esposito CJ, Banks SM: The sirens songs of confirmatory sepsis trials: selection bias and sampling error. Crit Care Med 1998;26:1927–1932.
6. Ehrlich P, Morganroth J: Ueber Hamolysins: Füntte Mittheilung. Berl Klin Wochenschr 1901;38:251–257.
7. Baue AE: The horror autotoxicus and multi-organ failure. Arch Surg 1992;127:1451–1462.
8. Dellinger RP: Post hoc analyses in sepsis trials: a formula for disappoinment? Crit Care Med 1996;24:727–729.
9. Danner RL, Cobb JP, Suffredini AF, Eichacker PO, Natanson C: Nitric oxide in sepsis: role in inflammation and shock. Shock 1995;3(Suppl):61–62.
10. Natanson C, Eichacker PO, Suffredini AF, Danner DL: Selected treatment strategies for septic shock based on proposed mechanisms of pathogenesis. Shock 1995;3(Suppl):62.
11. Suffredini AF, Natanson C, Danner RL, Suffredini AF: The neutrophil as a therapeutic target in septic shock. Shock 1995;3(Suppl):62–63.
12. Eichacker PO, Natanson C, Danner RL, Suffredini AF: The neutrophil as a therapeutic target in septic shock. Shock 1995;3(Suppl):62–63.
13. Tracey KJ, Fung Y, Hesse KR, et al: Anti-cachectin/TNF monoclonal antibodies prevent septic shock during letal bacteremia. Nature 1987;330:662–664.
14. Echtenacher B, Falk W, Mannel DN, Krammer PH: Requirement of endogenous tumor necrosis factor/cachectic for recovery from experimental peritonitis. J Immunol 1990;145:3762–3766.
15. Mancilla J, Garcia P, Dinarello CA: The interleukin-1 receptor antagonist can either reduce or enhance the lethality of Klebsiella pneumonia sepsis in newborn rats. Infect Immun 1993;61:926–932.
16. Cannon JG, Friedberg JS, Gelfand JA, et al: Circulating interleukin-1 beta and tumor necrosis factor-alpha concentrations after burn injury in humans. Crit Care Med 1992;20:1414–1419.
17. Luger A, Graf H, Schwartz H-P, Stummvoll H-K, Luger TA: Decreased serum interleukin 1 activity and monocyte interleukin 1 production in patients with fatal sepsis. Crit Care Med 1986;14:458–461.
18. Schatz A, Bugie E, Waksman SA: Streptomycin, a substance exhibiting antibiotic activity against gram-positive and gram-negative bacteria. Proc Soc Exp Biol Med 1944;4:66–69.
19. Hinshaw HC, Feldman WH: Streptomycin in treatment of clinical tuberculosis: a preliminary report. Proc Staff Meet Mayo Clin 1945;20:313–318.
20. Hinshaw HC, Plye MM, Feldman WH: Streptomycin in tuberculosis. Am J Med 1947;2:429–435.
21. McDermott W, Muschenheim C, Hadley SJ, et al: Streptomycin in the treatment of tuberculosis in humans. Ann Intern Med 1947;27:769–822.
22. Medical Research Council: Treatment of pulmonary tuberculosis with streptomycin and para-aminosalicylic acid. BMJ 1950;2:1073–1085.
23. Robitzek EH, Selikoff IJ: Hydrazine derivative of isonicotinic acid (Rimifon, Marsalid) in the treatment of acute progressive caseous-pneumonic tuberculosis: a preliminary report. Am Rev Tuberc 1952;65:402–428.
24. Committee on Treatment, International Union Against Tuberculosis and Lung Disease: Antituberculosis regimens of chemotherapy. Bull Int Un Tuberc Lung Dis 1988;63:60–64.
25. Tuberculosis Unit, Division of Communicable Diseases, World Health Organization: Guidelines for tuberculosis treatment in adults and children in national tuberculosis programs. World Health Organization 1991;WHO/TB91:161.
26. MacGregor RR: Treatment of myobacterial disease of the lungs caused by mycobacterium tuberculosis. In: A Fishman (ed) Pulmonary Diseases and Disorders. New York, McGraw-Hill, 1993;1869–1882.

27. Marchall EK Jr: Historical perspectives in chemotherapy. In: Golden A, Hawking IF (eds) Advances in Chemotherapy, vol 1. San Diego, Academic, 1964;1.
28. Alexander SF: Final report of Bari mustard casualties. Allied Force Headquarters, Office of the Surgeon. APO 512, June 20, 1944.
29. DeVita VA: The evolution of therapeutic research in cancer. N Engl J Med 1978;298:807.
30. DeVita VT Jr: Principles of cancer management: chemotherapy. In: DeVita VT Jr, Hellman S, Rosenberg SA (eds) Cancer Principles & Practice of Oncology, 5th ed, vol 1. Philadelphia, Lippincott-Raven, 1997;333–339.
31. DeVita VT Jr: The evolution of therapeutic research in cancer. Sounding Boards 1978;298:907–910.
32. DeVita VT Jr, Schein PS: Medical progress: the use of drugs in combination for the treatment of cancer, rationale and results. N Engl J Med 1973;288:988–1006.
33. Aasen AO, Naess E, Carlse H, et al: [abstract]. Shock 1995;3 (Suppl):65. Multi-agent therapy to protect against endotoxin.
34. Opal S, Cross AS, Sadoff JC, et al: Combined immunotherapy in the treatment of septic shock [abstract]. Shock 1995;3(Suppl):65.
35. Faist E: Immunomodulatory approaches in critically ill surgical patients [abstract]. Shock 1995;3(Suppl):65–66.
36. Fischer C: Unpublished discussion. Fifth Vienna Shock Forum, May 7–11, 1995.
37. Mannick JA, Lyons A, Kelly J, et al: Major injury induces increased production of IL-10 by cells of the immune system with a negative impact on resistance to infection. Ann Surg (in press).
38. Dalton JM, Gore DC, DeMaria EJ, et al: Combined administration of interleukin-1 receptor antagonist (IL-IRA) and soluble tumor necrosis factor receptor (STNF-R) decreases mortality and organ dysfunction following hemorrhagic shock. J Trauma (in press).
39. Knox J, Demling R, Wilmore D, et al: Increased survival after major thermal injury: the effect of growth hormone therapy in adults. J Trauma 1995;39:526–530.
40. Kirton O, Windsor J, Civetta JOV, et al: Persistent uncorrected intramucosal pH in the critically injured: the impact of splanchnic and antioxidant therapy [abstract]. Crit Care Med 1996;24:A82.
41. Gott JP, Cooper FE, Schmidt, et al: Documentation of risk naturalization for extracorporeal circulation in four limbed, 400 patient, risk stratified, prospective, randomized trial. J Surg Res
42. Fourrier F, Chopin C, Huart JJ, et al: Double-blind, placebo-controlled trial of antithrombin III concentrates in septic shock with disseminated intravascular coagulation. Chest 1993;104: 882–888.
43. Inthorn D, Hoffmann JN, Hartl WH, et al: Antithrombin III supplementation in severe sepsis: beneficial effects on organ dysfunction. Shock 1997;8:328–334.
44. Opal SM, Cross A, Jhung W, et al: Potential hazards of combination immunotherapy in the treatment of experiment septic shock. J Infect Dis 1996;173:1415–1421.
45. Dwenger A, Remmers D, Gratz M, et al: Aprotinin prevents the development of the trauma-induced multiple organ failure in a chronic sheep model. Eur J Clin Chem Clin Biochem 1996;30:204–214.
46. Redl H, Schlag G, Bahrami S, Yao YM: Animal models as the basis of pharmacologic intervention in trauma and sepsis patients. World J Surg 1996;20:487–492.
47. Moore E, Moore F, Franciose R, et al: The postischemic gut severes as a priming bed for circulating neutrophils that provoke multiple organ failure. J Trauma 1994;37:881.
48. Heslin MJ, Latkany L, Leung D, et al: A prospective: randomized trial of early enteral feeding after resection of upper GI malignancy. Ann Surg (in press).
49. Braga M, Gianotti L, Vignali A, et al: Artificial nutrition after major abdominal surgery: impact of route of administration and composition of the diet. Crit Care Med 1998;26:24–30.
50. Bryg DJ, Beale RJ: Clinical effects of enteral immunonutrition on intensive care patients: a meta-analysis. Crit Care Med 1998;26:A91.
51. Ivatury RR, Simon RJ, Islam S, et al: A prospective randomized study of end points of resuscitation after major trauma. J Am Coll Surg 1998;183:145–154.
52. Ljubanovic M, Calvin J, Peruzzi W: Meta-analysis of gastric pH as determinant of mortality in critically ill patients. Crit Care Med 1998;26:A123.
53. Dellinger RP, Zimmerman JL, Taylor RW, et al: Effects of inhaled nitric oxide in patients with acute respiratory distress syndrome: results of a randomized phase II trial. Crit Care Med 1998;26:15–23.
54. Mattay MA, Pittet JF, Jayr C: Just say NO to inhaled nitric oxide for the acute respiratory distress syndrome. Crit Care Med 1998;26:1–2.
55. Zapol WM: Nitric oxide inhalation in acute respiratory distress syndrome: it works, but can we prove it? Crit Care Med 1998; 26:2–3.
56. Mathisen DJ, Kuo EY, Hahn C, et al: Inhaled nitric oxide for adult respiratory distress syndrome following pulmonary resection. Ann Thorac Surg (in press).
57. Shoemaker WC, Appel PL, Kram HB, et al: Prospective trial of supranormal values of survivors as therapeutic goals in high-risk surgical patients. Chest 1988;94:1176–1188.
58. Durham RM, Neunaber K, Mazuski JE, et al: The use of oxygen consumption and delivery as endpoints for resuscitation in critically ill patients. J Trauma 1996;41:32–40.
59. Moore EE: Hypertonic saline dextran for post-injury resuscitation: experimental background and clinical experience. Aust NZ J Surg 1991;61:732–736.
60. Wade CE, Kramer GC, Grady JJ, et al: Efficacy of hypertonic 7.5% saline and 6% dextran-70 in treating trauma: a meta-analysis of controlled clinical studies. Surgery 1997;122:609–616.
61. Younes RN, Yin KC, Amino CJ, et al: Use of pentastarch solution in the treatment of patients with hemorrhagic hypovolemia: randomized phase II study in the emergency room. Word J Surg 1998;22:2–5.
62. Shackford SR, Bourguignon PR, Wald SL, et al: Hypertonic saline resuscitation of patients with head injury: a prospective, randomized clinical trial. J Trauma 1998;44:50–58.
63. Vassar JJ, Perry CA, Gannaway WL, et al: 7.5% Sodium chloride/ dextran for resuscitation of trauma patients undergoing helicopter transport. Arch Surg 1991;16:1065–1072.
64. Thangathurai D, Charbonnet C, Wo CCJ, et al: Intraoperative maintenance of tissue perfusion prevents ARDS. New Horiz 1996;4:466–474.
65. Wang P, Wheng FB, Zhou M, et al: Pentoxifylline restores cardiac output and tissue perfusion after trauma-hemorrhage and decreases susceptibility to sepsis. Surgery 1993;114:3520–3539.
66. Bacher A, Mayer N, Klimscha W, et al: Effects of pentoxifylline on hemodynamics and oxygenation in septic and nonseptic patients. Crit Care Med 1997;25:795–800.
67. Sun X, Wagner DP, Knaus WA: Does selective decontamination of the digestive tract reduce mortality for severely ill patients? Crit Care Med 1996;24:753–755.

68. Luiten EJ, Hop WCJ, Lange JF, Bruining HA: Controlled clinical trial of selective decontamination for the treatment of severe acute pancreatitis. Ann Surg 1995;222:57–65.
69. Baxby D, van Saene HKKF, Stoutenbeek CP, Zandstra DF: Selective decontamination of the digestive tract: 13 years on, what it is and what it is not. Intensive Care Med 1996;22:699–706.
70. Kolla S, Awad SS, Rich PB, et al: Extracorporeal life support for 100 adult patients with severe respiratory failure. Ann Surg 1997;226:544–566.
71. Hirasawa H, SugaI T, Oda S, et al: Continuous hemodiafiltration (Chdf) removes cytokine and improves respiratory index (Ri) and oxygen metabolism in patients with acute respiratory distress syndrome (ARDS). Crit Care Med 1998;26:A120.
72. Honore PM, James J, Wauthier M, et al: Reversal of intractable circulatory failure complicating septic shock with short time high volume haemofiltration (ST-HV-CWH) after failure of conventional therapy: a prospective evaluation. Crit Care 1998;2:62.

# 58
Maximizing Oxygen Delivery and Consumption: In Whom and For Whom?

Robert F. Wilson and James G. Tyburski

The importance of promptly providing optimal oxygen delivery to critically ill or injured patients, especially those who have been in shock, is based primarily on three observations: (1) during severe trauma or illness (especially with shock or any other impairment of tissue perfusion) an oxygen debt develops, and it is best treated by promptly providing extra oxygen to the tissues; (2) sepsis, surgery, trauma, and other critical illnesses are often hypermetabolic, and increased oxygen is needed; and (3) following shock and during many illnesses, especially sepsis, there is a shift of blood flow away from splanchnic organs, and these splanchnic perfusion deficits can often be corrected only by supplying more blood flow and oxygen than normal to the body as a whole.

Early Evidence That Improving Oxygen Transport Variables Is Beneficial

The hemodynamic effects of dibenzyline in clinical shock were reported in 1964.[1] Of three patients whose cardiac index was raised to 4.0 L/min/m² or more, two (67%) survived; and all six who did not achieve this cardiac index died ($p = 0.083$).

In a 1965 description of high cardiac output during septic shock (which was virtually unknown at the time), the survival rate was 75% (6/8) among patients with a cardiac index of 3.6 L/min/m² or more and 43% (10/23) among those with a lower cardiac index ($p = 0.220$).[2]

In 1972 we reported 100 critically ill patients in whom we directly measured oxygen consumption (by expired gas analysis). Of 46 patients who had an oxygen consumption (VO_2) more than 110% of the theoretic normal value calculated by age, sex, height, and weight, 29 (63%) survived; and of 20 with a VO_2 < 90% of normal, only 4 (20%) survived ($p = 0.001$).[3] Everyone with a VO_2I persistently < 100 ml/min/m² died.

During the 1970s Shoemaker and colleagues[4–6] reviewed the physiologic patterns of survivors and nonsurvivors in varying degrees of postoperative shock. In all of these studies, the survivors had significantly higher oxygen delivery (DO_2) and higher VO_2.

During the 1980s Shoemaker and colleagues[7,8] reported on large numbers of patients (300 and 220, respectively) with general surgical operations for life-threatening conditions. They repeatedly found that the highest survival rates were seen with a hematocrit of 33–40%, cardiac index > 4.0 L/min/m², DO_2 > 550 ml/min/m², and VO_2 > 140 ml/min/m².

In a 1985 study of 20 septic patients reported by Haupt et al.,[9] 8 patients responded to fluid loading with an increase in VO_2 (to 167 ± 15 ml/min/m²), five (63%) survived; and of the 12 who did not achieve an increase in VO_2, only 5 (42%) survived ($p = 0.650$). In another study on 42 pediatric patients with septic shock, Pollack et al.[10] noted that the survival rate was 75% (6/8) for a VO_2I of > 200 ml/min/m², 48% (10/21) with a VO_2I of 120–200, and 22% (2/9) with a VO_2I of < 120 ($p = 0.046$).

In 1987 Hankeln et al.[11] reported on 30 patients in shock. The final data in the 14 survivors (versus the 16 nonsurvivors) included a cardiac index of 4.6 ± 1.0 versus 3.61.1 L/min/m² ($p = 0.015$), DO_2I of 705 ± 143 versus 523 ± 152 ml/min/m² ($p = 0.002$), and VO_2I of 209 ± 77 versus 158 ± 31 ml/min/m² ($p = 0.021$).

In 1989 Edwards et al.,[12] from Manchester (UK), presented data on the use of therapeutic goals in septic shock in 29 patients, 14 of whom died. They noted that increases in DO_2 from 605 ± 245 (SD) to 843 ± 145 ml/min/m² were associated with increases in VO_2 from 130 ± 37 to 169 ± 33 ml/min/m² ($p < 0.001$). That same year Tuchschmidt et al.[13] reported on a retrospective study of patients with septic shock. Significant differences at 48 hours between 40 survivors (and 24 nonsurvivors) were in the cardiac index [4.1 ± 1.6 (SD) vs. 3.0 ± 1.2 L/min/m²] and DO_2 (15.6 ± 4.4 vs. 12.7 ± 3.9 ml/min/kg).

Scalea et al.[14] in 1990 reported on a study of 30 severely injured surgical patients who were more than 65 years of age. The major difference between the optimized values in the 17 who lived and the 13 who died was a cardiac output of 6.6 L/min versus 4.6 L/min (SD not given). They also noted that starting aggressive optimization, primarily with fluids and blood, within the first 1–2 hours of arrival in the emergency department was important for survival.

In a 1991 study of the change in oxygen transport induced with blood volume expanders, Shoemaker et al.[15] found that 500 ml of whole blood increased the DO_2 by an average of 78 ± 15 ml/min/m² and the VO_2 by 20 ± 6 ml/min/m². Two units of packed red blood cells (in spite of the increased viscosity) increased the DO_2 by 63 ± 20 ml/min/m² and the VO_2 by 11 ± 6 ml/min/m². A 100 ml bolus of 25% albumin increased the DO_2 by 26 ± 12 ml/min/m² and the VO_2 by 10 ± 4 ml/min/m², with the maximum changes generally occurring 45 minutes after the infusion.

Oxygen Debt

In 1932 Cuthbertson,[16] using indirect calorimetry, noted that the VO_2 was decreased in patients shortly after multiple long bone fractures but subsequently increased above normal. Crowell and Smith[17] and Guyton and Crowell[18] calculated cumulative VO_2 deficits in dogs subjected to hemorrhagic shock; they found essentially no mortality when the cumulative VO_2 deficit was <100 ml/kg, 50% mortality when the VO_2 deficit was 120 ml/kg, and > 95% mortality when the VO_2 deficit was >140 ml/kg.

In an evaluation of sequential VO_2 patterns in critically ill patients it was noted that VO_2 often falls before hypotension develops. If treatment is successful, though, there is a compensatory increase in VO_2 during the first day or two postoperatively.[4,8,19,20]

Shoemaker et al.[21] reported on cumulative tissue oxygen debts during and immediately after 100 consecutive high-risk surgical operations in 98 patients. The tissue VO_2 deficit was calculated as the measured VO_2 minus the estimated VO_2 requirements; the net cumulative VO_2 deficit was calculated as the integrated area under a VO_2 deficit–time curve. The maximum cumulative VO_2 deficit averaged 33.5 ± 36.9 (SD) L/m² in 21 nonsurvivors with organ failure, 26.8 ± 32.1 L/m² in 21 survivors with organ failure, and 8.0 ± 10.9 L/m² in 56 survivors without organ failure.

In a similar 1992 study, Shoemaker et al.[22] reported on 253 high risk patients. The 64 patients who died all had organ failure, and their maximum cumulative VO_2 deficit averaged 33.2 ± 32.0 L/m² (SD). For the 31 survivors with organ failure, the cumulative VO_2 deficit averaged 21.6 ± 20.6 L/m² ($p < 0.05$); whereas for the 158 survivors without organ failure or major complications, the maximum cumulative VO_2 deficit averaged 9.2 ± 16.3 L/m² ($p < 0.05$).

In 1993 Kreymann et al.[23] reported a study that measured VO_2 by expiratory gas analysis for 118 treatment days in 30 septic patients. They noted that as sepsis became more severe and progressed to septic shock there was a progressive decrease in VO_2, resulting in an increasing oxygen debt. In 15 patients with sepsis the mean VO_2 was 180 ± 19 (SD) ml/min/m²; in 11 patients with sepsis syndrome it was 156 ± 22 ml/min/m²; and in 8 patients with septic shock it was 120 ± 27 ml/min/m² ($p < 0.001$). Oxygen extraction (VO_2/DO_2) was highest with sepsis (0.39), next highest (0.33) with sepsis syndrome, and lowest (0.29) with septic shock.

Prospective O_2 Transport Studies

Randomized Studies

In a landmark study published in 1988 Shoemaker et al.[24] randomized 88 patients to have either central venous pressure (CVP) monitoring (30 patients), pulmonary artery wedge pressure (PAWP) monitoring without pursuing supernormal values (PA-control group, 30 patients), and a PA-protocol group in whom the goals of therapy were optimization of O_2 transport variables with a PA catheter (28 patients). The PA-protocol group was to be given fluid, blood, or inotropes (or a combination) until the cardiac index was >4.5 L/min/m², $DO_2 > 600$ ml/min/m², and $VO_2 > 170$ ml/min/m² (Table 58.1). Following these resuscitations, the combined CVP and PA-control groups (versus the PA-protocol group) had a significantly increased mortality rate (27% vs. 4%) and significantly increased complication rate (50% vs. 28%) ($p < 0.001$) (Table 58.2).

In 1990 Shoemaker et al.[25] combined the data from two clinical trials. Of 490 control patients from the two clinical trials, 142 (29%) died, a rate similar to the 30% mortality (32/107) of the preoperatively monitored PA-control patients. In contrast,

TABLE 58.1. Therapeutic Goals in Three Groups of High Risk Surgical Patients.

	Therapeutic goals		
Parameter	CVP	PA-control group	PA-protocol group
No. of patients	30	30	28
Blood pressure	>120/80	>120/80	>120/80
CVP (cmH₂O)	4–12	4–12	<15
PAWP (mmHg)	—	4–12	<18
Hematocrit (%)	>35	>35	>34
CI (L/min/m²)	—	2.8–3.5	>4.5
DO₂ (ml/min/m²)	—	400–550	>600
VO₂ (ml/min/m²)	—	120–140	>170

Adapted from Shoemaker et al.,[24] with permission.
CVP, central venous pressure; PAWP, pulmonary arterial wedge pressure; CI, cardiac index; DO₂, VO₂, oxygen delivery and utilization volumes.

TABLE 58.2. Results of Randomized Study.

	Complications		
Parameter	CVP	PA-control group	PA-protocol group
No. of patients	30	30	28
No. of deaths	7 (23%)	11 (37%)	1 (4%)*
Patients with complications	15 (50%)	15 (50%)	8 (28%)*
Patients with sepsis	6 (20%)	9 (30%)	0*

Adapted from Shoemaker et al.,[24] with permission.
See table 58.1 for abbreviations.
*$p < 0.01$.

the mortality rates of the PA-protocol patients from the two trials were only 14% and 4%, respectively ($p < 0.05$).

In another randomized study by the Shoemaker group, Fleming et al.[26] prospectively tested the effect of the early postinjury attainment of supranormal values. The cardiac index was significantly higher in the protocol group at 16 hours, the DO_2I higher at 16 and 48 hours, and the VO_2I significantly higher at 24 and 48 hours.

Eight (24%) of the protocol patients died, as did fifteen (44%) of the control patients ($p = 0.123$).[25] The protocol patients also had fewer mean (± SD) organ failures per patient (0.76 ± 1.21 vs. 1.59 ± 1.60) ($p = 0.02$).

Gutierrez et al.[27] studied 260 patients admitted to the intensive care unit (ICU) with Acute Physiology and Chronic Health Evaluation (APACHE II) scores of 15–25. The patients were randomly assigned to a control or protocol group. These groups were then subdivided according to the initial gastric intramural pH (pHi) to a normal group (pHi 7.35 or more) or low pHi group (pH < 7.35). The control groups in each pHi group were treated according to standard ICU practice. The protocol group was treated to increase the systemic oxygen transport or reduce the oxygen demand (or both) if the pHi fell below 7.35 or fell by more than 0.10 unit from the previous measurement. Among the protocol group, with normal or increased pHi on admission, the pHi fell in 67 (85%). For patients who had a low pHi initially, survival was similar in the protocol and control groups (37% and 36%); but for those admitted with a normal pHi which then fell, survival was significantly greater in the protocol group than among the controls (58% vs. 42%) ($p < 0.01$).

The benefits of preoperative optimization of high risk surgical patients were demonstrated by Boyd et al.[28] They randomized 107 patients into a control group ($n = 54$) who received "standard" perioperative care or to a protocol group ($n = 53$) who, in addition, had an oxygen delivery index that increased to more than 600 ml/min/m^2 after a dopexamine hydrochloride infusion.

The protocol group had a significantly higher DO_2 preoperatively (median 597 vs. 399 ml/min/m^2) ($p < 0.001$) and postoperatively ($p < 0.001$). There was also a 75% reduction in mortality (5.7% vs. 22.2%) ($p = 0.015$) and halving of the mean (± SEM) number of complications per patient (0.68 ± 0.16 vs. 1.35 ± 0.20) ($p = 0.008$).

In a prospectively randomized study by Bishop et al.[29] patients with severe trauma were randomized to "standard resuscitation" or resuscitation to supranormal values (cardiac index $\geq$ 4.5 L/min/m^2, $DO_2I \geq$ 670 ml/min/m^2, $VO_2I \geq$ 166 ml/min/m^2) within 24 hours of admission. The 50 protocol patients (versus the 65 control patients) had a significantly lower mortality rate (18% vs. 37%) and fewer organ failures per patient (0.74 ± 0.28 vs. 1.62 ± 0.45).

Prospective Nonrandomized Studies

Moore et al.[30] prospectively studied 39 severely injured patients who had known risk factors for multiple organ failure (MOF),

TABLE 58.3. Organ Failure Correlated with Baseline and 12-Hour VO_2.

	No. of patients with MOF		
12-Hour VO_2	Baseline VO_2 < 150 ml/min/m^2	Baseline VO_2 > 150 ml/min/m^2	Total
< 150 ml/min/m^2	9/11 (82%)	3/4 (75%)	12/15 (80%)
> 150 ml/min/m^2	3/10 (30%)	1/14 (7%)	4/24 (17%)

Adapted from Moore et al.,[30] with permission.
$p = 0.001$.

including: (1) major abdominal trauma (Abdominal Trauma Index > 15); (2) massive transfusion (>10 units of red blood cells during the initial 24 hours); (3) combined flail chest/pulmonary contusion with early hypoxemia (PaO_2/FiO_2 < 200 within 12 hours); (4) multiple severe fractures. The 39 patients were resuscitated according to a protocol aimed at attaining VO_2I > 150 ml/min/m^2 within 12 hours; 15 (38%) of these high risk patients did not meet this VO_2 goal. Of these 15 "nonresponding" patients, 12 (80%) developed MOF. Of the 24 patients who had VO_2 > 150 at 12 hours, only 4 (16%) developed MOF ($p < 0.001$) Table (58.3).

Bishop et al.[31] reported a series of 35 patients who had undergone emergency thoracotomy for chest trauma. The 14 survivors had a significantly higher cardiac index (4.2 ± 1.1 vs. 3.7 ± 0.9 L/min/m^2) ($p = 0.012$), DO_2I (631 ± 176 vs. 534 ± 130 ml/min/m^2) ($p < 0.001$), and VO_2I (165 ± 42 vs. 128 ± 49 ml/min/m^2) ($p < 0.001$).

Pathologic Supply-Dependent Oxygen Consumption During ARDS

Animal Data

Ronco et al.[32] and others[33] have pointed out that in healthy anesthetized dogs at normal and supranormal values of O_2 delivery, O_2 consumption remains relatively constant and independent of O_2 delivery. As O_2 delivery is gradually reduced to markedly low values, an increase in O_2 extraction maintains the O_2 consumption relatively constant until a critical value of O_2 delivery is reached. Below that critical value, O_2 extraction no longer can make up for further reductions in O_2 delivery. This phase of the O_2 delivery/consumption relation, in which there is direct dependence of O_2 consumption on O_2 delivery (below the critical O_2 delivery value) has been termed "supply-dependent O_2 consumption."[33]

In contrast to these healthy animals, which show supply-dependent O_2 consumption only at markedly low values of O_2 delivery (8 ml/kg/min), clinical studies of patients who have acute respiratory distress syndrome (ARDS) or sepsis have reported supply-dependent O_2 consumption at normal or even supranormal values of O_2 delivery, suggesting that the critical O_2 delivery value is increased in such patients.[34–37]

Nelson and various colleagues[33,38–40] hypothesized that it was sepsis, not the lung injury itself, that was responsible for the supply-dependent O_2 consumption in ARDS. In dog studies they demonstrated that both bacteremia and endotoxemia

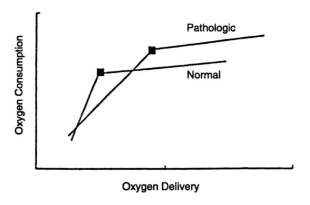

■ Critical oxygen-delivery

FIGURE 58.1. Normal and pathologic biphasic relations between oxygen delivery and oxygen consumption. Both bacteremia and endotoxemia caused a significant, pathologic increase in the critical oxygen-delivery value in septic animals. More importantly, the oxygen-extraction ratio at the point at which oxygen consumption became supply-dependent fell from 70% in healthy dogs to 51% in bacteremic dogs. This phenomenon has been termed pathologic supply-dependent oxygen consumption to distinguish it from the supply-dependent oxygen consumption seen below the critical oxygen-delivery value in healthy animals. (From Long et al.,[40] with permission.)

significantly increased the critical O_2 delivery value by 50% (i.e., from 8 to 12 ml/kg/min). More importantly, the oxygen extraction ratio (O_2ER) at the point at which O_2 consumption became supply-dependent fell from 70% to 51% in bacteremic dogs. They termed this phenomenon pathologic supply-dependent O_2 consumption to distinguish it from the supply-dependent O_2 consumption seen with an extremely low O_2 delivery in healthy animals (Fig. 58.1).

Human Data

Danek et al.[35] noted that one mechanism likely to contribute to the development of MOF in patients with ARDS is regional hypoxia in tissues rendered vulnerable by the high metabolic demands of ARDS. Furthermore, therapeutic interventions, such as increasing the positive end-expiratory pressure (PEEP), often cause severe decreases in cardiac output and delivery of O_2 and can induce changes in the distribution of peripheral blood flow. In 20 patients with ARDS they found a direct linear relation between DO_2 and VO_2. These authors commented that the supply-dependent VO_2 could be due to the inability to regulate peripheral blood flow, diffuse cellular dysfunction, or both, resulting in the inability to utilize available O_2.

Powers et al.[41] found an almost linear relation between cardiac output (Qt) and tissue O_2 consumption in 33 patients with ARDS. Subsequently, Rhodes et al.[42] demonstrated (in similar patients) that when O_2 delivery was increased with hypertonic mannitol, a corresponding increase in O_2 consumption occurred. In addition, King et al.,[43] in a study of 11 patients with ARDS, found that O_2 delivery decreased as PEEP was increased, but O_2 extraction did not increase.

Gutierrez and Pohil[44] studied the relation between DO_2 and VO_2 in 30 intensive care patients. One group of 20 patients had a well defined, linear relation between O_2 delivery and O_2 consumption, but they were unable to increase their O_2 extraction in response to decrease in DO_2. This group had severe sepsis and ARDS, with high mortality (70%). The other 10 less severely ill patients had a significantly lower mortality (30%) and were able to maintain their VO_2 independent of the DO_2 to low levels of O_2 supply by increasing O_2 extraction.

Mizock and Falk[45] noted that the linear relation that exists between the VO_2 and the DO_2 in the sickest ARDS patients results in a high value for the "critical DO_2." Sibbald et al.[46] thought that this phenomenon was related to a limited ability of tissues to extract oxygen as the result of microembolization of the nutrient capillary bed or tissue edema increasing the diffusion distance for oxygen from nutrient capillaries to the tissues. Bihari[47] thought it could also be related to consumption of oxygen by non-adenosine triphosphate (ATP)-producing metabolic pathways.

Ronco et al.[32] noted that all of the clinical studies reporting pathologic supply-dependent O_2 consumption used calculated values of VO_2. They and others[48-50] pointed out that the apparent linear relation between calculated DO_2 and calculated VO_2 could be the result of mathematic coupling of the shared variables (cardiac output and arterial oxygen content).

Abramson et al.[51] reported on 76 consecutive patients with multiple trauma admitted directly to the ICU from the operating room or emergency department. Their goal of resuscitation was to attain a state of non-flow dependent oxygen consumption and normal serum lactate levels (<2 mmol/L). All 27 patients whose lactate level normalized in 24 hours survived. If lactate levels cleared to normal between 24 and 48 hours, the survival rate was 75%. Only 3 of the patients who did not clear their lactate level to normal by 48 hours survived; only 10 of the 25 nonsurvivors (40%) achieved an optimal DO_2.

Data Not Supporting the Use of Optimizing Oxygen Transport

Bone et al.[52] reported on a multiinstitutional prospective randomized double-blind clinical trial designed to determine if patients with established ARDS [peak flow rate (PFR) < 150] would benefit from prostaglandin E_1 (PGE_1) infusion given at 30 ng/kg/min IV continuously for 7 days. There were 50 PGE_1 patients and 50 placebo patients. At 30 days after infusion, 30 PGE_1 and 24 placebo patients had died.

Although PGE_1 did not improve survival in patients with established ARDS, it did increase cardiac output, oxygen delivery, and oxygen consumption. Major adverse effects of PGE_1, included hypotension and nonfatal dysrhythmias. The average VO_2 was 156 ml/min/m^2 in the placebo group and only 136 ml/min/m^2 in the PGE_1 group (not significant). These patients with severe ARDS may have been too far along in their course to benefit from increased O_2 delivery, by PGE_1 especially if it was done at the expense of a significant drop in blood pressure (BP).

Silverman et al.[53] reported in more detail the oxygen consumption data from the prior PGE_1 study.[52] In the placebo survival group the VO_2 and DO_2 both decreased, whereas in the PGE_1 survival group the VO_2 and DO_2 increased. By day 6 the PGE_1 patients who survived had the highest cardiac output (9.9 ± 1.0 L/min) and the highest DO_2I (730 ± 100 ml/min/m^2). The authors concluded that although this trial failed to show an enhancing effect of PGE_1 on survival in patients with advanced ARDS, PGE_1 may still have a role in the treatment of early ARDS, alone or in combination with other agents.

Tuchschmidt et al.[54] reported a study of 25 patients in septic shock prospectively randomized to a normal treatment (NT) group and 26 randomized to an optimal treatment (OT) group. Resuscitation in the NT group was considered complete with systolic BP ≥ 90 mmHg and cardiac index (CI) ≥ 6.0 L/min/m^2. In the OT group the CI was to be increased to ≥ 6.0 L/min/m^2.

During treatment, the CI and DO_2 were much higher in the treatment group ($p < 0.01$); 72% of the OT patients died versus 50% of the NT patients ($p = 0.14$). Nevertheless, a significant correlation between DO_2 and survival was observed. The mortality rate was 100% for $DO_2 < 9.0$ ml/kg/min, 62% for DO_2 9.0–16.9 ml/kg/min, 47% for DO_2 17.0–24.9, and 33% for $DO_2 \geq 25$ ml/kg/min.

Although red blood cell transfusions have been used to augment systemic oxygen delivery to supranormal levels in patients with sepsis, Marik and Sibbald[55] reported on a prospective, controlled study of the effects of blood transfusions on 23 critically ill, mechanically ventilated patients with sepsis. VO_2 was measured by both indirect calorimetry and the Fick method. Gastric intramucosal pH, measured by tonometry, was used to assess changes in splanchnic oxygen availability.

The average hemoglobin level rose from 9.0 ± 0.8 to 11.9 ± 0.9 g/dl, but the cardiac index fell and the PAWP rose only minimally (16.0 ± 4.1 to 17.7 ± 3.9 mmHg). Thus it is not clear how much blood volume expansion occurred, if any. They found no increase in systemic oxygen uptake measured by indirect calorimetry in any of the patients studied for up to 6 hours after transfusion (including patients with elevated arterial lactate levels). An interesting observation was that in patients receiving blood stored for more than 15 days the gastric intramucosal pH consistently decreased following the red blood cell transfusions.

Yu et al.[56] reported a prospective, randomized, controlled trial on 67 patients with sepsis, septic shock, or ARDS (or some combination) to determine the effects of "optimizing" oxygen delivery. The 35 patients in the treatment group were assigned a therapeutic DO_2I goal of >600 ml/min/m^2 within 24 hours of entry into the study, and the control group was assigned a therapeutic goal of a "normal" DO_2I of 450–550 ml/min/m^2.

Although there were no statistical differences between the two groups in terms of mortality, incidence of organ failure, ICU days, or hospital days, further analysis showed that the patients comprised two clinically distinct subgroups based on the DO_2 achieved. Patients who achieved only normal values of oxygen delivery at 24 hours had a 56% mortality rate, whereas those who achieved the higher oxygen delivery values had a 14% mortality rate. In an editorial on this paper Nelson[57] pointed out that it again appears that patients who achieve higher than normal oxygen delivery during the early phases of their acute illness have a better outcome.

In a study reported by Hayes et al.[58] 109 critically ill patients were studied to determine if increasing the CI > 4.5 L/min/m^2, $DO_2 > 600$ ml/min/m^2, and $VO_2 > 170$ ml/min/m^2 was beneficial. If these goals were not achieved with volume expansion alone, patients were randomly assigned to a treatment group or a control group. The treatment group received intravenous dobutamine (5–200 µg/kg body weight per minute) until all three goals had been achieved. Dobutamine was administered to the control group only if the CI was < 2.8 L/min/m^2.

In nine patients the therapeutic goals were achieved with volume expansion alone, and all nine patients survived. Fifty patients were randomly assigned to the treatment group and fifty to the control group. During treatment there were no differences between the two groups in terms of mean arterial pressure or oxygen consumption, despite a significantly higher CI and level of oxygen delivery in the treatment group ($p < 0.05$). The in-hospital mortality was lower in the control group (34%) than in the treatment group (54%) ($p = 0.04$).

Further analysis revealed that in 35 of the 50 patients in the treatment group the three target values were not achieved simultaneously, and 25 (71%) of these 35 patients died. In 9 of the 50 patients in the control group and the 9 who were not randomized, the therapeutic goals were achieved; none of those 18 patients died.

In 1995 Gattinoni et al.[59] reported the results of a multiinstitutional, prospective, randomized study of goal-oriented hemodynamic therapy in critically ill patients already being treated in an ICU. A "control group" (252 patients) had a goal of a CI of 2.5 L/min/m^2; the "CI" group had a goal of a CI > 4.5 L/min/m^2; and the "oxygen saturation" group had the goal of a normal SvO_2 ($\geq 70\%$) or a difference of less than 20% between the arterial oxygen saturation and the venous oxygen saturation (SvO_2).

The mortality rates were 48%, 49%, and 52%, respectively ($p = 0.638$), in the three groups at the time of discharge from the ICU. Among the patients who survived, the number of dysfunctional organs and the length of the stay in the ICU were similar in all three groups; however, although the hemodynamic targets were reached by 94% of the control group, they were achieved in only 45% of the CI group, and 67% of the oxygen saturation group ($p < 0.001$). The authors indicated that background conditions, rather than intensity of treatment, were the major factors determining achievement of the hemodynamic goals and the outcome. The authors also noted that the treatments used by Shoemaker et al.[24] and Boyd et al.[28] were mainly preventive (i.e., preoperative and perioperative), making it difficult to compare results.

In 1995 Yu et al.[60] reported on another prospective, randomized study of critically ill surgical patients. The goal was to compare a "treatment group" reaching a high DO_2

(>600 ml/min/m^2) with inotropes versus a "control group" in which a "normal" DO_2 of only 450–550 ml/min/m^2 was required.

Among the 46 patients who achieved $DO_2 I > 600$ (regardless of the group to which they belonged), only 7 (15%) died. In contrast, among those unable to achieve that DO_2I, 28 of 43 (65%) died ($p < 0.001$). This study seems to support the concept that a high DO_2I is beneficial.

Durham et al.[61] randomly assigned 58 critically ill patients to treatment regimens that used either supranormal values ($DO_2I > 600$ ml/min/m^2 or $VO_2I > 150$ ml/min/m^2) or conventional clinical parameters as endpoints of resuscitation. All patients underwent vigorous volume resuscitation as required up to a maximum PAWP of 18 mmHg or right ventricular end-diastolic volume (RVEDVI) of 121 ml/m^2. Inotropic agents were added to achieve either the DO_2I or the VO_2I goal in the experimental group or to increase the CI to >2.5 L/min/m^2 or the mean arterial pressure to >60 mmHg (or both) in the control group.

The mortality rates were similar in the two groups (11% and 10%), as was the incidence of organ failure (68% and 73%). Among the patients responding adequately to fluid alone, only 6% died. In contrast, of the 10 patients requiring inotropic drugs, 9 (90%) developed organ failure and 3 (30%) died. Thus, in critically ill patients who cannot attain optimal O_2 delivery with fluids alone, excessive use of inotropes may be harmful.

Ivatury et al.[62] randomized trauma patients to two resuscitation protocols: (1) gastric mucosal pH (pHi) ≥ 7.3; or (2) $DO_2I \geq 600$ ml or $VO_2I \geq 150$ ml/min/m^2. After volume and red blood cell replacement, dobutamine was initiated if the target goal had not been met. Following treatment, the pHi was higher in the pHi group than it was in the DO_2I/VO_2I group, and there was a tendency toward greater organ failure and mortality in the DO_2I/VO_2I group. At 24 hours after injury, 77% of patients had pHi ≥ 7.3 and only 7% of these patients died. Of the 23% of patients with pHi < 7.3 at 24 hours, 54% died. Because the mean values for CI, DO_2I, and VO_2I were supranormal in the two resuscitation groups, the value of supranormal DO_2 cannot be evaluated in this series. Nevertheless, this study points out the importance of also correcting any evidence of regional hypoperfusion.

Hayes et al.[63] from St. Bartholomew's Hospital in London reported the results of a randomized, controlled trial on 78 patients with sepsis syndrome or septic shock. All patients underwent volume expansion to an optimal pulmonary artery occlusion pressure determined by plotting the left ventricular stroke work index (LVSWI) against the pulmonary artery occlusion pressure (PAOP). If the therapeutic goals (CI > 4.5 L/min/m^2, $DO_2 > 600$ ml/min/m^2, $VO_2 > 170$ ml/min/m^2) were not achieved with fluids alone, patients were randomized to a control group or a treatment group. In the treatment group of 36 patients, dobutamine (5–200 μg/kg/min) was administered to increase the CI and DO_2 until all three goals were achieved simultaneously. In the control group ($n = 36$) dobutamine was administered only if the CI was < 2.8 L/min/m^2.

The survival rate was better for the control group (67%) than for the treatment group (56%), although all six of the patients who achieved the therapeutic goals with fluids alone survived. In addition, the survivors from both groups significantly ($p < 0.001$) increased the CI, DO_2, and VO_2 in response to maximal resuscitation. In nonsurvivors from both groups the oxygen extraction decreased ($p < 0.01$) and VO_2 remained unchanged.

To avoid possible problems with mathematic coupling, several investigators[64-66] studied patients with ARDS or sepsis and measured VO_2 by analyzing respiratory gases. These groups found that the VO_2 measured by analyzing respiratory gases remained constant and independent of increases in O_2 delivery, whether the increase in O_2 delivery was produced by blood transfusion or dobutamine. In contrast, if the VO_2 was calculated from the cardiac output and arteriovenous oxygen differences, the VO_2 appeared to increase with increasing O_2 delivery, mimicking what others have called pathologic supply-dependent O_2 consumption.

Evidence of Persisting Splanchnic Hypoperfusion after Shock

Tonometric Studies

In 1984 Grum et al.[67] noted that the gut tolerated decreased oxygen delivery (down to 60% of baseline) before the intramural bowel pH (pHi) began to fall. Fink et al.[68] also used tonometry to demonstrate evidence of gut ischemia in lipopolysaccharide (LPS)-induced shock in pigs.

Doglio et al.[69] followed the gastric mucosal pH in 80 critically ill surgical patients, 26 of whom had a low gastric mucosal pHi (<7.35); 15 of the 26 continued to have a low pH despite treatment, and 13 (87%) died. Of the 11 who could be resuscitated to a normal pHi, only 4 (36%) died ($p < 0.01$).

Video-microscopy

Scalia et al.,[70] using in vivo video-microscopy, showed that there is persistent arteriolar constriction in the microcirculation of the terminal ileum in rats following moderate hemorrhage and volume restoration. Thus a blood volume and cardiac output larger than normal seemed to be required to reestablish adequate perfusion to the posthypovolemic gut.

Laser Doppler Flowmetry

Wang et al.,[71] using laser Doppler flowmetry, have shown that hemorrhage in rats causes a decrease in microvascular blood flow to the gut and other organs, and that it persists despite fluid resuscitation. They also found that resuscitation with four times the maximum bleedout increased the central venous pressure to more than twice normal, but it did not restore microvascular blood flow to the gut. They thought that the depressed gut mucosal blood flow following hemorrhage and resuscitation could be due to alterations in small blood vessel tone, shunting, maldistribution of cardiac output, blood vessel α-adrenergic receptors, increased plasma TNF or IL-6 levels (or both), and tissue acidosis.

Diebel et al.[72] studied splanchnic mucosal blood flow and the systemic effects of hypertonic versus isotonic crystalloid resuscitation in a porcine hemorrhagic shock model. Animals were bled to a mean arterial pressure of 40 mmHg for 1 hour and then resuscitated with equivalent sodium loads of lactated Ringer's solution (LR), 7.5% hypertonic saline (HSS), or 7.5% HSS with 6% dextran (HSD). Intestinal mucosal blood flow (IMBF) was measured by a laser Doppler flow probe placed on the mucosa of the small bowel.

Following resuscitation, the cardiac output (CO) (relative to baseline values) was significantly higher with HSD (158 ± 17%) and HSS (137 ± 24%) than with LR (84 ± 27%) ($p < 0.005$). There was prompt restoration of IMBF with both HSD (126 ± 31%) and HSS (106 ± 22%) (versus baseline). Resuscitation with LR was associated with a persistent reduction in IMBF (51 ± 16%) ($p < 0.05$) despite restoration of the mean arterial pressure and cardiac output to baseline levels. Thus cardiac outputs that are much higher than baseline appear to be needed to restore intestinal nutrient blood flow to normal levels.

Conclusions and Recommendations

We agree with Ronco et al.[32] and others who firmly believe that critically ill patients who, early in their course, have reduced oxygen delivery (or oxygen debt) should be resuscitated rapidly and aggressively. Serum lactate levels, base deficit, pHi, and alveolar-arterial CO_2 differences[73] may also help detect the individuals most apt to benefit from a supranormal DO_2. Certainly anyone who has been in shock and therefore is apt to have an oxygen debt and impaired splanchnic perfusion is particularly likely to benefit.

We also agree with Pasquale et al.[74] that many patients cannot cope with the increased metabolic requirements produced by trauma, stress, or sepsis because of an inadequate cardiac index and oxygen delivery. The resultant tissue hypoxia becomes a major metabolic deficiency; and the longer it persists, the more likely it is that complications such as organ failure or death will develop. It may or may not be associated with an abnormality of extraction (pathologic supply dependence) and may not be detectable by clinical criteria. Nevertheless, it seems prudent to optimize DO_2 and VO_2 as soon as possible, preferably with fluids.

The major criticism of the optimization studies has been the problem of mathematic coupling when calculating the DO_2 and VO_2 using a thermodilutional catheter. Although several investigators have not found an increased VO_2 in the presence of increasing DO_2 by direct measurement of respiratory gases,[64-66] very compelling data exist derived from direct gas analyses of a possibly reversible oxygen debt[23] and an advantage to increasing VO_2.[3]

Clearly, additional research is necessary to clarify a number of issues such as individual organ resuscitation, the relation between total body and individual organ resuscitation, issues of perfusion distribution within and between organs, the metabolic consequences of inadequate resuscitation, and their role in the pathogenesis of organ failure and effects on outcome. In the meantime, the current data support the position that early resuscitation is beneficial based on the principle of optimal (not necessarily supranormal) oxygen transport in critically ill patients. Indeed, even in studies that did not show a benefit to supranormal values, most survivors showed an improvement in DO_2. The "optimal" DO_2 for any particular patient cannot be readily predicted even though it may be important to the survival of that individual.

References

1. Wilson RF, Jablonski DV, Thal AP: The usage of dibenzyline in clinical shock. Surgery 1964;56:172–183.
2. Wilson RF, Thal AP, Kindling PH, et al: Hemodynamic measurements in septic shock. Arch Surg 1965;91:121–129.
3. Wilson RF, Christensen C, LeBlanc LP: Oxygen consumption in critically-ill surgical patients. Ann Surg 1972;176:801–804.
4. Shoemaker WC, Montgomery ES, Kaplan E, et al: Physiologic patterns in surviving and nonsurviving shock patients. Arch Surg 1973;106:630–636.
5. Shoemaker WC, Czer LSC: Evaluation of the biologic importance of various hemodynamic and oxygen transport variables: which variables should be monitored in postoperative shock? Crit Care Med 1979;7:424–431.
6. Czer LSC, Shoemaker WC: Myocardial performance in critically ill patients: response to whole blood transfusion as a prognostic measure. Crit Care Med 1980;8:710–715.
7. Shoemaker WC, Appel P, Bland R: Use of physiologic monitoring to predict outcome and to assist in clinical decisions in critically ill postoperative patients. Am J surg 1983;146:43–50.
8. Bland RD, Shoemaker WC: Probability of survival as a prognostic and severity of illness score in critically ill surgical patients. Crit Care Med 1985;13:91–95.
9. Haupt MT, Gilbert EM, Carlson RW: Fluid loading increases oxygen consumption in septic patients with lactic acidosis. Am Rev Respir Dis 1985;131:912–916.
10. Pollack MM, Fields AI, Ruttimann UE: Distributions of cardiopulmonary variables in pediatric survivors and nonsurvivors of septic shock. Crit Care Med 1985;13:454–459.
11. Hankeln KB, Senker R, Schwarten JU, et al: Evaluation of prognostic indices based on hemodynamic and oxygen transport variables in shock patients with adult respiratory distress syndrome. Crit Care Med 1987;12:1–7.
12. Edwards JD, Brown GCS, Nightingale P, et al: Use of survivors' cardiorespiratory values as therapeutic goals in septic shock. Crit Care Med 1989;17:1098–1103.
13. Tuchschmidt J, Fried J, Swinney R, et al: Early hemodynamic correlates of survival in patients with septic shock. Crit Care Med 1989;17:719–723.
14. Scalea TM, Simon HM, Duncan AO, et al: Geriatric blunt multiple trauma: improved survival with early invasive monitoring. J Trauma 1990;30:129–136.
15. Shoemaker WC, Appel PL, Kram HB: Oxygen transport measurements to evaluate tissue perfusion and titrate therapy: dobutamine and dopamine effects. Crit Care Med 1991;19:672–688.
16. Cuthbertson DP: Observations on disturbances of metabolism produced by injury to limbs. Q J Med 1932;1:233–238.

17. Crowell JW, Smith EE: Oxygen deficit and irreversible hemorrhagic shock. Am J Physiol 1964;106:313.
18. Guyton AC, Crowell JW: Dynamics of the heart in shock. Fed Proc 1961;10:51.
19. Bland RD, Shoemaker WC, Abraham E, et al: Hemodynamic and oxygen transport patterns in surviving and nonsurviving postoperative patients. Crit Care Med 1985;13:85–90.
20. Waxman K, Lazrove S, Shoemaker WC: Physiologic response to operation in high risk surgical patients. Surg Gynecol Obstet 1981;152:633.
21. Shoemaker WC, Appel PL, Kram HB: Tissue oxygen debt as a determinant of lethal and nonlethal postoperative organ failure. Crit Care Med 1988;16:1117–1120.
22. Shoemaker WC, Appel PL, Kram HB: Role of oxygen debt in the development of organ failure sepsis, and death in high-risk surgical patients. Chest 1992;102:208–215.
23. Kreymann G, Grosser S, Buggisch P, et al: Oxygen consumption and resting metabolic rate in sepsis, sepsis syndrome, and septic shock. Crit Care Med 1993;21:1012–1019.
24. Shoemaker WC, Appel PL, Kram HB, et al: Prospective trial of supranormal values of survivors as therapeutic goals in high-risk surgical patients. Chest 1988;94:1176–1186.
25. Shoemaker WC, Kram HB, Appel PL, et al: The efficacy of central venous and pulmonary artery catheters and therapy based upon them in reducing mortality and morbidity. Arch Surg 1990;125:1332–1338.
26. Fleming A, Bishop M, Shoemaker W, et al: Prospective trial of supranormal values as goals of resuscitation in severe trauma. Arch Surg 1992;127:1175–1181.
27. Gutierrez G, Palizas F, Doglio G, et al: Gastric mucosal pH as a therapeutic index of tissue oxygenation in critically ill patients. Lancet 1992;339:195–199.
28. Boyd O, Ground RM, Bennett ED: A randomized clinical trail of the effect of deliberate perioperative increase of oxygen delivery on mortality in high-risk surgical patients. JAMA 1993;270:2699–2707.
29. Bishop MH, Shoemaker WC, Appel PL, et al: Prospective randomized trial of survivors' values of cardiac index, oxygen delivery and oxygen consumption as resuscitation endpoints in severe trauma. J Trauma 1995;38:780–787.
30. Moore FA, Haenel JB, Moore EE, et al: Incommensurate oxygen consumption in response to maximal oxygen availability predicts postinjury multiple organ failure. J Trauma 1992;33:58–67.
31. Bishop M, Shoemaker WC, Landers S, et al: Survival from severe thoracic trauma is associated with supranormal circulatory function and increased fluid balance. Crit Care Med 1993;21:S245.
32. Ronco JJ, Fenwick JC, Tweeddale MG: Does increasing oxygen delivery improve outcome in the critically ill? No Controversies Crit Care Med 1996;12:645–659.
33. Nelson DP, Beyer C, Samsel RW, et al: Pathological supply dependence of oxygen uptake during bacteraemia in dogs. J Appl Physiol 1987;63:1487–1492.
34. Bihari D, Smithies M, Gimson A, et al: The effect of vasodilation with prostacyclin on oxygen delivery and uptake in critically ill patients. N Engl J Med 1987;317:397–403.
35. Danek SJ, Lynch JP, Weg JG, et al: The dependence of oxygen uptake on oxygen delivery in the adult respiratory distress syndrome. Am Rev Respir Dis 1980;122:387–395.
36. Fenwick JC, Dodek PM, Ronco JJ, et al: Increased concentrations of plasma lactate predict pathological dependence of oxygen consumption on oxygen delivery in patients with the adult respiratory distress syndrome. J Crit Care 1990;5:81–86.
37. Vincent JL, Roman A, De Backer D, et al: Oxygen uptake/supply dependency: effects of short-term dobutamine infusion. Am Rev Respir Dis 1990;141:2–7.
38. Nelson DP, Samsel RW, Wood LDH, et al: Pathological supply dependence of systemic and intestinal O_2 uptake during endotoxemia. J Appl Physiol 1988;64:2410–2419.
39. Samsel RW, Nelson DP, Sanders WM, et al: Effect of endotoxin on systemic and skeletal muscle O_2 extraction. J Appl Physiol 1988;65:1377–1382.
40. Long GR, Nelson DP, Sznajder I, et al: Systemic oxygen delivery and consumption during acute lung injury in dogs. J Crit Care 1988;3:249–255.
41. Powers SR, Mannal R, Neclerio M, et al: Physiologic consequences of positive end-expiratory pressure (PEEP) ventilation. Ann Surg 1973;178:265–272.
42. Rhodes GR, Newell JC, Shah D, et al: Increased oxygen consumption accompanying increased oxygen delivery with hypertonic mannitol in adult respiratory distress syndrome. Surgery 1978;84:490–497.
43. King EG, Jones RL, Patakas DA: Evaluation of positive end-expiratory pressure therapy in the adult respiratory distress syndrome. Can Anaesth Soc J 1973;20:546–558.
44. Gutierrez G, Pohil RJ: Oxygen consumption is linearly related to O_2 supply in critically ill patients. J Crit Care 1986;1:45–53.
45. Mizock BA, Falk JL: Lactic acidosis in critical illness. Crit Care Med 1992;20:80–93.
46. Sibbald WR, Calvin JE, Holiday RL, et al: Concepts in the pharmacologic and nonpharmacologic support of cardiovascular function in critically ill surgical patients. Surg Clin North Am 1983;63:455–482.
47. Bihari DJ: Prevention of multiple organ failure in the critically ill. In: Vincent JL (ed) Update in Intensive Care and Emergency Medicine. Berlin, Springer, 1987;26–39.
48. Archie JP: Mathematic coupling of data: a common source of error. Ann Surg 1981;193:296–303.
49. Stratton HH, Feustel PJ, Newell JC: Regression of calculated variables in the presence of shared measurement error. J Appl Physiol 1987;62:2083–2093.
50. Russell JA, Phang PT: The oxygen delivery/consumption controversy: approaches to management of the critically ill. Am J Respir Crit Care Med 1994;149:533–537.
51. Abramson D, Scalea TM, Hitchcock R, et al: Lactate clearance and survival following injury. J Trauma 1993;35:584–589.
52. Bone RC, Slotman G, Maunder R, et al: Randomized double-blind, multicenter study of prostaglandin E_1 in patients with the adult respiratory distress syndrome. Chest 1989;96:114–119.
53. Silverman HJ, Slotman G, Bone RC, et al: Effects of prostaglandin E_1 on oxygen delivery and consumption in patients with the adult respiratory distress syndrome. Chest 1990;98:405–410.
54. Tuchschmidt J, Fried J, Astiz M, et al: Elevation of cardiac output and oxygen delivery improves outcome in septic shock. Chest 1992;102:216–220.
55. Marik PE, Sibbald WJ: Effect of stored-blood transfusion on oxygen delivery in patients with sepsis. JAMA 1993;269:3024–3029.
56. Yu M, Levy MM, Smith P, et al: Effect of maximizing oxygen delivery on morbidity and mortality rates in critically ill patients: a prospective, randomized, controlled study. Crit Care Med 1993;21:830–838.

57. Nelson LD: All goals are not the same [editorial]. Crit Care Med 1993;21:815–817.
58. Hayes MA, Timmins AC, Yau EHS, et al: Elevation of systemic oxygen delivery in the treatment of critically ill patients. N Engl J Med 1994;330:1717–1722.
59. Gattinoni L, Brazzi L, Pelosi P, et al: A trial of goal-oriented hemodynamic therapy in critically ill patients. N Engl J Med 1995;333:1025–1032.
60. Yu M, Takanishi D, Myers SA, et al: Frequency of mortality and myocardial infarction during maximizing oxygen delivery: a prospective, randomized trail. Crit Care Med 1995;23:1025–1032.
61. Durham RM, Neunaber K, Mazuski JE, et al: The use of oxygen consumption and delivery as endpoints for resuscitation in critically ill patients. J Trauma 1996;41:32–40.
62. Ivatury RR, Simon RJ, Islam S, et al: A prospective randomized study of end points of resuscitation after major trauma: global oxygen transport indices versus organ-specific gastric mucosal pH. J Am Coll Surg 1996;183:145–154.
63. Hayes MA, Timmins AC, Yau EHS, et al: Oxygen transport patterns in patients with sepsis syndrome or septic shock: influence of treatment and relationship to outcome. Crit Care Med 1997;25:926–936.
64. Hanique G, Dugernier T, Laterre PF, et al: Significance of pathologic oxygen supply dependency in critically ill patients: comparison between measured and calculated methods. Intensive Care Med 1994;20:12–18.
65. Manthous CA, Schumacker PT, Pohlman A, et al: Absence of supply dependence of oxygen consumption in patients with septic shock. J Crit Care 1993;8:203–211.
66. Mira JP, Fabre JE, Baigorri F, et al: Lack of supply dependency in patients with severe sepsis. Chest 1994;106:1524–1531.
67. Grum CM, Fiddian-Green RG, Pittenger GL, et al: Adequacy of tissue oxygenation in intact dog intestine. J Appl Physiol 1984;56:1065–1069.
68. Fink MP, Chon SM, Lee PC, et al: Effect of lipopolysaccharide on intestinal intramucosal hydrogen ion concentration in pigs: evidence of gut ischemia in a normodynamic model of septic shock. Crit Care Med 1989;17:641–646.
69. Doglio GR, Pusajo JF, Egurrola MA, et al: Gastric mucosal pH as a prognostic index of mortality in critically ill patients. Crit Care Med 1991;19:1037–1040.
70. Scalia S, Burton H, Van Wylen D, et al: Persistent arteriolar constriction in microcirculation of the terminal ileum following moderate hemorrhagic hypovolemia and volume restoration. J Trauma 1990;30:713–718.
71. Wang P, Hauptman JG, Chaudry IH: Hemorrhage produces depression in microvascular blood flow which persists despite fluid resuscitation. Circ Shock 1990;32:307–318.
72. Diebel LN, Robinson SL, Wilson RF, et al: Splanchnic mucosal perfusion effects of hypertonic versus isotonic resuscitation of hemorrhagic shock. Am Surg 1993;59:495–499.
73. Wilson RF, Tyburski JG, Kubinec SM, et al: Intraoperative end-tidal carbon dioxide levels and derived calculations correlated with outcome in trauma patients. J Trauma 1996;41:606.
74. Pasquale MD, Cipolle MD, Cerra FB: Maximization of oxygen delivery: a plea for objective patient care and research [editorial]. J Trauma 1993;34:775–778.

59
Gut Decontamination: Prevention of Infection and Translocation

M. Poeze, J.W.M. Greve, and G. Ramsay

Multiple organ failure (MOF) remains the main cause of death and significant morbidity on the intensive care unit (ICU). The mortality varies from 40% to 100% depending on the number of organs failing.[1,2] In 60% of all patients dying in the ICU, MOF is the cause of death. This has a significant impact on the resources in the ICU regarding both cost and effort.

A substantial amount of experimental and human research has been performed to elucidate the mechanism responsible for the development of MOF. The presence of an infection or sepsis seemed to be an important contributor. In a study by Fry et al., 7% of the patients operated for penetrating trauma developed MOF.[3] Of these patients with MOF, 89% had clinical features of sepsis. MOF was seen as a "fatal expression of an uncontrolled infection." This research has led to an aggressive approach to patients developing MOF without a clear infectious source, including performance of multiple laparotomies to identify "occult abscesses." However, Norton showed that even adequate abscess drainage in 21 patients with MOF could not adequately treat these patients, as 16 of them died from MOF.[4] Moreover, Goris et al. showed that 33% of patients with multiple trauma and 65% of patients with an abdominal infection developed MOF.[2] If an occult abscess was the cause of MOF, these percentages should have been more or less similar. An occult abscess seemed to be able to promote the development of MOF but was not necessarily its cause.

Uncontrolled infection is still associated with an increased risk of MOF, but a noninfectious stimulus such as trauma or surgery can lead to a clinical picture identical to that caused by an infectious stimulus. In this case it is called the systemic inflammatory response syndrome (SIRS).[5] These patients display an exaggerated inflammatory response that can result in an autodestructive phenomenon, without an exogenous infectious source as the cause of this inflammatory response. A new hypothesis was postulated to explain the "septic" features of patients with SIRS dying from MOF. Although the presence of bacterial translocation has been known to occur in critically ill patients since the nineteenth century, it has only recently been shown to play a role in the development MOF with septic features.[6] The hypothesis states that the bacteria are assumed to be transported from the gut into the end-organ system, causing subsequent infection and inflammatory reaction.

The use of selective decontamination of the digestive tract (SDD) in the ICU was introduced by a group from Groningen, The Netherlands in 1983 to prevent deterioration of patients with SIRS.[3] Since then research into bacterial translocation and selective gut decontamination has attracted much attention.

Concepts and Pathophysiology

Bacterial Colonization and Translocation

The colon has been suggested to be a reservoir from which bacteria and bacterial products or parts (e.g., endotoxin) migrate across the intestinal mucosa, a process called bacterial translocation.[7] It was shown that bacteria can migrate across the mucosa pericellularly and transcellularly.[8,9] When bacteria pass through the lamina propria the bacteria can be cleared by macrophages and transported to the mesenteric lymph nodes. From there, invasion into the systemic circulation and lymphatic system has been described. In a study by Lemaire et al. the thoracic duct provided a route for translocation of endotoxin (unpublished observations). Other studies indicated that the bacteria and bacterial products are carried into the systemic circulation through the portal vein.[10,11] Whether these routes play a clinically important role in the development of MOF is questioned is these studies.[10,12]

In another hypothesis the oropharyngeal and gastric route are seen as the porte d'entrée for bacteria. The presence of an abnormal flora in the oropharynx and stomach has been implicated in the development of nosocomial pneumonia.[13,14] Aspiration of this abnormal flora has been found by many investigators to be an independent risk factor for the development of an end-organ infection, ventilator-associated pneumonia.[15] Pharyngeal aspiration in critically ill patients in the supine position with impaired reflexes is common,[16] but there is debate whether the oropharynx or stomach is the predominant site of colonization. At first, oropharyngeal colonization was considered the main risk factor for the development of infection.[17] Later the gastric reservoir emerged as a potential source of oropharyngeal colonization.[18] Studies have demonstrated that the oropharyngeal route seems to be the main origin of pathogenic bacteria to enter the lungs.[19] In a study by Garrouste-Orgeas et al. the median time for oropharyngeal colonization with potentially pathogenic organisms was 7 days, compared to 30 days for gastric colonization. In this study nosocomial pneumonia was detected after a median interval of 18 days, suggesting a primary role for the oropharyngeal route in the development of pneumonia.[20]

This main route for colonization seems to be dependent on the specific disease entity. In a study by Luiten et al. in patients with acute pancreatitis, colonization of the rectum was more predictive than colonization of the oropharynx for the development of pancreatic infection. This suggests that the lower intestinal tract serves as the most important reservoir from which translocation occurs in this specific patient group.[21]

Although abnormal colonization of the stomach and gut in critically ill patients may increase the likelihood of translocation from this portion of the gut, which in health is virtually sterile, it has been difficult to prove clinically whether the translocated bacteria eventually can cause an infection.[22] The liver may play an essential role by eliminating microorganisms.[23] The elimination of bacteria seems, however, to result in two seemingly opposing effects: elimination of toxic products from the circulation, but also induction of the systemic release of mediators into the systemic circulation from bacteria-activated Kupffer cells, thereby causing damage to the organs. The presence of such a systemic inflammatory response is receiving increasing attention. The presence of bacterial- or ischemia/reperfusion-induced release of mediators may be important in the systemic inflammation seen in patients with SIRS and MOF.[24]

Classification of Infections

The ICU infections have been classified as exogenous, primary endogenous, or secondary endogenous.[25] Exogenous infections may occur at any time during ICU admission. The term describes direct contamination of a normally sterile organ system by organisms from an external (exogenous) source. Primary and secondary endogenous infections are both caused by organisms carried in the oropharynx or gut of the patient prior to contamination and infection of adjacent organs. Primary endogenous infections are caused by organisms carried in the throat and gut on admission to the ICU, occurring early during ICU admission. Secondary endogenous infections are caused by organisms not carried by the patient on admission to the ICU. This infection is preceded by acquisition and subsequent colonization of the digestive tract. In critically ill patients the intestinal microbial flora frequently shifts from mainly anaerobic to aerobic gram-negative bacteria, colonizing the gastrointestinal tract of the patients prior to causing infection of an adjacent organ system. The percentages of patients who are colonized by staphylococci, gram-negative bacteria, and fungi can vary from 18% to 76%.[26] These differences may be caused by the detection methods, surveillance strategies, and antibiotics used. This bacterial colonization is crucial for the development of nosocomial infections. Most studies revealed an increase in colonization with pathogenic gram-negative bacteria from 10–40% on admission to 50–100% by 1 week.[27]

The above-mentioned classification is important because SDD has no role in the prevention of exogenous infections. The key to preventing exogenous infection is a high standard of hygiene, including hand-washing, careful aseptic techniques throughout the ICU stay, and disinfection measures. The effect of SDD is to reduce primary and secondary endogenous infections, and studies using SDD should therefore be evaluated in an ICU environment with a low exogenous infection rate.

Factors Influencing Bacterial Translocation

The numerous factors that can influence the occurrence of bacterial translocation may be grouped into those related to the bacteria themselves and those from the host. The host defense mechanisms directed against the invading bacteria are a mechanical barrier and an immunologic barrier. Bacteria can pass the mechanical barrier only when they adhere to the mucosa, when the intercellular junctions are broken down, or when transcellular transport of bacteria is possible.[28-30] The adherence of bacteria to the mucosa is an important event in the pathogenesis of bacterial translocation. The mucous layer overlying the intestinal epithelium is one of the most essential contributors to the mucosal barrier and is formed by the intestinal epithelium. The intestinal mucus modulates bacterial adherence. Such adherence has been shown to be enhanced after endotoxin challenge in rats.[29] Adherence also depends on the type of bacterium and the amount of commensal flora present. Normal anaerobic bacteria seldom translocate, in contrast to, for example, *Clostridium* and *Salmonella* species.[31,32]

The immunologic barrier is formed by the gastrointestinal lymphocytic system. The distinction between the development of a systemic inflammatory response or induction of tolerance against an antigen originates from this system, termed gut-associated lymphoid tissue (GALT).[33] Experimental data suggest that an antigen (including viruses, bacteria, and even small parasites) enter the intestinal mucosa via microfolded (M) cells in overlying lymphoid follicles called Peyer's patches, where the mucosal immune response starts. This initiation consists of uptake and processing of the antigen by macrophages and its presentation to T and B lymphocytes. Macrophage dysfunction has been associated with increased bacterial translocation.[34] The application of granulocyte colony-stimulating factor (G-CSF), which can stimulate macrophage function, decreases bacterial translocation.[35] Primed lymphocytes leave the mucosa and enter the mesenteric lymph nodes, where the primed lymphocytes proliferate. Subsequently, lymphocytes enter the circulation via the thoracic duct and migrate back to the intestinal mucosa, where their function is effected.

Adequate physiologic functioning of the mucosal epithelium therefore seems important[28] to withstand the translocation of bacteria from the gut. Many data have been gathered concerning a wide variety of stimuli that can disturb this normal immune function of the gut. It is dependent on perfusion and general gut function. Starvation and hemorrhage[36-38] with decreased visceral blood flow[39] increase the likelihood of bacterial translocation. Antibiotics can increase bacterial translocation by changing the bacterial flora from normal flora to widespread potentially pathogenic bacteria.

Experimental Data Indicating the Occurrence of Bacterial Translocation

The number of studies indicating the presence of bacterial translocation after experimental induction of shock, trauma, and burn injury are considerable. Most studies have focused on detecting bacteria in the mesenteric lymph nodes, as the first barrier station for the translocated bacteria.[7,40,41] Others have aimed at detecting bacteria and endotoxins in the portal or pheripheral blood.[42] Despite the fact that bacteria are frequently detected in the mesenteric lymph nodes, few studies have shown translocation of bacteria into the circulation and distant organs.[43-47] Critics have stated that the presence of bacteria in the mesenteric lymph nodes is merely the normal physiologic function of the GALT, not a pathologic response to injury.[48] Another explanation may be that the liver and lung, which comprise the largest portion of tissue lymphoid cells, efficiently eliminate all microorganisms from the circulation that escape the GALT. However, this elimination by liver and lung tissue can also activate an inflammatory response, which could lead to the development of MOF.[23]

Experimental studies have shown reduced bacterial translocation after the use of SDD[7] (Table 59.1). Most studies show that bacterial translocation occurs and that SDD is advantageous in that it reduces the frequency of translocation.[7,54,55,62] However, in a substantial number of studies the survival rate was not improved by SDD, despite the reduction in bacterial translocation.[50,53,55,58]

Human Data Indicating the Occurrence of Bacterial Translocation

Many clinical research studies detected bacteria in the mesenteric lymph nodes (MLNs).[63,64] For example, Ambrose et al. showed that the MNLs of patients with Crohn's disease were invaded by bacteria significantly more frequently than the MLNs of patients undergoing laparotomy for noninflammatory diseases.[63] Other studies have focused on detection of bacteria in peripheral blood. In a study by Rush et al. in patients with trauma accompanied by shock, the frequency of bacteria in the peripheral blood was increased compared to that in trauma patients without shock.[64] They concluded that the severity of illness correlated with the frequency of bacterial translocation.

In a second group of studies the presence of endotoxin in peripheral venous, arterial, or portal vein blood was measured as an indication of possible translocation of bacteria. The results from these studies have been inconsistent. Endo et al. compared the presence of endotoxin in the peripheral blood of patients with hemorrhagic shock to that of healthy volunteers. Endotoxin levels above 9.8 pg/ml were detected in 5 of 29 hemorrhagic shock patients using the *Limulus* amebocyte lysate (LAL) assay but were undetectable in 20 healthy volunteers.[65] Mason et al. could not detect endotoxin in either peripheral vein or portal

TABLE 59.1. Experimental Studies Using Gut Decontamination.

Study	Animal	Model	Antibiotics	Effect of treatment
Sorkine[49]	S-D rats	Intestinal ischemia/reperfusion	E/N	Decreased LPS and TNF levels; reduced lung injury
Deitch[7]	S-D rats	Hemorrhagic shock	S/P	Reduced bacterial translocation
Foitzik[50]	S-D rats	Acute pancreatitis	PeTA + C (IV)	No difference in survival; reduced bacterial translocation; reduced infection pancreas/kidney
Yao[51]	S-D rats	40% Thermal injury	PeTF	Reduced bacterial translocation and endotoxemia
Spath[52]	IS rats	TPN	PeT	Prevention of bacterial overgrowth and translocation; resotred intestinal IgA concentrations
Gianotti[53]	S-W mice	Acute pancreatitis	PbAbA	Reduced translocation; no difference in survival
Rosman[54]	Wistar rats	Zymosan peritonitis	PT	Prevention bacterial translocation; reduced endotoxin levels
Goris[55]	Wistar rats	Zymosan peritonitis	TrS	Prevention translocation; no effects on survival
Arai[56]	Fisher rats	Gut transplantation	Pb	Reduced portal vein endotoxins; reduced inflammation; liver damage
Lee[57]	Lewis rats	Gut transplantation	PeT	Prevention of translocation
Runyon[58]	S-D rats	CCl$_4$-induced ascites	No	Reduced bacterial peritonitis; no difference in overall translocation/survival
Barber[46]	Wistar rats	Diet-induced small bowel atrophy	N	Reduced translocation MLN; other organs no differences
Yao[59]	S-D rats	40% Thermal injury	PeTF	Reduced translocation; intestinal damage; improved survival
Jackson[60]	S-D rats	None	PeTA + C (IM)	Increased translocation of *Enterococcus* spp. during SBD
Marotta[61]	Wistar rats	Acute pancreatitis	R+/−L	Reduced translocation/pancreatic infection/damage

SD, Sprague-Dawley; TPN, total parenteral nutrition; SW, Swiss-Webster; IS, inbred strain; E, erythromycin; N, neomycin; S, streptomycin; P, penicillin; Pe, polymyxin E; T, tobramycin; Ab, amphotericin B; C, cefotaxime; F, 5-flucytosine; Pb, polymyxin B; A, amikacin; Tr, trimethoprim; No, norfloxacin; R, rifamixin; L, lactitol; LPS, lipopolysaccharide; TNF, tumor necrosis factor; IgA, immunoglobulin A; MLN, mesenteric lymph nodes.

vein blood 48 hours after trauma.[22] Similar results were found 2 hours after injury in a study by Hoch et al.[66] Van Goor et al. demonstrated endotoxin in the peripheral blood of 4 of 21 critically ill organ donors and detected viable bacteria in 11 patients, indicating that measuring only endotoxin may not be sufficient.[67] Shou et al. also detected endotoxin levels above 5 pg/ml in the peripheral blood of 4 of 40 healthy volunteers.[68]

In conclusion, although detection of endotoxin in the blood has been offered as proof of the occurrence of bacterial translocation, some problems were encountered with the sensitivity and specificity of the assay. The timing of assays is also important, as endotoxin is rapidly cleared from the circulation. In studies of trauma patients, full resuscitation prior to sampling may result in negative assays. Moreover, detection of translocated endotoxin does not necessarily seem to be correlated with the permeability of the gut for bacteria.

Effects of Selective Decontamination

There is a considerable literature about the use of SDD, which is a prophylactic regimen designed to prevent or minimize the impact of acquired colonization and infection. The principle of SDD is based on modulating the bacterial flora in stomach and gut through oral, enteral, and systemic application of antimicrobial agents aimed at maintaining the inert anaerobic intestinal flora, thereby inducing resistance to colonization of the intestinal tract by aerobic pathogenic bacteria. The original report on SDD in the ICU in Groningen described an oral regimen based on polymyxin E, tobramycin, and amphotericin B (PTA), the most widely studied regimen (Table 59.2).[69] This original regimen also included cefotaxime administered intravenously for the first 4 days of the ICU admission. In general, the PTA regimen was chosen, as these antibiotics are mostly not absorbed by the gut.

More than 50 controlled trials using SDD have been reported plus seven meta-analyses.[70-76] Despite this extensive evaluation, the role of SDD remains controversial.

The effects of SDD can be evaluated from different perspectives, all of which must be taken into account when judging the SDD regimen. Not only the effects on mortality and the incidence of infection but also the effects on bacterial colonization, microbial resistance, and costs should be taken into account. Furthermore, from a pathophysiologic point of view, the effects on the occurrence of bacterial translocation and MOF should be evaluated.

Effect on Colonization

Most but not all studies have reported sufficient surveillance cultures to allow definition of colonization rates. As reviewed earlier,[27] the trials have shown remarkably consistent results with regard to colonization rates despite variations in trial design. Typically, 50–100% patients are colonized with potentially pathogenic microorganisms after 1 week of ICU stay. In all studies reviewed, SDD achieved a reduction in colonization, with oropharyngeal colonization rates varying from 0 to 5% at 1 week. Rectal colonization with pathogenic gram-negative bacteria was also consistently reduced, but it took longer to achieve and was never as complete as oropharyngeal decontamination. Generally, 10–12 days of treatment were necessary for a significant improvement in rectal colonization rates, presumably related to various degrees of bowel paralysis with prolonged transit times for the intestinally administered antibiotics.

Gastrointestinal colonization with yeasts have been reported in some studies.[77-80] In these studies 10–20% of study patients had yeast colonization at admission. This level remained stable in the control group but was reduced to almost zero in the SDD-treated patients after 4–5 days.

These results indicate that SDD can indeed reduce colonization of the gastrointestinal tract with gram-negative bacteria and fungi. Reported data also suggest that this effect is selective to the extent the normal commensal organisms are not affected.

Effect on Infection

Throughout all of the reported meta-analyses and in most individual trials the effect of SDD on the occurrence of infections has been consistent. Of the trials reported, only two failed to show a significant reduction in infectious morbidity in the treatment group compared to the control group.

The meta-analyses report a significant reduction in the occurrence of infections. This is particularly true for the lower airways, where a reduction of up to 65% was found. However, the methodology used for the diagnosis of pneumonia in SDD trials has varied widely and been a source of criticism and controversy. In some early studies, such as the study by Ledingham et al., pneumonia was diagnosed on purely clinical grounds.[77] Although a gold standard for the diagnosis of pneumonia does not exist, it is clear that judgment based on clinical grounds alone undisputedly results in a relatively high incidence of pneumonia. It should be pointed out, however, that the difference between the SDD-treated and control groups remains valid because the criteria used were the same for the two groups. Critics of SDD have claimed that the diagnosis of pneumonia should be based on protected specimen techniques (protected specimen brush or bronchoalveolar lavage) and not on clinical and radiographic grounds alone. In total, five SDD trials have been reported in which protected brush catheters

TABLE 59.2. Prophylactic Regimen Based on a Combination of Topical and Systemic Antimicrobials.

Topical antimicrobials (PTA regimen): administered throughout the ITU stay.
  Oropharyngeal cavity: A small volume of a 2% mixture of polymyxin E, tobramycin, and amphotericin B in a paste with carboxymethylcellulose (Orobase) is applied to the buccal mucosa with a gloved finger 4 times daily.
  Gastrointestinal canal: A dose of 9 ml of a suspension of polymyxin E 100 mg, tobramycin 80 mg, and amphotericin B 500 mg is administered via the gastric tube 4 times daily.
Systemic antimicrobial: administered for the first 4 days of the ICU stay.

PTA, polymyxin E/tobramycin/amphotericin B; ICU, intesive care unit.

TABLE 59.3. Respiratory Infection in SDD trials Using Protected Catheter Techniques for Diagnosis.

Study	No. events/ no. entered in treatment	Controls	Odds ratio	95% CI
Brun-Buisson[81]	3/65	6/68	0.52	0.13–1.99
Ferrer[82]	7/39	9/41	0.78	0.26–2.32
Korinek[83]	20/96	37/95	0.42	0.23–0.78
Wiener[84]	8/30	8/31	1.04	0.34–3.24
Winter[85]	3/91	17/92	0.21	0.08–0.54
Total	41/321	77/327	0.46	0.31–0.70

From Ramsay and van Saene,[25] with permission.

were used to diagnose respiratory tract infection. In a meta-analysis the pooled data from these studies resulted in 321 patients in the SDD groups and 327 in the control groups.[81–85] Pneumonia was significantly reduced (by 54%) in the SDD group (Table 59.3).

Another point of debate may be the significant reduction of pneumonia in patients using the oral component of SDD alone.[86] These results were comparable to those found in studies using the "complete" SDD regimen. This indicates that oral SDD can sufficiently reduce the frequency of acquired infection and that application of the "gut decontamination" regimen is not necessary to achieve a reduction in infection. To what degree this makes the theory of reducing the frequency of bacterial translocation-induced pneumonia by SDD not plausible is unclear. The long-term effects looking at enteral development of antibiotic resistance in patients not receiving the enteral component of SDD must be examined.

Effect on Mortality

One of the main criticisms leveled at SDD is that despite producing a significant reduction in acquired infections it has, in most studies, not produced a reduction in mortality. This immediately raises the question to what extent acquired infections contribute to mortality on the ICU. It is clear that most patients dying from MOF die with infections present, but in some patients it is not clear whether the patients were dying *with* or *because of* an infection. The most common acquired infection on the ICU is pneumonia. Clear associations between the incidence of acquired pneumonia and increased mortality have been reported.[87–89] Despite these associations it remains uncertain whether the individual patient succumbs because of the acquired infection or the infection is merely a marker of the patient's physical deterioration eventually leading to death. One retrospective case–control study demonstrated an attributable or mortality risk ratio for acquired pneumonia of 2.0 (and 2.5 for *Pseudomonas* or *Acinetobacter* species acquired pneumonia).[90] In another study the increased risk of death in patients with pneumonia was related only to the presence of systemic release of inflammatory mediators.[91]

Most individual studies were not designed for or did not include enough patients to show any mortality difference, although a few studies did show a significant reduction in mortality. The study by Rocha et al. induced 101 patients with more than 3 days of mechanical ventilation and more than 5 days of ICU admission without infection at the time of randomization. This group showed a significant reduction in mortality using SDD.[92] The meta-analyses examining only randomized trials reported no reduction in mortality. However, the largest meta-analysis has been updated with a total of 33 evaluable trials included; the overall mortality reduction is now 12%, with odds ratio confidence intervals of 0.78–0.99. Thus a small but significant reduction in mortality could be demonstrated. Furthermore, a subanalysis of 16 trials in which the full topical plus systemic regimen was compared with a control group with no prophylaxis revealed a greater reduction in mortality (20% with odds ratio confidence interval of 0.68–0.93) (Table 59.4). Again, criticism has arisen in response to this meta-analysis. In comparison to the previous analysis not many reported randomized clinical trials have been added, and some

TABLE 59.4. Mortality in SDD trials Using Systemic and Topical Drugs for Prophylaxis.

Study	No. events/ no. entered in treatment	Controls	Odds ratio	95% CI
Aerdts[93]	4/28	12/60	0.68	0.22–2.17
Blair[94]	24/161	32/170	0.76	0.43–1.34
Boland[95]	2/32	4/32	0.48	0.09–2.57
Brun-Buisson[81]	14/65	15/60	0.97	0.43–2.20
Cerra[96]	13/25	10/23	1.40	0.46–4.29
Cockerill[97]	11/75	16/75	0.64	0.28–1.46
Ferrer[82]	15/51	14/50	1.07	0.45–2.52
Finch[98]	15/24	10/25	2.42	0.80–7.32
Gastinne[99]	88/220	82/225	1.16	0.79–1.70
Gaussorgues[100]	29/59	29/59	1.00	0.49–2.05
Hammond[101]	34/162	31/160	1.10	0.64–1.90
Jacobs (unpublished)	15/35	19/35	0.64	0.25–1.62
Jacobs[102]	14/45	23/46	0.46	0.20–1.06
Kerver[79]	14/49	15/47	0.85	0.36–2.03
Korinek[83]	22/96	17/95	1.36	0.67–2.74
Laggner[103]	9/33	14/34	0.54	0.20–1.46
Lenhart[104]	52/265	75/262	0.61	0.41–0.91
Lignau (unpublished)	13/90	17/177	1.62	0.73–3.62
Lignau (unpublished)	9/90	17/177	1.05	0.45–2.46
Quinio[105]	12/76	10/73	1.18	0.48–2.91
Palomar[106]	14/50	14/49	0.97	0.41–2.32
Pugin[86]	10/38	11/41	0.97	0.36–2.63
Rocha[92]	27/74	40/177	0.54	0.28–1.02
Rodriguez[107]	5/14	7/17	0.80	0.19–3.34
Sanchez-Garcia[108]	51/131	65/140	0.74	0.46–1.19
Stoutenbeek (unpublished)	42/201	44/200	0.94	0.58–1.51
Stoutenbeek[78]	2/49	8/42	0.22	0.06–0.82
Ulrich[80]	22/55	33/57	0.49	0.24–1.03
Unertl[109]	5/19	6/20	0.84	0.21–3.32
Verhaegen (unpublished)	45/220	40/220	1.16	0.72–1.86
Verhaegen[110]	47/220	40/220	1.22	0.76–1.95
Weiner[84]	11/30	15/31	0.62	0.23–1.71
Winter[85]	33/91	40/92	0.74	0.41–1.34
Total	723/2873	825/3099	0.88	0.78–0.99

From Ramsay and van Saene,[25] with permission.

trials were included in the previous meta-analyses but not included in the last one. The meta-analysis by Nathans and Marshall suggests that the mortality benefit from SDD is present in studies of surgical ICU patients but not medical ICU patients.[76]

There is currently considerable discussion about the use of mortality as an endpoint on the ICU. This discussion has arisen largely as a consequence of many trials of septic patients using antiinflammatory agents that did not diminish the mortality rate. The arguments against the use of mortality were set out by Petros et al.[111] Patients on a general ICU usually comprise a heterogeneous group in which each patient may have a different cause of their severe illness. Many factors contribute to mortality, and the death of a patient after an ICU stay of 30 days may be unrelated to the occurrence of an acquired infection early during the stay on the ICU. Therefore the use of infection-related death instead of a crude mortality rate may be a better marker for the effects of SDD in critically ill patients. It is remarkable that only a few studies have assessed this point.

Effect on Costs

Despite the large number of studies on SDD, until now only a few adequate cost-benefit analyses of the regimen were performed. In the study by Sanchez Garcia et al. a regimen of oropharyngeal paste (after cleansing the oral cavity with 0.1% hexedine solution) and a gastrointestinal suspension of gentamicin, polymyxin E, and amphotericin B combined with 3 days of ceftriaxone was used.[112] Using this regimen SDD was associated with significantly reduced morbidity at less cost. The mean cost per surviving patient was reduced by $4370. In a study by Bion et al. the cost for non-SDD antibiotics was significantly reduced in patients undergoing elective liver transplantation, although total antibiotics costs (including the SDD regimen) was higher in the SDD-treated patients.[113] The total cost of parenteral antibiotics required to treat acquired infections was reduced in a study by Korinek et al.[83]

The costs for topical nonabsorbable antibiotics vary from country to country. In some countries polymyxin E and tobramycin can be purchased in bulk amounts at relatively low prices. The drugs can be suspended in a paste or gel by the local hospital pharmacy. In the United Kingdom the current cost of the PTA antibiotics is £17 per patient per day. In other countries antibiotics designed for intravenous use are used to prepare the topical application, significantly increasing the cost.

Effect on Microbial Resistance

Since the early use of SDD there has been understandable concern about the possible development of microbial resistance as a result of the routine administration of large quantities of antibiotics. Evaluation of acquired antimicrobial resistance in the ICU is difficult. Calculating percentages of resistant strains may give a false impression. For example, if the total number of *Pseudomonas* isolates has been reduced by SDD, a few resistant strains might represent a substantial proportion of the total number of isolates, even though there is a decrease in absolute numbers. Furthermore, the number of isolates is counted in some studies, rather than the number of patients with a given isolate. A patient colonized with a resistant isolate staying on the ICU for several weeks may result in a large number of isolates being reported, but essentially it represents one organism in a single patient, a phenomenon known as "copy strains".

In one review 42 SDD trials were evaluated, in 24 of which resistance had been examined.[114] Of the 24 studies, 22 reported no increase in resistance. Two studies[92,115] reported the development of resistance against the parenteral component cefotaxime and the oral nonabsorbable tobramycin among *Staphylococcus areus* bacteria that were cultured from patients undergoing SDD. It is unclear from the two studies whether the analysis excluded copy strains.

The development of resistance has been reported and should not be regarded lightly. The PTA regimen is not active against coagulase-negative staphylococci and enterococci. Selection and possible overgrowth of such microorganisms is a known consequence of SDD. The PTA regimen also increases selection pressure on methicillin-resistant *Staphylococcus aureus* (MRSA), which is a potentially serious problem if the organism is present on the ICU. If early surveillance cultures reveal MRSA, two options are suggested: (1) addition of oral vancomycin to the PTA regimen and (2) withdrawal of the SDD regimen.[116] It is therefore important to maintain a high level of awareness. Certainly surveillance cultures play an essential role during application of an SDD regimen.

The threshold for the induction of resistance seems to be lowered when only oropharyngeal decontamination is used.

Specific Categories of Patients

Liver Transplantation

Several studies of SDD with liver transplantation have been reported. Arnow et al. reported a lower incidence of infection in patients undergoing the SDD regimen for 3 days or more prior to transplantation.[117] A problem in these patients is that the regimen is less applicable to urgent cases. In addition, it is usually thought necessary to add ampicillin or another agent to cover entercocci in these patients.

Ear/Nose/Throat Cancer

In patients with head and neck cancer, mucositis following therapeutic irradiation is a significant problem, leading to considerable morbidity. At least two studies have examined the use of SDD for preventing mucositis and reported a significant reduction in the incidence of this morbidity.[118,119]

Acute Pancreatitis

In patients with severe acute pancreatitis SDD has been used to prevent infection of pancreatic necrosis, which is believed due at least partly to translocation from the gastrointestinal tract. A controlled SDD trial was reported to reduce gram-negative colonization of the digestive tract, preventing subsequent pancreatic infection, with a reduction in morbidity and mortality.[120] However, whenever gram-negative intestinal colonization occurred, the risk of developing a pancreatic infection was independent of the use of SDD, emphasizing the importance of preventing colonization in ICU patients.

Surgery

There is currently interest in the role of gut-derived endotoxemia in SIRS. In a human volunteer study, SDD was shown to reduce significantly the intestinal endotoxin concentrations.[121] Although SDD causes destruction of gram-negative bacteria, which in theory could increase endotoxin levels, the endotoxin levels were reduced because of binding by polymyxin. The use of SDD has been reported in patients undergoing elective esophageal resection with a reported reduction in postoperative infections.[122] It was also used in a small study of patients undergoing cardiac surgery, resulting in reduced mortality.[123] The authors pointed out that the sample size in their study was small, but that the regimen seems worthy of further investigation. In the meta-analysis by Nathans and Marshall, which included 21 trials, it was suggested that SDD performs better in surgical ICU patients than in medical ICU patients.[76] Pneumonia was significantly reduced in both surgical and medical ICU patients. In contrast, bacteremia was significantly reduced only in the surgical ICU patients. Moreover, mortality was significantly reduced in trials including surgical ICU patients [odds ratio (OR) 0.70; 95% confidence interval (CI) 0.52–0.93] but not in medical ICU trials [OR 0.91, CI 0.53–1.06]. In the meta-analysis of D'Amico et al., no difference in effect was seen between the individual diagnostic groups (medical: OR 0.88, CI 0.61–1.27; surgical: OR 0.73, CI 0.52–1.03; trauma ICU patients: OR 0.78, CI 0.56–1.09).[74]

Effect on Bacterial Translocation and MOF

Surprisingly few studies report the effects of SDD on the occurrence of bacterial translocation and prevention of MOF. The effect of SDD on the presence of pancreatic infection was investigated by Luiten et al.[120] All pancreatic infections were preceded by intestinal colonization (monitored by surveillance cultures from the oropharynx and rectum) with the same microorganisms that caused the infection. This analysis provides clinical evidence that organ infection can originate from the gut by bacterial translocation,[21] probably related to direct extension of the inflammation to the transverse colon.

Martinez-Pellús et al. studied the effects of SDD in cardiac bypass patients regarding the presence of endotoxin in the peripheral blood 4 hours after surgery.[53] The endotoxin and interleukin-6 (IL-6) assays showed significantly lower levels in the SDD-treated group associated with a decrease in colony-forming units from rectal swabs. However, Bion et al. found no reduction of systemic endotoxemia, despite the fact that the pulmonary colonization with gram-negative microorganisms was decreased.[113]

In general, it is hypothesized that bacterial translocation and MOF are interrelated, so a reduction in the number of patients with MOF treated with SDD may be anticipated. Only a few studies focused on reducing the number of patients with MOF and acute respiratory distress syndrome (ARDS). Although one study found a 42% reduction in nosocomial infections, there was no difference in the number of patients with MOF. However, inadequate numbers of patients were entered in the study, and no severity indexing was used. On the other hand, the result of this study may indicate that the inflammatory response is more important in the development of MOF than the presence of bacteria.[92,124,125] The inflammatory response was not measured in this study. In a study by Ferrer et al. SDD could not reduce the number of patients dying of MOF.[82] In their placebo group 5 of 40 patients died of MOF or ARDS, whereas 6 of 39 died of MOF in the SDD group

Conclusions

The reported data regarding ICU patients seems to provide evidence that the SDD regimen can reduce acquired pulmonary infection on the ICU. It was shown by many individual trials and confirmed by all meta-analyses.

The results regarding mortality are less obvious, but the meta-analyses suggest that SDD produces a 10% overall reduction in mortality. The use of SDD seems to be cost-effective and does not seem to induce microbial resistance, although the discussion is ongoing.

Bacterial translocation can occur in the critically ill or surgical patient, and its occurrence is closely correlated with the degree of illness. Experimental data show that SDD can reduce the number of bacteria translocating to the mesenteric lymph nodes and reduce the systemic endotoxemia. A reduction of bacterial translocation to the end-organs has been proven clinically only in patients with acute pancreatitis. SDD seems to be effective in patients with acute pancreatitis for reducing both mortality and infection-related complications. Interesting work continues to be carried out in patients with pancreatitis.

It has been hypothesized that bacterial translocation plays a role in the development of MOF. Although the number of studies investigating a reduction in MOF and the number of patients included into these studies are small, there was no evidence for a reduction in MOF due to SDD. Based on the currently available data the hypothesis remains unproven. More recent data indicate that during the development of MOF the direct damage due to ischemia/reperfusion, with subsequent release of inflammatory mediators, may be more important than the translocation of bacteria.

References

1. Knaus WA, Draper EA, Wagner DP, et al: Prognosis in acute organ-system failure. Ann Surg 1985;202:685–693.
2. Goris RJ, te Boekhorst TP, Nuytinck JK, et al: Multiple-organ failure: generalized autodestructive inflammation? Arch Surg 1985;120:1109–1115.
3. Fry DE, Pearlstein L, Fulton RL, et al: Multiple system organ failure. Arch Surg 1980;115:136–140.

4. Norton LW: Does drainage of intraabdominal pus reverse multiple organ failure? Am J Surg 1985;149:347–350.
5. Bone RC, Balk RA, Cerra FB, et al: Definitions for sepsis and organ failure and guidelines for the use of innovative therapies in sepsis. Chest 1992;101:1644–1655.
6. Fine J, Ruteburg SH, Schweinburg FB: The role of the RES in hemorrhagic shock. J Exp Med 1959;110:547–551.
7. Deitch EA, Morrison J, Berg R, et al: Effect of hemorrhagic shock on bacterial translocation, intestinal morphology, and intestinal permeability in conventional and antibiotic-decontaminated rats. Crit Care Med 1990;18:529–536.
8. Deitch EA, Berg R, Specian R: Endotoxin promotes the translocation of bacteria from the gut. Arch Surg 1987;122:185–190.
9. Alexander JW, Boyce ST, Babcock GF, et al: The process of microbial translocation. Ann Surg 1990;212:496–511.
10. Moore FA, Moore EE, Poggetti R, et al: Gut bacterial translocation via the portal vein: a clinical perspective with major torso trauma. J Trauma 1991;31:629–636.
11. Olofsson P, Nylander G, Ollson P: Endotoxin: routes of transport in experimental peritonitis. Am J Surg 1986;151:443–446.
12. Lemaire LCJM: Immunological aspects of thoracic duct lymph in patients with and without multiple organ failure. Thesis, University of Amsterdam, 1998;52.
13. Johanson WG Jr, Pierce AK, Sanford JP, et al: Nosocomial respiratory infections with gram-negative bacilli: the significance of colonization of the respiratory tract. Ann Intern Med 1972;77:701–706.
14. Torres A, El-Ebiary M, Gonzalez J, et al: Gastric and pharyngeal flora in nosocomial pneumonia acquired during mechanical ventilation. Am J Respir Crit Care Med 1993;148:352–357.
15. Torres A, Serra-Batlles J, Ros E, et al: Pulmonary aspiration of gastric contents in patients receiving mechanical ventilation: the effect of body position. Ann Intern Med 1992;116:540–543.
16. Huxley EJ, Viroslav J, Gray WR, et al: Pharyngeal aspiration in normal adults and patients with depressed consciousness. Am J Med 1978;64:564–568.
17. Millership SE, Patel N, Chattopadhyay B: The colonization of patients in an intensive treatment unit with gram-negative flora: the significance of oral route. J Hosp Infect 1986;7:226–235.
18. Ephgrave KS, Kleiman-Wexler R, Pfaller M, et al: Postoperative pneumonia: a prospective study of risk factors and morbidity. Surgery 1993;114(4):815–819.
19. Bonten MJM, Gaillard CA, van der Geest S, et al: The role of intragastric acidity and stress ulcus prophylaxis on colonization and infection in mechanically ventilated ICU patients: a stratified, randomized, double-blind study of sucralfate versus antacids. Am J Respir Crit Care Med 1995;152:1825–1834.
20. Garrouste-Orgeas M, Chevret S, Arlet G, et al: Oropharyngeal or gastric colonization and nosocomial pneumonia in adult intensive care unit patients: a prospective study based on genomic DNA analysis. Am J Respir Crit Care Med 1997;156:1647–1655.
21. Luiten ET, Hop WJ, Endtz HP, et al: Prognostic importance of gram-negative intestinal colonization preceding pancreatic infection in severe acute pancreatitis: results of a controlled clinical trial of selective decontamination. Intensive Care Med 1998;24:438–445.
22. Mason CM, Dobard E, Summer WR, et al: Intraportal lipopolysaccharide suppresses pulmonary antibacterial defense mechanisms. J Infect Dis 1997;176:1293–1302.
23. Leeuwen van PAM, Boermeester MA, Houdijk APJ, et al: Clinical significance of translocation. Gut 1994;Suppl 1:S28–S34.
24. Hartung T, Sauer A, Hermann C, et al: Overactivation of the immune system by translocated bacteria and bacterial products. Scand J Gastroenterol Suppl 1997;222:98–99.
25. Ramsay G, van Saene RHKF: Selective gut decontamination in intensive care and surgical practice: where are we? World J Surg 1998;22:164–170.
26. Nyström B, Frederici H, von Euler C: Bacterial colonization and infection in an intensive care unit. Intensive Care Med 1988;14:34–38.
27. Reidy JJ, Ramsay G: Clinical trials of selective decontamination of the digestive tract: review. Crit Care Med 1990;18:1449–1456.
28. Deitch EA: The role of intestinal barrier failure and bacterial translocation in the development of systemic infection and multiple organ failure. Arch Surg 1998;125:403–404.
29. Katayama M, Xu D, Specian RD, et al: Role of bacterial adherence and the mucus barrier on bacterial translocation: effects of protein malnutrition and endotoxin in rats. Ann Surg 1997;225:317–326.
30. Fink MP: Effect of critical illness on microbial translocation and gastrointestinal mucosa permeability. Semin Respir Infect 1994;9:256–260.
31. Naaber P, Mikelsaar RH, Salminen S, et al: Bacterial translocation, intestinal microflora and morphological changes of intestinal mucosa in experimental models of Clostridium difficile infection. J Med Microbiol 1998;47:591–598.
32. Kops SK, Lowe DK, Bement WM, et al: Migration of Salmonella typhi through intestinal epithelial monolayers: an in vitro study. Microbiol Immunol 1996;40:799–811.
33. Köhne G, Schneider T, Zeitz M: Special features of the intestinal lymphocytic system. Baillieres Clin Gastroenterol 1996;10:427–442.
34. Reynolds JV, Murchan P, Redmond HP, et al: Failure of macrophage activation in experimental obstructive jaundice: association with bacterial translocation. Br J Surg 1995;82:534–538.
35. Agalar F, Iskit AB, Agalar C, et al: The effects of G-CSF treatment and starvation on bacterial translocation in hemorrhagic shock. J Surg Res 1998;78:143–147.
36. Qiu JG, Delany HM, Teh EL, et al: Contrasting effects of identical nutrients given parenterally or enterally after 70% hepatectomy: bacterial translocation. Nutrition 1997;13:431–437.
37. Nettelbladt CG, Katouli M, Volpe A, et al: Starvation increases the number of coliform bacteria in the caecum and induces bacterial adherence to caecal epithelium in rats. Eur J Surg 1997;163:135–142.
38. O'Brien R, Murdoch J, Kuehn R, et al: The effect of albumin or crystalloid resuscitation on bacterial translocation and endotoxin absorption following experimental burn injury. J Surg Res 1992;52:161–166.
39. Saydjari R, Beerthuizen GI, Townsend-CM J, et al: Bacterial translocation and its relationship to visceral blood flow, gut mucosal ornithine decarboxylase activity, and DNA in pigs. J Trauma 1991;31:639–643.
40. Deitch EA, Xu D, Naruhn MB, et al: Elemental diet and iv-TPN-induced bacterial translocation is associated with loss of intestinal mucosal barrier function against bacteria. Ann Surg 1995;221:299–307.
41. Shou J, Lappin J, Minnard EA, et al: Total parenteral nutrition, bacterial translocation, and host immune function. Am J Surg 1994;167:145–150.
42. Yao Y-M, Bahrami S, Leichtfried G, et al: Pathogenesis of hemorrhage-induced bacteria/endotoxin translocation in rats:

43. Runkel NS, Moody FG, Smith GS, et al: Alterations in rat intestinal transit by morphine promote bacterial translocation. Dig Dis Sci 1993;38:1530-1536.
44. Kueppers PM, Miller TA, Chen CY, et al: Effect of total parenteral nutrition plus morphine on bacterial translocation in rats. Ann Surg 1993;217:286-292.
45. Zhi-Yong S, Dong Y-L, Wang X-H: Bacterial translocation and multiple system organ failure in bowel ischemia and reperfusion. J Trauma 1992;32:148-153.
46. Barber AE, Jones WG, Minei JP, et al: Bacterial overgrowth and intestinal atrophy in the etiology of gut barrier failure in the rat. Am J Surg 1991;161:300-304.
47. Fukushima R, Gianotti L, Alexander JW, et al: The degree of bacterial translocation is a determinant factor for mortality after burn injury and is improved by prostaglandin analogs. Ann Surg 1992;216:438-444.
48. Wells CL, Maddaus MA, Simmons RL: Proposed mechanisms for the translocation of intestinal bacteria. Rev Infect Dis 1988;10:958-979.
49. Sorkine P, Szold O, Halpern P, et al: Gut decontamination reduces bowel ischemia-induced lung injury in rats. Chest 1997;112:491-495.
50. Foitzik T, Fernández-del Castillo C, Ferraro MJ, et al: Pathogenesis and prevention of early pancreatic infection in experimental acute necrotizing pancreatitis. Ann Surg 1995;222:179-185.
51. Yao YM, Lu LR, Yu Y, et al: Influence of selective decontamination of the digestive tract on cell-mediated immune function and bacteria/endotoxin translocation in thermally injured rats. J Trauma 1997;42:1073-1079.
52. Spath G, Hirner A: Microbial translocation and impairment of mucosal immunity induced by an elemental diet in rats is prevented by selective decontamination of the digestive tract. Eur J Surg 1998;164:223-228.
53. Martinez-Pellús A, Merino P, Bru M, et al: Endogenous endotoxemia of intestinal origin during cardiopulmonary bypass: role of type of flow and protective effect of selective digestive decontamination. Intensive Care Med 1997;23:1251-1257.
54. Rosman C, Wubbels GH, Manson WL, et al: Selective decontamination of the digestive tract prevents secondary infection of the abdominal cavity, and endotoxemia and mortality in sterile peritonitis in laboratory rats. Crit Care Med 1992;20:1699-1704.
55. Goris RJ, van Bebber I, Mollen RM, et al: Does selective decontamination of the gastrointestinal tract prevent multiple organ failure? An experimental study. Arch Surg 1991;126:561-565.
56. Arai M, Mochida S, Ohno A, et al: Selective bowel decontamination of recipients for prevention against liver injury following orthotopic liver transplantation: evaluation with rat models. Hepatology 1998;27:123-127.
57. Lee TK, Heeckt P, Smith SD, et al: Postoperative selective bowel decontamination prevents gram-negative bacterial translocation in small-bowel graft recipients. J Surg Res 1995;58:496-502.
58. Runyon BA, Borzio M, Young S, et al: Effect of selective bowel decontamination with norfloxacin on spontaneous bacterial peritonitis, translocation, and survival in an animal model of cirrhosis. Hepatology 1995;21:1719-1724.
59. Yao YM, Yu Y, Sheng ZY, et al: Role of gut-derived endotoxaemia and bacterial translocation in rats after thermal injury: effects of selective decontamination of the digestive tract. Burns 1995;21:580-585.
60. Jackson RJ, Smith SD, Rowe MI: Selective bowel decontamination results in gram-positive translocation. J Surg Res 1990;48:444-447.
61. Marotta F, Geng TC, Wu CC, et al: Bacterial translocation in the course of acute pancreatitis: beneficial role of nonabsorbable antibiotics and lactitol enemas. Digestion 1996;57:446-452.
62. Mainous MR, Tso P, Berg RD, et al: Studies of the route, magnitude, and time course of bacterial translocation in a model of systemic inflammation. Arch Surg 1991;126:33-37.
63. Ambrose NS, Johnson M, Burdon DW, et al: Incidence of pathogenic bacteria from mesenteric lymph nodes and ileal serosa during Crohn's disease surgery. Br J Surg 1984;71:623-625.
64. Rush BF, Sori AJ, Murphy TF, et al: Endotoxemia and bacteremia during hemorrhagic shock. Ann Surg 1988;207:549-554.
65. Endo S, Inada K, Yamada Y, et al: Plasma endotoxin and cytokine concentrations in patients with hemorrhagic shock. Crit Care Med 1994;22:949-955.
66. Hoch RC, Rodriguez R, Manning T, et al: Effects of accidental trauma on cytokine and endotoxin production. Crit Care Med 1993;21:839.
67. Van Goor H, Rosman C, Grond J, et al: Translocation of bacteria and endotoxin in organ donors. Arch Surg 1994;129:1063-1066.
68. Shou J, Lappin J, Daly JM: Impairment of pulmonary macrophage function with total parenteral nutrition. Ann Surg 1994;219:291-297.
69. Stoutenbeek CP, van Saene RHKF, Miranda DR, et al: A novel approach to infection control in the intensive care unit. Acta Anaesthesiol Belg 1983;34:209-221.
70. Vandenbroucke-Grauls CM, Vandenbroucke JP: Effect of selective decontamination of the digestive tract on respiratory tract infections and mortality in the intensive care unit. Lancet 1991;338:859-862.
71. Selective Decontamination of the Digestive Tract Trialist's Collaborative Group: Meta-analysis of randomised controlled trials of selective decontamination of the digestive tract. Chest 1993;307:525-532.
72. Kollef MH: The role of selective digestive tract decontamination on mortality and respiratory tract infections: a meta-analysis. Chest 1994;105:1101-1108.
73. Heyland DK, Cook DJ, Jaeschke R, et al: Selective decontamination of the digestive tract: an overview. Chest 1994;105:1221-1229.
74. D'Amico R, Pifferi S, Leonetti C, et al: Effectiveness of antibiotic prophylaxis in critically ill adult patients: systematic review of randomised controlled trials. BMJ 1998;316:1275-1285.
75. Hurley J: Prophylaxis with enteral antibiotics in ventilated patients: selective decontamination or selective cross-infection? Antimicrob Agents Chemother 1995;39:941-947.
76. Nathans AB, Marshall JC: Selective decontamination of the digestive tract in surgical patients: a systematic review of the literature. Arch Surg 1999;134:170-176.
77. Ledingham IM, Alcock SR, McDonald JC, et al: Triple regimen of selective decontamination of the digestive tract, systemic cefotaxime, and microbiological surveillance for prevention of acquired infection in intensive care. Lancet 1988;1:785-790.
78. Stoutenbeek CP, van Saene HK, Miranda DR, et al: The effect of selective decontamination of the digestive tract on colonisation

and infection rate in multiple trauma patients. Intensive Care Med 1984;10:185–192.
79. Kerver AJH, Rommes JH, Mevissen-Verhage EAE, et al: Prevention of colonisation and infection in critically ill patients: a prospective randomised study. Crit Care Med 1988;16(11):1087–1093.
80. Ulrich C, Hanrinck-de Weerd JE, Bakker NC, et al: Selective decontamination of the digestive tract with norfloxacin in the prevention of ICU-acquired infections: a prospective randomized study. Intensive Care Med 1989;15:424–431.
81. Brun-Buisson C, Legrand P, Rauss A, et al: Intestinal decontamination for control of nosocomial multi-resistant gram-negative bacilli. Ann Intern Med 1989;110:873.
82. Ferrer M, Torres A, Gonzalez J, et al: Utility of selective digestive decontamination in mechanically ventilated patients. Ann Intern Med 1994;120:389–395.
83. Korinek AM, Laisne MJ, Nicolas M, et al: Selective decontamination of the digestive tract in neurosurgical intensive care unit patients: a double-blind, randomized, placebo-controlled study. Crit Care Med 1993;21:1466–1473.
84. Wiener J, Itokazu G, Nathan C, et al: A randomized, double-blind, placebo-controlled trial of selective digestive decontamination in a medical-surgical intensive care unit. Clin Infect Dis 1995;20:861–867.
85. Winter R, Humphreys H, Pick A, et al: A controlled trial of selective decontamination of the digestive tract in intensive care and its effect on nosocomial infection. J Antimicrob Chemother 1992;30:73–87.
86. Pugin J, Auckenthaler R, Lew DP, et al: Oropharyngeal decontamination decreases incidence of ventilator-associated pneumonia: a randomized, placebo-controlled, double-blind clinical trial. JAMA 1991;265:2704–2710.
87. Craven DE, Kunches LM, Kilinsky V, et al: Risk factors for pneumonia and fatality in patients receiving continuous mechanical ventilation. Am Rev Respir Dis 1986;133:792–796.
88. Celis R, Torres A, Gatell JM, et al: Nosocomial pneumonia: a multivariate analysis of risk and prognosis. Chest 1988;93:318–324.
89. Rello J, Quintana E, Ausina V, et al: Incidence, etiology, and outcome of nosocomial pneumonia in mechanically ventilated patients. Chest 1991;100:439–444.
90. Fagon JY, Chastre J, Hance AJ, et al: Nosocomial pneumonia in ventilated patients: a cohort study evaluating attributable mortality and hospital stay. Am J Med 1993;94:281–288.
91. Bonten MJM, Froon AHM, Gaillard CA, et al: The systemic inflammatory response in the development of ventilator-associated pneumonia. Am J Respir Crit Care Med 1997;156:1105–1113.
92. Rocha LA, Martin MJ, Pita S, et al: Prevention of nosocomial infection in critically ill patients by selective decontamination of the digestive tract: a randomized, double blind, placebo-controlled study. Intensive Care Med 1992;18:398–404.
93. Aerdts SJ, van DR, Clasener HA, et al: Antibiotic prophylaxis of respiratory tract infection in mechanically ventilated patients: a prospective, blinded, randomized trial of the effect of a novel regimen. Chest 1991;100:783–791.
94. Blair P, Rowlands BJ, Lowry K, et al: Selective decontamination of the digestive tract: a stratified, randomized, prospective study in a mixed intensive care unit. Surgery 1991;110:303–309.
95. Boland JP, Sadler DL, Stewart W, et al: Reduction in nosocomial respiratory tract infections in the multiple trauma patients requiring mechanical ventilation by selective parenteral and enteral antisepsis regimen (SPEAR) in intensive care [abstract]. 1991, abstract 465.
96. Cerra FB, Maddaus MA, Dunn DL, et al: Selective gut decontamination reduces nosocomial infections and length of stay but not mortality or organ failure in surgical intensive care unit patients. Arch Surg 1992;127:163–167.
97. Cockerill FR, Muller SR, Anhalt JP, et al: Prevention of infection in critically ill patients by selective decontamination of the digestive tract. Ann Intern Med 1992;117:545–553.
98. Finch RG, Tomlinson P, Holliday M, et al: Selective decontamination of the digestive tract (SDD) in the prevention of secondary sepsis in a medical/surgical intensive care unit [abstract]. 1991.
99. Gastinne H, Wolff M, Delatour F, et al: A controlled trial in intensive care units of selective decontamination of the digestive tract with nonabsorbable antibiotics: the French Study Group on Selective Decontamination of the Digestive Tract. Engl J Med 1992;326:594–599.
100. Gaussorgues P, Salord F, Sirodot M, et al: Efficacité de la décontamination digestive sur la survenue des bactériémies nosocomiales chez les patients sous ventilation mécanique et recevant des betamimétiques. Rean Soins Intens Med Urg 1991;7:175.
101. Hammond JM, Potgieter PD, Saunders GL, et al: Double-blind study of selective decontamination of the digestive tract in intensive care. Lancet 1992;340:5–9.
102. Jacobs S, Foweraker JE, Roberts SE: Effectiveness of selective decontamination of the digestive tract (SDD) in an ICU with a policy encouraging a low gastric pH. Clin Intens Med 1992;3:52–54.
103. Laggner AN, Tryba M, Georgopoulos A, et al: Oropharyngeal decontamination with gentamicin for long-term ventilated patients on stress ulcer prophylaxis with sucralfate? Wien Klin Wochenschr 1994;106:15–19.
104. Lenhart FP, Unertl K, Neeser G, et al: Selective decontamination (SDD) and sucralfate for prevention of acquired infections in intensive care [abstract]. 1992, abstract K10.
105. Quinio B, Albanese J, Bues CM, et al: Selective decontamination of the digestive tract in multiple trauma patients: a prospective double-blind, randomized, placebo-controlled study. Chest 1996;109:765–772.
106. Palomar M, Alvarez F, Jorda R, et al: Nosocomial pnuemonia: selective digestive decontamination and sucralfate [abstract]. Intensive Care Med 1992.
107. Rodriguez RJ, Altuna CA, Lopez A, et al: Prevention of nosocomial lung infection in ventilated patients: use of an antimicrobial pharyngeal nonabsorbable paste. Crit Care Med 1990;18:1239–1242.
108. Sanchez-Garcia M, Cambronero JA, Lopez J, et al: Reduced incidence of nosocomial pneumonia and shorter ICU stay in intubated patients with the use of selective decontamination of the digestive tract (SDD): a multicenter, double blind, placebo-controlled study [abstract]. Intensive Care Med 1992.
109. Unertl K, Ruckdeschel G, Selbmann HK, et al: Prevention of colonization and respiratory infections in long-term ventilated patients by local antimicrobial prophylaxis. Intensive Care Med 1987;13:106–113.
110. Verhaegen J: Selective darm-decontaminatie in de preventie van nosocomiale pneumonie. Belg Tijdsch Geneesk 1994;50:563–566.
111. Petros AJ, Marshall JC, van Saene HK: Should morbidity replace mortality as an endpoint for clinical trials in intensive care? Lancet 1995;345:369–371.

112. Sanchez Garcia M, Galache JC, Diaz JL, et al: Effectiveness and cost of selective decontamination of the digestive tract in critically ill intubated patients: a randomized, double-blind, placebo-controlled, multicenter trial. Am J Respir Crit Care Med 1998;158:908–916.
113. Bion JF, Badger ILR, Crosby HA, et al: Selective decontamination of the digestive tract reduces gram-negative pulmonary colonization but not systemic endotoxemia in patients undergoing elective liver transplantation. Crit Care Med 1994;22:40–49.
114. Van Saene RHKF, Stoutenbeek CP, Hart CA: Selective decontamination of the digestive tract (SDD) in intensive care patients: a critical evaluation of the clinical, bacteriological and epidemiological benefits. J Hosp Infect 1991;18:261–277.
115. Konrad F, Schwalbe B, Heeg K, et al: Frequency of colonization and pneumonia and development of resistance in long-term ventilated intensive-care patients subjected to selective decontamination of the digestive tract. Anaesthesist 1989;38:99–109.
116. Rogers CJ, van SH, Suter PM, et al: Infection control in critically ill patients: effects of selective decontamination of the digestive tract. Am J Hosp Pharm 1994;51:631–648.
117. Arnow PM, Carandang GC, Zabner R, et al: Randomized controlled trial of selective bowel decontamination for prevention of infections following liver transplantation. Clin Infect Dis 1996;22:997–1003.
118. Symonds RP, McIlroy P, Khorrami J, et al: The reduction of radiation mucositis by selective decontamination antibiotic pastilles: a placebo-controlled double-blind trial. Br J Cancer 1996;74:312–317.
119. Spijkervet FK, van Saene HK, van Saene JJ, et al: Mucositis prevention by selective elimination of oral flora in irradiated head and neck cancer patients. J Oral Pathol Med 1990;19:486–489.
120. Luiten EJT, Hop WCJ, Lange JF, et al: Controlled clinical trial of selective decontamination for the treatment of severe acute pancreatitis. Ann Surg 1995;222:57–65.
121. Van Saene JJM, Stoutenbeek CP, van Saene RHKF, et al: Reduction of the intestinal endotoxin pool by three different SDD regimens in human volunteers. J Endotoxin Res 1996;3:337.
122. Tetteroo GW, Wagenvoort JH, Castelein A, et al: Selective decontamination to reduce gram-negative colonisation and infections after oesophageal resection. Lancet 1990;335:704–707.
123. Fox MA, Peterson S, Fabri BM, et al: Selective decontamination of the digestive tract in cardiac surgical patients. Crit Care Med 1991;19:1486–1490.
124. Koike K, Moore EE, Moore FA, et al: Gut ischemia/reperfusion produces lung injury independent of endotoxin. Crit Care Med 1994;22:1438–1444.
125. Yassin MMI, Barros D'Sa AAB, Parks TG, et al: Lower limb ischaemia-reperfusion injury causes endotoxaemia and endogenous antiendotoxin antibody consumption but not bacterial translocation. Br J Surg 1998;85:785–789.

60
Myocardial Depression: Is It Clinically Relevant?

Fred Bongard

Sepsis is the most common cause of death among patients in critical care units. Advances in respiratory support, hemodialysis, and nutrition have improved overall survival. When septic shock intervenes, however, deterioration may be rapid, with survival rates of 50% or less.[1]

The cardiac response to sepsis is central. Experimental and human studies have shown that septic shock can result from both gram-negative and gram-positive organisms, and that the severity of the physiologic derangement is proportional to the size of the microbial insult.[2] The classic cardiovascular response includes an elevated cardiac index and decreased systemic vascular resistance.[3] Although some early reports found that decreased cardiac output is present initially, it likely resulted from inadequate preload estimated by central venous pressure monitoring alone. Increased use of pulmonary artery catheters to measure pulmonary capillary wedge pressure in these situations has found that with adequate volume resuscitation a low cardiac index is unusual, even during the late stages of sepsis.[4]

The concept of myocardial depression in the face of an increased cardiac index seems contradictory. However, the cardiac index is a poor measure of cardiac function because it is sensitive to even small changes in preload, afterload, and contractility. Additionally, during the early stage of septic shock sympathoadrenal activation stimulates the myocardium both inotropically and chronotropically and may mask underlying cardiac depression. Hence a better measure of cardiac performance is needed before the extent and importance of such depression can be appreciated. Although a number of sophisticated parameters have been described, two of the most clinically useful are the ejection fraction and the stroke work index.

The left ventricular ejection fraction (LVEF) has classically been measured in humans using radionuclide techniques, which have found that the typical response is decreased LVEF occurring within 24 hours after of the onset of septic shock.[5] Associated with the decrease in LVEF is an increase in left ventricular end-systolic and end-diastolic volumes. These changes are reversible, with ventricular size and function returning to normal by 7–10 days. The increase in ventricular compliance can be thought of as a compensatory mechanism to maintain stroke volume in the face of altered contractility. Significantly, however, some authors have reported a decrease in compliance, which may be due to differences in the models or techniques of measurement.[6]

The left ventricular stroke work index (LVSWI) is defined as the product of the mean arterial blood pressure minus the pulmonary artery wedge pressure and stroke index. Stroke work declines during septic shock because of the decreases in blood pressure and stroke volume.[7] When left ventricular performance curves are created by plotting stroke work against pulmonary artery occlusion pressure, septic shock results in a downward and rightward displacement. Among survivors, this curve returns toward a normal position during the recovery phase, whereas it remains displaced in nonsurvivors (Fig. 60.1). Furthermore, because of the increased compliance of the left ventricle, there is a less steep slope (than in controls) when left ventricular stroke work is plotted against end-diastolic volume. Clinically, this is apparent by the decreased responsiveness to volume infusion compared to that in nonseptic controls. A study by Ognibene and colleagues found that in control patients a volume infusion led to increases in both end-diastolic volume index (EDVI) and LVSWI, whereas patients with septic shock had a poor response to volume infusion with only minor increases in both EDVI and LVSWI[9] (Fig. 60.2).

The depression in cardiac function, as evidenced by a decreased ejection fraction, occurs despite a decrease in systemic vascular resistance, which effectively reduces afterload. Parker et al. found that septic shock survivors experience a greater decrease in ejection fraction than do nonsurvivors.[10] The decreased systolic function in nonsurvivors is likely not offset by lower left ventricular afterload.

The end-systolic pressure–volume relation curve has been used as a load-independent measure of changes in cardiac contractility. The slope of this curve decreased in volunteers who were given endotoxin, even when hypotension was not present.[11]

Right ventricular performance also suffers as a result of the septic insult. Parker et al.[10] found that changes in the right ventricular ejection fraction were similar to those of the left

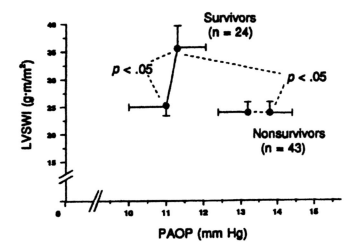

FIGURE 60.1. Plot of left ventricular stroke work index (LVSWI) and pulmonary artery occlusion pressure (PAOP). Nonsurvivors have greater downward and rightward shift than do survivors. (From Metrangolo et al.,[8] with permission.)

ventricle. Right ventricular afterload increases during sepsis because of the rise in pulmonary vascular resistance and pulmonary artery pressure. The right ventricular ejection fraction improves more often in patients who do not have pulmonary artery hypertension than in those who do. It is possible that afterload-induced right ventricular dysfunction may substantially contribute to left ventricular dysfunction by decreasing the preload and by shifting the intraventricular septum toward the left ventricle. Of additional concern is that dilation of the right ventricle increases wall tension and oxygen demand. Unlike the left ventricle, the right ventricle is normally perfused during both systole and diastole. When wall tension increases, it is possible that right ventricular perfusion is compromised during systole in the presence of hypotension. The resultant imbalance between oxygen supply and demand could embarrass right ventricular performance. An increase in systemic arterial pressure would reverse the process if such a change were not accompanied by an increase in pulmonary artery pressure.[12] Therefore rapid volume resuscitation of patients with a compromised right ventricle might further compromise the situation by increasing pulmonary artery hypertension and altering the septal geometry. In these patients right and left ventricular filling pressures increase rapidly, but cardiac output does not increase in parallel. This subset of patients may require vasopressors to increase coronary perfusion earlier than in those without this response.[13]

The etiology of septic myocardial depression has been under investigation for some time. The two most popular theories focus on: (1) coronary hypoperfusion; and (2) a circulating myocardial depressant factor.

Early studies on coronary hypoperfusion were based on animal models that were significantly different from the hemodynamic picture of human septic shock.[3,14] More recent work has found that coronary blood flow during septic shock is at least equal to, and perhaps greater than, that found in normal controls. Additionally, myocardial lactate extraction in patients with septic shock and myocardial depression was similar to that in septic patients without myocardial depression. This finding implies that *global* myocardial ischemia is unlikely to produce the observed effects.[15] Additional work in dogs, however, found that maldistribution of myocardial blood flow might occur. Limited vasodilatation may lead to transmural redistribution of blood flow and reduction in the endocardial/epicardial blood flow ratio. Because endocardial oxygen demand is fairly high, it could lead to selective focal ischemia even in the presence of normal global blood flow and oxygen delivery.[16] This maldistribution of coronary blood flow may be related to endothelial dysfunction, microembolization, and other ill-defined factors.[17] Coronary vessels from pigs that had been given endotoxin demonstrated altered endothelial-dependent, flow-induced vasodilation, which was in turn dependent on changes in the nitric oxide pathway.[17] Other potential causes include edema of the endothelial cells and cardiomyocytes plus neutrophil infiltrates, all of which may reduce regional blood flow. Refuting this potential mechanism is the finding that myocardial high-energy phosphate levels are preserved during septic shock, suggesting that there is an unchanged balance between energy production and consumption.[18]

A single circulating myocardial depressant factor (MDF) or group of myocardial depressant substances (MDS) has been

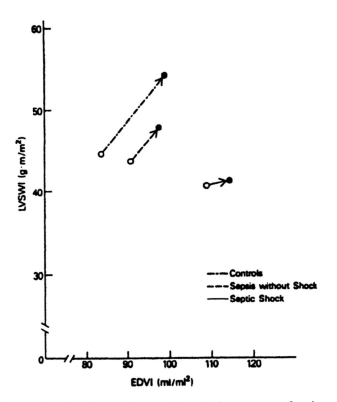

FIGURE 60.2. Results of volume infusion in three groups of patients. Note that the LVSWI/end-diastolic volume index (EVDI) relation is blunted and shifted downward and rightward among those with septic myocardial depression. (From Ognibene et al.,[9] with permission.)

suspected since the pioneering work of Lefer in 1970.[19] Development of the newborn rat myocyte assay improved the ability to assay for MDS.[20] When newborn rat myocytes are exposed in vitro to sera from patients during the acute phase of septic shock, the extent and velocity of myocyte shortening are significantly depressed. The degree of myocyte depression correlates with the decrease in clinically measured LVEF in vivo. Significantly, this depression does not occur with sera from normal volunteers or from nonseptic critically ill patients with reduced LVEF from other causes, or with the sera from patients recovering from septic shock.

A subsequent latex bead modification of the myocyte assay allowed improved quantification of myocyte shortening and confirmed earlier observations.[21] Using this methodology, patients are considered to have myocardial depression if their serum consistently depresses myocyte contractility by 20% or more. A study involving sera from 34 patients with septic shock found that 43% were positive for MDS.[22] Those patients who had evidence of MDS also had a higher pulmonary wedge pressure and a higher EDVI than those who did not. The presence of MDS was associated with a trend toward increased mortality.

Several compounds have been examined as potential myocardial depressants. It is likely that multiple substances are responsible, and that they work synergistically. For example, tumor necrosis factor-α (TNFα) has been shown to have an effect and time course similar to those of endotoxin in an experimental porcine model.[23] Of additional significance is the finding that TNFα is produced within the heart during endotoxemia, and that the myocardial depressant effect observed during sepsis may be associated more with local TNF production than with systemic release.[24] Additionally, interleukin-1β (IL-1β) has been found to cause myocardial cell depression in vitro and likely acts synergistically with TNF to produce more myocardial dysfunction than either cytokine alone.[25] When anti-TNF antibody was administered to patients in septic shock, a significant improvement in the LVSWI was observed.[26]

The possible role of nitric oxide in myocardial depression has been investigated. When isolated rat hearts are perfused with a nitric oxide donor, increased cyclic guanosine monophosphate (cGMP) production is associated with depressed contractility.[27] Because myocardial depression occurs early after the introduction of cardiodepressant cytokines, it is possible that constitutive rather inducible nitric oxide is responsible.[28] Nitric oxide also has an important effect on peripheral vascular smooth muscle, where it reduces tone and decreases systemic vascular resistance. Nitric oxide diffuses into smooth muscle cells and activates guanylate cyclase, which produces cGMP that in turn mediates vascular relaxation by activating cGMP-dependent protein kinase. A number of mediators produced during sepsis stimulate the production of inducible nitric oxide synthase (iNOS), which results in excessive vasodilatation and contributes to the hypotension of sepsis.[28] This vasodilatation is partly balanced by the release of vasoconstrictors, such as thromboxanes and endothelins.[28] Hence the degree of vasodilatation appears to be an imbalance between vasodilatation and vasoconstriction, rather than simple overproduction of vasodilators. A significant reduction in systemic vascular resistance has been shown to correlate with more severe sepsis and a worsened outcome.[29] It may be due to excessive mediator release, as nonsurvivors have been shown to have more circulating mediators than survivors.[30]

Clinical Implications

Clinical management of cardiovascular dysfunction accompanying septic shock begins with the diagnosis. Although definitions vary among investigators, commonly accepted criteria for septic shock include the following: prolonged (>1 hour) hypotension as evidenced by systolic arterial blood pressure less than 80 mmHg or a decrease in mean arterial pressure of at least 30 mmHg for more than 1 hour. These hemodynamic changes must be associated with signs of altered tissue perfusion, such as oliguria, altered mentation, or increased blood lactate concentration in the presence of signs of sepsis and a suspected source of infection or a documented bacteremia. Signs of sepsis include fever (temperature > 38.5°C), tachycardia (heart rate > 100 beats/min), tachypnea (respiratory rate > 20 breaths/min), or the need for mechanical ventilation.[8]

The initial step in management after adequate ventilation and oxygenation are ensured is to institute fluid resuscitation. Although debated in the past, most authorities now employ crystalloids only. During the initial resuscitation, survivors tend to have a more favorable blood pressure response than do nonsurvivors.[8] However, the use of blood pressure alone to gauge the adequacy of (initial) resuscitation is problematic because a number of other factors, such as activation of the sympathetic axis, can also increase blood pressure.[31]

Comprehensive hemodynamic monitoring is the cornerstone of competent clinical management. The need for real-time blood pressure information and the requirement for repeat blood gas analyses makes use of an indwelling intraarterial catheter mandatory. It must be accompanied by a urinary bladder catheter, a pulse oximeter, and end-tidal carbon dioxide monitoring, if available.

The utility of pulmonary artery catheterization has been debated.[32,33] Its use is certainly justified in those with septic shock and suspected myocardial depression. Pulmonary artery catheter monitoring is of paramount importance in those with preexistent or co-morbid factors, such as advanced age, cardiopulmonary disease, renal disease, or other potentially disabling systemic conditions such as diabetes. The pulmonary artery catheter serves several functions, including: (1) measurement of central venous and pulmonary artery pressures; (2) determination of thermodilution cardiac output; and (3) obtaining mixed venous blood gas for derived oxygenation variables. In addition, the newer pulmonary artery catheters can facilitate measuring continuous mixed venous hemoglobin oxygen saturation, right ventricular ejection fraction, and semicontinuous cardiac output.

An early stage of hypodynamic shock may precede the usual hyperdynamic picture in patients who are dehydrated.[31] In this group the central venous and pulmonary artery pressures are low (typically less than 8 mmHg), and a substantial volume of crystalloid solution is required. The more typical finding, however, is one of high cardiac output, low systemic vascular resistance, and elevated pulmonary artery pressure.

The extent of the myocardial depression during sepsis cannot be determined by measuring the cardiac output alone. Rather, alterations in ventricular stroke work and ejection fraction are better estimates. As noted previously, patients whose ejection fractions fall the most tend to have better outcomes. Until recently, bedside assessment of the ejection fraction has been difficult because radionuclide imaging techniques are cumbersome. Technologic developments have allowed incorporation of a fast response thermistor into a pulmonary artery catheter to permit direct measurement of the right ventricular ejection fraction. When used with a bedside computer, bolus thermodilution measurement of the right ventricular ejection fraction is possible. The device also provides information regarding stroke volume, right ventricular end-diastolic volume, and right ventricular end-systolic volume.

Fluid administration should be guided by the response to therapy. Any given patient may require more or less fluid than that required to produce the often cited target pulmonary artery pressure of 12–16 mmHg.[1] Higher pressures may be desirable in the face of preexistent coronary artery disease.[16] Because of the biventricular increase in compliance that accompanies myocardial depression, most patients require several liters of fluid before any appreciable increase in systemic blood pressure is observed. As previously noted, there is likely a subset of patients in whom pulmonary artery pressure increases disproportionately, and attempts at volume expansion may compromise right (and left) ventricular function even further.[13] This situation is evidenced by a rapid rise in pulmonary artery pressure without an accompanying increase in systemic blood pressure.

Persistent hypotension after volume expansion is usually due to low systemic vascular resistance in combination with myocardial depression. The clinical strategy at this point involves use of an α-adrenergic agent to increase systemic vascular resistance (Table 60.1).

Dopamine is typically chosen as the first agent for the support of blood pressure in patients with septic shock.[34] However, the α-mimetic effects of dopamine are disadvantageous because they may further perturb the microcirculation.[35] Among those who routinely seek to increase systemic oxygen delivery as part of the treatment for sepsis, dopamine is favored.[36]

Dopamine is the immediate precursor of endogenous norepinephrine, and its effects are due to the release of norepinephrine from sympathetic nerves and direct stimulation of α-, β-, and dopaminergic receptors. The effect of dopamine is less pronounced when endogenous norepinephrine stores have been depleted. At the infusion rates typically required for the patient in septic shock (>10 μg/kg/min), it has both chronotropic and inotropic effects, in addition to α-adrenegric mediation of vasoconstriction. Because it increases cardiac output, dopamine can adversely affect oxygenation by augmenting blood flow to poorly ventilated lung regions.

Research on the visceral effects of dopamine have had mixed results. A study by Lherm and colleagues found that low-dose dopamine increased urine output and creatinine clearance in patients with severe sepsis but had no effect on those with septic shock.[37] Giraud and MacCannell noted that when dopamine was given to dogs increased blood flow was detected in the superior mesenteric artery and in the muscularis of the gut, but that a decrease in flow was observed in the mucosa accompanied by a decrease in splanchnic oxygen consumption.[38] These and other studies suggest that although the use of dopamine may improve blood pressure by increasing afterload and systemic vascular resistance, its broader effects likely depend on individual baseline splanchnic flow, which varies markedly in septic patients.[39] Additionally, prolonged dopamine infusion has important effects on the concentrations of circulating pituitary-dependent hormones that affect metabolic and immunologic homeostasis.[40] Whether dopamine infusion should be increased or used at a lower dose in combination with other agents is debated, although most agree that beyond a dose of 20 μg/kg/min little additional effect is obtained.

When additional infusion of dopamine fails to elicit improved cardiac performance, norepinephrine is the next pharmacologic agent of choice. It should be used sooner in patients who respond to dopamine with excessive tachycardia.[41] Norepinephrine is the biosynthetic precursor of epinephrine and as such possesses both α- and β-adrenergic activity. In low doses its major effect is β-adrenergic. It increases cardiac contractility, conduction velocity, and heart rate. At higher doses, both α- and β-adrenergic effects occur, which include peripheral vasoconstriction and increased cardiac contractility, cardiac work, and stroke volume. In experimental models it increases splanchnic vascular resistance and decreases splanchnic blood flow,

TABLE 60.1. Pressors Useful for Treatment of Circulatory Depression.

Drug	Pharmacologic role	Clinical effect	Usual dose range
Epinephrine	Both α- and β-adrenergic agonist	Chronotropism, inotropism, vasoconstriction	5–20 μg/min
Norepinephrine	Both α- and β-adrenergic agonist*	Chronotropism, inotropism, vasoconstriction	5–20 μg/min
Dopamine	Dopamine and β-adrenergic agonist, progressive α-adrenergic effect with increasing doses	Chronotropism, inotropism, vasoconstriction	2–20 μg/kg/min
Dobutamine	β-Adrenergic agonist	Chronotropism, inotropism, vasodilation	5–15 μg/kg/min
Phenylephrine	α-Adrenergic agonist	Vasoconstriction	2–20 μg/min

*The α-adrenergic effect is greater than the β-adrenergic effect.

60. Myocardial Depression: Is It Clinically Relevant?

although these findings vary somewhat with the model being used.[42] When compared with dopamine, Marik and Mohedin found that patients who received norepinephrine had an increase in pHi, and those who received dopamine had a decrease in pHi.[43]

The use of dobutamine during septic shock with myocardial depression has been explored. Because of its predominantly β_1-receptor effects, some investigators believe that dobutamine is the catecholamine of choice for increasing myocardial contractility.[34] After volume resuscitation has been completed, dobutamine and norepinephrine, in combination, when compared with dopamine alone, were found to achieve a similar mean arterial pressure, lower heart rate, lower filling pressures, and decreased intrapulmonary shunting.[44] Vincent and colleagues have championed the use of dobutamine in this situation. In their initial study of 18 patients with septic shock treated with dobutamine 5 μg/kg/min, they found an overall increase in both cardiac index and heart rate that was associated with a significant increase in both systemic oxygen delivery and oxygen consumption.[45] Importantly, they found that patients

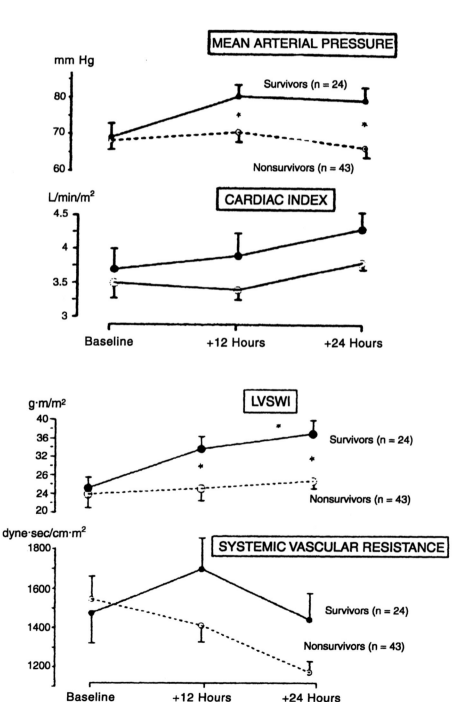

FIGURE 60.3. Improvements in the mean arterial pressure and left ventricular stroke work index were characteristic of survivors of septic shock. Cardiac index and systemic vascular resistance index (SVRI) were not significant predictors. (From Matrangolo et al.,[8] with permission.)

were disparate and identified a group of patients in whom blood pressure actually decreased with dobutamine use. Hence when dobutamine is used to increase cardiac performance and oxygen delivery, the response should be carefully monitored.

Dopexamine is a catecholamine with predominantly β_2 and dopaminergic activity. Like low-dose dopamine, dopexamine increases blood flow to both the kidneys and the viscera. Unlike dopamine, β_2-mediated vasodilatation is not counteracted by α_1-mimetic vasoconstriction. In patients with septic shock, dopexamine has been found to increase cardiac output and hepatosplenic flow.[1] In a septic canine model, Cain and Curtis found that the gut of dopexamine-treated dogs produced less lactate than controls.[46] The current use of dopexamine for the depressed myocardium during septic shock requires further investigation before recommendations can be made.

More important than the choice of "primary" or "secondary" agents is the patient's initial response to resuscitation. Metrangolo and coworkers examined the relative contributions of changes in vascular tone and cardiac function to hemodynamic recovery from shock.[8] Their study of 67 patients found that an initial improvement in blood pressure and left ventricular stroke work index (Fig. 60.3) distinguished survivors from nonsurvivors. The observed increase in cardiac index and systemic vascular resistance were greater in the survivors than in the nonsurvivors, but the difference was not statistically significant. Interestingly, oxygen-derived variables were not predictive of survival. The investigators routinely began dobutamine infusion at 5 µg/kg/min to increase cardiac output once the patient's blood pressure had stabilized. It was increased to as much as 15 µg/kg/min based on the clinical examination, measurement of cardiac output, and derived variables.

Several novel agents have been examined. The vasodilating prostaglandins (PGs)—prostacyclin, PGI_2 and PGE_1—may decrease pulmonary artery hypertension, improve cardiac performance, and augment tissue perfusion.[47] N-Acetylcysteine may help regenerate nitric oxide and glutathione. In both animal and human studies it has been found to improve cardiac function and oxygen extraction.[48] Nitric oxide inhibition has also been found to produce dose-dependent increases in blood pressure in patients with severe refractory hypotension unresponsive to fluid replacement or use of pressors.[49] Despite initial optimism, clinical trails of immunotherapeutic agents have generally failed to improve outcome.

Conclusions

Myocardial depression is a significant factor in septic shock. Because many variables determine cardiac performance, the use of measured cardiac output alone cannot reliably demonstrate its presence. Rather, depression of both stroke work and ejection fraction are more indicative. Investigation has shown that the extent of such depression and the response to therapy are predictive of survival. Modalities such as measurement of the right ventricular ejection fraction and the use of semicontinuous cardiac output catheters hold promise for improving diagnosis and treatment. Although a single myocardial depressant factor has been sought to explain the observed clinical findings, it is likely that a combination of circulating factors are responsible for these effects. Additionally, evidence indicates that redistribution, rather than an absolute decrease, in coronary blood flow may have an etiologic role.

The treatment of septic myocardial depression begins with volume resuscitation to overcome the biventricular compliance increase and to return preload to normal. If blood pressure and cardiac performance remain depressed, dopamine is the first pressor of choice, generally followed by norepinephrine to increase afterload and systemic vascular resistance. Some clinicians add dobutamine to improve oxygen delivery, but its benefit has not been clearly demonstrated. Newer pressors and pharmacologic interventions seem to hold promise, but further investigation and controlled clinical trials are warranted before they can be recommended.

References

1. Dhainaut JF, Cariou A, Gest V, et al: Cardiac dysfunction in sepsis. In: Fein AM, Abraham EM, Balk RA, et al. (eds) Sepsis and Multiorgan Failure. Baltimore, Williams & Wilkins, 1997; 209–219.
2. Natanson C, Danner RL, Fink MP, et al: Cardiovascular performance with E. coli challenges in a canine model of human sepsis. Am J Physiol 1988;254:H558–H569.
3. Snell RJ, Parillo WE. Cardiovascular dysfunction in septic shock. Chest 1991;99:1000–1009.
4. Braunwald E: Assessment of cardiac function. In: Braunwald E (ed) Heart Disease: A Textbook of Cardiovascular Medicine. Philadelphia, Saunders, 1988;457.
5. Parker MM, Suffrendini AF, Natanson C, et al: Response of left ventricular function in survivors and nonsurvivors of septic shock. J Crit Care 1989;4:19–25.
6. Natanson C, Danner RL, Fink MP, et al: Cardiovascular performance with E. coli challenges in a canine model of human sepsis. Am J Physiol 1988;254:H558–H569.
7. Stahl TJ, Alden PB, Ring WS, et al: Sepsis-induced diastolic dysfunction in chronic canine peritonitis. Am J Physiol 1990; 258:H625–H633.
8. Metrangolo L, Fiorillo M, Friedman G, et al: Early hemodynamic course of septic shock. Crit Care Med 1995;23:1971–1975.
9. Ognibene FP, Parker MM, Natanson C, et al: Depressed left ventricular performance response to volume infusion in patients with sepsis and septic shock. Chest 1988;93:903–910.
10. Parker MM, McCarthy KE, Ognibene FP, et al: Right ventricular dysfunction and dilation, similar to left ventricular changes, characterize the cardiac depression of septic shock in humans. Chest 1990;77:126–131.
11. Suffrendi AF, From RE, Parker MM, et al: The cardiovascular response of normal humans to the administration of endotoxin. N Engl J Med 1989;321:280–286.
12. Vincent JL, Reuse C, Frank N, et al: Right ventricular dysfunction in septic shock: assessment by measurements of right ventricular ejection fraction using thermodilution techniques. Acta Anaesth Scand 1989;33:34–38.
13. Schneider AJ, Teule GJJ, Groeneveld ABJ, et al: Biventricular performance during volume loading in patients with early septic

shock, with emphasis on the right ventricle: a combined hemodynamic and radionuclide study. Am Heart J 1988;116:103–112.
14. Adiseshiah M, Baird RJ: Correlation of the changes in diastolic myocardial tissue pressure and regional coronary blood flow in hemorrhagic and endotoxic shock. J Surg Res 1978;24:20–26.
15. Cunnion RE, Schaer GL, Parker MM, et al: The coronary circulation in human septic shock. Circulation 1986;73:637–644.
16. Groeneveld ABJ, Van Lambalgen AA, Van den Bos GC, et al: Maldistribution of heterogeneous coronary blood flow during canine endotoxin shock. Cardiovasc Res 1992;25:90–88.
17. Shibano T, Vanhoutte PM: Induction of NO production by TNF-α and lipopolysaccharide in porcine coronary arteries without endothelium. Am J Physiol 1993;264:H403–H407.
18. McDonough, Lanf CH, Spitzer JJ: The effect of hyperdynamic sepsis on myocardial performance. Circ Shock 1985;15:247–259.
19. Lefer M: Role of a myocardial depressant factor in the pathogenesis of circulatory shock. Fed Proc 1970;29:1836–1847.
20. Parillo JE, Burch C, Shellhammer JH, et al: A circulating myocardial depressant substance in humans with septic shock. J Clin Invest 1985;76:1539–1553.
21. Schuette JM, Burch C, Roach P, et al: Closed loop television tracking or beating heart cells in vitro. Cytometry 1987;8:101–103.
22. Reilly JM, Cunnion RE, Burch-Whitman C, et al: A circulating myocardial depressant substance is associated with cardiac dysfunction and peripheral hypoperfusion (lactic acidemia) in patients with septic shock. Chest 1989;95:1072–1080.
23. Leighton TA, Averbook AW, Klein SR, Bongard FS: Time course of cardiopulmonary effects of tumor necrosis factor and endotoxin are similar. Am Surg 1991;57:836–842.
24. Kapadia S, Lee J, Torre-Amione G, et al: Tumor necrosis factor-α gene and protein expression in adult feline myocardium after endotoxin administration. J Clin Invest 1995;96:1042–1052.
25. Waage A, Espevik T: Interleukin-1 potentiates the lethal effect of tumor necrosis factor/cachectin in mice. J Exp Med 1988;167:1987–1992.
26. Vincent JL, Bakker J, Marecaux G, et al: Administration of anti-TNF antibody improves left ventricular function in septic shock patients. Chest 1992;101:810–815.
27. Grocott-Mason R, Fort S, Lewis M, et al: Myocardial relaxant effect of exogenous nitric oxide in isolated ejecting hearts. Am J Physiol 1994;266:H1699–H1705.
28. Vincent JL: Cardiovascular alterations in septic shock. J Antimicrobial Chemother 1998;41:A9–A15.
29. Vincent JL, Gris P, Coffernils M, et al: Myocardial depression characterizes the fatal course of septic shock. Surgery 1992;111:660–667.
30. Pinsky MR, Vincent JL, Deviere J, et al: Serum cytokine levels in human septic shock: relation to multiple-system organ failure and mortality. 1993;103:565–575.
31. Wheeler AP, Berbard GR: Treating patients with severe sepsis. N Engl J Med 1999;340:207–214.
32. Pulmonary artery catheter consensus conference: consensus statement. Crit Care Med 1997;25:910–925.
33. Conners AF Jr, Speroff T, Dawson NV, et al: The effectiveness of right heart catheterization in the initial care of critically ill patients. JAMA 1996;275:889–897.
34. Meier-Hellman A, Reinhart K: Recommendations for the treatment of patients with septic shock. Acta Anaesthesiol Scand 1997;111:177–180.
35. Vincent JL, Van der Linden P, Domb M, et al: Dopamine compared with dobutamine in experimental shock: relevance to fluid administration. Anesth Analg 187;66:565–571.
36. Shoemaker WC, Appel PL, Kram HB: Oxygen transport measurements to evaluate tissue perfusion and titrate therapy; dobutamine and dopamine effects. Crit Care Med 1991;19:672–688.
37. Lherm T, Troche G, Rossignol M, et al: Renal effects of low dose dopamine in patients with sepsis syndrome or septic shock treated with catecholamines. Intensive Care Med 1997;23:31–37.
38. Giraud GD, MacCannell KL: Decreased nutrient blood flow during dopamine- and epinephrine-induced intestinal vasodilation. J Pharmacol Exp Ther 1984;230:214–220.
39. Meier-Hellman A, Bredle DL, Specht M, et al: The effects of low dose dopamine on splanchnic blood flow and oxygen uptake in patients with septic shock. Intensive Care Med 1997;23:31–37.
40. Van der Berghe G, de Zegher F: Anterior pituitary function during critical illness and dopamine treatment. Crit Care Med 1996;24:1580–1590.
41. Astiz ME, Rackow EC: Septic shock. Lancet 1998;351:1501–1505.
42. Bersten AD, Hersch M, Cheung H, et al: The effect of various sympathomimetics on the regional circulations in hyperdynamic sepsis. Surgery 1992;112:549–561.
43. Marik PE, Mohedin M: The contrasting effects of dopamine and norepinephrine used to treat septic shock patients. Crit Care Med 1990;18:282–285.
44. Hannemann L, Reinhart K, Grenzer O, et al: Comparison of dopamine to dobutamine and norepinephrine for oxygen delivery and uptake in septic shock. Crit Care Med 1995;23:1962–1970.
45. Vincent JL, Roman A, Kahn RJ: Dobutamine administration in septic shock: addition to a standard protocol. Crit Care Med 1990;18:689–693.
46. Cain SM, Curtis SE: Experimental models of pathologic oxygen supply dependency. Crit Care Med 1991;19:603–612.
47. Reinhart K, Bloos F, Spies C: Vasoactive drug therapy in sepsis. In: Sibbald WJ, Vincent JL (eds) Clinical Trials for the Treatment of Sepsis. Berlin, Springer, 1995;207–224.
48. Zhang H, Spapen H, Nguyen DN, et al: Protective effects of N-acetylcysteine in endotoxemia. Am J Physiol 1994;266:H1746–H1754.
49. Petros A, Bennet D, Vallance P: Effect of nitric oxide synthase inhibitors on hypotension in patients with septic shock. Lancet 1991;338:1557–1558.

61
Infection: Cause or Result of Organ Failure?

Donald E. Fry

Numerous publications have identified an association between clinical infection and emergence of the multiple organ dysfunction syndrome (MODS).[1-4] During the 1970s and 1980s the consensus was that overwhelming or uncontrolled infection is being the principal event that results in organ failure. More aggressive surgical strategies were advocated for managing pyogenic infections in the expectation that MODS could be reversed when such infections were effectively controlled.[5-7] During the latter part of the 1980s and into the 1990s, however, increased attention focused on the concept of the sepsis syndrome and the fact that the clinical and hemodynamic characteristics of human "sepsis" could in fact be the consequence of biologic events that were not invasive infection per se. The increased numbers of reports in the area of microbial gastrointestinal translocation then brought attention to the fact that even the presence of microbes in blood may not be invasive infection but, in fact, may represent failure of the host defense mechanisms.[8-13] The latter observations of bacteremia without a site of infection further kindled discussion that MODS was *associated* with infections but was not always *caused* by invasive infection.

As has been repeatedly emphasized by numerous authors in this book, the patient who develops the systemic inflammatory response syndrome (SIRS) and the transition to MODS, regardless of the etiologic factors associated with the process, ends up with numerous surgical and other clinical interventions. Frequent operations, the need for endotracheal intubation, and other invasions of the primary host defense mechanisms represent potential portals by which pathogens can gain access to the host, with infection the possible consequence. More recently, discussion has focused on whether SIRS and organ failure are in fact the precursors of clinical infection. The numerous infectious events seen in the intensive care unit (ICU) patient with MODS may be the consequence of the noninfectious organ failure syndromes or the attendant immunosuppression of hemorrhage and injury; that is, infection may not be the inciting event. This has led to the counterhypothesis that the SIRS and MODS patient may be dying *with* infection and not *from* infection.

Traditional Perspective: Infection Leading to Organ Failure

The traditional perspective of the relation of infection leading to MODS has been largely derived from the seemingly accurate but overstated observation that severe, acute bacterial infection leads to activation of a systemic process (SIRS) that if sustained for a critical period (or for critical levels of intensity) leads to inflammation-mediated organ damage (MODS). This traditional perspective has focused completely on the magnitude of the proinflammatory response: Once the summed effects of proinflammatory signaling exceeds its normal autocrine and paracrine domain within the infected site, the process is activated systemically.

Evidence to support this concept seemed apparent from the experiences of many physicians caring for critically ill and injured patients. We studied 553 emergency surgical patients, two-thirds of whom had operations for blunt or penetrating trauma.[1] Seven percent of these patients developed MODS, which was defined as failure of two or more of the organ systems being studied. Of the 38 MODS patients, 34 had sepsis or an associated event. These 34 MODS patients as a group developed clinical evidence of "sepsis" at about 2.5 days after emergency operation. The onset of sepsis and the first evidence of pulmonary failure occurred concurrently. About 50% of the infections were intraabdominal, and 50% were severe pulmonary infections. Thus the onset of sepsis from an anatomic site began temporally in conjunction with the emergence of clinical sepsis and MODS. All surgeons and critical care physicians have had experience with a rapid-onset septic event from severe infection that leads to the cascading events of organ failure. It is of interest that 123 patients in this study met the criteria for sepsis, but only 38 proceeded to MODS. The reasons selected patients had progression of the process and others did not remained undefined.

It was also apparent from these early data that there was a relation between hemorrhagic shock, sepsis, and organ failure. Patients with hemorrhagic shock due to injury were statistically more likely to develop a major septic event and then MODS.

Hemorrhage independent of the second septic event was not associated with subsequent organ failure. These data led to some speculation that hemorrhage had systemic consequences for the host defense mechanisms. An alternative conclusion after a perspective of years is that the hemorrhagic event, having provided the inflammatory response and the "second" hit of invasive infection, resulted in the exaggerated septic response. From these and many other studies, the concept of infection being a major activator of SIRS leading to MODS was accepted (see Chapter 10).

Counterinflammatory Response

As the understanding of inflammation and its effects has evolved, it is now appreciated that large array of counterinflammatory signals exist. These counterinflammatory cytokines and pathways are not as well understood as the proinflammatory ones at this time, and it is likely that the full array have yet to be defined. Interleukin-4 (IL-4), IL-10, IL-13, soluble IL-1 receptors, and many others appear to serve the role of antagonists or counter-control mechanisms to prevent excessive proinflammatory signaling.[14] It is also thought that the counterinflammatory effects serve the appropriate biologic purpose of downregulating inflammation once its purpose has been served. It is also clear that consequences of excessive antiinflammatory responses are immunosuppressive sequelae that place the host at considerable risk for intercurrent and poorly contained infection.[15] Detailed discussions about the counterinflammatory signals are present in Chapters 15, 17, 39 and 54.

The emergence of at least preliminary evidence about counterinflammatory signals has led to several different directions in thought about SIRS and MODS. A balance between pro- and counterinflammatory effects might explain why some patients have severe infection, including bacteremia and clear evidence of microbial dissemination, but do not develop severe SIRS and MODS. Whether consequences of the rapidity of onset, coexistence of other insults, or intrinsic differences in host responsiveness are at fault, it is likely that the balance between these opposing effects permits the host to tolerate the physiologic consequences. A quantitative or temporal disconnection between the proinflammatory signals and the counterinflammatory signals may explain the dominance of SIRS. Recognition of the counterinflammatory signals has kindled some hope that these natural biologic antagonists to inflammation might hold promise for new treatment strategies of the SIRS and MODS patient.[16]

Immunosuppression has been recognized for decades as a consequence of shock, severe trauma, sustained critical illness, and even infection. Measures of host responsiveness, including skin test hypersensitivity,[17] monocyte antigen presentation,[18] absolute lymphocyte counts,[19] and other surrogate measures of the immune response, show that sustained illness leads to immunosuppression. The aftermath of activation of the systemic inflammatory cascade leaves an immunosuppressed host who is vulnerable to intercurrent infectious events, which then further stimulate the inflammatory response.

Several other mechanisms have been proposed to explain or contribute to this immunosuppression. Catabolism due to the hypermetabolic consequence of SIRS is commonly cited with its attendant global protein-calorie malnutrition as contributing to impaired host responsiveness. Consumption of the activator mechanisms (e.g., coagulation proteins, kinins, complement) might create a refractory period of host responsiveness. With recognition of counterinflammatory mechanisms, there is now significant evidence to suggest that excessive counterinflammatory responses to the systemic inflammatory event leads to immunosuppression. The idea of a compensatory antiinflammatory response syndrome (CARS) has led to the proposal of exaggerated counterinflammatory signaling in the same way that excessive proinflammatory signaling led to SIRS.[20,21] Yet another proposed idea is that the temporal relations between proinflammatory and counterinflammatory signaling might lead to the mixed antagonist response syndrome (MARS).[20,21] Thus infection, trauma, injury, and shock as major activators of systemic inflammation become a pathway to the activation of SIRS and MODS. Similarly, SIRS and MODS with an overexuberant or dysregulated counterinflammatory response result in immunosuppression and infection as potential consequences.

Relation of Proinflammatory and counterinflammatory Responses

In the present environment of understanding, it appears to be the quantitative and temporal relation of the aggregate pro- and counterinflammatory signals that dictate the immunologic status of the patient who is severely ill. Overexpression of either response portends a negative outcome for the patient.

Balanced Response

The following case illustrates the balance response.

A 25-year-old man sustains a gunshot wound of the left lower quadrant. He was previously in very good health and is not in shock at the time of presentation. He receives preoperative antibiotics and undergoes an exploratory laparotomy, at which time a through-and-through injury of the sigmoid colon is identified. He is extubated at the end of the procedure. By the fifth postoperative day he has an intermittent fever up to 39°C and persistent ileus with poor oral intake and no colostomy function. His white blood cell (WBC) count is 18,000 cells/mm^3. He is lucid but somewhat diaphoretic. On the seventh postoperative day an abdominal computed tomography (CT) scan demonstrates a left pelvic abscess. Percutaneous drainage is performed with evacuation of 300 cc of pus. Within 48 hours he is afebrile, and his WBC count is down to 11,000 cells/mm^3. Oral intake is resumed and colostomy function is noted. On the twelfth postinjury day he is discharged from the hospital.

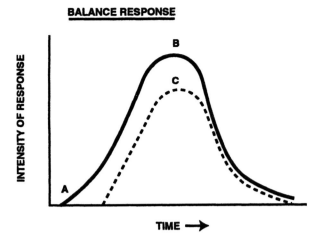

FIGURE 61.1. Theoretic relation of the intensity of the aggregate pro- and counterinflammatory responses seen in the balanced and appropriate response. A, Biologic insult of trauma, major soft tissue injury, or invasive infection, which initiates the pro- and counterinflammatory responses. B, Summed effects of proinflammatory signals. C, Summed effects of counterinflammatory signals.

This case is an example of the balanced response between pro- and counterinflammatory signals. The patient exhibits signs of infection and inflammation but without evidence of organ failure or hemodynamic instability. The abscess reflects appropriate containment by the host inflammatory response of a large density of pathogens that exceeded his phagocytic capacity to eliminate. Percutaneous drainage of the septic collection eliminates the activation drive of the inflammatory process. Drainage of pus and efficient elimination of residual pathogens permitted counterinflammatory signals to neutralize and downregulate the response. This balanced response is illustrated in Fig. 61.1.

Note that during the early phases of the host response proinflammatory responses occur more promptly and predominate over the counterinflammatory response. This response is required for the positive features of inflammation (e.g., eradication and containment) to be effective. During the resolution phase, after elimination of the activator stimulus the two antagonistic forces decline in concert.

SIRS-Dominant Response

The following case represents the rapid-onset, SIRS-dominant response.

> An otherwise healthy 30-year-old man sustains a small 1 cm diameter burn over the olecranon process of his right elbow. Within 24 hours of sustaining the burn the patient develops severe cellulitis of the area that rapidly progresses to massive edema and cellulitis of the entire right upper extremity. He develops orthostatic hypotension, becomes confused and delirious, and is brought to the emergency room for evaluation. Necrotizing fasciitis is diagnosed. A skin bleb is aspirated, and a Gram stain shows characteristic findings of group A streptococci. The patient undergoes massive resuscitation with Ringer's lactate solution and is given large doses of penicillin and clindamycin as he is taken to the operating room for débridement. He undergoes aggressive degloving débridement of the entire right upper extremity. Postoperatively he remains intermittently hypotensive and requires large volumes of crystalloid resuscitation and inotropic support to maintain his blood pressure. The patient has a clearly demonstrable pulmonary shunt and requires a fractional concentration of oxygen in inspired gas (FiO_2) of 0.5% and positive end-expiratory pressure (PEEP) of 15 cm H_2O to maintain arterial oxygenation. Postoperative laboratory studies identify the patient as having a WBC count of 28,000 cells/mm^3 with a mark shift to premature neutrophil forms. Liver enzymes demonstrate mark increases in aspartate aminotransferase (AST), alanine aminotransferase (ALT), and γ-glutamyl transferase (GGT). The patient's bilirubin level is 8 mg/dl, with 90% in the direct fraction. Despite the patient having abundant urine output during the early postoperative period, his normal preoperative serum creatinine is 2.1 mg/dl 24 hours after surgical débridement. He undergoes daily reoperations to débride and irrigate the wound on the right upper extremity. By the eighth postoperative day the infection is completely arrested and an ample bed of granulation tissue exists over the lower extremity, which permits reconstruction with split-thickness skin grafting. However, the patient's organ failure complex continues for a full 4 weeks after the onset of his disease, with final weaning from the ventilator on the 28th postinjury day.

The fulminant nature of rapidly progressing soft tissue infection with a pathogen capable of producing a potent exotoxin leads to the dominant proinflammatory state of SIRS. The

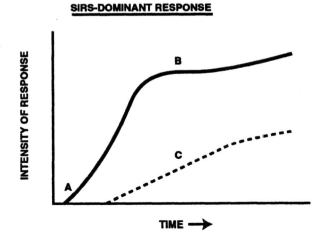

FIGURE 61.2. Theoretic relation of the intensity of the aggregate pro- and counterinflammatory response seen in the SIRS-dominant scenario. A, Biologic insult. Proinflammatory signaling (B) is far greater than counterinflammatory signaling (C).

rapidity of the SIRS development leaves counterinflammatory signaling in an inadequate role (Fig. 61.2) Clinically, these rapidly developing infections most commonly arise in soft tissues and in the intraabdominal compartment. Disease acuity becomes the important variable leading to the dominance of proinflammatory signaling and the emergence of organ failure.[22] The involvement of large amounts of tissue (e.g., necrotizing fasciitis) or large absorptive surfaces in the infection (e.g., acute peritonitis) results in the potential access of large numbers of bacteria, bacterial cell products, or proinflammatory cytokines into the systemic circulation.

This fulminant activation of systemic inflammation is clearly the scenario created in many animal models of endotoxemia and bacteremia. This combination of fulminant endotoxemia, bacteremia, and mediator dissemination has such a dominant proinflammatory effect that therapeutic antagonists such as anti-TNF antibodies and IL-1 receptor antagonists measurably affect the progression of the process in the experimental laboratory. It is this cohort of patients who may benefit from the various antimediator strategies that have not been successful in the unstratified trials of septic shock. The rapidly evolving invasive infection secondary to massive contamination or unusually virulent pathogens is clearly the setting where *infection is directly the protagonist of SIRS leading to MODS*. Failure to control the process by dramatic therapeutic interventions leads to relentless SIRS with end-organ failure or rapid circulatory collapse and septic shock.

CARS-Dominant Response

The following case illustrates the clinical scenario where SIRS due to a noninfectious event leads to MODS, which subsequently results in infection.

A 40-year-old patient is involved in a high speed motor vehicle accident that results in ejection of the patient from the vehicle. The patient sustains a host of severe injuries including a left flail chest, an open pelvic fracture with a large gaping peroneal wound, and a midshaft femoral fracture in addition to numerous other contusions and soft tissue lacerations. He is noted to have a pulse of 140 beats/min and a systolic arterial blood pressure of 70 mmHg. The patient's initial management requires endotracheal intubation to maintain oxygenation, vigorous resuscitation with intravenous Ringer's lactate solution, and placement of a chest tube to evacuate a hemopneumothorax. He is taken to the operating room after hemodynamic stabilization and appropriate overall systemic management at which time he undergoes an operative procedure that includes irrigation and débridement of the open wound leading into the pelvic fracture, a proximal diverting colostomy, and internal fixation of the fractured femur. He receives appropriate preoperative antibiotics. He is returned to the operating room on the second postinjury day at which time additional débridement is necessary for the open pelvic fracture wound. On the third postoperative day the patient is noted to have some fever and leukocytosis, necessitating reoperation for further irrigation of his pelvic wound and additional vigorous debridement and cleansing. He continues on antibiotics and remains on a ventilator. Because he is unable to ingest any calories and because of a protracted ileus associated with his pelvic fracture, total parenteral nutrition (TPN) is initiated. Continued irrigation and debridement of the open pelvic fracture wound are undertaken with bedside dressing changes and return trips to the operating room. Two weeks after the patient's injury and after multiple operative events the patient remains on a ventilator with an FiO_2 of 0.4% with 10 cm of PEEP. The bilirubin level is 4.0 mg/dl, and the AST, ALT, and GGT levels are mildly elevated. His serum creatinine is 1.8 mg/dl. Local debridement and cleansing of the wound shows only surface contamination at this point of the pelvic fracture. However, the patient has a persistent fever and leukocytosis and now is identified as having purulent sputum. Cultures of the lung identify moderate growth of *Pseudomonas aeruginosa*. Chest radiography shows an increasing area of infiltration in the lung on the side of the pulmonary contusion. Three of four blood cultures are positive for *Enterococcus faecalis*. Aggressive systemic antimicrobial therapy is required for treatment of both isolated pathogens (*P. aeruginosa* and *E. faecalis*). The patient has resumption of gastrointestinal function and is taken from his TPN strategy and starts receiving enteral feeding. Continued supportive care with ventilator management and enteral feeding ultimately results in resolution of the pneumonia and apparent clearing of the bacteremia. The patient is weaned from the respirator, and all liver enzyme abnormalities return to normal, as does the creatinine. The patient is discharged for rehabilitation some 5 weeks after the injury.

This patient represents a clinical scenario wherein a host of variables could potentially be implicated in his organ failure complex. The patient has severe soft tissue injury, direct pulmonary contusion, and long-bone fracture, shock; and he has undergone numerous resuscitations, multiple anesthetics, and surgical interventions.[23] Management of the perineal wound was largely mechanical; and although surface colonization could be identified, as would be expected in the perineal wound, in fact no septic events emanated from the perineal wound. Nevertheless, the patient developed criteria consistent with multiple organ failure. Evidence of bacteremia with enterococci and a ventilator-associated pneumonia occurred in the aftermath (or as a sequel to) organ failure.

One could logically argue that the "exhaustion" of host defenses created by the sustained illness, the hypermetabolic state of the severely injured patient, and the repeated insults of reoperation and multiple anesthetics rendered this patient unable to deal with the intercurrent contamination, which then led to invasive infection. Infection was doubtless the consequence of the CARS-dominant response following severe

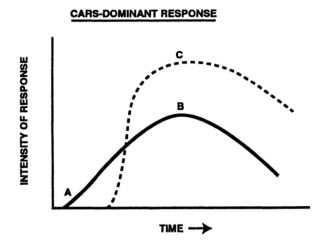

FIGURE 61.3. Theoretic relation of the intensity of the aggregate pro- and counterinflammatory response seen in the CARS-dominant scenario. A, Biologic insult. Counterinflammatory signaling (C) is far in excess of the proinflammatory signaling (B).

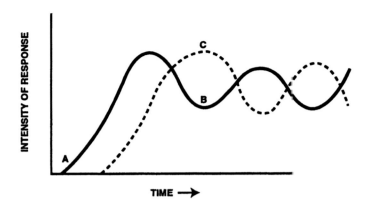

FIGURE 61.4. Theoretic relation of the intensity of the aggregate pro- and counterinflammatory response seen in the MARS scenario. A, Biologic insult. Fluctuations and a disordered relation between the proinflammatory (B) and counterinflammatory (C) signals create the "immunologic dissonance" seen during a sustained illness of the patient in the critical care unit.

injury (Fig. 61.3). Clearly, in this patient it seems that organ failure preceded emergence of the nosocomial bacteremia and the ventilator-associated pneumonia. Had the organ failure been severe enough from this life-threatening injury and had the nosocomial infections been somewhat more complex, what would have rightfully been viewed as the cause of death in such a patient? Would it be failure of the host defense and failure of critical organ system functions, or would it be preterminal clinical infection? This man certainly appears to have had infection as an accompanying event to organ failure, not as the instigating event that precipitated organ dysfunction.

Mixed SIRS/CARS Response

The mixed antagonist response, or MARS, is depicted in a theoretic construct in Fig. 61.4. Neither the SIRS-dominant nor the CARS-dominant scenario prevails; rather, an uncoordinated series of pro- and counterinflammatory responses are seen. Termed immunologic dissonance,[20] it may result from extreme, sustained SIRS or profound, sustained immunosuppression due to the dominant counterinflammatory forces. Measurements of specific cytokine signals at any point may identify increased proinflammatory signals,[24] increased counterinflammatory signals,[25] or fluctuating, confusing cytokine patterns.[26] It is likely to be the clinical scenario of repeated proinflammatory assaults with corresponding counterinflammatory responses that become dyscoordinated with respect to their balanced relation with each other. It is indeed the MARS scenario that is becoming a more common dilemma in the ICU, where contemporary support measures maintain the patient within the biologic limits between the two opposing antagonists. Achieving a coordinated, appropriate relation is a formidable therapeutic challenge.

Temporal Relation of Infection and Organ Failure

The temporal relation of the onset of clinical infection and subsequent MODS has been examined by numerous authors in an effort to define whether infection is the instigating event responsible for organ failure or part of the aftermath of systemic inflammation and immunosuppression. Clinical studies by Sauaia et al.[27] indicate that predictors of organ failure are present as early as within 12 hours of presentation in the trauma patient. They identified injury severity (determined by the Injury Severity Score), platelet counts, age of the patient, the need for transfused blood, inotrope utilization, and lactate concentrations early in the patient's course as predictors of organ failure. A natural extension of these results would be to say that the systemic consequences of the initial insult are the responsible events, and that infection, second operations, and other events in the critically ill patient are nonspecific secondary events. From these studies has emerged the construct that early organ failure, which is seen within the first week of the patient's injury or acute illness, may have a genesis different from that which is seen late in the evolution of the critically ill patient in the ICU.

The more closely one examines the temporal relation of systemic events (i.e., injury or hemorrhage) with the emergence of acute infection and the subsequent evolution of organ failure, the less clear the issue becomes. Acute injury creates cellular dyshomeostasis due to ischemia/reperfusion injury, tissue hypoxemia, and intracellular acidosis. The acute injury results in a component of systemic activation of inflammation and an obligatory immunosuppressive response. Infection may occur in the immediate aftermath of these global perturbations of the host; but was it infection that provoked the subsequent cascade of organ failure, was it the original event, or was it the consequence of all of these factors in concert?

Infection has been implicated more commonly in the late-onset emergence of organ failure. Patients develop infection 3–10 days following injury or major operation, and organ failure later ensues. The same issues exist here that were seen in the previous scenario. Was infection the primary or major event, or was it the consequence of immunosuppression?

Finally, in the late or sustained organ failure patient, determining the responsible clinical event becomes almost impossible. The ICU patient who requires sustained ventilator support usually has had a sequence of operations, infections, acute hemodynamic or oxygen delivery crises, sustained hypermetabolism, protein-calorie malnutrition, and other events that defy an organized sequencing to explain cause-and-effect relations. Bacterial infections at this stage of the illness are commonly with low-virulence microbes (e.g., *Enterococcus* sp.), and blood-borne infections in the aftermath of immunosuppression and catabolism may indeed reflect loss of the gut barrier.

Thus the arguments about temporal relations may be academic charades that only further obscure the true understanding of fundamental events in the critically ill or injured patient. The clinical variables of injury, shock, infection, and immunosuppression are so integrally intertwined that isolating them may be impossible with our current understanding.

Conclusions

It can be said that in selected patients infection is the stimulus for activation of the systemic inflammatory response. In other patients, severe injury and other noninfectious events activate systemic inflammation, which has immunosuppression as an attendant event and infection as a consequence. In many complex patients in the ICU the relation of infection, SIRS, and MODS become almost impossible to discern.

Current management of these patients remains independent of the argument about which event was the principal one. Early effective resuscitation, effective oxygen delivery, and precise management of injuries remain the hallmark of management. Diagnosis and treatment of clinical infections remain important determinants of patient outcome regardless of the relation to SIRS or MODS. Infection control practices are especially important for the immunosuppressed host. Early, effective enteral nutritional support strategies appear to play an important role in the reduction of infectious events in these patients. Continued aggressive supportive care will continue to be the hallmark of management until better diagnostic tools and a better understanding of this complex conundrum affords better mechanism-based therapy for the patient with SIRS and MODS.

References

1. Fry DE, Pearlstein L, Fulton RL, Polk HC Jr: Multiple system organ failure: the role of uncontrolled infection. Arch Surg 1980;115:136–140.
2. Fry DE, Garrison RN, Heitch RC, et al: Determinants of death in patients with intraabdominal abscess. Surgery 1980;89:517–523.
3. Fry DE, Garrison RN, Williams HC: Patterns of morbidity and mortality in splenectomy for trauma. Am Surg 1980;46:28–32.
4. Fry DE, Garrison RN, Polk HC Jr: Clinical implications in bacteroides bacteremia. Surg Gynecol Obstet 1979;149:189–192.
5. Eiseman B, Beart R, Norton L: Multiple organ failure. Surg Gynecol Obstet 1977;144:323–326.
6. Polk HC Jr, Shields CL: Remote organ failure: a valid sign of occult intraabdominal infection. Surgery 1977;81:310.
7. Hinsdale JG, Jaffe BM: Reoperation for intraabdominal sepsis: indications and results in modern critical care setting. Ann Surg 1984;199:31–36.
8. Rush BF Jr, Sori AJ, Murphy TF, et al: Endotoxemia and bacteremia during hemorrhagic shock: the link between trauma and sepsis? Ann Surg 1988;207:549.
9. Deitch EA: Simple intestinal obstruction causes bacterial translocation in man. Arch Surg 1989;124:699.
10. Marshall JC, Christou NV, Meakins JL: The gastrointestinal tract: the undrained "abscess" of multiple organ failure. Ann Surg 1993;218:111–119.
11. Van Leeuwen PA, Boermeester MA, Houdijk AP, et al: Clinical significance of translocation. Gut 1994;35(Suppl 1):S28–S34.
12. Nieuwenhuijzen GA, Deitch EA, Goris RJ: The relationship between gut-derived bacteria and the development of the multiple organ dysfunction syndrome. J Anat 1996;189:537–548.
13. Lemaire LC, van Lanschat JJ, Stoutenbeek CP, et al: Bacterial translocation in multiple organ failure: cause or epiphenomenon still unproven. Br J Surg 1997;84:1340–1350.
14. Goldie AS, Fearon KCH, Ross JA, et al: Natural cytokine antagonists and endogenous antiendotoxin core antibodies in sepsis syndrome. JAMA 1995;274:172–177.
15. Zedler S, Bone RC, Baue AE, et al: T-cell reactivity and its predictive role in immunosuppression after burns. Crit Care Med 1999;27:66–72.
16. Faist E, Schinkel C, Zimmer S: Update on the mechanisms of immune suppression of injury and immune modulation. World J Surg 1996;20:454–459.
17. Pietsch JB, Meakins JL, MacLean LD: The delayed hypersensitivity response: applications in clinical surgery. Surgery 1977;82:349–355.
18. Hershman MJ, Cheadle WG, Wellhausen SR, et al: Monocyte HLA-DR expression characterizes clinical outcome in the trauma paient. Br J Surg 1990;77:294.
19. Lewis RT, Klein H: Risk factors and postoperative sepsis: significance of preoperative lymphocytopenia. J Surg Res 1975;26:365–371.
20. Bone RC: Immunologic dissonance: a continuing evolution in our understanding of the systemic inflammatory response syndrome (SIRS) and the multiple organ dysfunction syndrome (MODS). Ann Intern Med 1996;125:680–687.
21. Bone RC, Grodzin CJ, Balk RA: Sepsis: a new hypothesis for pathogenesis of the disease process. Chest 1997;112:235–243.
22. Wickel DJ, Cheadle WG, Mercer-Jones NA, Garrison RN: Poor outcome from peritonitis caused by disease acuity and organ failure, not recurrent peritoneal infection. Ann Surg 1997;225:744–753.
23. Moore EE: Synergy of bone fractures, soft tissue disruption, and hemorrhagic shock in the genesis of postinjury immunochaos: the pathway to multiple organ failure. Crit Care Med 1998;26:1372–1378.

24. Pinsky MR, Vincent JL, Deviere J, et al: Serum cytokine levels in human septic shock: relation to multiple-system organ failure and mortality. Chest 1993;103:565–575.
25. Lehmann AK, Halstensen A, Sornes S, et al: High levels of interleukin 10 in serum are associated with fatality in meningococcal disease. Infect Immun 1995;63:2109–2112.
26. Marano MA, Fong Y, Moldawer LL, et al: Serum cachectin/tumor necrosis factor in critically ill patients with burns correlates with infection and mortality. Surg Gynecol Obstet 1990;170:32–38.
27. Sauaia A, Moore FA, Moore EE, et al: Multiple organ failure can be predicted as early as 12 hours after injury. J Trauma 1998;45:291–301.

62
Hypertonic Solutions

Mauricio Rocha e Silva and Luiz F. Poli de Figueiredo

Contemporary interest in the use of hypertonic solutions for the treatment of shock was triggered by our group in 1980.[1] We demonstrated that in a severely hemorrhaged dog a bolus injection of 7.5% NaCl (4 ml/kg, a volume equivalent to only 10% of the volume of shed blood) rapidly restored arterial pressure and cardiac output, resulting in long-term survival of all animals. In contrast, control animals, that received the same volume of isotonic saline did not respond with hemodynamic improvement or survival.

That same year, Fellipe et al. pioneered human studies with 7.5% NaCl solutions given to patients with refractory shock in an intensive care unit (ICU) and also observed hemodynamic benefits.[2] These papers stimulated hundreds of studies, including experimental studies and more than 60 clinical trials with 7.5% NaCl for treatment of several conditions (e.g., hemorrhagic, cardiogenic, and septic shock) and use of a volume-supporting solution during major surgical procedures.[3]

Several groups confirmed our findings that a small volume of 7.5% NaCl, infused into animals that have bled 40–50% of their blood volumes, rapidly restored arterial pressure, cardiac output, and vital organs' blood flow.[4–8] The cardiovascular improvement is instantaneous and has been attributed to plasma volume expansion, vasodilatation in several vascular beds, and a direct cardiac inotropic effect.[9,10]

We discuss here some current aspects of the mechanisms of action and the physiologic consequences of small-volume resuscitation with 7.5% NaCl solutions, including the issues of safety and potential limitations of use, based on the available published clinical experience (Table 62.1).

Mechanisms for Volume Expansion

A purely physical component causes the initial effect of a 4 ml/kg bolus injection of 7.5% NaCl (2400 mosm/L), which is volume expansion resulting from the osmotic gradient created, shifting fluid to the intravascular compartment. The 7.5% NaCl injection adds sodium at 5.13 mEq/L/kg body weight. Theoretically, this sodium load is distributed through the plasma volume (~40 ml/kg), resulting, also theoretically, in an increase in plasma sodium to 128 mEq/L above its basal level of 135–140 mEq/L (5.12 mEq in 40 ml of plasma). These events should result in plasma sodium levels of about 265 mEq/L, but such values have not been observed in either laboratory or clinical trials.

To reach these plasma levels of sodium, the sodium load should be administered within 10 seconds or less, with the plasma sodium level being estimated immediately after injection (Fig. 62.1). Such a rapid injection is feasible only if we employ a saturated solution of 30% NaCl, which reduces the volume to be injected to 1 ml/kg. The same sodium load, injected over 1 minute, produces a plasma sodium concentration of 165 mEq/L, similar to what is observed 1 minute after the 30% NaCl injection within 10 seconds. Thus the sodium dilution of 5.12 mEq/kg occurs throughout the extracellular compartment, representing about 200 ml/kg. This process increases the plasma sodium concentration by only 25 mEq/L above its normal value of 135–140 mEq/L. These observations explain why sodium levels above 165 mEq/L have not been observed in clinical and experimental studies. In fact, when an NaCl (7.5%) injection of 4 ml/kg is completed over 2 minutes a mean sodium peak of 155 mEq/L is normally observed, with a gradual decrease to 145 mEq/L during the first hours. Figure 62.1 demonstrates that at the end of this slower, 2-minute injection, which imitates the clinical scenario, the plasma sodium concentration is similar to that observed 2 minutes after the faster injections.[11]

The infusion of 250 ml of 7.5% NaCl solution to adult patients (the most commonly used dose) usually takes more than 2 minutes. This timing allows a second factor to exert its action: the osmotically driven fluid shift from the intracellular to the extracellular compartment, reducing the plasma sodium levels even more.

Using plasma volume measurements and hematocrit changes after 7.5% NaCl, we detected an 11 ml/kg increment in plasma volume, that disappeared after 6 hours.[1] The initial volume expansion represents about 2.75 ml of plasma for each milliliter of the injected solution, whereas with standard isotonic solutions an expansion ratio of 0.33 ml is observed for each milliliter injected as a consequence of the distribution of the isotonic solution into the extravascular compartment.

TABLE 62.1. Clinical Experience with 7.5% NaCl Solutions.

Setting	No. of Studies	HS	HSD	HSS	Total
Prehospital	9	202	495	16	713
Emergency room	8	138	326		464
Intraoperative	21	34	58	175	267
Intensive care unit	18	91	65	116	272
Clinical	4	18	19	4	41
Total	60	483	963	311	1757

HS, 7.5% NaCl; HSD, 7.5% NaCl/6% dextran 70; HSS, 7.5% NaCl/6% hetastarch.

The association of 6% dextran 70 to the 7.5% NaCl solution (HSD) does not add to the initial plasma expansion. It does contribute to maintenance of the fluid in the intravascular compartment for longer periods, thus prolonging the hemodynamic and metabolic benefits of the hypertonic solutions.[5,6,12] Dextran 70 exerts a colloid osmotic pressure two to three times greater than what is observed with a similar concentration of human albumin, being therefore hyperoncotic. Results similar to those seen with HSD have been demonstrated with the addition of 6% hetastarch to the 7.5% NaCl solution (HSS).[13]

The respective reflection coefficients of the endothelial barrier and cellular membrane must be considered when determining the osmotic force generated by the sodium gradient established after the use of hypertonic saline solution. The endothelial layer has a coefficient of 0.1, whereas the cell membrane coefficient is 1.0. Immediately after injection of 7.5% NaCl, a gradient of 25 mosm/L exerts an osmotic pressure of about 500 mmHg through the cellular membrane and only 50 mmHg through the endothelial membrane. Thus the equilibrium across the endothelial membrane is reached within seconds, whereas the equilibrium process across the cellular membrane requires a longer time.

The plasma expansion induced by hypertonic resuscitation is maximum during administration of the solution. It occurs from the intracellular compartment, not from the interstitial compartment, which is also expanded. This fluid shift from the intracellular to the extracellular compartment may be regarded as beneficial, as during shock states, ischemia/reperfusion, extracorporeal circulation, and sepsis, among other conditions, there is cellular edema due to the action of inflammatory mediators and sodium/potassium pump dysfunction in the cellular membranes.[14]

In all clinical studies performed to date with the use of 7.5% NaCl, isotonic fluids have been injected after the hypertonic solution, correcting an eventual loss of cellular volume. Clinical manifestations of cellular dehydration would be apparent first in the central nervous system, but there have been no reports of seizures or neurologic dysfunction in any of the more than 1700 patients who received hypertonic solutions.[3]

Effects on the Microcirculation

The main sources for the observed plasma expansion after 7.5% NaCl injection are the red blood cells and the endothelium, which are in close contact with the hypertonicity, losing about 8% of their volumes directly to the intravascular compartment. Apart from the volume expansion, these events result in important hemodynamic effects on the microcirculation, as the edema in the red blood cells and endothelium, as observed during shock and ischemia/reperfusion, are of critical importance in terms of viscosity and hydraulic resistance in the microcirculation, where the vascular lumen/red blood cells ratio approaches unity. Under these circumstances, cellular edema compromises the microcirculatory blood flow. Hypertonic, but not isotonic, solutions contribute to hemodynamic improvement at the microcirculatory level.[15]

These microcirculatory disturbances have been implicated in the origin of the sepsis and multiple organ dysfunction observed after an initially successful resuscitation from posttraumatic shock.[16] The resulting sustained splanchnic vasoconstriction may cause gut mucosal ischemia and consequent compromise of its integrity, with a predisposition to bacterial and toxin penetration from the intestinal lumen into the systemic circulation. The changes in the gut mucosa may be even more severe during the reperfusion period, mediated by oxygen free radicals, which also results in capillary lumen narrowing, leukocyte adhesion and activation, and stimulation of several inflammatory mediators and cytokines, which may cause local tissue and remote organ injury.[16–18]

Under these conditions, hypertonic solutions may produce several beneficial effects through rapid hemodynamic restoration at the macro- and microcirculatory levels. Based on these observed effects in posttraumatic shock, studies with 7.5% NaCl solutions, with and without dextran or hetastarch, have been

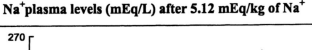
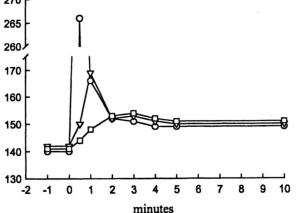

FIGURE 62.1. Plasma sodium levels after intravenous injections of Na$^+$ 5.12 mEq/kg to normovolemic anesthetized dogs. This sodium load was infused in three regimens: 30% 1 ml/kg 30% NaCl in 10 seconds (○), 4 ml/kg 7.5% NaCl in 1 minute (△), and 4 ml/kg 7.5% NaCl in 2 minutes (□).

performed using several models of sepsis and septic shock, and transient similar benefits have been observed in global and regional hemodynamics.[19-21]

Effects on Vascular Resistance

The hypertonicity induced by 7.5% NaCl injection is responsible for the increased blood flow in the peripheral circulation and in the microcirculation as a consequence of reduced vascular resistance, primarily by arteriolar vasodilatation. This response is caused by a direct relaxant effect of hypertonicity on vascular smooth muscle.

The reduction in blood viscosity, by the hemodilution rapidly induced by the hypertonic solution, also contributes to the reduction in vascular resistance and vasodilatation. The use of 7.5% NaCl in shock produces vasodilatation and increased regional blood flow to coronary,[22] renal,[23] intestinal,[8,9,24] and skeletal muscle[8] circulations.

Effects on Myocardial Contractility

The hemodynamic benefits observed after 7.5% NaCl have been partially attributed to a direct cardiac inotropic effect induced by hypertonicity.[25,26] However, an evaluation of left ventricular contractility after 7.2% NaCl/6% hetastarch in anesthetized, stable patients without cardiovascular disease did not demonstrate a clinically relevant positive inotropic effect. All hemodynamic benefits were therefore attributed to the combination of volume expansion and decreased afterload.[27]

Some authors showed no direct inotropic effect with hypertonic solutions in the treatment of hemorrhagic shock,[28] whereas others showed negative inotropic effects in normovolemic dogs.[29] Thus the question of whether hypertonic solutions have a direct positive inotropic effect via the hypertonicity contributing to the hemodynamic benefits remains controversial.

Additional Regional Effects

Improvements in renal function have been observed after HSD infusion to animals in shock. This benefit is probably multifactorial, resulting from volume expansion, general hemodynamic improvement, and increased renal blood flow.[30]

A great benefit with hypertonic resuscitation has been observed on cerebral hemodynamics during hemorrhagic shock, particularly in the presence of intracranial hypertension and systemic hypotension.[31-33] The rapid restoration of the arterial pressure associated with a reduction in intracranial hypertension induced by hypertonic solutions suggests a potential clinical application of these solutions for trauma victims with head injury and associated lesions with hypotension, a subset of trauma victims with poor prognosis. In the clinical trials, patients with a low Glasgow Coma Score and hypotension after trauma were benefited with an initial infusion of hypertonic solutions.[34]

Long-Term Effects

The immediate effects of hypertonic solutions in shock are dependent on the well demonstrated physical and physiologic effects of the hypertonicity. On the other hand, long-term effects of the hypertonic resuscitation have only recently been adequately evaluated.

The role of the dextran component as an oxygen free radical scavenger and the role of HSD as an inhibitor of leukocyte activation have been recognized.[35] More recently, a series of experiments by Coimbra et al. has shown that hypertonic saline solution, even without dextran, significantly interferes with the immune responses, both in vitro and in vivo.[36-40]

The addition of hypertonic saline solution to lymphocyte culture media in concentrations similar to those obtained with the infusion of 7.5% NaCl 4 ml/kg in humans produced a significant increase in lymphocyte proliferation.[36] The addition of prostaglandin E_2 (PGE_2) to the culture medium, in the absence of hypertonic saline, caused a reduction in T cell proliferation when compared to control cultures. On the other hand, when hypertonic saline was added to the culture medium containing PGE_2, there was a complete reversal on the PGE_2-induced immunosuppression.[39]

These in vitro findings were confirmed *in vivo* using a hemorrhagic shock model in mice in which infusion of 7.5% NaCl reversed the cellular immune function depression that occurs after hemorrhage. Plasma levels of several cytokines were determined, and the authors concluded that hypertonic saline solution prevents immunosuppression probably by decreasing plasma levels of interleukin-4 (IL-4) and PGE_2.[38] Using a hemorrhagic shock model in mice, followed by cecal puncture 24 hours later, these authors showed that with the use of 7.5% NaCl there was a significant decrease in mortality 72 hours after peritonitis induction compared to conventional isotonic resuscitation. Moreover, a significant reduction in pulmonary and hepatic changes after hypertonic solutions was observed.[39] We have described a significant reduction in bacterial translocation and pulmonary lesions in rats with hemorrhagic shock that were treated with hypertonic saline solution.[40]

Based on this evidence, it has been suggested that hypertonic saline solutions have significant potential as immunomodulating agents for resuscitating trauma victims.[41] Additional research and careful evaluation in clinical trials are required using these solutions.

Association with Oxygen Carriers

There is a great interest in the association of hypertonic saline, which causes hemodilution, with oxygen carriers, particularly modified cell-free hemoglobins. The latter are currently undergoing phase III clinical trials. It has been well demonstrated that small volumes of these solutions restore arterial pressure in animals in hemorrhagic shock. However, this benefit is achieved through marked vasoconstriction secondary to nitric oxide scavenging by the free hemoglobin.

Severe pulmonary hypertension and coronary, splanchnic and renal vasoconstriction also have been attributed to cell-free hemoglobin solutions.[42–45] The association of hypertonic sodium acetate solution (2400 mosm/L), with cell-free hemoglobin limited the potent arteriolar vasodilatory properties of this variety of hypertonic solution because of the marked hemoglobin-induced vasoconstriction. With this combination, it has been shown that the association of peripheral vasodilatation (induced by the hypertonic solution) with the pulmonary hypertension (induced by the hemoglobin) may result in severe hemodynamic instability.[44] Slower infusions of the combined hypertonic-hemoglobin solution, the use of inhaled nitric oxide to reverse pulmonary hypertension selectively,[45] and the use of encapsulated hemoglobin,[46] which is definitely less vasoconstrictive, are some of the potential alternatives that have been tested to expand the benefits of hypertonic saline resuscitation.

Clinical Experience

A substantial clinical experience has been accumulated regarding the use of 7.5% NaCl solutions (Table 62.1). Most patients have received these solutions as the initial treatment for posttraumatic hypotension followed by standard-of-care isotonic crystalloid solutions in the prehospital or emergency room environment, including those in several prospective and double-blind studies.[47–55] These patients have been submitted to extensive clinical and laboratory evaluation, demonstrating the complete safety of these solutions, even when infused into trauma victims, with immediate risk of death from hypovolemia, hemodynamic instability, and severe associated lesions. These same studies have provided valuable insights regarding the efficacy of these hypertonic saline solutions. The studies performed in patients undergoing cardiovascular surgery and in critically ill patients in ICUs units provide data regarding the effects of hypertonic saline solutions in patients presenting with associated preexisting diseases and organs and systems with limited reserve.

Efficacy

The ultimate test of efficacy for treatment of trauma plus shock is enhanced survival. Secondary, but equally important, endpoints are reduced complications and lower treatment costs. A number of reports have demonstrated significantly increased efficacy in patients treated with hypertonic saline followed by standard-of-care treatment when compared to equivalent patients receiving standard-of-care treatment only.

In the first trial, which included 105 patients in hypovolemic shock, the patients treated with hypertonic saline showed significant initial improvement of arterial pressure and reduced intravenous fluid requirements. No significant difference in mortality was detected.[47] In a subsequent study, in which 212 hypotensive patients were enrolled, Younes et al. showed that hypertonic saline as initial treatment caused a significant decrease in the long-term mortality rate for the subpopulation with an entry mean arterial pressure below 70 mmHg.[52]

A U.S. multicenter trial[51] (422 patients enrolled) showed a significant increase in survival for the HSD-treated patients in the subpopulation requiring surgery. It also showed a greater incidence of adult respiratory distress syndrome (ARDS), renal failure, and coagulopathy in the standard-of-care-alone treatment group.

Hypotensive patients sustaining a head injury with Glasgow Coma Scale scores of 8 or less who received hypertonic saline treatment had a higher survival rate up to hospital discharge. This was demonstrated in a multicenter trial[54] and in a meta-analysis of individual patients from all the known clinical trials.[55] A meta-analysis conducted on the individual patient records from controlled clinical studies on trauma demonstrated a significant increase in survival favoring HSD versus standard-of-care.[55]

Safety, Concerns, Controversies

Bleeding

Because hypertonic saline resuscitation induces an immediate restoration of cardiac output and arterial pressure, vasodilatation, and hemodilution, several investigators raised concerns that these effects could overcome homeostatic mechanisms, such as vasoconstriction and local tamponade, or even hypotension. It therefore represents a potential risk for increased internal bleeding.[56,57]

These concerns were highlighted by a controversial study that challenged the guidelines recommended by the Advanced Trauma Life Support Course,[58] for resuscitation of penetrating trauma victims and hypotension with large volumes of isotonic crystalloid solutions.[59] This study suggested that standard-of-care prehospital and emergency room fluid infusion for these patients resulted in higher mortality and morbidity than what was observed for patients in whom fluid resuscitation was delayed (i.e., after operative bleeding control).[59]

On the other hand, the U.S. multicenter trial compared standard-of-care fluid infusion to a regimen of HSD followed by standard-of-care for prehospital treatment of posttraumatic hypotension. The results demonstrated that penetrating trauma victims with hypotension who received HSD had a higher arterial blood pressure with a trend toward a higher survival rate and fewer complications than the patients treated by standard-of-care fluid treatment alone.[51] Similar results were observed in other studies, recently presented as a meta-analysis.[55] These data suggest that the negative effects of large-volume infusion of crystalloid solutions are not related to increased arterial pressure but to factors related to the isotonic solution itself. A trial comparing standard-of-care, HSD, and delayed resuscitation is needed to establish the best means to treat posttraumatic hypotension.

Patients receiving hypertonic solutions in these studies on posttraumatic hypotension underwent extensive laboratory investigations, which showed that the amount of dextran 70 in the HSD formulation did not alter the coagulation profile. Additionally, none of the studies with trauma victims or those conducted to test the intraoperative use of HSD demonstrated any association between hypertonic solutions and blood loss or with increased requirements of blood products. In all studies so far performed, blood product requirements have always been associated with the severity and mechanism of injury, not with the solution used. In fact, a reduction in subsequent fluid requirements is a common finding after the use of HSD.[55]

Neither was the use of HSD during complex cardiovascular surgical procedures, in which hemostasis alterations are common,[60] associated with increased blood loss or increased blood product requirements. Moreover, the use hypertonic solutions during cardiac and aortic surgery has been frequently associated with hemodynamic stability and less, rather than more, postoperative fluid requirement.[61-64]

Overall, the common observation of less fluid requirement, no increase in blood product requirement, and trends toward less morbidity and mortality with the use of hypertonic solutions suggest that there is no increase in bleeding associated with its use, even in patients sustaining penetrating trauma or during complex cardiovascular surgery.

Hypernatremia

A frequent concern with hypertonic resuscitation is that it might induce significant hypernatremia with potentially deleterious consequences. Such hypernatremia would of course result from cellular dehydration produced by the osmotic mechanisms already described. With severe hypernatremia, evidence of cellular dehydration manifests much earlier in the central nervous system than in other organs or systems. Symptoms of hypernatremia include lethargy, tremors, weakness, irritability, delirium, mental confusion, seizures, coma, and death. They occur in severe cases and particularly in small children and the elderly.

The use of hypertonic sodium solutions to correct hyponatremia rapidly in patients with severe malnutrition or alcoholism may result in central pontine myelinolysis, manifested through dysarthria, paraparesis, or paraplegia.[65] Another complication described with use of hypertonic sodium solutions to correct hyponatremia in neonates is rupture of cerebral veins and intracranial hemorrhage caused by retraction of the cerebral tissue.[66]

With these questions in the forefront of all clinical trials, patients receiving 7.5% NaCl were carefully evaluated for signs and symptoms of hypernatremia, particularly the associated neurologic alterations. It was especially true for patients at highest risk for neurologic dysfunction and intracranial hypertension (i.e., those sustaining head trauma and systemic hypotension).

Despite the fact that moderate hypernatremia and hyperosmolarity have been detected in most patients receiving 7.5% NaCl solutions, there was not a single case, among more than 1700 patients, of seizures, intracranial bleeding, or neurologic deterioration induced by the hypertonic solution.[55,67] Necropsies and careful anatopathologic studies of the brain tissues in trauma victims revealed no evidence of central pontine demyelination or of focal intracranial bleeding that could be attributed to the use of 7.5% NaCl.[55,67]

The short duration of the moderate hypernatremia, the absence of preexisting hyponatremia, and the exclusion of children and patients with chronic disabling diseases may have contributed to the lack of hypernatremia-related undesirable effects. On the other hand, hypotensive patients with head trauma and a low Glasgow Coma Scale comprised one of the subgroups who most benefited from 7.5% NaCl solution as the initial treatment, presenting better neurologic outcome and a significant increase in survival.[67] Thus 7.5% NaCl-induced hypernatremia and hyperosmolarity were associated with neurologic benefit, not neurologic dysfunction.

Although we cannot exclude the possibility that higher doses of hypertonic saline might induce hypernatremia-related side effects, the prescribed dose cannot result in such effects. However, it seems prudent to avoid these solutions in patients at the highest risk of severe neurologic disturbance induced by hypernatremia (i.e., patients with chronic debilitating diseases and children).

Cardiac Dysfunction

Experiments with anesthetized animals in shock have shown that rapid injection of 7.5 NaCl may cause hypotension and arrhythmia due to hypertonicity-induced vasodilatation and reduced peripheral vascular resistance.[68] These events may be particularly dangerous when the arterial pressure is markedly low before infusion of the solution. This hemodynamic instability is directly dependent on the speed with which the solution is infused and may be avoided with infusion times longer than 2 minutes.

Most trials with intraoperative use of 7.5% NaCl have demonstrated physiologic benefits and no side effects.[61-64] There is one study, however, in patients with myocardial dysfunction undergoing coronary artery bypass in which preoperative volume expansion with 250 ml of HSS caused hypotension and transient left ventricular failure.[69] This study showed that 7.5% NaCl solutions can be deleterious if rapidly infused in patients with ventricular dysfunction, in whom a fixed dose may be inadequate.[70] In a similar study of patients with cardiac dysfunction in which the volume of 7.5% NaCl solution was titrated to a target cardiac filling pressure, it was found that a lower dosage was enough to achieve the desired hemodynamic profile, with no hemodynamic instability.[70]

In a separate study, a fixed dose of HSD (250 ml) was used during extracorporeal circulation in a Jehovah's Witness, with no hemodynamic changes and reduced fluid requirements during the postoperative period.[64] A similar dose was used in surgical procedures for correction of thoracic and abdominal aortic aneurysms.[61,62,71] These procedures are normally associated with sudden hemodynamic changes, marked fluid loss to the third space, and a high incidence of postoperative complications.[72] The use of hypertonic saline solutions resulted in hemodynamic stability and fluid sparing during the postoperative period for these procedures. The use of 7.5% NaCl solution to patients with cardiogenic shock after right ventricular infarction also produced sustained hemodynamic benefits.[73]

When the entire population of 1700 patients in whom 7.5% NaCl solutions were used is examined, it is seen that there were no cardiac deaths. However, it seems prudent to recommend caution with the use of hypertonic solutions in patients with heart disease. Rigorous monitoring is mandatory, and gradual and slower infusions should be employed.

Hyperchloremic Acidosis

There is a significant increase in chloride plasma levels after 7.5% NaCl injection, which could predispose to hyperchloremic acidosis. Clinically relevant acidosis was observed in trauma victims who were moribund on arrival; the acidosis was associated with preexisting conditions such as cardiac arrest or severe hypothermia.[49] Despite hemodynamic and metabolic improvement after 7.5% NaCl solutions in most patients, based on the clinical evidence we suggest that these solutions should be avoided in patients with preexisting severe acidosis, which probably developed over longer periods of time.

Allergic Reactions

There is a small incidence of side effects associated with all colloids, including dextran; the incidence of anaphylactic reactions (preformed antibodies) or more common anaphylactoid (no preformed antibodies) is 1:2500.[73] Thus even though HSD and HSS solutions contain a limited amount of colloid, the use of hapten-dextran 1 (molecular weight 1000 daltons) is recommended preceding the elective use of HSD to reduce the risk of allergic reactions to levels similar to those observed with human albumin solution. On the other hand, among the hundreds of trauma patients receiving HSD without hapten-dextran-1, there were no reports of an allergic reaction.

Conclusions

Based on the available clinical experience with 7.5% NaCl solutions, we conclude that the use of hypertonic solutions is safe, but it is prudent to avoid their use in a well defined patient population (i.e., children, those who are moribund, or those with a chronic debilitating diseases). Efficacy has been suggested for this procedure as the first treatment for posttraumatic hypotension, particularly for penetrating trauma victims requiring surgery and those with head trauma. Elective intraoperative use of these solutions has been associated with hemodynamic stability and fluid sparing. However, titrated dosage and careful monitoring are required in patients with cardiac failure. Increased bleeding, clinically significant hypernatremia, and allergic reactions were not associated with hypertonic resuscitation. Although the safety issue has been well established, it appears that large prospective, multicenter trials are required to better define the patient population who can maximally benefit from hypertonic saline solutions.

References

1. Velasco IT, Pontieri V, Rocha e Silva M, et al: Hyperosmotic NaCl and severe hemorrhagic shock. Am J Physiol 1980;239:H664–H673.
2. De Fellipe JJ, Timoner J, Velasco IT, et al: Treatment of refractory hypovolaemic shock by 7.5% sodium chloride injections. Lancet 1980;2:1002–1004.
3. Poli de Figueiredo LF, Kramer GC: Safety concerns and contraindications of hyperosmolar small-volume resuscitation. In: Kreimeier U, Christ F, Messmer K (eds). Small-Volume Hyperosmolar Volume Resuscitation. Heidelberg, Springer, (1999, in press).
4. Nakayama S, Sibley L, Gunther R, et al: Small-volume resuscitation with hypertonic saline resuscitation (2400 mosm/L) during hemorrhagic shock. Circ Shock 1984;13:149–159.
5. Smith GJ, Kramer GC, Perron P, et al: A comparison of several hypertonic solutions for resuscitation of bled sheep. J Surg Res 1985;39:517–528.
6. Kramer GC, Perron PR, Lindsey DC, et al: Small-volume resuscitation with hypertonic saline dextran solution. Surgery 1986;100:239–247.
7. Poli de Figueiredo LF, Peres CA, Attalah AN, et al: Hemodynamic improvement in hemorrhagic shock by aortic balloon occlusion and hypertonic saline solutions. Cardiovasc Surg 1995;3:679–686.
8. Rocha e Silva M, Negraes G, Soares A, et al: Hypertonic resuscitation from severe hemorrhagic shock: patterns of regional circulation. Circ Shock 1986;19:165–175.
9. Kreimeier U, Bruckner U, Niemczyk S, Messmer K: Hyperosmotic saline dextran for resuscitation from traumatic-hemorrhagic hypotension: effect on regional blood flow. Circ Shock 1990;32:83–99.
10. Rocha e Silva M, Velasco IT, Nogueira da Silva RI, et al: Hyperosmotic sodium salts reverse severe hemorrhagic shock: other solutes do not. Am J Physiol 1987;253:H751–H762.
11. Rocha e Silva M: Evolving concepts in small volume resuscitation: the experimental basis. In: Kreimeier U, Christ F, Messmer K (eds). Small-Volume Hyperosmolar Volume Resuscitation. Heidelberg, Springer, (1999, in press).
12. Velasco I, Rocha e Silva M, Oliveira M, et al: Hypertonic and hyperoncotic resuscitation from severe hemorrhagic shock in dogs: a comparative study. Crit Care Med 1989;17:261–264.
13. Kramer GC, Elgjo GI, Poli de Figueiredo LF, et al: Hyperosmotic-hyperoncotic solutions. Ballieres Clin Anaesthesiol 1997;11:143–161.
14. Matteucci MJ, Wisner DH, Gunther RA, et al: Effects of hypertonic and isotonic fluid infusion on the flash evoked potential in rats: hemorrhage, resuscitation, and hypernatremia. J Trauma 1993;34:1–7.
15. Mazzoni M, Borgstron P, Intaglietta M, et al: Capillary narrowing in hemorrhagic shock is rectified by hyperosmotic saline-dextran reinfusion. Circ Shock 1990;31:407–418.

16. Border JR, Hassett J, Laduca J, et al: The gut origins septic states in blunt multiple trauma (ISS = 40) in the ICU. Ann Surg 1987;206:427–448.
17. Carrico CJ, Meakins JL, Marshall JC, et al: Multiple organ failure syndrome. Arch Surg 1986;121:196–208.
18. Deitch EA, Bridges W, Ma L, et al: Hemorrhagic shock-induced bacterial translocation: the role of neutrophils and hydroxyl radicals. J Trauma 1990;942–952.
19. Mullins RJ, Hudgens RW: Hypertonic saline resuscitates dogs in endotoxin shock. J Surg Res 1987;43:37–44.
20. Armistead CW, Vicent JL, Preiser JC, et al: Hypertonic saline solution-hetastarch for fluid resuscitation in experimental septic shock. Anesth Analg 1989;69:714–720.
21. Kreimeier U, Frey L, Dentz J, et al: Hypertonic saline dextran resuscitation during the initial phase of acute endotoxemia: effect on regional blood flow. Crit Care Med 1991;19:801–809.
22. Crystal GJ, Gurevicius J, Kim SJ, et al: Effects of hypertonic saline solutions in the coronary circulation. Circ Shock 1994;42:27–38.
23. Maningas P: Resuscitation with 7.5% NaCl in 6% dextran-70 during hemorrhagic shock in swine: effects on organ blood flow. Crit Care Med 1987;15:1121–1126.
24. Kreimeier U, Bruckner U, Schmidt J, et al: Instantaneous restoration of regional organ blood flow after severe hemorrhage: effect of small-volume resuscitation with hypertonic-hyperoncotic solution. J Surg Res 1990;49:493–503.
25. Ing RD, Nazeeri MN, Zelds S, et al: Hypertonic saline/dextran improves septic myocardial performance. Am Surg 1994;60:507–508.
26. Kien ND, Kramer GC: Cardiac performance following hypertonic saline. Braz J Med Biol Res 1989;22:2245–2248.
27. Goertz AW, Mehl T, Lindner KH, et al: Effect of 7.2% hypertonic saline/6% hetastarch on left ventricular contractility in anesthetized humans. Anesthesiology 1995;82:1389–1395.
28. Welte M, Goresch T, Frey L, et al: Hypertonic saline dextran does not increase cardiac contractile function during small volume resuscitation from hemorrhagic shock in anesthetized pigs. Anesth Analg 1995;80:1099–1207.
29. Constable PD, Muir WW, Binkley PF: Hypertonic saline is negative inotropic agent in normovolemic dogs. Am J Physiol 1994;267:H667–H677.
30. Sondeen JL, Gonzaludo GA, Loveday JA, et al: Hypertonic saline/dextran improves renal function after hemorrhage in conscious swine. Resuscitation 1990;20:231–241.
31. Prough DS, Johnson JC, Poole GV, et al: Effects on intracranial pressure of resuscitation from hemorrhagic shock with hypertonic saline versus lactated Ringer's solution. Crit Care Med 1985;13:407–411.
32. Prough DS, Johnson JC, Stump DA, et al: Effects of hypertonic saline versus lactated Ringer's solution on cerebral oxygen transport during resuscitation from hemorrhagic shock. J Neurosurg 1986;64:627–632.
33. Walsh JC, Zhuang J, Shackford SR: A comparison of hypertonic to isotonic fluid in the resuscitation of brain injury and hemorrhagic shock. J Surg Res 1991;50:284–287.
34. Wade CE, Grady J, Kramer GC, et al: Individual cohort analysis of the efficacy of hypertonic saline/dextran in patients with traumatic brain injury and hypotension. J Trauma 1997;42:S61–S65.
35. Bayer M, Nolte D, Lehr HA, et al: Hypertonic-hyperoncotic dextran solution reduces post-ischemic leukocyte adherence in post-capillary vessels. Langenbecks Arch Chir 1991;(Suppl 1):375–378.
36. Coimbra R, Junger WG, Hoyt DB, et al: Immunosuppression following hemorrhage is reduced by hypertonic saline resuscitation. Surg Forum 1995;46:84–87.
37. Coimbra R, Junger WG, Liu FC, et al: Hypertonic/hyperoncotic fluids reverse prostaglandin E_2 (PGE_2) induced T-cell suppression. Shock 1995;3:45–49.
38. Coimbra R, Junger WG, Hoyt DB, et al: Hypertonic saline resuscitation restores hemorrhage-induced immunosuppression by decreasing prostaglandin E_2 and interleukin-4 production. J Surg Res 1996;64:203–209.
39. Coimbra R, Hoyt DB, Junger WG, et al: Hypertonic saline resuscitation decreases susceptibility to sepsis after hemorrhagic shock. J Trauma 1997;42:602–607.
40. Coimbra R, Yada MM, Rocha e Silva M, et al: Hypertonic saline and pentoxifylline resuscitation reduce bacterial translocation and lung injury following hemorrhagic shock: lactated Ringer's does not [abstract]. In: Proceedings of the Fifty-Seventh Annual Meeting of the American Association for the Surgery of Trauma, 1997;285.
41. Junger WG, Coimbra R, Liu FC, et al: Hypertonic saline resuscitation: a tool to modulate immune function in trauma patients: Shock 1997;8:235–241.
42. Poli de Figueiredo LF, Mathru M, Solanki D, et al: Pulmonary hypertension and systemic vasoconstriction may offset the benefits of acellular hemoglobin blood substitutes. J Trauma 1997;42:847–854.
43. Poli de Figueiredo LF, Williams N, Mathru M, et al: Acellular hemoglobin blood substitutes impair nitroprusside-induced relaxation of rat aorta. Anesthesiology 1996;85:A571.
44. Poli de Figueiredo LF, Mathru M, Elgjo GI, et al: Hypertonic acetate-ααhemoglobin for small volume resuscitation of hemorrhagic shock. Artif Cells Blood Substit Immobil Biotechnol 1997;25:61–73.
45. Poli de Figueiredo LF, Mathru M, Jones J, et al: Inhaled nitric oxide reverses cell-free hemoglobin-induced pulmonary hypertension and decreased lung compliance: preliminary results. Crit Care 1997;1:111–116.
46. Rabinovici R, Rudolph AS, Vernick J, et al: A new salutary resuscitative fluid: liposome encapsulated hemoglobin/hypertonic saline solution. J Trauma 1993;35:121–126.
47. Younes RN, Aun F, Accioly CQ, et al: Hypertonic solutions in the treatment of hypovolemic shock: a prospective, randomized study in patients admitted to the emergency room. Surgery 1992;111:380–385.
48. Maningas PA, Mattox KL, Pepe PE, et al: Hypertonic saline-dextran solutions for the prehospital management of traumatic hypotension. Am Surg 1989;157:528–534.
49. Vassar MJ, Perry CA, Holcroft JW: Analysis of potential risks associated with 7.5% sodium chloride resuscitation of traumatic shock. Arch Surg 1990;125:1309–15.
50. Vassar MJ, Perry CA, Gannaway WL, et al: 7.5% Sodium chloride/dextran for resuscitation of trauma patients undergoing helicopter transport. Arch Surg 1991;126:1065–1072.
51. Mattox KL, Maningas PA, Moore EE, et al: Prehospital hypertonic saline/dextran infusion for post-traumatic hypotension: the USA multicenter trial. Ann Surg 1991;213:482–491.
52. Younes RN, Aun F, Ching CT, et al: Prognostic factors to predict outcome following the administration of hypertonic/hyperoncotic solution in hypovolemic patients. Shock 1997;7:79–83.
53. Vassar MJ, Perry CA, Holcroft JW: Prehospital resuscitation of hypotensive trauma patients with 7.5% NaCl versus 7.5%

NaCl with added dextran: a controlled trial. J Trauma 1993; 34:622–632.
54. Vassar MJ, Fisher RP, O'Brien PE, et al: A multicentre trial for resuscitation of injured patients with 7.5% sodium chloride: the multicenter group for the study of hypertonic saline in trauma patients. Arch Surg 1993;128:1003–1011.
55. Wade CE, Kramer GC, Grady JJ, et al: Efficacy of hypertonic 7.5% saline and 6% dextran-70 in treating trauma: a meta-analysis of controlled clinical studies. Surgery 1997;122:609–616.
56. Gross D, Landau EH, Klin B, et al: Is hypertonic saline resuscitation safe in "uncontrolled" hemorrhagic shock? J Trauma 1988;28:751–756.
57. Bickell WH, Bruttig SP, Wade CE: Hemodynamic responses to abdominal aortotomy in the anesthetized swine. Circ Shock 1989;28:321–332.
58. American College of Surgeons, Committee on Trauma: Advanced Trauma Life Support Program for Physicians, 5th ed. Chicago, American College of Surgeons, 1993.
59. Bickell WH, Wall MJ, Pepe PE, et al: Immediate versus delayed fluid resuscitation for hypotensive patients with penetrating torso injuries. N Engl J Med 1994;331:1105–1109.
60. Poli de Figueiredo LF, Coselli JS: Individual strategies of hemostasis for thoracic aortic surgery. J Cardiovasc Surg 1997;12:222–228.
61. Younes RN, Bechara MJ, Langer B, et al: Emprego da solução hipertônica de NaCl 7.5% na prevenção da hipotensão pós-desclampeamento da aorta abdominal. Rev Assoc Med Bras 1987;34:150–154.
62. Auler JOC, Pereira MH, Gomide-Amaral RV, et al: Hemodynamic effects of hypertonic sodium chloride during surgical treatment of aortic aneurysms. Surgery 1987;101:594–601.
63. Boldt J, Zickmann B, Ballesteros M, et al: Cardiorespiratory responses to hypertonic saline solution in cardiac operations. Ann Thorac Surg 1991;51:610–615.
64. Oliveira SA, Bueno RM, Souza JM, et al: Effects of hypertonic saline dextran on the postoperative evolution of Jehovah's Witness patients submitted to cardiac surgery with cardiopulmonary bypass. Shock 1995;3:391–394.
65. Sterns RH, Riggs JE, Schochet SS Jr: Osmotic demyelination syndrome following rapid correction of hyponatremia. N Engl J Med 1986;314:1535–1541.
66. Finberg L, Luttrell E, Redd H: Pathogenesis of lesions in the nervous system in hypernatremic states: II. Experimental studies of gross anatomic changes and alterations of chemical composition of the tissues. Pediatrics 1959;23:46–66.
67. Wade CE, Grady JJ, Kramer GC, et al: Individual patient cohort analysis of the efficacy of hypertonic saline/dextran in patients with traumatic brain injury and hypotension. J Trauma 1997;42: S61–S65.
68. Kien ND, Kramer GC, White DA: Acute hypotension caused by rapid saline infusion in anesthetized dogs. Anesth Analg 1991;73:597–602.
69. Prien T, Thulig B, Wuasten R, et al: Effects of hypertonic saline hyperoncotic hydroxyethyl starch infusion prior to coronary artery bypass grafting (CABG). Zentralbl Chir 1993;118:257–266.
70. Ellinger K, Fahnle M, Schroth M, et al: Optimal preoperative titrated dosage of hypertonic-hyperoncotic solutions in cardiac risk patients. Shock 1995;3:167.
71. Christ F, Niklas M, Kreimeier U, et al: Hyperosmotic-hyperoncotic solutions during abdominal aortic aneurysm (AAA) resection. Acta Anaesthesiol Scand 1997;41:62–70.
72. Coselli JS, Poli de Figueiredo LF, LaMarie SA: Impact of a previous thoracic aneurysm repair on the management of thoracoabdominal aortic aneurysm. Ann Thorac Surg 1997; 64:639–650.
73. Ramires JAF, Serrano CV, César LAM, et al: Acute hemodynamic effects of hypertonic (7.5%) saline infusion in patients with cardiogenic shock due to right ventricular infarction. Circ Shock 1992;37:220–225.
74. Ring J, Messmer K: Incidence and severity of anaphylactoid reactions to colloid volume substitutes. Lancet 1977;1:466–469.

63
Blood Substitutes

A. Gerson Greenburg and Hae Won Kim

The history of "blood substitutes" goes back nearly a century. Soon after the discovery of oxygen and the relation of oxygen and hemoglobin as life-delivering components of blood, efforts were undertaken to develop a solution to replace the red blood cell. Over the past century many avenues have been explored, many "solutions" postulated, and many blind alleys explored as the medical, scientific, and commercial communities sought the "ideal solution" to replace the red blood cell.[1-3] Developments in blood banking and transfusion medicine in general, yielding a greater appreciation of the functional capacity of blood and the indications for its replacement, continue to drive the effort to develop a substitute for blood.[2-4] The risks of red blood cell transfusion, considered a worldwide problem with specific reference to transmission of infectious disease, have caused the effort to become more assertive, resulting in a variety of red blood cell substitute solutions undergoing clinical testing.[5]

Transmission of infectious disease is not the only concern. There remains the issue of the effect of red blood cell or blood transfusion on the immune system. Conflicting data exist regarding immune suppression in terms of recurrence of malignancy or infectious complications from elective surgical interventions.[6,7] In response to these concerns various elements of the medical community have proposed guidelines to address the issue of when to use red blood cells and other blood components to limit risk and optimize benefit.[8-10] In this environment there appears to be a role for a red blood cell substitute that can provide oxygen-carrying capacity and increase the intravascular volume, two of the primary functions of blood.[11] Indeed, most of the solutions being tested today are capable of only those two functions. The question then arises: Can a solution with these traits and attributes be of benefit in the management of patients with multiple organ failure?

Red Blood Cell Substitutes and Multiple Organ Failure

The current crop of red blood cell substitutes replaces intravascular volume and affords a significant element of increased oxygen-carrying capacity. Being acellular they are more likely to perfuse capillary beds that might otherwise be avoided because of physiologic changes in the microcirculation related to the etiology of a hypoperfusion state, whatever the mechanism may be. As microcirculatory perfusion is an essential and critical element of survival to most, if not all, mammalian organisms, ensuring adequate tissue perfusion and oxygenation becomes a reasonable goal when dealing with organ failure.[12-15]

The pathophysiology underlying multiple organ failure (MOF) continues to be defined. There does not appear to be a single unifying process or mechanism to account for the rather specific patterns seen in a variety of illnesses with respect to the sequence of events. One can postulate that there is some element of organ failure that is related to poor perfusion and that altered or impaired oxygen delivery or utilization has in some way impaired organs and the organism as a whole. The theories behind MOF are explored elsewhere in this volume and are not reiterated here.

Much of the pathophysiology of MOF is thought to be initiated by poor or impaired tissue perfusion. The subsequent involvement of reactive oxygen species, the products of "reperfusion injury", plays an important role along with the cascades of cytokines and other mediators and messenger molecules.[12] One factor believed to be involved in the pathogenesis of sepsis hypotension and MOF deserves mentioning. Nitric oxide (NO), a potent vasodilator and cytotoxic agent, may have a particular relevance to hemoglobin-based oxygen carriers (HBOCs). In response to infection and sepsis, inducible NO synthase (iNOS), present in macrophages and other cells, is activated and produces large amounts of NO; excessive levels of NO could cause widespread vasodilation and systemic hypotension, resulting in poor organ perfusion. Because NO has a high affinity for hemoglobin (Hb), NO scavenging by HBOCs could alleviate the NO-mediated complications. Although HBOCs have been shown to be generally beneficial in various shock resuscitation studies, much is unknown about how they interact with various factors involved in MOF and affect the eventual outcome.

Red Blood Cell Substitutes: Traits and Characteristics

The current red blood cell substitutes are classified as perfluorocarbons (PFCs), or HBOCs. PFCs are essentially chemical solutions—emulsions of PFCs with added osmotic and oncotic agents—that carry oxygen in solution. They are totally synthetic and generally require a significant increase in inspired oxygen content to be effective. The first PFC emulsion in clinical trials was Fluosol-DA, a 20% (w/v) co-emulsion of perfluorodecalin and perfluorotripropylamine, with egg yolk phospholipid and Pluronic-68 as emulsifying agents. Breathing ambient air and having the normal arterial and venous oxygen tensions, Fluosol-DA could deliver only 0.4 ml oxygen per deciliter. To meet the metabolic demand, patients had to breathe pure oxygen (FiO_2, 1.0%). Not generally acceptable, this material failed to show efficacy. Furthermore, when used as an emulsifying agent, Pluronic-68 caused complement activation.

A 60% (w/v) emulsion of perfluorooctyl bromide has been developed using egg yolk phospholipid as the sole emulsifying agent.[16] Under normal arterial and venous oxygen tensions, this material can unload oxygen as much as 1.3 ml/dl. Although this improvement in oxygen delivery capacity, is remarkable, it still falls far short of the normal oxygen delivery capacity of blood (5 ml O_2/dl blood at 15 g Hb/dl). It may not deliver sufficient oxygen for normal organ function. To ensure adequate oxygen delivery, patients must still breathe 100% oxygen, a situation avoided whenever possible because of adverse effects on the lungs. Because of the shortfalls, currently PFC emulsions are being considered only as hemodilution agents for vascular or cardiac surgery.[17]

The HBOCs have been in development for some time and have been achieving success in a variety of clinical trials where the primary end point has been avoidance of allogeneic transfusion. Models have included elective surgical intervention and trauma, with similar results being reported by various investigators.[5] Few of the reports in the clinical arena have reported physiologically relevant endpoints such as improved oxygen delivery or tissue perfusion, as these variables are difficult to define and to measure in patients. There are, however, many well done laboratory studies in shock models that demonstrate effectiveness and efficacy, with improvement of tissue perfusion, using HBOCs generally and specifically by various products.[18–20]

TABLE 63.1. Variables of Hemoglobin-Based Red Blood Cell Substitutes.

Hemoglobin source
Hemoglobin concentration
   Methemoglobin content
   Oxygen-carrying capacity
Molecular weight distribution
   < 64 kDa
   64 kDa
   > 64 kDa
P_{50}
Cooperativity
Viscosity
pH
Electrolytes
Oncotic pressure
Additives
Metabolites
"Purity"
   Red blood cell stroma
   Endotoxin
   Nonhemoglobin protiens
   Sterility

Clearly, not all HBOCs are the same. They have different hemoglobin concentrations; the hemoglobin modification (if there is one) varies; and excipient carrier solutions differ with respect to pH, osmotic and oncotic pressures, electrolyte composition, viscosity, and so on. The variables that could contribute to the differences in the solutions are shown in Table 63.1. HBOCs currently in clinical testing and their physicochemical characteristics are listed in Tables 63.2 and 63.3. Comparisons of solutions, in terms of efficacy related to composition, has been difficult given the number of combinations and permutations possible to create points of difference.[3]

The HBOCs, by their very nature, have properties and traits that may be useful for managing patients with a variety of organ failure conditions. Hemoglobin in the native or modified state not only delivers oxygen, it acts as a "scavenger" of both carbon monoxide and nitric oxide, molecules of concern in patients with MOF. A significant body of knowledge from the experimental literature shows that HBOCs may be beneficial for

TABLE 63.2. Characteristics of HBOC Products in Clinical Testing.

Product	Company	Hb source	Modification	Testing phase
DCL-Hb	Baxter Healthcare	Human RBCs	Crosslinking between α subunits with bis-dibromosalicyl fumarate	III
HBOC-201	Biopure Corp.	Bovine RBCs	Polymerization with glutaraldehyde	III
PEG-Hb	Enzon	Bovine RBCs	Conjugation with polyethylene glycol	II
Hemolink	Hemosol	Human RBCs	Crosslinking and polymerization with o-raffinose	II
PolyHeme	Northfield Labs.	Human RBCs	Pyridoxalation followed by polymerization with glutaraldehyde	III
rHb1.1	Baxter Healthcare	*Escherichia coli*	Genetic engineering to produce crosslinked human Hb	II

HBOC, hemoglobin-based oxygen carriers; Hb, hemoglobin.

TABLE 63.3. Additional characteristics of HBOC Products.

Product	Hb (g/dl)	MW (kDa)	P50 (mmHg)	COP (mmHg)	MetHb (%)	pH	Viscosity (cP)	Plasma half-life (hours)[a]
DCL-Hb	9.5–10.5	64.5 (96–98%)	32–33	42–44	< 5	7.3–7.5	1	10.5
HBOC-201	13	68–500	34–38	17	< 15	7.6–7.9	1.3	20–24
PEG-Hb	6	64	9–16	118	< 10	7.5	3.4	48
Hemolink	10	126–600 (63%)	34	24	< 10	7.5	1.0	18
PolyHeme	8–10	Polymer (99%)	28–30	20–25	< 3	NR	1.9–2.2	24
rHb1.1	5–8	64	33	12	NR	NR	0.8	2.8–12.0

NR, not reported; MW, molecular weight; COP, capillary osmotic pressure; MetHb, methemoglobin.
[a] Values vary with Hb dose and plasma concentration.

management of sepsis and hemorrhagic shock situations,[21–26] presumed precursor etiologies of MOF. Indeed, in combination with NOS inhibition, hemoglobin solutions may effect improved survival in septic models; scavenging excess NO also has been demonstrated,[27] a trait that by itself may be beneficial in the management of critically ill patients.

Although little is known about the metabolism of the HBOCs, it seems logical that there is some significant increase in activity of the metabolic pathways that deal with hemoglobin, porphyrin, and iron. Released from Hb, heme is broken down to biliverdin and carbon monoxide (CO) by the action of heme oxygenase (HO). Increases in the enzymatic activity related to these processes may be beneficial to survival by dealing with potentially damaging interactions between heme iron and oxygen during toxic radical generation. Indeed, infusion of Hb to animals increased their HO activity, particularly HO-1, an inducible isoform that is also known as heat shock protein 32. Prior induction of HO-1 appears to protect cells from oxidant injury and improve survival after subsequent septic challenge.[26,28,29] On the other hand, HBOC-induced increased enzyme activity could be potentially detrimental by utilizing resources that could otherwise be directed at tissue recovery. The balance between these extremes is not clear. An answer is possible when the underlying mechanisms are made explicit and the pathways are defined to the extent that the interactions and intersections can be identified and interventions around them specified. Until all these factors and interactions are either appreciated or defined, the role of HBOCs in resuscitation and treatment of various shock states and MOF must remain speculative. However, as a therapy of the future, HBOCs have the potential to be powerful adjuncts in the prevention and active treatment of complex organ failure situations.

Hemoglobin Solutions

Great progress has been made since the late 1960s when the new generations of "ideal blood substitutes" appeared on the scene.[30] This sentinel effort was one of the first to use a "stroma-free hemoglobin", or pure hemoglobin, not modified to achieve promising results in a hemorrhagic shock resuscitation model. However, concern about the short intravascular persistence and possible altered oxygen affinity led to the concept of chemical modification as a means of addressing these issues.[31,32]

Chemically unmodified hemoglobin in the circulation dissociates rapidly into dimers, which are excreted in the urine. The concerns about nephrotoxicity related to hemoglobin go back almost 90 years when raw, crude, hemolyzed blood was infused as a "substitute", and renal failure resulted. It is now thought that nephrotoxicity is related to the circulating "stroma" or red blood cell membrane, not the hemoglobin per se. In all of the recently reported clinical studies where large doses of various modified hemoglobins have been infused, no nephrotoxicity has been observed.[2]

The scientific basis for the modification of hemoglobin is founded in an appreciation of the unique and specific hemoglobin function–structure relation, so well defined by Perutz.[33] Molecular modification to achieve improved oxygen delivery by maintaining low oxygen affinity was the objective. A means of substituting for the lost 2,3-diphosphoglycerate (DPG) was needed. DPG is the modifier that enables the hemoglobin molecule to make the transition from the deoxy to the oxy state. In the red blood cell it resides in the β pocket of the hemoglobin molecule and is extruded from this site during transition from one state to the next. While in the red blood cell the DPG stays in proximity to the hemoglobin and thus moves back and forth, participating in the overall function. Stripped of the red blood cell, the molecule floats free and is rapidly metabolized. With the loss of DPG, hemoglobin achieves increased oxygen affinity and so off-loads oxygen less easily.

Indeed, the approach directed at replacing the DPG in cell-free hemoglobin with analogues—producing a chemically modified hemoglobin—has been successful. A host of chemical modifiers have been evaluated, many with promising results relative to beneficial alteration of oxygen affinity or intravascular persistence.[31,34,35]

To address the issue of a "perceived" short intravascular persistence (the optimal duration has not been defined, as it may be context-sensitive), chemical modifications of hemoglobin have also been directed at altering the mechanism of renal clearance, the primary route of excretion for unmodified hemoglobin. Modifications to hemoglobin that alter renal clearance have included oligomerization, polymerization, and conjugation of the modified hemoglobin; more recently various forms of encapsulation have been proposed. Some of these lipid vesicles are large, and others are quite small.

As a matter of course, these modifications have their own routes of degradation and metabolic impact. Whether these processes are beneficial or detrimental to the survival of the organism is not clear. If upregulation of an enzymatic pathway allows the organ or organism to handle a challenge more effectively, it would be a positive effect. On the other hand, if the solution by its metabolic pathway significantly impairs one or more of the critical host defense mechanisms, that solution may not have a role in the management of critically ill patients. This point is considered a key issue for a solution that effects adequate resuscitation by affording improved perfusion to the microcirculation but also impairs one of the vital defense mechanisms. It may yield short-term gain at the expense of long-term benefit. Generally, the microencapsulated materials are cleared by the reticuloendothelial system (RES) to a greater or lesser extent. Hence microencapsulated materials may have limited application, as this is one host defense system that is needed to promote and effect survival in many of the situations associated with MOF.

The HBOCs can be considered part of a plan to manage acutely ill patients. Because of their ability to carry and deliver oxygen to tissues, they may have a role in the *resuscitation* phase of an illness. With their ability to act as scavengers of detrimental active metabolites (e.g., NO and CO) in combination with oxygen delivery, they may have a role in the management of a sequentially developing physiologic derangement such as MOF.

The HBOCs contribute to overall oxygen delivery, the product of oxygen content and cardiac output. Any variable that contributes or increases oxygen content, such as hemoglobin, increases oxygen delivery—the basic principle of any transfusion. Whether the addition of hemoglobin or red blood cells is the most effective mechanism for increasing oxygen delivery remains to be seen, as delivery can be increased by increasing cardiac output but there is a cost for that effort. Not every heart can increase output to match the need. Cardiac output is limited by heart rate and coronary flow, both of which contribute to stroke volume. In the presence of β-blockade a rate-responsive mechanism is eliminated as a means of increasing oxygen-delivery. In that instance the use of additional oxygen-carrying capacity—red blood cell transfusion or an HBOC—is indicated.

The field of HBOCs is related to the area of transfusion medicine. As more and more options for autologous transfusion evolve and weave their way into daily practice (e.g., hemodilution, cell salvage, autologous predeposit), the need for allogeneic transfusion wanes. In an analysis of the potential use of HBOCs in the surgical arena, fully 60–65% of the current use of allogeneic red blood cells could be replaced with an HBOC that simply provided oxygen-carrying capacity and some element of volume expansion.[11] With wider use of these unique solutions in combination with more judicious use of alternative techniques, as proposed by some of the newer guidelines for use of red blood cell transfusion, the risks of allogeneic red blood cell transfusion could be further minimized. As the science and clinical results progress, this outcome is likely. The use of HBOCs for trauma resuscitation and as adjunct therapy for the management of MOF awaits further development.

Hemoglobin Solutions: State of the Art

The broad classes of HBOCs are listed in Table 63.4. Additional issues in the development of these solutions relate to the source of the starting hemoglobin. The source may be outdated human red blood cells, bovine red blood cells, or recombinant hemoglobin. One product being tested uses *Escherichia coli* recombinant source hemoglobin as the source of a low-affinity hemoglobin with good retention time.[36] Indeed, this group is in pursuit of a genetically expressed, polymerized, crosslinked hemoglobin to meet the perceived needs of a solution that has a longer intravascular half-life. Recombinant sources include hemoglobin not only from *E. coli* but also from yeasts, transgenic plants, and animals. Hemoglobin from these sources is generally considered a purer starting material, but it is currently produced at great expense and so for the moment does not seem commercially feasible. That does not make these products undesirable, simply expensive for the moment. Any expression or separation technology on the horizon today could become reality tomorrow, making this approach a more probable scenario. For now, those in pursuit of a commercial license use either outdated red blood cells, *E. coli*-produced recombinant hemoglobin, or isolated bovine herds as their hemoglobin source.

Given the use of outdated red blood cells as starting material, the key processes during manufacture are isolation of a chemically pure hemoglobin A_0 with no stroma or other contaminants and a viral inactivation methodology that further reduces the risk of transmitting infectious disease. All of the current products using outdated human red blood cells as source material have reported effective viral inactivation processes that further reduce the risk of virus transmission. This step is thought

TABLE 63.4. Broad Classifications of Hemoglobin-Based Oxygen Carriers.

Stabilized (crosslinked) hemoglobins
   $\alpha\alpha$ Crosslinking
   $\beta\beta$ Crosslinking

Polymerized hemoglobins
   Glutaraldehyde
   o-Raffinose

Conjugated hemoglobins
   Inulix
   Dextran
   Polyethylene glycol

Encapsulated hemoglobins
   Lipid vesicles (liposomes)
      Stabilized (crosslinked) Hb vesicles
      Surface modified Hb vesicles
   Hb nanocapsules (< 0.2 μm)
      Lipid nanocapsules
      Polymeric nanocapsules (polylactides, polyglycolides)
   Heme-embedded liposomes

Genetically engineered human hemoglobins
   Recombinant *E. coli*/yeast
   Transgenic animals/plants

to be unnecessary for the materials that use bovine or recombinant technology.

Crosslinked, Tetrameric Stabilized Hemoglobin

Crosslinked, tetrameric stabilized hemoglobin is best represented by the efforts of Baxter in the development of an α crosslinked tetrameric hemoglobin solution. This solution has been tested extensively in many clinical trials, and during late 1997 and early 1998 it went into a phase III clinical efficacy trial. Unfortunately, during the early phases of the trial there was a higher mortality rate for patients who were given this solution than would be predicted from survival models. The solution was not effective, and the trial was aborted. The development of this material was thus halted.

Efforts by others using this approach continue as crosslinking agents are developed and evaluated. One constant in the evaluation of this class of modified hemoglobins appears to be the appearance of significant hypertension associated with the infusion. It is reported to be an increase in mean arterial pressure of as much as 40% within minutes of the infusion. The mechanism of the effect is poorly understood but thought to be related to NO depletion on the endothelial cell–smooth muscle interface. It is likely hypothesis, but proof that it is the mechanism has not been forthcoming. Alternative explanations include a central neurologic event or significant alterations in the microcirculation, with the hypertension related to small arteriolar vasoconstriction. There is some supporting evidence for the latter.[37]

The relevance of hypertension to the use of this class of materials for treatment of MOF or resuscitation is arguable, and many questions can be raised. Is it reasonable to increase the blood pressure and risk decreased organ perfusion? Is the hypertensive effect beneficial, or is it a significant detrimental side effect? Should a resuscitation fluid have a pressor effect? What would be the benefit of such a solution in a hypovolemic, underperfused patient? As the study was stopped because there was no efficacy, we may never learn the answers to these questions. On the other hand, while reviewing many of the studies that supported proceeding to a phase III trial in trauma patients, it became clear that groups treated with pressors were not part of the study design. Therefore it may have been possible to predict the outcome had the models explored the pressor effects of the agent, not only its oxygen delivery and vascular volume characteristics.

Recombinant hemoglobin, using *E. coli* to express a low-affinity hemoglobin with stabilization, has been studied in a variety of models and has completed some phase II clinical testing. It too has a pressor effect, but it is less pronounced and appears at somewhat higher doses than the Baxter product. This solution has excellent oxygen-delivery properties. Indeed, it appears to be as effective as red blood cells at 15 g Hb/dl when infused into human subjects at 5 g Hb/dl, a rather remarkable effect.[38] A similar effect has been shown with polymerized bovine hemoglobin.[39] This observation supports the concept that a cell-free solution may have better access to the microcirculation and effect better perfusion. It also speaks to the issue of what constitutes a "unit of red blood cell substitute."

Traditionally, a unit of red blood cells is considered to be about 50 g of hemoglobin. If the effective dose of a cell-free substitute is less than that, it may be reasonable to assume lower dosing with less potential for toxicity and greater use of the agent. Moreover, using hemoglobin by the gram and not the unit is more effective and precise treatment, with more controlled use of scarce resources.

The recombinant material was shown in the early phase I tests to induce some degree of esophagospasm, a bothersome adverse event beginning at doses around 150 mg Hb/kg.[40] Other investigators have reported this event as well.[41,42] It is poorly understood and not well explained. It can be obviated by pretreatment with muscle relaxants and can be treated with smooth muscle relaxants or calcium channel blockade once it occurs. This side effect is not observed in patients receiving the solution who are under general anesthesia. A similar effect was seen with the oligomeric solution (a mixture of stabilized tetramer and polymeric hemoglobin) of Hemosol in the phase I clinical test; the spasm was relieved with smooth muscle relaxants. This group observed mild hypertension at higher doses (500–600 mg Hb/kg), with an increased mean arterial pressure of 10–12%. Other smooth muscle activity was noted to be altered as well, especially with reference to the gastrointestinal (GI) tract.

One final issue is a perception of pancreatitis in patients who receive these HBOC solutions. Whether it is a clinical illness or hyperamylasemia has been debated. It does not appear to be clinical disease but, rather, part of a general GI disturbance in volunteer subjects that has been reported by some investigators. There are isolated reports of it occurring in some of the phase II patients, but an etiology has not been established. Again, the mechanism is not apparent.

Until the basis for some of these adverse events is defined, use of these hemoglobin solutions, despite their many positive attributes and potentials, should be guarded. As the spectrum of MOF is broad and the mechanisms not clear, it would be of some risk to add to the mix a solution with known side effects but unknown mechanisms. That approach should be avoided if possible.

Polymerized and Oligomeric Hemoglobins

The use of polymerized hemoglobin solutions has been advocated for years. As noted above, it is a technique for minimizing renal clearance that relates to dimerization of the hemoglobin tetramer. Many agents have been proposed to effect the crosslink.[43] Infusion of these solutions does not induce GI symptoms or hypertension. Large doses (up to 5000 ml) have been infused with no adverse effects reported. In the phase II study early use of allogeneic transfusion was avoided, although many of those who avoided the allogeneic transfusion early did have a transfusion before discharge from the hospital. Transfusion avoidance was not demonstrated but hinted at.[44] All of the stabilized tetramer is eliminated in this solution. The investigators believe this accounts for the absent GI and vasoconstriction events.

Polymerized bovine hemoglobin has also been evaluated extensively. Minimal side effects have been observed, and the material has been approved by the U.S. Food and Drug Administration (FDA) for use in veterinary practice.[45] The issue here is the impact of bovine hemoglobin on the human immune system. Is it recognized as a foreign protein, and does the risk of an allergic reaction exist? It is not clear just how antigenic hemoglobin or modified hemoglobins are, although some investigations have shown minimal antigenic potential for an intraspecies or interspecies response in multiple-dose models.[46-48]

The oligomeric solution of Hemosol, o-raffinose crosslinked human hemoglobin, is in phase II testing in at least three models. It has effectively in decreased red blood cell requirements during hemodilution for joint replacement and cardiac surgery. It is also being tested as a source of intravenous iron for patients with renal failure, as significant synergy with erythropoietin has been demonstrated (D. Bell, personal communication, 1998).

Conjugated Hemoglobin

The concept of conjugation of hemoglobin to insoluble polymers to prolong intravascular persistence has been explored by a number of investigators. The idea is to enlarge the molecule so it cannot be readily metabolized and removed from the circulation. Some clinical testing has been accomplished, but doses are low and patients are few in number. A variety of agents have been conjugated to human and bovine hemoglobins, including dextran and polyethylene glycol (polyoxyethylene). Initial applications include use as a means to increase oxygenation of hypoxic tumors, rendering them more radiosensitive,[49] and to scavenge NO in septic patients.[25]

Encapsulated Hemoglobins

The area of encapsulated hemoglobins is beginning to grow rapidly as lipid vesicle technology expands and the problems of creating stable uniform microcapsules are resolved. Moreover, the potential for using the capsule as a means of drug delivery, an additional adjunct in some situations, is appealing. A solid concept first proposed by Chang,[50] developments have brought this possibility closer to reality than one might have predicted. The mark against this approach is the fact that clearance from the circulation for foreign capsules is most assured via the RES. Numerous studies have confirmed that this is the primary mechanism of clearance for microcapsules of all sizes and content. The risk in the polytraumatized patient or the patient with MOF is compromise to the RES, a system needed by them to survive. It does not seem reasonable to compromise one system while supporting another without the details of the tradeoff resulting from the exchange.

Encapsulated hemoglobins come in a variety of configurations, as shown in Table 63.4. The first attempt to recreate the red blood cell by providing the necessary environment for hemoglobin was almost 50 years ago.[50] Much was learned from that experience, and subsequent developments included capsules with a lipid bilayer, synthetic biodegradable membrane capsules, and capsules that incorporate antioxidants to be effective during resuscitation from hemorrhagic shock.

Additional efforts aimed at creating capsules with longer circulatory persistence as a function of structure, size, and content have been described.[4] Although these materials have not been clinically tested yet, they are promising because they have many useful properties.

Hemoglobin Solutions and the Future

Predicting the future is a sensitive subject. Few investigators have been successful at the task, and we ourselves have not yet established a record in that area. How and when red blood cell substitutes can be useful in the management of MOF is not clear. It is clear, however, that one of the inciting factors for MOF is deficiency in oxygen delivery to tissues, with impaired tissue perfusion and localized hypoxia, which triggers a sequence of cellular and organ-specific metabolic and biochemical responses. When attempting to restore balance and homeostasis, some of the systems overshoot the control point, further discoordinating the system, which in turn provokes additional responses. If the initial event, the cellular hypoxia, can be minimized, the resulting cascade should be modulated and less damaging.

Hemoglobin-based red blood cell substitutes, in many forms, appear capable of achieving that desired improvement in cellular function in a variety of experimental models. Because of their many properties that relate to metabolism and cell function, they may be useful adjuncts to the care of patients who are candidates for MOF. In their current state of development, though, toxic effects and adverse events are still observed. Some of these adverse events and effects could compromise the patient who teeters on the brink of homeostatic dysfunction, altering the outcome. Nonetheless, the future appears bright for this class of therapeutic agents.

References

1. Winslow R: Hemoglobin-Based Red Cell Substitutes. Baltimore, Johns Hopkins University Press, 1992.
2. Chang T: Blood Substitutes: Principles, Methods, Products and Clinical Trials, vol I. Basel, Karger Landes Systems, 1997.
3. Greenburg A, Kim H: Current status of stroma-free hemoglobin. Adv Surg 1998;31:149–165.
4. Tsuchida E: Artificial Red Cells: Materials, Performances, and Clinical Study as Blood Substitutes. Chichester, Wiley, 1995.
5. Cutcliffe N, Carmichael F, Greenburg A: Blood substitutes: a review of clinical trials. In: Mathiowitz E (ed.). The Encyclopedia of Controlled Drug Delivery. New York: Wiley, 1999;94–112.
6. Greenburg A: Benefits and risks of blood transfusion in surgical patients. World J Surg 1996;20:1189–1193.

7. Klein H: Allogeneic transfusion risks in surgical patient. Am J Surg 1995;170:21S-26S.
8. American Society of Anesthesiologist Task Force on Blood Component Therapy: Practice guidelines for blood component therapy. Anesthesiology 1996;84:732-747.
9. Spence R: Surgical red cell transfusion practice policies. Am J Surg 1995;170:2S-15S.
10. American College of Physicians: Practice strategies for elective red blood cell transfusion. Ann Intern Med 1992;116:403-406.
11. Greenburg A: Clinical implications of blood substitutes. Artif Organs 1998;22(1):47-49.
12. Greenburg A, Simms H: Pathophysiology of shock. In: Miller T (ed) Modern Surgical Care: Physiologic Foundations and Clinical Applications. St. Louis, Quality Medical Publishing, 1998;197-219.
13. Fry D: Multiple system organ failure. Surg Clin North Am 1988;68:107-122.
14. Vincent J: Prevention and therapy of multiple organ failure. World J Surg 1996;20:465-470.
15. Rackow E, Astiz M: Pathophysiology and treatment of septic shock. JAMA 1991;266:548-554.
16. Faithful N: Mechanisms and efficacy of fluorochemical oxygen transport and delivery. Artif Cells Blood Substit Immobil Biotechnol 1994;22:687-694.
17. Habler O, Kleen M, Hutter J, et al: Hemodilution and intravenous perflubron emulsion as an alternative to blood transfusion: effects on tissue oxygenation during profound hemodilution in anesthetized dogs. Transfusion 1998;38:145-154.
18. Malcolm D, Kissinger D, Garrioch M: Diaspirin crosslinked hemoglobin solution as a resuscitative fluid following severe hemorrhage in the rat. Artif Cells Blood Substit Immobil Biotechnol 1992;20:495-498.
19. Chang T, Varma R: Effects of Ringer's lactate, albumin, stroma-free hemoglobin, o-raffinose polyhemoglobin, and whole blood on lethal hemorrhagic shock in rats. Artif Cells Blood Substit Immobil Biotechnol 1991;19:368-371.
20. Nho K, Glower D, Bredehoeft S, et al: PEG-bovine hemoglobin: safety in a canine dehydrated hypovolemic-hemorrhage shock model. Artif Cells Blood Substit Immobil Biotechnol 1992;20:511-524.
21. Kim H, Hughes J, Breiding P, Greenburg A: Nitric oxide scavenging: an alternative therapeutic approach to nitric oxide synthesis inhibition in nitric oxide mediated hypotension of sepsis. Surg Forum 1994;45:67-69.
22. Kim H, Breiding P, Greenburg A: Enhanced modulation of hypotension in endotoxemia by concomitant nitric oxide synthesis inhibition and nitric oxide scavenging. Artif Cells Blood Substit Immobil Biotechnol 1997;25:153-162.
23. Mourelatos M, Enzer N, Ferguson J, et al: The effects of diaspirin cross-linked hemoglobin in sepsis. Shock 1996;5:141-148.
24. Kilbourn R, Joly G, Cashon B, et al: Cell-free hemoglobin reverses the endotoxin-mediated hyporesponsivity of rat aortic rings to alpha adrenergic agents. Biochem Biophys Res Commun 1994;199:155-162.
25. De Angelo J: Clinical experience with pyridoxalated hemoglobin polyoxyethylene (PHP). Presented at the VII International Symposium on Blood Substitutes, Tokyo, 1997;33.
26. Otterbein L, Sylvester S, Choi A: Hemoglobin provides protection against lethal endotoxemia in rats: the role of heme oxygenase-1. Am J Respir Cell Mol Biol 1995;13:595-601.
27. Greenburg A, Kim H: Nitrosyl hemoglobin formation after intravenous administration of hemoglobin-based oxygen carrier. Artif Cells Blood Substit Immobil Biotechnol 1995;23:271-276.
28. Hauser G, Dayao E, Wasserloos K, et al: HSP induction inhibits iNOS mRNA expression and attenuates hypotension in endotoxin-challenged rats. Am J Physiol 1996;271:H2529-H2535.
29. Yet S, Pellacanti A, Patterson C, et al: Induction of heme oxygenase-1 expression in vascular smooth muscle cells. J Biol Chem 1997;272:4295-4301.
30. Peskin G, O'Brien K, Rabiner S: Stroma-free hemoglobin solution: the "ideal" blood substitute? Surgery 1977;66:185-193.
31. Greenburg A, Shooley M, Peskin G: Improved retention of stroma-free hemoglobin solution by chemical modification. J Trauma 1977;17:501-504.
32. Greenburg A, Hayashi R, Siefert I, et al: Intravascular persistence and oxygen delivery of pyridoxalated, stroma-free hemoglobin during gradations of hypotension. Surgery 1979;86:13-16.
33. Perutz MF: Stereochemical mechanism of oxygen transport by hemoglobin. Proc R Soc Lond B 1980;208-135.
34. Benesch R, Benesch R, Yung S, Edalji R: Hemoglobin covalently bridged across the polyphosphate binding site. Biochem Biophys Res Commun 1975;63:1123.
35. Chang T: Modified hemoglobin-based blood substitutes: cross-linked, recombinant and encapsulated hemoglobin. Vox Sang 1998;74(Suppl 2):233-241.
36. Looker D, Durfee S, Shoemaker S, et al: Production of recombinant hemoglobin specifically engineered to enhance delivery and circulating half-life: a recombinant cell-free blood substitute. Artif Cells Blood Substit Immobil Biotechnol 1991;19:418.
37. Intaglietta M: Hemoglobin and blood substitutes. Artif Cells Blood Substit Immobil Biotechnol 1994;22:137-144.
38. Caspari R: Recent progress in the development of Optro (recombinant human hemoglobin, rHb1.1). Presented at the VII International Symposium on Blood Substitutes, Tokyo, 1997;36.
39. Hughes G, Jacobs E: Hemodynamic responses to Hemopure 1(HIS), a polymerized bovine hemoglobin solution, in normal subjects. Presented at the Vth International Symposium on Blood Substitutes. San Diego, 1993.
40. Murray J, Ledlow A, Launspach J, et al: The effects of recombinant human hemoglobin on esophageal motor function in humans. Gastroenterology 1995;109:1241-1248.
41. Shorr R: Evaluation of polyethylene glycol-conjugated bovine hemoglobin in healthy human volunteers. Presented at the VII International Symposium on Blood Substitutes, Tokyo, 1977;34.
42. Adamson J, Bonaventura B, Er S, et al: Production, characterization, and clinical evaluation of Hemolink(tm), and oxidized raffinose cross-linked hemoglobin-based blood substitute. In: Rudolph A, Rabinovici R, Feuerstein G (eds) Red Blood Cell Substitutes: Basic Principles and Clinical Applications. New York, Marcel Dekker, 1997;335-352.
43. Greenburg A: Alternatives to conventional uses of blood products. Crit Care Med 1992;14:325-351.
44. Gould S, Moore E, Hoyt A, et al: The first randomized trial of human polymerized hemoglobin as a blood substitute in acute trauma and emergent surgery. J Am Coll Surg 1998; 187:113-122.
45. Biopure Corporation: Biopure Corp initiates phase III clinical trial of blood substitutes (news release: http://www.prenewswire.com). Cambridge, MA, 1998.
46. Feola M, Gonzalez H, Canizaro PC, et al: Development of a bovine stroma-free hemoglobin solutions as a blood substitute. Surg Gynecol Obstet 1983;157:399-408.
47. Chang T, Varma R: Pyridoxalated heterogeneous and homologous polyhemoglobin and hemoglobin: systemic effects of replace-

ment transfusion in rats previously received immunizing doses. Artif Cells Blood Substit Immobil Biotechnol 1987;15:443–452.
48. Chang T: Immunological and systemic effects of transfusion in rats using pyridoxalated hemoglobin and polyhemoglobin from homologous and heterologous sources. Artif Cells Blood Substit Immobil Biotechnol 1988;16:205–215.
49. Shorr R, Viau A, Abuchowski A: Phase 1B safety evaluation of PEG hemoglobin as an adjuvant to radiation therapy in human cancer patients [abstract]. Artif Cells Blood Substit Immobil Biotechnol 1996;24:407.
50. Chang T: Hemoglobin corpuscles. Report of Physiology BSc Honor's project, McGill University, 1957.

64
Growth Factors G-CSF and GM-CSF: Clinical Options

Thomas Hartung, Sonja von Aulock, and Albrecht Wendel

The body's immediate response to bacterial infection becomes clinically evident as an inflammatory reaction accompanied by an acute-phase response in the liver and hyperthermia. Activation of the immune system must be counterregulated to curb these processes and to prevent (or at least minimize) damage to the host tissue. The major part of this intricate regulation is performed by the cytokine mediator network, a relay of glycoprotein signals that first activate proliferation and host defense functions of immune cells and then control the return to a state of readiness when the infection is under control.

Septic shock encompasses fulminant, and self-destructive activation of the defense system that is now understood as a systemic inflammatory reaction followed by multiple organ failure. This extreme activation of the nonspecific immune system is followed, provided the patient can be stabilized by intensive medical care, by corresponding massive counterregulation. The patient, whose immune system is exhausted, is left almost defenseless in a state termed immune paralysis, or anergy. A patient in this state is particularly susceptible to life-threatening secondary infections.

Granulocyte (G-CSF) and granulocyte/macrophage colony-stimulating factors (GM-CSF) (Table 64.1), central mediators of the endogenous response to infection and inflammation, have been cloned and are commercially available in forms approved for clinical use (Table 64.2). Both stimulate the proliferation and release of immune cells from the bone marrow, and so they were originally approved for the treatment of leukopenia. G-CSF, when given prophylactically or as substitution in situations of deficiency, has also been attributed with improved host defense paired with antiinflammatory effects. GM-CSF, on the other hand, is considered a potent immunostimulator and proinflammatory agent.

Evidence from many animal studies and some clinical studies suggests that prophylactic treatment with G-CSF at the time a risk can be anticipated, such as before an operation, may offer protection from infections and lower the incidence of sepsis. GM-CSF therapy may find a place in reactivating the immune system of patients in a state of immune paralysis following septic shock, thereby reinforcing the patients' impaired defense system against secondary infections. (See Table 64.3 for approved and experimental indications.)

G-CSF

Endogenous G-CSF Response to Infection

The glycoprotein G-CSF is present at low concentrations (around 25 pg/ml) in the serum of healthy volunteers.[1] A significant increase in G-CSF secretion may be detected during the acute phase of a bacterial infection.[4–6] Patients may have peak concentrations as high as 200 ng/ml at the onset of septic shock.[7] These levels decrease significantly within a few days in survivors, but in nonsurviving sepsis patients the G-CSF levels remain persistently elevated.[8,9] Furthermore, patients who do not respond to infection with increased G-CSF production have a worse prognosis than patients who respond with G-CSF production.[10] These studies showed that patients with the best outcome are those who are able to respond appropriately to an infectious agent by increasing G-CSF levels and then decreasing them upon resolution of the infection. However, in patients with a fatal outcome, G-CSF levels tend to remain elevated, indicating an inability of the host to respond to circulating G-CSF, continued signaling for G-CSF production, or failure of the host to mount a sufficient G-CSF response.[11] The observation that injection of pharmacologic doses of G-CSF (10 μg/kg) into healthy volunteers elevated the serum G-CSF to levels in the upper range of those reached by endogenous production during infection[12] supports the hypothesis that administration of G-CSF under the conditions discussed above may be beneficial to the host by increasing or accelerating the response to infection.

Role of G-CSF in the Cellular Immune System

The central role of endogenous G-CSF lies in the maintenance and control of granulopoiesis, which is essential for efficient host defense, as demonstrated in knockout mice,[13] or in normal mice injected with anti-murine G-CSF antiserum.[14] Both sets of mice were severely neutropenic and unable to recruit additional

TABLE 64.1. Common Abbreviations and Synonyms for G-CSF and GM-CSF.

Abbreviation	Synonym
G-CSF, CSF-G	Granulocyte colony-stimulating factor
CSF-β, CSF-3	Colony-stimulating factor β or 3, respectively
MGI-1G, MGI-2	Macrophage/granulocyte inducer 1G or 2, respectively
G/M-CSA	Granulocyte/macrophage colony-stimulating activity
DF	Differentiation factor; pluripoietin
pCSF	Pluripotent colony-stimulating factor
GM-CSF, CSF-GM	Granulocyte/macrophage colony-stimulating factor
CSF-α, CSF-2	Colony-stimulating factor α or 2, respectively
MGI-1GM	Macrophage/granulocyte inducer 1GM
Eo-CSF	Eosinophil colony-stimulating factor
HCGF	Hematopoietic cell growth factor
KTGF	Keratinocyte-derived T cell growth factor
NIF-T	T cell-derived neutrophil migration inhibition factor

Modified from Ibelgaufts.[1]

TABLE 64.2. Commercial Formulations of G-CSF and GM-CSF.

Generic name	Trade name	Country
G-CSF		
Filgrastim	Neupogen	Europe, US, Canada, Australia
	Gran	Japan, Taiwan, Korea, China
Lenograstim	Neutrogin	Japan, China
	Granocyte	Europe, Australia
Nartograstim	Neu-Up	Japan
GM-CSF		
Molgramostim	Leukomax	Europe, Canada
Sargramostim	Leukine	US

Modified from Root and Dale,[2] with permission.

neutrophils from the bone marrow in response to an infectious challenge and were therefore more susceptible than controls to sublethal doses of infective agents.

Doses of G-CSF ranging from 1 to 60 μg/kg/day given to human volunteers for 6 days produced dose-dependent 1.8- to 12-fold increases in the absolute neutrophil count.[15] In a volunteer study, we found a dose-dependent increase of the polymorphonuclear neutrophil (PMN) count with a plateau lasting throughout the whole 12 days of treatment with G-CSF (filgrastim). Counts equal to those prior to treatment were seen 72 hour after the last injection, (unpublished observations; submitted for publication). Lesser increases in monocyte and lymphocyte counts have also been reported.[16] In addition to increasing the pool of circulating neutrophils, G-CSF primes these immune cells for enhanced effector functions by improving the oxidative burst, phagocytosis, and chemotaxis and by extending their lifetime by delaying apoptosis.[17-19] Thus G-CSF promotes the migration of increasing numbers of immunocompetent and highly potent neutrophils to the focus of infection in an effort to eradicate invading microbes.

Neutrophils pose the first line of defense against all particles identified as foreign; but they may cause damage to host tissues if they are activated prematurely or damaged or if the inflammatory reaction is not terminated on time.[20] Thus during the exploration of possible indications for G-CSF, it was necessary to consider whether the newly recruited neutrophils were functional or preactivated and whether application of G-CSF might unbalance the cytokine mediator network, resulting in exacerbation of the inflammatory reaction.

The in vitro studies discussed above showed that G-CSF does not directly activate but, rather, primes PMNs for increased responsiveness to subsequent stimulation. The implication of this priming effect of G-CSF on PMNs is that their functions are potentiated only in the case of stimulation by exogenous signals.

Effects of G-CSF on the Humoral Response

The inflammatory response is driven primarily by the cytokines tumour necrosis facor-α (TNFα), interleukin-1 (IL-1), and interferon-γ (IFNγ), which are produced by monocytes/macrophages and lymphocytes. Endogenous countermeasures include a reduction in their production or secretion and the release of their respective antagonists: soluble TNF receptors (sTNF-R) or IL-1 receptor antagonist (IL-1ra).

In vitro and ex vivo experiments indicated that G-CSF adjusts the response of rodent and human mononuclear cells to immunostimulatory agents, such as the gram-negative cell wall

TABLE 64.3. Approved and Experimental Indications of G-CSF and GM-CSF.

Indication	G-CSF	GM-CSF
Aplastic anemia	Approved in some countries	
Acute leukemia	Approved in some countries	Approved in some countries
Bone marrow transplantation	Approved	Approved
Chemotherapy-induced neutropenia	Approved	Approved
Diabetic foot infection	Experimental (phase II)	
Fungal infection, candidemia	Experimental (phase II)	
Myelodysplastic syndrome	Approved in some countries	
Nonneutropenic infection	Experimental (phase II–III)	
Neutropenia in HIV infection	Approved in some countries	Approved in some countries
Peripheral blood progenitor cell transplantation	Approved in most countries	Approved in some countries
Severe chronic neutropenia	Approved	

Modified from Frumkin and Dale,[3] with permssion.

component lipopolysaccharide (LPS), by causing a decrease in the production of proinflammatory cytokines and an increase in antiinflammatory cytokine release.[21-23] These results were substantiated in a series of ex vivo human volunteer studies: Whole blood from G-CSF-treated volunteers responded to a variety of immunostimuli, such as LPS, preparations from gram-positive bacteria, superantigens, or phorbol esters, with reduced TNF activity in comparison to blood from placebo-treated controls.[24,25] Neutrophils from these G-CSF-treated volunteers showed increased ex vivo LPS-inducible IL-1ra release, whereas the shedding of soluble TNF receptors was unaffected when calculated per PMN, though of course these cells were present in significantly higher numbers in the blood of the G-CSF-treated subjects.[25] Furthermore, the release capacity of the chemoattractive leukotriene B_4, when expressed per neutrophil, was decreased significantly. This finding can be interpreted as a further antiinflammatory effect of G-CSF unrelated to the cytokine network (unpublished observations). In addition, IFNγ formation by lymphocytes was attenuated in whole blood incubated in the presence of LPS. Thus the overall antiinflammatory effect of a single G-CSF injection consisted of the attenuated release of proinflammatory mediators by monocytes and lymphocytes and concomitant augmented formation and secretion of the respective antagonists by neutrophils.

In another study we examined the effects of daily G-CSF treatment for 12 days in 24 healthy volunteers. Compared to a placebo group, TNFα, IL-12, and IFNγ release in whole blood samples in response to ex vivo stimulation by LPS was reduced in the verum groups compared with the control group throughout treatment. Thus the antiinflammatory effect of G-CSF is also maintained under sustained treatment regimens. The in vitro addition of IL-12 to LPS-stimulated blood lessened the attenuation of IFNγ and TNFα release capacity, indicating that suppression of IL-12 release in pivotal is the antiinflammatory activity to G-CSF.

To assess the time window during which treatment with exogenous G-CSF might improve the course of an infection, a volunteer trial was held in which G-CSF was injected 2 or 24 hours before challenge with LPS in vivo.[26] Administration of G-CSF shortly before LPS boosted the levels of TNF, IL-6, IL-8, IL-1ra, and both kinds of sTNF-R. In comparison, G-CSF injection 1 day prior to challenge significantly decreased IL-8 levels and moderately attenuated the release of TNF and IL-6. The release of IL-1ra and sTNF-R had increased prior to LPS injection. Administration of LPS resulted in a further increase in the sTNF-R I and II levels, whereas IL-1ra release remained unaltered. Despite the different effects on cytokine release patterns, the two treatment regimens resulted in similar positive effects on neutrophil activation and similar changes in surface molecule expression. Moreover, both G-CSF pretreatments blocked LPS-induced granulocyte accumulation in the lung.

G-CSF in Sepsis Models

Many studies have been performed in diverse animal models to explore the relevance of these observations during sepsis and septic shock and to determine whether unacceptable side effects are associated with G-CSF treatment of these conditions. The efficacy of G-CSF, alone or in combination with antibiotics, has been explored in a wide variety of nonneutropenic infectious disease models including neonatal sepsis, pneumonia, infections complicated by ethanol intoxication, burn wound infection, intraabdominal sepsis, and intramuscular infection.[18,27] Results from these studies and those discussed below, in which the survival rate was increased significantly by G-CSF in most cases, indicated that prophylactic administration of G-CSF as a pretreatment when an increased risk of infection is foreseeable, (e.g., before an operation) may be beneficial prophylactically.

In all the animal studies discussed below, G-CSF treatment was initiated prior to or simultaneously with the infectious challenge. Results pertaining to the activity of neutrophils under G-CSF treatment in defense against infection were mostly uniformly positive: recruitment of neutrophils to the site of infection was improved in a pneumonia model[28] and infections seemed to remain more localized in infections with *Escherichia coli*, through cecal ligation and puncture (CLP) or with subcutaneous injections, than in control animals[29,30] as determined by histological evidence, myeloperoxidase activity, or glucose uptake in tissue adjacent to the site of infection. However, in a murine model where radionuclide-labeled *E. coli* were injected, no differences in the translocation through tissues were observed.[31] However, improved bactericidal activity was reported in each of these cases and in models of pneumonia and peritonitis.[32,33]

Regarding cytokine levels during infection, TNFα serum levels in G-CSF-treated animals were reported to be decreased compared to levels in controls in infection models in mice, rats and dogs.[21,34-36] G-CSF-treated galactosamine-sensitized mice exhibited reduced IL-2 serum levels without an effect on TNFα release.[37] Rabbits with immune complex colitis had lower levels of the proinflammatory leukotriene B_4 and thromboxane B_2, but levels of the antiinflammatory prostaglandin E_2 were not affected.[38]

Apart from the general improvement in the course and outcome of infections, there is evidence that prophylactic treatment with G-CSF would be beneficial in the specific treatment of septic shock. G-CSF was shown to protect rodents against endotoxin-induced hepatotoxicity and shock[21,39] and peritonitis-induced multiple organ failure and death.[6,40] It also improved cardiovascular function, endotoxin clearance, and survival in two canine models of septic shock.[6,41]

Neutrophils have been implicated as key mediators in the pathogenesis of acute lung injury due to sepsis or endotoxemia. Accordingly, deliberate augmentation of neutrophil production and activity might be deleterious in patients with sepsis. Several studies have addressed this issue by examining the effects of G-CSF treatment on acute lung injury in guinea pigs,[42] pigs,[29,43] and sheep[44] challenged with LPS. The data from these preclinical studies have been consistent in showing no evidence of exacerbation of lung injury as a consequence of treatment with G-CSF.

Use of G-CSF in Clinical Trials

The benefits of G-CSF treatment in nonneutropenic animal models of infection provided a basis for clinical studies on the effects of G-CSF in regard to the incidence and course of infections that might result in sepsis. G-CSF proved to be safe in intensive care unit (ICU) and septic patients,[10,45,46] who apparently also benefited from the therapy. Generation and function of neutrophils was improved in 20 postoperative/posttraumatic patients at risk of sepsis or with sepsis who were given continuous infusions of G-CSF (filgrastim) for 7 days. Furthermore, IL-8 decreased in all six patients whose initial IL-8 values were >90 pg/ml. IL-1ra increased in 10 patients, though there was no effect on the levels of TNFα or sTNF-R type I.[47]

When G-CSF treatment was commenced before an operation it significantly reduced the incidence of infectious complications in 19 cancer patients undergoing esophagectomy compared with 77 control patients.[7] G-CSF reduced the incidence of multiple organ failure in 756 pneumonia patients[48] and 37 liver allograft recipients.[49]

In conclusion, G-CSF showed antiinflammatory effects combined with improved host defense, not only in preclinical models but also in the clinical setting. Previous clinical experience has shown that the use of G-CSF is associated with a very low incidence of side effects, except mild bone pain. Therefore further trials of G-CSF given for prophylaxis of sepsis and septic complications are ratified, and widespread use of G-CSF in this setting might be considered a clinical option in the near future.

GM-CSF

The initial phase of the systemic inflammatory response syndrome (SIRS) is characterized by excessive production of proinflammatory cytokines by monocytes/macrophages and is therefore termed the hyperinflammatory phase.[50] Here, antiinflammatory therapy (e.g., anti-TNF antibodies, IL-1ra, IL-10) was proposed as the appropriate measure.[51] However, it has been found that this initial phase is followed by a so-called hypoinflammatory phase, also termed immune paralysis.[52,53] Many patients who survive the acute hyperinflammation owing to intensive medical care succumb to subsequent infections. In such patients a drastic change in monocyte activity was observed (i.e., in vitro): The monocytes are no longer able to respond to an inflammatory stimulus such as LPS with secretion of proinflammatory cytokines (e.g., TNFα).[52,54–59] The longer this state of immune paralysis continues, the more adverse is the prognosis.[52,56] Secondary infections during the condition of immune paralysis (i.e., when the organism's state of defense is insufficient) often determine the fate of a patient during septic multiple organ failure.

Therefore a therapeutic goal consists in the reconstitution of immune competence during the late phase of septic shock. For such an indication, immune stimulation with GM-CSF seems to represent a promising pharmacologic therapeutic principle. GM-CSF is a pluripotent hematopoietic growth factor involved in regulating the proliferation, differentiation, and mature functions of granulocytes and monocytes/macrophages,[60] the two key cell types of the nonspecific immune system. GM-CSF has been used to accelerate recovery of the granulocyte and monocyte counts after chemotherapy or bone marrow transplantation, thereby reducing the risk of infections from bacterial or fungal sources due to leukopenia.[61–64]

Role of Endogenous GM-CSF

The role of GM-CSF in vivo became evident in knockout animals. Mice with homozygous mutations of the GM-CSF gene showed no major deficits in hematopoiesis until 12 weeks of age, but they developed abnormal lungs and some suffered from subclinical bacterial or fungal infection.[65] These observations indicate that GM-CSF is not essential for maintenance of hematopoietic cells and their precursors but, rather, for normal pulmonary physiology and resistance to local infection. This conclusion was supported by the finding that the administration of neutralizing monoclonal antibodies specific for GM-CSF to *Cryptococcus neoformans*-infected normal mice increased mortality and induced rapid progresssion of the disease.[66]

To explore further the in vivo role of GM-CSF in infection, GM-CSF knockout mice were treated with endotoxin (LPS). Hypothermia and loss of body weight were markedly attenuated in LPS-treated GM-CSF-deficient mice compared with similarly treated control mice. Moreover, the levels of the circulating proinflammatory cytokines IFNγ, IL1α, and IL-6 were lower in LPS-treated GM-CSF-deficient mice than in LPS-treated control mice. Peak levels of TNFα in response to LPS treatment were the same in the serum of all the mice, but TNFα persisted longer in GM-CSF-deficient mice. LPS-stimulated peritoneal macrophages from GM-CSF-deficient mice produced significantly less IL-1α and nitric oxide than macrophages from wild-type mice, although there was no difference in TNFα production in vitro. These results indicate that GM-CSF contributes to cytokine production in LPS-mediated septic shock and that the attenuated production of these secondary cytokines (IFNγ, IL-1α, and IL-6) may contribute to the endotoxin-resistant phenotype of GM-CSF-deficient mice.[67]

GM-CSF as an Immunostimulatory Drug

The initiation of host defense in the form of an inflammatory reaction is mediated primarily by the cytokines TNFα and IL-1.[68–74] GM-CSF was found to potentiate LPS-induced TNFα and IL-1 production of murine and human monocytic cells.[58,75–77] We also found that GM-CSF is a potent enhancer of LPS-induced TNFα production in vivo in normal and experimentally immunocompromised (LPS-desensitized) mice.[78] Furthermore, in vitro and ex vivo experiments revealed that LPS-induced IL-1 release from bone marrow or spleen cells was also enhanced in GM-CSF-treated mice.[107]

GM-CSF Production: Strictly Controlled

GM-CSF is not detectable in the circulation of healthy animals or humans, though it may be found in the major organs at low concentrations.[79] Only small amounts of GM-CSF were measured in the serum of mice infected with *Listeria monocytogenes*.[80] Patients with experimental endotoxemia,[81] neutropenic fever,[82] or even sepsis[83] also do not normally have elevated serum GM-CSF levels. In patients with meningococcemia GM-CSF concentrations higher than 1 ng/ml were only briefly present in subjects with life-threatening septic shock and were strongly associated with fulminant infection.[6]

As no systemic GM-CSF levels can be detected in patients with infection, endogenous GM-CSF is thought to play its physiologic role in the immediate vicinity of the cells by which it is secreted.[84,85] The hypothesis is supported by the observation that in patients with meningitis only cerebrospinal fluid contained a measurable concentration of GM-CSF.[86]

In summary, it appears that the body highly restricts production of the powerful immunostimulator GM-CSF. Therefore it is not surprising that rats who underwent CLP with sepsis-induced organ injury, when given rmGM-CSF, showed no increased survival rates but, rather, earlier deaths than the control group. Early leukosequestration to the peritoneal cavity was inhibited, and severe liver injuries were observed,[87] that might have resulted from the stimulating activity of GM-CSF on the expression of TNF. One study found that survival in two mouse models of gut-derived sepsis was improved by pretreatment with GM-CSF because of better gut barrier function and better bacterial clearance.[88] However, we found that prophylactic administration of rmGM-CSF neither augmented leukocyte numbers nor protected mice from lethal fecal peritonitis.[14] Consequently, systemic application of GM-CSF may be detrimental if given before or during the proinflammatory phase of sepsis.[108]

GM-CSF in Models of Impaired Immune Competence

A number of studies have been performed in which neonatal rats (which are more vulnerable to infection than older animals) or animals first made susceptible to infection by trauma, burn, or myelosuppression were treated with exogenous GM-CSF and subsequently challenged by CLP or inoculation of infective agents. These studies may be considered models for the diminished status of the immune system experienced at the hypoinflammatory stage of sepsis.

Neonatal rats were found to have deficient PMN production and function during infection. Prophylactic rmGM-CSF given intraperitoneally 6 hours before a 90% lethal dose challenge with *Staphylococcus aureus* significantly improved survival in a neonatal rat model of infection.[89] In another study, neonatal rats with streptococcal sepsis were given rhGM-CSF after infection. A higher survival rate than in control animals not given rhGM-CSF was reported, apparently due to phagocyte priming or cellular influx into the peritoneum (or both),[90] even though human GM-CSF is generally believed not to be bioactive in mice. Furthermore, GM-CSF administered in conjunction with penicillin to neonatal rats with established group B streptococcal infection decreased the mortality rate substantially in comparison to penicillin alone.[91]

Mice made susceptible to infection by trauma were treated with GM-CSF for 5 days before induction of peritonitis. These mice had a significantly higher survival rate than control mice, which underwent the same regimen but received placebo instead of GM-CSF. Peritoneal cell yields were increased in the GM-CSF group, and harvested macrophages stimulated with phorbol ester released larger amounts of both superoxide anion and TNF and less nitric oxide than mice in the control group.[92]

In a murine model 20% surface burns plus CLP were applied. Survival was significantly better on day 10 after injury in animals treated with GM-CSF on days 5–9 after the burn.[93] Concanavalin A-stimulated T cell proliferation and IL-2 production, which were suppressed after burn injury, were also improved by treatment with GM-CSF.[93]

The infection of GM-CSF-pretreated, myelosuppressed mice with normally lethal doses of *Pseudomonas aeruginosa*, *Staphylococcus aureus*, or *Candida albicans* resulted in a significant dose-dependent improvement of survival.[94,95] There has also been research on combinations of GM-CSF with IL-6 or leukemia inhibitory factor (LIF), which are both potent inducers of the acute-phase response and can induce an increase in the platelet count.[95] The rationale for these combinations was that the synergism of the induction of opsonization of microorganisms by acute-phase proteins with activation of phagocytes by GM-CSF should increase resistance to infections. This hypothesis was proven correct when myelosuppressed mice were treated with either of the combinations and infected with *Pseudomonas aeruginosa*.[96]

Preclinical studies with recombinant human GM-CSF are limited by the lack of cross-species reactivity in mice.[97] The protein sequence homology between human and murine GM-CSF is only 60%.[98] Human GM-CSF does not affect canine PMNs in vitro;[99] and even in monkeys only-short-term studies can be undertaken because antibodies develop to human GM-CSF.[62] However, because of the dangers associated with immune stimulation, volunteer studies may be considered unethical. We have taken advantage of a dose-finding study of GM-CSF for wound healing of basalioma, where we investigated the change in white blood cell count and the cytokine production pattern ex vivo in blood from patients treated with low doses of GM-CSF. Patients responded to the treatment with a general leukocytosis, though only the eosinophil fraction was significantly increased relative to the other populations. Cytokine secretion from GM-CSF-treated patients in response to either LPS or lipoteichoic acid was characterized by decreased IFNγ and increased IL-10 and IL-1ra secretion and can therefore basically be considered an antiinflammatory reaction. Side effects were also relatively mild (unpublished observation; submitted for publication).

These results indicate that leukocytosis can be initiated by low doses of GM-CSF, with which the proinflammatory priming, observed in vitro and in animal models at higher doses, is replaced by a trend toward an antiinflammatory cytokine pattern.

Potential Application of GM-CSF for Human Sepsis

Although monocytes from septic shock patients exhibit greater baseline respiratory burst activity than monocytes from healthy subjects, the response to secondary stimulation with bacterial stimuli is attenuated.[100] GM-CSF restored the ability of monocytes to respond appropriately to secondary stimulation. Expression of certain integrin adhesion molecules, CD62L, and Fcγ receptors was increased on monocytes of septic shock patients; expression of CD11c was reduced. GM-CSF upregulated integrin expression and decreased CD62L, CD32, and CD16 expression. Priming monocytes with GM-CSF accelerated tissue factor activation following stimulation with LPS and bacterial culture supernatant.[100]

When a high dose (750 μg/m² day IV) of GM-CSF was administered to sarcoma patients with neutropenia for 2 weeks, no increase in basal release of TNFα or IL-1β by monocytes ex vivo was found, though the LPS-stimulated release of both factors reached 8-fold and 10-fold their respective values on day 0.[101] A single dose (2.5, 5.0, or 10.0 μg/kg) of GM-CSF resulted in a significant increase of in vivo plasma levels of IL-1ra and a trend toward increased IL-8 levels in cancer patients.[102] A case has been reported where a patient in the ICU with acquired agranulocytosis and sepsis experienced rapid neutrophil recovery and resolution of a clinical infection when treated with GM-CSF.[103]

Possible Adverse Effects

In humans, systemic administration of GM-CSF at doses sufficient to produce plasma levels comparable to endogenous levels seen during severe meningococcal septic shock induced vasodilatation, hypotension, and hypoxia.[6] In a model where GM-CSF was highly expressed in rat lung after intrapulmonary transfer of the gene coding for murine GM-CSF using an adenoviral vector, a sustained but self-limiting accumulation of eosinophils and macrophages was associated with tissue injury in the lung followed by varying degrees of irreversible fibrotic reactions observed at later stages, suggesting that GM-CSF plays a role in the development of respiratory conditions characterized by eosinophilia, granuloma, or fibrosis.[104] Increases in plasma GM-CSF in patients with inflammatory disorders such as asthma[86] or granulocytosis due to infection[105] indicate that GM-CSF should be used with caution in patients with respiratory diseases. However, in a patient with T lymphocytosis with granulocytopenia and severe perianal infection, the eosinophilia initiated by GM-CSF (12.5 μg/kg for 8 days) correlated with improvement of the perianal ulceration.[106]

Conclusions

A number of studies have indicated that the immunostimulatory properties of GM-CSF may be beneficial in reconstituting the compromised immune system, thereby improving the outcome after secondary infections or sepsis.

References

1. Ibelgaufts H: Lexikon der Zytokine, München: Medikon Verlag, 1992.
2. Root RK, Dale DC: G-CSF and GM-CSF: comparisons and potential for use in the treatment of infections in non-neutropenic patients. J Inf Dis 1999;149:5342–5352.
3. Frumkin LR, Dale DC: The role of colony-stimulating factors in HIV disease. AIDS Reader 1996;6:185–193.
4. Kawakami M, Tsutsumi H, Kamakawa T, et al: Levels of serum granulocyte colony-stimulating factor in patients with infections. Blood 1990;76:1962–1964.
5. Kragsbjerg P, Jones I, Vikerfors T, et al: Diagnostic value of blood cytokine concentrations in acute pneumonia. Thorax 1995;50:1253–1257.
6. Waring PM, Presneill J, Maher DW, et al: Differential alterations in plasma colony-stimulating factor concentrations in meningococcaemia. Clin Exp Immunol 1995;102:501–506.
7. Mansmann G, Engert A, Hübel K: Application of G-CSF in the nonneutropenic host. Onkologie 1998;21:124–127.
8. Kragsbjerg P, Holmberg H, Vikerfors T: Dynamics of blood cytokine concentrations in patients with bacteremic infections. Scand J Infect Dis 1996;28:391–398.
9. Tanaka H, Ishikawa K, Nishino M, et al: Changes in granulocyte colony-stimulating factor concentration in patients with trauma and sepsis. J Trauma 1996;40:718–725.
10. Gross-Weege W, Weiss M, Schneider M, et al: Safety of a low-dosage Filgrastim (rhG-CSF) treatment in non-neutropenic surgical intensive care patients with an inflammatory process. Intensive Care Med 1997;23:16–22.
11. Stoltz DA, Bagby GJ, Nelson S: Use of granulocyte colony-stimulating factor in the treatment of acute infectious diseases. Curr Opin Hematol 1997;4:207–212.
12. Lieschke GJ, Burgess AW: Granulocyte colony-stimulating factor and granulocyte-macrophage colony-stimulating factor (1). N Engl J Med 1992;327:28–35.
13. Lieschke GJ, Grail D, Hodgson G, et al: Mice lacking granulocyte colony-stimulating factor have chronic neutropenia, granulocyte and macrophage progenitor cell deficiency, and impaired neutrophil mobilization. Blood 1994;84:1737–1746.
14. Barsig J, Bundschuh DS, Hartung T, et al: Control of fecal peritoneal infection in mice by colony-stimulating factors. J Infect Dis 1996;174:790–799.
15. Dale DC: Potential role of colony-stimulating factors in the prevention and treatment of infectious diseases. Clin Infect Dis 1994;18 (Suppl 2):S180–S188.
16. Hartung T: Immunomodulation by colony-stimulating factors. Rev Physiol Biochem Pharmacol 1999;136:1–164.
17. Demetri GD, Griffin JD: Granulocyte colony-stimulating factor and its receptor. Blood 1991;78:2791–2808.
18. Dale DC, Liles WC, Summer WR, et al: Review: granulocyte colony-stimulating factor—role and relationships in infectious diseases. J Infect Dis 1995;172:1061–1075.

19. Hartung T, Wendel A: Immunomodulatory properties of Filgrastim (r-metHuG-CSF) in preclinical models. In: Morstyn G, et al (eds) Filgrastim (r-metHuG-CSF) in Clinical Practice. New York, Marcel Dekker, 1998;397–427.
20. Smith JA: Neutrophils, host defense, and inflammation: a double-edged sword. J Leukoc Biol 1994;56:672–686.
21. Görgen I, Hartung T, Leist M, et al: Granulocyte colony-stimulating factor treatment protects rodents against lipopolysaccharide-induced toxicity via suppression of systemic tumor necrosis factor-alpha. J Immunol 1992;149:918–924.
22. Kitabayashi A, Hirokawa M, Hatano Y, et al: Granulocyte colony-stimulating factor downregulates allogeneic immune responses by posttranscriptional inhibition of tumor necrosis factor-alpha production. Blood 1995;86:2220–2227.
23. Pan L, Delmonte J Jr, Jalonen CK, et al: Pretreatment of donor mice with granulocyte colony-stimulating factor polarizes donor T lymphocytes toward type-2 cytokine production and reduces severity of experimental graft-versus-host disease. Blood 1995;86:4422–4429.
24. Hartung T, Volk H-D, Wendel A: G-CSF: an anti-inflammatory cytokine. J Endotoxim Res 1995;2:195–201.
25. Hartung T, Docke WD, Gantner F, et al: Effect of granulocyte colony-stimulating factor treatment on ex vivo blood cytokine response in human volunteers. Blood 1995;85:2482–2489.
26. Pajkrt D, Manten A, van der Poll T, et al: Modulation of cytokine release and neutrophil function by granulocyte colony-stimulating factor during endotoxemia in humans. Blood 1997;90:1415–1424.
27. Nelson S: Role of granulocyte colony-stimulating factor in the immune response to acute bacterial infection in the nonneutropenic host: an overview. Clin Infect Dis 1994;18(Suppl 2):S197–S204.
28. Lister PD, Gentry MJ, Preheim LC: Granulocyte colony-stimulating factor protects control rats but not ethanol-fed rats from fatal pneumococcal pneumonia. J Infect Dis 1993;168:922–926.
29. Patton JHJ, Lyden SP, Ragsdale DN, et al: Granulocyte colony-stimulating factor improves host defense to resuscitated shock and polymicrobial sepsis without provoking generalized neutrophil-mediated damage. J Trauma 1998;44:750–758.
30. Lang CH, Bagby GJ, Dobrescu C, et al: Effect of granulocyte colony-stimulating factor on sepsis-induced changes in neutrophil accumulation and organ glucose uptake. J Infect Dis 1992;166:336–343.
31. Eaves-Pyles T, Alexander JW: Granulocyte colony-stimulating factor enhances killing of translocated bacterial but does not affect barrier function in a burn mouse model. J Trauma 1996;41:1013–1017.
32. Dunne JR, Dunkin BJ, Nelson S, et al: Effects of granulocyte colony stimulating factor in a nonneutropenic rodent model of *Escherichia coli* peritonitis. J Surg Res 1996;61:348–354.
33. Zhang P, Bagby GJ, Stoltz DA, et al: Enhancement of peritoneal leukocyte function by granulocyte colony-stimulating factor in rats with abdominal sepsis. Crit Care Med 1998;26:315–321.
34. Eichacker PQ, Waisman Y, Natanson C, et al: Cardiopulmonary effects of granulocyte colony-stimulating factor in a canine model of bacterial sepsis. J Appl Physiol 1994;77:2366–2373.
35. Lorenz W, Reimund KP, Weitzel F, et al: Granulocyte colony-stimulating factor prophylaxis before operation protects against lethal consequences of postoperative peritonitis. Surgery 1994;116:925–934.
36. Lundblad R, Nesland JM, Giercksky KE: Granulocyte colony-stimulating factor improves survival rate and reduces concentrations of bacteria, endotoxin, tumor necrosis factor, and endothelin-1 in fulminant intro-abdominal sepsis in rats. Crit Care Med 1996;24:820–826.
37. Aoki Y, Hiromatsu K, Kobayashi N, et al: Protective effect of granulocyte colony-stimulating factor against T-cell-meditated lethal shock triggered by superantigens. Blood 1995;86:1420–1427.
38. Hommes DW, Meenan J, Dijkhuizen S, et al: Efficacy of recombinant granulocyte colony-stimulating factor (rhG-CSF) in experimental colitis. Clin Exp Immunol 1996;106:529–533.
39. Vollmar B, Messner S, Wanner G, et al: Immunomodulatory action of G-CSF in a rat model of endotoxin-induced liver injury: an intravital microscopic analysis of Kupffer cell and leukocyte response. J Leukoc Biol 1997;62:710–718.
40. O'Reilly M, Silver GM, Greenhalgh DG, et al: Treatment of intra-abdominal infection with granulocyte colony-stimulating factor. J Trauma 1992;33:679–682.
41. Freeman BD, Quezado Z, Zeni F, et al: rG-CSF reduces endotoxemia and improves survival during *E. coli* pneumonia. J Appl Physiol 1997;83:1467–1475.
42. Kanazawa M, Ishizaka A, Hasegawa N, et al: Granulocyte colony-stimulating factor does not enhance endotoxin-induced acute lung injury in guinea pigs. Am Rev Respir Dis 1988;148:1030–1035.
43. Fink MP, O'Sullivan BP, Menconi MJ, et al: Effect of granulocyte colony-stimulating factor on systemic and pulmonary responses to endotoxin in pigs. J Trauma 1993;34:571–577.
44. Silver GM, Fink MP: Possible roles for anti- or pro-inflammatory therapies in the management of sepsis. Surg Clin North Am 1994;74:711–723.
45. Endo S, Inada K, Inoue Y, et al: Evaluation of recombinant human granulocyte colony-stimulating factor (rhG-CSF) therapy in granulopoietic patients complicated with sepsis. Curr Med Res Opin 1994;13:233–241.
46. Weiss M, Gross-Weege W, Schneider M, et al: Enhancement of neutrophil function by in vivo filgrastim treatment for prophylaxis of sepsis in surgical intensive care patients. J Crit Care 1995;10:21–26.
47. Weiss M, Gross-Weege W, Harms B, et al: Filgrastim (RHG-CSF) related modulation of the inflammatory response in patients at risk of sepsis or with sepsis. Cytokine 1996;8:260–265.
48. Andresen J, Movahhed H, Nelson S: Filgrastim (r-metHuG-CSF) in pneumonia. In: Morstyn G, et al (ed) Filgrastim (r-metG-CSF) in Clinical Practice. New York, Marcel Dekker, 1998;429–446.
49. Foster PF, Mital D, Sankary HN, et al: The use of granulocyte colony-stimulating factor after liver transplantation. Transplantation 1995;59:1557–1563.
50. Bone RC: Toward a theory regarding the pathogenesis of the systemic inflammatory response syndrome: what we do and do not know about cytokine regulation. Crit Care Med 1996;24:163–172.
51. Volk HD, Reinke P, Krausch D, et al: Monocyte deactivation—rationale for a new therapeutic strategy in sepsis. Intensive Care Med 1996;22(Suppl 4):S474–S481.
52. Döcke W-D, Syrbe U, Meinecke A, et al: Improvement of monocytic function—a new therapeutic approach? In: Reinhart K, Eyrich K, Sprung C (ed) Update in Intensive Care and Emergency Medicine. Sepsis—Current Perspectives in Pathophysiology and Therapy, vol 18. Berlin, Springer, 1994:473–500.
53. Von Baehr R, Lohmann T, Heym S, et al: Immunoparalysis in case of septicaemia. Z Klin Med 1990;45:1133–1137.

54. Faist E, Mewes A, Baker CC, et al: Prostaglandin E$_2$ (PGE$_2$)-dependent suppression of interleukin (IL-) 2 production in patients with major trauma. J Trauma 1987;27:837–848.
55. Faist E, Mewes A, Strasser T, et al: Alterations of monocyte function following major injury. Arch Surg 1988;123:287–292.
56. Munoz C, Carlet J, Fitting C, et al: Dysregulation of in vitro cytokine production by monocytes during sepsis. J Clin Invest 1991;88:1747–1754.
57. Volk HD, Thieme M, Ruppe U, et al: Alterations in function and phenotype of monocytes from patients with septic disease: predictive value and new therapeutic strategies. Z Kiln Med 1990;45:1133–1137.
58. Randow F, Döcke W-D, Bundschuh DS, et al: In vitro prevention and reversal of lipopolysaccharide desensitization by IFN-γ, IL-12, and granulocyte-macrophage colony-stimulating factor. J Immunol 1997;158:2911–2918.
59. Ertel W, Kremer JP, Kenney J, et al: Downregulation of proinflammatory cytokine release in whole blood from septic patients. Blood 1995;85:1341–1347.
60. Gabrilove JL, Jakubowski A: Hematopoietic growth factors: biology and clinical application. J Natl Cancer Inst Monogr 1990;10:73–77.
61. Scarffe JH: Emerging clinical uses for GM-CSF. Eur J Cancer 1991;27:1493–1504.
62. Morstyn G, Lieschke GJ, Sheridan W, et al: Pharmacology of the colony-stimulating factors. Trends Pharmacol Sci 1989;10:154–159.
63. Whetton AD: The biology and clinical potential of growth factors that regulate myeloid cell production. Trends Pharmacol Sci 1990;11:285–289.
64. Moore MA: The clinical use of colony stimulating factors. Annu Rev Immunol 1991;9:159–191.
65. Stanley E, Lieschke GJ, Grail D, et al: Granulocyte/macrophage colony-stimulating factor-deficient mice show no major perturbation of hematopoiesis but develop a characteristic pulmonary pathology. Proc Natl Acad Sci USA 1994;91:5592–5596.
66. Collins HL, Bancroft GJ: Cytokine enhancement of complement-dependent phagocytosis by macrophages: synergy of tumor necrosis factor-alpha and granulocyte-macrophage colony-stimulating factor for phagocytosis of Cryptococcus neoformans. Eur J Immunol 1992;22:1447–1454.
67. Basu S, Dunn AR, Marino MW, et al: Increased tolerance to endotoxin by granulocyte-macrophage colony-stimulating factor-defecient mice. J Immunol 1997;159:1412–1417.
68. Dinarello CA: Interleukin-1: amino acid sequences, multiple biological activities and comparison with tumor necrosis factor (cachectin). Year Immunol 1986;2:68–89.
69. Dinarello CA: An update on human interleukin-1: from molecular biology to clinical relevance. J Clin Immunol 1985;5:287–297.
70. Bone RC, Balk RA, Cerra FB, et al: Definitions for sepsis and organ failure and guidelines for the use of innovative therapies in sepsis: the ACCP/SCCM Consensus Conference Committee, American College of Chest Physicians/Society of Critical Care Medicine. Chest 1992;101:1644–1655.
71. Tracey KJ, Beutler B, Lowry SF, et al: Shock and tissue injury induced by recombinant human cachectin. Science 1986;234:470–474.
72. Tracey KJ, Cerami A: Tumor necrosis factor: an updated review of its biology. Crit Care Med 1993;21:S415–S422.
73. Damas P, Reuter A, Gysen P, et al: Tumor necrosis factor and interleukin-1 serum levels during severe sepsis in humans. Crit Care Med 1989;17:975–978.
74. Debets JM, Kampmeijer R, van der Linden MP, et al: Plasma tumor necrosis factor and mortality in critically ill septic patients. Crit Care Med 1989;17:489–494.
75. Cannistra SA, Vellenga E, Groshek P, et al: Human granulocyte-monocyte colony-stimulating factor and interleukin 3 stimulate monocyte cytotoxicity through a tumor necrosis factor-dependent mechanism. Blood 1988;71:672–676.
76. Sisson SD, Dinarello CA: Production of interleukin-1 alpha, interleukin-1 beta and tumor necrosis factor by human mononuclear cells stimulated with granulocyte-macrophage colony-stimulating factor. Blood 1988;72:1368–1374.
77. Cohen L, David B, Cavaillon JM: Interleukin-3 enhances cytokine production by LPS-stimulated macrophages. Immunol Lett 1991;28:121–126.
78. Bundschuh DS, Barsig J, Hartung T, et al: Granulocyte-macrophage colony-stimulating factor and IFN-γ restore the systemic TNF-α response to endotoxin in lipopolysaccharide-desensitized mice. J Immun 1997;158:2862–2871.
79. Metcalf D: The role of the colony-stimulating factors in resistance to acute infections. Immunol Cell Biol 1987;65:35–43.
80. Cheers C, Haigh AM, Kelso A, et al: Production of colony-stimulating factors (CSFs) during infection: separate determinations of macrophage-, granulocyte-, granulocyte-macrophage-, and multi-CSFs. Infect Immun 1988;56:247–251.
81. Granowitz EV, Porat R, Orencole SF, et al: Granulocyte-macrophage colony-stimulating factor synthesis during experimental endotoxemia in humans [letter, comment]. J Infect Dis 1992;166:1204–1205.
82. Cebon J, Layton JE, Maher D, et al: Endogenous haemopoietic growth factors in neutropenia and infection. Br J Haematol 1994;86:265–274.
83. Cebon J, Layton JE, Maher D, et al: Endogenous haemopoietic growth factors in neutropenia and infection. Br J Haematol 1994;86:265–274.
84. Gasson JC: Molecular physiology of granulocyte-macrophage colony-stimulating factor. Blood 1991;77:1131–1145.
85. Freund M, Kleine HD: The role of GM-CSF in infection. Infection 1992;20 (Suppl 2):S84–S92.
86. Sallerfors B: Endogenous production and peripheral blood levels of granulocyte-macrophage (GM-) and granulocyte (G-) colony-stimulating factors. Leuk Lymphoma 1994;13:235–247.
87. Toda H, Murata A, Oka Y, et al: Effect of granulocyte-macrophage colony-stimulating factor on sepsis-induced organ injury in rats. Blood 1994;83:2893–2898.
88. Gennari R, Alexander JW, Gianotti L, et al: Granulocyte macrophage colony-stimulating factor improves survival in two models of gut-derived sepsis by improving gut barrier function and modulating bacterial clearance. Ann Surg 1994;220:68–76.
89. Frenck RW, Sarman G, Harper TE, et al: The ability of recombinant murine granulocyte-macrophage colony-stimulating factor to protect neonatal rats from septic death due to Staphylococcus aureus. J Infect Dis 1990;162:109–114.
90. Wheeler JG, Givner LB: Therapeutic use of recombinant human granulocyte-macrophage colony-stimulating factor in neonatal rats with type III group B streptococcal sepsis. J Infect Dis 1992;165:938–941.
91. Givner LB, Nagaraj SK: Hyperimmune human IgG or recombinant human granulocyte-macrophage colony-stimulating factor

as adjunctive therapy for group B streptococcal sepsis in newborn rats. J Pediatr 1993;122:774–779.
92. Austin OM, Redmond HP, Watson WG, et al: The beneficial effects of immunostimulation in posttraumatic sepsis. J Surg Res 1995;59:446–449.
93. Molloy RG, Holzheimer R, Nestor M, et al: Granulocyte-macrophage colony-stimulating factor modulates immune function and improves survival after experimental thermal injury. Br J Surg 1995;82:770–776.
94. Tanaka T, Okamura S, Okada K, et al: Protective effect of recombinant murine granulocyte-macrophage colony-stimulating factor against *Pseudomonas aeruginosa* infection in leukocytopenic mice. Infect Immun 1989;57:1792–1799.
95. Liehl E, Hildebrandt J, Lam C, et al: Prediction of the role of granulocyte-macrophage colony-stimulating factor in animals and man from in vitro results. Eur J Clin Microbiol Infect Dis 1994;13(Suppl 2):S9–S17.
96. De Clerck F, De Brabander M, Neels H, et al: Direct evidence for the contractile capacity of endothelial cells. Thromb Res 1981;23:505–520.
97. Metcalf D: The molecular biology and functions of the granulocyte-macrophage colony-stimulating factors. Blood 1986;67:257–267.
98. Wong GG, Witek JS, Temple PA, et al: Human GM-CSF: molecular cloning of the complementary DNA and purification of the natural and recombinant proteins. Science 1985;228:810–815.
99. D'Alesandro MM, Gruber DF, O'Halloran KP, et al: In vitro modulation of canine polymorphonuclear leukocyte function by granulocyte-macrophage colony stimulating factor. Biotherapy 1991;3:233–239.
100. Williams MA, White SA, Miller JJ, et al: Granulocyte-macrophage colony-stimulating factor induces activation and restores respiratory burst activity in monocytes from septic patients. J Infect Dis 1998;177:107–115.
101. Perkins RC, Vadhan-Raj S, Scheule RK, et al: Effects of continuous high dose rhGM-CSF infusion on human monocyte activity. Am J Hematol 1993;43:279–285.
102. Aman MJ, Stockdreher K, Thews A, et al: Regulation of immunomodulatory functions by granulocyte-macrophage colony-stimulating factor and granulocyte colony-stimulating factor in vivo. Ann Hematol 1996;73:231–238.
103. Weiss J, Elsbach P, Shu C, et al: Human bactericidal/permeability-increasing protein and a recombinant NH_2-terminal fragment cause killing of serum-resistant gram-negative bacteria in whole blood and inhibit tumor necrosis factor release induced by the bacteria. J Clin Invest 1992;90:1122–1130.
104. Xing Z, Ohkawara Y, Jordana M, et al: Transfer of granulocyte-macrophage colony-stimulating factor gene to rat lung induces eosinophilia, monocytosis, and fibrotic reactions. J Clin Invest 1996;97:1102–1110.
105. Omori F, Okamura S, Shimoda K, et al: Levels of human serum granulocyte colony-stimulating factor and granulocyte-macrophage colony-stimulating factor under pathological conditions. Biotherapy 1992;4:147–153.
106. Krieger G, Kneba M, Vehmeyer K, et al: Use of recombinant human granulocyte-macrophage colony stimulating factor in T-lymphocytosis with granulocytopenia. Eur J Haematol 1990;44:205–206.
107. Tiegs G, Barsig J, Matiba B, et al: Potentiation by granulocyte macrophage colony-stimulating factor of lipopolysaccharide toxicity in mice. J Clin Invest 1994;93:2616–2622.
108. Hartung T, Doecke WD, Bundschuh D, et al: Effect of filgrastim treatment on inflammatory cytokines and lymphocyte functions. Clin Pharmacol Ther 1999;66:415–424.

65
Anabolic Effects of Growth Hormone in Critically Ill Patients

Douglas W. Wilmore

Injury, inflammation, and infection initiate dramatic metabolic changes in the body, characterized by hypermetabolism, glucose intolerance, mobilization and utilization of fatty acids, and net protein catabolism. Although most patients can withstand this altered metabolic state over the short term (7–10 days), more prolonged catabolism significantly erodes body tissue, reduces optimal function, and prolongs recovery.

The major metabolic concern following these stress states is the loss of protein, which represents the structural and functional components of the body. Progressive protein wasting results in decreased wound healing, reduced resistance to infection, attenuation of strength, and reduced activity. These factors contribute to increased morbidity, prolonged convalescent recovery, and increased mortality. Major therapeutic efforts have been made to reduce protein catabolism by providing adequate nutritional support to critically ill patients. Although this practice has reduced the weight loss and somewhat attenuated the protein loss that accompanies catabolic illness, the effects on protein loss and outcome have been disappointing.

For example, Plank et al. carefully studied a group of 12 adult patients with sepsis secondary to peritonitis.[1] Serial measurements of body composition were performed after initial laparotomy, while the patients were receiving optimal nutrition and state-of-the-art cardiorespiratory care and undergoing intensive care unit (ICU) monitoring. Despite successful provision of adequate energy, protein, vitamins, and minerals, the patients lost 1.12 kg of body protein (13.1% of total body protein) over the 21 days of the study. Others investigators, utilizing a variety of approaches, have concluded that it is difficult, if not impossible, to maintain or replete body protein during prolonged (>10 days) catabolic states.[2,3]

Many factors contribute to the protein-catabolic response. The production of cytokines is additive to the neurohumoral environment that initiates and propagates whole-body protein catabolism. However, treatment factors such as bed rest, sedation, mechanical ventilation and paralysis, inotropic support, other drug effects, and inadequate exercise are additive to the hormonal and inflammatory state. All of these factors contribute to the loss of protein from the body during critical illness. Modern intensive care relies on nutritional support of these subjects to attenuate the protein-catabolic response; and if enteral feeding is impossible, total parenteral nutrition (TPN) is provided. Yet an aggregate analysis of 26 randomized trials of TPN in critically ill patients found that this method of nutritional support does not influence the overall mortality rate in surgical or critically ill patients.[4] There was a trend toward fewer complications in TPN patients, but it occurred primarily in those who were malnourished, not in adequately nourished patients. Nevertheless, currently the only therapy available to counteract the catabolic events of critical illness is supportive nutritional care, even though the effects of this approach on outcome are minimal at best.

Investigators have explored other approaches to modify the catabolic state. One approach is to block the mediators of protein catabolism. Unfortunately, we do not know the primary mediator(s) of these events at the present time. Cytokines and other proinflammatory mediators undoubtedly play a major role, but these response systems are highly interconnected with multiple positive and negative feedback loops. Blocking one signal [e.g., tumor necrosis factor-α (TNFα) or interleukin-6 (IL-6)] has resulted in amplification of other proinflammatory mediators. Thus cytokine blockade has not been successful to date.

A second approach to this problem is to minimize events that enhance catabolism and provide an anabolic agent to balance the catabolic hormonal environment. This can be achieved by (1) providing adequate analgesia; (2) reducing environmental cooling in the war and operating room using a variety of warming techniques; and (3) providing adequate nutrition, preferably by the enteral route. In addition, an anabolic factor such as growth hormone (GH) can be provided to counterbalance the effect of the protein catabolic milieu. The relevant data related to studies of GH administration in critically ill patients is the basis for this chapter.

Normal Regulation of GH

Growth hormone is a large peptide hormone secreted by the anterior pituitary gland. Its elaboration is regulated primarily by hormones synthesized in areas of the hypothalamus that have multiple neural connections with other portions of the brain and peripheral nervous system and that respond to changes in the blood concentrations of various substances. In this manner, GH can be secreted to regulate growth, energy homeostasis, protein synthesis, and fluid balance.

Two primary hormonal messages are secreted at the median eminence and carried via the hypophyseal-portal system to the pituitary gland to control GH release.[5] The first hormone is growth hormone releasing hormone (GHRH), a polypeptide that has now been isolated, identified, and synthesized; it stimulates the synthesis and release of GH. The second regulatory hormone that inhibits GH release without affecting synthesis is somatostatin. The interplay between these two factors results in pulsatile release of GH, particularly during sleep. With critical illness, the mean constant elaboration of somatostatin greatly attenuates this pulsatile pattern.

In a normal individual the GH concentration rises periodically over a 24-hour period to levels frequently found only in individuals with acromegaly and a GH-secreting tumor. These concentrations gradually return to basal tonic concentrations. Because of this pulsatile pattern, single blood measurements of GH concentration are of little clinical diagnostic value. To determine the status of GH secretion accurately multiple samples must be obtained over an extended time (usually every 20 minutes over a 12-hour period at night); these data are then subjected to a mathematic technique referred to as deconvolution analysis.[6] Alternately, a stimulation test can be performed using insulin hypoglycemia or infusion of arginine, other secretogogues, or GHRH. Multiple blood samples are obtained over time, and the GH response is plotted. Criteria are then employed to determine if the response to the provocative stimulus is adequate or if a deficiency state exists.

The GH secretion rates for a normal adult range between 0.3 and 2.0 mg/day. This secretion rate decreases with age, and it has been suggested that a large proportion of elderly individuals are GH-deficient. This fall in GH secretion with age may account for the loss of muscle mass with aging and contribute to the prolonged recovery following severe illnesses.

When GH is liberated into the bloodstream, it is bound to its circulating carrier protein or exists in its free form. GH exerts its signal by attaching to the extracellular domain of a specific cell membrane receptor, which occurs on almost all cells; then, through a variety of intracellular transduction pathways, GH signals the cell to initiate a specific response. This response pattern is highly diverse and specific for certain cells. For example, GH causes fluid and sodium reabsorption in the kidney, stimulates the release of free fatty acids, and augments insulin resistance, bone growth, amino acid transport, and protein synthesis. Yet its major anabolic effects are manifested by liberation of a second hormone, insulin-like growth factor-1 (IGF-1). This hormone, which is synthesized in many tissues, is long-acting. The IGF-1 concentrations in the bloodstream primarily reflect hepatic synthesis of this hormone, but these levels are reasonably stable and have been used to determine nutritional status, the state of anabolism, and the quantitative effects of GH within the body.[7]

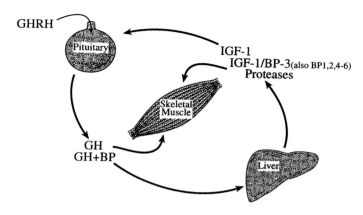

FIGURE 65.1. Physiologic basis of growth hormone (GH) actions. GH stimulates secretion of insulin-like growth factor-1 of (IGF-1) into the bloodstream, and it is then bound by BP-3. During inflammatory states this complex is attacked by proteases that free the IGF-1 and decrease its half-life. GHRH, growth hormone-releasing hormone; BP, binding protein.

The hormone IGF-1 has its own receptors and its own signaling pathway, although it can loosely bind to the insulin receptor and enhance glucose transport and protein synthesis in this manner. IGF-1 appears to exert its effects by acting as a circulating hormone and by exerting autocrine and paracrine activity. These effects include stimulation of protein synthesis and epiphyseal growth along with insulin-like effects and the generation of antilipolytic activity. Thus GH and IGF-1 work in concert to stimulate fuel mobilization and provide for protein synthesis and bone growth (Fig. 65.1).

Another element of IGF-1 control is the simultaneous synthesis and elaboration of binding proteins. There are six known proteins that bind IGF-1, and these proteins are primarily synthesized by the liver. The important binding protein associated with surgical illness is binding protein-3 (IGFBP-3).[8] This protein has a reasonably high affinity for IGF-1, and the highly anabolic circulating complex formed has a prolonged half-life when compared to free IGF-1. The binding of IGF-1 enhances plasma concentrations of this hormone and may augment its anabolic effects. During critical illness proteases are formed in the body that cleave IGF-1 from the binding protein, reducing its plasma concentration and thus decreasing anabolic activity.[9]

Alterations in the GH/IGF-1 Axis During Critical Illness

Most studies that have analyzed plasma GH concentrations in critically ill patients have found elevated levels. When a more formal analysis is performed by analyzing multiple blood samples[10] or performing stimulation tests,[11] it was found that the peaks of the response were lower than in normals, but that the interpulse levels were elevated (Fig. 65.2). Despite the elevated GH concentrations associated with critical illness,

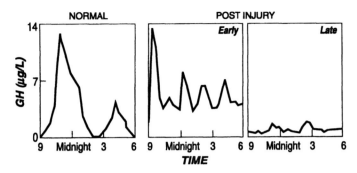

FIGURE 65.2. Pulsatile nature of GH release in normal subjects, acutely ill patients, and seriously ill patients >10 days after the illness.

IGF-1 levels were low. This state is referred to as GH resistance, and the attenuated IGF-1 response to GH occurs both in the basal state and following exogenous administration of GH.[12]

Associated with low levels of IGF-1 are reduced concentrations of IGFBP-3. Proteases, also present in the bloodstream, cleave the IGFBP-3 complex and reduce bioavailability.[9]

The fall in IGF-1 levels may also be related to alterations in the diet that occur with the onset of critical illness, as the effects of GH on IGF-1 elaboration are greatly modified by nutrient intake. For example, in normals GH administration can achieve a positive nitrogen balance and generate significant levels of IGF-1 when the subjects receive only 50% of their caloric needs but adequate protein and micronutrients.[13] With moderate caloric restriction in obese patients (24 kcal/kg ideal weight), GH caused a threefold increase in IGF-1 and a 135 mmol/day improvement in nitrogen balance.[7] Similar changes were observed during more severe dietary restriction (18 kcal/kg/day). When intake was decreased to 12 kcal/kg ideal weight and provided as a diet high in fat but adequate in protein, minimal effects of GH administration on IGF-1 and nitrogen balance were observed. When carbohydrate was substituted for the fat in this diet, improved nitrogen retention occurred. Thus both the quantity of energy provided and the type of energy (fat versus carbohydrate) modulated the GH effect on IGF-1 and protein metabolism.

Another possible cause of the reduced elaboration of IGF-1 is the presence of insulin resistance, which occurs in critically ill patients, as it has been demonstrated that insulin serves as a cofactor to the transcriptional step of IGF-1.[14] It has also been demonstrated that following the stress of a major operative procedure there is a decrease in GH receptor number,[15] which could also explain the occurrence of GH resistance.

If the catabolic illness persists (>10 days), subtle alterations occur in the GH/IGF-1 axis. Rather than the elaboration of GH by large pulsations, the pulsatile output is greatly reduced but the basal levels rise (Fig. 65.2). Evaluation of this response suggests that GH secretion falls within the low normal range. Because feedback mechanisms provide signals to the brain when GH and IGF-1 concentrations are low, it suggests uncoupling or block in this homeostatic feedback mechanism.[10]

During this chronic phase of catabolic illness the presence of GH resistance seems to have dissipated. If exogenous GH is administered or endogenous GH is stimulated, it appears to stimulate IGF-1 and IGFBP-3 appropriately.[16] Because GH levels are low in the nonstimulated basal state, concentrations of IGF-1 also remain low.

These data on the variation of IGF-1 production in response to GH over time are consistent with those from earlier trials, which demonstrated that major anabolic effects of GH occurred in burn patients during the chronic phase of recovery, not within the first 10 days following injury, the period associated with GH resistance.[17]

Factors Contributing to a Variable GH Response

Inflammation

The role the inflammatory response and the elaboration of proteases plays in IGF-1 elaboration and concentration has already been discussed and may be of significant importance in patients with critical illness. For example, Young and coworkers administered GH to patients with multiorgan failure (two or more failed organs) in a multicenter blinded trial.[18] The GH dose administered was gradually elevated (from 0 to 0.3 mg/kg/day) as additional patients were studied. The response of IGF-1 to 1–2 weeks of GH was highly variable and generally unrelated to the GH dose. Patients were grouped as those who could mount an IGF-1 response (defined as a concentration two standard deviations above the pretreatment baseline) and those who could not. IGF-1 responsiveness appeared to predict survival (Table 65.1), although the nonresponding group was slightly older and tended to have lower serum transferrin levels than the surviving group.

This study demonstrates the great variability of the IGF-1 response in critical illness. Such an approach could be utilized as a method of evaluating hepatic synthetic capacity; alternatively, it may indicate a requirement for IGF-1 infusions in selected critically ill patients. Further studies are necessary to address these issues.

Nutritional Status

It is often assume that all malnourished patients become anabolic in the presence of GH, but this is not the case. For example, Tayek and Brasel gave GH for 3 days to a group of 10 cancer patients.[19] The mean nitrogen balance for the entire

TABLE 65.1. Effect of the IGF-1 Response to GH on Outcome.

Parameter	IGF-1 response	No IGF-1 response	p
No.	13	9	—
Age (years)	45 ± 6	66 ± 5	0.016
Transferrin (mg/dl)	143 ± 14	111 ± 8	0.055
Bilirubin, total (mg/dl)	2.62 ± 1.45	4.73 ± 1.00	0.289
Survival (%, survivors/total)	69 (9/13)	22 (2/9)	0.04

Results are the mean ± SEM.

group did not change when controls were compared with patients given GH, but the nitrogen balance directly correlated with the percentage of the patient's ideal body weight. Seven of the ten patients were at or above 90% ideal body weight, and they had a significant improvement in nitrogen balance (-1.46 ± 0.99 g/day during the control period vs. 0.60 ± 1.03 g/day with GH; $p < 0.01$); the remaining three patients with weight loss showed no effect. Other studies of protein kinetics (leucine appearance and oxidation) also varied with body weight loss. The authors concluded that GH may be anabolic in cancer patients if there is no severe preexisting malnutrition.

Others have administered GH to specific groups of patients and observed variable results. For example, McNurlan and associates found that the rate of muscle protein synthesis in response to GH was highly variable and declined in relation to the severity of disease.[20] In another study, rapid weight loss was observed following discontinuation of GH in individuals with short bowel syndrome.[21] The authors concluded that the loss was due to excretion of retained water and that a protein anabolic response did not occur. In contrast, GH induced lean tissue gain in several studies, and the increase was maintained for several months in patients following colectomy,[22] in malnourished individuals with pulmonary insufficiency,[23] and in another series of patents with short bowel syndrome.[24]

The reasons for such variable responses to GH treatment are not known. The variability appears to be related to patient selection or the nutritional state of the individual at the initiation of therapy (or both).

GH–Nutrient Interaction

Many important interrelations exist between GH and nutrient intake. The relation between energy administration and IGF-1 responses have been discussed previously.

Animal studies indicate that important interactions occur between vitamin and mineral status and the production of IGF-1, the major anabolic signal stimulated by GH. If animals are rendered deficient in zinc[25,26] or manganese,[27] there is major attenuation of IGF-1 generation. Many patients with malnutrition, diarrhea, or both exhibit these deficiency states. [Such deficiencies are frequently observed in patients with malabsorptive disorders, Crohn's disease, and acquired immunodeficiency syndrome (AIDS)-related diarrhea.] It is possible that such nutrient deficiencies occur and limit the anabolic response to GH.

To optimize GH anabolic therapy in critically ill patients, a thorough nutritional assessment should be performed and sophisticated testing (tissue analysis or nutrient loading tests) undertaken to determine both mineral and vitamin status. If deficits are uncovered, these deficiencies should be restored before GH is initiated. Physicians must be aware that this point is especially important in that such deficiency states exist in specific populations such as those with Crohn's disease[28] and individuals on long-term TPN.[29]

Metabolic Effects of GH: Studies Following Elective Surgery

Negative nitrogen balance is a common postoperative response and reflects an imbalance between protein synthesis and protein breakdown within the body. Because of the predictable nature of this response, investigators have frequently utilized the postoperative patient as a model to evaluate anabolic therapy.

Ward and associates studied postoperative patients following laparotomy.[30] One-half of the subjects received GH (0.12 mg/kg/day), and the remaining patients received placebo injections. All subjects were given about 400 calories a day via infusion of 5% dextrose. GH treatment resulted in decreased nitrogen excretion from 42.7 g over 6 days in the controls to 24.0 g in the GH group. Fat oxidation was increased, and there was a rise in serum glucose, insulin, and IGF-1 concentrations. Similar findings were reported by Cardi et al., who utilized stable isotopic methodology to document enhanced protein synthesis in postoperative patients receiving GH.[31]

Jiang and associates infused a hypocaloric nutrient solution containing 20 kcal/kg/day and 1 g protein/kg/day to postoperative patients following gastrectomy or colectomy.[32] In this randomized placebo-controlled prospective study, GH was given at a dose of 0.06 mg/kg/day and compared with placebo. The subjects receiving GH lost significantly less weight over 7 days than controls (1.3 vs. 3.2 kg), and cumulative nitrogen loss over 8 days was only 7.1 g versus 32.6 g in controls.

Amino acid flux studies across the forearm demonstrated increased uptake of amino acids in the GH-treated patients, whereas the control subjects released amino acids from their forearm. This change in protein balance was translated into improved skeletal muscle function. Hand grip strength in controls decreased approximately 10% following operation, whereas patients who received GH maintained their grip strength throughout the perioperative period.

A variety of other metabolic studies have confirmed and extended the findings that protein synthesis can be enhanced with GH.[33,34] Because skeletal muscle breakdown and loss of strength are characteristic responses following operation, these data provide a method by which muscle strength can be preserved and possibly enhanced following elective operation. Spanish investigators reported that long-term low-dose GH administration is associated with a significant reduction in perioperative infections and a decline in postoperative fatigue.[35]

The effect of GH on protein-containing tissue is not transient in nature but appears to be maintained beyond the perioperative period. Jensen and coworkers administered GH (2.5 mg twice daily) or placebo during the postoperative period to individuals undergoing total colectomy.[22] By the seventh postoperative day the placebo-treated patents had lost 4.2 kg body weight, 3.6 kg lean body mass, and 0.5 kg fat mass. In contrast, the patients receiving GH had increased body weight 4.0 kg and gained 3.2 kg lean tissue (differences between groups were significant at $p = 0.001$). The patients were then discharged without further treatment but were restudied 3 months later. At that time the patients who had been given placebo had lost 2.4 kg more lean tissue than the treatment group. These changes occurred despite similar nutritional intake.

Another use of GH is to treat the patient preoperatively to enhance protein gain and minimize postoperative complications. Byrne et al. fed such patients 50 kcal/kg/day and 2 g protein/kg/day for 3 weeks; 10 subjects were given GH (0.14 mg/kg/day), and 4 served as controls.[36] Body composition studies demonstrated that the controls gained significant amounts of water and body fat, whereas the GH group gained significantly more protein-containing lean tissue. This study also demonstrated that GH enhanced the efficiency of the protein gain; the GH-treated patients gained 1.66-fold more body protein per available calories than those given standard therapy.

The GH doses administered to postoperative patients ranged from 0.03 to 0.14 mg/kg/day. In general, the higher the dose the greater was the nitrogen retention—but there was also a greater incidence of side effects. Administration of 0.1 mg/kg/day in uncomplicated patients approaches the upper limit of effects on protein metabolism without causing major side effects if contraindications to GH administration are not present. Only one-third to one-half of the targeted dose should be given initially, with the amount gradually increased over 7–10 days to achieve the final target dose. In convalescing patients, the total safe daily dose ranges between 2.5 and 6.0 mg/day depending on the patient's weight.

GH for Burn Patients and Wound Healing

During the late 1950s a series of studies were performed at the U.S. Army Burn Unit at Fort Sam Houston, Texas to evaluate the effect of GH on the protein catabolic response. A factorial design methodology was used to determine nitrogen balance, and individuals were studied at various times during their postburn course. Of note is the fact that the investigators analyzed all nitrogen losses from the body; in addition to analyzing losses in urine and stool, they collected all dressings and bed sheets and determined wound protein loss. The GH enhanced nitrogen retention, although the effect was much greater during the convalescent phase than during the first few weeks following injury.[37] Later, Liljedahl et al. also used GH for treatment of burn patients.[38] They reported beneficial results from administration of this anabolic agent and were the first to suggest that GH might accelerate healing of the cutaneous injury.

During the early 1970s Wilmore and colleagues studied burn patients on a fixed adequate diet.[39] The effect of either GH or no treatment on nitrogen loss was determined in this randomized crossover trial. The intake was fixed because previous investigations demonstrated that GH administration was associated with increased food intake, or studies were performed during inadequate food intake. Nitrogen loss decreased (balance improved) with GH, and hyperinsulinemia was observed. Nitrogen balance was found to be highly related to both nitrogen intake and basal insulin levels, determined at the end of the study.

With the availability of recombinant GH during the mid-1980s, additional trials in burn patients were undertaken. Sherman and associates examined the effect of this anabolic agent on wound healing.[40] Standard donor sites were created on the anterior thigh of burn patients during skin grafting, and the patients were randomized to receive GH or placebo. Food intake and wound care were similar in all patients. A single blinded observer examined the wounds twice daily. Donor site healing was improved by approximately 2 days in the subjects receiving GH. Herndon et al. confirmed this effect in young children (average age 9 years) receiving GH (0.2 mg/kg/day) or placebo.[41] The rate of wound healing was increased in the GH group by approximately 2 days, which accounted for a reduction in hospital stay of approximately 2 weeks.

In a follow-up study, Ramirez and associates compared the safety and efficacy of GH administration in 48 pediatric patients following thermal injury and 54 comparable individuals receiving placebo injections.[42] The groups were matched in terms of age (7 ± 5 vs. 8 ± 5 years, mean $\pm$ SD), total body surface burn ($59\% \pm 17\%$ vs. $62\% \pm 17\%$), and percent third-degree burn ($47\% \pm 22\%$ vs. $51\% \pm 22\%$). The mortality rate was 2% in each group. The total albumin requirement was 77 ± 71 g in the GH group and 190 ± 242 g in the controls ($p < 0.05$), and length of stay in hospital was reduced by 25% ($p < 0.01$). However, more hyperglycemia was observed in the GH group, and the requirement for insulin supplementation was almost doubled.

This study documents the safety of GH in thermally injured children. The reduction in length of hospital stay provides a significant cost saving even when calculating the expense of GH. Knox and colleagues provided similar information in adult burn patients.[43] In this open-label case–control study, GH was administered to 54 patients with poor wound healing following 1 week of initial observation. The results were compared with 27 comparable patients who did not receive GH. For the entire population the average age was 59 years; they sustained a 59% body surface area burn, and 30% of the group suffered from smoke inhalation. The groups were well matched with respect to injury extent, burn management, and pharmacotherapy (Table 65.2). The mortality rate for the group receiving GH was 11%, significantly less than the 37% mortality rate in patients not receiving GH.

These studies document a favorable outcome associated with GH in burn patients. Multicenter randomized blinded trials are now indicated in this area.

TABLE 65.2. Effect of GH on Outcome in Thermally Injured Adults.

Parameter	Control	GH
No.	27	27
Age (years)	57 ± 22	50 ± 24
% BSA burn	49 ± 21	62 ± 26
Smoke inhalation (%)	29	35
Mortality (%)	37	11*

Results are the mean $\pm$ SD.
BSA, body surface area.
*$p = 0.027$.

GH Therapy for Other Serious Illnesses

Metabolic studies have been performed in septic surgical patients receiving intravenous feedings. In one such study the effects of GH at approximately 0.1 g/kg were compared to those of placebo.[44] In the control group the net protein catabolism fell from 1.12 to 0.61 g protein/kg/day compared to a drop of 0.93 to 0.20 g protein/kg/day with GH ($p < 0.05$). Although the GH group achieved protein balance, no significant difference in outcome was reported.

Zeigler and associates observed that patients with respiratory muscle weakness secondary to spinal cord injury could improve in strength with GH.[45] Pape and associates tests this hypothesis by studying patients with stable chronic obstructive pulmonary disease (COPD).[46] They demonstrated enhanced pulmonary function, related to improved respiratory muscle strength, in patients receiving GH; this effect was not observed in the group receiving placebo. Others, however, have not reported an advantage of administering GH to patients with COPD who required respiratory support.[47]

Knox and associates administered GH to 53 respirator-dependent patients in a surgical ICU in an open label phase I trial.[48] These postoperative patients with complications were specifically selected because of decreased respiratory muscle strength, not COPD. All had failed ventilator weaning protocols. The mean age of the patients was 63 years, and the group presented with a wide variety of coexisting morbidities. The patients averaged 3.9 operative procedures per patient during the period of GH administration. GH was given for an average of 38 days; 81% of this population were weaned from mechanical ventilation, and the overall survival rate was 76%. This 24% mortality rate compared favorably with the overall predicted mortality of 42% using the Acute Physiology and Chronic Health Evaluation (APACHE II) scoring system and the 44% rate using the organ failure scoring system. The apparent improvement in survival occurred even though the patients had an average of 3.4 failed organs per individual. These results suggest that carefully selected ICU patients may benefit from GH therapy: A randomized, blinded trial is required to confirm this concept.

Growth hormone reduces the rate of urea generation; hence it may be a suitable agent for use in patients with renal insufficiency. To illustrate this effect, five clinically stable adults requiring chronic hemodialysis for end-stage renal failure were studied.[49] Dialysis prescription, pharmacologic therapy, and nutrient intake were kept constant over the 3 weeks of the study. Following an initial control week, subjects received GH (5 or 10 mg) after each dialysis session. Their blood urea nitrogen (BUN) fell 20–25%, and urea kinetic modeling demonstrated a significant reduction in urea generation (decrease of 32%) and protein catabolic rate (decrease of 23%) with GH. Such therapy may thus allow improved protein intake and lessen the need for dialysis therapy.

Complications

Growth hormone causes hyperglycemia (usually corrected by insulin administration) and fluid retention in patients with more chronic illnesses; arthralgia and myalgia often occur. Careful monitoring, attention to fluid balance and sodium adminstration, and judicious use of diuretics generally prevents or attenuates edema formation. Hypercalcemia is also a potential problem in adult patients with critical illness. Immobilization and suboptimal renal function are often associated with this complication.[50] By monitoring the plasma calcium levels, dietary calcium can be adjusted to prevent potential clinical problems.

Because of favorable reports from small short-term studies, a multicenter phase III trial was undertaken in Europe. Patients were entered into the study if they required ICU care for 5 days or more following open-heart surgery, laparotomy, multiple trauma, or acute respiratory failure. The individuals were randomized to receive GH (doses ranging from 5 to 8 mg/day depending on body weight) or placebo. The results of these trials have only recently been reported; the company terminated the study because mortality was approximately twice as high in the group receiving GH (42%) than among the placebo controls (19%).[51] Information concerning more details of these trials, such as type of nutritional support provided, associated pharmacologic intervention, and cause of death, have not been provided at this time. Until these data become available and are appropriately assessed, GH should not be administered to patients in a nonresearch setting. In addition, all research studies should include nonblinded observers to ensure patient safety.

The cause of the increased mortality is not known at this time, but several possibilities have been suggested. Because reasonably large initial doses of the drug were administered, the rapid mobilization of free fatty acids may have caused increased plasma levels of free fatty acids.[52] This situation may elicit toxic effects and would be amplified in a critically ill population with high circulating catecholamine levels (promoting fat mobilization), infusion of fat emulsion, and inability to elicit elaboration of insulin or IGF-1. The latter two anabolic hormones would serve to attenuate this fat-mobilizing response.

Another possible effect may be related to alterations that could occur in splanchnic oxygenation with GH administration. Dahn and Lange studied septic patients and showed that GH administration altered hepatic oxygen consumption, potentially contributing to regional tissue hypoxia.[53] Similar findings have been reported by Revhaug's group in animal models.[54] Others have utilized gastric tonometry to monitor splanchnic perfusion.[55] A persistently low gastric pH is reflective of splanchnic hypoxia; this low perfusion state has been associated with high mortality (risk ratio for death 4.5 with pH ≤ 7.32).[41] If a large GH dose was administered to patients with underperfused visceral organs, the hypoperfusion would probably persist for a longer time or become more severe. Thus a potentially useful drug therapy, because of its effects on redistribution of blood flow may exert untoward effects on morbidity and mortality.

We have administered GH to a variety of critically ill patients and have not observed the deleterious results reported in these randomized trials. In fact, we have reported improved outcomes in both burn patients[43] and postoperative surgical patients who could not be weaned from the ventilator[48] in our phase I studies. However, all of our patients were hemodynamically stable and were receiving adequate nutritional support; blood glucose was carefully monitored and maintained within safe limits. GH wasstarted at a low dose and gradually increased with time (over 7-10 days). The dose of GH was also titrated, depending on the clinical condition of the patients, an approach optimizing effects and reported by others.[56] Glutamine supplementation was also provided because GH limits glutamine efflux from skeletal muscle.[32]

A number of factors included in our clinical care protocols appear to have obviated the disastrous results observed in the European clinical trials. These approaches should be taken into consideration when designing further studies of GH in seriously ill patients.

Costs

If efficacy is demonstrated, costs become the next limiting factor to the utilization of GH. Agents such as testosterone and anabolic steroids, which are low cost, are being used more frequently despite the lack of scientific data that their administration enhances outcome. Side effects of these low cost drugs are rarely monitored, and data should be provided that the drugs are beneficial before they are prescribed.

A favorable cost-benefit analysis has been performed in some areas to confirm the justification for GH. The reduction in length of hospital stay for burned children more than justifies the use of GH in this population.[42] The ability to wean patients from parenteral nutrition for just 6 months more than pays for the cost of 4 weeks of GH treatment and bowel rehabilitation.[57]

More difficult economic justification is associated with administration of these agents to enhance recovery following major elective operations, such as total hip replacement coronary artery bypass, or valve replacement surgery. Depleted patients, the elderly, or those facing a major catabolic disease may require weeks or months following such operations to return to usual function; and GH and possibly other agents could accelerate this process. If such therapy could reduce overall hospital stay, their cost may be justifiable. However, because many of these patients are cared for at home, there is little economic incentive for an insurer to pay for an anabolic agent to enhance recovery, although there may be clear benefit to the patient by shortening the convalescent recovery. These issues must be resolved if widespread use of GH is to be initiated in this setting.

References

1. Plank LD, Connolly AB, Hill GL: Sequential changes in metabolic response in severely septic patients during the first 23 days after the onset of peritonitis. Ann Surg 1998;228:146-158.
2. Streat SJ, Beedoe AH, Hill GL: Aggressive nutritional support does not prevent protein loss despite fat gain in septic intensive care patients. J Trauma 1987;27:262-266.
3. Warnold I, Eden E, Lundholm K: The inefficiency of total parenteral nutrition to stimulate protein synthesis in moderately malnourished patients. Ann Surg 1988;208:143-149.
4. Heyland DK, MacDonald S, Keefe L, Drover JW: Total parenteral nutrition in the critically ill: a meta-analysis. JAMA 1998;280:2013-2019.
5. Hartman ML: Physiological regulations of growth hormone secretion. In: Juul A, Jorgensen JOL (ed) Growth Hormone in Adults, Cambridge University Press, Cambridge, 1996;5-35.
6. Veldhuis JD, Johnson ML: Deconvolution analysis of hormone data. Methods Enzymol 1992;210:539-575.
7. Thissen JP, Ketelslegers JM, Underwood LE: Nutrition regulation of the insulin-like growth factors. Endocr Rev 1991;15:80-101.
8. Botfield C, Ross RJM, Hinds CJ: The role of IGFs in catabolism. Baillieres Clin Endocrinol Metab 1997;11:679-697.
9. Gwyfan Hughes SC, Cotterill AM, Molloy AK, et al: The induction of specific proteases for IGFBPs following major heart surgery. J Endocrinol 1992;135:135-145.
10. Van de Berge G, de Zegher F, Bouillon RE: Acute and prolonged critical illness as different neuroendocrine paradigms. J Clin Endocrinol Metab 1998;83:1827-1834.
11. Wilmore DW, Orcutt TW, Mason AD Jr, Pruitt BA Jr: Alterations in hypothalamic function following thermal trauma. J Trauma 1975;15:697-703.
12. Ross RJM, Chew SL: Acquired growth hormone resistance. Eur J Endo 1995;132:655-660.
13. Manson MJCK, Wilmore DW: Positive nitrogen balance with human growth hormone and hypocaloric intravenous feedings. Surgery 1986;100:188-197.
14. Krishan A, Pao C, Thule B, Villafuerte B, Phillips L: Transcription initiation of the rat insulin-like growth factor gene in hepatocyte primary culture. J Endocrinol 1996;151:215-223.
15. Hermansson M, Wickelgren RB, Hammerquist F, et al: Measurement of human growth hormone receptor messenger ribonucleic acid by a quantitative polymerase chain reaction-based assay: demonstration of reduced expression after elective surgery. J Clin Endocrinol Metab 1997;82:421-428.
16. Van de Berghe G, de Zegher F, Veldhuis JD, et al: The somatotropic axis in critical illness: effect of continuous GHRH and GHRP-2 infusion. J Clin Endocrinol Metab 1997;82:590-599.
17. Sorroff HS, Pearson E, Green NL, Artz CP: The effect of growth hormone on nitrogen balance at various levels of intake in burn patients. Surg Gynecol Obstet 1960;111:259-273.
18. Young LS, Byrne TA, Wilmore DW: Organ specific nutrients and associated therapy: growth factors—growth hormone. In: Wilmore DW, Carpentier YA (eds) Metabolic Support of the Critically ill Patient. New York, Springer, 1993;252-264.
19. Tayek JA, Brasel JA: Failure of anabolism in malnourished cancer patients receiving growth hormone: a clinical research center study. J Clin Endocrinol Metal 1995;80:2082-2087.
20. McNurlan MA, Garlick PJ, Steigbigel RT, et al: Responsiveness of muscle protein synthesis to growth hormone administration in HIV-infected individuals declines with severity of disease. J Clin Invest 1997;100:2125-2132.
21. Scolapio JS: Effect of growth hormone, glutamine and diet on body composition in short bowel syndrome: a randomized controlled study [abstract 5]. JPEN 1999;23:52.

22. Jensen MB, Kissmeyer-Nielson P, Laurbug S: Perioperative growth hormone treatment increases nitrogen and fluid balance and results in short-term and long-term conservation of lean tissue mass. Am J Clin Nutr 1998;68:840–846.
23. Burdet L, deMuralt B, Schatz Y, Pichard C, Fitting JW: Administration of growth hormone to underweight patients with chronic obstruction pulmonary disease: a prospective randomized controlled trial. Am J Respir Crit Care Med 1997;156:1800–1806.
24. Ellegard L, Boseaus I, Nordgren S, Bengtsson BA: Low-dose recombinant human growth hormone increases body weight and lean body mass in patients with short bowel syndrome. Ann Surg 1997;225:88–96.
25. Droke EA, Spears JW, Armstrong JD, et al: Dietary zinc effects serum concentrations of insulin and insulin-like growth factor-1 in growing lambs. J Nutr 1993;13:12–19.
26. Ninh NX, Thissen J-P, Maiter D, et al: Reduced liver insulin-like growth factor-1 gene expression in young zinc-deprived rats associated with a decrease in liver growth hormone (GH) receptors and serum GH-binding protein. J Endocrinol 1995;144:449–456.
27. Clegg MS, Donovan M, Monaco MH, et al: The influence of manganese deficiency on serum IGF-1 and IGF binding proteins in the male rat. Proc Soc Exp Biol Med 1998;219:41–47.
28. Geerling BJ, Badart, Smook A, Stockbrugger RW, Brumma RJM: Comprehensive nutritional status in patients with long-standing Crohn's disease currently in remission. J Clin Nutr 1998;67:919–926.
29. Burnes JU, O'Keefe SJD, Fleming CR, et al: Home parenteral nutrition: a 3 year analysis of clinical and laboratory monitoring. JPEN 1992;16:327–332.
30. Ward HC, Halliday D, Sim AJW: Protein and energy metabolism with biosynthetic human growth hormone after gastrointestinal surgery. Ann Surg 1987;206:56–61.
31. Cardi F, Webster JD, Halliday D: A nitrogen-free hypocaloric diet and recombinant human growth hormone stimulates postoperative protein synthesis: fasting and fed leucine kinetics in surgical patients. Metabolism 1997;46:796–800.
32. Jiang SM, He GZ, Zhang SY, et al: Low-dose growth hormone and hypocaloric nutrition attenuate the protein-catabolic response after major operation. Ann Surg 1989;10:513–524.
33. Hammarqvist F, Strombereg C, von-der-Decken A, Vinnars E, Wernerman J: Biosynthetic human growth hormone preserves both muscle protein synthesis and the decrease in muscle-free glutamine, and improves whole-body nitrogen economy after operation. Ann Surg 1992;216:184–191.
34. Mjaaland M, Unneberg K, Larsson J, Milsson L, Revhaug A: Growth hormone after abdominal surgery attenuated forearm glutamine, alanine, 3-methylhistidine, and total amino acid efflux in patients receiving total parenteral nutrition. Ann Surg 1993;217:413–422.
35. Koea JB, Breier BH, Douglas RG, et al: Anabolic and cardiovascular effects of recombinant human growth hormone in surgical patients with sepsis. Br J Surg 1996;83:196–200.
36. Byrne TA, Morrissey TB, Gatzen C, et al: Anabolic therapy with growth hormone accelerates protein gain in surgical patients requiring nutritional rehabilitation. Ann Surg 1993;218:400–418.
37. Soroff HS, Rozin RR, Mooty J, et al: Role of human growth hormone in response to trauma. I. Metabolic effects following burns. Ann Surg 1967;166:739–752.
38. Liljedahl SO, Gemzell C, Plantin L, et al: Effect of growth hormone in patients with severe burns. Acta Chir Scand 1961;122:1–14.
39. Wilmore DW, Maylan JA, Bristow BP, et al: Anabolic effects of human growth hormone and high caloric feedings following thermal injury. Surg Gynecol Obstet 1974;138:875–884.
40. Shernan SK, Demling RH, LaLande S, et al: Growth hormone enhances re-epithelialization of human split-thickness skin graft donor sites. Surg Forum 1989;40:37–39.
41. Herndon DN, Barrow RE, Kunkel KR, Broemeling L, Rutann RL: Effects of recombinant human growth hormone on donor-sit healing in severely burned children. Ann Surg 1990;212:424–429.
42. Ramirez RJ, Wolf SE, Barrow RE, Herndon DN: Growth hormone is safe and efficacious in the treatment of severe pediatric burns. Ann Surg 228;439–446.
43. Knox J, Demling R, Wilmore D, Sarraf P, Santos A: Increased survival after major thermal injury: the effect of growth hormone in adults. J Trauma 1995;39:526–530.
44. Koea JB, Breier BH, Douglas RG, et al: Anabolic and cardiovascular effects of recombinant human growth hormone in surgical patients with sepsis. Br J Surg 1996;83:196–200.
45. Ziegler TR, Young LS, Ferrari-Balioeira E, Demling RH, Wilmore DW: Use of human growth hormone combined with nutritional support in a critical care unit. JPEN 1990;14:574–581.
46. Pape GS, Friedman M, Underwood LE, Clemons DR: The effect of growth hormone on weight gain and pulmonary function in patients with chemie obstructive pulmonary disease. Chest 1991;99:1495–1500.
47. Richard C, Kyle V, Chevrolet JC, et al: Lack of effects of recombinant growth hormone on muscle function in patients requiring prolonged mechanical ventilation: a prospective randomized, controlled study. Crit Care Med 1996;24:403–413.
48. Knox JP, Wilmore DW, Demling RH, Sarraf P, Santos AA: Use of growth hormone for postoperative respiratory failure. Am J Surg 1996;171:576–580.
49. Ziegler TR, Lazarus JM, Young LS, et al: Effects of recombinant human growth hormone in adults receiving maintenance hemodialysis. J Am Soc Nephrol 1991;2:1130–1135.
50. Knox JB, Demling RH, Wilmore DW, et al: Hypercalcemia associated with the use of human growth hormone in an adult surgical intensive care unit. Arch Surg 1995;130:442–445.
51. Takala J, Ruokonen E, Webster NR, et al: Increased mortality associated with growth hormone treatment in critically ill adults. N Engl J Med 1999;341:785–792.
52. Fleming RYD, Rutan RL, Jaboor F, et al: Effect of recombinant human growth hormone on catabolic hormones and free fatty acids following thermal injury. J Trauma 1992;32:698–703.
53. Dahn MS, Lange MP: Systemic and splanchnic metabolic responses to endogenous human growth hormone. Surgery 1998;123:528–538.
54. Unneberg K, Ralteskard L, Mjaaland M, Revhaug A: Growth hormone impaired compensation of hemorrhagic shock after trauma and sepsis in swine. J Trauma 1996;41:775–780.
55. Kirton OC, Windsor J, Wedderburn R, et al: Failure of splanchnic resuscitation in the acutely injured trauma patient correlates with multiple organ failure and length of stay in the ICU. Chest 1998;13:1064–1069.
56. Drake W, Coyte D, Camache-Huber C, et al: Optimizing growth hormone replacement therapy by dose titration in hypopituitary adults. J Clin Endocrinol Metab 1988;83:3913–3919.
57. Wilmore DW, Lacey JM, Soultanakis RP, Bosch RL, Byrne TA: Factors which predict a successful outcome after pharmacologic bowel compensation. Ann Surg 1997;226:288–293.

66
Immunoglobulin Therapy: Where Does It Stand Clinically?

Günter Pilz

There is increasing knowledge on the mechanisms of biologic efficacy of intravenous immunoglobulins (IVIGs), but their clinical effectiveness in septic patients remains a matter of controversy. At present, data suggest potential beneficial effects regarding a reduction in morbidity, particularly after IVIG prophylaxis or early treatment of selected patients. However, no large controlled clinical trial has yet been able to document a significant reduction in mortality after IVIG treatment for a population of adult septic patients.

Mechanisms of Biologic Efficacy

Classically, the potential effectiveness of polyvalent IVIGs in patients with sepsis had been attributed to three mechanisms: First is their content of various antibodies that can protect against bacterial endotoxins and exotoxins via direct antigen neutralization.[1] Second, opsonizing antibodies contained in IVIG can stimulate phagocytosis and enhance the bactericidal activity of human neutrophils.[2] Third, in vivo and in vitro results have shown that IVIGs can act synergistically with β-lactam antibiotics owing to their content of anti-lactamase antibodies and their ability to sensitize gram-negative bacteria by disorganizing their outer membranes.[3]

Modulation of cytokine production of monocytes and macrophages has emerged as a further putative protective mechanism of IVIG during sepsis and the systemic inflammatory response: Immunoglobulin G (IgG) inhibits production of the proinflammatory cytokines interleukin-1 (IL-1), IL-6, and tumor necrosis factor (TNF) in mononuclear cells,[4,5] and it influences the release of other cytokines.[6] In addition to the in vitro inhibition of lipopolysaccharide (LPS)-induced TNF production, IgG is also able to decrease TNF serum levels in vivo in animal models.[7] The anticytokine effect is mediated via the Fc fragment of the IgG molecule.[5] IgG interferes with T cell proliferation via regulation of IL-2 and IL-4 production.[8] It is also able to inhibit gram-positive superantigen-induced interferon-γ (IFNγ) and TNFβ synthesis.[6] Finally, IgG contains antibodies against IL-1[9] and increases production of the naturally occurring IL-1 receptor antagonist (IL-1ra) in human mononuclear blood cells.

Clinical Effectiveness: Controversy and Possible Explanations

Despite these findings and beneficial effects of prophylactic or early therapeutic administration of polyvalent IVIGs in animal sepsis models,[1-3] their effectiveness in treating septic patients remains controversial.[10] The main reason is the lack of a documented reduction in mortality induced by IVIG treatment, particularly within the two largest controlled trials available.[11,12] In fact, only a single small placebo-controlled trial (62 surgical patients) with a sepsis score of 20 or more was able to present solid data on a significant reduction in mortality by IVIG treatment (death rates: controls 67%, IVIG 38%).[13] A second study reporting a significantly improved prognosis[14] was subject to criticism because of uniquely low mortality rates and discrepant reports on the inclusion criteria.[15,16] The presently available information from the IVIG trials suggests at least three potential causes for the discrepancy between the promising experimental and disappointing clinical results: (1) the delayed application in patients compared to the experimental setting; (2) the observed inability to increase serum IgG levels in some patients; and (3) the use of remote and insensitive outcome measures in clinical trials, such as 28-day mortality.

Timing of IVIG Therapy

With regard to optimal timing to initiate IVIG therapy, both experimental and clinical results favor early or even prophylactic administration, as it has been used in the animal models. An indirect suggestion for early IVIG administration comes from the study of Cafiero et al.[17] In patients at risk for postoperative sepsis, the basal serum IgG levels were found to be significantly lower in patients who later developed postsurgical infections compared to patients with a regular outcome. The interventional studies seem to support prophylactic or early IVIG administration in at-risk patient populations in contrast to IVIG use for already established sepsis.

Using such a prophylactic approach, the prospective, double-blind IICSG study[11] was able to demonstrate a significant reduction in the incidence of postoperative infections in the IVIG group (36/109) compared to controls (53/112), the incidence of pneumonia (15 vs. 30 cases), and the number of days spent in the intensive care unit (ICU) (2 days fewer). Similarly, early (first postoperative day) IVIG administration was associated with a significant improvement in disease severity of score-identified postcardiac surgical patients at high risk for septic complications whose Acute Physiology and Chronic Health Evaluation (APACHE II) score was 24 or more on the first postoperative day compared to a historical control population of otherwise equivalent disease severity.[18] The hypothesis derived from this study is currently being prospectively challenged in an ongoing multicenter placebo-controlled trial (updated score threshold: APACHE II score of 28 or more[19]).

Serum IgG Levels

In patients with or at risk for sepsis, there seems to be an association between high serum IgG serum levels and a low incidence of postoperative infections[17] or even improved outcome.[13] Conversely, failure to achieve an increase in serum IgG during IVIG administration was associated with a significantly worse clinical course[17] or even survival.[13] This finding suggested that nonsurvivors either have greater IgG consumption or confine IgG in the extravascular space. Whether this hypothesis, together with the putative reduced serum IgG half-life during sepsis of about 5 days,[13] should lead to serial IgG measurements and a consecutive serum level-guided dosage regimen has not yet been investigated and so must be determined.

Study Design: Morbidity Measures as Efficacy Parameters

The need for more sensitive and biologically and clinically meaningful outcome measures in sepsis trials is increasingly recognized.[10,20] For IVIG, a specific marker of biologic activity seems unlikely in view of the complex mechanism of IVIG action. Rather than such a specific marker, morbidity measures such as disease severity assessment by scoring systems and their change over time could provide information on improvement or deterioration during therapy. Conceptually, such a quantitative measure for improvement under therapy would reflect the reversal of physiologic abnormalities, which have been shown to be the most important single predictor of outcome.[21] In the case of IVIG treatment, recording the changes in APACHE II scores[22] over 4 days in close temporal relation to treatment consistently displayed a significant correlation with prognosis in several studies.[10,18,23] The use of such measures as surrogate study endpoints in controlled treatment trials during sepsis as an indicator of therapeutic efficacy seems reasonable and has already been accomplished in the multicenter, randomized, prospective, placebo-controlled, double-blind Score-Based Immunoglobulin Therapy of Sepsis (SBITS) trial, which included 653 patients.[12] The prepublished concept of this study[10] included a priori the use of score-quantified changes in disease severity as prospectively defined secondary study endpoints. Another reported finding—that early IVIG application mitigates the severity of the critical illness polyneuropathy following sepsis[24]—might provide another morbidity marker for future trials. Similarly important, it emphasizes the need to continue the efforts for a better pathophysiologic understanding of the target organ systems involved and the mechanisms of biologic efficacy of the potentially beneficial effects of IVIG during sepsis.

References

1. Pollack M: Antibody activity against *Pseudomonas aeruginosa* in immune globulins prepared for intravenous use in humans. J Infect Dis 1983;147:1090–1098.
2. Fischer GW, Hunter KW, Hemming VG, et al: Functional antibacterial activity of a human intravenous immunoglobulin preparation: in vitro and in vivo studies. Vox Sang 1983;44:296–299.
3. Dalhoff A: In vitro and in vivo effect of immunoglobulin G on the integrity of bacterial membranes. Infection 1985;13(Suppl 2):S185–S191.
4. Andersson JP, Andersson UG: Human intravenous immunoglobulin modulates monokine production in vitro. Immunology 1990;71:372–376.
5. Horiuchi A, Abe Y, Miyake M, et al: Natural human IgG inhibits the production of tumor necrosis factor and interleukin-1 alpha through the Fc portion. Surg Today 1993;23:241–245.
6. Skansén-Saphir U, Andersson J, Björk L, et al: Lymphokine production induced by streptococcal pyrogenic exotoxin-A is selectively down-regulated by pooled human IgG. Eur J Immunol 1994;24:916–922.
7. Shimozato T, Iwata M, Tamura N: Suppression of tumor necrosis factor alpha production by a human immunoglobulin preparation for intravenous use. Infect Immun 1990;58:1384–1390.
8. Amran D, Renz H, Lack G, et al: Suppression of cytokine-dependent human T-cell proliferation by intravenous immunoglobulin. Clin Immunol Immunopathol 1994;73:180–186.
9. Svenson M, Hansen MB, Bendtzen K: Binding of cytokines to pharmaceutically prepared human immunoglobulin. J Clin Invest 1993;92:2533–2539.
10. Pilz G, Fateh-Moghadam S, Viell B, et al: Supplemental immunoglobulin therapy in sepsis and septic shock: comparison of mortality under treatment with polyvalent i.v. immunoglobulin versus placebo: protocol of a multicenter, randomized, prospective, double-blind trial. Theor Surg 1993;8:61–83.
11. Intravenous Immunoglobulin Collaborative Study Group: Prophylactic intravenous administration of standard immune globulin as compared with core-lipopolysaccharide immune globulin in patients at high risk of postsurgical infection. N Engl J Med 1992;327:234–240.
12. Werdan K, Pilz G, SBITS Study Group: Polyvalent immune globulins. Shock 1997;7(Suppl 1):5.
13. Dominioni L, Dionigi R, Zanello M, et al: Effects of high-dose IgG on survival of surgical patients with sepsis scores of 20 or greater. Arch Surg 1991;126:236–240.

14. Schedel I, Dreikhausen U, Nentwig B, et al: Treatment of gram-negative septic shock with an immunoglobulin preparation: a prospective, randomized clinical trial. Crit Care Med 1991;19:1104–1113.
15. Werdan K, Pilz G: Treatment of gram-negative septic shock with an immunoglobulin [letter]. Crit Care Med 1992;20:1364–1365.
16. Wortel CH, Dellinger P: Treatment of gram-negative septic shock with an immunoglobulin preparation: a prospective, randomized clinical trial [letter]. Crit Care Med 1993;21:163–165.
17. Cafiero F, Gipponi M, Bonalumi U, et al: Prophylaxis of infection with intravenous immunoglobulins plus antibiotic for patients at risk for sepsis undergoing surgery for colorectal cancer: results of a randomized, multicenter clinical trial. Surgery 1992;112:24–31.
18. Pilz G, Kreuzer E, Kääb S, et al: Early sepsis treatment with immunoglobulins after cardiac surgery in score-identified high-risk patients. Chest 1994;105:76–82. Erratum. Chest 1994;105:1924.
19. Kuhn C, Müller-Werdan U, Pilz G, et al: Early risk stratification of patients after cardiac surgery using extracorporeal circulation: identification of an escalating systemic inflammatory response syndrome. Eur Heart J 1997;18(Suppl):585.
20. Petros AJ, Marshall JC, van Saene HKF: Should morbidity replace mortality as an endpoint for clinical trials in intensive care? Lancet 1995;345:369–371.
21. Knaus WA, Wagner DP, Zimmerman JE, et al: Variations in mortality and length of stay in intensive care units. Ann Intern Med 1993;118:753–761.
22. Knaus WA, Draper EA, Wagner DP, et al: APACHE II: a severity of disease classification system. Crit Care Med 1985;13:818–829.
23. Pilz G, Appel R, Kreuzer E, et al: Comparison of early IgM-enriched immunoglobulin vs polyvalent IgG administration in score-identified postcardiac surgical patients at high risk for sepsis. Chest 1997;111:419–426.
24. Mohr M, Englisch L, Roth A, et al: Effects of early treatment with immunoglobulin on critical illness polyneuropathy following multiple organ failure and gram-negative sepsis. Intensive Care Med 1997;23:1144–1149.

67
Horizons in the Anesthetic Care of Injured, Operated, and Stressed Patients

Antonino Gullo, Giorgio Berlot, and Giovanni Galimberti

The physiologic response to a stressful event (e.g., acute disease, trauma, surgical procedures) includes a wide array of metabolic and cardiorespiratory alterations collectively known as the stress response (SR).[1] Teleologically, this response has been developed and maintained throughout evolution with the aim of setting up a number of changes capable of allowing the endangered subject to overcome a harmful situation and initiating the wound healing process.[1,2] Traditionally, the SR has been subdivided into Cuthbertson's "ebb and flow" phases, which are often used to describe the initial postinjury low flow status and the subsequent hemodynamic improvement induced by the volume resuscitation in trauma patients[3] (Table 67.1). The modern approach to stressed patients, especially trauma and postoperative patients, is aimed at reducing the "ebb" and promoting the early onset of the "flow" phase.[2] In contrast to immune reactions, the SR is rather nonspecific and is also triggered by noninfectious stimuli.[4] Although the most intimate mechanisms of the SR are yet to be elucidated, in recent years better understanding of these reactions has led to significant changes in the management of both perioperative and critically ill patients. At the same time, it has become clear that, as for inflammation, the SR exerts protective effects in and of itself, but if left uncontested it can kill the organism.[5]

For many years the SR was considered a relatively simple neuroendocrine reflex arc, whose triggers (e.g., painful stimuli), traveling along the peripheral and sympathetic nerves, prompted the hypothalamus-pituitary-adrenal axis (HPA) to produce and release a number of substances active on the target organs. Several discoveries have shown that this scheme is oversimplified.[1,6] Nevertheless, with the purpose of simplifying the description of this extremely complex reaction and the ways to manipulate it, its afferent and efferent limbs, its mediators, and the stress-induced modifications of the target organs are described separately.

Afferent Limb and Effectors

Investigations have provided new insights into both the activating pathways and the effector regions involved in the SR. First, the SR can be elicited by factors other than painful nervous stimuli [e.g., hypoxia, hypovolemia, circadian neurosensory signals, and sepsis mediators such as tumor necrosis factor (TNF) and interleukins (IL-1, IL-6)]. These cytokines are either transported to the SR effectors by peripherally activated immunocompetent cells permeating the blood-brain barrier or are produced locally by microglia.[7] Moreover, IL-1-containing nerve fibers have been identified in the hypothalamus.[8] Second, in addition to the HPA axis, adrenergic centers located in the brain stem participate actively in the reaction, and the final response is modulated by multiple positive and negative feedback loops existing between them and the involved structures.

There is reciprocal stimulation between corticotropin-releasing hormone (CRH) and norepinephrine-producing cells; CRH, arginine vasopressin (AVP), and norepinephrine production are stimulated by serotoninergic and cholinergic systems and are inhibited by the γ-aminobutyric acid (GABA) and opioid-peptide systems. The centrally produced substance P blocks CRH but not AVP neurons. In the paraventricular nuclei, specialized groups of neurons, in addition to producing AVP and CRH to be released into the pituitary portal system, stimulate the production of proopiomelanocortin and derived opioid peptides from the hypothalamus, in the hind brain, and in the spinal cord. The latter substances suppress CRH production and downregulate the stress response.[1]

Efferent Limb

In past years it appeared that the SR was driven essentially by stimulation of both the pituitary and adrenal glands. A deeper understanding of the mechanisms of the SR showed that other structures, including the immune system and endothelial cells, are involved.[9] The precise role played by these widely distributed cells in promoting and maintaining the SR is still, however, to be fully elucidated. The abnormal endocrine pattern, whose entity is roughly correlated with the severity of injury, returns toward normal when the patient recovers.[1,8,10] The subsequent biochemical, hemodynamic, and clinical alterations are easily recognized in stressed subjects (Table 67.2).

TABLE 67.1. Features of the Ebb and Flow Phases.

Ebb phase
  Hypometabolism
  Low body temperature
  Reduced energy expenditure
  Normal glucose production
  Mild protein catabolism
  Mild hyperglycemia
  Elevated catecholamine levels
  Elevated glucocorticoid levels
  Elevated glucagon
  Reduced insulin levels
  Low cardiac output
  Tissue hypoperfusion; oliguria
  Cold, clammy skin

Flow phase
  Hypermetabolism
  Normal/high body temperature
  Increased energy expenditure
  Gluconeogenesis
  Severe protein catabolism
  Normal or mildly elevated glycemia
  Normal or elevated catecholamine levels
  Normal or elevated glucocorticoid levels
  Normal or elevated glucagon
  Elevated insulin levels
  Increased cardiac output
  Normal tissue perfusion; normal diuresis
  Warm skin

After trauma or surgical procedures the pituitary gland exhibits a double pattern of hormonal secretion:[6] Whereas the levels of ACTH, prolactin, growth hormone (GH), and the endogenous opioids increase, the production of thyroid-stimulating hormone (TSH), luteinizing hormone (LH), and follicle-stimulating hormone (FSH) decreases. ACTH, which is the main regulator of the adrenal production of glucocorticoids, is produced mainly under stimulation by CRH; in the latter's absence, ACTH levels are low in both basal and stressful conditions. Upon pituitary stimulation, the cortical portion of the adrenal glands enhances the production of cortisol (see later), but it is not clear whether (1) there is a clear relation between the severity of the injury and the magnitude of the adrenal response or (2) its entity is correlated to the final outcome.[6]

Mediators of the Stress Response

Catecholamines

The serum levels of various catecholamines, including epinephrine, norepinephrine, and dopamine, increase during the SR. Epinephrine is secreted by the renal medulla under stimulation by the sympathetic nervous system, whereas norepinephrine is released by sympathetic nerve endings. In addition to the cardiovascular effects, increased catecholamine secretion is associated with a number of relevant metabolic effects, including glycogenolysis, lipolysis, increased hepatic gluconeogenesis, inhibition of insulin release, and induction of peripheral insulin resistance.[1,2,4]

Glucocorticoids and Related Compounds

Cortisol is the main glucocorticoid hormone produced during the SR. It has many actions, including a powerful antiinflammatory effect; it stimulates gluconeogenesis and increases proteolysis, insulin resistance, and the sensitization of adipose tissue to the action of lipolytic hormones. Cortisol is considered a major mediator of the SR, as adrenalized subjects tolerate even moderate stress poorly. The circadian rhythm of ACTH and cortisol secretion is disturbed but not abolished after trauma and surgery.[1,6] The production and release of aldosterone and enzymes of the renin-angiotensin system are increased.[1,6] During the SR the levels of other adrenally produced steroid hormones, such as testosterone and estradiol, are decreased: These changes could be ascribed to the decreased production of both FSH and LH or of their releasing factors.

Glucagon and Insulin

Glucagon and insulin levels are increased by many stressful conditions, and the final effect appears related to the balance of their actions. Glucagon exerts several physiologic actions, including an increase in gluconeogenesis, glycogenolysis, lipolysis, and hepatic ketogenesis. The release of glucagon is stimulated by catecholamines, hypoglycemia, protein meals, and GH. The effects of insulin are practically opposite to those of glucagon: Insulin stimulates glycogen production, inhibits lipolysis and hepatic ketogenesis, and increases both the rate of amino acid transport into the muscle and the consequent protein synthesis. The degree of gluconeogenesis is determined mainly by the glucagon/insulin ratio. The pattern of glucagon and insulin production varies according to the considered time frame; in fact, reduced insulin levels and increased glucagon levels have been observed in many, but not all, studies involving patients undergoing major surgery; the ultimate effect is increased gluconeogenesis. Postoperatively, the production of

TABLE 67.2. Clinical Effects of the Stress Response.

Mechanism	Target	Effects
Sympathetic discharge	Cardiovascular system	Tachycardia, hypertension
	Respiratory apparatus	Hypoventilation
	Coagulation cascade	Thrombophilia
	Gastrointestinal apparatus	Ileus
	Immune system	Suppression
	Central nervous system	Agitation, pain
Increased vasopressin and aldosterone production	Kidney	Oliguria, nitrogen retention
Increased growth hormone and ACTH production	Muscle, liver, pancreas, adrenal glands	Hyperglycemia, increased muscle catabolism, gluconeogenesis

both hormones increases, though that of insulin is disproportionately low for the elevated blood glucose levels.[1,5]

Growth Hormone

Growth hormone is secreted by the anterior pituitary gland, and most of its actions are indirect, being mediated by insulin-like factors. GH release is stimulated by hypothalamic releasing factors and inhibited by somatostatin. Its effects are time-dependent: Initially (during the initial 2–3 hours of exposure) there is an insulin-like effect, whereas later glucose intolerance supervenes, which is probably due to a postreceptorial effect, possibly associated with reduced splanchnic glucose uptake. In addition to these effects on carbohydrate metabolism, GH inhibits lipolysis and protein synthesis. The GH concentration increases after stressful events, including extensive surgical procedures, burns, and injuries.[5,6]

Thyroid Hormones

Disturbances of thyroid function are commonly seen in critically ill patients. The most common alteration, known as the "sick euthyroid syndrome," is characterized by reduced serum triiodothyronine (T_3) levels, low or normal thyroxine (T_4), normal free T_4, and elevated reverse-T_3, in the presence of normal TSH levels. In postoperative stressed patients, the serum TSH response after thyrotropin-releasing hormone (TRH) stimulation is normal, albeit with lower peak levels during the early postoperative phase. In intensive care unit (ICU) patients, thyroid function can be altered by administering dopamine, which reduces the TRH-induced production of TSH and decreases serum T_3 levels. Despite an apparent overall reduction of thyroid function, critically ill patients are hypermetabolic, probably under the influence of increased sympathetic discharge.[5,6,9]

Cytokines

Although the role played by cytokines as mediators of the SR in both limbs of the SR has emerged only recently, several years ago various investigators observed that a postinjury hypermetabolic phase was also present in spinally injured patients in whom both the ascending and descending pathways of the SR had been irreversibly interrupted.[11,12] More recently, a host of inflammatory and sepsis mediators have been identified as being involved in the postinjury SR,[4] but a precise mechanism of action has been identified for only some of them.

In addition to activation of the HPA axis, TNF causes a dose-dependent increase in whole-body muscle protein breakdown associated with a hypermetabolic state, increased hepatic gluconeogenesis, and increased lipolysis.[13] IL-1 has many effects in common with TNF, and the two act synergistically to determine the cardiovascular and metabolic alterations commonly observed in septic and injured patients.[14] Despite these observations, the systemic role of blood-borne cytokines released from injured regions in promoting and maintaining the SR should be limited, as (1) their effect, when they are injected into healthy volunteers, is usually short-lived and (2) measurement of their concentrations in the bloodstream of trauma patients has yielded controversial results, being elevated in some studies but normal in others.[8] On the other hand, it is probable that these substances do produce a sustained effect in tissues such as liver and muscle, where they are almost unmeasurable at the present time, acting as paracrine hormones and transducing signals coming from the higher centers.[8]

Counterregulatory Hormone Interactions

Despite the number of substances involved, it appears that the hydrocortisone–glucagon–catecholamine group plays a major role in the SR.[1] Their combined infusion was associated with increased gluconeogenesis and reduced glucose uptake, which was less sustained when only one or two of them were administered.[15] The possible causes of synergism include amplification of the epinephrine effect induced by the increased cAMP concentration determined by the glucagon and blockade of catecholamine reuptake induced by cortisol.[15,16] The above listed metabolic changes are also associated with a negative nitrogen balance, which is mainly ascribed to the action of the cortisol.[17] In clinical conditions the proteolytic effect of TNF and other cytokines amplifies that exerted by cortisol.[7,9]

Clinical Consequences of the Stress Response

Nutrition and Metabolic Aspects

Both metabolism and nutrition are heavily affected by the SR, with relevant influence on the clinical course of the stressed patients. All nutritional factors are involved. Carbohydrate metabolism is affected during the initial phase; the hyperglycemia commonly observed immediately after trauma is due to mobilization of the hepatic glycogen stores driven by sympathetic discharge. Later, when the glycogen has been exhausted, hyperglycemia is maintained by hepatic gluconeogenesis from various substrates, including amino acids (especially alanine, glutamine, and other glucogenic amino acids), glycerol, lactate, and pyruvate. Amino acids, lactate, and pyruvate derive from protein catabolism and glycogenolysis in the muscle, whereas glycerol is produced by the metabolism of triglycerides in adipose tissue. A major cause of the mobilization of glycogen and triglyceride stores is epinephrine, whose action is further enhanced by cortisol. Hyperglycemia persists owing to probable postreceptor resistance or epinephrine-associated reduction of insulin secretion (or both). The supply of exogenous glucose, which blocks gluconeogenesis in normal subjects, does not reduce the process greatly in stressed patients.[1,5,6] Fat can be used by the organism as a ready-to-use source of stored energy. Externally supplied or stored long-chain fatty acids are metabolized to free fatty acids (FFAs) and glycerol. In turn, FFAs can be used as fuel or can be reesterified with glycerol and stored again. Both glucagon and epinephrine promote lipolysis by activating tissue lipases, and their action is potentiated by cortisol. After trauma, patients develop marked lipolysis, and fat becomes a major fuel; blood FFA and glycerol levels are elevated. The main factors responsible for this increase are the lipoprotein lipases (LPLs), which are located in the capillary endothelial cells of muscle and fat; these enzymes mobilize FFAs and glycerol from circulating chylomicrons and very low density lipoproteins (VLDL). There is a marked difference between the roles played by the various LPLs in trauma and sepsis: In the former circumstance adipose tissue LPL activity is inhibited, whereas muscle LPL activity is increased; during sepsis the opposite occurs. Studies with isotope-labeled fatty substances demonstrated that there is an increased rate of reesterification within the adipose tissue, leading to a "futile cycle," which is considered a cause of the hypermetabolism. Because this process can be limited by administration of adrenergic blocking agents, it has been hypothesized that it could be ascribed to the intense catecholamine discharge.[18] Despite the high turnover of FFAs, the blood ketone level usually remains low; the elevated levels of both insulin and alanine probably account for this finding.[1,18] With trauma and in septic patients the overall lipogenic capacity is reduced, as demonstrated by failure of the respiratory quotient to rise 1.0 when a carbohydrate load is given. This finding can be ascribed to the effect of TNF and related cytokines.[18]

The SR is associated with increased protein breakdown, as indicated by the large urinary nitrogen losses, the increased release of amino acids, and inhibition of their uptake by the muscle. Amino acids derive from skeletal muscles or injured regions in the case of trauma. They are transported to the liver for gluconeogenesis and synthesis of other proteins, including the acute-phase reactants (APRs), whose synthesis is roughly proportional to both the lesion and the SR.[19] Many substances with relevant procatabolic effects include cortisol, glucagon, TNF, and IL-1; and their overall effect resembles that commonly observed in cachectic patients.[20]

Glutamine is the most abundant amino acid in the body, and its stores are rapidly depleted owing to its uptake by the liver to be used for gluconeogenesis and synthesis of APRs or to its peripheral use as a fuel by rapidly replicating cells, such as fibroblasts, lymphocytes, and enterocytes; the latter convert some glutamine to alanine, which is transferred to the liver for gluconeogenesis. The ammonia derived from deamination of the glutamine arrives at the liver in the portal bood and is transformed to urea. The use of glutamine in nutritional mixtures has been advocated to restore and maintain the viability of the intestinal epithelium in starved and parenterally fed patients,[21] and its administration to trauma patients has been associated with a reduced rate of infectious complications.[22]

Cardiovascular Effects

The SR-related release of epinephrine and norepinephrine is associated with an increase in heart rate, blood pressure, and inotropism, with a subsequent increase in myocardial oxygen demand.[23,24] At the same time, however, the myocardial oxygen supply can be reduced owing to coronary vasoconstriction or to coronary steal from ischemic myocardium.[25] A discrepancy between myocardial supply and myocardial oxygen demand can occur, resulting in postoperative ischemic events, including ST-segment changes, angina, myocardial dysfunction, and arrhythmias and increases in preexistent myocardial infarct size.[26,27]

Disturbances of Blood Coagulation

During the postoperative period there is an increased risk of vasoocclusive and thromboembolic events due to an increased concentration of coagulation factors, enhanced platelet activity,[28] and insufficient fibrinolysis.[29] During surgery the threshold to ADP-induced platelet aggregation is increased, and platelets are temporarily hypoaggregatable.[30] In contrast, during the postoperative period there is increased release of vasoactive substances with proaggregating action, such as thromboxane B_2, serotonin, and β-thromboglobulin.[31] The shift to a hypercoagulability state seems to be related to the endocrine-metabolic response elicited by surgery.[32,33] General anesthesia and parenteral opioid administration do not appear to modify this alteration.[34,35]

Respiratory Function

Several factors may affect lung function during surgery, including upper abdominal and thoracic incisions, postoperative pain, and the release of neuromediators form injured tissues.[36] This can evoke a sympathetic response with subsequent diaphragmatic inhibition, increased intercostal and abdominal work, and reduced chest wall compliance.[37] A respiratory pattern characterized by rapid, shallow breathing appears, and the cough mechanism becomes ineffective. This situation can stimulate dangerous reductions in the functional residual capacity and vital capacity that may result in atelectasis and ventilation-perfusion abnormalities, leading to perioperative pulmonary complications (e.g., hypoxemia, pneumonia, acute respiratory failure).[38]

Digestive Function

The SR, in association with pain and the effects of the anesthetic agents (e.g., opioids, nitrous oxide, inhalation agents) may lead to a reduction in gastrointestinal motility. Generally, sympathetic stimulation inhibits motility with an increased risk of postoperative ileus, whereas parasympathetic stimulation promotes bowel motility, assessed by the passage of flatus and feces. Postoperative ileus increases patient morbidity and health costs owing to prolonged hospitalization, costing an estimated $1500 per patient or $750 million per year in the United States.[39]

Immune Alterations

As stated above, the SR is associated with susbstantial changes in immune functions.[40,41] Postoperative immunosuppression after general anesthesia occurs early (after as short a time as 15 minutes) and persists for a long time (3–11 days), predisposing the patient to the development of postoperative infections, with subsequent increases in morbidity and duration of hospitalization.[42]

Anesthetic Technique and Patient Outcome: Many Problems and Few Solutions

Ideally, the choice of an anesthesia technique for an individual patient is based on evaluation of the most favorable risk/benefit ratio in terms of biologic impact on the SR, good tolerance, and economic costs. Studies using different anesthetic techniques have often produced conflicting conclusions, mainly due to the heterogeneity of patients enrolled and outcomes considered (Tables 67.3, 67.4). For example, a meta-analysis of randomized, controlled trials showed only that there was a significant reduction in deep venous thrombosis when regional rather than general anesthesia was used.[52] As a matter of fact, so many factors contribute to the outcome of surgical patients that the possible association of outcome with anesthesia technique is difficult to asses. Having said that, several investigators have tried to find associations between the anesthesia technique and the patients' outcome, but the results of the various studies are inconsistent, probably owing to the study design and type of statistical analysis used. So far, it seems that multiple factors acting in different time frames and through different mechanisms cooperate to determine the final outcome (Table 67.5).

TABLE 67.3. Risk factors for Surgical Patients.

Study	Study type	No. of patients	Identified risk
Marx[43]	Retrospective	34,145	American Society of Anesthesia; advanced age; emergency surgery
Farrow[44]	Retrospective	108,878	Age, sex; site of surgery; duration anesthesia; wrong choice of anesthesia
Holland[45]	Retrospective	5,262	Inadequate preparation and monitoring

TABLE 67.4. Impact of Various Anesthetic Techniques on Patient Outcome.

Study	Comparison	Surgery	Outcome
McQuay[48]	GA vs. GA + spinal (L)	Orthopedic	Preemptive analgesia
Salomaki[49]	GA vs. CEGA (F)	Thoracic	Modified hormonal response
Jayr[50]	GA vs. CEGA (L,M)	Abdominal	No differences
Galimberti[51]	GA vs. CEGA (L,F)	Abdominal	Shorter hospitalization
Tuman[52]	GA vs. CEGA (L,F)	Vascular (A,P)	Fewer thrombotic events
Davies[53]	GA vs. CEGA (L)	Vascular (A)	No differences

GA, general anesthesia; CEGA, combined epidural and general anesthesia; L, local anesthetic; F, fentanyl; A, aortic; P, peripheral.

TABLE 67.5. Factors Involved in the Postoperative Outcome.

Patient factors
  ASA
  Risk factors
  Monitoring
  Early mobilization
Anesthesia factors
  Anesthetic technique (GA, SA, EA, CSA, CSE, CEGA, nerve blocks)
  Analgesic technique (preemptive analgesia, wound infiltration, PCA, PACU, APS)
Surgical factors
  Site of surgery
  Surgical technique
  Surgeon's skill
  Traditions (nursing quality system, routine monitoring)
  Underlying pathology, expertise

ASA, American Society of Anesthesia; SA, spinal anesthesia; EA, epidural anesthesia; CSA, continuous spinal anesthesia; CSE, combined spinal and epidural anesthesia; PCA, patient-controlled analgesia; PACU, postanesthesia care units; APS, acute postoperative services. See Table 67.1 for other abbreviations.

The most significant of the various factors that can affect the patient's outcome seem to be preoperative block of afferent nociceptive pathways and effective control of acute postoperative pain. These factors can be eliminated from the SR only through a multimodal approach to anesthesia and analgesia.

Treatment of Acute Postoperative Pain: Hazards and New Perspectives

Wind-up and Neurochemical Memory of Pain

The continuous arrival of nociceptive stimuli appears to cause a prolonged increase in spinal cord hyperexcitability, the so-called "wind-up". This phenomenon is able to modify physiologic and anatomic neuronal characteristics ("neuroplasticity") and may be responsible, during the postoperative period, not only for an increased need of analgesic drugs but also for the pain itself, sometimes for prolonged periods. The mechanism of this neurochemical memory is not yet fully understood. In any case, a major contribution to this reaction seems to be related to the intracellular transduction of extracellular signals involving a cascade of phosphorylation-dephosphorylation events leading to modulation of the activity of several molecules. In fact, repeated nociceptive stimulation causes release of a variety of excitatory neurotransmitters, such as the amino acids glutamate and aspartate, activating N-methyl-D-aspartate (NMDA) and α-amino-3-hydroxy-5-methyl-4-isoxazoleproprionate (AMPA) receptors located in the dorsal horn neurons.[53,54] NMDA receptors in particular, induce the release of substance P and neurokinin A, maintaining spinal hypersensitivity and potentiating transmission of nociceptive messages.[55] As a consequence of this receptor activation, there is a double action at the level of neurons: a quick influx of calcium ions (Ca^{2+}) and proto-oncogene transcription. Following repeated sensory stimulation there is increased gene expression from some postsynaptic neurons. The c-*fos* and c-*jun* proto-oncogenes, for example, are part of this cell program that guarantees synaptic plasticity (i.e., the capacity of neurons to modify their synapses with activity and experience).[56] This activation of transcription factors by synaptic activity might be the link between neurotrophin and neuroplasticity in the developing peripheral and central nervous systems. Consequently, the appearance of new antigens in spinal cord neurons, as a phenotypic expression of the proto-oncogenes mentioned above, could be the first sign of a structural, chronic modification of protein synthesis, providing a persistent trace of pain. During the transition from acute to chronic pain, other factors, such as the nitric oxide level,[57] local blood flow regulation, and the glutamatergic mechanism,[58] seem to play an important role in the dorsal root ganglia and spinal cord.

Multimodal Approach to Pain Modulation

Since the development of balanced anesthesia, it has seemed clear that during anesthesia and analgesia it is better to use a combination of drugs with different mechanisms of action than to use only one. This synergistic interaction of the drugs is convenient because it increases the efficiency and safety of the treatment. In fact, the gains from drug and technique combination are twofold: The doses of the drugs can be reduced, and their side effects diminish. If the mechanism of action is distinct and the side effects of the drugs and techniques are different, it is possible to reduce the total drug dose and therefore the incidence and severity of side effects. Moreover, in the presence of synergism, the final effects are more than simply additive.[59] Thus at present most anesthesia and analgesia techniques, particularly those used in high risk patients, follow a multimodal approach to reduce afferent input to the spinal cord, block the autonomic response, and avoid the SR to surgery.

Wound Infiltration

Infiltration of local anesthetics (LAs) in the surgical wound, before or at the end of surgery, is a simple, attractive technique that has been recommended for postoperative pain relief after various surgical interventions.[60] When this technique is used alone and compared to placebo use, there is a significant decrease in postoperative pain at rest, during mobilization, and during cough, together with a reduction in total requirement for supplementary morphine.[61] No clinical differences in postoperative analgesic effects can be demonstrated between ropivacaine and bupivacaine for wound infiltration when they are used in equipotent doses. However, because large volumes of LAs are needed, ropivacaine may be preferred because it carries a lower risk of cardiovascular and cerebral side effects than bupivacaine.[62] It has been suggested that "preemptive administration" of incisional LAs in addition to general anesthesia may have a greater benefit than spinal anesthesia. It implies that the preemptive administration of LAs may have extended effects on postoperative pain due to interference with trauma-induced changes in the peripheral and central nervous systems.[63]

Preemptive Analgesia

Laboratory studies in rodents have demonstrated that prolonged stimulation or injury induces changes in central nervous system function and anatomy that may contribute to pain long after the offending stimulus has been removed; and it may influence responses to subsequent afferent inputs.[64] Moreover, studies of amputees demonstrated that the incidence of phantom limb pain was reduced by preoperative epidural block, demonstrating that noxious stimulus-induced neuroplasticity can be prevented or preempted by administration of analgesic agents before the injury.[65] Several studies have confirmed that pretreatment with opioids, local anesthetics, and nonsteroidal antiinflammatory drugs (NSAIDs) prevent the development of injury-induced spinal hyperexcitability.[66-68] The same treatments are significantly less effective when administered after injury.[69] Thus regional anesthesia, alone or in association with general anesthesia, seems to be the ideal tool for reducing postinjury hypersensitivity to pain.[70]

Peripheral Blocks

Role of Epidural Anesthesia and Analgesia

In recent years there has been increasing use of epidural anesthesia and analgesia (EAA), alone or in combination with general or regional anesthetic techniques. Combined anesthetic techniques, such as combined epidural and general anesthesia (CEGA) and combined spinal and epidural anesthesia (CSE), are examples of the role of EAA in clinical practice.

The use of EAA does, however, have some disadvantages during daily surgical activity, for example possible incomplete analgesic cover during surgery, delay in starting operations because of having to wait for the onset of the local anesthetic effect, the difficulty of patients remaining calm during long procedures, the need for additional muscle relaxation, and finally the unprotected airway and impairment of respiratory function particularly with blocks higher than T6. In addition, EAA may be associated with complications such as epidural abscesses, especially when local infection and septic conditions are present;[71] moreover, immunodeficiency states such as diabetes, renal failure, cancer, steroid administration, alcohol abuse, cachexia, and multitrauma may predispose to the formation of abscesses.[72] Another important complication of the use of EAA is intraspinal hematoma, particularly in patients with a positive family history of coagulopathy (e.g., von Willebrand's disease) or in those receiving low-dose, low-molecular-weight heparin (LMWH) associated with platelet-inhibiting drugs or potent NSAIDs and dextran.[73,74]

On the other hand, several studies have demonstrated that EAA reduces perioperative physiologic responses to surgery in addition to providing postoperative pain relief. Furthermore, compared to general anesthetic techniques, EAA is associated with less need for prolonged mechanical ventilation and recovery in intensive postanesthesia care units (PACUs); earlier postoperative mobilization, rehabilitation, and nutrition; shorter overall duration of hospital stay; and reduction of costs. The

TABLE 67.6. Proposed Advantages and Disadvantages of Epidural Anesthesia and Analgesia.

Epidural anesthesia/analgesia	Explanation
Pros	
Synergistic analgesia	Increased effectiveness and low incidence of side effects
Autonomic block	Decreased heart rate, blood pressure, myocardial oxygen consumption (MvO_2)
Modification of stress response	Decreased plasma levels of catecholamines, cortisol
Early nutrition	Increased gastric motility
Modification of postoperative hypercoagulopathy	Avoids reduction in fibrinolysis activity
Improved respiratory function	Improvement of diaphragmatic function and gas exchange
Cons	
Circulatory instability	Sympathetic block with variations in preload and afterload
Muscle weakness	Interference with motor function
Side effects due to epidural catheter	Infection, hematoma
Bladder dysfunction	Retention due to autonomic block
Respiratory depression	Central action of epidural opioids

proposed advantages and disadvantages of EAA are summarized in Table 67.6.

The use of EAA seems to influence early postoperative outcome, whereas long-term survival seems to be dependent on other factors, such as the patient's preoperative status and the surgical procedures. Consequently, the results emerging from the literature suggest that EAA should be used whenever possible. Several questions remain, however, about when epidural techniques are indicated (e.g., type of patient, drugs to use, and duration of analgesia after surgery). Moreover, the data are insufficient to assess the benefits EAA provides compared to optimal general anesthesia followed by intravenous analgesia with patient-controlled analgesia (PCA). Outcome studies should be multicentered and enroll thousands of patients to determine the effects of analgesic therapy, not only regarding early or intermediate complications but also ultimate patient outcome (e.g., death, reoperation, return to work).

Role of Combined Spinal and Epidural Anesthesia

Spinal anesthesia is an easy, economical technique that uses small doses of local anesthetic and produces an effective block with complete muscle relaxation. It also has some disadvantages, such as the risk of extensive autonomic block, fixed duration of anesthesia without the possibility of prolonging the regional block intra- or postoperatively, unpredictable hemodynamic side effects, and the risk of postdural puncture headache. On the other hand, CSE anesthesia is an effective alternative anesthetic technique because it has a rapid onset, offers good quality analgesia and motor block, carries a minimal risk of systemic toxic concentration, and allows the level of analgesia to be increased and the duration of the block to be prolonged.[75]

Various CSE techniques have been reported in the literature, the most popular being the single segment "needle-through-needle". Indications for the CSE technique include all surgery below the umbilicus, labor pain, and postoperative pain.

Role of Continuous Spinal Anesthesia

The continuous spinal anesthesia (CSA) technique has numerous advantages over epidural anesthesia and single-shot spinal anesthesia (SSA), including the more obvious endpoint for catheter placement (cerebrospinal fluid), careful titration of drugs minimizing cardiovascular instability, low doses of local anesthetic with minimal risk of toxicity, prolongation of anesthesia, and potential use for postoperative pain relief. On the other hand, it is a time-consuming technique and is associated with a risk of postdural spinal headache, catheter breakage, and potential serious neurologic complications such as persistent cauda equina syndrome.[76,77] CSA is indicated for lower abdominal and lower limb surgery in elderly and high risk patients. CSA is also used in trauma patients, in whom it is associated with fewer technical problems and faster onset than CSE,[78] and for long-term analgesia in cancer patients.

There are some adverse effects and technical problems associated with inserting the catheter into the subarachnoid space and injecting the local anesthetic. For these reasons, it is important to take some precautions for the safe practice of CSA, such as identifying preexisting neurologic dysfunction, limiting the distance of catheter advancement beyond the needle tip, carefully assessing the extent of anesthesia, and establishing the optimal position of the patient for catheter removal.

Pharmacologic Treatment

There is evidence that a multimodal analgesic therapy should be chosen to exploit logical drug interactions at the spinal cord. Combinations of drugs with different mechanisms of action increase safety and convenience during routine practice. Thus we can associate opioids and local anesthetics because local anesthetics block neuronal sodium channels, and opioids act on mu receptors, probably opening potassium channels. NSAIDs and opioids are suggested for minor to moderate pain and combinations of local anesthetics, opioids, and α_2-adrenergic agonists for severe pain.

Analgesia with NSAIDs inhibits cyclooxygenase-dependent prostanoid formation and intracellular phosphodiesterase and bradykinin levels. Opioids, on the other hand, provide effective analgesia through a central mechanism via opioid receptors. Other unconventional analgesics have been proposed (see Table 67.7). Adrenergic α_2 agonists such as clonidine are more effective when given epidurally rather than systemically and in association with local anesthetics or opioids rather than alone.[79] In addition, clonidine has some side effects, such as hypotension, bradycardia, and sedation, probably due to supraspinal mechanisms.[80] For this reason identification of more adrenergic receptor subtypes offers the possibility of using more selective, full agonists for the α_2-adrenergic receptors, such as dexmedetomidine.[81]

TABLE 67.7. Unconventional Analgesics Used for Multimodal Therapy.

Adrenergic blockade
  Norepinephrine
  Guanethidine
  Phentolamine
α_2-Agonists
  Clonidine
  Dexmedetomidine
NMDA antagonists
  Ketamine
  Amantadine
Other neuromodulators
  Neurokinin
  Tyrosine kinase receptors
  Sodium channel blockade
  Calcium channel blockade: ziconotide
  Galanin receptor
  5HT3 receptor antagonist: alosetron

The role of the *N*-methyl-D-aspartate (NMDA) receptor in the phenomenon of spinal cord hypersensitivity has created interest in NMDA antagonists, particularly ketamine. It was recently demonstrated that ketamine, a noncompetitive NMDA antagonist, potentiates the analgesic properties of morphine in postoperative patients.[82] Amantadine, another NMDA antagonist, has fewer side effects than ketamine and has also been used successfully in clinical studies in the form of an oral preparation.[83]

Organizational Aspects of Acute Postoperative Services

Although in recent years there has been widespread use of regional analgesic techniques for the relief of postoperative pain, the most common technique for providing postoperative analgesia remains the use of intramuscular opioids prescribed by ward surgeons and administered on an "as-needed" basis. It seems that to improve postoperative analgesic control it is necessary not to develop other analgesic techniques but, rather, to implement the organization of the existing structures.

Since 1988 acute postoperative services (APSs) have been developed in the United States[84] and are now present in almost all major hospitals. The main targets of these APS are frequent pain evaluation by the Visual Analogue Scale (VAS), monitoring the analgesic treatment, and bedside documentation of the pain. There is debate about the organization of APSs, particularly concerning their cost. The anesthesiology-based APS (U.S. style) ensures high level management of postoperative pain. The standard approach includes examining the patient every morning and questioning the patient about pain relief, satisfaction with analgesic technique (e.g., epidural, intravenous administration, continuous or PCA infusion), quality of sleep, opioid requirements, activity level, and side effects. The staff comprises anesthesiologists, resident anesthesiologists, specially trained nurses, pharmacists, and physiotherapists. The problems are the high cost ($100–300 per patient), the lack of continuity between the anesthesiologists (preoperative evaluation, anesthesia performance, postoperative pain management), and the small number of patients followed. For these reasons, the APSs in Europe have tried to develop different models to follow as many patients as possible, exploit existing structures, and consequently limit costs.[85] A possible basic organizational model of an APS involving few extra personnel is illustrated in Table 67.8.

TABLE 67.8. Proposed Basic Organizational Model of Acute Postoperative Services.

Health care member	Responsibility
Staff anesthesiologist	Responsible for perioperative care for his or her patients
"Pain representative" ward surgeon	Responsible for pain management on his or her ward and for implementing pain programs
"Pain representative" ward nurse	Responsible for management, pain guidelines, and monitoring
Resident anesthesiologist	Daily rounds of all surgical wards. Refers problem patients to staff anesthesiologist. Solve pain problems
Acute pain nurse	Daily rounds of all surgical wards. Checks VAS recording on charts. Solves technical problems (PCA, epidural, elastomeric pumps). Liaison between surgical ward and resident anesthesiologist
Acute pain anesthesiologist	Responsible for coordinating hospital acute pain services

VAS, Visual Analogue Scale; PCA, patient-controlled analgesia.

References

1. Weissman C: The metabolic response to stress: an overview and update. Anesthesiology 1990;73:308–327.
2. Stoner HB: Responses to trauma: fifty years of ebb and flow. Circ Shock 1993;39:316–319.
3. Cuthbertson DP: Post-shock metabolic response. Lancet 1942;1:233–246.
4. Mayers I, Johnson D: The nonspecific inflammatory response to injury. Can J Anaesth 1998;45:871–879.
5. Barton R, Cerra FB: The hypermetabolism-multiple organ failure system. Chest 1989;96:1153–1160.
6. Woolf PD: Hormonal response to trauma. Crit Care Med 1992;20:216–226.
7. Reichlin S: Neuroendocrine-immune interactions. N Engl J Med 1993;329:1246–1253.
8. Hill Ag, Hill GI: Metabolic response to severe injury. Br J Surg 1998;85:884–890.
9. Chrousos GP: The hypothalamic-pituitary-adrenal axis and immune mediated inflammation. N Engl J Med 1998;332:1351–1362.
10. Little RA, Kirkman E, Ohnishi M: Opioids and the cardiovascular responses to haemorrhage and injury. Intensive Care Med 1998;24:405–414.
11. Drucker WH, Craig JW, Hubary CA, Davis JH, Woodward HJ: The metabolic effect of trauma to denervated tissue in man. J Trauma 1961;1:306–321.
12. Wilmore DW, Taylor JW, Hander EW, Mason AD, Pruitt BA: Central nervous system following thermal injury. In: Wilkinson

AW, Cuthberson D (eds) Metabolism and the Response to Injury. London, Pittman, 1976;274-286.
13. Strieter RM, Kunkel SL, Bone RC: Role of tumour necrosis factor in disease states and inflammation. Cirt Care Med 1993;21 (Suppl):447-463.
14. Dinarello CA, Wolff S: The role of interleukin-1 in disease. N Engl J Med 1993;328:106-113.
15. Shamoon H, Hender R, Sherwin RS: Synergistic interaction among anti-insulin hormones in the pathogenesis of stress hyperglycemia in humans. J Clin Endocrinol Metab 1981;52:1235-1241.
16. Vaughan GM, Becker RA, Unger RH, et al: Nonthyroidal control of metabolism after burn injury: possible role of glucagon. Metabolism 1985;34:637-641.
17. Wise JK, Hendler R, Felig P: Influence of glucocorticoids on glucagon secretion and plasma aminoacid concentrations in man. J Clin Invest 1973;52:2774-2882.
18. Samra JS, Summers LKM, Frayn KN: Sepsis and fat metabolism. Br J Surg 1996;83:1186-1196.
19. Gabay C, Kushner I: Acute-phase proteins and other systemic responses to inflammation. N Engl J Med 1999;340:448-454.
20. Langstein HN, Norton JA: Mechanisms of cancer cachexia. Hematol Oncol Clin North Am 1991;5:103-123.
21. Grant JP: Nutritional support in critically ill patients. Ann Surg 1994;220:610-616.
22. Houdijk AP, Rijnsburger CA, Jansen J, et al: Randomized trail of glutamine-enriched enteral nutrition on infectious morbidity in patients with multiple trauma. Lancet 1998;352:772-776.
23. Slogoff S, Keats AX: Randomized trial of primary anesthetic agents on outcome of coronary artery bypass operations. Anesthesiology 1999;70:179-188.
24. Mangano DT, Hollenberg M, Pegert G, Meyer ML, London MJ, Tubau JF: Perioperative myocardial ischemia in patients undergoing non cardiac surgery: incidence and severity during the 4 day perioperative period. J Am Coll Cardiol 1991;17:843-850.
25. Heusch G, Deussen A, Thamer V: Cardiac sympathetic nerve activity and progressive vasoconstriction distal to coronary stenosis: feedback aggravation of myocardial ischemia. J Auton Nerv Syst 1985;13:311-326.
26. Klicks B: Influence of sympathetic tone on ventricular fibrillation threshold during experimental coronary occlusion. Am J Cardiol 1975;36:45-49.
27. Flately KA, DeFily DV, Thomas JX: Effects of cardiac sympathetic nerve stimulation during adrenergic blockade on infarct size. J Cardiovasc Pharmacol 1985;7:673-679.
28. O'Brien JR, Tulevski VG, Etherington M, Madgwick T: Platelet function studies before and after operative and the effect of postoperative thrombosis. J Lab Clin Med 1974;83:342-354.
29. Kluft C, Verheijen JH, Jie AFH, et al: The post-operative fibrinolytic shutdown: a rapidly reverting acute phase pattern for the fast-acting inhibitor of tissue type plasminogen activator after trauma. Scand J Clin Lab Invest 1985;45:605-610.
30. Naesh O, Friis JT, Hindberg I, Winther K: Platelet function in surgical stress. Thromb Haemost 1985;54:849-852.
31. Naesh O, Hindberg I, Friis J, et al: Platelet activation in major surgical stress: influence of combined epidural and general anaesthesia. 1994;8:802-825.
32. Murphy MG, Davies MJ, Eduardo A: The haemostatic response to surgery and trauma. Br J Anaesth 1993;70:205-213.
33. Harker LA, Malpass TW, Branson HE, Hesselli EA, Slichter SJ: Mechanism of abnormal transient platelet dysfunction associated with selective granule release. Blood 1980;56:824-834.
34. Lichtenfeld K, Schiffer D, Helrich M: Platelet aggregation during and after general anesthesia and surgery. Anesth Analg 1979;58:293-296.
35. Christopherson R, Beattie C, Frank SM, et al: Perioperative morbidity in patients randomized to epidural or general anesthesia for lower-extremity vascular surgery. Anesthesiology 1993;79:422-434.
36. Ali J, Weisel R, Layug A, Kripke B, Hechtman H: Consequences of postoperative alterations in respiratory mechanism. Am J Surg 1974;128:376-382.
37. Fratacci M-D, Kimball WR, Wain JC, Kacmarek RM, Polaner DM, Zapol WM: Diaphragmatic shortening after thoracic surgery in humans. Anesthesiology 1993;79:654-665.
38. Craig DB: Post-operative recovery of pulmonary function. Anesth Analg 1981;60:46-52.
39. Livingston EH, Passaro EP: Post-operative ileus. Dig Dis Sci 1990;35:121-132.
40. Salo M: Effects of anesthesia and surgery on the immune response. Acta Anaesthesiol Scand 1992;36:201-220.
41. Markovic SN, Knight PR, Murasko DM: Inhibition of interferon stimulation of natural killer cell activity in mice anesthetized with halothane or isoflurane. Anesthesiology 1993;78:700-706.
42. Moss NM, Gough DB, Jordan AI: Temporal correlation of impaired immune response after thermal injury with susceptibility of infection in a murine model. Surgery 1988;104:882-887.
43. Marx GF, Mateo CV, Orkin LR: Computer analysis of postanesthetic deaths. Anesthesiology 1973;39:54-58.
44. Farrow SC, Fowkes FGR, Lunn JN, Robertson IB, Samuel P: Epidemiology in anesthesia. II. Factors affecting mortality in hospital. Br J Anaesth 1982;59:834-841.
45. Holland R: Anaesthetic mortality in New South Wales. Br J Anaesth 1987;59:834-841.
46. McQuay HJ, Carroll D, Moore RA: Post-operative orthopaedic pain: the effect of opiate premedication and local anaesthetic blocks. Pain 1988;33:291-295.
47. Salomaki TE, Lappaluoto J, Laitinen JO, Vuolteenaho O, Nuutinen LS: Epidural versus intravenous fentanyl for reducing hormonal, metabolic, and physiologic responses after thoracotomy. Anesthesiology 1993;79:672-679.
48. Jayr C, Thomas H, Rey A, Farhat F, Lasser P, Bourgain J: Postoperative pulmonary complications: epidural analgesia using bupivacaine and opioids versus parenteral opioids. Anesthesiology 1993;78:666-676.
49. Galimberti G, Caristi D, Iscra F, Frassanito P, Gullo A: Blended anaesthesia vs general anaesthesia: is blended anaesthesia a really cheaper technique in decreasing post-operative costs? Br J Anaesth 1996;76:A227.
50. Tuman KJ, McCarthy RJ, March RJ, DeLaria GA, Patel RV, Ivankovic AD: Effects of epidural anesthesia and analgesia on coagulation and outcome after major vascular surgery. Anesth Analg 1991;73:696-704.
51. Davies MJ, Slibert BS, Mooney PJ, Dysart RH, Meads AC: Combined epidural and general anaesthesia versus general anaesthesia for abdominal aortic surgery. Anaesth Intensive Care 1993;21:790-794.
52. Sorensen RM, Pace NL: Mortality and morbidity of regional versus general anesthesia. Anesthesiology 1991;75:A1053.
53. Liu H, Mantyh PW, Basbaum AI: NMDA-receptor regulation of substance P release from primary afferent nociceptors. Nature 1997;386:721-724.

54. Harris JA, Corsi M, Quartaroli M, Arban R, Bentivoglio M: Upregulation of spinal glutamate receptors in chronic pain. Neuroscience 1996;74:7-12.
55. Schaible H-G, Jarrott B, Hope PJ, Duggan AW: Release of immunoreactive substance P in the spinal cord during development of acute arthritis in the knee joint of the cat: a study with antibody microprobes. Brain Res 1990;529:214-223.
56. Curran T, Margan JI: Fos: an immediate-early transcription factor in neurons. J Neurobiol 1994;26:403-412.
57. Meller ST, Gebhart GF: Nitric oxide (NO) and nociceptive processing in the spinal cord. Pain 1993;52:127-136.
58. Coderre TJ: The role excitatory amino acid receptors and intracellular messengers in persistent nociception after tissue injury in rats. Mol Neurobiol 1993;7:229-246.
59. Dickenson AH, Sullivan AF: Combination therapy in analgesia: seeking synergy. Curr Opin Anesthesiol 1993;6:861-865.
60. Ready LB: Acute Post-operative pain. In: Miller RD (ed) Anesthesia, 3rd ed. New York, Churchill Livingstone, 1990;2135-2146.
61. Dierking GW, Ostergaard E, Ostergard HT, Dahl JB: The effects of wound infiltration with bupivacaine versus saline on postoperative pain and opioid requirements after herniorrhaphy. Acta Anaesthesiol Scand 1994;38:289-292.
62. Erichsen CJ, Vibits H, Dahl JB, Kehlet H: Wound infiltration with ropivacaine and bupivacaine for pain after inguinal herniotomy. Acta Anaesthesiol Scand 1995;39:67-70.
63. Tverskoj M, Cozacov C, Ayache M, Bardley EL, Kissin I: Postoperative pain after inguinal herniorrhaphy with different types of anesthesia. Anesth Analg 1990;70:29-35.
64. Woolf CJ: Long-term alterations in the excitability of the flexion reflex produced by peripheral tissue injury in the chronic decerebrate rat. Pain 1984;18:325-343.
65. Jensen TS, Krebs B, Nielsen J, Rasmussen P: Immediate and long-term phantom pain in amputees: Incidence, clinical characteristics and relationship to pre-amputation pain. Pain 1985;21:268-278.
66. Page GG, McDonald JS, Ben-Eliyahu S: Pre-operative versus post-operative administration of morphine: impact on the neuroendocrine, behavioural, and metastatic-enhancing effects of surgery. Br J Anaesth 1998;81:216-223.
67. Gottschalk A, Smith DS, Jobes DR, et al: Pre-emptive epidural analgesia and recovery from radical prostatectomy. JAMA 1998;279:1076-1082.
68. Dahl JB, Daugaard JJ, Rasmussen B, Egebo K, Calrsson P, Kehlet H: Immediate and prolonged effects of pre- versus post-operative epidural analgesia with bupivacaine and morphine on pain at rest and during mobilisation after total knee arthroplasty. Acta Anaesthesiol Scand 1994;38:557-561.
69. Kundra P, Gurnani A, Bhattacharya A: Pre-empitive epidural morphine for post-operative pain relief after lumbar laminectomy. Anesth Analg 1997;85:135-138.
70. Blake DW: The general versus regional anaesthesia debate: time to reexamine the goals. Aust N Z Surg 1995;65:51-56.
71. Kindler CH, Seeberger MD, Staender SE: Epidural abscess complicating epidural anaesthesia and analgesia. Acta Anaesthesiol Scand 1998;42:614-620.
72. Breivik H: Neurological complications in association with spinal and epidural analgesia—again. Acta Anaesthesiol Scand 1998;42:609-613.
73. Horlocker TT, Heit JA: Low molecular weight heparin chemistry, pharmacology, perioperative prophylaxis, guidelines for regional anesthetic management. Anesth Analg 1997;85:874-885.
74. Lumpkin MM: FDA Public Health Advisory: reports of epidural or spinal hematomas with the concurrent use of low molecular weight heparin and spinal/epidural anesthesia spinal puncture. Anesthesiology 1998;88:27A-28A.
75. Flesby S, Juelsgaard P: Combined spinal and epidural anesthesia. Anesth Analg 1995;80:821-826.
76. Horlocker TT, McGregor DG, Matsushige DK, Schroeder DR, Besse JA: Perioperative Outcomes Group. A retrospective review of 4767 consecutive spinal anesthetics: central nervous system complications. Anesth Analg 1997;84:578-584.
77. Denny NM, Selander DE: Continuous spinal anaesthesia. Br J Aneasth 1998;81:590-597.
78. Wilhelm S, Standl T, Burmeister M, Kessler G, Schulte EJ: Comparison of continuous spinal with combined spinal-extradural anesthesia using plain 0.5% bupivacaine in trauma patients. Anesth Analg 1997;85:69-71.
79. Armand S, Langlade A, Boutros A, et al: Meta-analysis of the efficacy of extradural clonidine to relieve post-operative pain: an impossible task. Br J Anaesth 1998;81:126-134.
80. Kirno K, Landin S, Elam M: Epidural clonidine depresses sympathetic nerve activity in humans by a supraspinal mechanism. Anesthesiology 1993;78:1021-1027.
81. Dyck JB, Maze M, Haack C, Vuorilehto L, Shafer SL: The pharmacokinetics and hemodynamic effects of intravenous and intramuscular dexmedetomidine hydrochloride in adult human volunteers. Anesthesiology 1993;78:813-820.
82. Chih-Shung W, Chih-Chen L, Chen-Hwan C, Shung-Tai H: Pre-emptive analgesia with ketamine, morphine and epidural lidocaine prior to total knee replacement. Can J Anaesth 1997;44:31-37.
83. Eide PK, Jorum E, Stubhaug A, Bremmes J, Brevik H: Relief of post-herpetic neuralgia with N-methyl-D-aspartatic acid receptor antagonist ketamine: a double-blind, cross-over comparison with morphine and placebo. Pain 1994;58:347-354.
84. Ready LB, Oden Rollin Chadwick HS, Benedetti C, Rooke GA, Caplan R, Wild LM: Development of an anaesthesiology-based post-operative pain management service. Anesthesiology 1988;68:100-106.
85. Rawal N: Organization of acute pain services: a low-cost model. Pain 1994;57:117-123.

68
Integrative Biology and Genetic Variability: MODS' Next Frontiers

Timothy G. Buchman

> New frontiers of the mind are before us, and if they are pioneered with the same vision, boldness, and drive with which we have waged this war we can create...a fuller and more fruitful life.
> —Franklin Delano Roosevelt, to Vannevar Bush, November 17, 1944

Care of the critically ill patient has been revolutionized through advances in prehospital care, operative care, intensive care, and rehabilitative care. Systematic observation and dozens of rigorous clinical trials have yielded a complex picture of the patient in physiologic crisis who is at greatest risk for the multiple organ dysfunction syndrome (MODS). Widespread inflammation was suggested to be prerequisite to MODS, and a general hypothesis was articulated: that interruption of the biochemical cascade leading to this widespread inflammation would attenuate the progression and severity of MODS. More than two dozen clinical trials later, this simplistic hypothesis has been disproven. The purpose of this chapter is to explore the reasons why this apparently logical hypothesis concerning the pathogenesis of MODS might be incorrect and to consider alternative formulations of MODS pathogenesis.

Our approach to medicine in particular and science in general is rooted in the tradition of René Déscartes, the father of reductionism, who argued that the route to understanding all natural phenomena was to break each down into its component, irreducible parts.[1] This cartesian approach to inquiry has carried the natural sciences forward for nearly four centuries through its scale-independent application, ranging from the visible world to subatomic particles. Physiology had its greatest cartesian analyst in Claude Bernard, who in 1878 framed the idea that has guided investigators and clinicians alike for 120 years. He wrote.[2]

> It is the fixity of the milieu intérieur which is the condition of free and independent life; all of the vital mechanisms, however varied they may be, have only one object, that of preserving constant the conditions of life in the internal environment.

As J.B.S. Haldane later observed, "No more pregnant sentence was ever framed by a physiologist." Since that time investigators have charged themselves with identifying and unraveling those self-correcting mechanisms, and clinicians have set about restoring (insofar as possible) the measurable parameters of the milieu intérieur to their physiologic values.

The idea of providing external support to compensate for internal dysfunction permeates critical care medicine: Ventilators, dialysis machines, and inotropic drugs all aim to support patients until they can support themselves. Certainly such support is warranted when the internal dysfunction is life-threatening. However, many clinicians continue to interpret Bernard's idea of "preserving constancy" as a mandate to establish and maintain particular physiologic parameters, such as a hemoglobin of 10 g/dl, an oxygen delivery of 600 ml/min, or a serum potassium of 4 mEq/L. The Bernardian idea of "neutralizing the inflammatory response" to prevent MODS took root because unbridled inflammation was viewed as necessary and sufficient to cause MODS: If only the dysfunctional inflammatory system could be brought under pharmacologic control, MODS would never evolve.

Support for this idea emerged from animal studies. Mice, rats, and rabbits were used to test the modulators of inflammation in the laboratory. Models of sepsis, including endotoxemia and bacteremia, were created; and the modulators apparently improved outcome in many cases. The first clinical trial of a modulator, the anti-endotoxin antibody HA-1A, was reported to be successful.[3] New antiinflammatory molecules were then sought, developed, and tested.

We now know those several strategies that appeared so promising in the animal models are problematic in humans. Indeed, there is some evidence that aggressive control of inflammation can actually worsen outcome in human clinical sepsis. Does this mean that MODS is neither predictable nor controllable? Or are there lessons to be gleaned from the failure of the antiinflammatory therapies that suggest alternative formulations?

Genes and Development: Cascades and Networks

Much of the excitement surrounding modulation of the inflammatory response emerged from the notion that there existed an inflammatory "cascade"; that is, the idea that activation of a relatively few proximal triggers set into motion a series of amplification events. Even when it became clear that there existed a parallel set of antiinflammatory molecules, clinicians and investigators alike clung to the notion that these sets of molecules behaved like so many dominoes—their activation could be predictably controlled at a small number of distinct points. Implicit in this notion is the idea that human biology is organized in "blueprint" fashion: One gene codes for one enzyme, one enzyme serves one particular function, and the performance of a particular function can be readily inferred from the performance of each enzyme that contributes to that function. Indeed, attribution of certain diseases to single gene defects (e.g., hemoglobinopathies, cystic fibrosis) and their management by replacing the missing gene product supports this "blueprint" model. What is often missed is that, given the infinite genetic variation manifest among living humans, such single gene defects of clinical significance are decidedly rare: Nature and evolution have conspired to build a substantial redundancy into mammalian physiology. We now know that seemingly critical genes, such as those coding for specific antiinflammatory gene products, can be "knocked out" in experimental animals, often with negligible effect on their phenotype.

The simplest explanation for this systems redundancy is that inflammatory and antiinflammatory systems are not cascades at all. Rather, they are networks whose individual components may well vary with respect to their activation level without affecting the overall state of the network. Put differently, genetic variation is so widespread that critical biochemical pathways must be robust to this variation or we would not survive as a species.

This is not to say that genetic variation has no relation to inflammatory responses or survival. Evidence from the experimental laboratory and from clinical series is accumulating to suggest that genetic variation may play an enormous role in predicting recovery from severe inflammation. In the experimental laboratory, DeMaio, Reeves, and their colleagues have studied inbred strains of mice, all commonly used as experimental subjects.[4] Each of these strains is thought to be "representative", each is thought to be robust to most experimental manipulations, and, importantly, each strain is genetically distinct. What these investigators have observed is that in the face of a uniform inflammatory challenge (administration of a carefully defined endotoxin) the strains behave quite differently. One strain (A/J) has a survival that exceeds 91%, whereas another (C57BL6) has a survival below 19%.

Murine endotoxemia may indeed be a poor surrogate for clinical MODS. However, Stuber and colleagues have identified markers in the human genome that appear to correlate with outcome in similarly severe cases of sepsis. Variants in the gene coding for the lymphokine tumor necrosis factor-β (TNFβ) appear to predict outcome in MODS.[5] This is not to say that TNFβ activity itself modulates the outcome but, rather, the product(s) of gene(s) near the TNFβ gene may influence outcome. The distinction is subtle but important: The fact that a genetic marker may correlate with outcome in no way establishes a link between the product of that gene and the outcome. The best that a marker can do is provide a measure of how robust the inflammatory/antiinflammatory network is to (a particular) perturbation.

We introduced the concept of "network" but left it undefined. For our purposes, a network is a biologic system of nodes (organelles, cells, tissues, organs) and connections (second messengers, gap junctions, hormones and cytokines, peripheral nervous system). Two features of networks are immediately apparent. First, large (biologic) networks contain smaller networks (the architecture is "nested"); and second, changing the state of a single node or the strength of a single connection may or may not affect the state of the network.

A third feature of biologic networks is their capacity to organize themselves.[6] Given that the zygote and every daughter cell contain all the genetic information necessary to create an adult human, our complex structure and differentiated functions must be the product of a temporal succession of network states. We are less the product of a blueprint in which every molecular and cellular function is specified and organized into an exhaustively detailed plan than we are the product of a starting network that, once released from its initial state, creates new networks that organize themselves in specific ways according to distances from one another (chemical gradients) and time (number of cell divisions).[7]

The capacity for self-organization of dividing cells into an intact human form speaks to a fourth feature of biologic networks: They are generally fairly robust to perturbation. The program of human development in which ontogeny recapitulates phylogeny is generally difficult to derail. Variation in structural and regulatory gene products are commonplace, yet development proceeds. Maternal stresses ranging from malnutrition to substance abuse to direct invasion of the amniotic sac (amniocentesis) are amazingly well tolerated. To use the jargon of the informatics industry, the developing human is "fault-tolerant".

What is not well tolerated, however, is wholescale resequencing of events. Put differently, the initial regulatory state of the fertilized ovum is both necessary and sufficient to trigger development of an intact human despite wide genetic variation. That development, however, always proceeds in a precisely defined order. Unlike building by blueprint, in which the order of most events (save for a new critical steps) is irrelevant to the final product, building by program requires that a temporal pace and sequence be maintained. For example, the final stages of fetal maturation always begin with renal maturation, followed by gut and liver maturation, and ending with lung maturation. We note the sequence of organ dysfunction in what used to be called multiple *sequential* organ failure: The lung fails first, the gut and liver follow, and finally the kidneys quit. In the weave of organ development and the unraveling of organ function, sequence and event are not readily separable.

Multiple organ dysfunction syndrome almost never occurs de novo. Rather, it is a common response to a spectrum of stresses, each of which perturbs organs and the networks that connect them to the point that support of one or more organs is required to sustain vital functions. Our approach to care of the patient with impending or fully developed MODS is sequence-blind. We typically impose supports to force several systems simultaneously into particular performance regimens. Should additional organ systems fail, we search for missed diagnoses even while instituting additional supports. Our aim for "stability" seems intended to terminate the progressive loss of integration of physiologic networks.

At first glance, this clinical intention appears entirely logical. Analysis of physiologic data obtained from critically ill children and adults suggest that during physiologic illness the coupling among biologic systems weakens. In studies of brain-injured children, Goldstein and colleagues observed that the coupling between heart rate and blood pressure diminished with decreasing Glasgow Coma Score.[8] Godin and colleagues observed the same loss of fine physiologic variability in experimental human sepsis[9] that Kim and colleagues observed in clinically septic humans.[10] Indeed, Winchell and Hoyt showed that loss of heart rate variability is tightly linked to a mortal outcome in critically ill adults without cardiac disease.[11] Deliberate attempts to "restore the network," by physically supporting the nodes or the coupling among them, is an attractive therapeutic goal. Whether this approach leads to improved outcomes is open to question.

Integrative Biology and Complex Systems

We have so far suggested that critical illness is associated with perturbation and decoupling of biologic networks. There are at least two ways such an association might exist. One possibility is that there is one principal healthy state for biologic networks at each level of granularity ("healthy" cells make a "healthy" tissue, "healthy" tissues makes a "healthy" organ, and so on), and that the "criticality" of illness is linked to how far the patient appears to have drifted from this principal healthy state. This line of thought leads to the therapeutic idea that we can "nudge" the patient back toward health by correcting various physiologic irregularities. Such therapeutic ideas are pervasive and are reflected in the notion that there exists a preferred pH, an optimal heart rate, a desirable (if supranormal) oxygen consumption, and so on. The problem with this reasoning is that patients appear to get "stuck" in what appear to be "unhealthy" states where even aggressive care fails to budge them from their critical illness. John Siegel has formalized this idea through unbiased analysis of physiologic parameters measured in critically ill patients. The technique, formally called k-means cluster analysis, shows that what clinicians recognize as "sepsis," "respiratory failure," and "cardiogenic shock" exist as well defined, stable, but unfortunately unhealthy states.[12]

The other possibility linking critical illness with perturbation of biologic networks is the idea that perturbations are commonplace and in fact are required to sustain normal integrative physiology. This link embeds the robustness to external perturbation in the tendency of perturbed networks to couple, uncouple, and recouple. With this formulation, the problem during critical illness is not that the patient (and his networks) have departed from the healthy state but, rather, that the patient (and his networks) are having difficulty finding the sequence of couplings that can return them to health after the inciting stimulus has been neutralized. If this formulation is correct, the classic approach to critical care—imposing a set of arbitrary parameters by aggressive intervention—may actually retard the patient's return to health.

Pictures of Health

Despite obvious anatomic and endocrinologic connections among the major organ systems, it has been difficult to demonstrate physiologic coupling. Standard references typically describe the coupling between essential systems (e.g., cardiac and respiratory systems) as "weak".[13] This description persists in part because the classic mathematic tools recruited to investigate this coupling limit the types of coupling that are detected. For example, several of the methods estimated coupling between the cardiac and respiratory systems based on crude integer synchrony (synchronous states of integer order n), which provides only the number of heartbeats contained within a single respiratory cycle.

One of the reasons such crude tools were employed is that the definition of synchrony is elusive. For example, the definition of noninteger synchrony requires that the method go beyond merely recognizing the completion of a physiologic cycle to define explicitly what is meant by "phase" at each point in that cycle. A series of reports from Schäfer and colleagues described the analysis of synchronization between the cardiac and respiratory systems based on new, powerful definitions of phase and, more importantly, phase locking.[14] The mathematics, based on the analytic signal concept and the Hilbert transform, are daunting, but the general method is more or less readily grasped.

Measurable parameters of cardiac and respiratory function are clearly periodic; plotted as parameter versus time, they appear as oscillating signals. The signals, however, are not "clean." First, there is often a fair bit of noise associated with the biologic system itself, the measurement technique, or both. Second and more problematic is that the measurement conditions are not stationary; that is, over the period of measurement external and internal factors influence the two signals and their relation with one another. Whatever definition of phase is used, it must be robust to these two noisome aspects of the biologic signals. The Hilbert transform fulfills these requirements. The general method, then, is to obtain a time series of measurements

$s(t)$. Such measurements might be simultaneously obtained from an electrocardiography (ECG) trace, blood pressure trace, pneumotachograph, capnograph, and so on, sampling at a rate sufficiently fast that at least 20 samples are collected in the fastest oscillation. For each of these signals $s(t)$, one constructs an analytic signal $\zeta(t)$, which is a complex function of time defined as $\zeta(t) = s(t) + j\tilde{s}(t) = A(t)e^{j\phi(t)}$, where the function $\tilde{s}(t)$ is the Hilbert transform of $s(t)$, namely $\tilde{s}(t) = \pi^{-1} \text{P.V.} \int_{-\infty}^{+\infty} \frac{s(\tau)}{t-\tau} d(\tau)$ where P.V. indicates that the integral is taken in the sense of the Cauchy principal integral. (Operationally, the Hilbert transform is accomplished by a digital infinite impulse response filter[15] 256 points in length.) The $A(t)$ component of the analytic signal is the instantaneous amplitude, and $\phi(t)$ defines the instantaneous phase. If two signals, $s_1(t)$ and $s_2(t)$, are recorded for the same times t, and if those two signals have instantaneous phase, $\phi_1(t)$ and $\phi_2(t)$, at a particular time t, it is possible to calculate a variety of metrics from those instantaneous phases. One such metric is displayed as the cardiorespiratory synchrogram, which is a plot of the normalized relative phase of the heartbeat within two respiratory cycles.[14]

When data were obtained from the healthiest humans (trained athletes at rest), the cardiorespiratory synchrograms revealed substantial coupling between the cardiac and respiratory systems. Importantly, the systems would be coupled at one synchrony (e.g., five heartbeats for two respiratory cycles) for a few minutes, uncouple, and then recouple with an identifiably different synchrony (e.g., six heartbeats for two respiratory cycles) with phase locking for as long as 20 minutes before again uncoupling and recoupling.[16] The data support the hypothesis that health is characterized by a constant search through the space of available couplings.

A separate line of investigation has focused on the average strength of coupling within epochs of time. The analytic technique is based on the concept of signal entropy. This esoteric sounding concept is, in fact, familiar to intensivists and refers to the disappearance of "runs" of data in a data set. In the intensive care unit, we often encounter this idea embedded in analysis of cardiac rhythms. For example, a fibrillatory rhythm with an average ventricular response rate of 100 has precisely the same number of beats per unit time as a bigeminal rhythm with an average ventricular response rate of 100. The timing of the nth beat in the bigeminal rhythm can be predicted with fair certainly so long as the timing of the first and second beats is known. In contrast, the timing of the nth beat of the fibrillatory rhythm can never be predicted based on the timing of the first and second beats. The bigeminal rhythm has less uncertainty and therefore less signal entropy.

Two facts make such signal entropy a useful analytic tool for biologists and clinicians. The first fact is that all biologic signals include a stochastic or random component. The second fact is that, for large classes of signals, interaction of one random component with another random component leads to increased randomness in each of the interacting signals.[17] In other words, randomness or entropy in a signal can be used as a proxy for connectedness of the node producing that signal to a network. Although entropy cannot be measured precisely in a discrete time series $s(t)$, an approximation (approximate entropy, or ApEn) serves well.[18] ApEn measures the logarithmic likelihood that in the series of data $s(t)$ runs of patterns that remain close over a set number of observations (m) remain "close" (within an absolute value, r) on the next incremental comparison ($m + 1$). A more formal definition is that, given the time series of data $s(t)$ containing N data points,

$-$ ApEn $\approx$ average over the entire data series $s(t)$ from $t = 1$ to $(N - m + 1)$ of the

$$\ln \begin{bmatrix} \text{conditional probability that} \\ |s(t+m) - s(t'+m)| \leq r \text{ given that} \\ |s(t+k) - s(t'+k)| \leq r \text{ for } k = 0, 1, \ldots, m-1 \\ \text{where } t \text{ and } t' \text{ represent all of the values of } t \\ \text{from } t = 1 \text{ to } (N - m + 1) \end{bmatrix}$$

This statistic has been used to demonstrate loss of system connectedness as premonitory to such disparate critical events as systemic responses to endotoxemia and ventricular tachyarrhythmias. ApEn and other measures of variability that may provide insight into system connectedness have been reviewed elsewhere.[19]

Transition from the "Cascade" View to the "Network" View of Pathobiology in MODS

We now recognize at least three characteristics of human biology that are not well addressed in existing models of MODS. The first characteristic is that humans are products of programs not blueprints. We are constructed as self-organizing, nesting networks that become increasingly stable as interconnection increases. Whereas the cascade concept—a process that proceeds unidirectionally over time—may reflect the development of these networks, the consequence of perturbing these networks is not well represented by that cascade concept. The second characteristic is that human "health" appears to require ongoing self-organization and rearrangement of the connections that link one vital system to the next. Current therapies that fix physiologic performance to specific values may retard recovery from severe illness by inhibiting that self-organization. The third idea is that the experimental approach to understanding and treating MODS should follow conventional cartesian logic, isolating each node and connection to understand its contribution to the organism as a whole. Neither node nor connection may have a particular meaning once taken out of context. We suggest that a complex systems approach integrating genetics, developmental biology, cell biology, and integrative physiology may prove useful for unraveling the pathogenesis of MODS.

References

1. Descartes R: Rules for the Direction of the Mind, Rule IX.
2. Bernard C: Leçons sur les Phénomènes de la Vie Communs aux Animaux et aux Végétaux. Paris, Ballière, 1878. This translation is

in Fulton JF: Selected Readings in the History of Physiology. New York, Charles C Thomas, 1930;307.
3. Ziegler EJ, Fisher CJ Jr, Sprung CL, et al: Treatment of gram-negative bacteremia and septic shock with HA-1A human monoclonal antibody against endotoxin: a randomized, double-blind, placebo-controlled trial. N Engl J Med 1991;324:429–436.
4. De Maio, Mooney ML, Matesic LE, Paidas CN, Reeves RH: Genetic component in the inflammatory response induced by bacterial lipopolysaccharide. Shock 1998;10:319–323.
5. Stuber F, Petersen M, Bokelmann F, Schade U: A genomic polymorphism within the tumor necrosis factor locus influences plasma tumor necrosis factor-alpha concentrations and outcome of patients with severe sepsis. Crit Care Med 1996; 24:381–384.
6. Chauvet GA: Hierarchical functional organization of formal biological systems: a dynamical approach. I. The increase of complexity by self-association increases the domain of stability of a biological system. Philos Trans R Soc Lon B. 1993;339:425–444.
7. Kauffman SA: The Origins of Order: Self-organization and Selection in Evolution. New York, Oxford University Press, 1993;173–235.
8. Goldstein B, Toweill D, Lai S, Sonnenthal K, Kimberly B: Uncoupling of the autonomic and cardiovascular systems in acute brain injury. Am J Physiol 1998;275:R1287–R1292.
9. Godin PJ, Fleisher LA, Eidsath A, et al: Experimental human endotoxemia increases cardiac regularity: results from a prospective randomized crossover trial. Crit Care Med 1996; 24:1117–1124.
10. Kim R, Hsu J, Kacin M, Morgan L, Szaflarski N, Seiver A: Low-frequency, periodic fluctuations in physiologic variables of critically-ill patients. Crit Care Med 1995;23:A27.
11. Winchell RJ, Hoyt DB: Spectral analysis of heart rate variablity in the ICU: a measure of autonomic function. J Surg Res 1996; 63:11.
12. Goldwyn RM, Friedman HP, Siegel JH: Iteration and interaction in computer data bank analysis: a case study in the physiologic classification and assessment of the critically ill. Comput Biomed Res 1971;4:607.
13. Glass L, Mackey MC: From Clocks to Chaos: The Rhythms of Life. Princeton, Princeton University Press, 1988;136.
14. Schäfer C, Rosenblum MG, Abel H-H, Kurths J: Synchronization in human cardiorespiratory system. Phys Rev 1999 (in press).
15. Hahn SL: Hilbert Transforms in Signal Processing. Boston, Artech House, 1996;226.
16. Schäfer C, Rosenblum MG, Kurths J, Abel HH: Heartbeat synchronized with ventilation. Nature 1998;392:239–240.
17. Pincus SM: Greater signal regularity may indicate greater signal isolation. Math Biosci 1994;122:161–181.
18. Pincus SM, Goldberger AL: Physiological time-series analysis: what does regularity quantify? Am J Physiol 1994;266:H1643–H1656.
19. Goldstein B, Buchman TG: Heart rate variability in intensive care. J Intensive Care Med 1998;13:252–265.

69
Are We Making Progress in Preventing and Treating MOF?

Arthur E. Baue

We like to think that we are improving the care of injured and operated patients so more patients survive and recover.[1] Certainly regional trauma centers, better monitoring and intensive care, new drugs, improved operative surgery, and minimal surgical procedures have improved the possibilities of survival of our patients.[2] During an era in which "evidence-based medicine"[3] and "evidence-based research"[4] are stressed, can we document objectively such improvements in patient care if they truly have occurred? Prospective, randomized, double-blind clinical trials are required to document the efficacy of various therapeutic efforts. Unfortunately, many, if not all, such studies of a single "magic bullet" have been negative.[5] It is difficult to measure and document whether general resuscitation, operations, and intensive care have made an impact on survival and well-being. Controlled randomized trials are not possible. What would be the variable? Randomized to what?

Our science is powerful, but our ability to apply such science to patient care is much weaker. There are amazing scientific revelations in our understanding of infection, sepsis, stress, trauma, and cell and organ injury. Despite this understanding, our clinical efforts continue haltingly and sputter along with difficult-to-measure clinical advances. We are told that animal models would contribute more to patient care if they were more relevant. What is clinical relevance? Is there ever relevance of normal animals undergoing a single perturbation or treatment after an insult in a well controlled experiment to an elderly, complex, uncontrolled, sick patient. If the treatment affects the critical problem of the illness, you may be able to document improvement. If, the perturbation is one of many factors involved in the illness of this elderly sick patient, however, do not make the effort.[6] You can never document anything other than being sick [systemic inflammatory response syndrome (SIRS)], sicker (severe SIRS), very sick [multiple organ dysfunction syndrome (MODS)], or dying [multiple organ failure (MOF)]. What makes a difference in improving the care of patients? Molecular biology? Shock research? Clinical trials? Technologic advances? Evidence-based medicine or research? All of the above? These factors all contribute to our scientific knowledge base and fill the empty spaces of a complex puzzle. Eventually, they may contribute directly to clinical therapy.

Comparison of Results Over the Years

There have been several important reviews of experiences to document change or progress. Zimmerman et al. compared risks and outcomes for intensive care unit (ICU) patients with organ system failure from 1982 to 1990.[7] They found that the incidence of organ system failure was 48% among patients treated form 1979 to 1982. An identical proportion (14%) of patients developed multiple organ system failure (MOSF) during both time periods. They found significant improvement, however, in the hospital mortality rate for patients with three or more organ system failures on day 4 or later in the ICU. Despite this, overall hospital mortality rates due to MOSF were not different over this 8-year period, but there was improved survival of patients with persistent severe organ system failure. This report confirms again our contention that (1) better intensive care is helping, and (2) the secret to MOF is prevention.[1] Once MOF is evident, mortality is high, and other problems occur. There are several problems with the comparisons of these authors, however. One is that during their early experience with the Acute Physiology and Chronic Health Evaluation (APACHE) scoring system, there was no gastrointestinal (GI) component or hepatic organ failure. Also, platelet counts are now included, which may have some prognostic significance.

Christou et al. reported a 20-year follow-up of 4292 patients in which they studied the delayed-type hypersensitivity (DTH) skin test.[8] They found that, overall, hospital surgical mortality was 11.4% during the 1970s, 10.2% during the 1980s, and fell to 4.0% during the 1990s. They concluded that this decrease in overall hospital surgical mortality was due to improved preoperative, intraoperative, and postoperative care. However, there was no change in the mortality of patients who required intensive care. They also reviewed septic-related mortality and found that during the 1970s patients who reacted to the DTH skin test had 4.2% mortality, whereas those who were anergic or nonreactive had 34% mortality. During the 1980s these rates were 2.8% and 28.1%, respectively. During the 1990s they had fallen to 1.7% for reactive patients and 7.4% for those who were anergic. This was no longer a significant difference. These authors also found that walk-in elective patients, whether reactive or nonreactive, had similar outcomes, so being nonreactive or anergic made no difference if the patient was ambulatory and in otherwise reasonable health. They suggested that the reason the incidence of ICU deaths did not change is that there is a continuing bacterial challenge in these patients. They concluded that over the last 5 years of the study, with a reduction in overall patient mortality, the contribution of a reduced DTH skin test response to septic-related mortality was no longer important. However, a reduced DTH skin test response maintained a strong association with sepsis-related mortality in ICU/trauma patients.

In their Hannover, Germany trauma unit, Regel et al. compared the morbidity and mortality rates for the decade 1972–1981 with rates for the decade 1982–1991.[9] They found that during the second decade prehospital care had improved immensely. Most patients received intravenous fluids for resuscitation in the field (98%), intubation was carried out in 91% of patients, and chest tube insertions were done in 76% of patients. Rescue times were shorter, and ultrasonography had replaced abdominal peritoneal lavage. CT scans were also used routinely for head injuries. They found an increase in head and thoracic injuries during the second decade, but the improvement in patient outcome was considerable. Renal failure greatly decreased in trauma patients, almost to the point of disappearing. The incidence of acute respiratory distress syndrome (ARDS) also decreased significantly. Overall mortality decreased from 37% to 22%; but the incidence of MOF increased from 15.4% during the earlier decade to 28.2% during the second decade. In addition, lethal MOF increased from 13.8% to 18.6%. They concluded that more severely injured patients stayed alive longer to develop MOF and then died. This, then, is the group to focus on to try to improve the mortality rate by decreasing the possibility of developing MOF. Prevention is the key.

Offner et al. reviewed the temporal trends and postinjury MOF incidence and outcome over a 5-year period in the trauma center in Denver.[10] They found that the annual incidence of postinjury MOF and MOF case mortality did not change significantly over a 5-year period at their institution using a consistent definition of MOF. The incidence of MOF was 17% with an overall mortality of 37% in those patients. They recommended continued efforts to identify effective clinical interventions in patients at risk for MOF. Again, the question must be raised as to whether more seriously ill patients are surviving and develop MOF, so the overall patient mortality rate may be improving, although it is not demonstrated in this kind of study.

Ali et al., in Trinidad and Tobago, carried out a study of trauma patient outcome after several changes were instituted.[11] One was use of the Advanced Trauma Life Support program (ATLS) and the other was use of the Prehospital Trauma Life Support program (PHTLS). They found that mortality and morbidity were significantly decreased after institution of these programs, suggesting a positive impact on trauma patient outcome. They found also that age, injury severity score, and mechanism of injury were positively correlated wit mortality both before and after these changes. Controls were historic, however, and there were several limitations to the study. Other changes in trauma care, resuscitation, and intensive care may have influenced these improvements as well.

O'Keefe et al. reviewed 10-year trends in costs, resource utilization, and survival outcome in an established trauma center in Seattle.[12] They found no change in mean age or Injury Severity Score (ISS) over the 10-year period. Crude mortality, which was 8% overall per year, did not change. Length of stay, however, decreased significantly from 9.5 days to 6.8 days. Costs increased by 16.7%, likely related to more expensive and sophisticated monitoring and diagnostic studies. When they adjusted their patient population for ISS and the Abbreviated Injury Score (AIS), they found that mortality decreased by 3% per year in patients with an ISS > 16.

Hudson-Civetta et al. used a three-armed treatment strategy in trauma patients that included administering agents to block free oxygen radical production, providing scavengers for these radicals, and bolstering natural defenses.[13] Along with this protocol they tried to normalize gastric intramucosal pH (pHi) by circulatory support. Using historic controls, they found that patients receiving this treatment program had a higher severity of illness but, despite this fact, had the same mortality rate and ICU stay. Their results seem promising and require confirmation in a randomized trial. The details of this regimen are described in a later section on multiple therapeutic agents (Chapter 57).

Are Some Clinical Problems Decreasing in Frequency?

Regel et al. described a decrease in renal failure and ARDS in trauma patients in recent years.[9] Other problems that are no longer severe threats to survival or represent improvements are shown in Table 69.1. Christou et al. documented a decreased mortality rate for elective surgery.[8] That development of trauma centers and teams has improved results for trauma victims has been well documented in the literature. Other examples can be cited. The threat of GI stress bleeding has decreased,[14] possibly due to better general patient care. Prophylaxis, which seems best with sucralfate or omeprazole, is still used commonly in severely injured or sick ICU patients.[18] Ranitidine may increase infectious complications in trauma patients.[19] Methods to control GI bleeding by nonoperative endoscopic means have also improved. How do we document these improvements? The only documentation is from reports of clinical experience. ARDS had been frequent in elderly patients with hip or long bone fractures treated by bed rest and traction. There was a revolution in patient care when early or immediate fixation or joint replacement was carried out.[15] The patients could get out of bed, and they did not require ventilator support for long; they were much better off. Then it was learned that reaming a long bone fracture to put in a nail damaged the lung, so reaming was

TABLE 69.1. Improvements in Care that Should Increase Survival: What Is Disappearing?

Gastrointestinal stress bleeding has decreased.[14]
The number of intraabdominal abscesses has decreased, and there is a greater possibility of percutaneous (nonoperative) drainage.
Peritoneal lavage is performed less often (still used in selected patients) (ultrasonography and computed tomography are more accurate).
Anesthesia-related complications are decreased (fewer accidents and errors, better techniques and monitoring).
There is decreased elective surgical mortality.[8]
There is decreased acute renal failure and acute respiratory distress syndrome (ARDS)[9] after injury and operation.
There is decreased ARDS and the need for prolonged ventilatory support with early fixation of long bone fractures.[15]
Reaming of long bone fractures is avoided.[16,17]
Earlier and rapid resuscitation after injury is done.
Trauma centers and trauma teams are designated.
There is recognition and discussion of errors in medicine in the intensive care unit (ICU), and with drug monitoring and programs to control them.[18]
Thromboembolism prophylaxis is available.
ICU monitoring and critical care are improved.
Minimal cardiac, thoracic, and abdominal procedures by video-assisted techniques are available.

stopped. Also, early fixation was not as well tolerated in those with pulmonary contusions due to trauma.[16,17]

Intraabdominal and liver abscesses have decreased in frequency. When they do occur, it is much more likely that they can be drained percutaneously without operation using computed tomography (CT) control of the catheter insertion.

Resuscitation after injury is often initiated in the field and is much more vigorous in the hospital. Complete resuscitation cannot be completed until sites of blood loss are controlled.

There have always been errors in medicine. On surgical services these errors are routinely reviewed weekly or monthly at a conference called the morbidity and mortality conference. Now there is a general move to recognize and document errors, particularly medication errors, and to find methods to decrease them.[18] This is a healthy move and should improve patients' well-being.

Thromboembolism prophylaxis by minidose heparin, or calf compression, or both has reduced the likelihood of pulmonary emboli. Better monitoring techniques such as right ventricular function measurement, venous oxygen values, and other measures are helpful.

Finally, minimal surgical procedures decrease the metabolic and neuroendocrine (stress) response to operations, improve safety, and decrease risk. Anesthesia techniques such as epidural anesthesia also decrease the response to injury, improve comfort, and help the patient get well faster.

These clinical advances may be difficult to document by an improvement in overall mortality. In fact, a patient may avoid some of these problems only to survive longer and develop other complications. This situation could increase the incidence of MOF.

Some clinical advances seem to contribute to better patient care and then fall into disuse or are never used extensively simply because they did not make enough difference. There are a number of examples, such as the use of low-molecular-weight dextran, tris(hydroxymethyl)aminomethane (THAM) 2,3 diphosphoglycerate (2,3-DPG), $NaHCO_3$, and others. Some of these methods represent modern clinical controversies, such as driving oxygen transport and oxygen consumption to supranormal values, selective gut decontamination, and vasoactive agents. Which one should be used, when, and why? They are reviewed later.

Clinical Advances That Seem to Be Important or Have Benefited Some Patients But May Not Have Produced a Decrease in Mortality

There are therapeutic contributions that make good sense clinically, but the evidence is divided over the worth of the effort. They may help in some patients with specific problems but not in all. Some are also controversial, with some trials reporting clinical improvement and others failing to document such changes. Some improve a patient's condition but do not decrease mortality. None has been accepted universally. All have active supporters and some distractors. Some of these techniques are shown in Table 69.2.

Gut

In a randomized trial of early enteral nutrition in patients having major operations, Heslin et al. found no benefit.[59] Most of these patients had no nutritional deficiencies. Braga et al. in a randomized trial after abdominal surgery[20] and Bryg et al. in a meta-analysis,[30] however, found that enriched enteral nutrition decreased severity of infection, length of stay, and days on a ventilator, but there was no change in mortality. Immediate postoperative enteral feeding may decrease morbidity and

TABLE 69.2. Areas with Clinical Advances (and Controversies).

Enteral nutrition[20,21] (immunomodulation of diet, RNA, glutamine, omega-3 fatty acids, arginine)
Gastric pH (pHi) for resuscitation[22-24]
Inhaled NO for ARDS[25-33]
High DO_2 and VO_2 during resuscitation and support[34-37]
Hypertonic/hyperoncotic solutions[38-42]
Pentoxifylline[43-45]
Selective gut decontamination[25-29]
Extracorporeal membrane oxygenation[46,47]
Abdominal compartment syndrome[48]
Staged laparotomy for trauma[49]
Abdominal reexploration for peritonitis or severe contamination, bacterial translocation, gut permeability
Techniques of ventilatory support: prone position, rotation partial liquid ventilation, permissive hypercapnia[50-55]
Hemodiafiltration by polymyxin columns[56,57]
Resuscitation by measuring of right ventricular function
Intraoperative maintenance of tissue perfusion[58]
Omeprazole suspension for stress mucosal damage[18]

impair respiratory mechanics.[60] In general, most of us believe that early immune-enhanced enteral feeding is worthwhile when tolerated by the patient.

Measurement of gastric intramucosal pH (pHi) has been found to be helpful for resuscitation and patient care, but the technique is cumbersome and has not been universally adopted.[22,23] Those who have used this monitoring technique have found it helpful for improving blood flow to the gut (perhaps microcirculatory flow) and for improving outcome. Failure to increase the pHi to normal has been associated with increased mortality.[24] Some have found selective gut decontamination to be worthwhile in general ICU patients,[25] whereas others have not found benefit in trauma ICU patients.[26] Sun et al., in a meta-analysis, determined that the possibility of this therapy reducing mortality is significantly better in patients with a high mortality risk at study entry.[27] Selective gut decontamination seems to be a therapy searching for the right patient. When this modality was used in patients with a specific disease process, such as acute pancreatitis where gut bacteria may play a role, there was reduced-mortality and general improvement.[28] Baxby et al. reviewed the 13-year history of selective decontamination and 46 trials. They recommended treating specific problems: patients with liver disease and burns and medical patients after some days in the ICU.[29] The best method for preventing stress bleeding and perforation now seems to be a simplified omeprazole suspension, particularly in ventilated ICU patients.[50]

Lungs

Another example of help in some patients is the result of a randomized phase III trial of inhaled nitric oxide (NO) for patients with ARDS. Dellinger et al. found that NO was well tolerated and produced a significant improvement in oxygenation ($PaO_2 > 20\%$) in 60% of patients, but there was no change in overall mortality or the number of days alive and off mechanical ventilation.[30] A similar result has been reported in surgical patients.[31] One editorialist group described it as a negative study,[32] whereas Zapol described the results as potentially positive.[33] He urged the use of NO in the future in patients with ventilatory failure alone (no other problems). This raises the question as to whether ARDS is truly a syndrome; it is not a disease. Perhaps some diseases that produce respiratory failure are susceptible to inhaled NO and others are not. It is worth trying. Mathison et al. have reported on early use of inhaled NO in patients developing ARDS after lung resection (a homogeneous group).[61] Previously, the mortality was 85.7%. With NO, the PaO_2/FiO_2 ratio and chest radiograph improved progressively in all patients. Seven of ten patients survived; the other three died of sepsis). None died of ARDS.

Extracorporeal membrane oxygenation (ECMO) has provided survival for some patients with severe respiratory failure not alleviated by any other means.[46,47] These patients would certainly have died otherwise.

Patients with ARDS who require ventilator support seem to benefit from rotational kinetic therapy and positioning from time to time in the prone position.[50–52] Other ventilator strategies that seem to help include inverse-ratio ventilation[53,54] and permissive hypercapnia.[55]

Circulation

Patients who achieve an adequate or high oxygen transport (DO_2) and oxygen consumption (VO_2) after an injury or operation or with an illness are more likely to survive.[34,35] Some believe that if treatment can drive the DO_2 and VO_2 to supranormal values, the chances of survival are increased.[36] Others have found evidence to the contrary.[37] All in all, a sick patient is better off having a high DO_2 and VO_2 unless these are artificially increased by catecholamines. It has been known for many years that patients after injury or operation or with sepsis must be able to increase the cardiac index to survive.

Hypertonic solutions (saline-dextran) have been found to be of great benefit in animal experiments[38] and in some clinical trials.[39,40] However, the benefit has not been great enough that these solutions have been used commonly or routinely. The same is true for synthetic colloids such as pentastarch, which is safe and efficient and reduces the intravenous volumes required for resuscitation.[41] The one area where hypertonic solutions may be of specific value is in patients with head injury. Such solutions do not increase the intracranial pressure and tend to decrease it.[42]

Thangathurai et al. maintained intraoperative tissue perfusion by giving nitroglycerin and fluids to high risk patients. None of 155 patients, developed ARDS.[58] This is a promising, physiologic approach to patient care. Its use requires verification.

Pentoxifylline has a number of admirable qualities demonstrated in experimental animals, such as restoring cardiac performance and tissue perfusion and decreasing susceptibility to sepsis.[43] Thus it should be worthwhile clinically. Two clinical trials have suggested some hemodynamic improvement (e.g., increased DO_2 and VO_2).[44,45] Whether these changes are enough for this agent to be used more widely must be determined.

Recognition of the abdominal compartment syndrome and then decompression certainly benefits patients with this problem.[48] Staged laparotomy for trauma patients who developed hypothermia acidosis and a coagulopathy in the operating room provided survival in some.[49] The patients would otherwise have died in the operating room.

Hirasawa et al. continue to use hemodiafiltration in ICU patients.[56] Recently they found decreased cytokine mediators and an improved respiratory index and tissue oxygenation in patients with ARDS who received this treatment. Honore et al. also found it to be beneficial.[57]

Hypothermia does not protect trauma patients and should be corrected rapidly.[62] Maintaining a normal temperature intraoperatively seems to decrease wound infections.[63] Friedman et al. reviewed 131 studies of patients with septic shock and concluded that there was a slight reduction in mortality from 1958 to 1997.[64] However, the heterogeneity of the patients and the absence of severity scores limit the usefulness of this result. Gram-positive causative organisms become more common and the site of origin was more commonly in the chest than in the abdomen. These findings indicate the ICU problem of resistant gram-positive organisms and nosocomial pneumonia. An accompanying editorial by Cohen emphasized the ICU problem of nosocomial infection and drug resistance.[65]

There are certainly many other experiences and therapies that may be worthwhile and could be cited. In this survey we have given only some examples that seem to us to be important. We have not tried to be exhaustive in this review.

Are these then negative or positive studies? Some help is provided to the patient but not enough to decrease the death rate among those treated. There is another interpretation, which I now favor. In complex clinical situations in very sick patients, an adjunctive or supplementary therapy may help the patient, but it requires more than that single intervention to avoid mortality. It is also possible that such an intervention could be helpful in a certain group of patients but not in others. If you spread a wide net for entry into a study, the results may be negative because of the many different disease processes in the sick patients in the study.

Treatment of Symptoms or Manifestations of Disease: Lumpers and Splitters

Previously we argued that treatment of symptoms or the manifestations of a disease would be only palliative. Stehben urged us to focus on the causes of diseases.[66] He stated: "It is essential to differentiate between specific diseases and those conditions which represent a class of disorders, complications common to many diseases and merely symptoms, signs, a physical state or laboratory findings. Treatment of a disease, when based on symptoms or clinical manifestations, is at best palliative and nonspecific." Aspirin for the flu may make the patient feel better, but it does nothing to deter the underlying disease. This is exemplified by therapeutic efforts to treat SIRS. What would you do?

We tend to lump sick patients together in various classifications of categories based on severity, the possibility of death, clinical manifestations, ICU admissions, and other criteria such as the APACHE, SAPS, SIRS, MODS, MOF, and ISS. If such classifications of patients are used as the entry criteria for therapy trials, we may miss important treatments. Some therapies may be excellent for certain diseases or abnormalities and worthless for others even though the disease severity may be similar in both.

Some clinical advances seem to contribute to better patient care and then fall into disuse simply because they did not make *enough* difference. They are not worth the trouble.

Finally, how do we measure the impact or overall improvement in survival when 50% of patients with ARDS who are put on ECMO survive? The predicted mortality without ECMO would be 100%. The same is true of other approaches, such as staged laparotomy.

Conclusions

Levine, with us, described MOF and raised the question as to whether it was disappearing.[67] He found that the incidence of MOF during the last decade was reported variously as 2% to 25%, depending on the patient population. The mortality rates from this devastating complication ranged from 40% to 80%. Although the incidence does not seem to have changed during the last decade, it does not mean that there has been no progress. Tertiary centers are now seeing trauma and nontrauma patients who have more extensive underlying disease and injury. In the past, these patients would not have survived long enough to reach the hospital, operating room, or ICU—or to develop MOF.

A higher percentage of our trauma patients are now referred from outside institutions that do not have the facilities to provide the complex rapid resuscitation these patients require. We believe that prevention of MOF remains its best treatment. Rapid, adequate volume resuscitation, adequate nutrition, appropriate antibiotic usage, and aggressive pulmonary management are important for reversing the downward physiologic spiral that leads to MOF and death. In surgical and trauma patients, it is critical to have the correct diagnosis, optimal preparation of the patient, best time for the operation, appropriate anesthesia and monitoring, a technically correct procedure with no defects or technical errors, and careful postoperative monitoring with no errors, minimizing risk. Aggressive support of normal organ function and prevention of complications are the best hope for preventing MODS and MOF. Once MOF has occurred, it is not clear that these same measures can alter outcome as effectively.

There is evidence of decreased mortality in patients undergoing elective surgical procedures and of increased survival of patients after injury. The incidence of MOF does not seem to have changed, however, and may have increased in some situations. Mortality, once MOF develops, remains high. Despite this fact, there has been progress. We are slowly and carefully winning the battle, but it is far from over. There are many advances and improvements in the care of patients. It is difficult to document their overall benefit except for individual patients or small groups of patients.

Christou et al. found no decrease in ICU mortality over the years.[8] Offner et al. found the same.[10] They believe that more severely injured patients are reaching the ICU alive; hence there has been improvement, but it is difficult to document. If sicker patients reach the ICU or higher risk patients survive, the incidence of MOF and the mortality would remain as they had been. Zimmerman et al. found that there had been a significant decrease in mortality among patients who develop MOF in ICUs, an encouraging finding.[7]

Major advances with reduced mortality will accompany injury and disease prevention. Many of the risk factors for death due to trauma and illness are beyond our control. They are present when we first see the patients. Each of us should actively practice disease and injury prevention. Have we stood up to be counted on gun control, drunken driving, auto safety, smoking and prevention of home fires that result from smoking, obesity, stroke, and cardiac risk factors?

Finally, we raise the question as to whether mortality can be reduced in patients who require ICU care for a prolonged period. Such reduction is not easy, and it cannot happen quickly. Perhaps we must do a number of things, each of which improves an ICU patient's condition to some extent and collectively improves survival. These steps forward have been called "critical care creep." It is difficult to document. Large databases, such as those of Zimmerman et al.[7] and Knaus et al.,[68] may be able to quantitate this phenomenon. Petros and Van Saene have asked whether mortality is the best or only endpoint for prolonged care in an ICU.[69] In the meanwhile, we continue to fine-tune our efforts to alleviate a gross problem.

References

1. Baue AE, Durham RM, Faist E: Systemic inflammatory response syndrome (SIRS), multiple organ dysfunction syndrome (MODS), multiple organ failure (MOF): are we winning the battle? Shock 1998;10:79–89.
2. Baue AE: Multiple organ failure. multiple organ dysfunction syndrome and the systemic inflammatory response syndrome: where do we stand? Shock 1994;2:385–339.
3. Sackett D, Rosenberg W: The need for evidence-based medicine. J R Soc Med 1995;88:620–624.
4. Piper R, Cook D, Bone R, Sibblad W: Introducing critical appraisal to studies of animal models investigating novel therapies in sepsis. Crit Care Med 1996;24:2059–2070.
5. Baue AE: Multiple organ failure, multiple organ dysfunction syndrome, and the systemic inflammatory response syndrome: why no magic bullets? Arch Surg 1997;132:703–707.
6. Baue AE: What is clinical relevance? In: Baue AE, Berlot E, Gullo A, Vincent JL (ed) Sepsis and Organ Dysfunction. Milano, Springer, 1997;95–104.
7. Zimmerman J, Knaus W, Wagner D, et al: A comparison of risks and outcomes for patients with organ system failure: 1982–1990. Crit Care Med 1996;24:1633–1641.
8. Christou N, Meakins J, Gordon J, et al: The delayed hypersensitivity response and host resistance in surgical patients 20 years later. Ann Surg 1995;222:534–548.
9. Regel G, Lobenhoffer P, Grotz M, et al: Treatment results of patients with multiple trauma: an analysis of 3406 cases treated between 1972 and 1991 at a German level I trauma center. J Trauma 1995;38:70–78.
10. Offner P, Moore F, Sauaia A, Moore E: Temporal trends in postinjury MOF incidence and outcome. J Trauma (in press).
11. Ali J, Adam R, Gana T, Williams J: Trauma patient outcome after the prehospital trauma life support program. J Trauma 1997;42:1018–1022.
12. O'Keefe GE, Jurkovich GJ, Maier RV: 10-Year trends in costs, resource utilization, and survival outcome in an established trauma center. Surg Forum 1997;48:595–597.
13. Hudson-Civetta J, Civetta J, Kirton O, et al: Mitigating increased severity of illness in trauma patients. Crit Care Med 1998;26:A94.
14. Shuman RB, Schuster DP, Zuckerman GR: Prophylactic therapy for stress bleeding: a reappraisal. Ann Intern Med 1987;106:562–567.
15. Goris RJA, Gimbrere JSF, van Niekerk JLM, et al: Early osteosynthesis and prophylactic mechanical ventilation in the multitrauma patient. J Trauma 1982;22:895.
16. Pape HC, Auf'm Kolk M, Paffrath T, et al: Primary intramedullary femur fixation in multiple trauma patients with associated lung contusion: a cause of post-traumatic ARDS? J Trauma 1993;34:540–548.
17. Pelias ME, Townsend C, Flancbaum L: Long bone fractures predispose to pulmonary dysfunction in blunt chest trauma despite early operative fixation. Surgery 1992;111:576–579.
18. Phillips JO, Metzler MH, Palmieri MTL, et al: A prospective study of simplified omeprazole suspension for the prophylaxis of stress-related mucosal damage. Crit Care Med 1996;24:1793–1800.
19. O'Keefe GE, Gentilello LM, Maier RV: Incidence of infectious complications associated with the use of histamine$_2$-receptor antagonists in critically ill trauma patients. Ann Surg 1998;227:120–125.
20. Braga M, Gianotti L, Vignali A, et al: Artificial nutrition after major abdominal surgery: impact of route of administration and composition of the diet. Crit Care Med 1998;260:24–30.
21. Bryg DJ, Beale RJ: Clinical effects of enteral immunonutrition on intensive care patients: a meta-analysis. Crit Care Med 1998;26:A91.
22. Ljubanovic M, Calvin J, Peruzzi W: Meta-analysis of gastric pH as determinant of mortality in critically ill patients. Crit Care Med 1998;26:A123.
23. Kirton O, Civetta J, Hudson-Civetta J, et al: Gastric intramucosal pH (pHi) driven resuscitation and anti-oxidants: normalized pHi is associated with high survival. Crit Care Med 1998;26:A142.
24. Ivatury RR, Simon RJ, Islam S, et al: A prospective randomized study of end points of resuscitation after major trauma. J Am Coll Surg 1996;183:145–154.
25. Vandenbrouke-Grauls CMJ, Vandenbroucke JP: Effect of selective decontamination of the digestive tract on respiratory infections and mortality in the intensive care unit. Lancet 1991;338:859–862.
26. Lingnau W, Berger J, Javorsy F, et al: Selective intestinal decontamination in multiple trauma patients: prospective controlled trial. J Trauma 1997;42:687–694.
27. Sun X, Wagner DP, Knaus WA: Does selective decontamination of the digestive tract reduce mortality for severely ill patients? Crit Care Med 1996;24:753–755.
28. Luiten EJ, Hop WCJ, Lange JE, Bruining HA: Controlled clinical trial of selective decontamination for the treatment of severe acute pancreatitis. Ann Surg 1995;222:57–65.
29. Baxby D, van Saene HKF, Stoutenbeek CP, Zandstra DF: Selective decontamination of the digestive tract: 13 years on, what it is and what it is not. Intensive Care Med 1996;22:699–706.
30. Dellinger RP, Zimmerman JL, Taylor RW, et al: Effects of inhaled nitric oxide in patients with acute respiratory distress syndrome: results of a randomized phase II trial. Crit Care Med 1998;26:15–23.
31. Johannigman JA, Davis K Jr, Campbell RS, et al: Inhaled nitric oxide in acute respiratory distress syndrome. J Trauma 1997;43:904–910.
32. Matthay MA, Pittet JF, Jayr C: Just say NO to inhaled nitric oxide for the acute respiratory distress syndrome. Crit Care Med 1998;26:1–2.
33. Zapol WM: Nitrix oxide inhalation in acute respiratory distress syndrome: it works, but can we prove it? Crit Care Med 1998;26:2–3.

34. Moore FA, Haenel JB, Moore EE, Whitehill TA: Incommensurate oxygen consumption in response to maximal oxygen availability predicts postinjury multiple organ failure. J Trauma 1992;33:58-66.
35. Durham RM, Neunaber K, Mazuski JE, et al: The use of oxygen consumption and delivery as endpoints for resuscitation in critically ill patients. J Trauma 1996;41:32-40.
36. Shoemaker WC, Appel PL, Kram HB, et al: Prospective trial of supranormal values of survivors as therapeutic goals in high-risk surgical patients. Chest 1988;94:1176-1188.
37. Gattinoni L, Brazzi L, Pelosi P, et al: A trial of goal-oriented hemodynamic therapy in critically ill patients. N Engl J Med 1995;333:1025-1032.
38. Moore EE: Hypertonic saline dextran for post-injury resuscitation: experimental background and clinical experience. Aust NZ J Surg 1991;61:732-736.
39. Vassar JJ, Perry CA, Gannaway WL, Holcroft JW: 7.5% Sodium chloride/dextran for resuscitation of trauma patients undergoing helicopter transport. Arch Surg 1991;126:1065-1072.
40. Wade CE, Kramer GC, Grady JJ, et al: Efficacy of hypertonic 7.5% saline and 6% dextran-70 in treating trauma: a meta-analysis of controlled clinical studies. Surgery 1997;122:609-616.
41. Younes RN, Yin KC, Amino CJ, et al: Use of pentastarch solution in the treatment of patients with hemorrhagic hypovolemia: randomized phase II study in the emergency room. World J Surg 1998;22:2-5.
42. Shackford SR, Bourguignon PR, Wald SL, et al: Hypertonic saline resuscitation of patients with head injury: a prospective, randomized clinical trial. J Trauma 1998;44:50-58.
43. Robinson DA, Wang P, Chaudry IH: Pentoxifylline restores the depressed cardiac performance after trauma-hemorrhage and resuscitation. J Surg Res 1996;66:51-56.
44. Staubach K-H, Schroder J, Stuber, et al: Effect of pentoxifilline in severe sepsis. Arch Ital Surg 1998;133:94-100.
45. Bacher A, Mayer N, Klimscha W, et al: Effects of pentoxifylline on hemodynamics and oxygenation in septic and nonseptic patients. Crit Care Med 1997;25:795-800.
46. Kolla S, Awad SS, Rich PB, et al: Extracorporeal life support for 100 adult patients with severe respiratory failure. Ann Surg 1997;226:544-566.
47. Peek GJ, Moore HM, Moore N, et al: Extracorporeal membrane oxygenation for adult respiratory failure. Chest 1997;112:759-764.
48. Meldrum DR, Moore FA, Moore EE, et al: Prospective characterization and selective management of the abdominal compartment syndrome. Am J Surg 1997;174:667-673.
49. Moore EE: Staged laparotomy for the hypothermia, acidosis and coagulopathy syndrome. Am J Surg 1996;172:405-410.
50. Stiletto R, Bruck E, Bittner G: Low cost prone positioning of critically ill ARDS patients with MPS (modular prone positioning system). Crit Care 1998;2:59.
51. Raguin O, Rusterholtz T, Berton C, et al: Use of a clinical protocol to assess the respective indications of prone position and nitric oxide in patients with ARDS. Crit Care 1998;2:58.
52. Stiletto RJ, Bruck E, Ziering E, Gotzen L: The role of positioning in the prevention of ALI and ARDS in polytrauma patients. Crit Care 1998;2:58.
53. Abraham E, Yoshihara G: Cardiorespiratory effects of pressure controlled inverse ratio ventilation in severe respiratory failure. Chest 1989;96:1356-1359.
54. Poelart JI, Visser CA, Everaert JA: Acute hemodynamic changes of pressure controlled inverse ratio ventilation in the adult respiratory distress syndrome. Chest 1993;104:214-219.
55. Schmidt GA, Wood LDH: Critical care medicine. JAMA 1993;270:192-196.
56. Hirasawa H, Sugai T, Oda S, et al: Continuous hemodiafiltration (CHDF) removes cytokines and improves respiratory index (RI) and oxygen metabolism in patients with acute respiratory distress syndrome (ARDS). Crit Care Med 1998;26:A120.
57. Honore PM, James J, Wauthier M, Dugernier T: Reversal of intractable circulatory failure complicating septic shock with shock with short time high volume haemofiltration (ST-HV-CVVH) after failure of conventional therapy: a prospective evaluation. Crit Care 1998;2:62.
58. Thangathurai D, Charbornnet C, Wo CCJ, et al: Intraoperative maintenance of tissue perfusion prevents ARDS. New Horiz 1996;4:466-474.
59. Heslin MJ, Latkany L, Leung D, et al: A prospective, randomized trial of early enteral feeding after resection of upper GI malignancy. Ann Surg (in press).
60. Watters JM, Kirkpatrick SM, Norris SB, et al: Immediate postoperative enteral feeding results in impaired respiratory mechanics and decreased mobility. Ann Surg 1997;226:369-380.
61. Mathisen DJ, Kuo EY, Hahn C, et al: Inhaled nitric oxide for adult respiratory distress syndrome after pulmonary resection. Ann Thorac Surg 1998;65:1894-1982.
62. Gentielelo LM, Jurkovich GJ, Stark MS, et al: Is hypothermia in the victim of major trauma protective or harmful? Ann Surg 1997;226:439-449.
63. Kurz A, Sessler DI, Lenhardt R: Perioperative normothermia to reduce the incidence of surgical-wound infection and shorten hospitalization. N Engl J Med 1996;334:1209-1215.
64. Friedman G, Silva E, Vincent JL: Has the mortality of septic shock changed with time? Crit Care Med 1998;23:2078-2086.
65. Cohen NH: Reduced mortality from septic shock: lessons for the future. Crit Care Med 1998;26:1956-1958.
66. Stehben WE: Causality in medical science with particular reference to heart disease and arteriosclerosis. Perspect Biol Med 1993;36:97-119.
67. Levine JH, Durham RM, Moran J, Baue A: Multiple organ failure: is it disappearing? World J Surg 1996;20:471-473.
68. Knaus W, Draper E, Wagner D, Zimmerman J: Prognosis in acute organ-system failure. Ann Surg 1985;202:685-693.
69. Petros A, Van Saene R: Is reduction in mortality in intensive care just another Holy Grail? In: Gullo A (ed) Critical Care Medicine A.P.I.C.E. 12. Milan, Springer, 1998;495-498.

70
Ethical Considerations of MODS, SIRS, and MOF

Rosemary Dysart Baue

Physicians, particularly surgeons and intensivists who work on the cutting edge of technology and in areas of quick decisions, not only must remember that their patients are persons but they must stay current with legislative and managed care parameters affecting the essence of treatment, the doctor–patient relationship. In this chapter the "technologic imperative," patients' rights, and professional and administrative responsibility are discussed. A case study involving multiple ethical-moral issues illustrates the considerations.

Our current use of impersonal language when discussing medical "cases" points to the first ethical consideration. People are reduced to "thing-hood" when we refer to futile cases; human beings disappear when we speak of health care professionals and managed care organizations. The "case study" below describes a desperately ill wife and mother of seven children who needed compassionate doctors and nurses in a hospital with ethically responsible administrators.

Case Study*

Mrs. Smith underwent a right upper lobectomy for carcinoma of the lung at age 53. A year later she had an endarterectomy, and the phrenic nerve was injured on the same side. Shortly afterward Mrs. Smith experienced an episode of severe shortness of breath and thereafter was subject to mild panic attacks but did not cease smoking. Four years after the thoracotomy tiny malignant polyps were found in Mrs. Smith's colon. She underwent colon resection at St. Cecelia Hospital where the chest radiographs revealed no metastases from either colon or lungs. While in the hospital Mrs. Smith completed an advance directive notarized by the St. Cecelia notary that was placed on file at the hospital. The directive, a copy of which she gave to her sister, stated that Mrs. Smith was to have no extraordinary means of treatment, and should she be in a terminal state Mrs. Smith was not to be intubated.

Seven years after the thoracotomy, Mrs. Smith began to have great difficulty breathing and was unable to sleep in a supine position. She also had severe left anterolateral chest pain. Dr. Johnson, the family internist for 20 years, primarily prescribing by telephone, was apparently convinced that fear of panic attacks caused Mrs. Smith's breathing problems. He sent her for both breathing therapy and treatment of an old leg injury. After several weeks of sleeping with her head on a table, Mrs. Smith's breathing difficulty was so severe one night her husband Ben took her to the St. Cecelia emergency room (ER). Mrs. Smith was admitted to the intensive care unit (ICU) for 2 weeks, where she acquired bacterial endocarditis from a central line and thus had to remain in the hospital for another 2 months. Dr. Johnson ordered several tests, including a computed tomography (CT) scan, none of which disclosed a malignancy. Although a consultant suggested a biopsy, it was not ordered, and Mrs. Smith was discharged. Her smoking finally ceased during her hospital stay.

Two months later Mrs. Smith was again admitted for the same breathing problems and severe chest pain. After more negative tests a biopsy was ordered. A minithoracotomy was performed that revealed multiple tumor implants on the pleura, diaphragm, and mediastinum. Only palliative treatment was feasible. Dr. Johnson had shifted responsibility to a number of specialists, none of whom provided continuity of care. During the following 2 weeks, no radiotherapy or chemotherapy was instituted to allow Mrs. Smith her fervent wish to return home despite the recommendation by a consultant that it be done, nor was she appraised of the fact that recovery was not possible. The window of opportunity for therapy or returning home closed when, experiencing difficulty breathing one night, Mrs. Smith was intubated and taken to the ICU on a ventilator. No one, including her immediate family, had checked for an advance directive. The sister with a copy of her directive was in another state and, like Mrs. Smith and her family, was unaware of the terminal condition. Mrs. Smith was intubated, ventilated, and restrained.

Mrs. Smith had six children in the same city. Her oldest daughter was not convinced of her vegetative state, nor was her sister who came into town. Using one finger to respond to questions, Mrs. Smith was able to communicate her wish for patient autonomy. Now, contrary to her advance directive, Mrs. Smith indicated that she wanted to stay alive. Therefore within a few days, she had a tracheotomy for ventilation, a long-term

---
*Only names were changed in this case study.

epidural catheter for pain relief, and a percutaneous gastrostomy for feeding. Neither Mrs. Smith's sister, who reminded the hospital of the advance directive, nor Ben Smith, whose law firm represented the hospital, were inclined to go to court; nevertheless, Mrs. Smith was kept in the ICU for 2 months before the insurance company refused to reimburse further and for another 2 weeks at the hospital's expense. By this time she was seldom fully conscious, and other manifestations of the disease were appearing. Mrs. Smith was taken to the only nursing home in the area that accepted ventilated patients.

After a month the family, finally in complete consensus, authorized gradual removal of the ventilator. Although the physician for the nursing home gave the order, one nurse objected strenuously, personally unable to allow death. Mrs. Smith's family was with her for the removal of the ventilator. She did not regain consciousness and was pronounced dead within a few hours.

This case study demonstrates a number of considerations and some actual violations of ethical medical practice within the realms of the physician–patient–family relationships. Using ethics terminology, the problems are the physician–patient relationship, benefit versus burden, economic distributive justice, allocation of scarce resources, professional responsibility, administrative responsibility, informed consent, advance medical directives, and consensus about ethical principles by caregivers. The leap from ethical theory to treating a particular person whose therapy involves systemic inflammatory response syndrome (SIRS), multiple organ dysfunction syndrome (MODS), and multiple organ failure (MOF) is never short or easy. The right to care with excellence in the art and science of medical practice requires an understanding of pertinent ethical considerations by all persons involved in a patient's care.

"I Can, Therefore I Must"

Technologic imperatives—"I can, therefore I must"—or the intellectual equivalent—"I know, therefore I must"—need to be balanced with moral and ethical imperatives.[1] Prolongation of life or prevention of death is no longer the recognizable overriding factor in health care. The development of medical, or health care ethics has increased physician awareness for the moral domain, the rights of patients, and the needs and religious parameters of patients and their families. An acceptable definition of "futility of care" becomes increasingly important. O'Rourke defined futile therapy as that which prolongs physiologic function when "one has lost the capacity to pursue the goods of life, when the power to think, love and relate to others will never be restored."[2] In our case study there was no compelling definition guiding patient, physicians, nurses, or hospital and managed care administrators. Mrs. Smith, although ventilator-dependent, did not meet O'Rourke's definition for many weeks, regardless of how extraordinary or expensive was her treatment. Medical technology is enabling startling numbers of patients to straddle life, death, and futile therapy.

Physicians are doubtless aware of factors driving debates over clear criteria for responsibility, such as the shift of insistence for further interventions, from physicians to patients and their families. Patient autonomy and advances in patients' rights are pitted against the conscience of physicians; and managed care practices to reduce health care expenditures are changing the definition of nonbeneficial interventions. The notion of rationing underlies much of the concern in ethical futility debates. Levinsky argued that society has the right to ration care "provided that the limitation of appropriate, effective care is openly revealed."[3] He concluded that Americans are willing to pay the price necessary to avoid undisguised rationing of medical care, a conclusion supported by the actions taken in the case study and the length of Mrs. Smith's stay in the ICU. Less nobility of public conscience is seen in the acceptance of the rationing of medical care for the poor in the Oregon Plan.[3]

For Mrs. Smith, the technologic imperative was implemented too late in the process of care, calling attention to timing as well as ability. Simpler, less expensive radiotherapy instituted immediately by her physician might have enabled Mrs. Smith to return home for her remaining weeks or months. Such decisions, best made prospectively, fall into an increasingly large "gray" area of treatment that was once "black and white." What must a physician do who deems futile the care insisted on by a patient or a patient's family? The issue of physician refusal of requested care has not been resolved by law or legal statute; it is supported only by ethical principles. Luce wrote that physicians are not ethically required to provide futile or unreasonable care, especially to patients who are brain-dead, vegetative, critically or terminally ill, or unlikely to benefit from resuscitation.[4] Civetta claimed that "the ideal case is resolutions of conflict between the family and providers before any outsiders need to be involved."[5]

Ethical problems increase for physicians when patients in advanced stages of Alzheimer's disease or senility are in various stages of unresponsiveness. At what point is treatment futile when quality of life is not improved and the patient will be returned to custodial or institutional care? These patients are brought to ERs with surgical emergencies, such as a perforated ulcer, perforated diverticulitis, acute cholecystitis, or a perforated colon cancer; and a surgeon performs an operation to correct the acute problem. After the fact, with the patient in the ICU, the family and surgeon agree on "do not resuscitate" (DNR) when an advance directive, properly stated and made known, might have prevented the senseless operation. Frequently when a family insists on treatment, against the judgment of a physician, the insistence is motivated by guilt. For example, a son refused an autopsy on his father when a physician wished to determine the cause of death because the son had not seen his father in 10 years but was now going to "protect my father from further suffering."[6]

Those things which science must expurgate from consideration—the personal, the ambiguous—are the very things which the humanities recognize as universal qualities of human experience, the very things especially heightened in confrontation with death or disease."   —Barger (cited by Pellegrino[7])

The positive effect of technology for Mrs. Smith, the "good" in ethical terminology, was quantitative rather than qualitative. The technology that placed her in the ICU for an extended time was also the technology that enabled her to be intubated through her body instead of her face—with a relatively lower discomfort level. Pellegrino wrote that medicine has "failed to yield an earthly paradise while extracting a price man may not wish to pay."[7] Technology in itself cannot be ethical, but ethical human control of technology can mitigate the technologic imperative. Proportional benefits versus burdens require clear, reasonable institutional standards on which to base the ethics of care. Two questions in regard to drawing up standards need answers: Who must live with the consequences? Why?

The Patient and Patient Rights

The progression of events in the care of Mrs. Smith demonstrates the many ways in which patients' rights can be violated. Although Dr. Johnson did not uphold the principles that are or should be inherent in doctor–patient relationships, Mrs. Smith's rights were also violated in other ways. In this era of managed care, Americans are urging Congress to legislate their rights. A poll conducted in Spring 1998 found that more than 90% of Americans would support legislation that requires health care providers to give their patients full information about their conditions and treatment options, access to in-network specialists, the right to a speedy appeal when a plan denies coverage, and provision of a complete list of benefits and costs.

Above all, the patient is a person—not a consumer. The first imperative is the Golden Rule ("Do unto others as you would have others do unto you"), which has a counterpart in every major religion and culture. A unique definition for compassion emerged in a project I once did for Henri Nouwen when he was on the faculty of the Yale Divinity School. I solicited the admissions committee for the medical school and some of the department chairmen for their definition of compassion. Several replied that, in relation to patient care, excellence was a better definition than the Latin derivative of com + pati, to bear or suffer with. Certainly, as a patient, and particularly with a surgeon or an intensivist, excellence has priority. Excellence without empathy, however, may not be effective. The patient needs to feel the imaginative projection of the physician's state of mind into his or her own state. It is a mistake for a physician to underestimate the power of a patient's psyche.

A clinical example of the power of empathy was given by Bellet and Maloney[8] to caution against a hasty remark of reassurance that increases anxiety. The mother of a boy suspected of meningitis initially refused the diagnostic lumbar puncture.

Physician: What concerns you about the spinal tap?
Mother: I refuse to give consent.
Physician (*calm and interested*): Tell me more about why you are worried.
Mother: I think my son will get better without that long needle.
Physician (*using active listening to reflect the mother's concern and his understanding without lecturing*): You are concerned about the length of the needle.
Mother: Yes, I'm concerned. It could make him bleed into his back.
Physician (*understanding the fear rather than repeating the explanation*): What do you mean?
Mother: My neighbor's father had a bad time with headaches after a spinal tap, and Johnny is sick enough already.
Physician (*verbalizing his understanding of the fear*): You don't want your sick child to suffer more discomfort. It is difficult for you to put him in that painful situation.
Mother (*relaxing and now able to listen to the physician and his advice*): Yes, I'm confused. Maybe it wouldn't hurt him like it did my neighbor's father. How long is the needle?

Time for empathy that decreases anxiety and increases the feeling that the physician understands is both time- and cost-effective. In the words of Peabody, "the secret of the care of the patient is in caring for the patient."[9]

Physician paternalism has shifted to respect for autonomy of patients in which patients make decisions about care in consultation with their physicians. Physicians, as personal examples[5] and as a lobbying group, must ensure all patients the right to treatment information, the right to privacy and dignity, the right to refuse care, the right to emergency care, and the right to an advocate.[10] During the early 1970s there was an effort to regulate health care, but physicians and health care administrators vowed to voluntarily honor regulations and directives. O'Rourke maintained that there have been too many different people and institutions involved for initiatives to regulate health care voluntarily to succeed. The President's Advisory Commission on Consumer Protection and Quality in the Health Care Industry declined to endorse the use of legislation to define and enforce the rights of patients as consumers in relation to activities of insurance companies and employers. O'Rourke stated that "opting for voluntary directives to protect patients' rights will once again put the fox in charge of the hen house."[10] President Clinton in 1997, appointed an advisory commission for protection and quality of the health care industry, which provided an outline of what could be a National Bill of Rights for patients. Then in the President's State of the Union message on Jan. 28, 1998 he proposed a National Bill of Rights in Health Care in which he stated "You have the right to know all of your medical options, not just the cheapest. You have the right to choose the doctor you want for the care you need. You have the right to emergency care, wherever and whenever you need it. You have the right to keep your medical records confidential." This is now the subject of debate by many groups. Recently, a Federal Appeals Court ruled that Medicare patients are entitled to immediate hearings and other protection when they are denied care by Health Maintenance Organizations (HMO's). Pear in his discussion of this, pointed out that "the decision of Medicare is significant because it holds that its beneficiaries have rights that are rooted in the Constitution, not merely in statues or regulations subject to change by Congress and the President.[12] This was the result of a class actions suit filed in Arizona on behalf of nearly six million medicare patients and HMO's around the country. There will very likely be more such legal actions in the near future." This court decision along with the Presidents push indicates that the final shape of a bill for Patients Rights should come from a wide ranging public and congressional debate and the important ingredients should be:

1) The right to treatment information.
2) The right to privacy and dignity.
3) The right to refuse treatment.
4) The right to emergency care.
5) The right to an advocate.

Such action, if and when approved, will be good for you, the patient and hopefully will protect you in your options for care. What this does not address is the access to health care for all Americans and that is another matter that should be taken up nationally. Each hospital should provide for you when you are admitted a brochure on Advanced directives and patients' rights. The Yale New Haven Hospital in Connecticut and many hospitals give each patient a brochure describing their rights, responsibilities and ethical decisions. Rights include respect, privacy, a full explanation of care, knowing who is taking care of you, confidentiality, emotional support and informed decision making. So far such legislation has not been passed by the Congress. The physician, already stretched, must also be cognizant of both the effect of his or her patient's medical coverage for the amount of care covered and the patient's attitude toward care as a result of the coverage.

Primary decisions are made by the patient, the patient's family, and the physician. Mrs. Smith's primary decision team was not functioning because her primary physician did not provide continuity, her advance directive was not in her chart, and the family either did not know of it or did not think to request it. Before her middle of the night trip to be ventilated and put in the ICU, Mrs. Smith was perfectly capable of declaring her wishes. Once consultants were called, there was no clear authority to monitor Mrs. Smith's privacy, dignity, and willingness to undertake her care. After the endotracheal tube allowed her to communicate, it was unclear whether Mrs. Smith understood how terminal was her condition or how capable she was of making decisions. At the same time there was a wide range of reactions and opinions in her large family.

The Patient Self-Determination Act was passed in 1991. A recent study by Teno and colleagues of George Washington Center to Improve Care for the Dying revealed that only 14% of 4804 terminally ill patients had written medical directives.[13] Fewer than 30 of the 569 documents contained specific instructions about the use of life-sustaining treatment, and only 22 directives matched the actual situation, with care consistent with the instructions in only 11 cases.[14] The bottom line for Mrs. Smith and patients in general is that advance directives have been ineffective. A physician needs to know—ethically and legally—whether one exists, particularly when one has been prepared by the physician's institution.

Surrogate or proxy decision makers who are effective must make decisions by bonds of love rather than by legal documents proving their power of attorney. "From an ethical perspective the surrogate is the person who promotes the dignity of the patient and ensures respect for the patient, even when the patient cannot speak for himself or herself."[14] The closest family member becomes the surrogate in the absence of a legal proxy.

Mr. Smith decided that he and the children should be in consensus when the decision to remove the ventilator was made. In general, such an approach; is a loving, ethical approach; but physicians should seek assistance from helpful agents who can assist them if there are issues of benefits versus burdens and futile therapy. Helpful agents are clergy, hospital chaplains, and members of ethics committees. It is essential to understand the parameters set by the patient's religious beliefs and to know if they conflict with those of physicians, members of the family, and other caregivers, as manifested by the nurse who objected to the withdrawal of Mrs. Smith's ventilator until the end (Table 70.1).

Advance directives were meant to allow the utmost patient autonomy. They attracted attention because of the impression that medical technology and knowledge could and would exceed patients' competence to exercise their will for their health care decisions. Furthermore, "true autonomy implies a freedom of choice that is only possible when patients, their loved ones, and physicians act jointly in addressing immediate and ultimate goals."[14] In the environment of providers and consumers, such autonomy is lost. Although an advance directive should enable the physicians and families to feel comfortable about decisions, they are of no benefit if they do not reflect true autonomy. They are completely useless if, as in the case of Mrs. Smith, they are filed away in a hospital never to be seen or heard of again. Advance directives have failed to live up to their potential because there have been low completion rates, physicians have been reluctant to initiate discussions regarding them, they seldom represent *informed* consent, they have been inaccessible when needed and for both valid and invalid reasons they have not been honored by physicians.[15,16] Desperate measures, such as the Kevorkian "mercy killings" and increased membership in the Hemlock Society are simply further proof of people's fears for their end-of-life wishes.

A small but positive study to counteract disappointment in the effectiveness of SUPPORT (Study to Understand Prognoses and Preferences for Outcome and Risks of Treatment) reports a proactive ethics consultation program that improves communication and shortens the stay of ventilated patients who die in the ICU. A group of professionals at Bon Secours St. Mary's Hospital developed a program to educate the staff of individual hospitals about ethics and the need for concrete plans to improve terminal care: Two clinicians trained in clinical ethics review the patient's chart and discuss it with the care team but not the patient, surrogate, or family. They raise questions to stimulate decision making and communication about the patient's "diagnosis, prognosis, treatment objectives, availability of an advance directive, capacity to make decisions, availability of surrogate decision makers, and any issues that were not

TABLE 70.1. Religious Views on the Right to Die.

Religion	Treatment termination	Feeding tubes	Assisted suicide/active euthanasia
Adventist (Seventh-Day Adventist)	Informal consensus in favor of passive euthanasia (allowing to die) in some cases.		No official denominational position.
Baptist American Baptist Churches	The individual's right to make his/her own decisions regarding life-sustaining treatment or measures should be enhanced through relevant advance-directive legislation.		
Southern Baptist Convention (Christian Life Commission)		Supports efforts to discourage designation of food and/or water as "extraordinary" medical care for some patients.	Active euthanasia is held to violate the sanctity of human life.
Christian Church (Disciples of Christ)	Strong affirmation of liberty of conscience and freedom of individual choice on moral-ethical questions related to personal behavior.		The customary reasons for euthanasia—patient suffering and irreversible condition—are nullified by the Biblical witness to meaningful suffering and to possible healing.
Church of Christ, Scientist (Christian Scientist)	The restoration of health and well-being comes best through spiritual regeneration rather than through material methods. A choice for medical treatment is a free choice of conscience.		Christian Science teachings regarding life, death, and illness and a century-long experience of healing entail that euthanasia and assisted suicide are not a genuine expression of the faith. Euthanasia and assisted suicide are a denial of God's presence and power.
Church of Jesus Christ of Latter-Day Saints (Mormonism)	When dying becomes inevitable, it should be seen as a blessing and purposeful part of eternal existence. No obligation exists to extend mortal life by unreasonable means.		A person who participates in euthanasia—deliberately putting to death a person suffering from incurable conditions or diseases—violates the commandments of God.
Eastern Orthodox Churches Greek Orthodox Orthodox Church	Extraordinary mechanical devices may be withheld or removed when the major physical systems have broken down and there is no reasonable expectation of restoration. The spiritual welfare of the patient in some instances is best served by removing life—support machinery. Hospice and advanced directives are encouraged.	Removing feeding tubes and withholding liquids may be appropriate for a terminally ill patient if such deprivation does not cause suffering.	Euthanasia constitutes the deliberate taking of human life and as such is to be condemned as murder. Any procedure that makes active euthanasia a preferred alternative is by its very nature immoral and should be rejected.
Episcopal Church	No moral obligation to prolong dying by extraordinary means and at all costs if the dying person is hopelessly ill and has no hope of recovery. Such decisions should ultimately rest with the patient or proxy, as expressed in advance directives.	Advice of the church community should be sought in cases of persons in a comatose state from which there is no hope of recovery and for whom the withholding or removing of life-sustaining systems, including nutrition and hydration, is contemplated.	It is morally wrong to intentionally take a human life to relieve the suffering caused by incurable illness; including a lethal dose of medication or poison, use of lethal weapons, homicidal acts, and other forms of active euthanasia.

TABLE 70.1. (Continued)

Religion	Treatment termination	Feeding tubes	Assisted suicide/active euthanasia
Jehovah's Witnesses	When there is clear evidence that death is imminent and unavoidable, the Scriptures do not require that extraordinary (and perhaps costly) means be employed to stretch out the dying process.		Active euthanasia is murder and violates the sanctity of life, Christian conscience, and obedience to governmental laws.
Judaism			
Reformed	Removing the cause of delay of death or refraining from doing what will prevent dying, when death is otherwise imminent, is permitted.		The sanctity of human life means life may not be shortened or terminated because of considerations of patient convenience or usefulness, or sympathy with the patient's suffering. Positive steps that hasten death are prohibited.
Conservative		Some rabbis permit withholding or withdrawing medications, including artificial nutrition and hydration, from an incurably ill patient (trefah), including patients in a persistent vegetative state.	
Orthodox	All life-prolonging measures are required unless a person cannot be kept alive for more than 3 days (goses).		
Lutheran Churches			
Missouri Synod	Discontinuing extraordinary or heroic means for prolonging life belongs to proper medical care. Administering pain-killing medications, even at the risk of hastening death, is permissible. Advance directives are encouraged.		Euthanasia is a synonym for mercy killing, which involves suicide and/or murder, and is contrary to God's law.
Evangelical Lutheran Church[a]	Treatment may be withdrawn, withheld, or refused if the patient is irreversibly dying or the treatment imposes disproportionate burdens.		Active euthanasia deliberately destroys life created in the image of God and is contrary to Christian conscience and stewardship of life. Deliberate injection of drugs or other means of terminating life are acts of intentional homicide.
Mennonite Church	Informal approval of removing an obstacle that impedes a natural death.		As human life is a sacred trust from God, participation in hastening the death process would not be approved.
United Methodist Church	Every person has a right to die with dignity, with loving personal care and without efforts to prolong terminal illnesses merely because the technology is available to do so.	Support for withdrawing artificial nutrition in the *Cruzan* case (1990) is consistent with the tradition of conscience.	Washington Initiative 119 to legalize physician-assisted suicide and voluntary euthanasia was endorsed by the Pacific Northwest Conference of the United Methodist Church.
Church of the Nazarene	Decisions about withdrawal of life-support systems should consider quality of life and prospects for recovery. Personal dignity can be served by allowing a patient to die.	Allowing a terminally ill patient to die by withdrawing artificial feeding and hydration can be a Christian decision in some instances.	Euthanasia—the intentional and overt merciful termination of life of a patient for whom death is imminent—is categorically rejected.

TABLE 70.1. (Continued)

Religion	Treatment termination	Feeding tubes	Assisted suicide/active euthanasia
Pentecostal (United Pentecostal)	An informal acknowledgment that life-sustaining treatment can appropriately be terminated for patients with incurable terminal illness or in a persistent vegetative state.	No consensus about disconnecting artificially supplied food and water.	Strong (informal) opposition to assisted suicide and active euthanasia.
Reformed			
Presbyterian Church	It is unnecessary to prolong life during the dying process of a person who is gravely ill with little or no hope for remission.		A study document will examine "all sides" of the euthanasia debate but will not offer a denominational position. Life should not be unreasonably prolonged by artificial means or heroic measures, but it also should not be directly taken.
Reformed Church in America	Permits withholding or withdrawing life support systems to allow a patient's natural progress toward death.		
Roman Catholicism	"Extraordinary" measures that provide little or no benefit to the patient or result in disproportionate burdens can be discontinued. The rule of double effect permits the use of medication with the intent to relieve pain, even if death may be hastened. The patient should not be so sedated as to lose consciousness.	For some theologians and ecclesiastical leaders, "extraordinary" measures can include medical nutrition and hydration.	Euthanasia is an act or an omission with the intent to cause death to eliminate suffering. The killing of an innocent human being violates divine law, offends the dignity of the human person, and is a crime against life and an assault of humanity.
Unitarian Universalist Association	Each person has an inviolable right to determine in advance the course of action if there is no reasonable expectation of recovery from extreme physical or mental disability.		Advocacy of the right to self-determination in dying and the release from legal penalties of those who, under proper safeguards, honor the rights of terminally ill patients.
United Church of Christ	Ethically and theologically proper for a person to wish to avoid artificial and/or painful prolongation of terminal illness and to execute an advance directive.		Affirms individual freedom and responsibility. It is not claimed that euthanasia is the Christian position, but the right to choose is a legitimate Christian decision. Government should not close off options that belong to individuals and families.
Baha'i	Freedom to make personal decisions about terminating life-sustaining treatment for terminally ill patients within the boundaries of the civil law.		Baha'i faith teaches that suicide is prohibited by God, which would encompass prohibitions of assisted suicide and active euthanasia.
Islam	Prolongation of breathing by artificial life-supports would be strongly disapproved of by the Qur'an. If life cannot be restored, it is futile to maintain a person in a vegetative state by heroic means of animation.		Suicide is forbidden in Islamic law. Physicians must not take positive measures to terminate a patient's life.

From Campbell CS: Kennedy Inst Ethics J 1992, with permission.
*The Evangelical Lutheran Church was formed in 1988 from a merger of three Lutheran Churches; the ELC currently relies on statements from these predecessor bodies as the basis for its positions.

addressed about patient care, preferences, and communication."[17]

The challenge for physicians, members of ethics committees, nurses, and other caregivers is to understand patient values regarding terminal care and dying and then to be able to bridge any gulf between their own values and those of the patients. The literature indicates that there is a gap in the fulfillment of patient rights, autonomy, and informed consent that is not, and perhaps cannot be, filled by any of the present structures of care.

Ethical Professional Responsibility

Fidelity was the essential norm lacking in the physician–patient relationship for Mrs. Smith. Dr. Johnson had an obligation to respect the principles of autonomy, justice, and utility that he did not respect. He was the internist who had sent her to a vascular surgeon for an endarterectomy following the thoracotomy; he had supervised her care for the colon resection; he had prescribed therapy for her breathing difficulties and an earlier leg injury. As a primary care physician, he should not only have known the contents of her directive but have discussed the contents with her and later been prepared to discuss the contents with the family.

The ethics of all physicians are dependent on their own moral character. "Almost all great ethical theories converge to the conclusions that the most important ingredient in a person's moral life is a developed character that provides the inner motivation and strength to do what is right and good." The only way for physicians to maintain their own integrity while respecting patients' and families' wishes is to have full, open discussions at every stage of care. No physician can carry out all beneficial procedures for patients, nor can they meet all family and patient expectations in many instances; but physicians do have a specially mandated role in society "first, because it requires a special fidelity to the patient, and, second, because clinicians can be shown to hold special values that patients would not want used in decisions to allocate medical services."[18]

There are divisions of fidelity in the art and practice of medical care at present because of managed health care regulations "that have produced divided loyalties in many areas of medical practice, nursing and clinical research.... The issuing of orders and the assignments of duties create some forms of divided loyalty." Physicians need to rise to the challenge of such divisions of fidelity rather than use them as an excuse for less than the best possible care.

The basic cause of premature morbidity for Mrs. Smith was tobacco misuse. Unhealthy behavior supercedes access to medical treatment as the major health care problem in the United States and frustrates physician care. The Centers for Disease Control and Prevention estimate that only 10% of premature morbidity from the 10 leading causes of death in the United States could have been avoided through improved access to medical treatment. Environment and genetics were the contributing factors in 20%, and the 50% of premature deaths remaining resulted from behavioral factors such as tobacco use, alcohol misuse, poor eating habits, sedentary life style, unsafe sexual practices, drugs, physical violence and abuse, and other risk-taking behaviors.[19] There is no magic formula for the way in which physicians must deal with behavior modification as part of medical care, but it is the ethical responsibility of each physician to educate himself or herself about behavioral factors and how best to incorporate them into medical care.

The religion or faith beliefs of patients and their families—often interfaith—can assist a physician's care. The central question in all religions is: What constitutes life? Although there is not a consensus, much medical practice is consistent with Christian faith: sanctity of human life, alleviation of suffering, truth telling, informed consent, and confidentiality. Recognition of the enormous influence of mental and emotional states over one's physical state has led to at least one legitimate scientist proclaiming the healing power of belief. Herbert Benson, a Harvard cardiologist, wrote: "In my scientific observations, I have learned that no matter what name you give the Infinite Absolute you worship, no matter what theology you ascribe to, the results of believing in God are the same... because faith seems to transcend experience and base reality, it is supremely good at quieting distress and generating hope and expectancy... and remembered wellness."[20]

Distributive Justice and Informed Consent

Mrs. Smith's situation falls in the nonsystematic allocation of distributive justice in the United States, which is based on the ability to pay for health care or insurance.[21] Until or unless there are established cooperative agreements, ICU time will be allocated to many by the bottom-line ability to pay. Mrs. Smith's time on the ventilator was her good or bad fortune, depending on the point of view. Decisions for Mrs. Smith were optional rather than obligatory, and it can be argued that the burden outweighed the minimal benefits on a distributive justice basis. Once mistakes were made, however, it can also be argued that patient autonomy and the wishes of the family prevailed. On an economic basis, it would be difficult to argue that Mrs. Smith's situation represents a just allocation of scarce resources.

Managed Care and HMOs have changed the principle of the greatest good for the greatest number to the greatest good for the greatest number *within the budget*, thereby creating distributive ethics as well as distributed justice. Jerome Kassirer, the editor of the *New England Journal of Medicine*, said that "intentionally providing minimally acceptable care to some for the benefit of others in an arbitrary group—let alone for the benefit of the bottom line—is wrong.... When patients are sick and vulnerable, they expect their physicians to be their advocates for optimal care, not for some minimalist standard."[22] By definition, professionals conform to both the technical and ethical standards of their occupation. For physicians, the welfare of their patients must take priority over any imposed group ethic.

"Distinguished physician-ethicists have argued that teaching clinical ethics improves the quality of patient care by acknowledging that a serious medical decision involves two essential and necessary components: a technical decision that requires application of basic scientific and clinical knowledge and a moral decision that takes into account what ought to be done for an individual patient."[6] Although ethics is part of the curriculum of all the medical schools in the United States, most surgical residencies do not include ethics instruction on a regular basis. A multiauthored book entitled Surgical Ethics, edited by McCullough, Jones, and Brody fills a vacancy in the ethical literature for surgeons that will hopefully be followed by others in the straightforward language surgeons prefer.[23]

The discussion of ethical considerations at every step of surgical patient care might seem reasonable during this time of sensitivity to ethics. Again, however, residents participate only to the extent that the ethical considerations are important to the teaching staff. Even then, the personal ethical behavior and morality of the instructor and the residents are most influential. Resolution of ethical conflict, as depicted in the case study, becomes difficult on any basis without continuity of care and an overt effort on the part of the caregivers. Disparity of ethical awareness on the part of physicians is not just, and such disparity leaves informed consent in doubt.

Truly informed consent was in doubt after Mrs. Smith had the tracheotomy for ventilation, the long-term epidural catheter for pain, and percutaneous gastrostomy for feeding. Did she understand her situation? Did the staff, for fear of legal repercussions minimize her situation to the family? What happens to informed consent when Alzheimer's and senile patients are taken from an institution, or even the family home, to an ER for emergency surgery? In our diverse society, can we understand the multicultural factors in addition to any possible language barriers influencing informed consent?

To be informed is to understand for the patient; and for the ethical physician to understand within the patient's ethical parameters is critical for the care of the patient. The complexity of conscientious practice was stated eloquently in a 1992 presidential address to the Southern Thoracic Surgical Society: "Each gene can be thought of as a point in a Seurat painting or as a note in a Mozart symphony. Neither can be understood outside its relation to all the other parts of the work, and changing the iota changes the meaning and function of the overall design."[24]

References

1. Barger-Lux MJ, Heaney RP: For better and worse: the technological imperative in health care. Soc Sci Med 1986;22:1313–1320.
2. O'Rourke K: Court decisions on futile therapy. Health Care Ethics 1995;3:4.
3. Levinsky NG: Truth or consequences. N Engl J Med 1998;338:913–915.
4. Luce JM: Physicians do not have the responsibility to provide futile or unreasonable care if a patient or a family insists. Crit Care Med 1995;23:760–766.
5. Civetta JM: A practical approach to futile care. Bull Am Coll Surg 1996;81:24–29.
6. Baue AE, Baue RD: Medical decision making in critical care. In: Gullo A (ed) Anaesthesia, Pain, Intensive Care and Emergency Medicine. Milan, Springer, 1997;969–974.
7. Pellegrino ED: Contempo. JAMA 1992;268:214–220.
8. Bellet PS, Maloney MJ: The Importance of empathy as an interviewing skill in medicine. JAMA 1991;266:1831–1832.
9. Williams TF: Cabot, Peabody and the Care of the Patient. Bull Hist Med 1950;24:462–481.
10. O'Rourke K: From the director. Health Care Ethics 1998;6:1, 8.
11. Annas GJ: A national bill of patient's rights. N Engl J Med 1998;338:695–699.
12. Pear R: Rights expanded Medicare case. NY Times, Friday, August 14, 1998.
13. Teno JM, Lynn J, Phillips RS, et al: Do formal advance directives affect resuscitation decisions and the use of resources for seriously ill patients? J Clin Ethics 1994;5:23–30.
14. Lears L: Advance directives revisited: ethical instruments or useless documents. Health Care Ethics 1997;98:2–3.
15. Tonelli MR: Pulling the plug on living wills: a critical analysis of advance directives. Chest 1996;110:816–822.
16. Silverman HJ, Lanken PN: Advanced directives: are they fulfilling their purpose? Curr Opin Crit Care 1996;2:337–343.
17. Dowdy MD, Robertson L, Bander JA: A study of proactive ethics consultation for critically in patients with extended lengths of stay. Crit Care Med 1998;26:252–259.
18. Mansheim BJ: What care should be covered? Kennedy Inst Ethics J 1997;7:14–24.
19. Foster HW Jr: The enigma of low birth weight and race. N Engl J Med 1997;337:1232–1233.
20. Benson H, Stark M: Timeless Healing: Wired for God. New York, Simon & Schuster, 1997.
21. Beauchamp TL, Childress JF: Principles of Biomedical Ethics. New York, Oxford University Press, 1994.
22. Kassirer JP: Managing care: should we adopt a new ethic? N Engl J Med 1998;339:397–398.
23. McCullough LB, Jones JW, Brody BA (eds) Surgical Ethics. New York, Oxford University Press, 1998.
24. Sade RM: Presidential address to the Society of Thoracic Surgeons. Ann Thorac Surg 1992;53:183–190.

71
Socioeconomic Impact of Multiple Organ Failure

Carol R. Schermer and Donald E. Fry

Advances in intensive care have made it possible to prolong life or delay death in patients with low expectations of survival. Despite progress in intensive care management, the outcome after multiple organ dysfunction syndrome (MODS) appears relatively unchanged over time.[1-3] The time-honored surgical principles of aggressive resuscitation, timely operative intervention, and adequate drainage of infection and débridement of devitalized tissue are used to prevent MODS. If MODS develops, organ dysfunction is potentially recoverable when the factors responsible for progression of the syndrome can be reversed. Progression of MODS may occur despite optimal intensive care unit (ICU) support, as the prognosis appears to be directly related to the underlying severity of organ dysfunction.

Physician estimates of survival vary greatly when asked about identical patients.[4] Severity of illness scoring systems such as the Acute Physiology and Chronic Health Evaluation (APACHE II and III),[5,6] Simplified Acute Physiology Score (SAPS II),[7] and Mortality Probability Model (MPM)[8] estimate the probability of death in the hospital and allow comparisons of groups of patients. Despite the vast literature on ICU morbidity and mortality, prognostic indicators are of limited applicability and are rarely applied to the individual patient. Outcome data are generated using large numbers of patients, so their usefulness for predicting individual outcome is questionable. In fact, the most common mode of death for patients with advanced MODS is withdrawal of life support in the face of failure of the patient to respond to full, aggressive support.[4] Factors for withdrawal of support that are taken into consideration include the premorbid health of the patient, the underlying disease, the wishes of the patient and family, prospects for independent functioning, and the potential reversibility of the driving forces for MODS.

Many clinical studies have been performed that describe the morbidity and mortality of MODS. What has not been significantly addressed is the societal and economic impact of multiple organ failure (MOF). How quickly functional recovery is attained and how well the patient is reintegrated into society and occupation truly determines the ultimate societal impact of MODS. The impact ranges from the direct costs in the ICUs to the days of work lost, to the long-term sequelae of organ dysfunction. High cost surgical patients make up only 10% of the surgical patient population but occupy 35–50% of total resources.[9] It is reasonable to ask, then, whether such high costs are warranted if the patients are limited in their social and occupational quality of life after MODS.

Outcome from Individual Organ Failures

Pulmonary Failure

Studies attempting to look at whether the duration of mechanical ventilation is predictable have shown that a lung injury score of more than 1.0 predicts a duration of mechanical ventilation for more than 15 days.[10] Fewer than half of patients with acute respiratory distress syndrome (ARDS) die of progressive pulmonary failure. MOF is a contributory cause of death in 33%.[11] Early improvement in gas exchange portends better survival.[12]

In a multivariate analysis of mechanically ventilated patients, only the Organ System Failure Index and APACHE II score independently predicted outcome after mechanical ventilation (Table 71.1). In the same study, 52 survivors of mechanical ventilation over the age of 70 were observed after hospital discharge. Nearly 10% required care in a nursing home or a rehabilitation hospital until their deaths. ICU length of stay was the sole predictor of this outcome.[13]

Injured patients with pulmonary failure have been followed for the recovery of residual pulmonary dysfunction. Despite markedly abnormal pulmonary function tests shortly after injury, rapid improvement has been documented at 4 months after discharge with a return to almost normal by follow-up at 6 months. In this particular study, nearly all patients who were employed prior to injury had returned to work by 6 months. Long-term disability after severe blunt chest trauma has been reported in fewer than 5% of patients.[14]

Ghio and colleagues have looked at pulmonary function tests in survivors of ARDS.[15] They found that among patients examined a year or more after ARDS, 67% of subjects showed some degree of respiratory impairment, although most were only mildly impaired. Fifty percent had reductions in forced vital capacity (FVC) and 61% in forced expiratory volume in 1

TABLE 71.1. Potential Predictors of Mortality among 240 Consecutive ICU Patients with 246 Episodes of Mechanical Ventilation.

Variable	p
Age	< 0.025
Gender	NS
Hospital length of stay	NS
ICU length of stay	< 0.01
Duration of mechanical ventilation	< 0.0001
APACHE II score	< 0.0001[a]
Age-independent APACHE score	< 0.0001
Organ system failure index	< 0.0001
Diagnostic category	< 0.001
Presence of cancer	< 0.01
Cardiac arrest event	NS
Use of pulmonary catheter	NS
ICU readmission	NS

Modified from Koffef,[13] with permission.
With stepwise logistic regression, only the organ system failure index and the APACHE II scores independently predicted deaths.
NS, not statistically significant.
[a] Variables that independently predicted a fatal outcome by stepwise logistic regression.

TABLE 71.2. Univariate Analysis of Variables Evaluated as Predictors of Death in Patients Treated with Hemofiltration.

Variable	p
Binary variables	
Gender	NS
Surgical diagnosis	NS
Ventilator requirement	< 0.001[a]
Fever	< 0.001
Positive blood culture	NS
Antibiotics	< 0.025
Abdominal sepsis	0.001
Total parenteral nutrition	< 0.01
Prior chronic renal failure	NS
Prolonged prothrombin time	< 0.001
Continuous variables	
Age	NS[a]
Mean arterial pressure	NS
Hemoglobin	NS
White blood cell count	NS
Platelet count	NS
Bilirubin concentration	< 0.001[a]
Alanine aminotransferase (ALT) concentration	NS
Albumin concentration	NS
Creatinine concentration	< 0.001[a]
Sodium concentration	NS
Potassium concentration	NS
Arterial pH	NS
Base deficit	0.01
Inotrope score	< 0.001[a]
Urine volume score	< 0.001[a]

Modified from Barton et al.,[20] with permission.
[a] Variables independently significant following stepwise logistic regression analysis.

second (FEV_1), and 82% had abnormal diffusing capacity. In addition, abnormalities that persisted after 1 year were unlikely to resolve. Similar to the study done on posttraumatic lung dysfunction, more than 50% of the patients demonstrated severe impairment 1 month after ARDS.

Elliot and colleagues have documented restrictive pulmonary physiology in ARDS survivors characterized by a reduction in the FEV_1 and FVC with a normal FEV_1/FVC ratio.[16] Peters and colleagues demonstrated an abnormally low FVC in 43% of patients and abnormally low total lung capacity (TLC) in 21% of patients studied at least 6 months after their acute episode of ARDS.[17] Elliot and colleagues prospectively followed survivors of ARDS to determine the timing of pulmonary function recovery. Pulmonary function improved considerably after the first 3 months following extubation with only slight addition improvement at 6 months. No further changes were evident at 1 year. Patients with more severe ARDS had significantly lower results of their pulmonary function tests than did other survivors throughout the period of follow-up. Some ARDS survivors experience normal gas exchange at rest but have evidence of hypoxemia with exercise.[18]

Renal Failure

Survival after acute renal failure (ARF) does not appear to have improved over several decades,[19] although patient age has increased and the severity of illness has worsened. Previous health, co-morbid disease, patient age, and the number of failed organ systems appear to influence outcome. The need for artificial ventilation significantly worsens the outcome of ARF[20] (Table 71.2). Bellomo et al. reported a 29% survival rate at hospital discharge among ventilated patients with ARF.[21]

Creatinine clearance may remain significantly reduced for up to 3 months in ARF patients, but few patients fail to recover enough renal function to lead normal lives. In one study only 8% of patients had persistent azotemia.[22] Renal failure occurs in 1–2% of severely injured trauma patients; and sepsis is responsible for two-thirds of these outcomes. The mortality associated with posttraumatic ARF is approximately 60%.[23] Over the past four decades there has been only a 10% reduction in mortality due to renal failure following surgery or trauma.[24]

Although continuous renal replacement therapy (continuous venovenous hemodialysis, or CVVHD) benefits the patient by improving hemodynamic stability with gradual control of the metabolic environment, it does not appear to alter survival when compared to intermittent dialysis. Continuous therapy may be less expensive owing to the reduction in personnel and supervision time required. A study with a mean follow-up of 2.5 years looked at outcomes measured by quality of life and long-term survival in patients who underwent CVVHD for renal failure due to MODS (Table 71.3). Of 85 patients who had survived the hospitalization during which they had undergone CVVHD, 38% were lost to follow-up, 20% were dead, and 42% responded to the questionnaire. Two-thirds of the respondents were satisfied with their present state of health, although in 60% their mobility had been affected and 42% were unable to walk more than 200 meters. Using an overall 2.5-year survival of

TABLE 71.3. Variables Associated with Nonsurvival in Patients Undergoing CVVHD in the ICU.

Variable	p
Age	NS
Gender	NS
APACHE II score	< 0.0001
No. of failing organs	NS
Duration of hemofiltration therapy	NS
ICU length of stay	NS
Hospital length of stay	< 0.0001
Requirement for inotropic support	< 0.0001
Requirement for mechanical ventilation	< 0.0001
Presence of septic shock	< 0.0001
Postoperative cardiac surgery	< 0.05

Modified from Gopal et al.,[25] with permission.
CVVHD, continuous venovenous hemodialysis.

20% after MODS with renal failure, the approximate cost for each year of survival was estimated at $ 50,000 (US).[25]

Another study of CVVHD for renal failure secondary to MODS that looked to ICU stay, hospital stay, and 6-month follow-up found that the ICU, hospital, and 6-month survivals were 48%, 38%, and 36%, respectively.[26] Again, 8% of survivors required long-term renal replacement therapy. This study showed that patient survival appears to be related to the primary diagnosis. For example, renal failure after liver disease carried a mortality of 69%, whereas after obstetric complications or trauma the mortality was 40%. Patients with liver failure due to alchol abuse who then progressed to renal failure had 100% mortality as did patients with hematologic malignancy combined with sepsis that was responsible for their ARF.

A study from the Cleveland Clinic showed that even octagenarians with MOF and renal failure requiring dialysis have a 33% chance of overall survival and a 28% chance of renal recovery. This study also revealed a high rate of withdrawal of care from the octagenarian (42% versus 8% in younger patients) requiring dialysis.[27]

Predicting Death and Resource Utilization

Although there appears to be a uniform sequence of organ failure,[28,29] and failure of at least three organs for 4 days uniformly predicts death in some series,[30] early prediction of death in the ICU patient remains elusive. Most ICU deaths are due to MODS and sepsis. Admission APACHE II scoring (severity of illness scoring), which incorporates patient physiologic derangements on admission, does not predict resource utilization, nor does it predict the development of MODS in surgical patients.[31] Among ICU patients whose stay is longer than 2 weeks, 7% of patients generate 36% of the total charges, yet 44% of those 7% survive.[32] The organ failures are generally treated by supportive measures, stimulus control, and appropriate observation. Thus containing hospital costs during organ failure is restricted to decreasing the number of frequent tests. The desire to influence outcome often increases medical costs and the number of manipulations which we allow sufficient time to see if the patient can resolve the abnormalities.

Admission APACHE II scoring helps allow comparisons of patients and permits continuous quality improvement evaluation but does not allow clinical decision making. Patients who are moribund or minimally injured require the least amount of time to reach an outcome. An example is the sickest patient admitted to the ICU who dies within 1 day and has low costs that are comparable to those of patients with the lowest APACHE scores. None of the current scoring systems accurately predicts the risk for development of MODS.[33] A study from Miami reported that if physiologic stability was not achieved quickly continued therapy became futile. A nonsurvival pattern of response was identified by the requirement of similar or greater number of interventions on each day of monitoring to achieve adequate cardiovascular function.[34] The value of identifying problems may be to identify and immediately treat those who need additional interventions so these patients are provided the best opportunity of survival and to recognize when continued efforts are likely to be futile owing to the lack of improvement.

Physical, Occupational, and Psychiatric Outcomes after ICU and MODS

In a study from Finland patients were followed for 5 years after their ICU discharge. After the first 6 months, when 15% of the patients had died, the survival curves paralleled those for the general population. Mortality was greatest among patients who had experienced cardiac arrest: Only 30% were alive 6 months after discharge.[35] A study from Germany[36] looked at rehabilitation results of trauma patients with MOF and long-term intensive care. The mean follow-up was nearly 5 years. Of the 69 survivors, 50 were willing to participate in the study. All patients who were alive at 5 years had normal laboratory results for liver, kidney, and hematologic function. Altogether 91% of patients had age-correlated normal values determined by spirometry and 83% by plethysmography; 81% had normal diffusion capacity. Nineteen percent of the patients had combined clinically insignificant abnormalities seen by spirometry, body plethysmography, and diffusing capacity tests. More than 25% of patients had decreased range of motion of the elbow, hip, or ankle; in one-third of patients these joints were not originally injured. About 40% had permanent motor nerve lesions, only 14% of which had been diagnosed prior to the present illness.

The return to work rate in the German trauma study was 60%. As far as occupational rehabilitation is concerned, 38% had no change in workplace, 15% changed their workplace, 7% changed jobs, 17% were unemployed, 17% were retired, and 6% were still on sick leave. Unskilled workers were less likely to be employed. Among those working, the level of maximal physical work was significantly decreased. The nonworking group had spent a longer time in the ICU and rehabilitation centers.[36]

A Finnish study showed that among severely injured trauma patients who had worked prior to injury, 72% were able to return to work and were still working at 5–20 years of follow-up.[37] A similar study in Switzerland looked at a 5-year follow-up of ICU patients: 5.6% of patients died after hospital discharge, 89% of survivors were healthy or slightly disabled, 9% were severely disabled, 2% were vegetative. A total of 79% of survivors were working after 5 years.[38] In the Swiss study patients experienced reduced social well-being and changed professional and recreational activities.[38] In the outcome study after venovenous hemofiltration for MODS[25] depression was reported in 66% of patients, with a strain in family relationships in 47%.

TABLE 71.4. Economic Loss and Mortality Rates of Age-Stratified Diagnosis-Related Groups in a Large Study ($N = 2898$) of Hospitalized Patients.

Age (years)	No. of patients	$ Loss per case	Mortality rate (%)
≤ 54	153	—	5.2
55–60	153	1033	8.5
65–69	592	992	8.3
70–74	633	1566	11.7
75–79	573	1096	10.6
80–85	408	1874	12.5
> 85	386	2408	20.2

Modified from Munoz et al.,[46] with permission.

Predicting Survival and Cost

The cost of medical and surgical critical care in the United States was estimated to be $34 billion, or about 20% of all inpatient hospital costs in 1990.[39] Care plans and management protocols have been advocated to decrease costs and length of stay in the ICU, but to our knowledge no care plan has been shown to affect directly the progression of organ failure or limitation of cost in the most critically ill patients. The percentage of the gross domestic product occupied by ICU costs in 1986 and 1988 was 0.7% and was up to 0.9% in 1992.[40] More than 15 years before that the economic costs of trauma due to care and lost income were estimated to be $61 billion.[41] No current prognostic indicator can resolve whether a patient has a 0.1%, 1.0%, or 10% chance of survival, so the cost per survivor cannot be determined.

Barton and Cerra reported a study in 1989 that linked organ failure with prolonged stay and high costs in the surgical ICU. The total cost of hospitalization and rehabilitation for survivors averaged $385,000 per patient.[42] Barie et al. showed that MODS is a more powerful predictor of prolonged stay than is severity of illness.[43] They later showed that the MODS score on day 2 in the ICU predicted survival versus nonsurvival in patients who stayed more than 21 days. Similar to the study in Miami,[34] nonsurvivors developed MODS progressively through their ICU stay, but survivors began to improve almost immediately.

Predicting organ failure has proven difficult. The scenario of a patient with a ruptured abdominal aortic aneurysm has been looked at extensively to try to reduce costs by evaluating preoperatively who is likely to do poorly. There appear to be no good preoperative predictors of who will do poorly, although one study of 99 patients who reached the ICU alive after surgery demonstrated that MODS was responsible for 93% of late deaths. When an organ system failure score was used for each patient at 48 hours after operation, there was a strong positive correlation between organ failure score and mortality. All patients with failure of more than two organ systems died. If the score had been used for decision making at 48 hours, 43% of ICU days associated with late mortality would have been saved.[44]

In another study looking at visceral ischemia and organ dysfunction after thoracoabdominal aneurysm repair, postoperative organ dysfunction was not related to preoperative organ dysfunction but was entirely related to aortic cross-clamp time. There was a significantly higher incidence of pulmonary, renal, hepatic, and hematopoietic failure with cross-clamp times of more than 40 minutes. Along with more organ failures there was a more than twofold increase in hospital and ICU costs. The overall mortality in this study was 17%. Patients developing MODS had mortality rates of 33% compared to 10% of those not developing MODS; this was entirely predicted by the cross-clamp time. The average length of hospital stay was 35 days in the MODS patients compared to 17 days in those with shorter cross-clamp times.[45] This study demonstrated what is all too common. More money and time are spent on patients with high mortality rates.

The highest priced hospital care is that of the very elderly in the ICU[46] (Table 71.4). ICU outcome in the very elderly (over age 85) has been studied. As a group the very elderly had ICU, 30-day posthospital discharge, and 1-year mortality rates of 30%, 43%, and 64%, respectively. Mortality rates of the very elderly with two or more organ system dysfunctions had an 88% thirty-day posthospital discharge mortality rate and 100% one-year mortality rate. There was also 100% mortality for the very elderly admitted to the ICU after cardiopulmonary arrest.[47]

Among patients with major complications after coronary artery bypass surgery, 64% survived hospitalization. When 42 patients were surveyed 22 months after surgery, one-half had excellent independent function, seven were moderately impaired but living at home, and six were institutionalized with severe limitations; eight had died. Patients with severe cardiac or neurologic dysfunction 1 week after surgery had extremely poor outcome and little chance for independent recovery.[48]

Ethics and the Futility of Care

The point of futility in care arrives when life cannot be extended with value, dignity, and meaning as defined by the patient's wishes. Ethical principles support the physician in futile care where "the physician is not ethically required to provide futile or unreasonable care, especially to patients who are brain-dead, who are vegetative, critically, or terminally ill with little chance of recovering, and who are unlikely to benefit from cardiopulmonary resuscitation."[49] Unfortunately, futility in care has not been resolved by legal statute. A retrospective study looking at the process of death in three university-affiliated ICUs in Canada found that 70% of patients who died in the ICU did so because of withdrawal or withholding of life support.[50] Such patients were older and had a longer length of stay than patients dying of other causes. Poor prognosis was given as the most common reason for withdrawal, generally due to significant organ dysfunction at the time of withdrawal. Future quality of life was given less often as a reason.

The ability to prolong life in the critically ill along with the rising costs of ICU care creates a need to recognize those patients who will die despite treatment. One study looked at the relation of "do not resuscitate" (DNR) orders and ICU deaths at 13 U.S. hospitals: 39% of all ICU deaths were preceded by DNR orders; and 94% of patients with DNR orders died in the hospital. The mean interval from ICU admission to DNR orders was 5.4–24.0 days.[51]

The identification of futility in care is a difficult issue. A modification of the APACHE II score was tested to make daily predictions of individual outcome in 3600 patients. By following an algorithm based on daily APACHE II score calculations and number of organ failures, 95.6% of patients expected to die did so within 90 days of discharge from the hospital. Patients predicted to die stayed 1492 days in the ICU and incurred 16.7% of all ICU expenditures and 46.4% of the cost of all patients who died. The authors recommended that the algorithm has the potential to indicate futility of continued ICU care but at the cost of 1 in 20 patients who would survive if intensive care were continued.[52]

In a Canadian study[53] the issue of withdrawal of care was addressed via a poll of physicians, nurses, and housestaff. Clinical scenarios were given; in only 1 of 12 scenarios did more than 30% of the respondents make the therapeutic decision. In 8 of 12 scenarios, more than 10% of respondents chose diametrically opposed care plans (e.g., full aggressive care versus comfort measures only). This problem of the discrepancy of expected outcomes will continue until accurate predictors of outcome are available and a consensus is developed, rather than relying on idiosyncratic values of health care professionals.

Conclusions

There is much ICU literature that predicts outcome in large groups of patients, but these data are of limited use in the individual patient. Outcome studies have primarily focused on the severity of illness and its relation to survival or death. Interventions that cure the disease are limited, and care is primarily supportive.

In the studies referred to in this chapter, one-half to two-thirds of patients were satisfied with their outcomes after MODS and major complications and were reasonably independent during activities of daily living. In some of the monoclonal antibody and receptor antagonist sepsis studies, the cost per survivor was as much as $100,000. The cost of each survival appears to range from $50,000 to $385,000. However 20–40% of patients never return to work after they had received the most costly care.

To have better prognostic indicators of an individual patient's outcome we need more information on social, financial, and health outcomes. What is needed are adequate data based on a combination of life-threatening diseases, finite resources, and level of social outcome and function to make clinical decisions for the individual patient.

The physician's desire to influence outcome often increases medical costs while allowing the patient to declare the outcome. We need the ability to recognize progressive organ dysfunction early in order to withdraw care that has already begun but will ultimately prove futile.

Although it is difficult to put a price on survival, patients undergoing withdrawal or withholding of life support tend to be older and have a longer length of hospital stay than patients dying of other causes. Thus small numbers of patients use significant resources with little chance of survival. Physicians still withdraw patients from life support because of what they believe is a poor prognosis for the individual due to organ dysfunction. Physicians still have trouble withholding and withdrawing care, and there appears to be significant disagreement on how aggressive care should be. We now have a small amount of data on future quality of life but are lacking good, early predictors of death and adverse outcome on which to base decision that can decrease the economic impact of MODS and ICU care.

References

1. Barie PS, Hydro LJ, Fischer E: A prospective comparison of two multiple organ dysfunction/failure systems for prediction of mortality on critical surgical illness. J Trauma 1994;37:660.
2. Regel G, Grotz M, Weltner T, et al: The pattern of organ failure following severe trauma. World J Surg 1996;20:422.
3. Sauaia A, Moore FA, Moore EE, et al: Early predictors of postinjury multiorgan failure. Arch Surg 1994;129:39.
4. Pearlman RA: Variability in physician estimates of survival for acute respiratory failure in chronic obstructive pulmonary disease. Chest 1987;91:515.
5. Knaus WA, Draper EA, Wagner DP, et al: APACHE-II: a severity of disease classification system. Crit Care Med 1985;13:818.
6. Knaus WA, Wagner DP, Draper EA, et al: The APACHE III prognostic sytem: risk prediction of hospital mortality for critically ill hospitalized patients. Chest 1991;100:1619.
7. LeGall JR, Lemeshow S, Saulnier F: Development of a new scoring system, the SAPS II, from a European/North American multicenter study. JAMA 1993;270:2957.
8. Lemeshow S, Teres D, Klar J, et al: Mortality probability models (MPM II) based on an international cohort of intensive care unit patients. JAMA 1993;270:2478.
9. Drucker WR, Gavett JW, Kirsckner R, et al: Toward strategies for cost containment in surgical patients. Ann Surg 1983;198:284.
10. Troche G, Moine P: Is the duration of mechanical ventilation predictable? Chest 1997;112:745.
11. Montgomery AB, Stager MA, Carrico CJ, et al: Causes of mortality in patients with the adult respiratory distress syndrome. Am Rev Respir Dis 1985;132:485.

12. Sloane PJ, Gee MH, Gottlieb JE, et al: A multicenter registry of patients with acute respiratory distress syndrome. Am Rev Respir Dis 1992;146:419.
13. Kollef MH: Do age and gender influence outcome from mechanical ventilation? Heart Lung 1993;22:442.
14. Livingston DH, Richardson JD: Pulmonary disability after severe blunt chest trauma. J Trauma 1990;30:562.
15. Ghio AJ, Elliot CG, Crapo RO, et al: Impairment after adult respiratory distress syndrome: an evaluation based on American Thoracic Society recommendations. Am Rev Respir Dis 1989;139:1158.
16. Elliot CG, Rasmusson BY, Crapo RO, et al: Prediction of pulmonary function abnormalities after adult respiratory distress syndrome (ARDS). Am Rev Respir Dis 1987;135:634.
17. Peters JI, Bell RC, Prihoda TJ, et al: Clinical determinants of abnormalities in pulmonary functions in survivors of the adult respiratory distress syndrome. Am Rev Respir Dis 1989;139:1163.
18. Elliot CG, Morris AH, Cengiz M: Pulmonary function and exercise gas exchange in survivors of adult respiratory distress syndrome. Am Rev Respir Dis 1981;123:492.
19. Turney JH, Marshall DH, Brownjohn AM, et al: The evolution of acute renal failure, 1956–1988. Q J Med 1990;74:83.
20. Barton IK, Hilton PJ, Taub NA, et al: Acute renal failure treated by haemofiltration: factors affecting outcome. Q J Med 1993;86:81.
21. Bellomo R, Farmer M, Boyce N: Combined acute respiratory and renal failure management by continuous haemodiafiltration. Resuscitation 1994;28:123.
22. Eliahou HE, Boichis H, Bott-Kanner G, et al: An epidemiologic study of renal failure. II. Acute renal failure. Am J Epidemiol 1975;101:281.
23. Morris JA, Mucha P, Ross SE, et al: Acute postraumatic renal failure: a multicenter perspective. J Trauma 1991;31:1584.
24. Finn WF: Recovery from acute renal failure. In: Brenner BM, Lazarus JM (eds) Acute Renal Failure. Philadelphia, Saunders, 1983.
25. Gopal I, Bhonagiri S, Ronoco C, Bellomo R: Out of hospital outcome and quality of life in survivors of combined acute multiple organ and renal failure treated with continuous venovenous hemofiltration/hemodiafiltration. Intensive Care Med 1997;23:766.
26. Jones CH, Richardson D, Goutcher E, et al: Continuous venovenous high flux dialysis in multiorgan failure: a 5 year single center experince. Am J Kidney Dis 1998;31:227.
27. Baldyga AP, Paganini EP, Chaff C, Higgins TL: Acute dialytic support of the octagenarian: is it worth it? ASAIO 1993;39:M805.
28. Fry DE, Pearlstein L, Fulton RL, Polk HC: Multiple system organ failure: the role of uncontrolled infection. Arch Surg 1980;115:136.
29. Baue AE: Multiple, progressive, or sequential system failure. Arch Surg 1975;110:779.
30. Knaus WA, Draper EA, Wagner DP, Zimmerman J: Prognosis in acute organ system failure. Ann Surg 1985;202:685.
31. Cerra FB, Negro F, Abrams J: APACHE II score does not predict multiple organ failure or mortality on postoperative surgical patients. Arch Surg 1990;125:219.
32. Civetta JM, Hudson Civetta JA: Maintaining quality of care while reducing charges in the ICU: 10 ways. Ann Surg 1985;202:524.
33. Knaus W, Wagner D, Draper E, et al: The APACHE III prognostic system risk prediction of hospital mortality for critically ill hospitalized adults. Chest 1991;100:1619.
34. Kirton OC: Cost effectiveness in the intensive care unit. Surg Clin North Am 1996;76:175.
35. Niskanen M, Kari A: Five year survival after intensive care: a comparison of 10,976 patients with general population. Crit Care Med 1995;23(Suppl A):A20.
36. Grotz M, Hohensee A, Remmers D, et al: Rehabilitation results of patients with multilple injuries and multiple organ failure and long term intensive care. J Trauma 1997;42:919.
37. Kivioja AH, Myllynen PJ, Rokkanen PU: Is the treatment of the most severe multiply injured patients worth the effort? A follow-up examination 5 to 20 years after severe multiple injury. J Trauma 1990;30:480.
38. Frutiger A, Ryf C, Bilat C, et al: Five years' follow-up of severely injured ICU patients. J Trauma 1991;31:1216.
39. Jacobs P, Noseworthy TW: National estimates of intensive care utilization and costs: Canada and the United States. Crit Care Med 1990;18:1282.
40. Halpern NA, Bettes L, Greenstein R: Federal and nationwide intensive care units and healthcare costs: 1986–1992. Crit Care Med 1994;22:2001.
41. Munoz E: Economic costs of trauma, United States, 1982. J Trauma 1984;24:237.
42. Barton R, Cerra FB: The hypermetabolism organ failure syndrome. Chest 1989;96:1153.
43. Barie PS, Hydo LJ, Fischer E: Utility of illness severity scoring for prediction of prolonged surgical critical care. J Trauma 1996;40:513.
44. Tromp Meesters RC, van der Graff Y, Vos A, Eikelboom BC: Ruptured aortic aneurysm: early postoperative prediction of mortality using an organ system failure score. Br J Surg 1994;81:512.
45. Harward TRS, Wellnorn MB, Martin TD, et al: Visceral ischemia and organ dysfunction after thoracoabdominal aortic aneurysm repair: a clinical and cost analysis. Ann Surg 1996;223:729.
46. Munoz E, Rosner F, Chalfin D, et al: Financial risk and hospital cost for elderly patients. Arch Intern Med 1988;148:909.
47. Kass JE, Castriotta RJ, Malakoff F: Intensive care unit outcome in the very elderly. Crit Care Med 1992;20:1666.
48. Wahl GW, Swinburne AJ, Fedullo AJ, et al: Long term outcome when major complications follow coronary artery bypass graft surgery: recovery after complicated coronary artery bypass graft surgery. Chest 1996;110:1394.
49. Luce JM: Physicians do not have a responsibility to provide futile or unreasonable care if a patient or family insists. Crit Care Med 1995;23:760.
50. Keenan SP, Busche KD, Chen LM, et al: A retrospective review of a large cohort of patients undergoing the process of withholding or withdrawal of life support. Crit Care Med 1997;25:1324.
51. Zimmerman JE, Knaus WA, Sharpe SM: The use and implications of do not resuscitate orders in intensive care units. JAMA 1986;255:351.
52. Atkinson S, Bihari D, Smithies M, et al: Identification of futility in intensive care. Lancet 1994;344:1203.
53. Cook DJ, Guyatt GH, Jaeschke R, et al: Determinants in Canadian health care workers of the decision to withdraw life support in the critically ill. JAMA 1995;273:703.

72
Future Directions in the Treatment of SIRS and MODS

Donald E. Fry

The patient with systemic inflammatory response syndrome (SIRS) and evolving organ failure has been managed in an aggressive fashion within the scope of available strategies in the contemporary intensive care unit (ICU). Supportive care to maintain tissue perfusion and appropriate systemic oxygenation is the goal in every patient, although it remains unclear as to how much oxygen delivery is truly enough. Nutritional support has evolved through numerous iterations of intravenous-to-parenteral administration and formulation strategies. Patients with surgical problems associated with SIRS, of which intraabdominal infection is the prototype,[1] undergo aggressive surgical management of the primary source of infection and timely reintervention with minimally invasive methods or repeated open surgical reoperation when appropriate. When the assumed cause, or consequence, of SIRS is infection, systemic antimicrobial chemotherapy is vigorously applied for documented or anticipated pathogens.

Despite the application of these conventional treatment strategies, the clinical results in the severe SIRS/multiple organ dysfunction syndrome (MODS) patient have continued to be a disappointment.[2-4] Although improved overall patient management has likely reduced the frequency of MODS, once multiple systems are dysfunctional or are failing the mortality rates remain higher than 50%, patient morbidity is severe, and health care costs are enormous. Sustained application of supportive care methods, reoperation, and systemic antibiotics not only reach a point of seeming futility but may become potentially damaging to the patient. Repeated systemic stress is sequentially administered to the host with multiple reoperations.[5,6] Portals of nosocomial infection are increased. The continued and worrisome evolution of antimicrobial resistance among nosocomial pathogens is active, occurring within the ICU during treatment and waging a hopeless battle in the compromised host. The legacy of antimicrobial resistance is not only a consequence for the SIRS/MODS patients but for other patients within the hospital environment as well.

It is clear that future new treatments must be developed that constitute more than supportive measures of organ function and be more than current nutritional support strategies. New treatments must be other than newer antibiotics to attack would-be infections that may or may not be responsible for the self-destructive processes leading to the death of the patient. Future therapies require a mechanistic approach to abort the fundamental mechanisms of the systemic inflammatory process. It is not enough to manage the activating events (e.g., shock, infection, soft tissue injury), but modification or enhancement of elements of the host response must be the treatment objective. Finally, the new treatment agenda should learn from the early failed attempts at patient management by manipulating the inflammatory response.

General Directions of Future Treatment

As has been detailed in other chapters of this book, many directions are being actively pursued for potential treatment modalities in the SIRS/MODS patient. Most of the current directions are linked to our present understanding of the process, and most are focused on blocking, inhibiting, or modifying a component of the inflammatory response at some point in the cascade. For organizational purposes, the therapeutic directions are categorized as: (1) blocking inflammation activation; (2) inhibiting phase I of inflammation; (3) inhibiting phase II of inflammation; (4) inhibiting the effector mechanisms of inflammation; (5) augmenting counterinflammatory responses; (6) managing immunosuppression; (7) gene therapy strategies; and (8) others.

Blocking Inflammation Activation

The activation events of inflammation are those clinical events that provoke the response. They include shock, trauma, burns, pancreatitis, and most notably infection. Endotoxins and exotoxins from bacteria have been the most commonly studied activators of inflammation and certainly are the most commonly used in laboratory studies. The role of endotoxin in activating inflammation and proinflammatory cytokine release has been frequently documented in vivo and in vitro from isolated monocytes/macrophages. Blockade of endotoxin effects seems to make good sense as a therapeutic strategy.

Chelation with an agent such as polymyxin[7] and hemofiltration[8] have been explored, but their effectiveness has yet to be tested in prospective trials. The use of bacterial permeability-inducing protein is another idea being actively pursued,[9,10] but the promise appears removed from the reality of it becoming a treatment strategy anytime soon. Endotoxin in blood binds to lipopolysaccharide (LPS)-binding protein, and this complex binds to the CD14 receptor on the monocyte or macrophage, resulting in production of the proinflammatory cytokines. A soluble CD14 has been used on a preliminary basis in patients as a means of blocking endotoxin effects, but additional studies are needed.[11]

The most advanced efforts to blunt or neutralize the endotoxin effect have been achieved using anti-endotoxin antibodies. The common target of lipid A in most gram-negative endotoxins, in experimental studies[12] and in initial trials of a polyclonal antibody preparation in human studies, seemed to have promise of clinical efficacy.[13] However, the clinical trial of a human monoclonal anti-endotoxin antibody failed to demonstrate an improved clinical outcome among patients with septic shock.[14,15] The cohort of patients with culture-positive gram-negative bacteremia on post hoc analysis appeared to have a favorable therapeutic effect. An effort to study this monoclonal antibody in a prospective fashion resulted in abandonment of the study before completion owing to adverse clinical events. Studies with a murine-derived anti-endotoxin antibody have similarly showed some promised when cohorts of patients within the study population have been examined, but overall results have shown no benefit.[16,17] Among the many issues raised by the failed but tempting results of the anti-endotoxin antibody studies is the primitive nature of our current diagnostic ability to detect endotoxin or bacteremia in the ICU.

Inhibiting Phase I of Inflammation

Inhibiting phase I of inflammation is specifically an attempt to alter those mechanisms that promote vasodilation, increased vascular permeability, edema formation, and chemoattractant production. Blockade of the biologically active products released by each of the five initiators of SIRS have been contemplated, and attempts have been made to alter the effects of each. Activation of the hemostatic mechanism assumes a seminal role in inflammation. Activation of coagulation proteins and platelets leads to the release of proinflammatory proteins, which initiate inflammation. Antithrombin III and heparin have been examined as modulating mechanisms to counterbalance excessive systemic activation of the coagulation and platelet pathways.

Inhibition of the coagulation cascade as a prime initiator of inflammation has been attempted by several methods. Inhibiting factor XII experimentally affected the outcome in septic baboons[18] but would obviously have negative effects relative to hemostasis.

Antithrombin III is the natural inhibitor of thrombin. It also has important functions as a serine protease inhibitor that interferes with other coagulation steps, including inhibition of factor XII activation. In the presence of heparin its effects are dramatically amplified. Experimental studies have demonstrated potential benefits from treatment models of sepsis or endotoxemia with antithrombin III alone,[19] antithrombin III plus heparin, or heparin alone.[20–22] Heparin effects alone are dependent on endogenous antithrombin III but may also have direct antiaggregation effects on platelets. Early clinical evidence has not been consistent, but supporting evidence has shown some favorable outcomes with antithrombin III treatment.[23] A large trial of antithrombin III therapy is presently being pursued for patients with disseminated intravascular coagulation (DIC) due to sepsis or shock. The timing of administration, the dose, the value of adding heparin, and the risks of anticoagulation therapy are all considerations with this potential new treatment.

Inhibition of the contact activating system by inhibiting bradykinin has now undergone a prospective, randomized clinical trial after encouraging results from animal experimentation.[24] These data have demonstrated no improvement in clinical outcome with a specific bradykinin antagonist.[25] Various antagonists of bradykinin with different modes of action are being explored.

The principal mechanism for the bradykinin effect has been through the release of nitric oxide via the endothelial cell. Specific receptors are bound by bradykinin, which induces nitric oxide synthase; and the vasoactive consequences of nitric oxide are the result. This has led to investigation of blocking nitric oxide production in the septic shock patient.[26] Most efforts to block nitric oxide production have been with N-methyl-L-arginine. It is of interest that blood pressure has been stabilized but without improving patient outcome. Among considerations with this treatment strategy is whether nitric oxide synthase inhibition may affect both inducible and constitutive forms of nitric oxide. Furthermore, global inhibition of nitric oxide effects may alter cardiac performance in the septic state and may have adverse host effects on the other nonvasoactive roles of nitric oxide.

Yet another initiating event that is a focus of inhibition therapy is the complement cascade. Experimental studies have explored inhibition of specific complement protein activation, and others have explored the use of antibodies to specific activation products of complement (anti-C5a antibodies).[27–30] Clinical trials have not been pursued at this point.

Antihistamine therapies have been examined over the years in models of shock and infection, but histamine has not been demonstrated consistently in the circulation of injured and septic patients.[31] Histamine antagonists have yielded limited if any value in animal experiments of endotoxemia.[32,33] To the author's knowledge, no active treatment strategies for inhibiting histamine effects are currently being pursued.

Inhibiting Phase II of Inflammation

For purposes of this discussion, phase II of inflammation is the process of phagocytic cell margination to endothelial cells, migration into tissues, and elaboration of cytokine and cellular products that effect tissue destruction. Phase II deals with the activity of neutrophils and monocytes/macrophages within the inflammatory milieu. It is in this area where the largest number of clinical trials have been undertaken and where the greatest disappointments of new therapeutic strategies have been realized. Specific cytokine blockade has failed. The central role of tumor necrosis factor (TNF) has led to development of an anti-TNF monoclonal antibody. This antibody has shown considerable promise, with favorable outcomes seen in several animal models of sepsis and endotoxemia.[34,35] However, several clinical trials have now been completed, and specific TNF blockade has not improved outcome in septic patients.[36-38] Soluble TNF receptor and anti-TNF receptor antibodies have similarly had promise of being clinically beneficial. A prospective trial of a novel fusion protein of soluble TNF receptor with the Fc component of immunoglobulin G (IgG) antibody has not only been shown to not be of benefit but in high doses may be detrimental.[39]

Interleukin-1 (IL-1) as a proinflammatory cytokine has similarly been studied. Experimental studies with blockade of IL-1 effects with a recombinant receptor antagonist showed promise,[40] but clinical benefits have not been identified in human trials.[41,42] The potential value of an anti-IL-6 antibody is currently being explored.[43]

The realm of leukocyte–endothelial cell adhesion molecules are now being evaluated for potential therapeutic advantages. Anti-CD18 monoclonal antibodies have been demonstrated to have benefits in animal models of shock and ischemia.[44-47] Some potential for negative effects on the host have also been recognized with this potential strategy.[48-50] Specific antibodies for functional blockade of other cell adhesion molecules are being explored.[51] The clear concern of such strategies is that margination and adverse events mediated by neutrophil activation may be attenuated, but if the host can marginate neutrophils as part of the salutary response of the host in an area of local infection is in question.

Platelet-activating factor (PAF) is another lipid signal important for facilitating neutrophil–endothelial cell adhesion in the microcirculation. A vast array of antagonists to PAF have been identified for use in possible therapeutic strategies.[52] The use of antagonists to PAF have shown promise in the experimental laboratory, but clinical trials with specific blocking agents have been unsuccessful.[53,54] The complex nature of the leukocyte–endothelial cell adhesion process and the complex molecular biology of the transendothelial migration process can doubtlessly open numerous opportunities for therapeutic intervention.

Neutralization of Effector Signals

The tissue destructive events of inflammation appear to be primarily mediated by reactive oxygen intermediates and by potent digestive enzymes released by neutrophils that have infiltrated soft tissues. The release of these destructive effectors of tissue injury also are responsible for endothelial injury and potentially microcirculatory arrest. Considerable interest has focused on the use of antioxidant therapies, which can hopefully neutralize the destructive effects of oxygen radicals released by

TABLE 72.1. Antioxidants Studied in Animal Models and Found to Have Potential Benefit Against Infection.

Allopurinol
Ascorbic acid
β-Carotene
Butylated hydroxyanisole
Butylated hydroxytoluene
Canthaxanthin
Catalase
Glutathione
Lazaroids
Melatonin
Nordihydroguaniaritic acid
Propyl gallate
Silymarin
Superoxide dismutase
Vitamin E

The number of potential antioxidants is large, and this list is not complete.

neutrophils. (Table 72.1) Superoxide dismutase and catalase have been used investigationally in models of shock,[55,56] endotoxemia,[57,58] and sepsis.[59,60] Lazaroids reduce lipid peroxidation.[61] Nitrones appear to be free radical scavengers of both oxygen and nitrogen (i.e., nitric oxide) reactive intermediates.[62] Clinical trials during human sepsis have not been undertaken but are being pursued for inflammation-mediated injury within the central nervous system.

Augmentation of the Counterinflammatory Response

A yin-yang relation exists among mediator signals of all physiologic and metabolic responses. For insulin, there is glucagon. For vasoconstrictors, there are vasodilators. Evidence is now accumulating that for the summed effects of the proinflammatory signals there is a corresponding antiinflammatory set of biologic signals. Most research in human sepsis and organ failure has focused on the proinflammatory signals and their deleterious effects. More recently, the counterinflammatory signals of IL-4,[63] IL-10,[64] and IL-13[65] have been identified. Exogenous administration of these counterinflammatory cytokines in the experimental situation have benefits for the host with a bacterial infection and other inflammatory events.[66-74] Soluble receptors for the proinflammatory signals of TNF and IL-1 have been identified and may be part of the counterinflammatory response. Transforming growth factor-β (TGFβ) is another counterinflammatory signal.[75] Endogenous catecholamines and glucocorticoids have counterinflammatory effects as part of the neuroendocrine response to severe injury and infection. Prostaglandin E (PGE) production has far-reaching immunosuppressive and antiinflammatory effects.[76] Even heparin release from mast cells can be viewed appropriately as a counterinflammatory signal.

A future direction in the therapeutic quest to treat SIRS and MODS is better definition of the counterinflammatory response.

For each SIRS event, there must be a corresponding compensatory antiinflammatory response (CARS).[77] An inadequate or delayed antiinflammatory response means that SIRS is unchecked, and systemic injury to the host is the result. In this scenario, the administration of counterinflammatory mediators at the apex of the proinflammatory response may be the appropriate treatment strategy. Thus IL-4, IL-10, and IL-13 are being explored for their antiinflammatory benefit to the host. It is clear that future research must focus on the quantitative and temporal relation of the summed proinflammatory and the summed counterinflammatory responses as a coordinated series of events within the host. Exogenous use of counterinflammatory therapies is in its experimental infancy.

Management of Immunosuppression

If the counterinflammatory response of the host is delayed, or it is predominant because of the summed effects of all potential antiinflammatory signals, a situation of immune suppression may exist. Reduced monocyte responsiveness and the development of skin test anergy reflect immune suppression of the host, which may then lead to an evolving microbial infection being unchecked by the salutary benefits of human inflammation. This has led to interest in immune stimulation or augmentation as a necessary requirement in the very patient in whom an excessive and robust host inflammatory response was paradoxically the inciting event that precipitated the entire initial SIRS. Interferon-γ (IFNγ),[78] levamisole,[79] muramyl dipeptide,[80] granulocyte colony-stimulating factor (G-CSF),[81] and granulocyte/monocyte colony-stimulating factor (GM-CSF),[82] have been examined as potential treatments in the patient with advanced, prolonged SIRS and critical illness. The concept of a mixed or dysfunctional relation between proinflammatory events (SIRS) and counterinflammatory events (CARS) can lead to the mixed antagonist response syndrome (MARS).[77] A mixed or intermittent, but dyscoordinated, relation between the pro- and counterinflammatory forces in the complex ICU patient clearly means that our level of understanding is inadequate to make immune stimulation a meaningful therapeutic effort at this time.

Finally, inflammatory "exhaustion" of the host is yet another area that requires future exploration. In our experimental studies of complement activation due to trauma or sepsis,[83,84] it has become apparent that the host who has experienced a severe insult undergoes systemic activation of the complement cascade, which leads to a period of reduced residual total hemolytic complement reserves. When an animal has only 30% of the total hemolytic complement remaining after hemorrhage or experimental trauma, it is relatively refractory to an intervening event (e.g., infection). This "exhaustion" of complement, prekallikrein, coagulation proteins (e.g., DIC), or platelets may be an internal control to temporize the excessive systemic inflammatory response. During the period of being refractory to inflammatory stimulation, the risk of intercurrent infection being unchecked is real. Conversely, the response of the host to inflammatory events may result in a "rebound" state of hypercoagulability, increased prekallikrein, or increased complement proteins (as an acute-phase response), which primes the host for a "second hit" and an inappropriate proinflammatory consequence. The important point is that longitudinal studies of the pro- and counterinflammatory signaling and the capacity of the host to respond to an intercurrent event (e.g., another infection, another operation) is fundamental for understanding the process and formulating both preventive and therapeutic strategies.

Gene Therapy

Is there intrinsic biologic variability among patients in their capacity to respond to a proinflammatory "activator" event? Is there similarly host variability in responding to proinflammatory events with an appropriate, balanced antiinflammatory response? Biologic variability among hosts is likely. Every clinician has had the patient with a bacteremic event who was lucid, was conversant, and appeared to tolerate the episode with a seemingly mild response. All have also had the patient who, in an apparently a similar situation, had a florid septic response leading to MODS and a fatal outcome. Although accepting the clear understanding that apparently analogous clinical scenarios are in reality never analogous, one cannot but believe that the intrinsic responsiveness of the host must contribute to a well compensated response to bacteremia in one setting and to fulminant SIRS, MODS, and death in another.

Gene therapy may pose a treatment strategy to restore a balanced host response. Using viral vectors of liposomal gene delivery vehicles, it may be possible to deliver the necessary genetic capacity to counteract an exaggerated inflammatory response in the host. Of the numerous therapies proposed as exogenous treatments in this chapter, gene therapy affords the opportunity to provide an endogenous source of treatment. Thus gene transfer into experimental animals for encoding antiinflammatory cytokines (e.g., IL-4, IL-10),[85] antioxidants,[86] and antiproteases[87] has been successfully done. Enhanced cellular responsiveness to improve stress tolerance by enhancing the heat shock response also appears feasible.[88] Such therapies imply that the host's capacity to respond appropriately is defective. A defective or dyscoordinated response clearly requires an overall understanding of the interaction of pro- and counterinflammatory signaling, which does not exist at the present time.

Molecular blockade of excessive cytokine production is being explored through the use of antisense oligodeoxynucleotides. The "antisense" strand of nucleotide could bind to the mRNA for TNF[89] or the mRNA for IL-1[90] and eliminate or dramatically reduce the proinflammatory response. Although the potential of such a therapeutic strategy defies the imagination, molecular engineering may well pose avenues for modification, enhancement, or ablation of specific responses of the host that are deemed inconsistent with an optimum outcome.

Other Therapies

Other therapeutic strategies will undoubtedly emerge. Nutritional support has been one such area where dramatic new

TABLE 72.2. Current Prospective Randomized Trials Collectively Demonstrating the Benefit of Immune-Enhanced Enteral Nutrition Formulas.

Study	No. of patients	Pathology	Clinical results
Gottschlich[91]	50	Burns	Reduced infections; reduced length of stay
Daly[92]	85	Upper GI-cancer	Reduced infections; reduced length of stay
Bower[93]	296	Surgical ICU	Reduced infection; reduced length of stay
Daly[94]	60	Esophageal, gastric, pancreatic cancer	Reduced postoperative infection; reduced wound complications
Moore[95]	98	Torso trauma	Fewer intraabdominal abscesses; less organ failure
Senkal[96]	154	Upper GI malignancy	Late complications less; reduced total costs
Kudsk[97]	35	Trauma	Reduced infections; reduced length of stay; reduced antibiotic use; reduced intraabdominal abscesses
Schilling[98]	41 (three-arm study)	Major abdominal surgery	Reduced infections

directions are being explored. So-called immunonutrition with additions of arginine, omega-3 fatty acids, and nucleotides to the nutritional support strategy has been an approach to supply nutritional elements that are currently thought to enhance host responsiveness. Early evidence indicates that immunonutrition has reduced infection morbidity in the severely ill patient, although survival has not been favorably influenced[91-98] (Table 72.2). These initial reports are encouraging because of the new vistas that may be opened by nutritional manipulation of the host. Are there nutritional support regimens favorable to proinflammatory or counterinflammatory responses? Certainly efforts to nullify the hypermetabolic response have not been reported by nutritional support, but efforts should continue. Furthermore, immunonutrition may prove to provide neither direct "immune" enhancement nor "nutrition" in terms of its salutary benefits. The regulation/control of splanchnic blood flow by intraluminal nutrients raises the interesting idea that immunonutrition is actually vasotherapy. The role of intraluminal nutrients in the improvement of splanchnic perfusion, true immunonutrients, and substrates to enhance the gut barrier become exciting future directions.

Yet another component of the nutritional riddle is the role of the host gut microflora. Some nutritional supports regimens support normalization of gut colonization, which may be of critical value for supporting the gut barrier. Systemic antibiotics commonly ablate this microbial component of the barrier. The role of preserving normal gut colonization through nutritional support, alternative antimicrobial strategies such as selective gut decontamination (Table 72.3), or perhaps in giving bacteria to the patient is certainly an interesting area for continued evaluation. What a novel idea—giving bacteria to the patient to prevent infection.

Back to the Future

The failure of the numerous clinical trials of "silver bullet" therapy to contain and treat SIRS, sepsis, and septic shock should have a sobering effect on practicing clinicians. Efforts to block, inhibit, or neutralize any one stimulus, mediator, or effector

TABLE 72.3. Prospective Randomized Trials of Various Regimens of Selective Gut Decontamination Since 1990.

Author Year	Condition	No. of patients	Antibiotic choices employed
Godard[99] (1990)	Surgical ICU	181	Tobramycin, colistin, amphotericin to all patients; no IV antibiotics
Rodriguez-Roldan[100] (1990)	Ventilated	28	Tobramycin, polymyxin, amphotericin; no IV drugs
Blair[101] (1991)	Mixed ICU	256	Polymyxin, amphotericin, tobramycin, IV cefotaxime
Pugin[102] (1992)	Ventilator	52	Polymyxin, neomycin, vancomycin; no IV drugs
Aerdts[103] (1991)	Ventilator	56*	Norfloxacin, polymyxin, amphotericin, IV cefotaxime
Rocha[104] (1992)	Surgical ICU	101	Polymyxin, amphotericin, tobramycin, IV cefotaxime
Cerra[105] (1992)	Surgical ICU	46	Norfloxacin, nystatin; no IV drugs
Cockerill[106] (1992)	Mixed ICU	150	Gentamicin, polymyxin, nystatin, IV cefotaxime
Hammond[107] (1992)	Mixed ICU	239	Amphotericin, colistin, tobramycin; all patients IV cefotaxime
Gastinne[108] (1992)	Ventilator	445	Tobramycin, colistin, amphotericin; no IV drugs
Winter[109] (1992)	Mixed	183	Polymyxin, amphotericin, tobramycin, IV ceftazidime
Korinek[110] (1993)	Neurosurgical ICU	123	Tobramycin, polymyxin, amphotericin, vancomycin; no IV drugs
Ferrer[111] (1994)	Ventilator	80	Polymyxin, amphotericin, tobramycin; all IV cefotaxime
Wiener[112] (1995)	Ventilator	61	Polymyxin, gentamicin, nystatin; no IV drugs
Quinio[113] (1996)	Mixed	148	Colistin, polymyxin, gentamicin, amphotericin; no IV drugs
Verwaest[114] (1997)	Ventilator	660*	One group: ofloxacin, amphotericin, IV ofloxacin Second group: polymyxin, tobramycin, amphotericin, IV cefotaxime

Most results demonstrate reduced infection rates but no difference in survival. This table illustrates differences in the size of populations that have been studied and the various antibiotic regimens used.
IV, intravenous.
*Three arms in the study.

mechanism of the human inflammatory response and its regulation is destined to fail. How many additional billions of dollars of wasted research resources are necessary to prove this point? It is time for a fundamental reappraisal of what is being done during the formulation of clinical trials. Just because a good idea (e.g., anti-TNF monoclonal antibodies) can be shown to work in a short-term experimental animal model that has few of the features seen in the human septic response (parenteral endotoxin with results at 24–48 hours) should not be the foundation for a multimillion dollar clinical trial of poorly stratified, heterogeneous patients with a disease that resembles sepsis, septic shock, or SIRS. Eager efforts to capture the "quick fix" have now created an atmosphere and attitude of cynicism and resignation, such that meaningful investigative efforts are potentially impaired. It is time to "back up" to the mid-1980s in our intellectual mind-set and reevaluate what is being done.

The clinical trials of the last 10 years are reminiscent of the use of preventive antibiotics in surgery. After World War II and the clinical introduction of antibiotics into clinical practice, many surgeons thought that the millennium of infection-free surgery was at hand. Operations could be done, antibiotics could be given, and excellent results would be the consequence. The euphoria of the new treatment yielded to the skepticism of unchanged clinical outcomes. Prospective clinical trials failed to show improved outcomes in terms of postoperative infection rates, and in some studies the results actually indicated poorer outcomes.[115–117] Preventive antibiotics were either abandoned altogether or were used in a half-hearted fashion by surgeons expecting results where clinical prudence would dictate otherwise. However, the basic animal research experiments by Miles et al.[118] and Burke[119] in clinically relevant models identified the critical importance of timing when administering preventive antibiotics.

Clinical studies by Bernard and Cole[120] and by Polk and Lopez-Mayor[121] translated the experimental findings into clinical reality by further demonstrating the importance of risk stratification. Patients of similar risk were compared with the appropriate timing. Risk stratification without *preoperative* administration of the antibiotic would have failed. Preoperative administration of preventive antibiotics but in a hodge-podge of patients with elective inguinal hernia repair, abdominoperineal resection, and gunshot wounds of the abdomen would have yielded no differences in outcome. In the sepsis trials with multiple agents, enrollment into the studies has occurred when the patient is recognized to meet "entry criteria," therapeutic doses and duration are given for uncertain reasons, and the case mix of patients is so diverse as to defy the imagination. Thus patients with leaking anastomoses after operations with uncertain adequacy of source control are included. Young patients with acute events are included with older patients that have recurrent and chronic events. Surgical disasters are compared to bacteremia due to urinary retention. The effort to enroll adequate numbers of these patients within a defined time period to meet study goals has destroyed the process of meaningful evaluations. In the pursuit of better future trials and study design, we should learn from the preventive antibiotic studies that have gone before. The fundamentals of our trial strategies must be revisited.

Forward to the Future

In my view, there are at least seven areas for reevaluating future directions as new therapies are formulated for the treatment of SIRS, MODS, and their sequelae.

1. *Development and use more clinically relevant animal models.* Much has been learned about host responsiveness and the cytokine responsiveness of inflammation using animal models, but most of these models have employed hyperacute administration of endotoxin or bacteria to otherwise healthy animals. Interventions in these hyperacute models with proposed antagonists or new treatment strategies have yielded results that have become the foundation of clinical trials. For animal models to be useful for the development of effective treatment, they must truly mirror the disease process being treated in the clinical setting. Porcine models of peritonitis that lasts for days and has hemodynamic and metabolic features consistent with the human septic condition are more appropriate for examining the utility of a new therapy. Although the use of such models will be expensive, nothing is more expensive that an inexpensive mouse experiment with endotoxin that paves the way for a 100 million clinical trial of human disease that has no resemblance to the animal experiment.

2. *Better definition of the counterinflammatory response.* The proinflammatory signals, though probably not fully defined, have been recognized and studied for a full 15 years. The rapidity of the TNF response to specific activating stimuli has been characterized. Sustained IL-6 elevation as a predictor of outcome has been examined. However IL-4, IL-10, IL-13 and others are only now being fully characterized as counterinflammatory signals. The appropriateness of their release and action with respect to the proinflammatory signals is clearly important. Both the quantitative and temporal responses must be characterized. Premature and excessive counterinflammatory signals could impair the salutary effects of the proinflammatory signals and lead to unchecked, aggressive infection. Delayed or weak responses could lead to unchecked inflammation, with SIRS as the immediate consequence. The normal dose of insulin necessary to avoid ketoacidosis is inadequate to abort the process once it is activated. Rapid expression of spiking proinflammatory signals may exceed normal counterinflammatory responsiveness. A therapeutic window may present itself as we better understand the coordinated or dyscoordinated responses of the pro- and counterinflammatory relations.

3. *Better refinement of bedside diagnostic capabilities.* It could be argued that prior clinical trials have treated a heterogeneous group of diseases that have some common characteristics (i.e., inclusion criteria). Is endotoxin a significant participant in a given patient's septic response? Rapid, sensitive endotoxin determinations at the bedside would allow inclusion of patients into appropriate trials for neutralizing antibody, hemofiltration, and other chelating strategies (e.g., polymyxin). The current

number of patients without endotoxin or with intermittent endotoxemia as a contributor but not sole "activator" of SIRS cannot be determined; thus we see nonsignificant clinical outcomes or draw dubious, post hoc conclusions about potential efficacy. The diagnostic capacity to identify circulating endotoxin or bedside polymerase chain reaction (PCR) studies to define microbial DNA will hopefully confirm when microbial cell products are participating in the process, or if the patient is even infected. The totally promiscuous use of antibiotics in the ICU as a desperate measure by clinicians who are treating something that looks like an infection will not be viewed favorably by the post hoc analysis of future generations.

Better quantification of proinflammatory and counterinflammatory signals will also be a diagnostic requirement for anticytokine or cytokine administration therapy. It is probably naive to believe that circulating cytokine concentrations have relevance to the interactive biologic conundrum of SIRS and MODS. Cytokines surface-bound to receptors is certainly the critical determinant, with circulating concentrations being simply an "overflow" from excessive signaling. Detectable circulating cytokine concentrations may reflect saturation kinetics at the receptor site. Hence any measured quantity may have uncertain significance. Bedside or other rapid diagnostic methodologies will allow real-time determination of the patient's current status, allow better mapping of the natural history of the disease, and permit stratification of interactions at common points in the evolution of the host's response.

4. *Better understanding of patient variability.* It is reasonable to expect that the proinflammatory and counterinflammatory responses of the population follow a standard distribution. A given challenge may provoke an overexuberant proinflammatory response in one patient or an excessive counterinflammatory response in another. A balance between these opposing cytokine responses may likely define the patient who will develop an excessive inflammatory response and the patient who may have immune suppression due to excessive or ill-timed counterinflammatory signaling.

Although intrinsic variability is of interest, acquired variability or dyscoordinated responsiveness between the pro- and counterinflammatory responses may have particular relevance in the evolution of SIRS and MODS. The role of acquired illness (e.g., malnutrition) or the consequence of sequential systemic insults may alter the coordinated relations of a balanced host response. Certainly some evidence in the "two-hit" response favors the idea that a second biologic insult during a window of a "primed" proinflammatory response or a refractory counterinflammatory response may create an imbalance of responsiveness and provoke SIRS. Surrogate markers reflective of net pro- and counterinflammatory influences might permit accurate predictors of which patient is at risk for a SIRS response.

5. *Better clinical staging systems of SIRS and MODS.* A consistent failure of clinical trials of therapeutic interventions for the "septic" or "septic shock" patient has been poor stratification of patients. Patients with evidence of early organ failure are commonly excluded. Sepsis and septic shock are viewed as binary events that patients either have or do not have.

During trauma care the combination of the trauma score and the injury severity score (ISS) have been used to establish a national database that permits determination of "expectation of survival." The trauma score is a physiologic measure, and the ISS is an estimate of the degree of anatomic injury. Such a methodology allows stratification of patients into populations at risk for anticipated outcomes. The relation between MODS and the blood lactate concentration reflects organ system injury, and lactate reflects a biochemical measure that could permit stratification. The heterogeneous groups of patients with different activator events and different host responses that are currently being studied means that a valuable, innovative therapy may be discarded as worthless because of the failed stratification by risk.

6. *Failure to appreciate the complex and redundant processes of human inflammation.* Whether it is the proinflammatory cytokines, counterinflammatory cytokines, chemokines for leukocyte trafficking, or initiators of human inflammation, it is overwhelmingly evident that each step in the unfolding of human inflammation and its regulation are governed by complex and redundant pathways. It should be evident that the search for a "silver bullet" is fruitless. Perhaps multimodality therapy is a more prudent strategy where efforts to comprehensively block one step of the process or to attempt multiple "tandem" modulation at sequential steps in the process will be more effective. The search for multiphasic therapy will prove to be difficult and will likely have many deadends in clinical trials.

7. *Inflammation evolved for the benefit of the host.* Comprehensive blockade of inflammatory signals may be of benefit for breaking the SIRS process but leaves a host who is unable to respond to an intervening local infection. Clinical trials of would-be treatments must carefully monitor patients for nosocomial infectious morbidity. Again, patient stratification for risk of death and probability of nosocomial infection becomes essential to "unmask" significant differences that may be obscured by heterogeneous treatment populations.

In summary, future directions require forward thinking. The failures of past therapeutic efforts must be sources of learning for how *not* to do things. The enormous complexity of the human inflammatory response poses a riddle that cannot be easily solved. A serious reappraisal of past failures with an eye toward understanding the normal and coordinated responses of all elements of the inflammatory response should lead to meaningful treatment strategies.

References

1. Fry DE, Garrison RN, Heitsch RC, et al: Determinants of death in patients with intra-abdominal abscess. Surgery 1980;89:517-523.
2. Barie PS, Hydro LJ, Fischer E: A prospective comparison of two multiple organ dysfunction/failure systems for prediction of mortality on critical surgical illness. J Trauma 1994;37:660.
3. Regel G, Grotz M, Weltner, et al: The pattern of organ failure following severe trauma. World J Surg 1996;20:422.
4. Sauaia A, Moore FA, Moore EE, et al: Early predictors of postinjury multiorgan failure. Arch Surg 1994;129:39.

5. Sautner T, Gotzinger P, Redl-Wenzl EM, et al: Does reoperation for abdominal sepsis enhance the inflammatory host response? Arch Surg 1997;132:250–255.
6. Van Goor H, Hulsebos RG, Bleichrodt RP: Complications of planned relaparotomy in patients with severe general peritonitis. Eur J Surg 1997;163:61–66.
7. Flynn PM, Shenep JL, Stokes DC, et al: Polymyxin B moderates acidosis and hypotension in established, experimental gram-negative septicemia. J Infect Dis 1987;156:706–712.
8. Hirasawa H, Sugai T, Ohtake Y, et al: Blood purification for prevention and treatment of multiple organ failure. World J Surg 1996;20:482–486.
9. Lechner AJ, Lamprech KE, Johanns CA, Matuschak GM: The recombinant 23-kDa N-terminal fragment of bactericidal/permeability-increasing protein (rBPI23) decreases *E. coli*-induced mortality and organ injury during immunosuppression-related neutropenia. Shock 1995;4:218.
10. Elsbach P: The bactericidal/permeability-increasing protein (BPI) in antibacterial host defense. J Leukoc Biol 1998;64:14–18.
11. Landmann R, Reber AM, Sansano S, Zimmerli W: Function of soluble CD14 in serum from patients with septic shock. J Infect Dis 1996;173:661–668.
12. Burd RS, Cody CS, Raymond CS, Dunn DL: Anti-endotoxin monoclonal antibodies protect by enhancing bacterial and endotoxin clearance. Arch Surg 1993;128:145–150.
13. Ziegler EJ, McCutchan JA, Fierer J, et al: Treatment of gram-negative bacteremia and shock with human antiserum to a mutant *Escherichia coli*. N Engl J Med 1982;307:1225.
14. Ziegler EJ, Fischer CJ, Sprung CL Jr, et al: Treatment of gram-negative bacteremia and septic shock with HA-1A human monoclonal antibody against endotoxin: a randomized, double-blind, placebo-controlled trial. N Engl J Med 1991;324:429.
15. McCloskey RV, Straube RC, Sanders C, et al: Treatment of septic shock with human monoclonal antibody HA-1A: a randomized, double blind, placebo-controlled trial: CHESS Trial Study Group. Ann Intern Med 1994;121:1–5.
16. Greenman RL, Schein RMH, Martin MA, et al: A controlled clinical trial of E5 murine monoclonal IgM antibody to endotoxin in the treatment of gram-negative sepsis. JAMA 1991; 266:1097.
17. Bone RC, Balk RA, Fein AM, et al: A second large controlled study of E5, a monoclonal antibody to endotoxin: results of a prospective, multicenter, randomized, controlled trial: the E5 Sepsis Study Group. Crit Care Med 1995;23:994–1006.
18. Jansen PM, Pixley RA, Brouwer M, et al: Inhibition of factor XII in septic baboons attenuates the activation of complement and fibrinolytic system and reduces the release of interleukin-6 and neutrophil elastase. Blood 1996;87:2337–2344.
19. Dickneite G: Antithrombin III in animal models of sepsis and organ failure. Semin Thromb Hemost 1998;24:61–69.
20. Hau T, Simmons RL: Heparin in the treatment of experimental peritonitis. Ann Surg 1978;187:294.
21. O'Leary JP, Malik FS, Donahoe RP, et al: The effects of a minidose of heparin on peritonitis in rats. Surg Gynecol Obstet 1979;148:571.
22. Schirmer WJ, Schirmer JM, Naff GB, et al: Heparin's effect on the natural history of sepsis in the rat [abstract]. Circ Shock 1987;21:363.
23. Eisele B, Lamy M: Clinical experience with antithrombin III concentrates in critically ill patients with sepsis and multiple organ failure. Semin Thromb Hemost 1998;24:71–80.
24. Ridings PC, Blocher CR, Fisher BJ, et al: Beneficial effects of a bradykinin antagonist in a model of gram negative sepsis. J Trauma 1995;39:81–88.
25. Fein AM, Bernard GR, Criner GJ, et al: Treatment of severe systemic inflammatory response syndromes and sepsis with a novel bradykinin antagonist, deltibant (CP-0127): results of a randomized, double-blind, placebo-controlled trial; CP-1027 SIRS and Sepsis Study Group. JAMA 1997;277:482–487.
26. Ketteler M, Cetto C, Kirdorf M, et al: Nitric oxide in sepsis-syndrome: potential treatment of septic shock by nitric oxide synthase antagonists. Kidney Int 1998;53(Suppl 64):S27–S30.
27. Lindsay TF, Hill J, Oritz F, et al: Blockade of complement activation prevents local and pulmonary albumin leak after lower torso ischemia reperfusion. Ann Surg 1992;216:677.
28. Hack CE, Voerman HJ, Eisele B, et al: C1-esterase inhibitor substitution in sepsis. Lancet 1992;339:378.
29. Jansen PM, Eisele B, de Jong IW, et al: Effect of C1 inhibition on inflammatory and physiologic response patterns in primates suffering from lethal septic shock. J Immunol 1998;160:475–484.
30. Mohr M, Hopken U, Opperman M, et al: Effects of anti-C5a monoclonal antibodies on oxygen use in a porcine model of severe sepsis. Eur J Clin Invest 1998;28:227–234.
31. Neugebauer E, Lorenz W, Rixen D, et al: Histamine release in sepsis: a prospective, controlled, clinical study. Crit Care Med 1996;24:1670–1677.
32. Neugebauer E, Lorenz W, Beckurts T, et al: Significance of histamine formation and release in the development of endotoxic shock: proof of current concepts by randomized controlled studies in rats. Rev Infect Dis 1987;9(Suppl 5):S585–S593.
33. Leeper-Woodford SK, Carey D, Byrne K, et al: Histamine receptor antagonists, cyclooxygenase blockade, and tumor necrosis factor curing acute septic insult. Shock 1998;9:89–94.
34. Beutler B, Milsark IW, Cerami AC: Passive immunization against cachectin/tumor necrosis factor protects mice from lethal effect of endotoxin. Science 1985;229:869.
35. Tracey KJ, Fong Y, Hesse DG, et al: Anticachectin/TNF monoclonal antibodies prevent septic shock during lethal bacteraemia. Nature 1987;330:662.
36. Abraham E, Wunderink R, Silverman H, et al: Efficacy and safety of monoclonal antibody to human tumor necrosis factor alpha in patients with sepsis syndrome: a randomized controlled, double-blind, multicenter clinical trial. JAMA 1995;273:934–941.
37. Cohen J, Carlet J: Intersept: an international, multicenter, placebo-controlled trial of monoclonal antibody to human tumor necrosis factor-alpha in patients with sepsis: International Sepsis Trial Study Group. Crit Care Med 1996;24:1431–1440.
38. Reinhart K, Wiegard-Lohnert C, Grimminger F, et al: Assessment of the safety and efficacy of the monoclonal anti-tumor necrosis factor antibody-fragment, MAK 195F, in patients with sepsis and septic shock: a multicenter, randomized, placebo-controlled, dose-ranging study. Crit Care Med 1996;24:733–742.
39. Fisher CJ Jr, Agosti JM, Opal SM, et al: Treatment of septic shock with the tumor necrosis factor receptor: Fc fusion protein: the Soluble TNF Receptor Sepsis Study Group. N Engl J Med 1996;334:1697–1702.
40. Wakabayashi G, Gelfand JA, Burke JF, et al: A specific receptor antagonist for interleukin 1 prevents *Escherichia coli*-induced shock in rabbits. FASEB J 1991;5:338.
41. Fisher CJ Jr, Dhainaut JF, Opal SM, et al: Recombinant human interleukin 1 receptor antagonist in the treatment of patients with sepsis syndrome: results from a randomized, double-blind,

placebo-controlled trial; phase III rhIL-1ra Sepsis Syndrome Study Group. JAMA 1994;271:1836–1843.
42. Opal SM, Fisher CJ Jr, Dhainaut JF, et al: Confirming interleukin-1 receptor antagonist trial in severe sepsis: a phase III, randomized, double-blind, placebo-controlled, multicenter trial; the interleukin-1 Receptor Antagonist Sepsis Investigation Group. Crit Care Med 1997;25:1115–1124.
43. Van der Poll T, Levi M, Hack CE, et al: Elimination of interleukin 6 attenuates coagulation activation in experimental endotoxemia in chimpanzees. J Exp Med 1994;179:1253.
44. Vedder NB, Winn RK, Rice CL, et al: A monoclonal antibody to the adherence promoting leukocyte glycoprotein CD18, reduces organ injury and improves survival from hemorrhagic shock and resuscitation in rabbits. J Clin Invest 1988;81:939.
45. Walsh CJ, Carey D, Cook DJ, et al: Anti CD18 antibody attenuates neutropenia and alveolar capillary membrane injury during gram negative sepsis. Surgery 1991;110:205.
46. Winn RK, Ramamoorthy C, Vedder NB, et al: Leukocyte-endothelial cell interaction in ischemia reperfusion injury. Ann NY Acad Sci 1997;832:311–321.
47. Cornejo CJ, Winn RK, Harlan JM: Anti-adhesion therapy. Adv Pharmacol 1997;39:99–142.
48. Ramamoorthy C, Sasaki SS, Su DL, et al: CD18 adhesion blockade decreases bacterial clearance and neutrophil recruitment after intrapulmonary E. coli, but not after S. aureus. J Leukoc Biol 1997;61:167–172.
49. Redl H, Schlag G, Davies J, Robinson M: Detrimental effects of the application of anti-CD18 antibodies in baboon live E. coli sepsis. Circ Shock 1993;2(Suppl):33.
50. Eichacker P, MacVittie T, Farese A, et al: Antibody agonist leukocyte CD18 membrane protein does not improve outcome in a canine model of human sepsis. 1992;20:S51.
51. Seekamp A, Till GO, Mulligan MS, et al: Role of selectins in local and remote tissue injury following ischemia and reperfusion. Am J Pathol 1994;144:592.
52. Fink MP: Therapeutic options directed against platelet activating factor, eicosanoids, and bradykinin in sepsis. J Antimicrob Chemother 1998;41(Suppl A):81–94.
53. Froon AM, Greve JW, Buurman WA, et al: Treatment with the platelet-activating factor antagonist TCV-309 in patients with severe systemic inflammatory response syndrome: a prospective, multi-center, double-blind, randomized phase II trial. Shock 1996;5:313–319.
54. Dhainaut JF, Tenaillon A, Hemmer M, et al: Confirmatory platelet-activating factor receptor antagonist trial in patients with severe gram-negative bacterial sepsis: a phase III, randomized, double-blind, placebo controlled, multicenter trial: BN 52021 Sepsis Investigator Group. Crit Care Med 1998;26:1963–1971.
55. Kapoor R, Kalra J, Prasad K: Cardiac depression and cellular injury in hemorrhagic shock and reinfusion: role of free radicals. Mol Cell Biochem 1997;176:291–306.
56. Simon HM, Scalea T, Paskanik A, Young B: Superoxide dismutase (SOD) prevents hypotension after hemorrhagic shock and aortic cross clamping. Am J Med Sci 1996;312:155–159.
57. Harris NR, Russell JM, Granger DN: Mediators of endotoxin-induced leukocyte adhesion in mesenteric postcapillary venules. Circ Shock 1994;43:155–160.
58. Abello PA, Fidler SA, Bulkley GB, Buckman TG: Antioxidants modulate induction of programmed endothelial cell death (apoptosis) by endotoxin. Arch Surg 1994;129:134–140.
59. Rose S, Baumann H, Jahreis GP, Sayeed MM: Diltiazem and superoxide dismutase modulate hepatic acute phase response in gram-negative sepsis. Shock 1994;1:87–93.
60. Rose S, Sayeed MM: Superoxide radical scavenging prevents cellular calcium, dysregulation during intraabdominal sepsis. Shock 1997;7:263–268.
61. Krysztopik RJ, Bentley FR, Spain DA, Wilson MA, Garrison RN: Free radical scavenging by lazaroids improves renal blood flow during sepsis. Surgery 1996;120:657–662.
62. Pou S, Keaton L, Surichamorn W, et al: Can nitric oxide be spin trapped by nitrone and nitroso compounds? Biochim Biophys Acta 1994;1201:118–124.
63. Maher DW, Davis I, Boyd AW, Morstyn G: Human interleukin-4: an immunomodulator with potential therapeutic application. Prog Growth Factor Res 1991;3:43–56.
64. De Waal Malefyt R, Abrams J, Bennet B, et al: Interleukin 10 inhibits cytokine synthesis by human monocytes: an autoregulatory role of IL-10 production by monocytes. J Exp Med 1991;174:1209.
65. De Vries JE: Molecular and biological characteristics of interleukin-13. Chem Immunol 1996;63:204–218.
66. Matsumoto T, Tateda K, Miyazaki S, et al: Effect of interleukin-10 on gut-derived sepsis caused by Pseudomonas aeruginosa in mice. Antimicrob Agents Chemother 1998;42:2853–2857.
67. Lubberts E, Joosten LA, Helsen MM, van den Berg WB: Regulatory role of interleukin 10 in joint inflammation and cartilage destruction in murine streptococcal cell wall arthritis: more therapeutic benefit with IL-4/IL-10 combination therapy than with IL-10 treatment alone. Cytokine 1998;10:361–369.
68. Nicoletti F, Mancuso G, Ciliberti FA, et al: Endotoxin-induced lethality in neonatal mice is counteracted by interleukin-10 and exacerbated by anti-IL-10. Clin Diagn Lab Immunol 1997;4:607–610.
69. Mulligan MS, Warner RL, Foreback JL, et al: Protective effects of IL-4, IL-10, IL-12, and IL-13 in IgG immune complex-induced lung injury: role of endogenous IL-12. J Immunol 1997;159:3483–3489.
70. Muchamuel T, Menon S, Pisacane P, et al: IL-13 protects mice from lipopolysaccharide-induced lethal endotoxemia: correlation with down-modulation of TNF-alpha, IFN-gamma, and IL-12 production. J Immunol 1997;158:2898–2903.
71. Nicoletti F, Mancuso G, Cusumano V, et al: Prevention of endotoxin-induced lethality in neonatal mice by interleukin-13. Eur J Immunol 1997;27:1580–1583.
72. Hogaboam CM, Vallance BA, Kumar A, et al: Therapeutic effects of interleukin-4 gene transfer in experimental inflammatory bowel disease. J Clin Invest 1997;100:2766–2776.
73. Inobe JI, Chen Y, Weiner HL: In vivo administration of IL-4 induces TGF-beta-producing cells and protects animals from experimental autoimmune encephalomyelitis. Ann NY Acad Sci 1996;778:390–392.
74. Kato T, Murata A, Ishida H, et al: Interleukin 10 reduces mortality from severe peritonitis in mice. Antimicrob Agents Chemother 1995;39:1336–1340.
75. Wahl SM, McCartney-Francis N, Mergenhagen SE: Inflammatory and immunomodulatory roles of TGF-beta. Immunol Today 1989;10:258–261.
76. Faist E, Schinkel C, Zimmer S: Update on the mechanisms of immune suppression of injury and immune modulation. World J Surg 1996;20:454–459.

77. Bone RC, Grodzin CJ, Bulk RA: Sepsis: a new hypothesis for pathogenesis of the disease process. Chest 1997;112:235-243.
78. Polk HC Jr, Cheadle WG, Livingston DH, et al: A randomized prospective clinical trial to determine the efficacy of interferon-gamma in severely injured patients. Am J Surg 1992;163:191-196.
79. Meakins JL, Christou NV, Shizgal HM, MacLean LD: Therapeutic approaches to anergy in surgical patients: surgery and levamisole. Ann Surg 1979;190:286-296.
80. Brown GL, Foshee H, Pietsch J, Polk HC Jr: Muramyl dipeptide enhances survival for experimental peritonitis. Arch Surg 1986;121:47-49.
81. O'Reilly M, Silver GM, Greenhalgh DG, et al: Treatment of intra-abdominal infection with granulocyte colony-stimulating factor. J Trauma 1992;33:679-682.
82. Stern AC, Jones TC: Role of human recombinant GM-CSF in the prevention and treatment of leukopenia with special reference to infectious disease. Diagn Microbiol Infect Dis 1990;13:391-396.
83. Schirmer WJ, Schirmer JM, Townsend MC, Fry DE: Femur fracture with associated soft tissue injury produces hepatic ischemia. Arch Surg 1988;123:412-415.
84. Schirmer WJ, Schirmer JM, Naff GB, Fry DE: Complement activation in peritonitis: association with hepatic and renal perfusion abnormalities. Am Surg 1987;53:683-687.
85. Xing Z, Ohkawara Y, Jordana M, et al: A transient transgenic model of IL-10 functional studies in vivo: adenoviral-mediated intramuscular IL-10 gene transfer inhibits cytokine responses in endotoxemia. Gene Ther 1997;4:140-149.
86. Ezurum SC, Lemarchand P, Rosenfeld MA, et al: Protection of human endothelial cells from oxidant injury by adenovirus-mediated transfer of the human catalase cDNA. Nucleic Acids Res 1993;21:1607-1612.
87. Canonico AE, Conary JT, Meyrick BO, Brigham KL: Aerosol and intravenous transfection of human alpha-1 antitrypsin gene to lungs of rabbits. Am J Respir Cell Mol Biol 1994;10:24-29.
88. De Maio A: The heat-shock response. New Horiz 1995;3:198-207.
89. Rojanasakul Y, Weissman DN, Shi X, et al: Antisense inhibition of silica-induced tumor necrosis factor in alveolar macrophages. J Biol Chem 1997;272:3910-3914.
90. Maier JAM, Voulalas P, Roeder D, Maciag T: Extension of the life-span of human endothelial cells by an interleukin-1 alpha antisense oligomer. Science 1990;249:1570-1574.
91. Gottschlich MM, Jenkins M, Warden GD, et al: Differential effects of three enteral dietary regimens on selected outcome variables in burn patients. JPEN 1990;14:225.
92. Daly JM, Lieberman MD, Goldfine J, et al: Enteral nutrition with supplemental arginine, RNA, and omega-3 fatty acids in patients after operation: immunologic, metabolic, and clinical outcomes. Surgery 1992;112:56.
93. Bower RH, Cerra FB, Bershadsky B, et al: Early enteral administration of a formula supplemented with arginine, nucleotides, and fish oil in intensive care patients: results of a multicenter, prospective, randomized, clinical trial. Crit Care Med 1995;23:436.
94. Daly JM, Weintraub FN, Shou J, et al: Enteral nutrition during multimodality therapy in upper gastrointestinal cancer patients. Ann Surg 1995;221:327.
95. Moore FA, Moore EE, Kudsk KA, et al: Clinical benefits of an immune-enhancing diet for early postinjury enteral feedings. J Trauma 1994;37:607.
96. Senkal M, Mumme A, Eickhoff U, et al: Early postoperative enteral immunonutrition: clinical outcome and cost comparison analysis in surgical patients. Crit Care Med 1997;25:1489-1496.
97. Kudsk KA, Minard G, Croce MA, et al: A randomized trial of isonitrogenous enteral diets following severe trauma: an immune-enhancing diet (IED) reduces septic complications. Ann Surg 1996;224:531.
98. Schilling J, Uranjes N, Fierz W, et al: Clinical outcome and immunology of postoperative arginine, omega-3 fatty acids, and nucleotide-enriched enteral feeding: a randomized preoperative comparison with standard enteral and low calorie/low fat i.v. solutions. Nutrition 1996;12:423-429.
99. Godard J, Guillaume ME, Bachmann B, et al: Intestinal decontamination in a polyvalent ICU: a double-blind study. Intensive Care Med 1990;16:307-311.
100. Rodriquez-Roldan JM, Altuna-Cuesta A, Lopez A, et al: Prevention of nosocomial lung infection in ventilated patients: use of an antimicrobial pharyngeal non-absorbable paste. Crit Care Med 1990;18:1239-1242.
101. Blair P, Rowlands BJ, Lowry K, et al: Selective decontamination of the digestive tract: a stratified, randomized, prospective study in a mixed intensive care unit. Surgery 1991;110:303-310.
102. Pugin J, Auckenthaler R, Lew DP, Suter PM: Oropharyngeal decontamination decreases incidence of ventilator-associated pneumonia: a randomized, placebo-controlled, double-blind clinical trial. JAMA 1991;265:2704-2710.
103. Aerdts SJA, van Dalen R, Clasener HAL, et al: Antibiotic prophylaxis of respiratory tract infection in mechanically ventilated patients. Chest 1991;100:783-791.
104. Rocha LA, Martin MJ, Pita S, et al: Prevention of nosocomial infection in critically ill patients by selective decontamination of the digestive tract: a randomized, double blind, placebo-controlled study. Intensive Care Med 1992;18:398-404.
105. Cerra FB, Maddaus MA, Dunn DL, et al: Selective gut decontamination reduces nosocomial infections and length of stay but not morality or organ failure in surgical intensive care unit patients. Arch Surg 1992;127:163-169.
106. Cockerill FR, Muller SR, Anhalt JP, et al: Prevention of infection in critically ill patients by selective decontamination of the digestive tract. Ann Intern Med 1992;117:545-553.
107. Hammond JM, Potgieter PD, Saunders GL, Forder AA: Double-blind study of selective decontamination of the digestive tract in intensive care. Lancet 1992;340:5-9.
108. Gastinne H, Wolff M, Delatour F, et al: A controlled trial in intensive care units of selective decontamination of the digestive tract with non-absorbable antibiotics. N Engl J Med 1992;326:594-599.
109. Winter R, Humphreys H, Pick A, et al: A controlled trial of selective decontamination of the digestive tract in intensive care and its effect on nosocomial infection. J Antimicrob Chemother 1992;30:73-87.
110. Korinek AM, Laisne MJ, Nicolas MH, et al: Selective decontamination of the digestive tract in neurosurgical intensive care unit patients: a double-blind, randomized, placebo-controlled study. Crit Care Med 1993;21:1466-1473.
111. Ferrer M, Torres A, Gonzalez J, et al: Utility of selective digestive decontamination in mechanically ventilated patients. Ann Intern Med 1994;120:389-395.
112. Wiener J, Itokazu G, Nathan C, et al: A randomized, double-blind, placebo-controlled trial of selective decontamination in a

113. Quinio B, Albanese J, Bues-Charbit M, et al: Selective decontamination of the digestive tract in multiple trauma patients. Chest 1996;109:765–772.
114. Verwaest C, Verhaegen J, Ferdinande P, et al: Randomized, controlled trial of selective digestive decontamination in 600 mechanically ventilated patients in a multidisciplinary intensive care unit. Crit Care Med 1997;25:63–71.
115. Sanchez-Ubeda R, Fernand E, Rousselot LM: Complication rate in general surgical cases: the value of penicillin and streptomycin as postoperative prophylaxis. N Engl J Med 1958;259:1045–1050.
116. Barnes J, Pace WG, Trump DS, Ellison EH: Prophylactic postoperative antibiotics. Arch Surg 1959;79:190–196.
117. Johnstone FRC: An assessment of prophylactic antibiotics in general surgery. Surg Gynecol Obstet 1963;116:1–10.
118. Miles AA, Miles EM, Burke JM: The value and duration of defense reactions of the skin to the primary lodgment of bacteria. Br J Exp Pathol 1957;38:79–96.
119. Burke JF: The effective period of preventive antibiotic action in experimental incisions and dermal lesions. Surgery 1961;50:z161–167.
120. Bernard HR, Cole WR: The prophylaxis of surgical infection: the effect of prophylactic antimicrobial drugs on the incidence of infection following potentially contaminated operations. Surgery 1964;56:151.
121. Polk HC Jr, Lopez-Mayor JF: Postoperative wound infection: a prospective study of determinant factors and prevention. Surgery 1969;66:97–103.

73
Summary and Overview: What Does the Future Hold?

Arthur E. Baue, Donald E. Fry, and Eugen Faist

This volume provides information that is on the leading edge of the care of critically ill patients. Each author is an expert in the field about which they write. They have written extensively on their subjects previously and now update the information about where support and treatment are clinically feasible. Although basic concepts have been reviewed in many chapters, the thrust of this book is clinical patient care. The basic science underlying these therapies is important and is reviewed briefly but in depth; background information may be found in other books and journals.

Despite the extensive reviews contained herein, it was inevitable that we could not include everyone who has made an important contribution to this field. To you we apologize. It was not an oversight, simply due to a limitation of space. Our many colleagues in the basic sciences who have made an important contribution to our knowledge could not be included. We maintained the focus on what is known and what can be done for patients. We can name many surgeons, intensivists, and other colleagues from Tel Aviv to Montreal to Amsterdam to Buenos Aires to New Zealand and from San Francisco to Boston and elsewhere who continue to contribute to our knowledge of MOF, MODS, and SIRS. Our thanks to you. You have indeed contributed to this book through your work. We hope that the information in this book will help readers provide even better care for their patients.

Remaining Weak Links in the Chain

A remaining weak link in the chain of injury is central nervous system (CNS) injury or failure. It has been well documented—by Faist et al. at the University of Munich[1] and by Baker and our group at Yale[2]—that 50% of patients who die after accidental injury do so from primary CNS causes. This is true whether the trauma was due to gunshot or knife wounds or to high speed accidents on the Autobahn, and it is consistent with other experience. It provides a major challenge to prevention of injury and care of the injured. Patients with primary CNS injury may die from that injury alone or may develop multiple organ problems; but at the present time the CNS, when injured, remains the major single limiting organ system after injury. Hence it is a challenge for those who attempt to decrease the impact of accidental injury and death.

Another weak link in the chain is the prolonged stay in the intensive care unit (ICU).[3] First, patients in the ICU become immunosuppressed with an injury or operation. We understand how but not why this occurs. It results in increased nosocomial infections and increased resistant organisms, a problem that seems to be a one-way street.[4] Nursing homes send patients to the hospital and to the ICU with an extended spectrum of beta-lactamases on plasmids. Ventilator dependence leads to ventilator-acquired infection and pneumonia. Moreover, the ICU is contaminated. It is not an operating room. In a way, it is a bacteriologic nightmare, with tubes, catheters, and organisms. Nosocomial infections are often due to methicillin-resistant *Staphylococcus aureus* or *Staphylococcus epidermidis*; penicillin-resistant *Streptococcus pneumoniae*; vancomycin-resistant *Enterococcus faecium*, *S. aureus*, or *S. epidermidis*; *Pseudomonas aeruginosa*; and *Candida albicans*.

The warning signs of these hazards is that mortality for long-term ICU patients has not decreased in recent years. There is a bacteriologic cesspool in most ICUs. Nosocomial infection is difficult to prevent. Antibiotic resistance develops; and once antibiotics have lost their effectiveness, they do not become powerful agents again. Patients who require prolonged ICU stays frequently develop problems that limit their survival. Jasny and Bloom recently said, on the subject of nosocomial infection: "To have invested in science, achieved understanding of the steps that need to be taken, and then fail to act on that knowledge would be folly of the highest order."[5]

We have made a modest proposal that there be two kinds of ICUs. One would be a short-term unit for overnight or 2- to 3-day standard care—a standard facility that is clean, requiring the use of handwashing and gloves. The second unit would be a long-term ICU similar to an operating room facility, with vertical air handling, ultimate filters and exchange of air from high to low, and scrub clothing (gowns and masks for all personnel and gloves for all patient contact). Such a unit would be for patients who must be in an ICU for some period of time or who are ventilator-dependent (or both). In today's world this

ICU division would increase costs, which is a problem. However, it may be the only way to lower the high mortality of patients with MOF who are in ICUs. In a presentation to the Society of Intensive Care Medicine in January 1999, Barie et al. reported using an intermediate ICU for patients who required close observation after an operation for several days.[6] This, they believed, optimized critical care resources.

Limitations: Year 2000—The Millennium

1. Limitations imposed by chronic illness brought on by deleterious life habits: smoking producing lung cancer and chronic obstructive pulmonary disease (COPD)/emphysema; alcohol causing liver disease; obesity; food fads; and untreated hypertension.
2. Limitations imposed by lack of adequate health care for the poor, causing infant mortality, and neglected disease.
3. Limitations imposed by lack of social responsibility: drugs, violence; lack of gun control due in part to the efforts of the National Rifle Association; alcohol-related traffic deaths; road rage.
4. Limitations imposed by extensive injury, extensive operations, or serious illnesses that were previously uniformly fatal.
5. Limitations imposed by uncontrollable world population growth. Genesis 5:25: "Methuselah was 187 years old when he begot Lamech. After the birth of Lamech he lived for 782 years and had other sons and daughters. He lived to 969 years and then he died." The cause of death was not given—it was during pre-ICU days.

Unsolved Clinical Problems

A number of unsolved problems require clinical and investigative attention: (1) The bioenergetic failure of increased venous oxygen content and altered oxygen consumption (VO_2) during sepsis; (2) fluid accumulation, producing generalized edema in severely injured and septic patients; (3) modulating the inflammatory response without doing harm; (4) the presence of infection and determining if it is due to invasive bacteria, saprophytic bacteria, or host defense failure; (5) why there is immunosuppression after injury and the problem of controlling all aspects of it; (6) the severity of injury and age remain major risk factors; (7) prevention of MOF.[7]

New and Exciting Science

Who would have thought that atherosclerosis would be accelerated by an infectious agent. Stephens et al. detected *Chlamydia trachomatis* in as many as 70% of atheromatous lesions in blood vessels.[8] There is also evidence that patients with infection in the body exhibit accelerated atherosclerosis. Where will it end? This finding seems similar to the evidence that *Helicobacter pylori* is the major agent producing duodenal ulcer, and gastric ulcer, and gastritis and perhaps is related to gastric carcinoma.

Occult herpes family viruses may increase mortality in critically ill patients. Such viruses have immunosuppressive effects that predispose chronic surgical ICU patients to subsequent bacterial and fungal infections.[9]

There is an Unexplained Illness Working Group in California that is cooperating closely with the Centers for Disease Control and Prevention in Atlanta.[10] They found that no pathogen was detected in 14% of patients who died seemingly due to infections in patients ages 1–49. They now are using state-of-the-art methods of molecular biology to detect similar responses: polymerase chain reaction (PCR) (detection of microbial DNA in blood is more sensitive than blood cultures), consensus PCR-shared conserved genetic sequences representational difference analysis, pathogen detection chips, DNA microarray techniques, and gene expression and immune cells. New infectious agents have been found using some of these techniques: enteroviruses, Ebola virus, Hanta virus, herpes virus-producing encephalitis, a herpes virus called KSHV that causes Kaposi's sarcoma, and a bacterium that causes Whipple's disease. Kane et al. found that detection of microbial DNA in the blood is a more sensitive method for diagnosing bacteremia or bacterial translocation in surgical patients.[11] Could it be that sepsis with negative bacteria blood cultures is not due to inflammation but that the organisms simply have not been cultured or identified.

Inflammation After Insertion of Prosthetic Devices

Zimmer et al. provide evidence of an inflammatory syndrome that follows endovascular aortic prosthesis insertion in patients. Thus although the severity of the operative repair is greatly reduced by an endovascular prosthesis, the inflammatory reaction may be a hazard.[12] Long-term implanted left ventricular assist devices (LVADs) have also caused difficulty.[11] The LVAD is an implanted immune-inflammatory device that provides, according to Spanier et al., sustained proinflammatory and prothrombotic stimuli with significant impact on the host beyond its mechanical function as a pump.[13]

Complexities of Our Biologic Systems

We give only one example of the complexity of biologic systems. Nitric oxide synthase inhibition during septic shock has been evaluated clinically, and we understand that a recent clinical trial in 900 patients was stopped because of some deleterious effects (see Chapter 18). Thus nitric oxide, nitric oxide synthase, and nitric oxide synthase inhibition all have some deleterious effects (maladaptive), some positive effects (adaptive), and as pointed out by Deutschman some nebulous effects.[14] Can we ever understand these phenomena?

In a review of nitric oxide synthase inhibition in septic shock, Bone said that the problem is "a question of the right time, the right drug, and the right model?."[15] When the timing, correct agent, and dose are critical, how can it ever be clinically useful? It is a highly complex problem. De Boisblanc reviewed a study and editorialized about the complexities of the effects of nitrogen oxide on microbes:[16] "These studies may have no relevance in vivo. The agents may be protective; they may immunomodulate, be bactericidal, or have no effect whatsoever."

The lessons of chaos theory may be helpful. Goodwin stated that the chaos theory does not attack the established findings of traditional science; it simply points out the limitations of the linear, reductionist approach in our attempt to describe natural phenomena. He went on to say that "When complete understanding is abandoned as a goal, the traditional tasks of the physician—listening, witnessing, relieving suffering—will no longer be relegated to a small corner of medicine, the so-called art of medicine, but will be returned to the core of medical practice and medical education." Traditional science cannot predict complex systems.[17] We in today's medical establishment still believe that somehow or other we can understand everything. The complexities, if approached by the chaos theory, may help us understand more but probably never everything.

Conclusions

We can reduce the stress and metabolic response to injury or operation and increase the well-being of patients by using minimally invasive procedures, epidural anesthesia, pain control, other agents such as fentanil and morphine (which decrease the stress response), and other agents in specific circumstances. Once MOF develops, however, mortality is high, and support of organ function is difficult.

Prevention is critical. Each organ or system—cardiovascular, pulmonary, hepatic, gastrointestinal, metabolic, musculoskeletal, central nervous system, blood, coagulation—must be supported. MOF often begins with single organ failure and progresses with deleterious relations among the various organs and systems. These interrelations are still not completely understood. Gradually, however, we believe that we are preventing MOF more frequently.

References

1. Faist E, Baue AE, Dittmer H, Heberer G: Multiple organ failure in polytrauma patients. J Trauma 1983;17:389–393.
2. Baker CC, Miller ID, Baue AE: Predictors of outcome. J Trauma 1983;23:627.
3. Baue AE: Prevention and treatment of sepsis: present and future problems. In: Baue AE, Berlot G, Gullo A, Vincent JL (eds) Sepsis and Organ Function. Milan, Springer, 1999;69–82.
4. Uknis ME, Dunn DL: Nosocomial infections and sepsis syndrome in critically ill surgical patients. Curr Opin Crit Care 1996;2:304–310.
5. Jasny K, Bloom R: Nosocomial infection. Science 1998;280:1507.
6. Barie PS, Eachampati SR, Hydo LJ: Impact of a new intermediate care unit on utilization and outcomes of a surgical intensive care unit. Crit Care Med 1999;27:A28.
7. Baue AE: Multiple organ failure, multiple organ dysfunction syndrome and the systemic inflammatory response syndrome: where do we stand? Shock 1994;2:385–397.
8. Hatch T: Chlamydia: old ideas crushed, new mysteries bared (review of Stephens et al). Science 1998;282:638–639.
9. Cook CH, Yenchar JK, Kraner TO, et al: Occult herpes family viruses may increase mortality in critically ill surgical patients. Am J Surg 1998;176:357–360.
10. Balter M: Molecular methods fire up the hunt for emerging pathogens. Science 1998;282:219–221.
11. Kane PD, Alexander JW, Johannigman JA: The detection of microbial DNA in the blood. Ann Surg 1998;227:1–9.
12. Zimmer S, Heiss MM, Schardey HM, et al: Inflammatory syndrome after endovascular aortic prothesis: a comparative study. Langenbecks Arch Chir J 1998;1:13–17.
13. Spanier TB, Mehmet C, Oz HC, Stern DM, et al: Long term implanted left ventricular assist devices function as immune inflammatory organs. J Thorac Cardiovasc Surg (in press).
14. Deutschman CS: Acute-phase responses and SIRS/MODS: the good, the bad, and the nebulous. Crit Care Med 1998;26:1630–1631.
15. Bone HG: Nitric oxide synthase inhibition in septic shock: a question of the right time, the right drug, and the right model? Crit Care Med 1998;26:1945–1946.
16. De Boisblanc BP: What do the bugs think about inhaled NO? Crit Care Med 1998;26:1785–1786.
17. Goodwin JS: Chaos, and the limits of modern medicine. JAMA 1997;278:1399–1400.

Index

A

Abdominal compartment syndrome, 291–302, 659–660
  mortality rate in, 277
Abdominal wall, effect on, of intraabdominal hypertension, 293, 296
Abscess
  abdominal, and reoperation in peritonitis, 270
  percutaneous drainage of, 306
  as a response to peritonitis, 265
Acetaminophen
  acute liver failure caused by, 462
  toxicity of, effect of N-acetylcysteine on, clinical trial, 549
N-Acetylcysteine, effect on cardiac performance, 596
Acetylhydrolase, degradation of platelet activating factor by, 197
Acidosis
  carbon dioxide partial pressure as a measure of, 258
  lactic, in trauma patients, 274
  systemic, in shock, 411
Acinetobacter, nosocomial pneumonia due to, 309
Acronyms, brave new world of, 14–22
Acute acalculous cholecystitis (AAC), in surgical patients, 62
Acute hepatic failure, defined, 462
Acute lung injury (ALI)
  defined, 353
  nonspecific nitric oxide synthase inhibition in, 180
  oxidative stress in, 172
Acute-phase protein (APP), monitoring in infection and sepsis, 477
Acute-phase response (APR), to trauma or surgery, 420–421, 644
Acute Physiology and Chronic Health Evaluation (APACHE)
  development of, 9–10
  scores on

    and eligibility for clinical trials, 563
    in intestinal ischemia, correlation with endotoxin concentration, 87
    and organ failure, 45–46, 389
    of patients in surgical intensive care, 54
    utilization of, 36
Acute postoperative services (APSs), pain evaluation as a target of, 648
Acute renal failure (ARF), management of acute respiratory distress syndrome due to, 365
Acute respiratory distress syndrome (ARDS), 353–361
  from capillary leak syndrome, injuries associated with, 75–76
  effect on, of inhaled nitric oxide, 180
  glucocorticoid treatment for, 514–523
  Inhaled Nitric Oxide in ARDS Study Group, 180
  injuries associated with
    head and systemic, 404
    due to oxidative stress, 172
  liver damage associated with, 460
  soluble complement receptor 1 treatment in, clinical trials, 217–218
  susceptibility to, effect of IL-10, 147
Acute tubular necrosis (ATN), 365
  in hypovolemic shock, 369–370
  in intraabdominal hypertension, 295, 298
  in renal failure, 367
Adhesion molecules
  blockade of, for preventing polymorphonuclear-mediated tissue injury, 235
  deficiency of, clinical syndromes, 234
  endothelial and leukocytic, 227–232
  role in organ injury, 224–240
α-Adrenergic agents, for increasing systemic vascular resistance, 594
α-Adrenergic agonists, for reversing septic shock, 374–375
β-Adrenergic receptor blocking agents, 326–327
  in myocardial dysfunction, 343

Adrenocorticotropic hormone (ACTH), regulation of glucocorticoid secretion by, 517
Adult respiratory distress syndrome (ARDS)
  in chest trauma, after reamed intramedullary nailing, 285
  chronic alcohol abuse associated with, 39
  eicosanoid plasma levels in, 200–202
  injuries associated with, 34
  mortality in, 46
  outcomes of treatment, 672–673
  patterns in, 39
    cardiac output and oxygen consumption, 574
    pathologic supply-dependent oxygen consumption, 573–574
    and systemic inflammatory response syndrome, 305
  pulmonary hypertension associated with, 342
Advance directives, effectiveness of, 666
Advanced Trauma Life Support program, 657
Afferent limb, role in stress response, 641
Age
  growth hormone secretion changes with, 631
  as a risk factor for mortality in multiple organ failure, 38–39, 675
Airflow resistance, in acute respiratory distress syndrome, 356
Alcohol abuse, as a risk factor for adult respiratory distress syndrome, 39
Algal fibers, nutritional characteristics of, 452
Algorithms, utility of, 14
Allergic reactions, to injected colloids, 610
Alveolar deadspace, measuring to evaluate the need for intensive postoperative monitoring, 286–287
Alveoli, overinflation of, limiting in acute respiratory distress syndrome, 358
Amantadine, analgesic properties of, 648
American College of Chest Physicians (ACCP), 30, 44

American Society of Health-System
    Pharmacists (ASHSP), 417
Aminoglycoside, dosage of, in septic patients,
    269
Amrinone, effect on end-systolic elastance in
    endotoxin shock, 345
Anabolic steroids, in hypermetabolic response
    to trauma and burns, 327
Anaphylatoxins
    biologic effects of, 214
    C5a, inhibition of, 218
    complement, as stimulants for polymor-
        phonuclear leukocytes (PMNs), 73
    filtering from blood, 345
Anatomic profile (AP), for rating injury
    severity, 35
Anergy. See Immune paralysis
Anesthesia
    epidural, 646–647
    selecting a technique for, and patient
        outcome, 645
Anesthetic care, 641–650
Aneurysm, ruptured, progressive organ system
    failure following, 4
Aneurysmal subarachnoid hemorrhage
    (SAH), treating with nimodipine, 402
Angioedema, hereditary, in C1 inhibitor-
    deficient individuals, 216
Angiogenesis, promotion of, by mast cells,
    192–193
Angiotensin-converting enzyme inhibitor,
    clinical trial, effect on stress response,
    549
Antacids, for reducing stress gastritis, 415
Antagonists, to platelet activating factor,
    207–208
Antibiotics
    effect of
        on gastrointestinal microflora,
            455–456
        on release of endotoxin from gram-
            negative bacteria, 115–118
    β-lactam, release of bacterial endotoxin in
        response to, 116
    for treating acute bacterial peritonitis, 269
    for treating bacterial peritonitis, 261
    for treating nosocomial pneumonia, 310
Antibodies
    anti-complement C5, therapeutic effects of,
        218
    anti-tumor necrosis factor, therapeutic
        effects of, 156–157
Anticytokine therapy, 156–157
    effect on muscle cachexia, 384–385
Antigen presentation, defined, 135
Antiinflammatory response
    balance with proinflammatory
        response, 53
    See also Antithrombin III; Cytokines;
        Granulocyte colony-stimulating
        factor

Antioxidants/antioxidant systems
    cardiac effect in septic shock, 345
    cellular, 170–171
    consumption during acute-phase response,
        431
    defense function reduction with age, 423
    natural, 169–170
Antithrombin III
    administration of, in disseminated
        intravascular coagulation, 443,
        565, 679
    characterization of, and role in the
        coagulation system, 505–509
    effect in trauma, 394
Antithromboplastin. See Tissue factor pathway
    inhibitor
Anti-tumor necrosis factor
    antibodies for therapy, 156–157
    effect on myocardial function, 345
Anuria, in intraabdominal hypertension,
    294–295
Apoptosis
    cytokine role in, after sepsis and burns,
        149–150
    effect on
        of interleukin-10, 160
        of proinflammatory cytokines, 158
    hepatic, effect of selective nitric oxide
        synthase inhibition on, 181
    in human development, 131
    immune cell, role of interleukin-1 in, 159
    induction by attachment through integrins,
        232
    neutrophil, plasma mediator roles in,
        131–132
    polymorphonuclear response termination
        by, 74
    tumor necrosis family in, 147–148
    untimely, 131–133
Aptamers, inhibition of complement proteins
    by, 218
Arachidonic acid (AA)
    eicosanoid synthesis from, 196–197
    metabolites of, role in renal dysfunction,
        371–372
Arginine, 324
L-Arginine
    binding site for, on nitric oxide synthase,
        177–178
    blocking of nitric oxide synthesis with
        analogues of, 345
Arterial blood pressure, in intraabdominal
    hypertension, 293
Arterial ketone body ratio (AKBR), as an
    indication of hepatic function, 460,
    467
Arthralgia, in response to growth hormone,
    635
Arthritis
    association with transmembrane form of
        tumor necrosis factor-α, 151

rheumatoid
    effect of interleukin-11 on inflammatory
        response in, 542
    neopterin levels in, 482
Aspirin, effect on cyclooxygenase COX-1,
    198–199
Atrial natriuretic peptide (ANP), in septic
    shock, 343
Autocoids. See Eicosanoids
Autoimmune disorders, procalcitonin levels in,
    480–481
Aztreonam, release of endotoxin from bacteria
    by, 116

B

Bacteremia
    causes of, uncommon, 456
    defined, 101, 367
Bacterial infections, neopterin levels in, 484
Bacterial translocation
    evaluation of role in systemic inflammatory
        response, 35–36
    experimental data, 582
    human data, 582–583
        effect of SDD on multiple organ failure
            in, 586
Barbiturates, effect on intracranial
    hypertension, 403
Baroreceptor activation, in septic shock,
    343–344
Betafectin (PGG-glucan), clinical trials,
    548–549
Bioartifical liver support system, 467–470
Biochemistry
    of antithrombin III, 505–506
    of endotoxin, 492–493
    of interferon-γ, 531–538
    of interleukin-11, 539–540
    of neopterin, 482–483
    of platelet activating factor, 204–206
    of tissue factor pathway inhibitor, 509
Biology
    complexity of, future questions, 690–691
    integrative, and genetic variability, 651–655
Bleeding
    in disseminated intravascular coagulation,
        clinically significant, 441
    in fulminant hepatic failure, 466–467
    as a potential effect of volume expansion,
        608–609
    in stress gastritis, clinically significant, 412
    See also Shock, hemorrhagic
Blood
    hemostatic component replacement, in
        disseminated intravascular
        coagulation, 443–444
    substitutes for, 613–620
    supply after nailing, reamed versus
        unreamed, 284
Blood flow
    autoregulation of

by endothelial-derived nitric oxide, 178–179
by platelet activating factor in kidney and brain, 204–205
coronary, in septic shock, 592
gastric mucosal, in stress gastritis, 411–412
See also Circulation; Microcirculation
Blood purification therapy, in multiple organ failure, 501–504
See also Hemofiltration
B lymphocytes, effect of interferon-γ on, 531
Bone marrow
injected, effect on coagulation and pulmonary permeability, 282
transplant of, acute respiratory distress syndrome following, 354
Bradykinin, future therapy using to inhibit the contact activating system, 679
Brain-immune axis, 391–392
Brain injury
emergency care for
in the emergency department for, 249
in the field for, 243–244
infection-related, oxidative stress in, 171
transcranial near-infrared spectroscopy for monitoring oxygenation in, 261
Bronchoalveolar lavage (BAL), for diagnosing pneumonia, 310
Burns
apoptosis following, blocking, 150
chemotherapy for, multiagent, 565
complement C1 inhibitor treatment for, 217
effect of anisodamine on splanchnic vasoconstriction in, 88
growth hormone treatment for, 634
hypermetabolic response to, 322–329
immunosuppression after, flow cytometry data for characterization of, 527
mechanism of muscle breakdown in, 380
neopterin levels in, 485
size of, and systemic endotoxemia, 87
stress gastritis accompanying, 412

C

Calcium, dependence on
of nitric oxide generation, neuronal and endothelial NOS reactions, 176
of phospholipases, 196–197
Calcium channel blocking agents
for aneurysmal subarachnoid hemorrhage treatment, 402–404
as platelet activating factor antagonists, 208
Calories, restricting, effect on immune function, 433–434
Calpains, expression of, in sepsis-induced muscle protein degradation, 383
Cancer
colon, peritonitis from perforations associated with, 268
head and neck, effect of SDD on mucositis in, 585

multiagent chemotherapy for, 564
organ failure associated with treatment for, 49
Candida albicans, bacteremia from an intravascular device due to, 312
Capillary leakage syndrome (CLS), complement C1 inhibitor for treating, 217
Capnography, in intensive care, 260
Carbon dioxide, partial pressure of, as a measure of intramucosal acidosis, 258
Cardiac function
failure of
defined, 7
and mortality from noncardiac causes, 47–48
in hypertonic saline administration, 609–610
and nitric oxide synthase inhibition, 180–181
in severe sepsis and septic shock, 374
Cardiac index
as a measure of cardiac performance, 591–597
and survival, in septic shock, 571
Cardiac output
Doppler versus thermodilution measurement, in transesophageal echocardiography, 260
effect on oxygen delivery, 336
in intraabdominal hypertension, 293
measuring in intensive care, 255
and oxygen delivery, survivors of injury, 571
thoracic bioelectric impedance cardiography for estimating, 259
Cardiogenic circulatory failure, defined, 333
Cardioprotection, by complement C1 inhibitor, animal studies, 217
Cardiopulmonary bypass
for cardiac surgery, systemic inflammation associated with, 82–84, 547–548
long-term outcomes of, 675
risk reduction with multiagent therapy, 565
systemic inflammation associated with, 76–77, 354
Cardiopulmonary resuscitation (CPR), peak exhaled or end-tidal carbon dioxide in, 260
Cardiovascular system
failure of
defined, 5
in surgical patients, 59–60
role in the stress response, 644
support for, in acute respiratory distress syndrome, 356
synchrony with the respiratory system, 653–654
Case study, in ethical considerations, 663–664
Caspase-3 pathways, role in apoptosis after burn injury, 149
Catabolism, in critical illness, preventing, 630

Catalase, as a natural antioxidant, 169–170
Catecholamines
interactions with the immune system in trauma, 104
mediation of stress response by, 642
reduced responsiveness to, and vasoplegia, 75
role in burn injury, 326–327
Catheter-related infections (CRIs), nosocomial, 311–313
Ceftazidime (CAZ)
comparison with imipenem for treating urosepsis, 118
release of lipopolysaccharide from bacteria by, 116
Ceftriaxone, effect of dexamethasone on treatment with, meningitis clinical trial, 118
Cefuroxime, endotoxin release from bacteria by, 116
Cell-mediated responses, immunomodulation of, 389–397
Cellular activation, role of adhesion molecules in, 232
Cellular hydration, effects on protein synthesis and degradation, 104–105
Cellular infiltration, after injury, 553
Cellular stress response, 74
Central nervous system (CNS)
disorders of, association with organ failure, 48
dysfunction of, and mortality, 60–61
effect on
of intraabdominal hypertension, 296
of mediators from immunocompetent cells, 391–392
failure of, 398–410
defined, 6–7
injury to, as a cause of death after accidental injury, 5, 689
Central venous pressure
catheter for monitoring in intensive care, 255–256
in intraabdominal hypertension, 293
Cerebral blood flow (CBF), autoregulation of, 398–399
Cerebral systems
edema of, in fulminant hepatic failure, 465
hemodynamics of, effect of hypertonic resuscitation on, 607
perfusion pressure management, 399–401
See also Encephalpathy; Head injury
Cerebrospinal fluid (CSF), neopterin levels in, diagnosis of infectious diseases using, 484
Chemical structure, of platelet activating factor, 204–205
Chemoattractants, systemic distribution of, in systemic inflammatory response syndrome, 97
Chemokines, 93–94

Chemokines (*Continued*)
  interaction with adhesion molecules, 233
  production in mast cells, 191–192
Chemotherapy
  effect of interleukin-11 on bone marrow recovery after, 541
  historical development, 564
Chest
  severe injury to, mortality in, 285
  severe trauma to, mortality in, 243
  surgery of, video assisted, 545–546
  trauma to, management in the multiply-injured patient, 285–286
Chronic obstructive pulmonary disease (COPD)
  effect of growth hormone on, 635
  prognosis in, 48
Cimetidine, evaluation of, in stress gastritis, 415
Circulatory system, 333–339
  failure of, defined, 333
  hyperdynamic, in hypotension with septic shock, 369–371
  treating oxygen transport, and survival, 659–660
Cirrhosis, endotoxemia associated with, and mortality in hepatic encephalopathy, 121
Classification
  of cytokines, 104
  of multiple organ failure, 7–9
  of patients, for clinical trials, 660
Clinical considerations
  in evaluating circulatory failure, 337
  frequency of problems, change over time, 657–658
  in intraabdominal hypertension, 297–298
Clinical studies/trials
  of antithrombin III, 507–509
  of diet effects, on multiple organ failure after gastrointestinal surgery, 453–455
  of endotoxin antagonists, 496–498
  of glucocorticoid treatment, for septic shock or ARDS, 514
  of granulocyte colony-stimulating factor, 624
  of immunomodulation, 392–394
  of inflammation, multiple therapeutic agent evaluation, 565
  of interleukin-11, 543
  of laparoscopic procedures, 546–547
  of prophylactic therapy for stress gastritis, meta-analyses, 413–414
  of therapeutic agents in minimum surgical procedures, 548–550
  of tissue factor pathway inhibitor, 511
Clinical therapy, in severe trauma, 247–250
Clostridium difficile, antibiotic-associated pseudomembranous colitis due to, 316
Clotting cascade, enzymes of, temperature sensitive, 274

Coagulation systems
  activation in cardiopulmonary bypass, 82–83
  dysfunction of, 61
    in the stress response, 644
  failure of, defined, 6–7
  inflammation initiated by proteins of, 93
  protease inhibitors of, 505–513
  response after fat intravasation, 282
Coagulopathy
  with fulminant hepatic failure, 466
  from hypothermia, 274
  See also Disseminated intravascular coagulation
Cobra venom factor, complement depletion by, 219
Cofactors, for nitric oxide synthases, 176
Colitis, experimental, treatment with diet, 453
Collagen
  synthesis of, by wound-derived fibroblasts, 555
  type III, in wound matrix formation, 555–556
Colloids, for prehospital fluid resuscitation, emergency care, 245
Colon cancer, peritonitis from perforations associated with, 268
Colonic mucosa, nutrients for, 424
Colonization, effect on, of selective decontamination of the digestive tract, 583
Colony-stimulating factors, immunomodulating effects of, 393–394
  See also Granulocyte colony-stimulating factor; Granulocyte macrophage colony-stimulating factor
Comorbidity, as a risk factor for trauma mortality, 39
Compartment syndrome, risk of, in reamed nailing, 284
Compensatory antiinflammatory response syndrome (CARS), 17
  clinical scenario, 599
  delayed immunosuppression associated with, 37
  differentiation of components of, 528
  as the dominant response to illness or injury, 601–602
  response to cytokines, 526
  role of mast cells in, 192
Complement
  analysis of, prognostic value, 215
  therapeutic inhibition of, 214–223
Complement anaphylatoxins, as stimulants for polymorphonuclear leukocytes (PMNs), 73
Complement cascade, role in inflammation, 93
Complications
  of growth hormone administration, 635–636
  of liver failure, 463–464

Compstatin, inhibition of complement C3 activation by, 218
Computed tomography
  abdominal, for evaluating abscess, 270, 305–306
  for assessing lung contusion damage, 282–283
  cranial, in emergency therapy for trauma, 247–250
  for evaluating trauma patients in the emergency department, 249
Computer simulation, of intraoperative heat loss, 276–277
Consumption coagulopathy. *See* Disseminated intravascular coagulation
Contact activating system, role in inflammation, 93
Continuous cardiac output catheter, 257
Continuous hemodiafiltration (CHDF), 501
Continuous mixed venous oximetric catheter, 257
Continuous renal replacement therapy (CRRT), 501
Coronary insufficiency, in septic shock, 344
Corticotropin-releasing hormone (CRH), interaction with norepinephrine-producing cells, 641
Cortisol
  binding to corticosteroid-binding globulin, 517
  effect on arterial blood pressure, 516
  mediation of the stress response by, 642
Corynebacterium jeikeium, bacteremia from an intravascular device due to, 312
Cost
  of acute postoperative services, 648
  of intensive care, as a percentage of gross domestic product, 675
  of survivals, after multiple organ dysfunction syndrome, 676
Cost/benefit calculation
  for growth hormone administration, 636
  for pharmaceutical intervention in stress gastritis, 417–418
  and predicting survival, 675
  for selective decontamination of the digestive tract, 585
Counterinflammatory response to infection, 599
  augmentation of, future research in, 680–681
  definition of, future work on, 683
Counterregulatory hormone interactions, in the stress response, 643
Cournand–Euler mechanism, in acute embolization, 282
C-reactive protein (CRP), blood levels of, after trauma, 477
Critical illness polyneuropathy, 61
Cryoprecipitate (Cryo), for treating disseminated intravascular coagulation, 443

Index

Crystalloids, for prehospital fluid resuscitation, emergency care, 245
Cultures, blood, analysis for identifying source of infection, 306
Curling ulcers, 412
Cushing ulcers, 412
Cyanosis, acral, as an indication of disseminated intravascular coagulation, 441
Cycling processes, in microcirculatory arrest, 98
Cyclooxygenase, role in synthesis of prostaglandins, 197–198
Cyclooxygenase-2 (COX-2), 196, 198–199
Cytochrome A, A_3, redox potential of copper of, as a measure of oxygen supply, 261
Cytokine antagonists, trials of, for treating systemic inflammation therapy, 78
Cytokine cascade, induction of, following hemorrhage, 87
Cytokines
  adhesion molecule CD11-B levels, in aneurysm repair, 109–110
  antiinflammatory, 157–158, 159–160
    failure to modulate in nonsurvivors of sepsis, 518–519
  classification by type, 104
  control of collagen synthesis and lysis by, 556
  endotoxin-induced inflammatory, antibodies to, 114
  in host responses to insult, 514–516
  increase in serum levels, after trauma, 111–112
  induction by lipoteichoic acid, 119–120
  inflammatory, levels after trauma, 136
  interaction of
    with endotoxin, 494
    with glucocorticoids, 379
  involvement of
    in disseminated intravascular coagulation, 439–440
    in systemic hyperinflammation, 35
  levels of, after trauma, 390
  as markers of the inflammatory state, 45
  mediation of the stress response by, 643
  from natural immunity cells, 525
  predicting organ damage from levels of, 71
  predicting outcomes of multiple organ failure from levels of, 37
  production by mast cells, 190–191
  proinflammatory
    cascade after injury, 74
    cascade in sepsis, 477
    downregulation by interleukin-11, 540
    effect of granulocyte colony-stimulating factor on, 622–623
    effect of immunoglobulin G on, 638
    mediation of the catabolic response to injury by, 378
    role in apoptosis, 159
    in systemic hyperinflammation, 155
  release from macrophages after trauma and hemorrhage, 134–135
  removal from blood, using continuous hemofiltration, 502
  role of
    in organ apoptosis after sepsis and burns, 149–150
    in the sepsis response, 145–154
  Th1 and Th2 patterns of secretion of, 524–530
  See also *Interleukin* entries
Cytolytic membrane attack complex, pathways leading to formation of, 214
Cytotoxic lymphocyte maturation factor (CLMF). See Interleukin-12

D

Damage control, in trauma organs, 273–275
Dantrolene, effect on skeletal muscle degradation in sepsis, 383
Database
  Cornell, APACHE III evaluation using the ROC curve, 56
  Denver, for multiple organ failure, 33–34
  multiple organ failure, for analyzing the relationship with blood transfusion, 37–38
D-dimer testing, in diagnosis of disseminated intravascular coagulation, 442
Death effector molecules, apoptosis activated by, 149–150
  See also Apoptosis
Débridement, in peritonitis, 268–269
Decompression, abdominal, for treating intraabdominal hypertension, 298–299
Deep core lipid A (DCLA) antibodies, binding to lipopolysaccharides, 495
Defibrination syndrome. See Disseminated intravascular coagulation
Dehydroepiandrosterone (DHEA), modulation of glucocorticoid action by, 125
Delayed-type hypersensitivity (DTH) reaction, depression of, and mortality from, sepsis, 135
Delayed-type hypersensitivity (DTH) skin test, predicting septic-related mortality from reactions to, 656–657
Deoxyribonucleic acid (DNA), bacterial, immunostimulation by, 120
Development, human
  apoptosis in, 131
  robustness of, 652–653
Dexamethasone, effect on morbidity
  in lethal experimental infection, 519
  in meningitis treated with ceftriaxone, 118
Dextran, addition to hypertonic saline, 606
Diacylglycerol (DAG), induction by platelet activating factor, 205–206
Diagnosis
  of abdominal compartment syndrome, 298
  of acute bacterial peritonitis, 266–267
  of antibiotic-associated pseudomembranous colitis, 316
  bedside, future improvement in, 683–684
  of catheter-related nosocomial infections, 312–313
  of disseminated intravascular coagulation, 441–442
  of fungal urinary tract infections, in the intensive care unit, 315
  of infection and inflammation, 477–491
  of need for therapy, after cardiac surgery, 346–347
  of nosocomial pneumonia, 310
  of septic shock, criteria, 593
  of sinusitis, in intensive care unit patients, 316
  of stress gastritis, 412
  of systemic inflammatory response syndrome and renal failure, 367–368
  in trauma, identification of life-threatening injuries, 248
  of urinary tract infections, 314
  in ventriculitis or meningitis, nosocomial, 317
Dibenzyline, hemodynamic effects of, in clinical shock, 571
Differential diagnosis
  of disseminated intravascular coagulation, 442–443
  of viral and bacterial infections, using procalcitonin assay, 478–479
Diffuse intravascular coagulation (DIC), in trauma or infection, 75. See also Disseminated intravascular coagulation
Digestive function, in the stress response, 644
2,3-Diphosphoglycerate (DPG), oxygen affinity balance maintained by, in hemoglobin, 615
Disease, defined, 14
Disseminated intravascular coagulation (DIC), 438–446
  antithrombin III treatment for, 507, 565
  in fulminant hepatic failure, 466
  inhibition by monoclonal antibodies against FVII/FVIIa, 510
  pathophysiology in, 372
Distributive circulatory failure, defined, 333
Distributive justice, and informed consent, 670–671
Dobutamine
  for failure of volume expansion to improve oxygen consumption, clinical trials, 575–576
  for treating circulatory failure, 336, 595–596
"Do not resuscitate" orders, analysis of mortality rate after, 676
Dopamine
  for treating circulatory failure, 335–336, 594

Dopamine (*Continued*)
  for treating renal dysfunction, 374–375
Dopexamine, effect of, on blood flow, 596
Doppler flowmetry, laser, for studying microvascular blood flow in hemorrhage, 576–577
Drugs
  anticoagulant, for treating disseminated intravascular coagulation, 444
  hepatotoxic, 463
  See also Pharmacology
Dysbiosis, causes of, 447
Dyslipidemia, metabolic syndrome X associated with, 422–423

E

Echocardiography, transesophageal, 259–260
Effectors, of the stress response, 641
Effector signals, neutralizing, as a future therapy in inflammation, 680
Efferent limb, role in stress response, 641–642
Eicosanoid pathways, 196
Eicosanoids, 196–203
  plasma levels of, following shock, 137
Ejection fraction
  left ventricular, measuring, 591
  and myocardial depression, 594
  right ventricular
    prediction of survival in trauma and coronary artery disease using, 257
  in sepsis, 591–592
Elastase, as a marker for severity of ARDS, MOF and sepsis, 76
Elastase α_1-protease inhibitor (EPI), prediction about multiple organ failure from levels of, 484–485
Emboli, in reamed nailing versus unreamed nailing, 284
Embryogenesis, interleukin-11 activity in, 540
Emergency care
  field, long-term follow-up of outcomes, 657
  for injured patients, 243–253
  in the emergency department, 247–250
Enalaprilat, effect of, on stress response, 549
Encephalopathy
  complicating hepatic failure, 462, 464–466
    criterion for clinical study, 468–469
  See also Cerebral entries
Endocrine system, roles in postinjury inflammation, 158
Endoscopy, for diagnosing stress gastritis, 412
Endothelial cell adhesion molecules (ECAMS), in reperfusion injury, 110
Endothelial cells
  interactions with leukocytes, 224–240
  regulatory function during inflammation, 439–440
  role in wound healing, 555
Endothelial-derived relaxing factor, nitric oxide as, 176
Endothelin
  in pulmonary hypertension, postoperative, 347
  release in septic shock, 343
Endothelin-1, in renal dysfunction, 371
Endothelium, regulatory function during inflammation, 72–73
  and PAF production, 207
Endothelium-derived factors, multiple organ failure associated with, 45
Endotoxemia
  in burn patients, 87
  neutrophil adhesion and injury after, 235
  systemic
    effects of nitric oxide on liver in, 181
    endotoxin translocation from the intestine in, 121
Endotoxicity, effect on, of hemoglobin, 125
Endotoxin
  absorption from gastrointestinal tract, 86
  antagonists to, 492–500
  in blood
    as evidence of bacterial translocation, 582–583
    removal with hemoperfusion, 501–502
  defined, 115
  effect on the end-systolic pressure–volume relation curve, 591
  in human disease, 114–130
  IL-10 stimulation of, 146
  plasma levels of, effect of ibuprofen on, 88
Enteral nutrition
  inhibition of proinflammatory cytokine release through, 386
  perioperative, 426–427
  for preventing stress gastritis, 414–415
  support for the gut in critically ill patients through, 420–437
Environment, manipulating, in treating trauma and burns, 324
Eosinophilic neutrophils, appearance in wounds, 553–554
Epidemiology
  of inflammatory conditions of the heart, 340–345
  of postinjury multiple organ failure, 33–39
Epidural anesthesia, stress response to, 547
Epidural anesthesia and analgesia (EAA), complications of, 646–647
Epinephrine, antiinflammatory effects of, 158
Epithelial cells, effects of interleukin-11 on, 541
Errors, medical, documenting, 658
Erythropoietin, immunomodulating effects of, 393–394
E-selectin levels, and prognosis in sepsis, 45
Esophagospasm, response to recombinant hemoglobin injection, 617
Estrogen, effect of, on the immune response, 139
Ethical questions, 663–671
  in futile care, 675–676
Etiology, of fulminant hepatic failure, 462
Euthyroid sick syndrome, following cytokine release, 74
Excitatory amino acid (EAA), inhibitors of, neurotrauma management trials using, 403–404
Extracorporeal gas exchange, in treating acute respiratory distress syndrome, 359
Extracorporeal membrane oxygenation (ECMO), for severe respiratory failure, 567, 659

F

Famotidine, evaluation, for stress gastritis, 416
FasL, role in response to injury, 147–149
Fat
  intravasation of
    in fixation of long bones, 281
    metabolic effects, 282
  for nutritional support in trauma and burns, 324–325
  saturated, and immunodepression, 423–424
  utilization of
    in normal and critically ill patients, 102
    in trauma and burns, 323
Fat embolism syndrome, mortality rate in, 279
Feeding tubes, efficiency of, 427–428
Femoral fractures
  stabilization in patients with severe chest injury, 285
  studies of treatment timing, 280
Fenton reaction
  formation of reactive hydroxyl radical in, 167
  role of ascorbic acid in, 171
Fermentation, of foods, by lactic acid bacteria, 448
Ferritin, levels of, and risk for acute respiratory distress syndrome, 355
Fever
  and energy expenditure, 102
  role of prostaglandin E_2 in, 198
Fiber, nutrient, 451–452
Fibrinogen cascade, 505
Fibrinolytic inhibitors, for treating disseminated intravascular coagulation, 444
Fibroblasts, role in wound healing, 555
Fibronectin, in wound matrix formation, 555–556
Fick equation, for analyzing oxygen consumption, 255
Fluconazole, for treating urinary tract infections, 315
Fluids
  to correct hypovolemia, in field treatment of trauma, 244–245
  replacement in circulatory failure, 335
Follow-up
  rehabilitation results, Finland, 674–675
  return to work

German trauma study evaluation, 674
Swiss trauma study evaluation, 675
twenty-year study of surgical mortality, 656–657
Fracture, early fixation
outcomes, 657–658
with polytrauma, 279–290
severe head injury accompanying, outcomes, 404
Free radicals (oxygen), defined, 167
Fulminant hepatic failure (FHF), 462
intracranial hypertension in, 465
Fungal infections
nosocomial, in the intensive care unit, 314–315
procalcitonin levels in, 479
Future, in systemic inflammatory response syndrome and multiple organ failure treatment, 678–688

G

Gastrectomy, for treating a perforated peptic ulcer, 268
Gastric intramucosal tonometry, for monitoring in intensive care, 254
Gastric secretion, as a protection against microorganisms, 428–429
Gastritis, stress, 411–419
Gastrointestinal system
dysfunction of, 61–62
bleeding associated with fulminant hepatic failure, 467
effect on
of interleukin-11, 541
of intraabdominal hypertension, 295
of nitric oxide synthase inhibition, 181–182
failure of, defined, 6–7
tonometry for monitoring in intensive care, 258
Genes
antithrombin III deficiency, 506
effect of, on response to infection, 44
expression of ubiquitin-proteasome, in cachectic muscle, 380–381
Gene therapy, to counteract exaggerated inflammatory response, 681
Genetic variability, and effective therapy, 651–655
Glasgow Coma Scale (GCS)
predictive power of, 60
use in acute respiratory distress syndrome, 355
use in severe head injury, 399
Glomerular filtration rate (GFR)
effect on, of nitric oxide, 370
intrarenal regulation of, 368–369
Glomerular thrombosis, from nonselective nitric oxide synthase inhibition, 179
Glucagon
effect on phenylalanine oxidation, 104

mediation of the stress response by, 642–643
Glucocorticoid/hormonal regulation, in sepsis, 124
Glucocorticoid receptor antagonist, RU38486, effect on muscle proteolysis, 384
Glucocorticoid resistance, in sepsis or acute respiratory distress syndrome, 520
Glucocorticoids
effect of
catabolic, 104
on the heart, clinical studies, 345
on host defense responses, 516–517
on immune cell apoptosis, 160
in septic shock, 158
inhibition of NFκB activation by, 75
interaction with cytokines, 379
mediation by
of muscle cachexia in injury and sepsis, 378–379
of stress response, 642
for sepsis treatment, clinical trials, 15, 78
for septic shock treatment, 514–523
Glucose, energy yield from, in critically ill patients, 102
Glucose intolerance, metabolic syndrome X associated with, 422–423
Glutamine, consumption during acute-phase response, 431
Glutathione peroxidase, in the antioxidant system, 169–170
Glycomannans, nutritional characteristics of, 452
Glycoproteins
granulocyte colony-stimulating factor, 621–624
immunoglobulin superfamily, 231–232
integrins, 230–231
selectins, 227–230
soluble complement receptor 1, 217–218
vascular cell adhesion molecule-1, 232
Granulocyte colony-stimulating factor (G-CFS)
immunomodulation by, 392
responses to infection, 621–624
Granulocyte colony-stimulating factor (G-CSF), administering in sepsis, 78
Granulocyte macrophage colony-stimulating factor (GM-CSF), 624–626
release of, effects on leukocytes, 73
Growth factors
in infection and inflammation, 621–629
role in hypermetabolic response in trauma and burns, 325
role in wound healing, 556–557
Growth hormone
anabolic effects of, in critically ill patients, 630–637
mediation of the stress response by, 643
regulation of, 630–631

for treating burn patients, 325–326, 383–384
Growth hormone/insulin-like growth factor-1 axis, alterations in critical illness, 631–632
Growth hormone releasing hormone (GHRH), 631
Gut
in acute-phase response, 421–422
decontamination of
for preventing infection and translocation, 580–590
selective, 567
effect on, of enteral nutrition after abdominal surgery, 658–659
endotoxins from, 86–91
immune system of, 420–437
ischemia/reperfusion in, effect on systemic inflammatory response, 35–36
refunctionalization of, 447–458
Gut-associated lymphoid tissue (GALT), immunologic barrier formed by, 581–582

H

Head injury
hypertonic solution administration in, 567, 608
immunity suppression in, 392
pathophysiology of, 398–399
See also Cerebral entries; Encephalopathy
Health, pictures of, 653–654
Health care, provision without regard to income, 690
Heart
effect of inflammatory conditions on, 340–352
right, monitoring function of, 256–257
transplantation of, procalcitonin levels in, 480
See also Cardiac entries; Ejection fraction
Heat-shock proteins (HSPs)
role in downregulating the inflammatory response, 75
upregulation of, in response to stress, 74
Helicopter transport, emergency, and outcome in trauma, 246–247
Hematogenous spread, as a source of catheter-related nosocomial infections, 312
Hematologic conditions, multiple organ failure associated with, 48–49
Hematopoietic cells, effects of interferon-γ in, 541–542
Hemodiafiltration, effect on tissue oxygenation, 659
Hemodynamic monitoring
in intensive care, 254
of septic shock, 593
Hemodynamic optimization
clinical trial, 575
in intensive care, 254–255

Hemodynamic parameters
  in circulatory failure, indicators for
    treatment, 337
  in consequences of systemic inflammatory
    response syndrome, 97
Hemofiltration
  depression following, outcome study, 675
  in renal failure, 375
  for treating acute respiratory distress
    syndrome, 568
Hemoglobin
  arterial, oxygen saturation of, 260–261
  conjugated, as an oxygen carrier, 618
  crosslinked, tetrameric stabilized, clinical
    trial, 617
  effect of
    on endotoxicity, 125
    on oxygen delivery, 336
    on peritonitis, 265
  encapsulated, 618
  liposome-encapsulated, use in emergency
    field care, 246
  as a nitric oxide carrier/donor, 177
  polymerized, as an oxygen carrier, 617–618
  recombinant, 616
  solution of
    as a blood substitute, 613–618
    polymerized pyridoxilated stroma-free,
      38
  stroma-free, use in emergency field care,
    246
Hemoglobin-based oxygen carriers, 616
  as nitric oxide scavengers, 613–615
Hemorrhage, in fulminant hepatic failure,
  466–467
  See also Bleeding; Shock, hemorrhagic
Hemostasis, as an early phase of wound
  healing, 553
Heparin
  effects of, in disseminated intravascular
    coagulation, 444
  as an inhibitor of the complement system,
    219
  interaction with antithrombin III,
    505–506
  low-molecular-weight, for treating
    disseminated intravascular
    coagulation, 444
  roles of, 190
Heparin-binding domain, of chemokines, 233
Hepatic system
  dysfunction of, in surgical patients, 62–63
  effects on, of nitric oxide synthase
    inhibition, 181
  failure of, defined, 5
  See also Fulminant hepatic failure; Liver
Hepatitis
  A and B, hepatic failure in infection by, 462
  chemical, treating with diet, 453
  non-A non-B non-C, hepatic failure in
    infection by, 463

Hepatocytes, porcine, in a bioartificial liver
  support system, 467–470
Hetastarch, for reducing reperfusion injury
  from cell adhesion molecules, 110
Histamine, biologic effects of, 189–190
History of multiple organ failure, 3–13
Hormones
  adrenocorticotropic hormone, glucocorti-
    coid regulation by, 517
  anabolic
    effect on muscle cachexia, 383–384
    in hypermetabolic response to trauma
      and burns, 327
  of the hypothalamic-pituitary-adrenal
    (HPA) axis, 392
  stress
    modulating in trauma and burns, 325
    in systemic inflammatory response
      syndrome, 104
  testosterone, effect on macrophage function
    in males, 139, 391
  See also Growth hormones
Host, role in clinical signs of infection, 92–100
Host response
  defense, components of, 515–516
  to endotoxin, 493–494
  to insults, 514–516
Human immunodeficiency virus (HIV)
  bacterial sepsis associated with, procalcito-
    nin marker for, 479
  neopterin levels associated with infection
    by, 484
  organ failure associated with, 49
Hyaluronic acid and wound healing, 558
Hydrocortisone, protection against endotoxin
  by injection of, 519
Hydrogen peroxide, 167–168
Hydrogen-receptor antagonists, for controlling
  stress gastritis, 415–416
Hydroxyl radical, 167–168
Hydroxyperoxyeicosotetraenoic acids
  (HPETEs), conversion of arachidonic
  acid to, 199
Hyperalgesia, role of prostaglandins in, 198
Hypercalcemia, in response to growth
  hormone administration, 635
Hypercapnia, permissive, to prevent
  overinflation of lung units, 358
Hyperchloremic acidosis, following hypertonic
  saline administration, evaluation, 610
Hyperglycemia
  in burn injury, 322
  effect of growth hormone on, 635–636
  in burn patients, 325, 634
  in the stress response, 643–644
Hypermetabolism
  defined, 101
  mediators of, 104–105
  response to trauma and burns, 322–329
Hypernatremia, from hypertonic saline
  administration, evaluations, 609

Hypertension
  arterial, effect in severe head injury,
    400–401
  in eNOS knockout mice, 178
  intraabdominal, consequences of, 293–297
  pulmonary, accompanying septic shock,
    342
  pulmonary artery, 180, 592
  See also Intracranial hypertension
Hypertonic solutions
  for field resuscitation in trauma, 245
  saline, for resuscitating trauma victims, 404,
    567, 659–660
  for treating shock, 605–612
Hyperventilation, for reducing intracranial
  pressure, 402, 465
Hypochlorous acid (HOCl), formation of, 167
Hypoperfusion
  organ, in shock, 334
  splanchnic, in shock, 576
Hypotension
  defined, 24
  effect of nitric oxide on, 178–179
  and renal dysfunction, 370–371
  macrophage antigen presentation depres-
    sion following, 135
  risk of wound infection following, 138
  as a sign of circulatory failure, 333–334
  in trauma patients due to hemorrhage, 248
  treatment of, in systemic inflammatory
    response syndrome, 372
Hypothalamic–pituitary–adrenal (HPA) axis
  activation of, and control of the host defense
    response, 516–517
  hormones of, role in cell-mediated
    immunity, 392
  role in stress reaction, 641
  sensitization to, in metabolic syndrome X,
    422–423
Hypothalamus
  growth hormone regulation originating in,
    630–631
  interleukin-1 in nerve fibers of, 641
  response to trauma and burns, 322
Hypothermia
  avoiding while treating intraabdominal
    hypertension, 299
  for cerebral protection, 401–402
  physiologic effects of, 274, 659
Hypothermia-coagulopathy-acidosis
  syndrome, 273–278
Hypovolemia
  as a contraindication for decompression in
    intraabdominal hypertension, 299
  fluid resuscitation for, 254–255
Hypovolemic shock, 333
Hypoxemia, tissue
  and cardiac complications of surgery, 261
  in uncompensated vasoplegia, 75
Hypoxia
  regional

Index

in acute respiratory distress syndrome, 574
and macrophage antigen-presentation, 135
role in shock, 77
tissue, detecting with gastric tonometry, 258
See also Oxygen debt

I

Ibuprofen, clinical trial
  effect in burn patients, 88
  effect in renal failure, 372
Iliac vascular injuries, factors affecting survival in, 275
Imipenem (IMP)
  comparison with ceftazidime, for treating urosepsis, 118
  release of lipopolysaccharide from bacteria by, 116
Immune system
  activation of
    in association with anemia, cachexia, and multiple organ failure, 487
    by lactic acid bacteria, 450
  cellular, role of granulocyte colony-stimulating factor in, 621-622
  and commensal flora establishment, 449
  depression of, and saturated fat, 423-424
  deterioration after trauma and surgery, 135
  enhancement by postoperative diets, 432-433
  failure of, defined, 7
  function of, and nutritional status, 421
  granulocyte macrophage colony-stimulating factor in, 624-626
  modulation to reduce inflammatory response, 345
  regulation of, role of interferon-γ in, 531-533
  response of
    gender-specific, after trauma and hemorrhage, 138-139
    protective, role of endotoxin proteins in, 119
  suppression of
    after thermal injury or sepsis, 147
    after trauma and burns, 322
Immunoassay, of procalcitonin, 478
Immunoglobulins
  E (IgE), as an activation signal for mast cells, 188-189
  G (IgG)
    effect on proinflammatory cytokines, 638
    serum levels of, and risk of sepsis, 639
  intravenous administration of
    efficacy of, 638-640
    for treating inflammatory and autoimmune diseases, 219
  M (IgM)
    antibodies to, for gram-negative bacterial infection, 496-498

as a predictor of mortality after cardiac surgery, 76
mixed lymphocyte reaction and graft-versus-host disease involving, 232
platelet-endothelial cell adhesion molecule-1, 232
superfamily of, 231-232
Immunology, of endotoxin, 492-493
Immunomodulation
  of cell-mediated responses, 389-397
  by hypertonic saline solutions, 607
Immunonutrients
  and enteral nutrition, 420-437
  future therapy for inflammation using, 682
  See also Enteral nutrition; Nutrients
Immunosuppression
  delayed, after multiple insults, 33, 37
  by interleukin-10, 392
  management of, future therapy in inflammation, 681
  postoperative, in the stress response, 644-645
  in sustained illness, 599
  transfusion as a cause of, 37-38
  trauma as a cause of, 134-142
Immunotherapy, anticytokine, clinical trials, 122-123
Indomethacin, effect on cell-mediated immunity, 393
Infections
  acute renal failure following, 365
  association with organ failure, 598-604
  classification of, 581
  defined, 92, 367
  effect on, of selective decontamination of the digestive tract, 583-584
  eliminating, effect on the host, 71
  and immune response following trauma, effect on multiple organ failure, 137
  neopterin assays in, 483-487
  nosocomial
    in postoperative and trauma patients, 421-422
    systemic inflammatory response syndrome associated with, 303
  role in systemic inflammation, 76-77
  as symptoms of multiple organ failure, 37
  See also Sepsis
Inflammation
  activators of, 96-97
  benefits of, future clinical trial attention to, 684
  biology of, 23
  blocking activation of, future interventions, 678-679
  after cardiopulmonary bypass, 82-83
  circulation and organ function associated with, 5
  dysregulation of, organ failure as a mark of, 44
  after fat intravasation, 282

fulminant hepatic failure associated with, 466
future understanding of complexity of, 684
inhibiting, future therapies, 679-680
mediation of, by platelet-activating factor, 209-210
metabolism during, 101-103
modulating, 562-563
multiple agent therapy for, studies of, 565
and nitric oxide, 179
response to
  in critical illness, 15-17
  effect of integrin blockade on, 230-231
severe, counterregulation of, 155-166
variable response to growth hormone in, 632
whole-body, multiple organ failure as a result of, 75-77
Inflammatory mediators, circulating, after cardiopulmonary bypass, 346-347
Informed consent, and distributive justice, 670-671
Inhaled Nitric Oxide in ARDS Study Group, 180
Initiator events, for activation of systemic inflammatory response, 96-97
Injury
  effect of, on cytokine responses, 534
  host response to, 72-75
  initial, risk factors for multiple organ failure following, 34-35
  liver damage following, 459
  risk factors for multiple organ failure following, 34
  second, risk factors for multiple organ failure following, 37-39
  severity rating, and effect of early intubation in the field, 243-244
  See also Trauma
Injury Severity Score (ISS), 10
  and inflammation, 389
  trends in, and crude mortality, 657
  with and without multiple organ failure, 34-35
Inotropic drugs
  for increasing oxygen delivery and consumption, clinical trials, 576
  for patients with septic shock, 26
  for treating systemic inflammatory response syndrome, 374
Insulin, mediation of the stress response by, 642-643
Insulin-like growth factor-1 (IGF-1)
  interaction with growth hormone, in protein synthesis and bone growth, 631
  for treating burn patients, 326
  effect on catabolism of skeletal muscle, 384

Insulin resistance
  in catabolic conditions, 383–384, 632
  metabolic syndrome X associated with, 422–423
Integrin adhesion molecule β_2, role in adhesion of polymorphonuclear leukocytes to endothelial cells, 227
Integrins, 230–231, 235
Intensive care unit (ICU) patients
  duration of stay, and mortality, 689
  monitoring of, 254–263
  nosocomial infections in, 309–321
  systemic inflammatory response in, 36
  tertiary care, studies of multiple organ dysfunction syndrome in, 53–56
Intercellular adhesion molecule (ICAM), 232
  levels of
    as a predictor of multiple organ failure in hemorrhagic shock, 111
    in response to ischemia/reperfusion, 110
    receptor for, on the endothelial cell surface, 94
  role in adhesion of polymorphonuclear leukocytes to endothelial cells, 227
  and survival in multiple organ failure, 45
Interferon-γ (IFNγ)
  biologic roles of
    and outcomes of excessive production, 156
    in synthesis of neopterin, 483
  immunomodulation by, clinical studies, 392–393
  interaction with neopterin and tumor necrosis factor-α, 485–486
  pathophysiologic and clinical role of, 531–538
  role in lethal shock, 120
Interleukin-1 (IL-1)
  biologic roles of, and outcomes of excessive production, 155–156
  future inflammation inhibition trials using, 680
  role in immune cell apoptosis, 159
Interleukin-1β (IL-1β)
  effect on myocardial cell depression, 592
  role in initiation of host defense response, 515–516
Interleukin-1 receptor antagonist (IL-1ra), evaluating therapeutic use of, 157
Interleukin-3 (IL-3), for maturation and maintenance of mast cells, 188
Interleukin-4 (IL-4)
  biologic roles of, and use as a therapeutic agent, 157–158
  effect on apoptosis, 160
Interleukin-6 (IL-6)
  biologic roles of, and outcomes of excessive production, 156
  effect of
    on acute-phase protein synthesis, 422
    on immune cell apoptosis, 159

interaction with granulocyte macrophage colony-stimulating factor, 625
  levels of, in septic shock, 477
Interleukin-8 (IL-8)
  biologic roles of, and outcomes of excessive production, 156
  role of, in immune cell apoptosis, 159
Interleukin-10 (IL-10)
  biologic roles of
    pro- and antiinflammatory mediation by, 534
    and therapeutic use of, 158
  effect of, on apoptosis, 160
  roles in sepsis, 146–147
Interleukin-11, effect of, in systemic inflammatory states, 539–544
Interleukin-11 receptor, molecular biology of, 540–541
Interleukin-12 (IL-12)
  biochemistry of, 532–533
  biologic roles of, and outcomes of excessive production, 156
  therapeutic administration of, in trauma-induced immunodeficiency, 393
  triggering of, by interferon-γ, 531–538
Interleukin-18 (IL-18)
  biologic roles of, 534–536
  and outcomes of excessive production, 156
  triggering of, by interferon-γ, 531–538
Intervention, in bacterial translocation, 87–89
Intraabdominal hypertension, consequences of, 293–297
Intraabdominal infection, experimental, treatment with diet, 453
Intraabdominal pressure (IAP)
  defined, 291
  measuring, 297
Intracellular mechanisms, for muscle cachexia during injury and sepsis, 379–383
Intracranial hypertension
  effect on
    of barbiturates, 403
    of hypertonic saline, 567, 607
  in fulminant hepatic failure, 465
Intracranial pressure monitoring, after severe brain injury, 249
Intramedullary fixation, of long bones, 281–282
Intramedullary nailing (IMN), for long bone fractures, 280
Intravascular volume expansion, for treating systemic inflammatory response syndrome, 373–374
Intubation, endotracheal, 243–244
  in the emergency department, 248
Ion channels, effects of insulin and glucagon on, 105
Iron-heme complex, interaction of nitric oxide through, 177

Ischemia
  depletion of phosphocreatine in, measuring, 261–262
  regional, hemodynamic monitoring to prevent, 254
  renal
    in systemic inflammatory response syndrome, 369–370
    and thromboxane production, 372
Ischemia/reperfusion
  acute coronary syndromes associated with reactive oxygen species in, 172
  in cardiopulmonary bypass, 346
  as a cause of multiple organ failure, 108–113
  intestinal, treatment with soluble complement receptor 1, 217–218
  mediation of, by complement activation, 214–215
  myocardial, treatment with soluble complement receptor 1, 217–218
  oxidative damage to the liver, 172
  platelet activating factor release in, 207
  reducing injury from, by IL-10 pretreatment, 146–147
  as a risk factor for postinjury multiple organ failure, 35–36
  in sepsis, effect on the heart, 344
Isoeicosanoids, association with oxidative stress and free radical damage, 200
Italian Sepsis Study, 36

J
Jet ventilation, high-frequency, 359

K
Kallikrein-kinin system, bradykinin from, role in microcirculatory leakage, 72–73
Kallikrein, activation in systemic inflammatory response syndrome, 93
Kallikrein cascade, activation in cardiopulmonary bypass, 82–83
Ketamine, interaction with morphine, 648
Ketoconazole, clinical trial, response in acute respiratory syndrome, 550
Ketorolac trimethamine (Toradol), effect on stress response to surgery, 547
Kidney
  effect on, of intraabdominal hypertension, 294–295
  failure of, defined, 7
  See also Renal entries
K-means cluster analysis, of physiologic parameters in critically ill patients, 653
Kupffer cells, proinflammatory cytokines produced by, in shock, 136–137

L
Laboratory markers, for diagnosis of infection and inflammation, 477–491

Lactate, levels in the blood
  in circulatory failure, 337
  of critically ill patients, 102
Lactic acid bacteria (LAB)
  immunoactivation by, 450
  restoring in dysbiosis, 448
Lactic acidemia, in systemic inflammatory response syndrome, state B, 27
Lactic acidosis
  effect in the heart, 344–345
  in systemic inflammatory response syndrome, 77
Lactobacillus plantarum, 450–451
  treating patients with, 453–455
Lactulose therapy, in liver failure, 465
Lamotrigine, effect on stress response to surgery, 547
Lansoprazole, for treating stress gastritis, 416
Laparoscopy, for diagnosing peritonitis, 267
Left ventricular ejection fraction (LVEF), measuring, 591
Left ventricular stroke work index (LVSWI), in septic shock, 591
Leukemia inhibitory factor (LIF), 540
  interaction with granulocyte macrophage colony-stimulating factor, 625
Leukocyte adhesion deficiency (LAD), effects of, 234
Leukocyte filtration, to reduce reperfusion injury, 109
Leukocytes
  diapedesis into infection sites, 191
  as effector cells in acute inflammation, 73–74
  interactions with endothelial cells, 224–240
  migration of, 227
Leukocytosis, in peritonitis, 266
Leukopenia, as a prognostic marker for multiple organ failure, 75–76
Leukotrienes
  biosynthesis of, 199–200
Life style
  limitation on medical care's effectiveness imposed by, 690
  and microbial flora, 448–449
Limitations
  on effective medical care, 690
  in treating multiple organ failure, 6–7
Limulus amebocyte lysate (LAL), assay for lipopolysaccharide, 116
Lipid peroxidation, 168–169
Lipid peroxides
  decomposition in the presence of iron complexes, 169
  levels of, in sepsis, 170–171
Lipids, products of, from mast cells, 191
Lipolysis, in the stress response, 643–644
Lipopolysaccharide (LPS)
  effects on tumor necrosis factor-α, 123
  neopterin synthesis associated with, 483
  purified versus spontaneously shed, 115

  role of, in macrophage activation, 493
  sepsis induced experimentally by administration of, 506–507
  toxic portion of, 114, 492–493
  translocating, local effects of, 87
Lipoprotein lipases (LPLs), roles of, in trauma and sepsis, 644
Lipoteichoic acid
  induction of cytokines by, 119–120
  interaction with peptidoglycan to cause multiple organ failure, 119
Lipoxygenase pathway, 191, 199–200
Lisophylline, clinical trial, 548
Liver
  in acute-phase response, 421–422
  bioartificial support system for, 467–470
  neutrophil adhesion in, after endotoxemia, 235
Liver failure, 459–461
  defined, 7
  hepatic support and the bioartificial liver, 462–473
  in induced shock, effect of matrix metalloproteinase inhibitors on, 150
  mortality in, 48
  reactive oxygen species associated with, 172
Liver transplantation (OLT), orthotropic
  effect of selective decontamination of the digestive tract on infection in, 585
  for fulminant hepatic failure patients, 467
  postoperative morbidity in, effect of prostaglandin E_1, 202
Loculation, of microbes in secondary peritonitis, 265
Lung, 353–363
  contusion of, progressive, 283
  effects on, of modified treatments, 659
  injury to
    after blunt trauma, 280–281
    responses of selectin blockade in, 229–230
  neutrophil adhesion in, after endotoxemia, 235
  transplantation of, complement C1 inhibitor pretreatment in, 217
Lymphatic system, effect on, of intraabdominal hypertension, 296–297
Lymphocele, peritoneal cavity as, 265
Lymphocytes
  B, effect of interferon-γ on, 531
  function after hemorrhagic shock, trauma and burns, 135–136
  interleukin-11 in, 541
  role of, in wound healing, 554–555
Lysophospholipids, conversion to inflammatory mediators, 196–197

M
Macroendocrine counterregulation, 158
Macroendocrine molecules, role in immunocyte apoptosis, 160

Macrophage-activating factors (MAFs), interferon-γ, 531
Macrophage colony-stimulating factor (M-CSF), effect on leukocytes, 73
Macrophage inflammatory protein (MIP), 233
Macrophages
  activation following injury, 73–74, 515–516, 554
  dysfunction of, and bacterial translocation, 581–582
  function following trauma and hemorrhage, 134–135
  interaction with endotoxin, mouse model, 117
Magnetic resonance spectroscopy, phosphorus, 261–262
Major histocompatibility complex-I (MHC-I), effect of interferon-γ on, 531
Malaria, procalcitonin levels in, 479
Malassezia furfur, bacteremia from an intravascular device due to, 312
Mannitol, for reducing intracranial pressure, 465–466
Margination, defined, for polymorphonuclear lymphocytes, 224
Mast cells, 188–195
  interaction with adhesion molecules, 233–234
  role in wound healing, 554
  stimulation of, and vascular permeability, 93
Measurement, of neopterin in biologic fluids, 483
Mediators
  antiinflammatory, synthesis of, 532
Mediators (*Continued*)
  of catabolic response to injury and sepsis, 378–379
  inflammatory
    circulating, after cardiopulmonary bypass, 346–347
    ideal multiagent therapy in the presence of, 565–568
    in myocardial dysfunction, 342–345
    neutralizing or blocking, 372–375
    removing from blood, 502–503
    proximal, of host defense responses, 515–516
  of the stress response, 642–643
Melatonin, effect on immune function following trauma or hemorrhage, 392
Meningitis, nosocomial, 317
Mesenteric lymph, evaluation of microbial translocation in, 36
Metabolic syndrome X, morbidity in, 422–423
Metabolic system
  depletion and failure of, 378–388
  effect on
    of bioartificial liver support in fulminant hepatic failure, 470

Metabolic system (*Continued*)
of growth hormone, after elective surgery, 633–634
of the stress response, 643–644
failure of, defined, 6–7
in inflammation and sepsis, 101–103
Metalloproteinase, matrix, tumor necrosis factor-α converting enzyme, 150
Methionine-enkephalin, effects on immune function, 392
Methylprednisolone, effect on mortality in sepsis, 519
Metoprolol, for treating hypermetabolic response to trauma and burns, 327
Microbe organ, bacterial cells of the human body, 447–448
Microbial resistance, effect on, of selective decontamination of the digestive tract, 585
Microbiology, of peritonitis, 265
Microcirculation
effects on, of hypertonic solution administration, 606–607
injury to, in systemic inflammatory response syndrome, 27–28, 98
leakage of, in reaction to inflammation, 72–73
Microcirculatory arrest, 92–100
in systemic inflammatory response syndrome, 96–99, 303
Mifepristone (RU486)
for blocking of apoptosis after burn injury, 150
effect on septic shock, rat model, 518
Migration inhibitory factor (MIF), macrophage, and glucocorticoid resistance, 124–125
Milk, for nutritional support in trauma and burns, 325
Misoprostol, inhibition of gastric secretion by, 416–417
Mitochondrial oxidative dysfunction, near-infrared spectroscopy to demonstrate, 35
Mitogen-activated protein (MAP) kinases, role in lethal shock, 119–120
Mixed antagonistic response syndrome (MARS), 17, 599
diagnosis using flow cytometry, 526–527
as immunologic dissonance, 602
Models
for clinical testing, future emphasis, 683
of postinjury multiple organ failure, 32–33
predictive, for multiple organ failure, 35
for testing combinations of therapeutic agents, 565
ZIGI, for sterile peritonitis, 76
Modulation, of hypermetabolic response to trauma and burns, 324
Monoclonal antibody
for blocking inflammation activation, clinical trial, 679
for cytokines, clinical trials, 680
protecting nephrons with, during endotoxemia, 372
Monocytes
circulating, role in systemic inflammatory response syndrome, 97
immune response functions of, 94
Monoethylglycinexylidide (MEGX), measuring, as a test of liver function, 63
Morbidity
in metabolic syndrome X, 422–423
organ dysfunction as a measure of, 19–20
premature, related to behavioral factors, 670
Mortality
in abdominal compartment syndrome, 277, 300
in acute renal failure, 365, 375
in acute respiratory distress syndrome (ARDS), 46
in burn patients treated with growth hormone, 384
in coagulopathy, 275
effect on
of melatonin treatment in hemorrhage, 392
of selective decontamination of the digestive tract, 584–585
in gram-negative bacterial sepsis, 492
in growth hormone trials, 635
in head injury, 400
in hypothermia, severely wounded patients, 274
in meningococcal bacteremia, prediction from tumor necrosis factor-α levels, 494
in multiple organ failure, 7, 28
in nosocomial infection in the intensive care unit, 309
in operative fracture treatment, historic record, 286
organ dysfunction as a measure of, 19–20
predicting
in adult respiratory distress syndrome, 355–356
from gastric tonometry measurements, 258
resource utilization affected by, 674
reduction in, 690
in severe chest injury, dependence on day of surgery, 285
in severe chest trauma, effect of early intubation, 243
in stress gastritis, 413
with active bleeding, 417
Mortality Probability Models (MPM II), 10
Mucosa, role in the immune system, 449–450
Multiagent approach, inflammatory response to cardiopulmonary bypass, 83–84
Multimodal analgesic therapy, pharmacologic treatment, 647
Multiple organ dysfunction (MOD), in limb surgery and limb injury, 111–112
Multiple Organ Dysfunction Score (MODS), defined, literature sources, 10
Multiple organ dysfunction syndrome (MODS)
acute respiratory distress syndrome associated with, 353
defined, 24, 367
consensus conference, 30–31
literature sources, 9
describing, 18
indications for surgical intervention in, 303–308
procalcitonin levels in, 479–480
role of mast cells in, potential, 191–193
in surgical patients, 52–67
triggered by therapy for intraabdominal hypertension, 299
Multiple organ failure (MOF)
clinical applications for reducing, 234–235
defined, literature sources for classification, 9
origin of the term, 5
Multiple organ failure score (MOF), defined, Denver score, 31–32
Muscle, respiratory, growth hormone effect on strength of, 635
Muscle cachexia
during injury and sepsis, 378–388
and negative nitrogen balance, 381–382
Musculoskeletal system, failure of, defined, 6
Myalgia, from growth hormone administration, 635
Myeloperoxidase, formation of hypochlorous acid by, 167
Mylanta, evaluation, in stress gastritis, 415
Myocardial depressant factor (MDF), 342
circulating, 592–593
Myocardial dysfunction
clinical relevance of depression, 591–597
effect of inflammatory conditions in, 340–345
and pathogenesis of multiple organ dysfunction syndrome, 59
after surgery, 346–347
Myocardial infarction
monoclonal anti-C5a immunoglobulin G treatment in, 218
soluble complement receptor 1 treatment in, clinical trials, 217–218
Myocardium
changes associated with inflammatory conditions, 344
contractility of, effects of hypertonic solutions on, 607
ischemic, multiple organ failure associated with reperfusion in, 109

Index

Myofilaments, calcium-dependent release of, 383

N

N-Acetylcysteine (NAC)
  cardiac effect in septic shock, 345
  clinical trial, effect on stress response in surgery, 549
  effect on acetaminophen toxicity, 549
  treating sepsis patients with, 171
Nafamostat mesylate, anticoagulant, in continuous hemodiafiltration, 501
Nailing, reamed versus unreamed, systemic burden of, 283–286
Natriuresis, dopamine-mediated, 374–375
Natural killer cell stimulatory factor (NKSF). See Interleukin-12
Near-infrared spectroscopy (NIR), transcutaneous and transcranial, for monitoring oxygenation, 261
Necrosis, focal, in systemic inflammatory response syndrome, 95–96, 98
N-endrule pathway, and muscle protein breakdown, 382–383
Neoplasias, neopterin levels in, 482
Neopterin
  as a marker
    for cellular immunity, 482–487
    for severity of ARDS, MOF and sepsis, 76
  monitoring of, 477
Nephrotoxicity, drug-induced, 171
Networks versus cascades, in biologic systems, 652–653
Neural network model, for predicting outcome in hyperthermia-coagulopathy-acidosis syndrome, 275
Neurochemical memory of pain, 645–646
Neuroendocrine system
  antiinflammatory effect of reactions of, 74
  failure of, defined, 7
Neurohormones, effect on, of intraabdominal hypertension, 297
Neurologic effects, of bioartificial liver support, 469–470
Neurotrauma, trials for managing, 399–404
Neutrophils
  activation of, 97, 224, 226
  apoptosis in the normal biology of, 131–132
  eosinophilic, appearance in wounds, 553–554
  inhibition of, for treating sepsis, 77–78
  margination of, in systemic inflammatory response syndrome, 97
  priming of
    by complement activation, 215
    by granulocyte colony-stimulating factor, 622
    by platelet activating factor, 207
    in severe injury, 36–37
    by stored blood for transfusions, 38
  role in tissue injury, 224
  surface rolling of, in inflammation, 94
New Injury Severity Score (NISS), 35
Nimodipine, for aneurysmal subarachnoid hemorrhage (SAH) treatment, 402
Nitric oxide (NO)
  in the contact activating system, 93
  effect of
    on blood pressure, 75
    on gastrointestinal motility and blood flow, 429–431
    on oxidant damage to the liver, 172
  hemoglobin-based oxygen carriers as scavengers for, 613
  inhaled, in acute respiratory distress syndrome treatment, 360–361, 566–567, 659
  molecular action of, 177
  in myocardial dysfunction, 593
    following ischemia/reperfusion, 346
  nitrosyl generation, 168
  in renal impairment related to systemic inflammatory response syndrome, 370–371
  sepsis modulation by, 176–187
  synthesis by wound fibroblasts, 555
Nitric oxide synthase
  coronary artery, response to sepsis, 344
  in the endothelium, 72–73
  inducible, 72
    mediation of bacterial translocation by, 87
    in myocardial dysfunction, 342–343
    in the inflammatory cascade, 170–171
    transcriptional regulation of, 176
  inhibitors of, 177–178
    and mortality in clinical trials, 182
    vascular permeability suppression by, 88
Nitrite, ingested, effect on bacteriostasis in the stomach, 429–430
Nitrogen balance
  negative, in muscle cachexia, 381–382
  in trauma and burns, 323–324
Nitrogen oxides, free radical, 167–168
S-Nitrosylation, control of nitric oxide biosynthesis through, 177
N-methyl-D-aspartate (NMDA) receptor, role in spinal cord hypersensitivity, 648
Nonsteroidal antiinflammatory drugs (NSAIDs), analgesia with, 647
Norepinephrine
  antiinflammatory effects of, 158
  for treating circulatory failure, 336, 594–595
Normothermia, maintaining in surgery, 547
Nuclear factor-κB (NF-κB), 74–75
  activation level in sepsis and adult respiratory distress syndrome, 517–518
Nutrients
  immunomodulatory, 431
  interaction with growth hormone, 633
  in preserved foods, 450–451
  release in the colon by commensal flora, 447
  sources of, 424–425
  See also Immunonutrients
Nutrition
  calorie restriction, effect on immune function, 433–434
  and growth hormone response, 632–633
  parenteral, and thrombosis, 421–422
  and stress response, 643–644
  See also Enteral nutrition; Total parenteral nutrition (TPN)
Nutritional support
  for burn patients, effect on gastrointestinal dysfunction, 61
  effect of continuous hemodiafiltration on, 504
  effect on muscle catabolism after injury, 385–386
  in liver failure, 464
  for modulating the hypermetabolic response to trauma and burns, 324–325

O

Oat gum
  components of, 451
  treating patients with, after gastrointestinal surgery, 453–455
Obstructive circulatory failure, defined, 333
Oligofructans, nutritional characteristics of, 452
Oliguria, in intraabdominal hypertension, 294–295
Omeprazole, for treating stress gastritis, 416
Opioids
  for analgesia, 647
  immune modulation by, 392
  in septic shock, 343
Organ failure, relation to infection, temporal, 602–603
Outcomes
  of depression following hemofiltration, 675
  of early fracture fixation, 657–658
  of excessive production
    of interferon-γ (IFNγ), 156
    of interleukin-8 (IL-8), 156
  measures of, in clinical trials of sepsis treatment, 639
  predicting, 9–10
  of pulmonary system failure, 672–673
Oxidative metabolism, and systemic inflammatory response syndrome, 95–96, 111
Oxidative radicals, in sepsis and trauma, synthesis of PAF-like oxidized phospholipids using, 205
Oxidative stress
  mechanisms of, 170
  neopterin levels in, 486–487

Oxygen
  partial pressure of, raising in shock, 336
  reactive, formation in the body, 167–168
Oxygen carriers
  blood
    association with hypertonic saline, 607–608
    substitutes for emergency field care, 245–246
  hemoglobin-based, 616
    as nitric oxide scavengers, 613–615
  See also Oxygen transport
Oxygen consumption
  effect of continuous hemodiafiltration on, 503–504
  effects associated with, in trauma, 567
  maximizing, 571–579
  measuring in intensive care, 255
  by tubular cells, 368
  uptake in circulatory failure, 334–335, 659–660
Oxygen debt
  multiple organ failure associated with, 46
  and survival in organ failure, 572
  tissue, as a determinant of organ failure, 35–36
  See also Hypoxia
Oxygen probes, fiberoptic, 261
Oxygen transport
  effect on, of intraabdominal hypertension, 296
  monitoring in intensive care, 255
  prospective studies of, 572–573
  See also Oxygen carriers, blood

P

Pain
  modulation of, and anesthetic care, 646
  postoperative, treatment of, 645–648
Pancreas, characteristics of organ failure involving, 7
Pancreatitis
  experimental, preventing with diet, 453
  neopterin levels in, 485
  preventing infection in, with selective decontamination of the digestive tract, 585–586
  procalcitonin levels in, 480
  pulmonary failure associated with, 97
  reactive oxygen species associated with, 172
  response to recombinant hemoglobin injection, 617
  severe acute, phases of systemic inflammatory response syndrome in, 304
  treatment of
    with complement C1 inhibitor, 216
    with platelet activating factor antagonists, 210
Paracentesis, for diagnosing peritonitis, 267
Parasitic infections, neopterin levels in, 484
Parenteral nutrition, and thrombosis, 421–422
  See also Total parenteral nutrition
Pathobiology, cascade-to-network transition in viewing, 654
Pathogenesis
  of antibiotic-associated pseudomembranous colitis, 316
  of catheter-related nosocomial infections, 311–312
  of myocardial dysfunction
    after cardiac surgery, 346–347
    septic, 342–345
  of sinusitis in the intensive care unit, 315–316
  of urinary tract infections, nosocomial, 313–315
  of ventriculitis or meningitis, in the intensive care unit, 317
Pathophysiology
  of adult respiratory distress syndrome, 353–354
  of bacterial colonization and translocation, 580–581
  of disseminated intravascular coagulation, 439–441
  of nosocomial pneumonia, in the intensive care unit, 309–310
  of peritonitis, 264–266
  renal, in systemic inflammatory response syndrome, 369–372
  of severe head injury, 398–399
  of stress gastritis, 411–412
Patients
  medical, risk for multiple organ failure in, 44–51
  rights of, 665–671
  surgical, risk for multiple organ failure, 52–67
Patient Self-Determination Act, 666
Peak exhaled or end-tidal carbon dioxide ($PETCO_2$), and cardiopulmonary resuscitation, 260
Pectin, nutritional advantages of, 429, 451–452
Pentastarch, for resuscitating trauma victims, 567
Pentoxifylline
  effect of
    on neopterin levels, 486
    in sepsis, 394, 567, 659–660
    in sepsis, clinical trial, 549–550
  selective inhibition of tumor necrosis factor-α by, 392
Peptic ulcers, treating, in peritonitis, 267
Peptidoglycan, effects on lymphocytes and immune cells, 119
Percutaneous drainage, of an abscess, 306
Perfluorocarbons (PFCs)
  as artificial oxygen carriers, 245–246
  as red blood cell substitutes, 613
  for treating acute respiratory distress syndrome, 361
Perfusion, nonpulsatile, in cardiopulmonary bypass, 82
Perioperative therapy, to decrease the stress response, 547
Peritonitis
  experimental, role of mast cells and chemokines in response to, 233–234
  multiple organ failure and systemic inflammatory response syndrome in, 264–272
  P-selectin antibody for treating, 228–229
  tertiary, management of, 270–271
  tissue factor pathway inhibitor for treating, 510–511
Permeability
  intestinal, 86–91
  of the pulmonary system, after reamed nailing of the femur, 234
  vascular, and stimulation of mast cells, 93
Peroxisome proliferating activated receptors (PPARs), role in macrophage activation, 125
pH, gastric intramucosal, 566
  clinical trial of effect in trauma patients, 576
  for evaluating circulatory failure, 337, 659
  in stress gastritis, 412
Phagocytic response, to injury, 94
Pharmacoeconomic issues, in treating stress gastritis, 417–418
Pharmacology
  multimodal analgesic therapy, 647
  of neurotrauma management, 402–404
  of platelet activating factor, 206–207
  See also Drugs
Phosphatidylinositol (PI), induction by platelet activating factor, 205–206
Phosphodiesterase inhibitors, as inodilators, for treating circulatory failure, 336
Phospholipases, role in eicosanoid synthesis, 196–197
Phospholipids, platelet activating factor as a mediator for, 204–213
Physiologic envelope
  and damage control in surgery for trauma, 273
  quantitative analysis of, 275–276
Physiologic supply dependence, defined for oxygen, 334–335
Physiology, of the hypermetabolic response after trauma and burns, 322–324
Plasma, fresh frozen, for treating disseminated intravascular coagulation, 443
Plasma mediators, roles in human neutrophil apoptosis, 131–132
Platelet activating factor (PAF), 204–213
  degradation by acetylhydrolase, 196–197
  in ischemia/reperfusion, 35
  from the mast cell, 191

role in renal dysfunction in septic shock, 371
Platelet activating factor antagonists, 207–208
Platelet-derived growth factor, role in hypermetabolic response in trauma and burns, 325
Platelet-endothelial cell adhesion molecule
role in adhesion of polymorphonuclear leukocytes to endothelial cells, 227
transmigration across the endothelial layer promoted by, 232
Platelets
activated, effect on inflammatory response, 93
aggregation of, following disruption of endothelial tissue, 72
concentrate administration, in disseminated intravascular coagulation, 443
Pneumonia
effect on, of selective decontamination of the digestive tract, 583–584
nosocomial, 37
mortality rate in, 46
mortality with stress gastritis, 414
in the intensive care unit, 309–311
prevention of, in systemic inflammatory response syndrome and ARDS, 357
Poiseuille's law, 398
Polyclonal antibodies, anti-endotoxin, production in host immune response, 494–495
Polymorphonuclear neutrophils (PMNs)
activation of, 33
after intramedullary nailing, 282
preventing with monoclonal antibodies, 112
complement anaphylatoxins as stimulants for, 73
effects on, of interferon-γ, 531
roles in tissue injury, 224–226, 553
Polymyxin B
clinical trial of, 497
as an endotoxin antagonist, 496
use in hemoperfusion, 501
Polytrauma, fracture treatment for patients with, 279–280
Polytrauma Score (PTS), in acute respiratory distress syndrome, 355
Polyunsaturated fatty acids, oxidation of, stages, 168–169
Population growth, limitations on medical care imposed by, 690
Porin, shock induced by, 119
Positioning, prone, in acute respiratory distress syndrome, 359–360
Positive end-expiratory pressure (PEEP)
managing in acute respiratory distress syndrome, 357
reduction of, for treating intraabdominal hypertension, 298

Preclinical studies
of antithrombin III in sepsis, 506–507
of interleukin-11, in systemic inflammatory states, 542–543
of tissue factor pathway inhibitor, 509–511
Prediction
of acute respiratory distress syndrome, scoring systems for, 355
of mortality
in acute respiratory distress syndrome, 355–356
from gastric tonometry measurements, 258
resource utilization affected by, 674
in septic shock, from interleukin-18 levels, 536
Preemptive analgesia, to prevent spinal hyperexcitability, 646
Pregnancy
acute fatty liver of, 463
acute respiratory distress syndrome in, 354
Prehospital Trauma Life Support program, 657
Preload status, and resuscitation, in intensive care, 257
Pressure, external, effect on intraabdominal pressure, 293
Prevention
of abdominal compartment syndrome, 300–301
of antibiotic-associated pseudomembranous colitis, 317
of catheter-related nosocomial infections, 313
importance of, 660
of multiple organ failure, 3, 6–7
of muscle cachexia, 383
of nosocomial pneumonia, 310–311
of sinusitis, in the intensive care unit, 316
of urinary tract infections, nosocomial, 314–315
of ventriculitis or meningitis, nosocomial, 317
Procalcitonin (PCT), 477, 478–482
Professional responsibility, ethical, 670
Prognosis, in organ system failure, 17–18
See also Outcomes; Prediction
Programmed cell death (PCD), in immunocyte regulation, 159
See also Apoptosis
Proinflammatory responses, relation to counterinflammatory responses, 599–600
Prolactin, effect on immune response, 139, 392
Proliferative phase of wound healing, 553
Propanolol, effect in hypermetabolic response to trauma and burns, 327
Prophylaxis
preoperative, immunoglobulin therapy for at-risk patients, 638–639
for stress gastritis, 414–417

Propofol, reducing stress responses in the intensive care unit with, 547
Prostacyclin, vasodilation by, 198
Prostaglandin D, from activated mast cells, 191
Prostaglandin E_1 (PGE_1), for treating the inflammatory response associated with ARDS, 201–202
for treating the inflammatory response associated with ARDS, clinical trial, 574–575
Prostaglandin E_2 (PGE_2), inhibition of cell-mediated immune function by, 137
Prostaglandins
biosynthesis of, 197–199
metabolism of, and bacterial translocation, 87
vasodilating, effect on cardiac performance, 596
Prostheses
hazards of, evaluating, 690
for open management treatment in intraabdominal hypertension, 299
Protease inhibitors
C1, 215–216
for treating disseminated intravascular coagulation, 444
Proteases
activation through actions of integrin v_3, 232
neutral, of mast cells, 190
release on degranulation of mast cells, 192
tissue damage associated with, 226
Proteasome inhibitors
effect of, on muscle protein breakdown, 381
selective, for treating hypermetabolism, 105
Protected specimen brushing (PSB), for diagnosing pneumonia, 310
Protein C
activated, role in coagulation, 505
for treating disseminated intravascular coagulation, 444
Protein C1 inhibitor, clinical trial of effect on stress response, 549
Proteins
acute-phase, downregulation by cytokines, 104
denaturation of, in cardiopulmonary bypass, 82–83
effect of insulin-like growth factor-1 on synthesis of, 326
loss of, in the stress response, 644
penicillin-binding, 116
porin, shock induced by, 119
regulatory, to control complement activation, 215–218
total body, loss in critically ill patients, 102–103
Proteoglycans, of the human mast cell, 190
Proteolysis
intracellular pathways for, 379

Proteolysis (Continued)
    muscle, in response to trauma and burns, 322–323
    in the ubiquitin/proteasome-dependent pathway, 103, 380
Proteolysis-inducing factor (PIF), effect on skeletal muscle, 379
Prothrombin time (PT), for detecting disseminated intravascular coagulation, 441
Prothrombotic state, metabolic syndrome X associated with, 422–423
Protocol, for severe head injury management, 406
Proton-pump inhibitors for stress gastritis, 416
Pseudomembranous colitis, antibiotic-associated, 316–317
Pseudomonas aeruginosa
    bacteremia from an intravascular device due to, 312
    nosocomial pneumonia due to, 309
Psychotropic substances, as platelet activating factor antagonists, 208
Pulmonary artery catheter, information from, 256
Pulmonary artery hypertension, and right ventricular ejection fraction, 592
Pulmonary capillary pressure, in intraabdominal hypertension, 293
Pulmonary system
    complications in, of fulminant hepatic failure, 466
    dysfunction of
        after cardiopulmonary bypass, 82
        in fat embolism syndrome, 279
        in surgical patients, 63
    edema in, after prevention of renal failure, 71
    failure of
        defined, 7
        effects of eicosanoids in, 200–202
        effects of nitric oxide in, 179–180
        mortality in, 48
        outcomes, 672–673
        posttraumatic, 4
    hypertension in, accompanying septic shock, 342
    permeability of, after reamed nailing of the femur, 284
    reactions of vasculature, in trauma, 282
Pulse oximetry, in intensive care, 260–261
Pyridinyl imidazoles, inhibition of cytokine biosynthesis by, 89

Q

Quality of care, in emergency treatment for trauma, 250
Quincke edema, in C1 inhibitor-deficient individuals, 216

R

Radiocontrast-induced injury, renal, 63
Radiography, in the initial phase of emergency treatment for trauma, 248
Radiologic assessment, of acute respiratory distress syndrome, 355
Ranitidine, evaluation, for stress gastritis, 416
Rationing of medical care, 664
Reactive oxygen metabolites (ROMs), tissue damage associated with, 226
Reactive oxygen species (ROSs)
    in clinical practice, 167–175
    stress on mitochondria, 72–75
Receiver operator characteristic (ROC) curve, for evaluating a variable predicting a dichotomous outcome, 55–56
Receptor antagonists, IL-1ra, in antiinflammatory response, 74
Receptors, for platelet activating factor, 205–206
Red blood cells, outdated, as a source of hemoglobin, 616–617
Redundancy, in inflammatory systems, 652–653
Regulation, normal, of growth hormone, 630–631
Relevance, clinical, process of defining, 656
Remodeling pathway, synthesis of platelet activating factor in, 204
Remote organs, damage to accompanying inflammation, 562
Renal system
    acute failure of
        after cardiopulmonary bypass, 83
        reactive oxygen species involvement, 171–172
    blood flow in, maintenance by prostaglandins, 198
    damage to
        and mortality, 3–4
        from stroma-free hemoglobin administration, 246
    dysfunction of
        in multiple organ failure, 365–377
        in surgical patients, 63–64
    effect on
        of hypertonic solutions, 607
        of nitric oxide synthase inhibition, 179
    failure of, 365
        defined, 5
        in fulminant hepatic failure, 466
        Korean War data, 53
        mortality in, 48
        and multiple organ failure syndrome, 365–366
        prevalence in at-risk patients, 366
        socioeconomic impact, 673–674
        with intraabdominal pressure rise, 291
    normal function of, 368–369
Reoperation
    in peritonitis, indications for, 269–270
    planned, 306–308
    in systemic inflammatory respiratory syndrome, selecting patients for, 304–306
    in trauma, as part of damage control, 275, 277
Reperfusion, controlled, in isolated limbs after clot removal, 109
Reperfusion syndrome, lethal, in decompression to treat intraabdominal hypertension, 299
Resource utilization
    organ dysfunction scores as an estimate of intensity of, 19, 56
    and prediction of death, 674
Respiratory system
    failure of
        association with intraabdominal hypertension, 296
        association with peritonitis, 5
        granulocyte macrophage colony-stimulating factor in, 626
    function in the stress response, 644
    synchrony with the cardiovascular system, 653–654
Resting energy expenditure, in intensive care unit patients, 101–102
Resuscitation
    in the field, after injury, 243–247
    after initial therapy in multiple trauma treatment, 273
Reticuloendothelial system (RES), inactivation of external pathogens in, in shock, 281
Rhabdomyolysis
    acute respiratory distress syndrome associated with, 44
    renal failure associated with, 365
    renal failure secondary to, 171
Rheumatic fever, neopterin levels in, as an indicator of valve lesions, 484
Rheumatoid arthritis
    effect of interleukin-11 on inflammatory response in, 542
    neopterin levels in, 482
Right heart function monitoring catheter, 256–257
Right to die, religious views on, 667–669
Right ventricular ejection fraction (LVEF)
    prediction of survival in trauma and coronary artery disease using, 257
    in sepsis, 591–592
Risk factors
    for acute respiratory distress syndrome, 353
    for catheter-related infections, 311
    for coagulopathy after transfusion, 275–276
    versus injury severity score, for acute respiratory distress syndrome, 354–355
    for multiple organ dysfunction syndrome, 54
    for multiple organ failure, 10–11, 30–43
        in medical patients, 44–51

organ dysfunction as, 18–19
  prospective studies of oxygen consumption maximization, 573
  for stress gastritis, 413
  for ventriculitis or meningitis in the intensive care unit, 317
Risk stratification, in evaluating preoperative antibiotic administration, 683
Roentgenographic studies, for diagnosing peritonitis, value of, 266–267

S

Saliva, immune function of, 428
Schwartzman reaction, 372
Score-Based Immunoglobulin Therapy of Sepsis (SBITS), 639
Scoring systems
  for acute respiratory distress syndrome prediction, 355
  for organ failure, 8
  See also Classification
Selectins, 228–230
  blockade of, for preventing polymorphonuclear-mediated tissue injury, 235
  P-, as a requirement for polymorphonuclear migration, 233
  role in cellular activation, 232
Selective decontamination of the digestive tract (SDD), 583–586
  effects on bacterial translocation, 582
Sepsis
  antithrombin III treatment for, 565
  apoptosis associated with, 132
  control of, enteral nutrition in, 421–422
  cytokines in, 145–154
    deficient production of T cells, 485–486
  defined, 15, 24, 367
  effect on
    of antithrombin III, 506–507
    of antithrombin III, clinical trials, 507–509
    of insulin-like growth factor, 384
  effect on the heart, 340–346
  endotoxin response to, 146–147
  granulocyte colony-stimulating factor levels in, 621
  granulocyte macrophage colony-stimulating factor for treating, 626
  immunoglobulin therapy in, 638
  interleukin-18 levels in, 536
  liver function changes in, 459–460
  models of, evaluation of granulocyte colony-stimulating factor, 623
  muscle proteolysis induced by, 380
  neopterin levels in, 485–486
    predictive value of, 484–485
  nosocomial, in critically ill patients, 46
  outcome measures in clinical trials of immunoglobulin G, 639
  oxygen uptake and cardiac index indicators in survivors of, 571
  platelet activating factor antagonist treatment in, 208–209
  polymicrobial, 137–138
  procalcitonin levels in, 479–480
  reactive oxygen species involved in responses to, 170–171
  survival of, 15–16
Sepsis-related Organ Failure Assessment Score (SOFA), 10
Sepsis Severity Score (SSS)
  in acute respiratory distress syndrome, 355
  in intestinal ischemia, correlation with endotoxin concentrations, 87
Sepsis syndrome, 15–16, 101–107
  antiinflammatory response in, 146
  defined, 32, 496
  reproduction of sequelae of, by endotoxin, 114
Septic shock. See Shock, septic
Sequence, importance in biological development, 652–653
Sequential system failure, in survivors of initial trauma, 26
Sequestration
  defined, for polymorphonuclear lymphocytes, 224
  regulation of, for polymorphonuclear lymphocytes, 227
Serine protease inhibitor
  antithrombin III as, 505
  for managing inflammation, 75
  synthetic, 219
Severe sepsis
  defined, 24, 367
  inotropic drugs for improving cardiac contractility in, 374
Shock
  acidosis in, monitoring, 274
  blood flow changes in, 412
  Brussels study, mortality rate and severity of, 44–45
  circulatory failure in, 333
  defined, 7
  hemorrhagic
    as a cofactor in organ failure, 282–283
    decision for surgery in, 273
    effect of hypertonic saline in, 607
    endotoxin levels in, 582–583
    immunoglobulin suppression following, 136
    prototype for systemic ischemia/reperfusion injury, 110–111
    sepsis and organ failure associated with, 598–599
    septic complications in, 389–390
    treating, 110–111, 565
  hypotension in, 25
  hypovolemic, 369–370
  measures of efficacy of treatment of, hypertonic saline administration, 608
  mortality rate in, 3–4
  postoperative, oxygen uptake and delivery in, 571
  resuscitation in, 254–255
  as a risk factor for postinjury multiple organ failure, 35–36
  septic
    antithrombin III treatment for, 508–509
    bacterial components having roles in, 118–121
    complement C1 inhibitor treatment for, clinical trial, 216
    defined, 367, 496
    effect of norepinephrine on mortality in, 60
    effect on the heart, 340–346
    glucocorticoid therapy for, 16, 514–523
    from gram-negative and gram-positive bacteria, 118
    hemofiltration in, 502
    left ventricular stroke work index in, 591
    management of patients with, 25
    nitric oxide role in, 179
    nosocomial infection and drug resistance in, 660
    oxygen debt in, 572
    oxygen delivery therapy, prospective clinical trial, 575
    oxygen uptake and delivery in, 335
    predictive value of interleukin-18 levels in, 536
    renal response to hypotension in, 369–370
    reversing, 374
    short-term treatment with methylene blue, 429
  in surgical patients in intensive care units, 54
  following trauma and burns, 322
Sick euthyroid syndrome, 643
Signaling
  by cell-associated tumor necrosis factor-α, 150–151
  immunomodulatory and counterinflammatory, in mast cells, 192
  by integrins, 232
Signal transduction
  after injury, role of endothelial cell-associated PAF synthesis in, 204
  role of tumor necrosis factor-α in, 493–494
Simplified Acute Physiology Score (SAPS), 10
  correlation with endothelium-derived factors and multiple organ failure, 45
Sinusitis, nosocomial, in the intensive care unit, 315–316
Skin, effect of growth hormone on, 326
Small-volume fluid resuscitation, in field emergency care, 245
S-nitroso-amino-penicillamine (SNAP), as a nitric oxide donor, 180–181

Social responsibility, limitations on health care outcomes imposed by, 690
Society of Critical Care Medicine (SCCM), 30, 44
Socioeconomic impact, of multiple organ failure, 672–677
See also Cost/benefit calculations
Soluble complement receptor 1 (sCR1), 217–218
Somatostatin, role in growth hormone regulation, 631
Spectroscopy, near-infrared, 261
Spinal anesthesia, 647
Staging systems, improving, for systemic inflammatory response syndrome and MODS, 684
Staphylococcus aureus
  bacteremia from an intravascular device due to, 312
  methicillin-resistant, nosocomial pneumonia due to, 309
Staphylococcus epidermidis, bacteremia from an intravascular device due to, 312
Starling's law, 255
Steal phenomenon, in coronary insufficiency, 344
Stem cell factor, for maturation and maintenance of mast cells, 188
Stenotrophomonas maltophilia, nosocomial pneumonia due to, 309
Steroids
  anabolic, 327
  cerebral edema management using, clinical trials, 403
  sex, effect on cell-mediated immune function, 391
Stress gastritis, 411–419
Stress response
  anesthetic care and, 641–650
  levels of, to define stages of systemic inflammatory response, 23–25
  metabolic, in minimum surgical procedures, 546
  perioperative therapy for decreasing, 547
  Th1/Th2 T cell shifts induced in, 524–530
Study to Understand Prognoses and Preferences for Outcomes and Risks of Treatment, 666
Sucralfate, for treating stress gastritis, 416
Superoxide dismutase (SOD)
  forms of, 169–170
  protective role of, 167–168
  for treating systemic reperfusion injury, 112
Superoxide radical, formation of, at physiologic pH, 167–168
Supranormal oxygen delivery, in circulatory failure, 336–338
Surgery
  chest, video-assisted, 545–546
  minimal, to decrease stress response, 545–552

multiple organ dysfunction syndrome following, 598
oxygen delivery and consumption following, prospective study, 575–576
in peritonitis, for source control, 267–268
postcardiac, 346–347
procalcitonin levels following, 481
secondary operative procedures, multiple organ failure following, 38
selective decontamination of the digestive tract for reducing infection after, 586
systemic burden of, in primary fracture fixation, 283–286
timing of, for trauma patients, 249–250
urgent, for trauma patients, 248–250
Syndrome, defined, 14–15
Systemic inflammation
  clinical applications for reducing, 234–235
  after trauma, infection and cardiopulmonary bypass, 71–81
Systemic inflammatory response syndrome (SIRS)
  acute respiratory distress syndrome inducing, 353
  antithrombin III treatment in, 508
  characterization of, 477, 526
  complement activation in, 214–215
  in critical illness, 15–17, 600–601
  defined, 16, 24, 367, 496
  development of a system to describe, 9–10
  diagnostic criteria for, 30
  dominant response in illness, 600–601
  hypoinflammatory phase of, granulocyte macrophage colony-stimulating factor in, 624
  immunomodulatory intervention in, 390–391
  indications for surgical intervention in, 303–308
  microcirculatory arrest theory of, 92–100
  and multiple organ dysfunction syndrome, 23–29, 44–45, 52
    measuring correlation between, 56–58
  nonsepsis-related, in acute respiratory distress syndrome, 354
  role of mast cells in, potential, 191–193
  selective decontamination of the digestive tract in, 580
  severity of, and organ failure, 36–37
  soft signs of, 307
Systemic lupus erythematosus (SLE)
  neopterin levels in, 482
  procalcitonin levels in, 480–481
Systemic vascular resistance, hypotension after volume expansion as evidence of, 594

T

T cells
  CD4+ and CD8+, differentiation of, 525–526

maintaining a balance of
  effect of interferon-γ on, 531
  Th1/Th2, 449
  stress-induced Th1/Th2 shifts in, 524–530
Technologic imperatives, balance with ethical imperatives, 664–665
Testosterone, effect on macrophage function in males, 139, 391
Therapeutic Intervention Scoring System (TISS), 10
  as an estimate of intensity of resource utilization, 19
Therapeutic window, in acute-phase response, 425–426
Thoracic bioelectric impedance cardiography, for estimating cardiac output, 259
Thoracic tube insertion, in field emergency care, 246
Thrombin
  inhibitor of, effect in trauma, 394
  role in co-activation of inflammation by coagulation, 75
Thromboembolism, preventing, 658
Thrombosis
  microcirculatory, role in inflammation, 95
  microvascular, renal failure associated with, 372
  venous, effect of parenteral nutrition on, 421–422
Thromboxanes
  biosynthesis of, 197–199
  renal ischemia associated with, 372
Thymopentin, effect on cell-mediated immunity, 393
Thyroid
  calcitonin synthesis in, 478
  mediation of stress response by hormones of, 643
  role in hypermetabolic response to trauma and burns, 325
Tissue factor (TF), exposure of circulating blood to, in disseminated intravascular coagulation, 439
Tissue factor pathway inhibitor, 505
  for treating disseminated intravascular coagulation, 444
Tissue oxygen debt, as a determinant of organ failure, 35–36
Tissue perfusion
  intraoperative, nitroglycerin and fluids for, 567, 659–660
  role in multiple organ failure, 613
Tissue repair, mechanisms of, 74
Tolerance, to endotoxin, early, 121–123
Toll-like receptors, role in lipopolysaccharide-dependent responses, 114
Total parenteral nutrition (TPN)
  in acute respiratory distress syndrome, 357
  in critically ill patients, 630

Index

Toxic liver syndrome, treating, 470
Toxic shock syndrome, streptococcal. clinical trial of complement C1 inhibitor for treating, 216
    See also Shock, toxic
Toxins
    affecting the heart, 59
    drug-induced nephrotoxicity, 171
    liver failure caused by, 463
    See also Endotoxin
Transcription factors, activation in inflammation
    cytoplasmic, 514–516
    nuclear factor κ-B, 74–75
Transcutaneous oxygen tension, 261
Transesophageal echocardiography, 259–260
Transforming growth factor-β (TGFβ), levels in plasma after trauma and hemorrhage, 137
Transfusion
    acute respiratory distress syndrome associated with, 354
    and multiple organ failure, 111
    mortality rate associated with, in circulatory failure, 335
    red blood cell, effect on oxygen uptake in sepsis, 575
    renal insufficiency following, 71
    risk for postinjury multiple organ failure after, 37–38, 248
Translocation
    bacterial
        factors influencing, 581–582
        from the gut, 86–91, 323
    of endotoxins, and sepsis syndrome, 77
Transplantation
    heart, procalcitonin levels associated with, 480
    liver, 467
    renal, procalcitonin levels associated with, 480
Trauma
    acute respiratory distress syndrome in, 354
    chest, emergency care in the field, 243
    immune response to, 389–390
    modulation of hypermetabolic response to, 322–329
    neopterin levels in, 484–485
    platelet activating factor levels in multiple organ failure following, 207
    procalcitonin levels following, 481
    resuscitation to supranormal oxygen delivery and consumption, 573
    See also Injury
Trauma center, criteria for admission to, 247
Trauma Score (TS), 355
Treatment
    of acute respiratory distress syndrome, 357
    of antibiotic-associated pseudomembranous colitis, 316
    of bacterial peritonitis, 267–268
    of catheter-related nosocomial infections, 313
    of circulatory failure, 335–338
    of disseminated intravascular coagulation, 443–444
    of inflammatory complications of cardiopulmonary bypass, 83–84, 347
    of inflammatory diseases, by complement inhibition, 214–223
    of inflammatory response leading to systemic inflammatory response syndrome, 372–375
    of intraabdominal hypertension, 298–299
    of liver failure, 460
    multiagent, future trials in inflammation control, 562–570
    of nosocomial pneumonia, 310
    of nosocomial urinary tract infections, 315
    objectives of, in hepatic encephalopathy, 465
    of septic patients, with platelet activating factor antagonists, 210
    of sinusitis, in the intensive care unit, 316
    of urinary tract infections, 314
    of ventriculitis or meningitis, nosocomial, 317
Trephination, emergency, 249
Triazolobenzodiazepines, inhibition of platelet activating factor by, 208–209
Tricarboxylic acid cycle (TCA cycle), in trauma and burns, 322–323
Tuberculosis, multiagent therapy for, 563–564
Tumor necrosis factor-α (TNFα)
    biologic roles of, and outcomes of excessive production, 155
    cell-associated, signaling by, 150
    correlation with severity of illness and mortality, 76
    inhibition by peroxisome proliferating activated receptors, 125
    interaction with neopterin and interferon-γ, 485–486
    as a mediator of porin-induced toxic shock, 119
    neopterin synthesis associated with, 483
    plasma levels of, after trauma and hemorrhage, 136
    pleiotropic effects of, 104
    production in response to ceftazidime treatment, 117
    role of
        in initiation of host defense response, 515–516
        in myocardial depression in septic shock, 592
Tumor necrosis factor family, 147–149
Tumor necrosis factor receptors (TNFRs), soluble, effectiveness in therapy, 157
Two-hit model of multiple organ failure, 33, 52, 97

U

Ubiquitin/proteasome-dependent pathway, proteolysis in, 103, 380
Ulcer, stress, trials of prophylaxis, 414
Ultrasound, for early diagnosis in severe trauma treatment, 248
Urea, effect of growth hormone on generation of, 635
Urinary tract infections, nosocomial, 313–314
Urokinase, for treating reperfusion injury, 108–109

V

Variability, individual, future work on understanding of, 684
Vascular cell adhesion molecule-1 (VCAM-1), 232
Vascular reactivity, and nitric oxide synthase inhibition, 179
Vascular tone
    effect of hypertonic solutions on, 607
    nitric oxide as a mediator of, 178–179
Vasoactive agents, titration of, with a continuous cardiac output catheter, 257
Vasoconstriction
    enhancing with drugs, in severe sepsis and septic shock, 374–375
    role of isoeicosanoids in, 200–202
Vasodilation
    by histamine, 191–193
    by prostacyclin, 198
Vasomotor nephropathy, and renal failure, 371–372
Vasopressors, administration with fluids, in circulatory failure, 335–336
Ventilation
    in circulatory failure, 335
    emergency, in the field, 243–244
    inverse ratio, in treating acute respiratory distress syndrome, 359
    partial liquid, 361
Ventilation-associated pneumonia (VAP), associated with acute respiratory distress syndrome, 357
Ventilatory-associated pneumonia (VAP), diagnosing, 310
Ventilatory system, failure of, defined, 5
Ventriculitis, nosocomial, 317
Virus infection
    neopterin levels in, 483–484
    oxidant stress in, 171
Volume, of abdominal contents
    extraanatomic, and intraabdominal hypertension, 293
    and intraabdominal pressure increase, 292
Volume expanders
    blood, effect on oxygen transport, 572
    hypertonic solution, 605–606

W

Water, extracellular, in trauma or sepsis, 102
Wegener's granulomatosis, procalcitonin levels in, 481
Wilson's disease, liver damage in, 463
Wind-up (spinal cord hyperexcitability), 645–646
Wounds
  biology of, 92–95
  closure of, in surgery for peritonitis, 269
  failure of, defined, 7
  healing of, 553–561
    effect of growth hormone, 634
    fetal, 557–558
    promotion by mast cells, 192–193
  infection of, 138
  infiltration of local anesthetics in, 646

X

Xenotransplantation, complement inhibition during, 219

Z

Z-disks, sepsis-induced disintegration of, 383